DIAGNOSIS AND MANAGEMENT OF OVARIAN DISORDERS

SECOND EDITION

DIAGNOSIS AND MANAGEMENT OF OVARIAN DISORDERS

SECOND EDITION

Edited by

ALBERT ALTCHEK, M.D.
Clinical Professor with Tenure
Department of Obstetrics, Gynecology and Reproductive Science
The Mount Sinai School of Medicine
Attending Obstetrican-Gynecologist and Chief of Pediatric and Adolescent Gynecology
The Mount Sinai Hospital
Obstetrics-Gynecology Staff
Lenox Hill Hospital
Attending Gynecologist
Beth Israel Hospital North
New York, New York 10029

LIANE DELIGDISCH, M.D.
Professor
Department of Obstetrics, Gynecology and Reproductive Science
Director
Division of Gynecological Pathology
Department of Pathology
The Mount Sinai School of Medicine and Hospital
New York, New York 10029

NATHAN G. KASE, M.D.
Dean Emeritus and Professor
Department of Obstetrics, Gynecology and Reproductive Science
The Mount Sinai School of Medicine and Hospital
New York, New York 10029

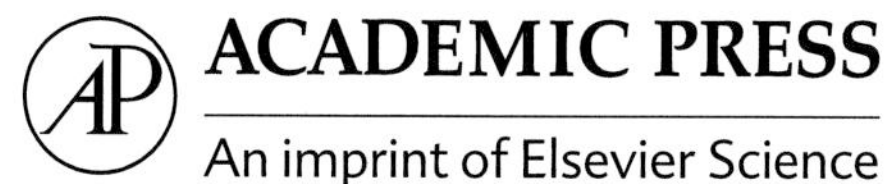

Amsterdam Boston Heidelberg London New York Oxford
Paris San Diego San Francisco Singapore Sydney Tokyo

Cover photo credit: © 2003 Digital Stock.

This book is printed on acid-free paper. ♾

Academic Press
An imprint of Elsevier Science
525 B Street, Suite 1900, San Diego, California 92101-4495, USA
http://www.academicpress.com

Academic Press
84 Theobald's Road, London WC1X 8RR, UK
http://www.academicpress.com

Library of Congress Catalog Card Number: 2003105446

International Standard Book Number: 0-12-053642-0

PRINTED IN CHINA
03 04 05 06 07 8 7 6 5 4 3 2 1

Dedicated to Our Families, Our Patients, and Our Colleagues.

Dedicated to my beloved wife
Miriam Estelle Schargel Jawitz Altchek

Albert Altchek

Contents

4. Pathology of Non-Neoplastic Ovarian Enlargements

FRÉDÉRIQUE PENAULT-LLORCA, CATHERINE VAURS BARRIÈRE, MICHEL CANIS, JACQUES DAUPLAT

5. Precancerous Lesions of the Ovary

LIANE DELIGDISCH

6. Epithelial Ovarian Neoplasms

LIANE DELIGDISCH

7. Germ Cell Tumors of the Ovary

ALEKSANDER TALERMAN

8. Gonadal Sex Cord-Stromal Tumors

DOROTA POPIOLEK AND RITA DEMOPOULOS

9. Metastatic Tumors of the Ovary

TAMARA KALIR

10. Peritoneal Lesions Related to Ovarian Neoplasms

LIANE DELIGDISCH

11. The Genetic Etiology of Sporadic Ovarian Cancer

JOHNATHAN M. LANCASTER, LAURA J. HAVRILESKY, AND ANDREW BERCHUCK

PART
II
DIAGNOSTIC PROCEDURES AND NEW APPROACHES

12. Diagnostic Tests for Evaluation of Ovarian Function

MICHAEL ZINGER AND JAMES H. LIU

13. Premature Ovarian Failure

LISA KOLP

14. Ultrasound of the Ovary

KAREN JERMY AND TOM BOURNE

15. CA125 and Other Tumor Markers in Screening and Monitoring of Ovarian Cancer

USHA MENON AND IAN JACOBS

16. BRCA1 and BRCA2 Mutations in Ovarian Carcinoma

GEORGE COUKOS AND STEPHEN C. RUBIN

17. Epidemiology of Ovarian Cancer

M. STEVEN PIVER AND TOM S. FRANK

18. Early Diagnosis and Screening for Ovarian Cancer

MARK H. EINSTEIN AND CAROLYN D. RUNOWICZ

19. Clues to Tumors: New Concepts of Symptoms, Signs, Syndromes, Paraneoplastic Syndromes, and Predisposition to Ovarian Cancer

ALBERT ALTCHEK

20. A Geneticist Looks at Ovarian Cancer

FRED GILBERT

21. Gene Therapy of Ovarian Cancer—State-of-the-Art and Future Perspectives

DIRK G. KIEBACK, ANNETTE HASENBURG, INGO B. RUNNEBAUM, XIAO W. TONG, AND DAGMAR-C. FISCHER

22. Speculation and Deductive Reasoning About Ovarian Epithelial Carcinogenesis and New Horizons

ALBERT ALTCHEK, LIANE DELIGDISCH, AND FRÉDÉRIQUE PENAULT-LLORCA

23. *In Vitro* Fertilization, Stem Cells, Cloning, and the Future of Assisted Reproductive Technologies

LISA SPIRYDA, AMY ANTMAN, AND ELIZABETH S. GINSBURG

PART III
CONTEMPORARY MANAGEMENT

24. Polycystic Ovarian Syndrome

ALAN B. COPPERMAN, TANMOY MUKHERJEE, AND NATHAN G. KASE

25. General Concepts of Endocrine Manipulation of Assisted Reproduction

SOZOS J. FASOULIOTIS AND NERI LAUFER

26. Endometriosis

W. PAUL DMOWSKI

27. Menopause

NATHAN G. KASE

28. Laparoscopic Surgery of Benign Ovarian Disorders

M. CANIS, A. WATTIEZ, R. BOTCHORISHVILI, B. RABISCHONG, C. HOULLE, H. MANHES, G. MAGE, J. L. POULY, AND M. A. BRUHAT

29. The Management of Malignant Ovarian Neoplasms in the Young Patient

LYNDA ROMAN

30. Ovarian Carcinoma Complicating Pregnancy

HUGH R. K. BARBER

31. Ovarian Cancer: The Initial Laparotomy

JAMAL RAHAMAN AND CARMEL. J. COHEN

32. Surgical Management of Large Ovarian Carcinoma Tumor Masses

DANIEL DARGENT AND PATRICE MATHEVET

33. The Long-Term Management of Ovarian Cancer

JAMAL RAHAMAN AND CARMEL J. COHEN

34. The Laparoscopic Management of Adnexal Masses and Ovarian Cancer

FARR NEZHAT AND TANJA PEJOVIC

35. Chemotherapy of Ovarian Cancer

MARTEE L. HENSLEY AND WILLIAM J. HOSKINS

36. Intraperitoneal Chemotherapy

MAURIE MARKMAN

37. Prevention of Ovarian Serous Epithelial Carcinoma

ALBERT ALTCHEK

38. Psychological Aspects of Ovarian Cancer and BRCA Testing

JENNIFER LIU AND JIMMIE C. HOLLAND

Contributors

Numbers in parentheses indicate the pages on which the authors' contributions begin.

Albert Altchek, M.D. (231, 305, 515) Clinical Professor with Tenure, Department of Obstetrics, Gynecology and Reproductive Science, The Mount Sinai School of Medicine; Attending Obstetrican-Gynecologist and Chief of Pediatric and Adolescent Gynecology, The Mount Sinai Hospital; Obstetrics-Gynecology Staff, Lennox Hill Hospital; Attending Gynecologist, Beth Israel Hospital North, New York, New York 10029

Amy Antman, B.A. (325) Resident and Medical Student, Harvard Medical School, Boston, Massachusetts 02115

Hugh R.K. Barber, M.D. (439) Professor, Department of Clinical Obstetrics and Gynecology, Cornell University Medical College, New York, New York 10021

Catherine Vaurs Barrière, Ph.D. (61) Service d'Anatomie et Cytologie Pathologiques, Clermont-Ferrand Cedex 01, France

Andrew Berchuck, M.D. (139) Professor, Department of Obstetrics and Gynecology, Division of Gynecologic Oncology, Duke University Medical Center, Durham, North Carolina 27710

R. Botchorishvili (415) Department of Obstetrics, Gynecology, and Reproductive Medicine, Polyclinique CHU, 63003 Clermont-Ferrand, France

Tom Bourne, Ph.D. (181) Consultant, St. Georges Hospital and Medical School, London SW1 70QT, United Kingdom

M.A. Bruhat, M.D. (415) Professor, Department of Obstetrics, Gynecology, and Reproductive Medicine, Polyclinique CHU, 63003 Clermont-Ferrand, France

Vladimir Bychkov, M.D. (3) Visual Pathology, LLC, Chicago, Illinois 60605

Michel Canis, M.D. (61,415) Associate Professor, Department of Obstetrics, Gynecology, and Reproductive Medicine, Polyclinique CHU, 63003 Clermont-Ferrand, France

Carmel J. Cohen, M.D. (445, 467) Professor and Vice-Chairman, Director, Division of Gynecologic Oncology, The Mount Sinai School of Medicine and Hospital, New York, New York 10029

Alan B. Copperman, M.D. (337) Director, Division of Reproductive Endocrinology, Department of Obstetrics, Gynecology and Reproductive Science, The Mount Sinai School of Medicine and Hospital, New York, New York 10029

George Coukos, M.D., Ph.D. (201) Assistant Professor, Division of Gynecologic Oncology, University of Pennsylvania Medical Center, Philadelphia, Pennsylvania 19104

Daniel Dargent, M.D. (453) Professor, Department of Gynecology, Hopital Edouard Herriot, 69437 Lyon, France

Jacques Dauplat, M.D. (61) Professor, Department of Oncologic Surgery, Clermont-Ferrand Cedex 01, France

Liane Deligdisch, M.D. (75, 83, 133) Professor, Department of Obstetrics, Gynecology and Reproductive Science; Director, Division of Gynecological Pathology, Department of Pathology, The Mount Sinai School of Medicine and Hospital, New York, New York 10029

Rita Demopoulos, M.D. (111) Professor, Department of Pathology, Division of OB/GYN Pathology, New York University School of Medicine, Bellevue Hospital Center, New York, New York 10016

W. Paul Dmowski, M.D., Ph.D. (369) Director, Institute for the Study and Treatment of Endometriosis, Oak Brook, Illinois 60523 and Professor, Department of Obstetrics and Gynecology, Rush Medical College, Chicago, Illinois 60612

Mark H. Einstein, M.D. (219) Assistant Professor, Division of Gynecologic Oncology, Department of Obstetrics, Gynecology, and Women's Health, Montefiore Medical Center and Albert Einstein Cancer Center, Bronx, New York 10461

Sozos J. Fasouliotis, M.D. (357) Department of Obstetrics and Gynecology, Hebrew University–Hadassah Medical Center, Jerusalem, 91120, Israel and Clinical Fellow, Center for Reproductive Medicine and Infertility, Weill Medical College of Cornell University, New York, New York 10021

Dagmar-C. Fischer, Ph.D. (277) UD Molecular Oncology, Department of Obstetrics and Gynecology, Maastricht University Medical Center, NL 6202 AZ Maastricht, Netherlands

Tom S. Frank, M.D. (Deceased) (209) Medical Director, Myriad Genetics Laboratories, Salt Lake City, Utah 84108

Fred Gilbert (271) Associate Professor, Department of Pediatrics, Division of Human Genetics, Weill College of Medicine of Cornell University and Human Cancer Genetics, Strang Cancer Prevention Center, New York, New York 10021

Elizabeth S. Ginsburg, M.D. (325) Medical Director, Assisted Reproductive Technologies Programs, Brigham & Women's Hospital, Boston, Massachusetts 02115

Annette Hasenburg (277) Department of Obstetrics and Gynecology, Freiburg University Medical Center, D-79106 Freiburg, Germany

Laura J. Havrilesky, M.D. (139) Department of Obstetrics and Gynecology, Division of Gynecologic Oncology, Duke University Medical Center, Durham, North Carolina 27710

Martee L. Hensley, M.D., M.Sc. (487) Developmental Chemotherapy Service, Department of Medicine, Memorial Sloan-Kettering Cancer Center, New York, New York 10021 and Novartis Pharma AG, Oncology, CH-4002 Basel Switzerland

Jimmie C. Holland, M.D. (545) Chief, Department of Psychiatry, Memorial Sloan-Kettering Cancer Center, New York, New York 10021

William J. Hoskins, M.D. (487) Curtis & Elizabeth Anderson Cancer Institute, Memorial Health University Medical Center, Savannah, Georgia 31404

C. Houlle (415) Department of Obstetrics, Gynecology, and Reproductive Medicine, Polyclinique CHU, 63003 Clermont-Ferrand, France

Ian Jacobs (193) Professor, Gynecology Oncology Unit, St. Bartholomew's and The London Queen Mary's School of Medicine and Dentistry, London EC1M 6GR, United Kingdom

Karen Jermy (181) St. Georges Hospital and Medical School, London SW1 70QT, United Kingdom

Tamara Kalir, M.D., Ph.D. (127) Assistant Professor, Department of Pathology, The Mount Sinai School of Medicine, New York, New York 10029

Nathan G. Kase, M.D. (11, 33, 337, 387) Dean Emeritus and Professor, Department of Obstetrics, Gynecology and Reproductive Science, The Mount Sinai School of Medicine and Hospital, New York, New York 10029

Dirk G. Kieback, M.D., Ph.D. (277) Professor and Chairman, Department of Obstetrics and Gynecology, Maastricht University Medical Center, NL 6202 AZ Maastricht, Netherlands

Lisa Kolp, M.D. (169) Assistant Professor, Department of Gynecology and Obstetrics, Johns Hopkins Medical Institution, Baltimore, Maryland 21287

Johnathan M. Lancaster, M.D. (139) Department of Obstetrics and Gynecology, Division of Gynecologic Oncology, Duke University Medical Center, Durham, North Carolina 27710

Neri Laufer, M.D. (357) Professor and Chairman, Department of Obstetrics and Gynecology, Hebrew University–Hadassah Medical Center, Jerusalem, 91120, Israel

James H. Liu, M.D. (159) Arthur H. Bill Professor, Chair, Department of Obstetrics and Gynecology, University Hospitals of Cleveland, Department of Reproductive Biology, Case Western Reserve University, Cleveland, Ohio 44106

Jennifer Liu, M.D. (545) San Francisco Veteran's Affairs Medical Center, University of California, San Francisco, San Francisco, California 94121

G. Mage (415) Professor, Department of Obstetrics, Gynecology, and Reproductive Medicine, Polyclinique CHU, 63003 Clermont-Ferrand, France

H. Manhes (415) Polyclinique "La Pergola," 03200 Vichy, France

Maurie Markman, M.D. (505) Chairman, Department of Hematology/Medical Oncology, The Cleveland Clinic Taussig Cancer Center, The Cleveland Clinic Foundation, Cleveland, Ohio 44195

Patrice Mathevet, M.D., Ph.D. (453) Department of Gynecology, Hopital Edouard Herriot, 69437 Lyon, France

Paul G. McDonough, M.D. (51) Professor, Departments of Obstetrics and Gynecology, Pediatrics and Physiology, Medical College of Georgia, Augusta, Georgia 30912

Usha Menon, M.D. (193) Senior Lecturer/Consultant, Gynecology Oncology Unit, St. Bartholomew's and The London Queen Mary's School of Medicine and Dentistry, London EC1M 6GR, United Kingdom

Tanmoy Mukherjee, M.D. (337) Assistant Clinical Professor, Department of Obstetrics, Gynecology and Reproductive Science, The Mount Sinai School of Medicine and Hospital, New York, New York 10029

Farr Nezhat, M.D. (477) Professor, Division of Gynecologic Oncology, The Mount Sinai School of Medicine and Hospital, New York, New York 10029

Tanja Pejovic, M.D. (477) Instructor, Division of Gynecologic Oncology, Yale University School of Medicine, New Haven, Connecticut 06520

Frédérique Penault-Llorca, M.D., Ph.D. (61) Associate Professor, Service d'Anatomie et Cytologie Pathologiques, Clermont-Ferrand Cedex 01, France

M. Steven Piver, M.D.LLD(hc) (209) Senior Gynecologic Oncologist, Sisters of Charity Hospital, Buffalo, New York 14214 and Director, Gilda Radner Familial Ovarian Cancer Registry, Roswell Park Cancer Institute, Buffalo, New York 14263

Dorota Popiolek, M.D. (111) Assistant Professor, Department of Pathology, Division of OB/GYN Pathology, New York University School of Medicine, Bellevue Hospital Center, New York, New York 10016

J. L. Pouly (415) Professor, Department of Obstetrics, Gynecology, and Reproductive Medicine, Polyclinique CHU, 63003 Clermont-Ferrand, France

B. Rabischong (415) Department of Obstetrics, Gynecology, and Reproductive Medicine, Polyclinique CHU, 63003 Clermont-Ferrand, France

Jamal Rahaman, M.D. (445,467) Assistant Professor, Division of Gynecologic Oncology, The Mount Sinai School of Medicine and Hospital, New York, New York 10029

Lynda Roman, M.D. (431) Associate Professor, Department of Obstetrics and Gynecology, University of Southern California School of Medicine and USC Women's and Children's Hospital, Los Angeles, California 90033

Stephen C. Rubin, M.D. (201) Director, Division of Gynecologic Oncology, University of Pennsylvania Medical Center, Philadelphia, Pennsylvania 19104

Ingo B. Runnebaum, M.D. (277) Professor, Department of Obstetrics and Gynecology, Freiburg University Medical Center, D-79106 Freiburg, Germany

Carolyn D. Runowicz, M.D. (219) Professor, Department of Obstetrics and Gynecology, Columbia University College of Physicians and Surgeons at the St. Luke's-Roosevelt Hospital Center, New York, New York 10019

Lisa Spiryda, M.D., Ph.D. (325) Department of Obstetrics and Gynecology, Brigham & Women's Hospital, Boston, Massachusetts 02115

Aleksander Talerman, M.D., Ph.D. (95) Professor, Department of Pathology and Cell Biology, Thomas Jefferson University, Philadelphia, Pennsylvania 19107

Xiao W. Tong, M.D. (277) Professor and Chairman, Department of Obstetrics and Gynecology, Tongi University Shanghai, Shanghai, 200065 PR China

A. Wattiez (415) Department of Obstetrics, Gynecology, and Reproductive Medicine, Polyclinique CHU, 63003 Clermont-Ferrand, France

Michael Zinger, M.D. (159) Department of Obstetrics and Gynecology, University of Cincinnati, Cincinnati, Ohio 45267

Foreword to the First Edition

Anyone interested in women's health, especially those who offer care specifically to women will be refreshed and rewarded by this volume about the ovary. Authored and edited by a clinician and a pathologist, with contributions from experts in various aspects of the structures and functions of this multidimensional organ, this book is unique in its eclectic content and style.

Because it bases clinical diagnosis and treatment on a foundation of embryology, anatomy, physiology and steroid endocrinology, if offers a valuable translation of basic "bench" phenomena for use at the bedside in the care of patients. This wide-ranging text encompasses the functional, the dysfunctional and the neoplastic, from childhood to advanced age.

This book is a modern presentation of the scientific basis of health and diseases in a clear, practical style that will be appreciated by physicians and students alike. It will take an important place in the library of everyone responsible for the health care of women, for ovarian function is central to reproduction and health.

I congratulate the editors for this excellent contribution, and take some pride in their sometime work under my aegis.

S. B. Gusberg, M.D., D.Sc.
Distinguished Service Professor Emeritus
The Mount Sinai School of Medicine
Past President and Present Consultant
American Cancer Society
Founder and Former Chief Editor
Gynecologic Oncology

Foreword to the Second Edition

The second edition of *Diagnosis and Management of Ovarian Disorders* by Albert Altchek, Lianne Deligdisch, and Nathan Kase is a unique contribution to literature. What this group has done is taken one organ (the ovary) and written an entire book on its function and dysfunction. The book is divided into three basic categories:

Part I: Physiology, Pathology, and Basic Science
Part II: Diagnostic Procedures and New Approaches
Part III: Contemporary Management

The book is expanded, up-to-date, and cutting edge in regards to new techniques and therapies. The editors have brought together the leading authorities in the field to discuss their various disciplines and how it relates to ovarian pathology and physiology. Each chapter is well written and illustrated and there is editorial consistency.

In the patho-physiology and basic science area, an encyclopedic discussion occurs about the various tumors, both benign and malignant. This is coupled with introductory chapters on ovarian embryology, anatomy and histology, function of the normal ovary and ovarian steroid hormones, and recent progress in organogenesis. Special attention should be directed towards the important chapter on the Genetic Etiology of Sporadic Ovarian Cancer.

In the diagnostic techniques and investigation portion of the text, a broad spectrum of clinical areas are elaborated including new work on premature ovarian failure, ultrasonic evaluation of the ovary, the epidemiology of ovarian cancer and early diagnosis and screening for ovarian cancer. Included is a chapter on *in vitro* fertilization, stem cell cloning, and the future of assisted reproductive technologies. In the unique section on Contemporary Management, Polycystic Ovary Syndrome is covered in depth including the newer therapeutic approaches utilizing the principals of treatment impacting on insulin resistance, areas of laparoscopic surgery of benign ovarian disorders, long-term management of ovarian cancer and psychological aspects of ovarian cancer, and BRCA testing.

At first, one would think a book only about the ovary would be a bit contrived. Yet the editors and contributors have carried this off with aplomb. It is an extremely interesting read with new and old insights eloquently elaborated. It draws in all factors of a single organ, but also teaches many other aspects of pathology and physiology. Of course, the authors could not have taken a more interesting organ to study than the ovary, since this is such an active and complex organ. The key, of course, is that in this book you can find "everything you wanted to know about the ovary."

Alan H. DeCherney, M.D.
Professor of OBGYN
David Geffen School of Medicine
UCLA
Los Angeles, California
Editor
Fertility and Sterility
April, 2003

Preface to the First Edition

Most gynecology textbooks deal with only one aspect of a problem. This book is different—it is a multidisciplined panorama, ranging from molecular biology to psychiatry. It was developed for clinicians as a practical review and update, with useful new concepts, as well as a reference for sharpening both their practice and their surgical skills.

Each chapter is contributed by an experienced subspecialist who emphasizes essential basic knowledge and evaluates new findings which have clinical relevance to improved quality of care. This research would be an impossible task for the busy practicing physician.

Part I covers pathology and basic science including embryology; the recently appreciated self-regulating ovarian hormonal microenvironment and the adventures of the follicle; premature ovarian failure; cystic ovaries; cancer susceptibility; ovarian neoplasms; ovarian intraepithelial neoplasia (OIN) and computerized image analysis; the different germ cell neoplasms; the dramatic functioning neoplasms; the surprisingly high incidence of metastatic cancer; the confusing peritoneal endosalpingiosis and provocative serous papillary peritoneal carcinoma; the new technology of flow cytometry finding its role; and the developing understanding of oncogenes, tumor suppressor genes and carcinogenesis.

Part II deals with clinical diagnosis—signs, symptoms, and syndromes; the early diagnosis of cancer; the use of transvaginal color Doppler ultrasound; and serves as a practical guide for hormone testing.

Part III concerns contemporary management, and offers direct help in patient care. This includes reproductive endocrinology techniques using GnRH analog therapy for uterine myomas and endometriosis, and the "threshold" and "add back" concepts; assisted reproduction presented step by step; management of the problems of the common polycystic ovarian syndrome; and advanced laparoscopy with "how to" advice; the different ovarian tumors of the young patient, with the possibility of preserving fertility even with ovarian malignancy; the realization that most torsed ovaries can be salvaged and the concept of pexy or plication of both ovaries; the management of ovarian tumors in pregnancy; what is involved in the initial laparotomy for ovarian cancer and its significance in prognosis and management planning; a French view of surgery for advanced cancer; determining the role of intraperitoneal chemotherapy with its high local concentration; the use of laparoscopy for ovarian cancer, the long term course of cancer (despite good results of platinum combination chemotherapy the frequent eventual cancer recurrence, the pros and cons of second-look surgery, and the atypical late metastases); and finally the thing that all dread—the shattering emotional impact of progressive ovarian cancer with its recurrent stressful episodes on the patient, her family, and the physician, and what to do about it.

The need to have a practical and readily available book required informative but concise chapters containing appropriate references and helpful illustrations.

I owe a debt of gratitude to my co-editor Dr. Liane Deligdisch, a world authority on gynecologic pathology, to the enthusiastic contributors who are leaders in their fields, to the encouragement of Lila Maron of Igaku-Shoin and to Fortune Uy, B.S.N., R.N. for her secretarial assistance.

Albert Altchek, M.D.

Preface to the Second Edition

The first edition of *Diagnosis and Management of Ovarian Disorders* was published in 1996 and was received with resounding enthusiasm. The *New England Journal of Medicine* offered a very favorable book review in its December 19, 1996 issue (volume 335, no. 25, pp. 1929–1930). The reviewer described the first edition as "... a comprehensive overview of the biology of the ovary that cannot be found elsewhere ..." done by "... a distinguished panel of authors from many fields..." It was considered helpful for clinicians, especially to general obstetricians and gynecologists as well as subspecialists, particularly regarding cross-specialty ready access "... to material related to their practice that is not generally covered in their own highly specialized literature." In addition to the quality of its content, some of its success was attributed to the division into pathology, basic science, molecular biology, physiology, diagnostic approaches, and contemporary management.

Encouraged by the reception of the first edition, the editors felt this second edition, published by Academic Press (division of Elsevier Science), was essential to keep up with expanding knowledge of ovarian function and the new insights that have influenced evolving practice patterns. Experts from various disciplines and from different institutions have again presented a broad spectrum, multidiscipline approach in a comprehensive update and review of selected aspects of ovarian function and problems. Ovarian cancer continues to be a major problem and has again been emphasized in pathology, molecular biology, speculation on etiology, management, and the role of laparoscopy. New authors and chapters have been added including prevention of ovarian cancer especially with the realization that as much as 13% may be due to hereditary predisposition together with the association with breast cancer. We have been fortunate in having the leading authors review their fields, retrieve and analyze significant concepts and crystallize them for the clinician.

The basic purpose of this book is to teach and inspire the clinician to continue to give quality care. The broad range of chapters was selected for pertinent background understanding and for practical clinical usage. Written in a clear, concise and easily understood fashion we hope it will have great appeal not only for generalist obstetrician-gynecologists and subspecialists, but also for medical students, house staff, research fellows, and medical generalists. The book may be picked up, opened to any section, and read at any time whenever the reader has a few minutes and wants an update by an outstanding expert.

The second edition again has three sections:

I. Physiology, Pathology, and Basic Science
II. Diagnostic Procedures and New Approaches
III. Contemporary Management

New chapters have also been included. The presumed precursor of epithelial ovarian carcinoma was originally described by Dr. Liane Deligdisch who has refined the diagnosis by objective morphometric analysis. Such dysplasia is found in prophylactic removed ovaries as well as early occult carcinoma in high-risk women.

A new chapter on speculation about ovarian carcinogenesis, dynamic testing, and inter-institutional collaboration may stimulate new concepts. The chapter on paraneoplastic syndromes suggests clues to early detection, mechanisms of carcinogenesis, and the possibility that the ubiquitous "dyspepsia" often present several months before ovarian cancer is identified may be an identifiable paraneoplastic syndrome. The chapter on prevention of ovarian cancer indicates that salpingo-oophorectomy rather than oophorectomy alone is now recommended. Early prophylactic ovarian surgery may give as much as a 50% chance of reduction of later breast cancer. The preventive value of long-term oral contraceptives may be due to the progestin component which suggests the possibilities of short-term prevention.

The multidiscipline, relatively novel approach to medical education is now being incorporated in many medical schools and teaching programs at all levels to make it more interesting, inspiring, relevant, and to give it perspective. In that regard, we welcome our new co-editor, Dr. Nathan G. Kase, who brings many years of experience as an author and educator to this edition.

We believe that the second edition, featuring a larger format, will make the text more reader friendly. Furthermore the publishers have provided the superb printing, reproduction of illustrations, and quality of paper necessary for comfortable as well as edifying reading.

Accordingly, we wish to thank the Acquisition Editor Tari Paschall, the Developmental Editor Judy Meyer, and the Production Editor Paul Gottehrer for their encouragement and assistance.

Most importantly this book would not be possible without the dedicated, conscientious, and distinguished contributing authors. We, the medical profession, and patients everywhere are indebted to them.

Albert Altchek, M.D.
Liane Deligdisch, M.D.
Nathan G. Kase, M.D.
April, 2003

PART I

PHYSIOLOGY, PATHOLOGY, AND BASIC SCIENCE

CHAPTER

1

Embryology, Anatomy, Histology

VLADIMIR BYCHKOV

Visual Pathology, LLC
Chicago, Illinois 60605

I. EMBRYOLOGY

In its embryonic development an ovary passes through a number of stages. It begins with the formation of a genital ridge at approximately 30 days post conception, followed by an indifferent gonad at 35 days, an embryonic ovary at 42 days (6 weeks), an early fetal ovary at 8 weeks, a late fetal ovary at 16 weeks, and a perinatal ovary at 28 weeks.

Genital ridges are formed on the medial border of the mesonephros by the proliferating cells of mesodermally derived coelomic epithelium (mesothelium). As the genital ridges continue to progress as multilayered structures, the basement membrane between the coelomic epithelium and the mesenchyme disappears and the cell cords invade the underlying mesoderm.

The indifferent gonad appears when primitive germ cells join the other two components—the coelomic epithelium and the mesenchyme. The germ cells can be traced in an embryo because of their large size and the presence of alkaline phosphatase. They become visible at 4 weeks post conception in the wall of the yolk sac near the allantoic region. Then they migrate around the allantois and the gut into the part of the mesentery adjacent to the mesonephros and into the gonadal ridges, perhaps with "assisted passage" due to expansion of tissues through which they migrate.[1] Presence of the germ cells is necessary for the development of a functional ovary, but their absence does not completely suppress the formation of the gonad.[2]

Two waves of the proliferation of coelomic epithelium occur in the indifferent gonad.[3] The first wave produces sex cords which are arranged radially within the gonad. In male embryos they link up with other cell cords originating from the mesonephros to establish the urogenital connection. In phenotypic females the second wave establishes the basis of the ovarian cortex. At about 6 weeks post-conception, the gonadal sex of an embryo becomes apparent.

The early fetal stage spans the 8–16 weeks after conception. During this stage the oogonia are arranged in clusters, each cluster being enclosed within aggregates of coelomic epithelial cells. After the 12th week epithelial cells surround some ova and form primordial follicles (Fig. 1.1).

The late fetal stage begins after 16 weeks of gestation. At this stage oocytes, which are incompletely surrounded by epithelial cells, degenerate.

By the 28th week of gestation, a number of growing follicles surrounded by several layers of cuboidal epithelial cells begin to emerge. The stroma adjacent to these follicles differentiate into theca interna consisting of crowded oval cells and theca externa formed by slender cells interspersed with numerous collagen fibers. As gestation progresses, some of the growing follicles become vesicular, and the cells of the theca interna demonstrate features of steroidogenesis, that is, well-developed smooth endoplasmic reticulum and presence of $3B$-hydroxysteroid dehydrogenase.[4]

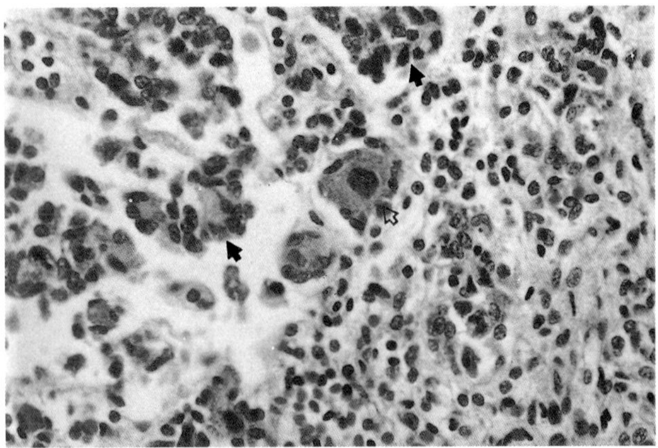

FIGURE 1.1 Fetal ovary between 12th and 16th week. Clusters of oogonia (dark arrow) and early primordial follicle (light arrow) are seen.

II. ANATOMY

Adult ovaries are ovoid structures measuring from $0.6\times1.5\times3$ to $1\times2.5\times4.5$ cm. It is normal to see cystic follicles and corpora lutea protruding under the surface. The ovarian artery arises from the abdominal aorta below the renal artery. The right gonadal vein joins the inferior vena cava directly, while the left vein reaches the ipsilateral renal vein.

The lymphatics accompany the ovarian arteries and drain to the para-aortic nodes at the level of the second lumber vertebra. Some ovarian lymphatics follow the round ligament and drain to the inguinal lymph nodes.

The nerves derive mainly from the aortic plexus and accompany the ovarian artery.

III. HISTOLOGY

A. Surface Epithelium

The surface of the ovary is covered by a single layer of cuboidal epithelium containing some ciliated cells. With advancing age it becomes flattened.

The surface epithelium focally invades the underlying stroma, forming small cysts which usually do not exceed a few millimeters in diameter. These structures are not pathological since they are found even in the fetal ovaries and at any period of life.[5] Their linings are prone to metaplastic changes, and mainly produce a pattern similar to the epithelium of fallopian tubes. The other metaplastic patterns (mucinous, endometrioid) are rarely seen.[6]

Electron microscopy reveals uniform closely apposed small cells with terminal bars, prominent desmosomes and numerous, often branching, microvilli. The cytoplasm contains scattered ribosomes, occasional rough endoplasmic reticulum, elongated mitochondria, and rare lipid droplets.[7] This pattern, which is neither proliferative nor secretory, reflects the protective function of the surface epithelium.

B. Cortex

The cortical stroma of the ovary consists of closely packed spindle cells with scant cytoplasm and slender nuclei which are capable of transforming into functionally active oval cells with plump nuclei and well-developed cytoplasm. These cells constitute the "theca interna."

Theca interna evolves around growing follicles and persists in corpora lutea, and, sometimes, around atretic follicles. It may exist without any relation to the follicular structures in pregnancy and in some pathological conditions. The other cortical stromal cells constitute a poorly defined layer around follicles that may be called "theca externa." The term "theca" embraces both "interna" and "externa" as one system differing only in functional capacity.

Theca cells differentiate continuously from stromal cells at the periphery of developing follicles, a process beginning during fetal life and ending at menopause.[8] The theca interna is usually three or four layers thick and is separated from adjacent granulosa by a basement membrane.

The theca interna layer of the growing follicles contains a rich vascular plexus consisting of dilated capillaries enmeshed in the dense reticulum network surrounding each cell.

The cells of the theca interna vary from round to polygonal, measure 12–20 μm in diameter and have well-developed, eosinophilic to clear vacuolated cytoplasm, and centrally located vesicular nuclei. They display features of steroidogenesis.[9–11] The lipid they contain is anisotropic when polarized, a feature characteristic of steroid hormones. The ultrastructural features of steroidogenesis include abundant smooth endoplasmic reticulum and mitochondria with tubular cristae.

C. Primordial Follicles

When a primitive ovum in the developing ovary becomes enclosed by a single layer of epithelial cells, the newly formed small structure is called a "primordial" or "primary" follicle. The cells of the single layer surrounding the oocyte are termed "follicular epithelial cells" or "granulosa." Each primordial follicle present in the cortical stroma at puberty consists of a primary oocyte measuring approximately 25–30 μm in diameter and is enclosed by a single layer of flattened follicular epithelium (Fig. 1.2).

The younger the individual, the more numerous the primordial follicles; the ovaries at birth have 1 to 2 million follicles and the puberty, about 380,000.[12] By the age of forty their number is reduced to about 8000, and after menopause they are extremely difficult to find, although a few follicles may persist into old age.

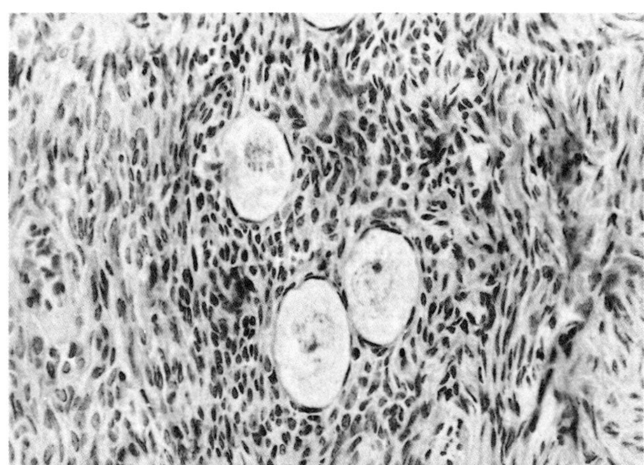

FIGURE 1.2 Primordial follicles at puberty. Each oocyte is surrounded by a single layer of flattened follicular epithelium.

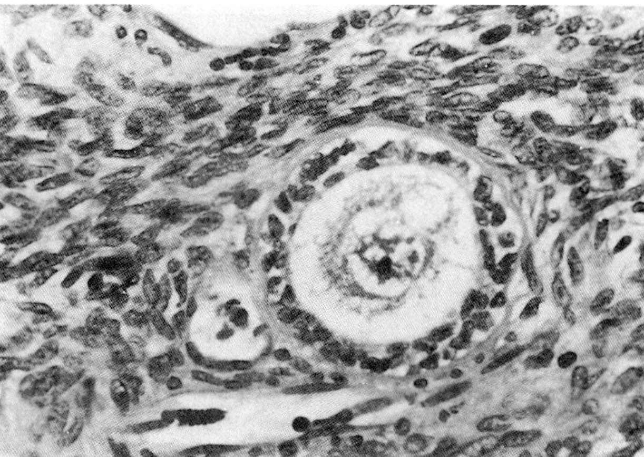

FIGURE 1.3 Growing follicle (preantral). Oocyte is surrounded by several layers of follicular epithelial cells, but there is no cavity.

Soon after primary oocytes are formed, they enter the prophase of their first meiotic division, which they will complete after puberty. This will occur only in those follicles ready for ovulation. The pool of primordial follicles in a fetus reaches its maximum at about 20 weeks of gestational age and then decreases throughout life until complete depletion occurs around the time of menopause. Reproductive life begins when less than 10% (near 500,000) of primordial follicles are left. The entire process of maturation of the follicles takes at least 3 months. Follicle growth up to the antral stage occurs during fetal life and infancy.[13]

The active corpus luteum locally suppresses neighboring follicular growth, with the most pronounced effect in the middle and late luteal phases.[14]

D. Growing Follicles

The growth of the follicles begins in the fetus at 28 weeks of gestation and continuous until menopause. There is always about 10% of the follicles in a growing stage, while the others remain inactive. Growth of the follicles occurs in stages to which unstandardized terminology is applied in the literature. Inactive follicles are called "primordial" and also "primary," but sometimes the term "primary" is applied to the early stage of growth.[15] The term "secondary follicle" always means a growing phase. The term "tertiary follicle" is used for the definition of the preovulatory stage. Follicles at this stage are often referred to as "Graafian," but this term is also used for the secondary follicles.

It would be appropriate to call all growing follicles "secondary" and to reserve the term "primary" to the non-growing/primordial/follicles. The secondary follicles may be divided into "preantral," which have no cavities and whose enlargements depend on proliferation of the granulosa; "antral," when the cavities are formed, and the enlargements depend mostly on the accumulation of fluid; and "preovulatory" which contain cumulus oophorus and bulge under the surface.

The earliest sign of growth is manifested in the follicular cells which become cuboidal and form two or more layers (Fig. 1.3).

After the proliferating follicular cells form a multilayered structure, fluid starts to accumulate between them. An increase in osmotic pressure caused by the mucopolysaccharides secreted by the granulosa is a contributing factor in the formation of follicular fluid. In this way the preantral follicles enter the antral stage (Fig. 1.4). Minute cavities among granulosa cells filled with PAS-positive material are known as the Call-Exner bodies.[16]

The oocyte continues to grow together with the follicle and, in the antral stage, it is surrounded by a well-defined, dark-stained membrane called "zona pellucida." Electron microscopy shows that the microvilli and the cytoplasmic processes of the granulosa extend through the zona pellucida to the oocyte. These contacts form areas of low-resistance, facilitating passage of the nutrients to the oocyte. These areas are known as "gap junctions" or "nexuses." The oocyte contains many coated vesicles indicating that it absorbs protein from the surface. Thus, the maturation of the follicle and the oocyte is synchronized.[17]

With continued accumulation of fluid, the oocyte assumes an eccentric position at one pole of the follicle. At this site, granulosa cells proliferate to form a cumulus oophorus (Fig. 1.5).

During each menstrual cycle, only one or two growing follicles attain the preovulatory stage. At this stage, the oocyte, the surrounding zona pellucida, and a layer of radially disposed granulosa cells (corona radiata) are separated from the cumulus oophorus and float in the antral fluid. The preovulatory follicle, which may be more than 1 cm in diameter, bulges under the ovarian surface, and the point where it will

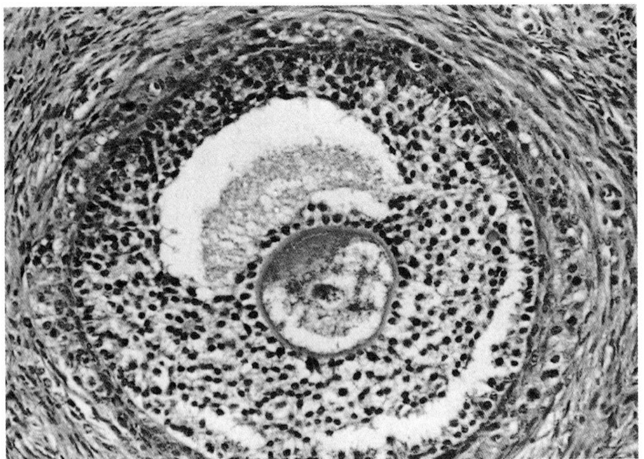

FIGURE 1.4 Growing follicle (antral). Cavity is formed in the multilayered follicular epithelium.

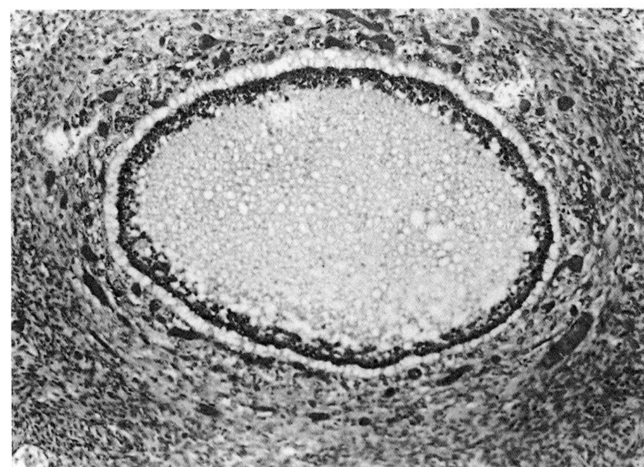

FIGURE 1.6 Early follicular atresia. Separation of granulosa from underlying theca and degenerative changes in follicular epithelium are present.

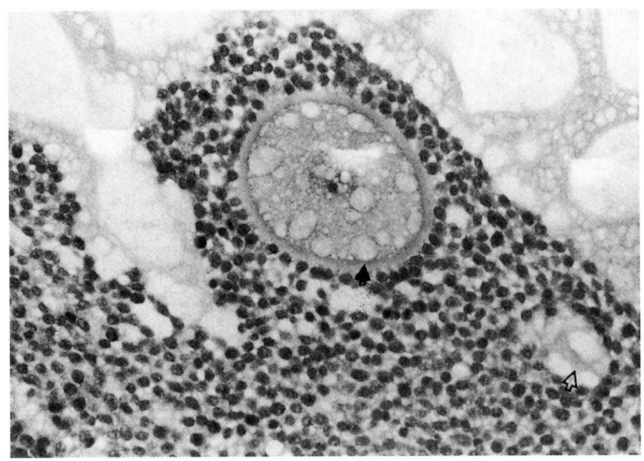

FIGURE 1.5 Cumulus oophorus with oocyte surrounded by zona pellucida (dark arrow). Call-Exner body (light arrow) is seen in granulosa.

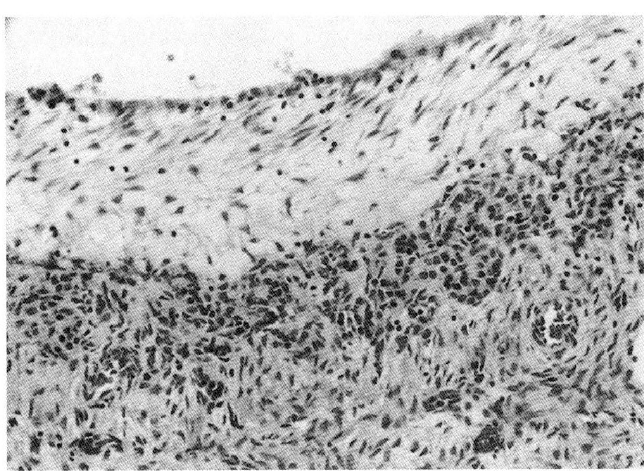

FIGURE 1.7 Atertic follicle with disintegrated granulosa and invasion of fibroblasts into the cavity.

rupture (the stigma) is characterized by the degeneration of the surface epithelium and underlying stroma. Simultaneously, the oocyte completes the first meiotic division, and is now termed a "secondary oocyte."

Ultrastructurally, granulosa cells of the maturing follicles are characterized by the growing number of mitochondria with lamelliform cristae, granular endoplasmic reticulum, and a large Golgi complex suggesting active protein synthesis.[18] The features of steroidogenesis (abundant smooth endoplasmic reticulum and mitochondria with tubular cristae) are absent until a short time before ovulation.[9–11]

E. Atretic Follicles

Of the original 1–2 million primordial follicles present at birth only 400 ovulate. The remaining 99.9% of the follicles disappear throughout the stages of maturation. This process is called atresia. The process continues long after maturation, explaining the predominance of atretic follicles in the histological picture.

The early signs of atresia include the separation of granulosa from the underlying theca and the degeneration of follicular cells (Fig. 1.6). Later granulosa cells disappear and the fibroblasts invade the cavity (Fig. 1.7). The basement membrane between theca and granulosa becomes thick and hyalinized, but the theca interna persists for a while. This pattern is more pronounced in premenarche, pregnancy, and in polycystic ovary syndrome.

Compact structures formed by the theca interna cells at the site of atresia are known as "interstitial glands," justifiably a criticized term.[19]

The theca interna cells produce androstenedione, which, in the absence of granulosa, is not transformed into estradiol, and their microenvironment is predominantly androgenic.

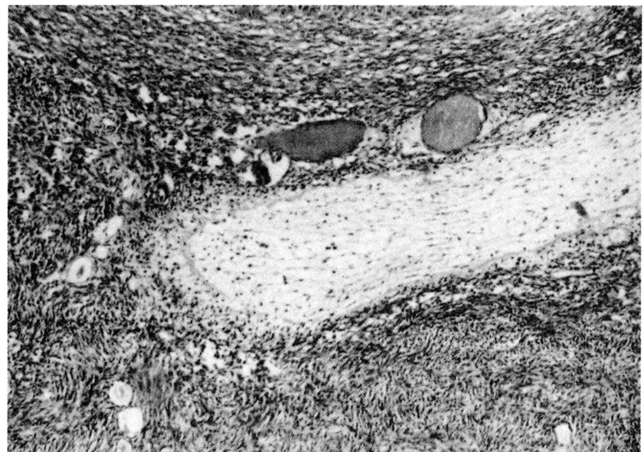

FIGURE 1.8 Corpus atreticum.

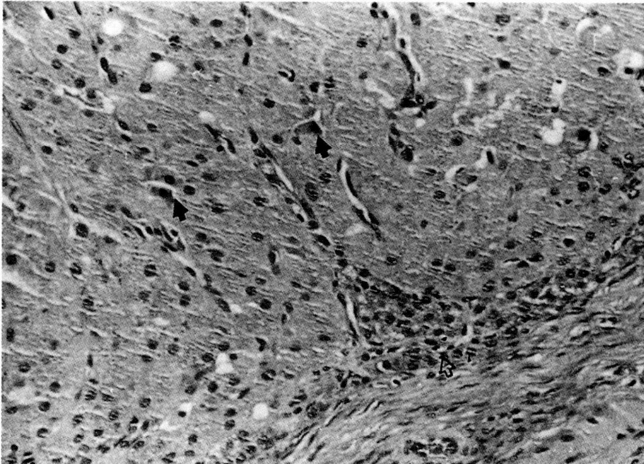

FIGURE 1.9 Active corpus luteum. K cells (dark arrow) are scattered among granulosa lutein cells, which constitute the bulk of the specimen. Theca (light arrow) is located at the periphery.

This is in contrast to a high concentration of estrogens in the growing follicles.[20]

In preantral follicles, atresia is primarily manifested by the pyknosis and fragmentation of the oocyte. In the antral stage, atresia is supplemented by the degeneration of granulosa. Sometimes granulosa cells persist and continue to secrete mucopolysaccharides maintaining high enough osmotic pressure to attract fluid, so the cavity of the atretic follicle expands despite the fact that the follicle is not growing. As a result, small cystic structures representing a cystic stage of the atretic process are frequently seen in the normal ovary. They are "cystic atretic follicles," and not "cysts," as they are commonly called, because "cyst" defines a pathological condition to which these structures do not belong.

The final product of atresia of the larger follicles is a slender scar termed "corpus atreticum" (Fig 1.8). A small follicle disappears without a trace.

F. Active Corpora Lutea

After ovulation and discharge of the oocyte, the ruptured follicle collapses and the blood forms an inner coagulum in its folded cavity. Immediately, the granulosa cells acquire an appearance quite distinct from that seen in the preovulatory follicle. They increase in size, accumulate lipids, and develop abundant cytoplasm containing fat soluble yellow pigment (lipochrome). The result is the new structure called the "corpus luteum."

Maturation of the corpus luteum involves the growth of vessels from the periphery, resorption and organization of the coagulum, and formation of the folds that consist of closely packed granulosa lutein cells. These cells are surrounded at the periphery by the theca interna which remain from the preexisting follicle (Fig. 1.9).

The corpus luteum exists for 14 days after ovulation and begins to degenerate if pregnancy does not occur. Its degeneration causes menstrual discharge, and correspondingly, it is called the "corpus luteum of menstruation." This structure attains complete maturity 8–10 days after ovulation when the blood vessels reach the central coagulum, and fibroblasts invade.

The luteinized granulosa cells of the mature corpus luteum are large (30–35 μm) with abundant pale eosinophilic cytoplasm containing small lipid droplets. The theca interna cells form a thin layer at the periphery of the corpus luteum and along the blood vessels. They are discernible by their smaller size and more deeply stained cytoplasm.

Other cells, the "K cells," appear within the granular lutein layer of the early corpus luteum. These stellate cells are characterized by deeply eosinophilic cytoplasm and irregular hyperchromatic nuclei (see Fig 1.9). K cells do not show histochemical features of steroidogenesis and are considered to be degenerative forms of the granulosa lutein cells or the theca cell.[21]

At the ultrastructural level, granulosa lutein cells have all the features of metabolically active steroid producers.

G. Involuting Corpora Lutea

In the absence of fertilization, the corpus luteum begins to disappear after 14 days post ovulation. The involution is marked by an increased density of the cytoplasm together with the appearance of the coarse lipid deposits, and pyknosis of the nuclei. After the granulosa lutein cells degenerate, fibroblasts invade the corpus luteum which continues to persist as a partially homogenized structure surrounded by a rim of still viable theca interna (Fig. 1.10). Finally, the regressing corpus luteum is converted to a hyalinized scar known as the "corpus albicans" (Fig 1.11). Most corpora albicantia are eventually resorbed. Some become dark brown or black due to the depositon of hemosiderin and form the "corpus nigricum."

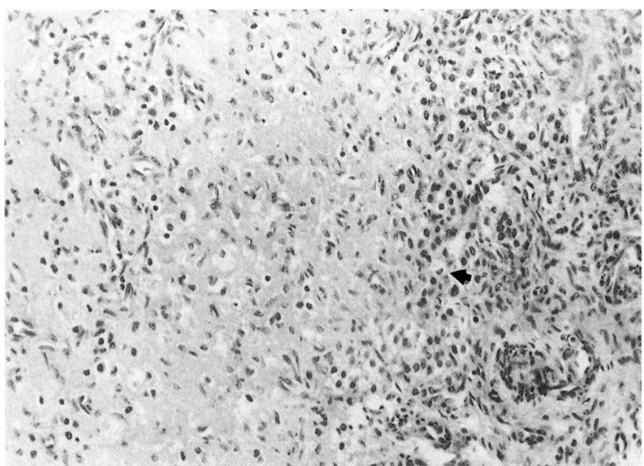

FIGURE 1.10 Involuting corpus luteum. Viable theca interna (arrow) is present at the periphery.

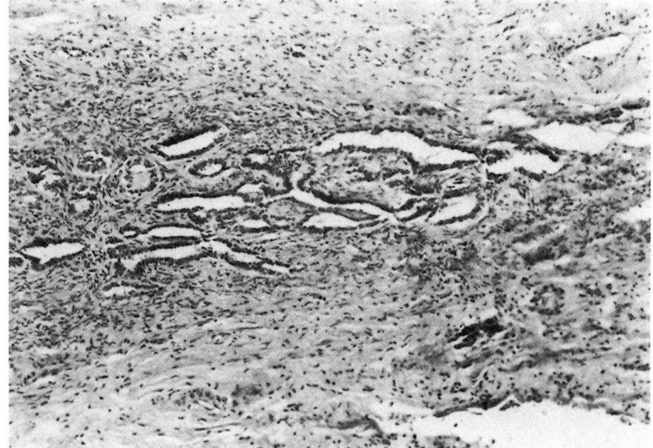

FIGURE 1.12 Rete ovarii.

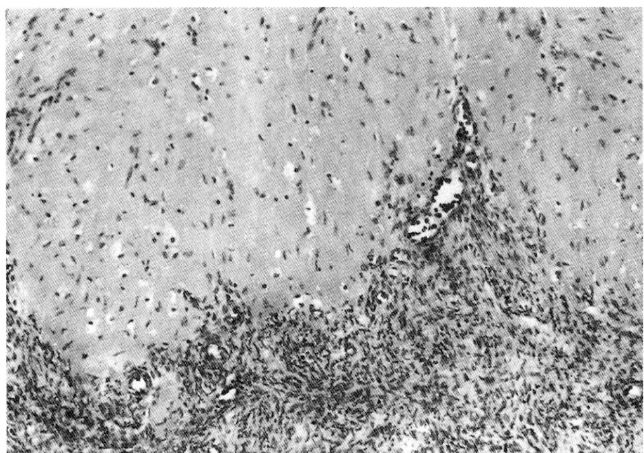

FIGURE 1.11 Corpus albicans.

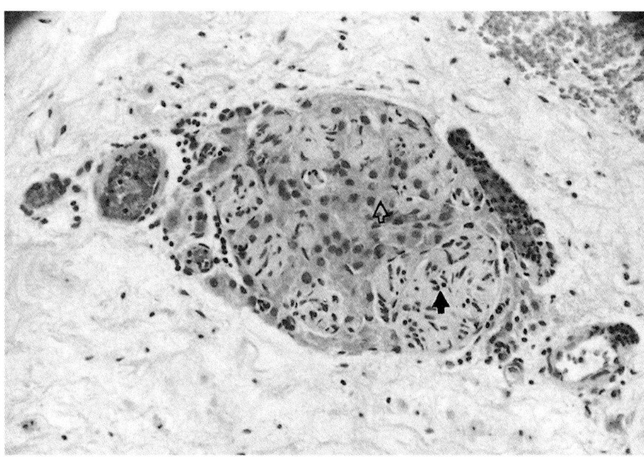

FIGURE 1.13 Hilus cells (light arrow) adjacent to the nerves (dark arrow).

The medulla of the mature ovary contains large tortuous vessels among which the spiral arteries constitute a special arrangement. These arteries provide the flow of blood as determined by the functional needs of the ovary. The flow is regulated by estrogens.[22]

H. Rete Ovarii and Hilus Cells

Two structural elements of the ovary represent the vestiges of that part of the undifferentiated gonad which could have become a testicle in a male fetus. They are the rete ovarii and the hilus cells.

The rete consists of anastomosing slit-like channels within the hilus of the ovary (Fig. 1.12). The channels are lined with the low cuboidal epithelium and represent the ducts which, in the male, transform into seminiferous tubules.

Ovarian hilus cells are morphologically identical to the testicular Leydig cells. They are located predominantly in the medulla, and their number varies significantly, being higher during pregnancy and after menopause.

The hilus cells form aggregates which are typically found in proximity to the nerve fibers (Fig. 1.13). Occasionally, the hilus cells surround the rete ovarii. They measure 15–25 μm in diameter, are round to oval, and have well-developed eosinophilic cytoplasm. The latter may contain rod-shaped homogenous crystalloid structures ("crystals of Reinke") characteristic of the testicular Leydig cells.

The ultrastructure of the ovarian hilar cells shows evidence of steroid hormone synthesis.

References

1. Snow, M. H. L., and Monk, M. (1983). Emergence and migration of primordial germ cells. *In* "Current Problems in Germ Cell differentiation" (A. McLaren, and C. C. Wylie, eds.), p. 115. Cambridge University Press, Cambridge.
2. Merchant, H. (1975). Rat gonadal and ovarian organogenesis. *Dev. Biol.* 44, 1–21.

3. Zuckerman, S., and Baker, T. G. (1977). Development of the ovary and oogenesis. *In* "The Ovary," Vol. 1, 2nd ed. (S. Zuckerman, and B. G. Weir, eds.), pp. 41–67. Academic Press, London.
4. Jirasek, J. E. (1977). Morphogenesis of the genital system in humans. *In* "Morphogenesis and Malformation of the Genital System," (R. J. Blandau, and D. Bergsma, eds), pp. 13–39. Alan R. Liss, New York.
5. Blaustein, A., Kantius, M., Koganowicz, A. *et al.* (1982). Inclusions in ovaries of females aged day 1–30 years. *Int. J. Gynecol. Pathol.* 1, 145–153.
6. Mulligan, R. M. (1976). A survey of epithelial inclusions in the ovarian cortex of 470 patients. *J. Surg. Oncol.* 8, 61–66.
7. Gondos, B. (1980). Surface epithelium of the developing ovary. *Am. J. Pathol.* 81, 303–320.
8. Dennfors, B. L., Janson, P. O., Knutson, F. *et al.* (1980). Steroid production and responsiveness to gonadotropin in isolated stromal tissue of human postmenopausal ovaries. *Am. J. Obstet. Gynecol.* 136, 997–1002.
9. Deane, H. W., Lobel, B. L., and Romney, S. L. (1962). Enzyme histochemistry of normal human ovaries of the menstrual cycle, pregnancy, and the early puerperium. *Am. J. Obstet. Gynecol.* 83, 281–294.
10. Feinberg, R., and Cohen, R. B. (1965). A comparative histochemical study of the ovarian stromal lipid band, stromal theca cell, and normal ovarian follicular apparatus. *Am. J. Obstet. Gynecol.* 92, 958–969.
11. Jones, C. E. S., Goldberg, B., and Woodruff, J. D. (1968). Histochemistry as a guide for interpretation of cell function. *Am. J. Obstet. Gynecol.* 100, 76–83.
12. Hammond, C. B., and Ory, S. J. (1985). Endocrine aspects of menopause. *In* "Clinical Reproductive Endocrinology" (R. P. S. Scherman, ed.), pp. 185–208. Churchill Livingstone, Edinburgh.
13. Macklon, N. S., and Fauser, B. C. (1999). Aspects of ovarian follicle development throughout life. *Horm. Res.* 52, 161–170.
14. Fukuda, M., Fukuda, A., Yiding Andersen, C., and Byskov, A. G. (1997). Does corpus luteum locally affect follicular growth negatively? *Hum. Reprod.* 12, 1024–1027.
15. Baker, T. G., and Franchi, L. L. (1986). The ovary including its development. *In* "Scientific Foundations of Obstetrics and Gynecology" (E. Philipp, J. Barnes, and M. Newton, eds.), p. 166. Year Book Medical Publishers, Chicago.
16. Russell, P., and Bannatyne, P. (1989). "Surgical Pathology of the Ovaries," p. 14. Churchill Livingstone, Edinburgh.
17. Motta, P. M., and Hafez, E. S. E. (1980). "Biology of the Ovary," p. 176. Martinus Nijhoff, The Hague.
18. Clement, P. B. (1987). Anatomy and histology of the ovary. *In* "Blaustein's Pathology of the Female Genital Tract." (R. Kurman, ed.), p. 450. Springer-Verlag, New York.
19. Balboni, G. C. (1976). Histology of the ovary. *In* "The Endocrine Function of the Human Ovary" (M. Serio, and G. Giusti, eds.), pp. 1–24. Academic Press, London.
20. McNatty, K. P., Smith, D. M., Markis, A. *et al.* (1979). The microenvironment of the human antral follicle. *J. Clin. Endocrinol. Metab.* 49, 851–860.
21. Gillim, S. W., Christensen, A. K., and McLennan, C. E. (1969). Fine structure of the human menstrual corpus luteum at its stage of maximum secretory activity. *Am. J. Anat.* 126, 409–428.
22. Baker, T. G., and Franchi, L. L. (1986). The ovary including its development. *In* "Scientific Foundations of Obstetrics and Gynecology" (E. Philipp, J. Barnes, and M. Newton, eds.), p. 175. Year Book Medical Publishers, Chicago.

CHAPTER

2A

The Normal Human Ovary Part I
Reproductive and Endocrine Functions

NATHAN G. KASE

Department of Obstetrics, Gynecology and Reproductive Science
The Mount Sinai School of Medicine and Hospital
New York, New York 10029

I. INTRODUCTION

The major functions of the human ovary are the nurture, development, and release of a mature oocyte ready for fertilization and achievement of successful propagation of the species. In support of these processes the ovary secretes steroid hormones which stimulate growth and development of secondary sexual characteristics, are critically involved in an elaborate endocrine interchange which directs orderly, repetitive cyclic ovulations, and finally supports successful uterine implantation and the early phase of pregnancy.[1–3] A description of how the ovary and its secretions achieve these reproductive functions is the focus of this chapter.

In addition, it is now clear from observations in prolonged physiologic (menopause) and nonphysiologic (gonadal failure) hypofunctional states that ovarian steroid secretions have important influences on a variety of nonreproductive organ systems which influence the quality of life as well as the life expectancy of women. A more complete treatment of these issues is dealt with in Chapter 27, Menopause, as well as Part II of this chapter.

II. REPRODUCTION

The physiologic responsibilities of the ovary are the periodic release of gametes (oocytes or "eggs") and the timely sequential secretion of the hormones estradiol, progesterone, and the inhibins A and B. These endocrine signals integrate the hypothalamus, anterior pituitary, and ovaries in

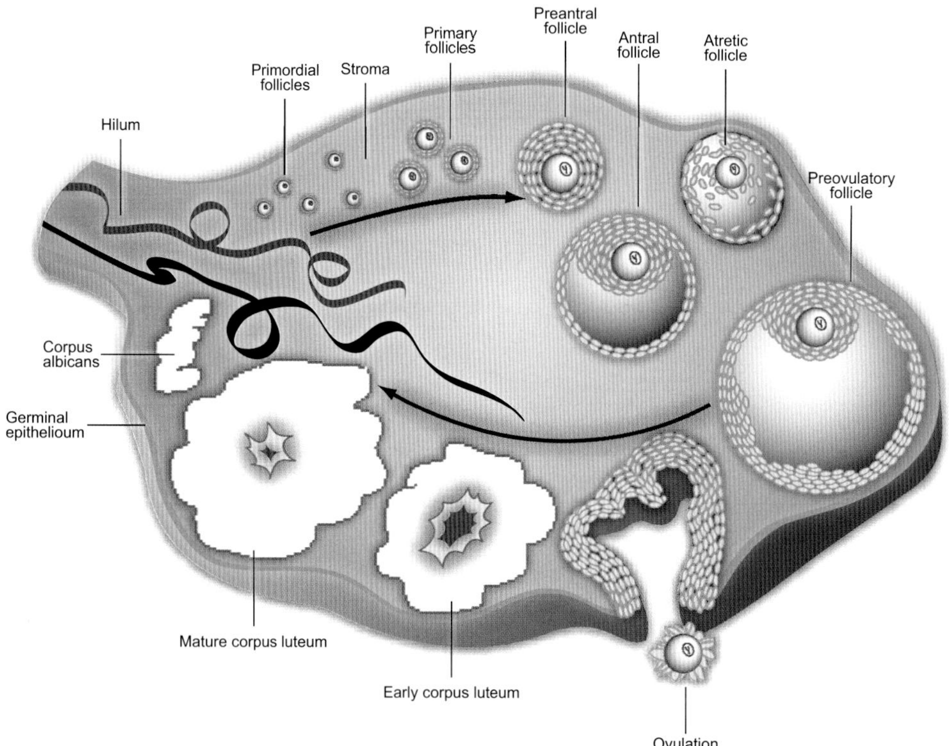

FIGURE 2A.1 Extrinsic and intrinsic factors direct folliculogenesis beginning with emergence from a resting pool of primordial follicles, follicle recruitment, rescue or atresia, selection of the dominant follicle, ovulation, corpus luteum function, and regression. The ovary is a heterogeneous constantly changing organ, and each phase of its function is governed by a specific anatomic subunit—either the dominant follicle or the corpus luteum. (From Speroff *et al.* 1999, p. 119).

a continuous repetitive process of follicle rescue, maturation, ovulation, and corpus luteum formation, function, and regression (Fig 2A.1).[4, 5] The ovary cannot be viewed as a relatively static purely endocrine organ whose size and function waxes and wanes depending on the stimulatory input of tropic hormones. Rather the female gonad is a heterogeneous, constantly changing organ with cyclicity measured in days and weeks rather than hours with each phase governed by a specific anatomic subunit. Functionally the ovary is an envelope the function of which in any month in adult menstrual life is defined by a single dominant follicle and after ovulation its transformation into a corpus luteum.

A. Human Follicle Endowment, Development, and Depletion

1. The Fixed "Pool" and "Resting Reserve" of Primordial Follicles

Three sequential partially overlapping processes—oogonial proliferation, initiation of meiosis I with conversion of oogonia to primary oocytes, encapsulation of the oocyte by pregranulosa cells forming the primordial follicle—establish the reservoir of ovarian primordial follicles.[6]

In humans, primordial germ cells arise in the yolk sac endoderm and migrate to the gonadal ridge (they do not survive elsewhere) by the seventh week of gestation. Oogonia proliferate by mitosis during migration and at a greatly accelerated pace once in the gonadal ridge resulting in a peak germ cell content in excess of 6–7 million at 20 weeks of fetal life. Thereafter oogonial division dramatically declines, in effect ending at midgestation thereby creating a "fixed endowment" of germ cells which cannot be replenished.[7, 8] Transformation of individual oogonia into primary oocytes (entry into the first stages of meiosis) is initiated at 11–12 weeks and continues over the remainder of fetal life. Also around midgestation primordial follicle formation begins as a single layer of pregranulosa cells envelopes each oocyte in a process that continues until just after birth (Fig. 2A.2). After oocytes are enclosed within the primordial follicles they remain arrested for variable time intervals in the dictyate state of meiosis I and remain in this condition in a "resting pool." Oocytes not surrounded by pregranulosa cells are lost presumably by extrusion beyond the ovarian capsule or more likely by programmed cell death (apoptosis).[9]

The variable duration of the period of arrest and the factors which modify it are not understood. However, from within minutes or even decades after formation, a primordial follicle may leave the resting pool and initiate oocyte enlargement and granulosa cell differentiation and proliferation to a variety of preantral or antral stages (Fig. 2A.3). At any point during this process atresia may take place. As a result, from a peak oocyte number of 6–7 million at 20 weeks, only 1–2 million exist at birth and at puberty an average of 200,000 follicles remain in the ovary.[7] During reproductive life, in addition to the monthly ovulation of a single dominant follicle, continuing reactivation, growth, and atresia of follicles at the rate of about 1000 per month results in an unrelenting decrease in the original follicle reserve pool. Approximately 8–10 years before menopause, concomitant with rising levels of follicle stimulating hormone (FSH) and diminished inhibins, increasing percentages of follicles are lost from the resting pool.[10] This terminal acceleration in follicle depletion rate "serves as a ticking clock to time the onset of menopause." Eventually as a result of ovarian follicle exhaustion menopause occurs at about 51 years of age, "a time point that has remained constant for centuries."[11]

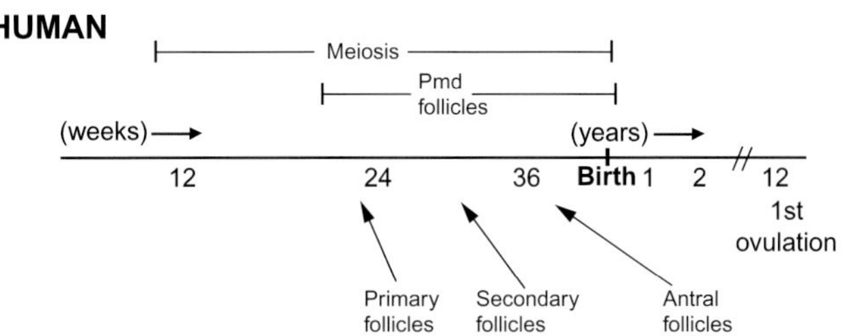

FIGURE 2A.2 Follicle development during fetal and neonatal life in humans. Before birth oocyte meiosis I has been initiated and arrested, primordial follicles are generated, and the resting pool of primary follicles is established. Also, before birth initiation of follicle development occurs, expressed in generation of large numbers of secondary follicles and various stages of preantral and antral follicles—all lost in a follicle reserve reducing wave of atresia. (From McGee, E. A., and Hsueh, A. J. W., (2000). *Endocr. Rev.* 21, Issue 2, Fig. 3, p. 203.)

B. The Dynamics of Normal Human Follicle Activation, Recruitment, Selection, or Atresia [11]

1. "Timeline" of Follicle Activation, Recruitment, Selection, and Dominance

Initial recruitment of a primordial follicle into the growing pool of primary follicles is protracted but the exact duration is unknown (Fig. 2A.4). Clearly longer than previously imagined, more than 120 days is required to pass from primary to the secondary follicle stage and 71 days are needed for the secondary group to enter the early antral stages.[13] At the 2–5 mm antral stage, *cyclic recruitment* intervenes as the menstrual and postmenstrual increase in FSH stimulates

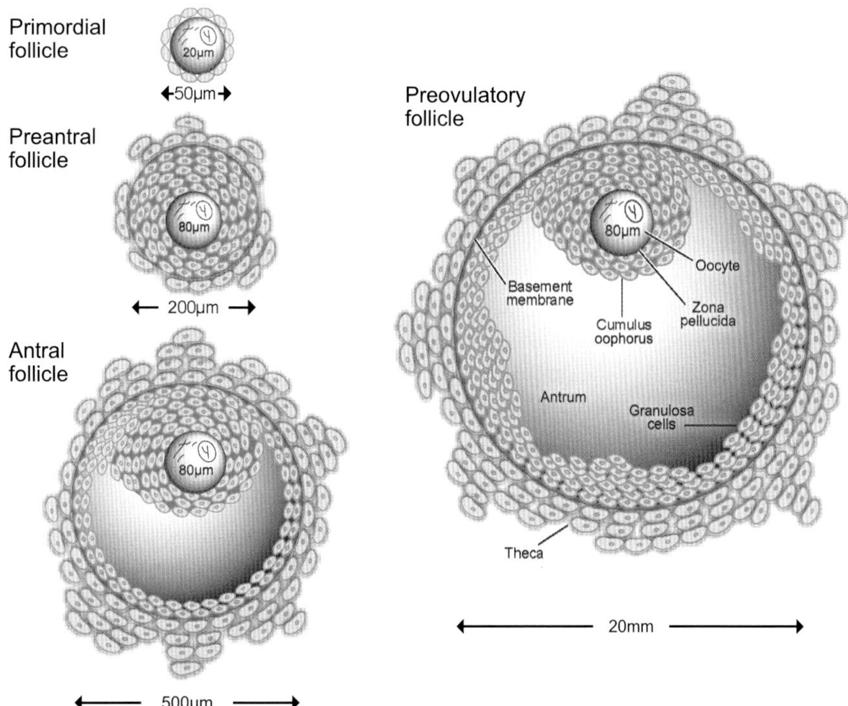

FIGURE 2A.3 The various stages of preovulatory follicle development. (From Speroff *et al.* (1999). "Clinical Gynecologic Endocrinology and Infertility," pp. 203, 6th Ed. Williams & Wilkins, Baltimore, MD.)

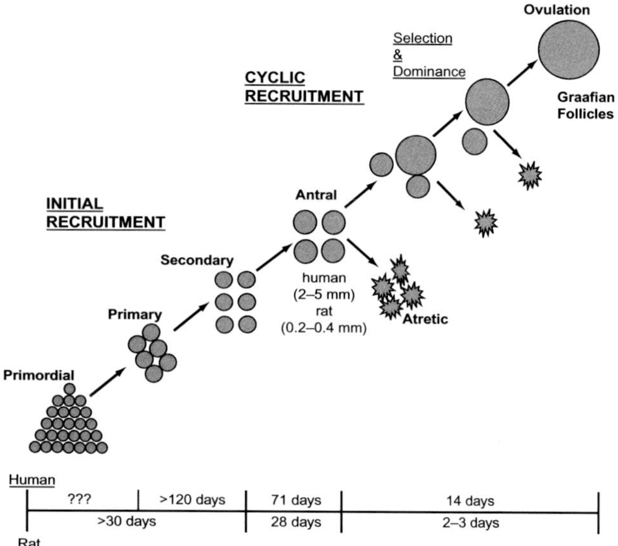

FIGURE 2A.4 The "timelines" of establishment of the resting pool of follicles, follicle activation, recruitment, select or atresia, and ovulation, in the human and rodent ovary. (From McGee, E. A., and Hsueh, A. J. W. (2000). *Endocr. Rev.* 21, Issue 2, Fig. 2, p. 202.)

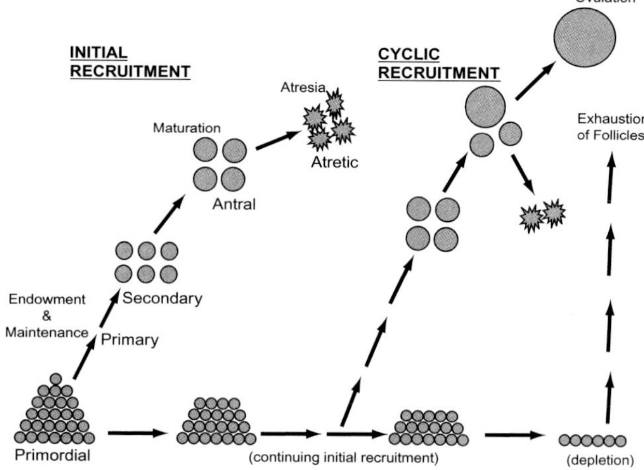

FIGURE 2A.5 The distinction between "initial" and "cyclic" follicle recruitment. Large numbers of follicles undergo *initial recruitment* from the resting pool (activation) and proceed through various stages of development even into antral stages only to cease further maturation and become atretic. On the other hand, a small portion of initially recruited antral stage follicles are "rescued" from atresia at a particular phase of the menstrual cycle by FSH by a process defined as cyclic recruitment. FSH and LH combined with a variety of intrinsic factors stimulate a selected follicle to ovulatory readiness. (From McGee, E. A., and Hsueh, A. J. W. (2000). *Endocr. Rev.* 21, Issue 2, Fig. 1, p. 201.)

a cohort of these follicles to resist apoptotic degeneration and escape demise.[14] Among this group, a "selected" follicle emerges as dominant and is readied for ovulation.[15] The duration of this selection and dominance phase is comparatively brief lasting only 14 days.

C. Gonadotropin- and Follicle-Dependent Factors Determine Follicle Destiny

1. General Principles [11]

The fate of each follicle is controlled by endocrine as well as intrafollicular factors (Fig 2A.5). In the human, regulation of the continuous process of activation and preliminary growth up to the small antral stage (initial recruitment) occurs independent of gonadotropin stimulation. Only at advanced antral stages do follicles unequivocally become dependent on FSH for avoidance of apoptosis and receipt of the impetus to further development. Whereas initial recruitment is cycle- and gonadotropin-independent, rescue and further development (cyclic recruitment) depends on the cyclic increase in circulating FSH during the menstrual and early follicle phases of the menstrual cycle. In simplest form, the development of follicles is divided into gonadotropin-independent and -dependent stages.

Gonadotropin involvement in follicle development can be refined further into gonadotropin and other *survival factor (antiatretic) dependent* and *gonadotropin plus other growth factor follicle responsive* (dominant follicle selection) stages. The lead follicle is *selected* from the rescued cohort of antral follicles by a combination of *extrinsic* (endocrine) and *intrinsic* (autocrine, paracrine) mechanisms. For example, by secreting increasingly high levels of estradiol and inhibin B, the selected follicle suppresses FSH availability. The result is a negative selection influence on the remaining cohort which lapses into atresia due to diminished availability of anti-apoptotic FSH.[16, 17] On the other hand, through *intrinsic* processes [18] such as increased FSH receptors, local growth factors and thecal vascular enhancement, the lead follicle is able to maximize utilization of dwindling FSH which fosters not only survival/positive selection, but stimulation of further growth, differentiation, and ultimately, ovulation.[19–22]

In summary, whereas preantral growth displays increasing degrees of *FSH responsiveness*, the events governing the fate of the selected follicle reflect *complete dependence* on FSH and the intrafollicular (*intrinsic*) mechanisms that maximize and ensure follicle survival and further development.

The complex events that yield an oocyte for fertilization and the ovarian processes that protect and support follicle function involve practically every regulatory mechanism in human biology. These include classic endocrine signals, intracrine, autocrine, paracrine regulation, probably neuronal input, and immune system contributions. With the single exception of FSH none of these systems alone is either sufficient or absolutely necessary for achievement of final growth and ovulation. Rather, these should be looked upon as interactive participants in a collective, synergistic mutually facilitating response mechanism, which maximizes FSH and luteinizing hormone (LH) instructions (Fig 2A.6).[23]

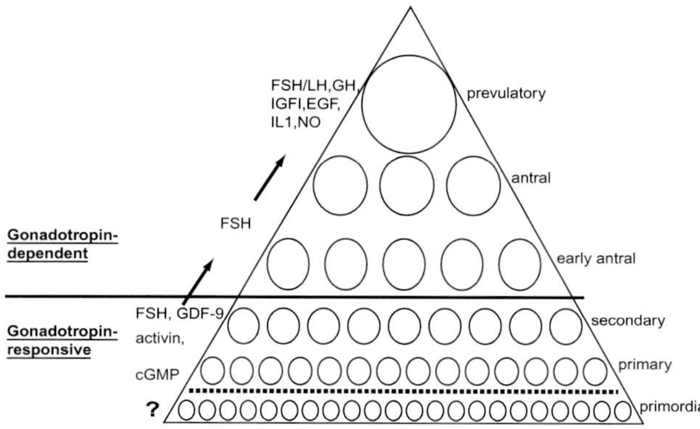

FIGURE 2A.6 Stage specific endocrine and intrinsic factors involved in the survival and development of follicles. The crucial importance of FSH not only in the gonadotropin dependent antral through preovulatory stages (rescue from atresia in cyclic recruitment), but also in the earlier gonadotropin responsive phases of follicle development is emphasized. (From McGee, E. A., and Hsueh, A. J. W. (2000). *Endocr. Rev.* 21, Issue 2, Fig. 4, p. 208.)

2. Specific Regulators

a. Intrinsic Control Factors in Follicle Development [24]

Any consideration of the microenvironment factors and events involved in the control and promotion of follicle function must begin with a review of the various modes of action of these molecules and examination of the properties and function of the major elements in this system.

Whereas in the classic endocrine pathways regulatory molecules (hormones) are secreted into the blood stream and transported to distant target tissues whose function they modify, at least three modes of local action are understood.

1. *Paracrine* modality: Regulatory molecules are secreted by one cell and influence functions of contiguous neighboring cells
2. *Autocrine* modality: A cell regulates its own function by secreting factors which then interact with receptors on its own plasma membrane
3. *Intracrine* (or ultracrine) modality: A cell regulates its own function without secretion and without interaction with a plasma membrane receptor; rather, unsecreted factors bind with intracellular receptors or other modulating mechanisms

b. Major "Intrinsic" Follicle Regulators

i. Inhibin, Activin, Follistatin [25–28] This family of peptides is synthesized by granulosa cells in response to FSH and is secreted into follicle fluids. In addition, each possesses endocrine hormonal action as they are secreted into the ovarian vein. As such inhibins (A and B) are important inhibitors of FSH secretion. Activin stimulates FSH release in the pituitary and augments FSH action in the ovary. Follistatin suppresses FSH activity *in vitro* but seems less important in clinical conditions. Its demonstrated suppression of FSH is probably achieved by inactivating binding of activin.

ii. Growth Factors These polypeptides modulate cell proliferation and differentiation by binding to specific cell membrane receptors. Some have important endocrine functions but most work locally in autocrine and paracrine fashion. Multiple growth factors exist and most cells of the body have receptors for these peptides. Those of importance in the ovary include:

1. Insulin-Like Growth Factors (IGF-I and -II).[29] Formerly called somatomedins, IGF-I and -II are peptides that have structural and functional similarity to insulin and mediate growth hormone (GH) action. IGF-I mediates the growth-promoting action of GH. The majority of circulating IGF-I is synthesized and secreted by the liver in response to GH. However, IGF-I can be made in many tissues in response to factors other than GH and has important autocrine/paracrine activities. IGF-II is the major IGF in the ovary and has little GH dependence. Like IGF-I, it is expressed in many tissues and works locally to modulate cell proliferation and differentiation.
   - *Insulin-Like Growth Factor Binding Protein (IGFBP).*[30] Of the six known IGFBPs, 1 and 3 are the most important. These proteins transport IGF in blood, prolong their half-lives, and regulate tissue effects of the IGFs. Generally they prevent IGF access to cell membrane receptors.
   - *Insulin-Like Growth Factor Receptors.*[31, 32] The physiologic effects of IGF-I are mediated by its receptor while IGF-II binds to both its receptor and the IGF-I receptor with equal affinity. In humans IGF-I and IGF-II receptors are present in granulosa, theca, and in the luteinized granulosa cells of the Corpus luteum. Ovarian stroma contains IGF-I receptors.
2. *Epidermal Growth Factor.*[33] Epidermal growth factor is a mitogen for a variety of cells, and its action is potentiated by other growth factors. Granulosa cells, in particular, respond to this growth factor in a variety of ways related to gonadotropin stimulation, including proliferation. Epidermal growth factor suppresses the upregulation of FSH on its own receptor.
3. *Transforming Growth Factors.* TGF-α is a structural analog of epidermal growth factor and can bind to the epidermal growth factor receptor. TGF-β utilizes a receptor distinct from the epidermal growth factor receptor. These factors are thought to be autocrine growth regulators. Inhibin and activin are derived from the same gene family. TGF-β, secreted by theca cells, enhances FSH induction of LH receptors on granulosa cells, an action which is opposite that of epidermal growth factor. In the theca, TGF-β has a negative action, inhibiting androgen production.

4. *Fibroblast Growth Factor*.[34, 35] This factor is a mitogen for a variety of cells and is present in all steroid-producing tissues. Important roles in the ovarian follicle include stimulation of mitosis in granulosa cells, stimulation of angiogenesis, stimulation of plasminogen activator, inhibition of FSH upregulation of its own receptor, and inhibition of FSH-induced LH receptor expression and estrogen production. These actions are opposite of those of TGF-β.
5. *Platelet-Derived Growth Factor*.[24] This growth factor modifies cyclic AMP pathways responding to FSH, especially those involved in granulosa cell differentiation. Both platelet-derived growth factor and epidermal growth factor may also modify prostaglandin production within the follicle.
6. *Angiogenic Growth Factors*.[36, 37] Blood flow within the ovary is most intense in the theca surrounding the dominant follicle and in luteinized granulosa cells of the corpus luteum. This vascularization is induced by angiogenic peptides, especially vascular endothelial growth factor (VEGF), a cytokine produced in granulosa cells in response to LH. Luteal cells respond to human chorionic gonadotropin (HCG) with even greater VEGF output, thereby maximizing substrate delivery and corpus luteum progesterone production during early pregnancy. This is also the probable mechanism contributing to the increased vascular permeability associated with HCG during exogenous gonadotropin ovulation induction and development of the hyperstimulation syndrome.

iii. Cytokines

1. *Interleukin-1 System*.[38] Leukocytes are a prominent component of the ovarian follicle and a major source of interleukins. Interleukin-1 is a member of this cytokine family of immunomediators. The human ovary contains the complete interleukin-1 system (ligand and receptor). In the rat, interleukin-1 stimulates ovarian prostaglandin synthesis and perhaps plays a role in ovulation.
2. *Tumor Necrosis Factor-α (TNF-α)*. TNF-α is also a product of leukocytes (macrophages). It is a key player in the process of apoptosis, follicle atresia, and luteolysis of the corpus luteum.

iv. Other Peptides

1. *Anti-Müllerian Hormone (AMH)*. Is best known for its production by Sertoli cells and its crucial influence on the internal genitalia phenotype of the developing male fetus. In female granulosa cells AMH is expressed later in life and may act as a meiosis-inhibiting factor as well as an inhibitor of granulosa cell and luteal cell proliferation.
2. *Oocyte Meiosis (or Maturation) Inhibitor (OMI)*. Is secreted by granulosa cells into the follicle fluid. It may also cross directly to the oocyte by gap junction channels which connect granulosa cell and the oocyte. Oocytes not exposed to follicle fluid or not in contact with granulosa immediately resume meiosis and degenerate. The LH surge overcomes or represses OMI allowing acceleration and completion of meiosis I at ovulation.
3. *Endothelin I*. This peptide made in vascular endothelial cells in reaction to hyproxia, is emerging as a major factor in luteolysis. It inhibits luteinization, reduces LH-induced progesterone production, and probably induces prostaglandin F2α release.[39]

3. Ovarian Actions of Intrinsic Factors

a. Estradiol

Although the central stimulatory role of estradiol in granulosa cell growth and differentiation in the *rodent* is unquestioned, recent observations in the primate have cast doubt on whether estradiol is a participant, let alone required, for human ovarian folliculogenesis, oocyte maturation, and ovulation. While its endocrine role in the HPO axis is undisputed, lessons learned from successful exogenous gonadotropin induction of follicle enlargement (antral expansion), retrievable and fertilizable oocytes, as well as with cleavable and apparently transferable embryos in women with markedly reduced to nonexistent intrafollicular and circulating concentrations of estradiol are the basis for this uncertainty. These clinical demonstrations include women with steroid synthesis abnormalities such as 3β-hydroxysteroid dehydrogenase deficiency, aromatase deficiency, and in particular the 17α-hydroxylase/17–20 lyase deficiency, as well as profoundly hypogonadotropic women or those treated with GnRH agonist gonadotropin suppression.

Palter *et al*.[40] have reviewed the literature on this important subject and have framed their analysis of the available data in four key categories:

1. Human granulosa cells *do* possess the subtype ERα and ERβ receptors. There *is* both reception and activity induced by estrogen in the human ovary and represents the net impact generated by the relative contributions of these receptors at both the nuclear and "nonclassical" nongenomic level (Tables 2A.1 and 2A.2).
2. The human oocyte does *not* display clear evidence of expression or immunohistochemical presence of either ER subtype. However, given the apparent importance of estradiol to normal cytoplasmic gametogenic maturation and efficient rates of fertilization and embryogenesis, an indirect estrogen impact via a granulosa-oocyte gap junction transfer must be considered. Similarly non-genomic, non-ER mediated estrogen influenced membrane agents may also play an important role in oocyte biology.
3. An estrogen-free intrafollicular environment *is* compatible with antral enlargement (if not full granulosa proliferation or differention), ovulation, and corpus luteum formation.
4. An estrogen free/poor intrafollicular environment is probably *not* compatible with full gametogenic maturation in either primates or humans. As shown in a number of primate studies, an estrogen free/poor follicle is associated

Table 2A.1 Compilation of Evidence that the Primate/Human Ovary is a Site of Estrogen Reception and Action by Molecular Probing

Species	Developmental stage	Imaging technology	ERα status	ERβ status
Baboon cyonomolgus/rhesus	Mature	NB	Whole ovary (+)	NA
	Mature	RT-PCR	Whole ovary (+) GE(+) CL(–) GC(–) GC*(–)	NA
Rhesus	Mature	RT-PCR ISH	Whole ovary (+) GH(+)	Whole ovary (+) GH(+)
Rhesus	Mature	RT-PCR	GC(+) GC*(+)	GC(+) GC*(+)
Cynomolgus	Mature	ISH	NA	GC (+) TC (+) GE (+) CL (+)
Human	Mature	RT-PCR/SB	Whole ovary (+) Oocyte (+) GC*(–)	NA
Human	Mature	RT-PCR/SB	GC*(+)	NA
Human	Mature	ISH	GC (+) TC (+) CL (+) Stroma (+) Oocyte (–)	NA
Human	Fetus	RT-PCR	Whole ovary (+)	Whole ovary (+)
Human	Mature	ISH RT-PCR	NA	Stroma (+) GC*(+)
Human	Mature	RT-PCR/SB	Whole ovary (+)	Whole ovary (+) GC*(+)
Human	Mature	RT-PCR NB	GC*(+)	GC*(+)

ISH, *in situ* hybridisation; GC, granulosa cell; (+), positive result; NB; Northern blot analysis; GC*, luteinized granulosa cell; (–), negative result; SB, southern blot analysis; CL, corpus luteum, TC, theca cell; NIA, not applicable/available; GE, germinal epithelium.

Source: From Palter, S. F., Tavares, A. B., Hourvitz, A., Veldhuis, J. D., Hyashi, E. Y. (2001). *Endocr. Rev.* 22, Table 3, p. 398.

with marked decrements in the rates of meiotic maturation and fertilization efficiency.

In summary, it appears that while intrafollicular estradiol is neither necessary nor sufficient, it plays a significant contributory role in development of the selected dominant follicle's maturation leading to ovulation and an essential role in oocyte maturation. In this regard, the importance of nonclassical modes of hormone action should be emphasized. Furthermore, in addition to nongenomic mechanisms, ligand-independent steroid receptor activation by signaling pathways stimulated by growth factors such as EGF, TGF-α, and IGF-I should be considered in the paradoxical generation of activity in follicles equipped with estrogen receptors but without significant presence of the provocative ligand estradiol.[24]

b. IGF [41–44]

IGF-II stimulates granulosa cell proliferation, aromatase activity and progesterone synthesis in the human follicle and corpus luteum. In the *early proliferative* phase IGF-II is produced in the theca in response to LH. IGF-II acts in an autocrine mode through its receptor and augments the LH-induced steroidogenesis of testosterone and androstenedione. Furthermore, in a paracrine mode IGF-II again through its receptor on the granulosa cell augments FSH-directed cell proliferation, aromatase availability, and also induces synthesis of inhibin and activin. In the preovulatory follicle, when LH receptors are now active in the granulosa cell, thecal IGF accelerates granulosa cell proliferation and assists LH in the initiation of progesterone synthesis, a property that continues into the Corpus Luteum phase. That successful induction of ovulation in IGF-I-deficient women can be accomplished with exogenous (human menopausal gonadotropin) HMG/HCG places the IGF system in a facilitatory supportive role in follicle maturation and emphasizes, as in enzymatic impaired hypoestrogenism, the genetic survival pressure to equip the follicle with multiple enhancing but not uniquely essential systems to achieve ovulation.

TABLE 2A.2 Compilation of Evidence that the Primate/Human Ovary is a Site of Estrogen Reception and Action by Immunohistochemistry

Species	Developmental stage	Antibody	Immunoreactivity
Rhesus/cynomolgus	Mature	H222/D75	ER (+) in GE, all others structures negative
Baboon	Mature	H222/D75	ER (+) in GC of AF, TC (+), stroma (–)
Rhesus	Mature	H222	ER (+) in GC of AF, TC (+), GE (+), interstitium (+)
Marmoset	Mature	ERα=NCL-ER-6F11	ERα=GC (+) (M/L follicles) TC (+) GE (+)
		ERβ=P3/P4/P7	ERβ=GC (+) (S/M/L follicles) TC (+) GE (+)
Human	Mature	H222	ER (+) in GC of AF/DF
			CL (–) GC* (–) GE (NA)
Human	Mature	H222	ER (+) in GC of AF/DF
			GC* (+) GE (NA)
Human	Mature	EDR_{1d5}	ER (+) in GC of AF/DF
			TC (–) stroma (–) CL (–) oocytes (–)
Human	Mature	N/A	ER=GC (+) (S/M/L follicles) TC (+), stroma (+), CL (+)
Human	Mature	ERα=anti-bovine ERα (05-394)	ERα=GC (+) TC (–) CL (–)
		ERβ=anti-rat ERβ (06-629)	ERβ=GC (+) (S/M/L follicles) TC (+), CL (+)
Human	Mature	ERα=NCL-ER-6F11	ERα=GC (+) (M/L follicles) TC (+) GE (+)
		ERβ=P3/P4/P7	ERβ=GC (+) (S/M/L follicles) TC (+) GE (+)
Human	Mature	ERα=HC-20	ERα=TC (+) GE (+) interstitum (+)
		ERβ=directed to a SP (aa 46-63 of ERβ)	ERβ=GC (+) (S/M/L follicles) GE (+), interstitium (+)

ER, estrogen receptor; ERα, estrogen receptor subtype α; GE, germinal epithelium; GC, granulosa cell; AF, antral follicle; CL, corpus luteum; TC, theca cell; DF, dominant follicle; N/A, not applicable/available; ERβ, estrogen receptor subtype β; (+), positive result; (–), negative result; SP, synthetic peptide; GCS', luteinized granulosa cell; S, small; M, medium; L, large; aa, amino acid.

Source: From Palter, S. F., Tavares, A. B., Hourvitz, A., Veldhuis, J. D., Hyashi, E. Y. (2001). *Endocr. Rev.*, Table 4, p. 401.

c. Inhibin/Activin System [24]

This system possesses critically important intrinsic as well as extrinsic endocrine functions in follicle development in humans (Fig. 2A.7).[45, 46] Inhibin is an important circulating signal which inhibits FSH secretion. Activin stimulates FSH release from the pituitary and augments FSH action in the ovary. The broad out line of this system's promotion of human follicle development follows.

FSH stimulates inhibin and activin production by granulosa cells.[27] By autocrine mode, activin increases FSH functional impact by accelerating granulosa cell proliferation, aromatase capacity, and upregulating FSH receptors in these cells. Granulosa cell inhibin, acting in a paracrine mode augments *theca* cell androgen synthesis, whereas activin modifies that stimulation.[47] As follicle maturation progresses granulosa cell inhibin B continues to stimulate androgen synthesis in the theca and now is of sufficient quantity to be secreted as a hormone and act in a negative feedback endocrine mode decreasing FSH. Activin, while continuing to exert its important antiapoptotic control of androgen synthesis in the theca, begins to prepare the granulosa cell for luteal phase function by assisting FSH in the induction

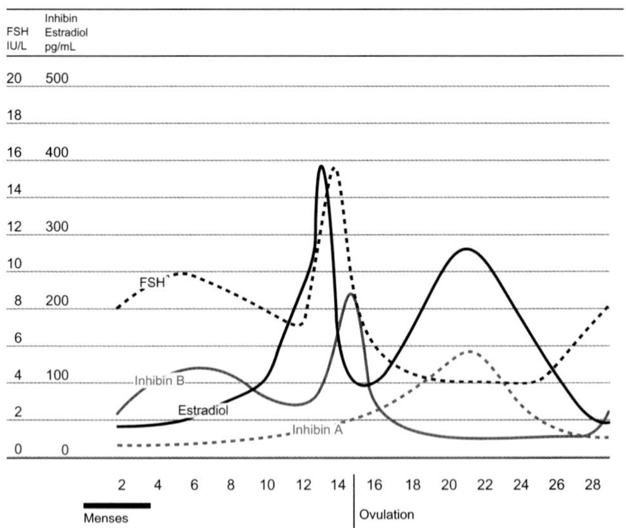

FIGURE 2A.7 Concentrations of FSH, E2, and inhibin A and B throughout the human menstrual cycle. During the late follicle phase, the combination E2 and inhibin B reduce FSH through negative feedback. In the luteal phase, E2, inhibin A, and progesterone (not shown) suppress FSH and LH. (From Speroff *et al.* (1999). "Clinical Gynecologic Encodcrinology and Infertility," p. 212, 6th Ed. Williams & Wilkins, Baltimore, MD).

of LH receptors on these cells.[48] However, activin modifies the synthesis of progesterone in the preovulatory ovary. Finally, and in a crucial step in selection of the dominant follicle, activin stimulates further induction of FSH receptors in granulosa cells thereby maximizing the dominant follicle's capacity to survive and continue to flourish despite the dwindling supply of FSH (inhibin induced).

III. INTEGRATIONS OF ENDOCRINE AND INTRINSIC FACTORS: GONADOTROPINS, INTRAOVARIAN FACTORS, AND THE OOCYTE IN THE SPECTRUM OF FOLLICLE FUNCTION

A. Initial Recruitment and Primary Follicle Growth

Although the mechanisms controlling the earliest stages of follicle growth, i.e., initial recruitment and primary follicle growth are understandably difficult to study, these steps are generally believed *not* to be absolutely gonadotropin or steroid dependent.[49, 50] Receptors for these hormones cannot be detected at this stage of follicle development. Furthermore, initial recruitment and growth is seen in gonadotropin-deficient mutant mice and in anencephalic human fetuses. However, the rates of depletion of the follicle reserve pool are highest when fetal FSH concentrations are maximal such as in midgestation and in the adult perimenopause suggesting a possible influence of this tropic hormone. Nevertheless, thyroid hormone, corticoid and estrogen replete hypophysectomized women can achieve follicle maturation and ovulation with exogenous HMG/HCG.

Because pregranulosa cells of the primordial follicle can respond to activators of cyclic AMP pathways by increased expression of aromatase and FSH receptors, nongonadotropin activators may participate in the first stages of initial recruitment.[51] Finally, factors derived from oocyte-granulosa cell communication in these early follicles may also be involved. Table 2A.3 [11] shows examples of alterations in preantral follicle development which result from granulosa cell and oocyte dysfunction in mutant mouse models. Mice that are genetically deficient in growth differentiating factor-9 (GDF-9), a peptide synthesized only in the oocyte, are infertile because follicular development cannot proceed beyond the primordial follicle stage.

B. Preantral Follicle Growth and Differentiation

In this stage granulosa cells differentiate and multiply, the oocyte continues to grow, the zona pellucida is formed, and thecal cells enlarge and multiply as they condense to form a distinct theca interna which becomes increasingly vascularized. Through studies in the rodent, somewhat more is known about the regulation of this stage of follicle differentiation and growth.

TABLE 2A.3 Mutant Mouse Models which Display Alterations in Preantral Follicle Development

Gene	Ovarian expression pattern	Phenotype of mutant mice
GFD-9	Growing oocyte	No normal follicle growth beyond the primary stage
Kit ligand	Granulosa cells	Soluble from necessary for follicle growth beyond primary stage
Connexin 37	Oocyte-granulosa gap junction	Defective oocyte/granulosa interaction. Small oocytes not meiotically competent. Antral follicles formed but are small in size.
Cyclin D2	Granulosa cells	Reduced number of granulosa cells by secondary stage, small antral follicles

Source: From McGee, E. A., and Hsuen, A. J. W. (2000). Endocr. Rev., 21, Table 2, p. 205.

Interaction between oocyte and granulosa cells through connecting gap junctions are important to normal primary and secondary follicle and oocyte growth.[52] Without these interaction channels oocytes cannot undergo meiosis. Granulosa cell mitosis, receptor accession, and steroidogenesis are also adversely affected.

Because preantral follicle development is much slower than larger antral follicles, it is possible that gradually diminishing levels of a suppressor of ovarian growth and differentiation may be involved.[53, 65] High levels of Wilms' tumor gene WT-1 expression in granulosa cells gradually wane during follicle growth and are almost nonexistent in antral follicles. WT-1 gene product proteins suppress the expression of several growth factors and their receptors including inhibin and FSH receptor, genes essential for follicle development. Thus, WT-1 may act as a stasis factor on small follicles, but falling levels allow progression of early follicle development. *Granulosa theca cell* [54, 55] steroidogenesis may also have a role in development of early follicles. Although the number and size of preantral follicles may increase as a result of steroid-receptor interactions as noted earlier, the influence of androgens and estrogen in these early stages remains unclear. Estrogen receptor knockout studies show significant alterations in follicle maturation. Similarly studies in mutant mice models, cultures of rodent follicles, and dispersed follicle cells demonstrate involvement of inhibin, activin, IGF-I, and IGF receptors in augmenting FSH responsiveness and FSH receptor expression.[56–58]

As a result, preantral follicles do respond to gonadotropins with cell division and differentiation. However, it is clear that follicles can progress even to the antral stage in the *absence* of gonadotropins. A clinical demonstration of this fact is seen in ovulation induction efficiency in women with hypogonadotropic hypogonadism. Treatment with exogenous gonadotropins leads to preovulatory follicles within two weeks, indicating that despite lack of endogenous FSH preantral and early antral follicles are present and available for swift cyclic recruitment, selection, and ovulation.[23]

In summary, these early phases of initial follicle recruitment up to the small antral stage reflects two processes: (1) The emergence from the restraints of stasis, arrest, and growth inhibitory or repressive factors, and (2) the gradual but accelerating emergence of *intrafollicular* growth promotion and endocrine assisted survival factors preparing for increased FSH *responsiveness* of the growing follicles.

C. The Antral Follicle: Cyclic Recruitment, Escape from Atresia, and Selection of the Dominant Follicle

Under normal conditions in a lifetime only about 400 follicles are selected from the continuously available initial recruitment cohort (perhaps 1000 a month) or the smaller cyclic recruitment group of antral follicles (3–10 per cycle) and for one to reach the dominant, preovulatory follicle stage and ovulate. Accordingly, loss of follicles due to atresia rather than growth and subsequent ovulation should be considered the "normal" fate of ovarian follicles.

As previously noted the lead follicle is selected by a combination of extrinsic (endocrine) and intrinsic mechanisms. By day 8–10 of the menstrual cycle, the lead follicle secretes increasingly high levels of estradiol and inhibin B which suppress anterior pituitary FSH release and availability. The result is a negative selection influence on the remaining cohort, which becomes atretic due to diminished availability of antiapoptotic FSH. Once apoptosis is initiated, TNF produced in these granulosa cells inhibits FSH stimulation of estradiol secretion. Thus, follicles with a failing response to gonadotropins increase TNF production, which accelerates their demise.

On the other hand, through continued FSH availability (albeit reduced) increasing LH concentrations, and by progressively increasing *intrinsic* processes such as FSH receptor capacity, local growth factors and enhanced theca vascularization, the lead follicle is able to maximize utilization of dwindling FSH which promotes not only survival but positive selection for further growth stimulation, functional differentiation, and ultimate ovulation (Fig. 2A.6).

1. The Extrinsic System: Gonadotropins

Stimulation by cyclic gonadotropins FSH and LH is essential for survival and continued growth of only a limited number of antral follicles which reach the preovulatory stage. Loss of gonadotropins after hypophysectomy leads to atresia and apoptosis of developing follicles and oocytes. Clinical *in vivo* and *in vitro* studies demonstrate that *FSH is the survival factor* that prevents this follicle demise and induces the escape mechanisms which avoid atresia. *FSH is both necessary and sufficient as the endocrine agent for selected follicle survival.*[17] In this regard recombinant human FSH is sufficient to produce a dominant follicle in therapy of hypogonadotropic-hypogonadal women. However, follicle estradiol production is dependent on both FSH stimulation of aromatase in granulosa cells and LH stimulation of androstenedione precursor production by the theca.[59] Therefore LH plays an important facilitatory role in the continuing survival of growing follicles and ovulation of the dominant follicle. Gonadotropin therapy, which includes both FSH and LH, requires shorter duration and lower doses to achieve readiness for ovulation.

2. The Intrinsic Systems

FSH rescues the selected follicle and with LH promotes its development to dominance largely but not exclusively by stimulation of two principles [18–22]—*intrinsic follicle mechanisms*—the IGF system and the inhibin/activin system.[24]

a. IGF

Since there are no detectable changes in serum concentrations of IGF-I or -II throughout the ovulatory cycle, the important effects of this system must be limited to the microenvironment of the selected follicles.

IGF-I has been demonstrated to stimulate the following events in theca and granulosa cells: DNA synthesis, steroidogenesis, aromatase actuivity, LH receptor synthesis, and inhibin/activin synthesis and secretion. As seen in Fig. 2A.8, LH stimulates synthesis of IGF-II in theca cells. By an autocrine effect IGF-II acts through its thecal cell receptor to enhance LH-driven steroidogenesis. Through a paracrine effect on its receptors on the granulosa cell it induces cell proliferation and aromatase enzyme capacity as well as FSH-driven synthesis of inhibin and activin. With further follicle development and accession of LH receptors on the granulosa (Fig. 2A.9) IGF promotes LH synthesis of follicle progesterone. IGF-II levels in the granulosa cell increase with growth and maturation of the follicle by the same process.

b. Inhibin/Activin

FSH is both necessary and sufficient for the stimulation of folliculogenesis and in the primate this gonadotropin action is relayed through activation of the intrinsic inhibin/activin system as depicted graphically in Figs. 2A.10 and 2A.11. FSH stimulates inhibin and activin production in granulosa cells. With IGF, activin in the early follicle augments all FSH activities including FSH receptor expression,

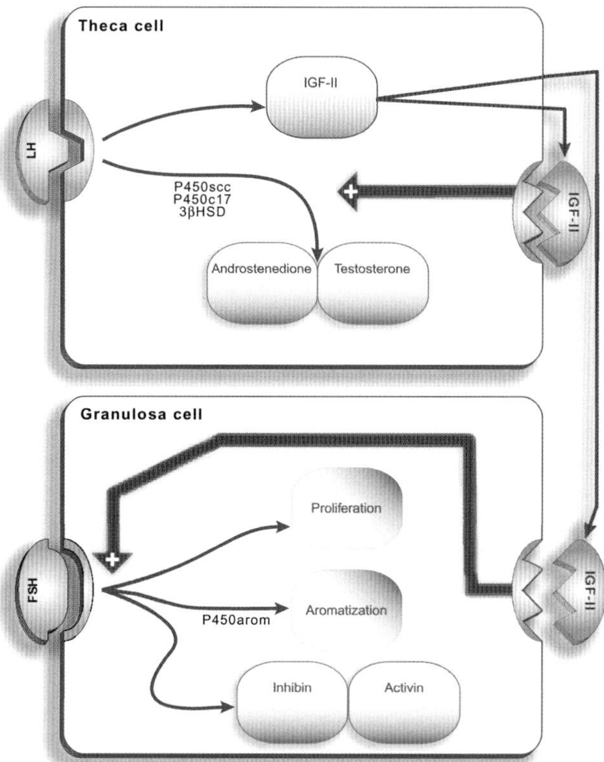

FIGURE 2A.8 In the early follicle phase FSH stimulation of granulosa cell proliferation and function (i.e., aromatase, production of inhibin, and activin) is augmented by the paracrine action of IGF-II produced in the theca cell. By an autocrine function LH stimulated IGF-II augments steroid biosynthesis of the androgens androstenedione and testosterone.

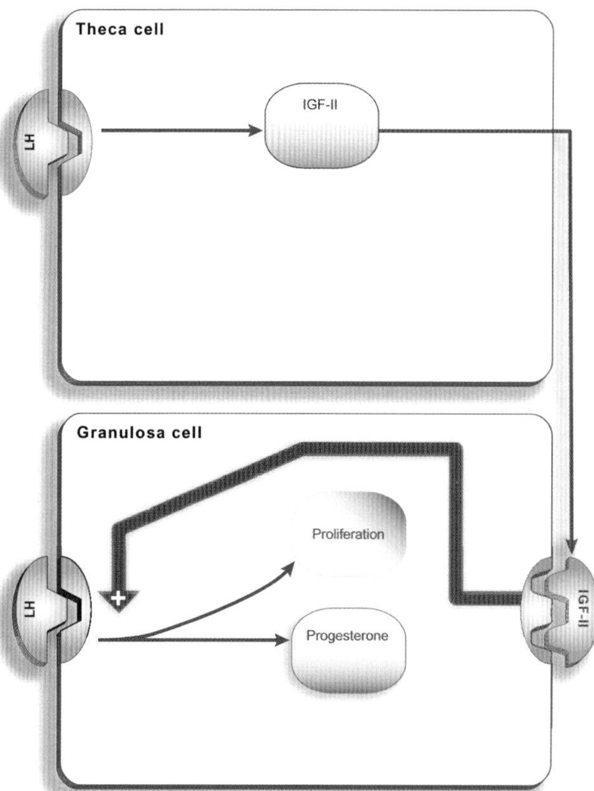

FIGURE 2A.9 In the preovulatory follicle, with the accession of LH receptors on both theca and granulosa cells, IGF-II promotes synthesis of small amounts of progesterone which is active in the follicle microenvironmental changes leading to ovulation, follicle rupture and ovum extrusion. (From Speroff, L., Glass, R., and Kase, N. (1999). "Clinical Gynecologic Endocrinology and Infertility," pp. 201–231, 6th Ed. Williams & Wilkins, Baltimore, MD.)

aromatase capacity, and stimulates additional activin/inhibin. Through paracrine action inhibin stimulates androgen synthesis in the theca ensuring adequate substrate for granulosa cell aromatization to estradiol. Activin modifies that local androgen synthesis. As the follicle matures and while inhibin production increases, activin levels diminish, androgen substrate rises, and with accession of LH receptors on the granulosa, steroidogenesis is further enhanced with massive production of estradiol and initial synthesis of progesterone. Inhibin B is secreted and as an endocrine hormone imposes negative feedback on FSH (see Fig. 2A.7).

In summary, the successful selected follicle is the one that acquires the highest level of FSH and LH receptors despite diminishing levels of FSH. Furthermore it is characterized by the highest estradiol secretion (for central positive feedback) and the greatest local inhibin and IGF-II production for maximizing the FSH rescue and "snowballing" acceleration of follicle development as it approaches ovulation.

D. The Preovulatory Follicle

As the result of the increasing concentrations of LH and the preovulatory follicle's abundant (both theca and granulosa) LH receptor capacity, a cascade of endocrine and intrinsic factor events occur as the Graafian follicle achieves ultimate maturity. Estrogen secretion becomes sufficient to achieve and sustain circulating concentrations required for positive feedback on LH and induction of the LH surge.[60, 61] Acting through its receptor LH induces luteinization of granulosa cells and promotes progesterone production.[62] Similarly LH stimulates further VEGF release for maximal thecal vascularity. Early progesterone secretion *adds* to positive feedback on LH.[63]

With respect to intrinsic mechanisms, with continued LH stimulation the inhibin/activin and IGF systems remain active. The orderly transition from an androgen/activin dominant to an estrogen/inhibin A dominant microenvironment is critical to dominant follicle development.[64] In addition, cultured preovulatory follicles are prevented from undergoing apoptosis by not only the presence of FSH and LH, but also GH, IGF-I, epidermal growth factor, TGF-α, fibroblast growth factor-2, IL-2, and its imposed generation of nitric oxide (NO).[18–22]

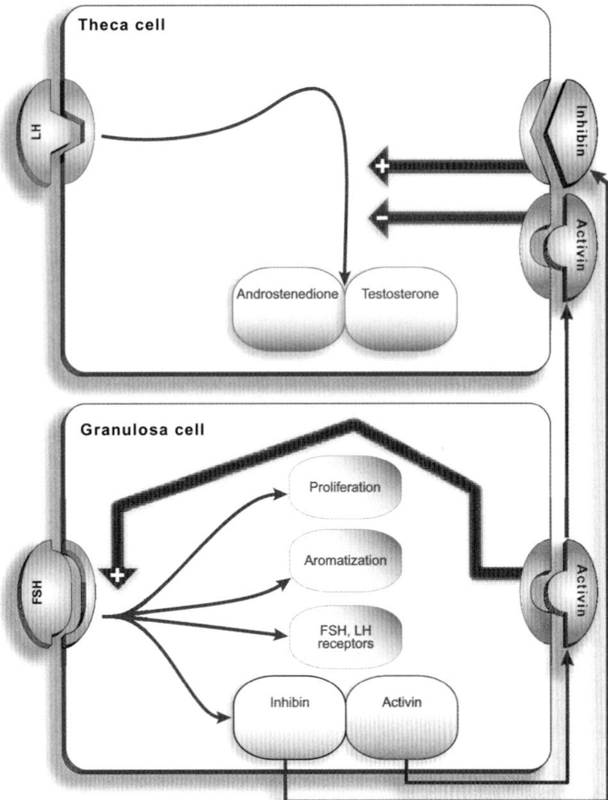

FIGURE 2A.10 The intrinsic function of the inhibin/activin system in follicle development. In the early follicle phase, whereas inhibin produced in the granulosa stimulates LH induced androgen synthesis, activin inhibits this thecal cell process. On the other hand, activin produced in the granulosa cell, similar to IGF-II, augments FSH actions in that compartment. (From Speroff *et al.* (1999). "Clinical Gynecologic Endocrinology and Infertility," pp. 222, 6th Ed. Williams & Wilkins, Baltimore, MD.)

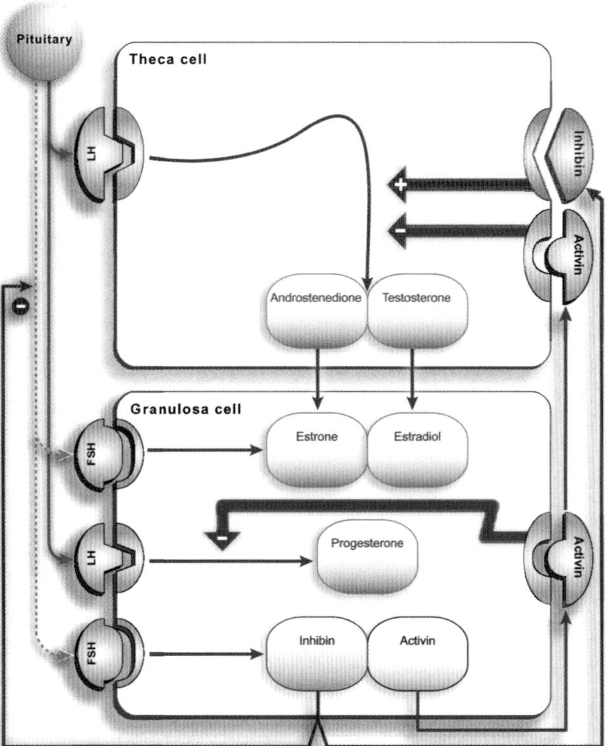

FIGURE 2A.11 In the late follicle phase, activin inhibits LH-induced granulosa cell synthesis of progesterone, thereby modifying the IGF-II stimulation of this process. FSH-induced inhibin B synthesis and now secretion acts as an endocrine humoral negative feedback signal to the anterior pituitary which diminishes circulating levels of FSH. (From Speroff, L. *et al.* (1999). "Clinical Gynecologic Endocrinology and Infertility," pp. 201–231, 6th Ed. Williams & Wilkins, Baltimore, MD.)

E. Ovulation

The Graafian follicle signals its readiness to ovulate by maximal secretion of estradiol. As circulating concentrations of estradiol reach 200–400 pcg/ml range, a midcycle rapid increase in LH (i.e., the onset of LH surge) begins. Within 14–24 h after peak estradiol levels, the maximal secretion of LH (the LH surge) occurs. Ten to twelve hours later, as LH levels decline, ovulation, the physical extrusion of the oocyte and its cumulus through the weakened follicle wall, and the completion of meiosis I are all realized. From the beginning of the LH surge, 34–36 h later, usually in the early morning hours, follicle rupture occurs.[66–68]

The LH surge accelerates the final steps in meiosis I, expands the granulosa cell cumulus, luteinizes the granulosa cells, and induces synthesis of prostaglandins. LH-induced cyclic AMP activity overcomes the local inhibitory action of OMI and luteinization inhibitor LI (endothelin I).[39]

With the LH surge intrafollicular progesterone levels rise. In addition to its endocrine effects, progesterone changes the elastic properties of the follicle compensating for the vast increase in antral fluid volume. FSH, LH, and progesterone stimulate the activity of proteolytic enzymes resulting in digestion of the collagen in the follicle "envelope."[69] Postaglandins, which rise markedly in preovulatory follicle fluids also enhance release of proteolytic enzymes, induce hyperemia and fluid accumulation, and stimulate perifollicular smooth muscle contractions to aid in the extrusion of the oocyte.[70, 71] Plasminogen activators activate plasminogen to produce plasmin. Plasmin in turn activate collagenase which serves to free the oocyte and the cumulus from its follicular attachments.

Finally, FSH induces abundant LH receptors in the remaining granulosa cells thereby insuring normal duration and steroid output of the corpus luteum.

F. Corpus Luteum

1. The Importance of Progesterone [24]

Within 3 days after ovulation granulosa cells enlarge and luteinize, vessel ingrowth and full vascularization is underway, the basal lamina separating the granulosa from theca disappears, and theca cells become incorporated into this last form of follicle evolution and function—the corpus luteum (Fig. 2A.12). This new anatomic unit must quickly fulfill its major endocrine responsibility by massive secretion of progesterone and this steroid's effect on the endometrium. Progesterone by 3–4 days post ovulation must (1) induce secretion of nutrients from the endometrial glands in sufficient quality and quantity to meet the needs of the morula/blastocyst as it enters and remains unattached in the uterine cavity, (2) stimulate endometrial superficial capillary and arteriolar complexity through VEGF, (3) prepare and support the endometrium for trophoblast attachment, implantation, and development of a rudimentary hemochorial placentation, (4) induce nutritive factors and mechanical stability by decidualization of superficial stroma cells, (5) with estrogen suppress gonadotropins to avoid supernumerary ovulation, and (6) with estrogen stabilize the endometrium to avoid premature tissue dissolution and disruption. All this must be accomplished within its programmed life span of 14 days and until the corpus luteum is rescued by rising levels of HCG. Without this salvage mechanism luteolysis occurs, its hormone product is withdrawn, and menses begins.

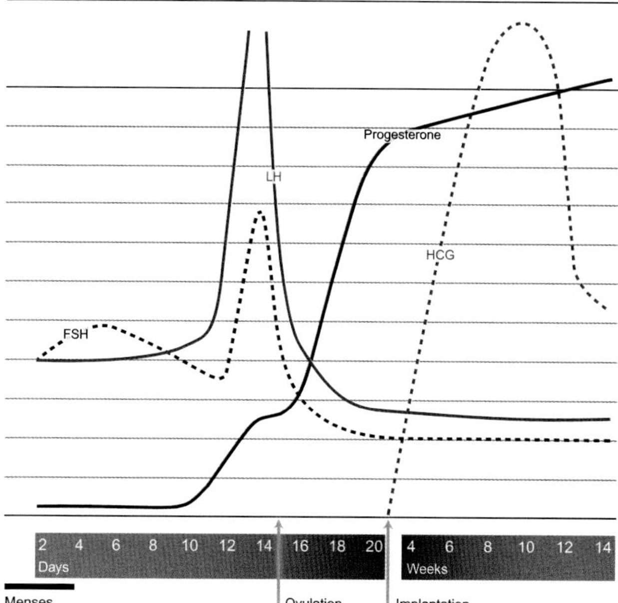

FIGURE 2A.12 The function of the corpus luteum. After ovulation, low levels of LH stimulate massive progesterone biosynthesis and secrtion of progesterone, but only for the programmed life span of the Corpus luteum, roughly 14 days. Should a significant mass of trophoblastic cells emerge as a result of successful placentation capable of production of dramatic increases in HCG concentrations required to sustain luteal cells, the luteolytic process is postponed for 6–8 weeks. Thereafter, as the placenta takes over progesterone (and estradiol) production from the Corpus luteum, HCG levels diminish and the luteolytic process is completed. (From Speroff *et al.* (1999). "Clinical Gynecologic Endocrinology and Infertility," p. 235, 6th Ed. Williams and Wilkins, Baltimore, MD.)

2. The Importance of Gonadotropins

Although negative feedback of serum estradiol and progesterone leads to suppression of FSH and LH during the luteal phase, continued availability of LH even at low levels is essential (Figs. 2A.12 and 2A.13).[72] This LH dependence is graphically demonstrated in ovulation induction practices in hypophysectomized women. Either the longer acting HCG or daily administration of LH is necessary to sustain corpus luteum function. GnRH agonist suppression of LH promptly induces luteolysis substantiating the importance of gonadotropin and the reduced frequency but increased amplitude of the GnRH pulses that direct their secretion during the luteal phase.[73]

LH plays the critical role in progesterone biosynthesis and secretion by its classic induction of cholesterol side chain cleavage and upregulation of a variety of steroidogenic enzymes which insures continued high-level progesterone secretion. In addition LH, through its receptor on the luteinized granulosa cell, sustains adequate cholesterol substrate by inducing LDL receptor expression and expanding LDL cholesterol internalization and processing by which cholesterol is delivered to appropriate steroid synthesis sites on the mitochrondria.[74] Finally, LH insures delivery of these precursors and their product by upregulating VEGF and inducing extensive corpus luteum angiogenesis and vascularization. As a result the midluteal phase corpus luteum at maximum steroid production has one of the highest blood flows per unit mass in the body. Finally, LH induces the secretion of inhibin A which joins estrogen and progesterone in negative feedback restraint of maturation of other follicles.[75]

FSH also provides important activity in the corpus luteum. In addition to the midcycle surge of FSH which is crucial to enhanced granulosa cell capacity and function, the low level of FSH throughout the luteal phase continues to support granulosa cell integrity and most important, sustains adequate numbers of LH receptors.

3. The Cells of the Corpus Luteum

The corpus luteum should not be viewed solely as a luteinized granulosa cell organ.[24] Besides luteal cells, the total cell population is made up of endothelial cells, leukocytes, and fibroblasts. Only 15–30% of the corpus luteum is involved in steroidogenesis. Together the nonsteroid producing cells provide prostaglandins, growth factors, angiogenic factors, and blood flow controls. "Cross talk" between the various cell groups is crucial to luteal function. For example, FSH and LH and the cytokines TGF-β_1 and M-CSF are involved in suppression of apoptosis whereas TNF-α and PGF2α contribute to luteal cell regression. The chemokine IL-8 is involved in repair of the ruptured follicle and the

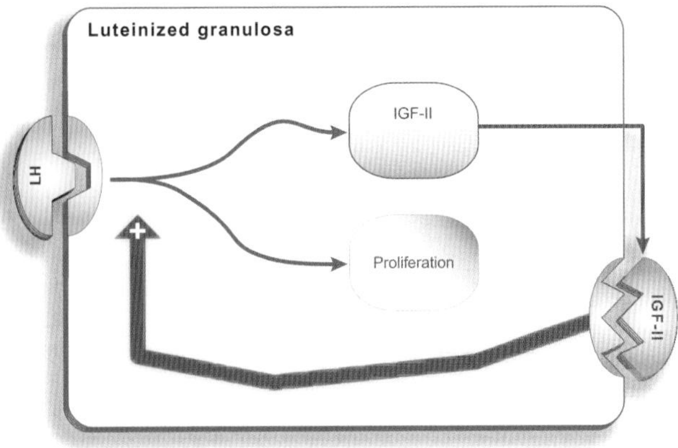

FIGURE 2A.13 The luteinized granulosa of the corpus luteum proliferates and generates massive progesterone synthesis despite the low luteal levels of LH by intrinsic autocrine augmentation of LH process by IGF-II. (From Speroff *et al.* (1999), "Clinical Gynecologic Endocrinology and Infertility," p. 217, 10th Ed. Williams & Wilkins, Baltimore, MD.)

structural integrity of the subunit during its extensive vascularization.[76] BCL-2 and BAX play important diverse and competitive roles in regulation of corpus luteum cell competence. LH (and HCG) increase BCL-2 (antiapoptotic) and decrease BAX (apoptotic) expression in human corpus luteum cells.[77] Finally, VEGF and its receptors [78] stimulate angiogenesis in the corpus luteum and the angiopoietins (Ang-1 and Ang-2) through their common receptor (Tie-2) modulate VEGF function in the luteal phase and in luteolysis.[79]

Not even the luteal cells are homogenous.[80] Rather "large" cells exist which are the producers of progesterone and estrogen as well as inhibin A, oxytocin, relaxin, prostaglandins, and tissue stabilizers such as tissue inhibitor of metaloproteinases (TIMPS).[81] These large cells are connected to smaller corpus luteum cells by gap junctions (supported by large cell oxytocin). Unlike large cells, these more abundant small cells possess the LH/HCG receptor response system.[82]

G. Luteolysis

In the normal cycle the life span of the corpus luteum is tightly controlled. The interval between the midcycle LH surge and menses is consistently close to 14 days with a "normal" range of 11–17 days. Cycle length varies as the follicle phase duration varies; the luteal phase remains constant in all nonpregnancy ovulatory cycles.

Luteolysis (programmed death of the corpus luteum) is an active process. The corpus luteum can be preserved for no more than 8 weeks into gestation and only because of the availability of massive and rapidly increasing rescuing levels of HCG secreted from a large mass of healthy trophoblasts. Uterine bleeding in ectopic gestations occurs due to corpus luteum demise despite elevated but plateauing levels of HCG.

Neither the tightly conserved life span of the corpus luteum nor the mechanism of human luteolysis is understood. Speculations have centered on a $PGF_{2\alpha}$ induced process because of its luteolytic activity in ruminants. Endothelin I has been investigated as an initiator of luteolysis. ET-I from endothelial cells inhibits progesterone synthesis in luteal cells.[83] In addition ET-I has been shown to increase synthesis and release of $PGF_{2\alpha}$ from these cells [84] and induces apoptosis by release of TNF-α.[85] Finally, downregulation of LH receptors by a combination of elevated estrogen and a local GnRH peptide may also be involved in this process.

With secretion of HCG from an implanted embryo 8 days after ovulation, the luteolytic program is temporarily arrested and the corpus luteum temporarily rescued. Progesterone secretion persists at peak luteal levels until 6–8 weeks gestation. Thereafter the human corpus luteum regresses and is no longer an important source of steroid.

H. The Luteal-Follicular Transition

The events which occur following luteolysis during an interval that is called the luteal follicular transition phase have crucial bearing on the success of the next follicle phase. Specifically, the decline of the corpus luteum sets in motion cyclic recruitment of available antral follicles for the next cycle's ovulation.[11]

The demise of the corpus luteum results in a steep decline of serum estradiol and progesterone as well as inhibin A (Fig. 2A.14). The withdrawal of the combined inhibitory influences of E_2, P, and inhibin A eliminates the strong negative feedback on FSH (and LH) that prevails throughout the luteal phase. In the absence of negative feedback, GnRH pulses gradually return to typical follicle phase frequency and amplitude leading to increased synthesis and secretion of FSH. The combination of withdrawal of inhibin A and the low levels of E_2 typical of menses and the early follicle phase magnify the FSH secretory response to GnRH.[24]

The resulting rise in FSH, should it meet the dual physiologic requirements of a concentration threshold and an appropriate duration of availability, will rescue a cohort of small antral follicles from apoptosis, and from this cyclically recruited group a dominant follicle will be selected.

IV. THE REGULATION OF THE MENSTRUAL CYCLE

A. Endocrine Extrinsic Controls

Thus far this chapter has focused largely on the chronicle of ovarian follicle events that reflect intrinsic intracrine, autocrine, and paracrine events involved in follicle arrest,

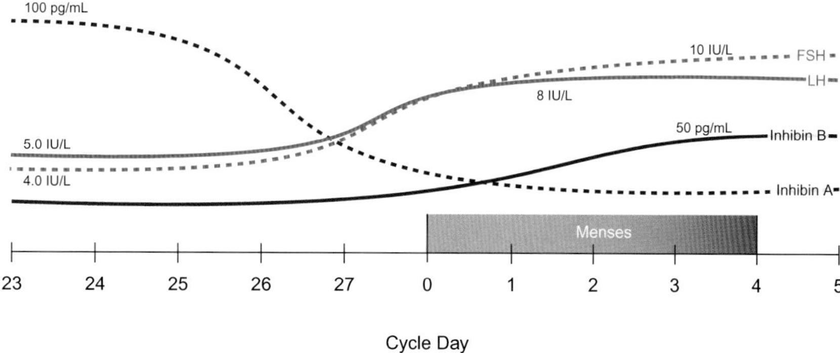

FIGURE 2A.14 The luteal–follicular phase transition. The withdrawal of the combined negative feedback of inhibin A, estradiol, and progesterone upon the demise of the Corpus luteum, FSH and to a lesser extent LH resume secretion from the anterior pituitary. The impact of this renewed tropic hormone endocrine stimulus on the "rescued" initially recruited follicles can be seen in the increased concentrations of inhibin B and estradiol (not shown). (From Speroff *et al.* (1999). "Clinical Gynecologic Endocrinology and Infertility," p. 237, 6th Ed. Williams & Wilkins, Baltimore, MD.)

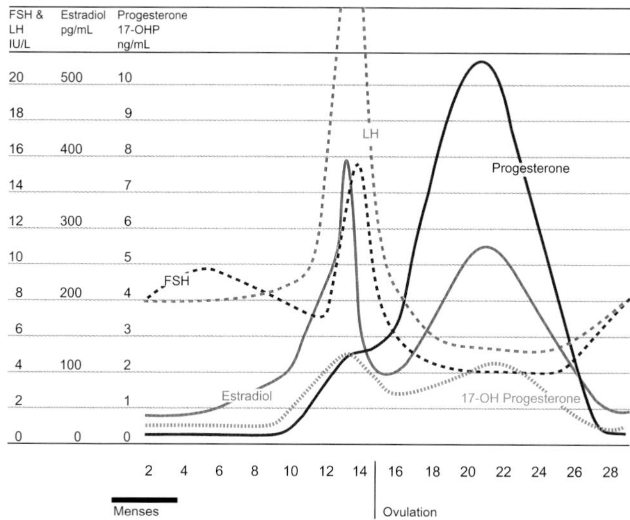

FIGURE 2A.15 Depiction of the integrated peptide–steroid hormone endocrine signaling activities during an ovulatory menstrual cycle. Mandatory recycling event #1 is the renewal of FSH cyclic recruitment which results form the withdrawal of negative feedback from the demise of the previous cycle's Corpus luteum. Mandatory recycling event #2 requires sufficient concentration and duration of circulating estradiol to achieve maximum positive feedback and stimulate ovulation inducing LH surge. Mandatory recycling event #3 occurs whether luteolysis takes place (with resumption of event #1) or is postponed by HCG levels of early pregnancy. After 10 weeks of pregnancy and to term high negative feedback levels of placental estradiol and progesterone further delay resumption of recycling event #1. Even after parturition, with breast feeding, prolactin inhibits FSH secretion despite low postpartum E_2 and absent P. (From Speroff *et al.* (1999), "Clinical Gynecologic Endocrinology and Infertility," p. 209, 10th Ed. Williams & Wilkins, Baltimore, MD.)

activation, recruitment, selection and dominance, ovulation, and corpus luteum function (Fig. 2A.15). In this description the crucial importance of the timely appearance, concentrations, and sequence of the gonadotropins FSH and LH was emphasized. In this section, the endocrine—long distance, blood-borne humoral signals—that direct, integrate, and perpetuate the events that define the ovary will be reviewed.

As seen in Fig. 2A.15, this integration involves interactions between steroid and peptide hormones. The feedback loops from the ovary (O) to the hypothalamus (H) and gonadotropes of the anterior pituitary (P) include both negative and positive feedback instructions, a circumstance unique to the HPO. The efferent portion of the link involves FSH and LH. The sustaining importance of GnRH pulses in the synthesis, packaging, transport to the cell membrane and timely secretion of gonadotropin is an absolute requirement for the normal function of the system.

The influence of corticotropin releasing hormone (CRH), opioides, TSH/thyroid hormone, ACTH, prolactin, and insulin, among others on the integrity of the basic system and the perturbations each cause in dysfunction and disease are recognized but are beyond the scope of this analysis of fundamental ovarian function.

It is helpful to view the process as a sequential series of three mandatory recycling events by which the ovary asserts its readiness to proceed successfully into the next phase of the cycle.

1. Recycling Event #1

This crucial early cycle (early proliferative phase) step provides sufficient FSH to rescue and recruit an available group of antral follicles. As corpus luteum function declines, GnRH and FSH are freed from intense negative feedback induced by luteal P, E_2, and inhibin A. These factors must fall to levels low enough and over a sufficient period of time to allow FSH to meet the concentration and duration requirements for follicle rescue and promotion. Note that a rise in potentially inhibiting levels of E_2 and inhibin B are delayed to achieve this goal but not so long as to permit super ovulation.

2. Recycling Event #2

This step involves the positive feedback of E_2 and the initiation of an ovulatory LH surge. The dominant follicle signifies its readiness to ovulate by this endocrine message since it directly reflects the number and function of the granulosa cells of the preovulatory follicle but also indirectly the entire array of support factors involved in dominant follicle generation and oocyte preparation.

The parameters of E_2 feedback, the threshold for LH stimulation, and duration of signal directing the magnitude of the response (48 h) occur within a very narrow window. Experiences with exogenous gonadotropin stimulation have underlined the detrimental effects of too early or excessive delay in LH (HCG) provision.

If all these elements are in correct alignment then mandatory recycling event #2—ovulation and the formation of the corpus luteum—is completed. The decline in inhibin B and the delay in inhibin A well into the luteal phase permits an FSH secretory surge with clear benefit to the corpus luteum.

3. Recycling Event #3

The corpus luteum has a programmed life span of roughly two weeks. Luteolysis will take place *unless* rescue by HCG becomes available. Recycling event #3 depends upon whether the life of the corpus luteum is extended and the suppressive feedback of E_2, progesterone, and inhibin A is sustained, i.e., a source of HCG. In the absence of a pregnancy, luteolysis proceeds and the events associated with mandatory recycling event #1 return.

V. SUMMARY

In this portion of the chapter the advances in ovarian endocrinology, molecular biology, molecular genetics, and the powerful transgene and knockout technologies which have provided a new and exciting insight into the life history of a human ovarian follicle, ovulation, and corpus luteum formation and function have been reviewed. Both the intrinsic intrafollicle and extrinsic endocrine factors controlling these events have been emphasized. Accordingly, the emphasis has been less on morphology and more on the molecular events which drive the crucial elements of folliculogenesis, i.e., oocyte maturation, angiogenesis, controls of cell growth and differentiation, receptor expression and activity which, combined with extrinsic endocrine direction culminate in the exquisite microenvironmental control of the fate of the ovarian follicles.

VI. ENDOCRINE FUNCTIONS OF OVARIAN STEROID SECRETION

A. Ovarian Biosynthesis of Steroids [86, 87]

The steroid biosynthesis in the ovarian follicle, corpus luteum, and stroma cells proceeds via a fundamental pathway (Fig. 2A.16) in which cholesterol, a 27 carbon sterol, is delivered to the cell(s) involved in biosynthesis by LDL-cholesterol entry via its cell membrane receptor, incorporation within the cell (endocytosis), processing to generate cholesterol and transport to the mitochondria where it is stored prior to steroid synthesis. Thereafter cholesterol substrate is transformed by a sequence of enzymatic hydroxylations, lyase-induced reductions in carbon number, rearrangement of electron densities (double bonds) via oxidation/reduction processes to yield the 21 carbon Δ4-3 ketone steroid progesterone, and the 19 carbon androgens dihydroepiandrosterone (DHA), androstenedione (AD), and testosterone (T). Finally, through loss of yet another carbon appendage and aromatization of ring A the production of the 18 carbon estrogens, estradiol, and estrone is achieved. The crucial synthetic portal of entry to this steroidogenic cascade is the side chain cleavage of cholesterol by enzyme P450scc at the mitochondrial inner membrane which is induced by LH. In summary, LH activity, via generation of cyclic AMP frees cholesterol from its storage-esterified form, assists in transport of cholesterol to the mitochondria site, and upregulates downstream steroidogenic enzymes and associated proteins.

In the estrogen secreting maturing follicle steroid synthesis proceeds through an integration of theca and granulosa (the two-cell system).[88, 89] LH stimulates theca cell synthesis of precursor androgens which are delivered to the granulosa cell for aromatization to corresponding estrogens by the FSH-induced aromatase system. Thecal cells and stroma cells secrete androgens exclusively since this cell compartment is devoid of aromatase capability. Finally, the fully luteinized granulosa cell of the *corpus luteum*, equipped with abundant cholesterol reserves and LH receptors, generates large quantities of progesterone as well as modest amounts of estradiol.

B. Circulating Concentrations of Ovarian Steroids

The day to day (indeed minute to minute) concentrations of ovarian steroid secretions depend on the phase of the cycle (menstrual, early and late follicle phase, ovulation, and the luteal phase), the extent of shared secretion rates (i.e., androstenedione is secreted by the adrenal cortex in reaction to ACTH and is thereby substantially modified by circadian rhythms and stress), and the degree of extragonadal conversion of a steroid substrate to circulating levels

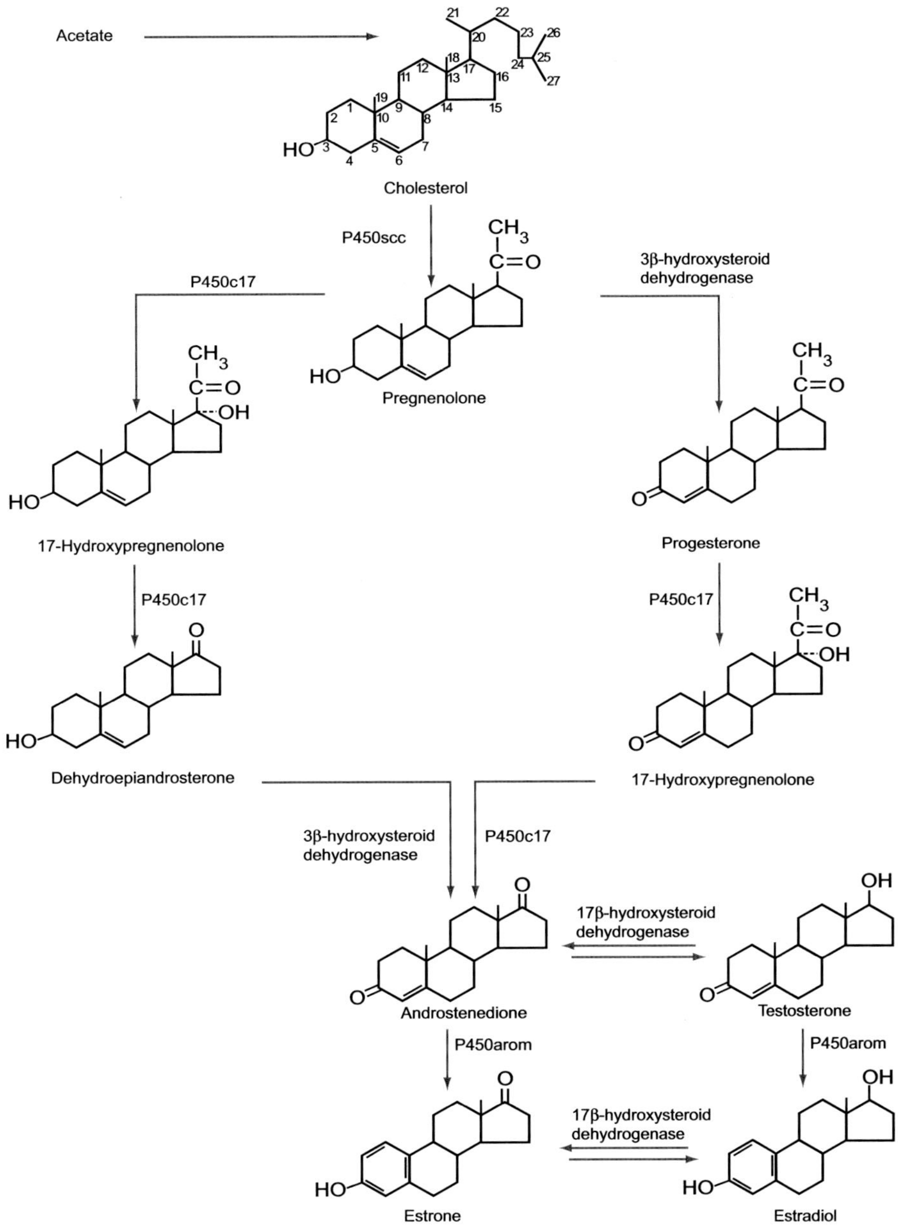

FIGURE 2A.16 The biosynthesis of gonadal steroids proceeds through a cascade of events induced and accelerated by LH induction and enhancement of various enzyme systems. Through these steps reduction in carbon numbers, rearrangement of double bonds, specific hydroxylations and finally aromatization is achieved.

of a steroid product with potentially different biologic activity. Given these limits, the "normal" ranges of steroid concentrations are provided in Table 2A.4.

1. Blood Transport of Steroids

While circulating in blood a majority of the principal sex steroids such as estradiol and testosterone are bound to a specific protein carrier produced in the liver called sex hormone binding globulin (SHBG). An additional 10–30% is loosely bound to albumin leaving only 1% unbound and free for diffusion into target cells. The specific binding characteristics of selected steroids are depicted in Table 2A.5.

Hyperthyroidism, pregnancy, and estrogen administration all *increase* SHBG whereas corticoids, androgens, progestins, GH, insulin, and IGF-I *decrease* SHBG.[90] Dysfunction or disease in any organ leading to abnormal availability of these controls on SHBG concentration can disrupt the integrity of the fine tuned narrow windows for steroid feedback on FSH and LH secretions and as a consequence result in discordant ovarian follicle function. Furthermore, the distribution of body fat has a strong *negative* influence on SHBG concentrations.

TABLE 2A.4 Circulating Concentrations of Gonadal Steriods

Estrogens	
estradiol	20–400 pcg/ml
estrone	5–200 pcg/ml
Androgens	
A	60–300 ng/dl
T total	20–80 ng/dl
Free	100–200 pcg/ml
Progrestrone	
follicle phase	<0.3 ng/ml
luteal phase	5–30 ng/ml

TABLE 2A.5 Steroids Circulate in Free (Biologically Active) and Protein Bound States

	Free (unbound)	Albumin-bound	SHBG-bound
Estrogen	1%	30%	69%
Testosterone	1%	30%	69%
DHA	4%	88%	8%
Androstenedione	7%	85%	8%

Accordingly, small increases in the concentration of free steroid may have biologic and clinical importance but will not be appreciated if only total steroid (free and bound) concentrations are measured. For example, increased androgen levels (as in PCOS, adrenal cortical disease, or endocrinologically active tumors) may increase free androgen by both excess secretion and/or production and androgen induced reduction of SHBG. Combined oral contraceptives at once suppress gonadal secretion of androgen in PCOS but also reduces free T further by increasing SHBG.

Android or central fat deposition located in the abdominal wall and visceral mesentery is associated with insulin resistance, hyperinsulinemia, hyperandrogenemia, and decreased SHBG.[91] Combining these properties with the ability of this fat to aromatize androgen to estrogen it is clear why morbidly obese women are prone to dyslipidemia, cardiovascular disease, anovulation, hirsutism, and breast and endometrial cancer.

Progesterone on the other hand circulates bound to corticosteroid-binding globulin (CBG). The binding distributions are 18% bound to CBG, 80% to albumin, and a minor quantity to SHBG.

C. Metabolism and Clearance of Ovarian Steroid Secretions

Before describing the specific metabolic and clearance mechanisms governing each class of ovarian steroid secretion, certain important generalities are worthy of mention.

The conversion of active steroids in peripheral tissues can either lead to "detoxification," i.e., conversion to permanently inactive forms prior to excretion (metabolic clearance) *or* conversion to another class of steroids with the same or different biologic activity. For example, significant inactivation of estradiol occurs as the steroid is converted to estriol and other metabolites. However, estradiol may also be processed to estrone which, though less active, still retains substantial biologic activity. Similarly, free androgens are converted to free estrogens in central adipose tissue. In this circumstance where free androstenedione (a weak androgen) is aromatized in fat to estrone (an estrogen with considerable activity) not only the class of the steroid is changed but the type and strength of biologic activity as well. A further complication arises as the tropic and feedback controls of substrate and product differ. In the example of androstenedione conversion to estrone, ACTH controls substrate availability but the product estrogen cannot exert modifying negative feedback on ACTH. Stress in an obese postmenopausal woman can produce vaginal bleeding and endometrial hyperplasia by this process.

1. Estrogen [90]

In the normal nonpregnant female, estradiol is produced at the rate of 100–300 μg/day. Given the considerations noted above in normal women the bulk of that production derives from secretion by a dominant follicle. In healthy women, the contributions from androgen precursor, while potentially important in dysfunction states of excess substrate or aromatase, are small. This insures "clarity" of endocrine feedback signals to the hypothalamus and anterior pituitary as to the "state" of follicle maturity.

2. Progesterone

Peripheral conversion of steroids to progesterone does not exist in the nonpregnant female; rather the progesterone production rate almost entirely reflects secretion from the corpus luteum plus minute quantities originating in the adrenal cortex. As a result, the secretion rate of progesterone and its production rate are virtually equal. Production rate of progesterone in the follicle phase is less than 1 mg/day but during the luteal phase it rises to 20–30 mg/day and as high as 100 mg in the last trimester of pregnancy.

Progesterone is metabolized (inactivated) to a variety of saturated and reduced forms such as pregnanediol. Progesterone metabolism is swift and very efficient; one pass through the liver essentially clears active progesterone from the effluent blood. To be active orally large quantities of micronized steroid must be administered frequently over the day. Progesterone derivatives such as medroxy progesterone acetate (MPA) possess substituents located on the basic progesterone molecule which substantially delay progestin inactivation thereby increasing the half-life of the biologically active principal.

TABLE 2A.6 Production Rates per 24 h and Interconversion of Metabolic Products of Gonadal Steroids

Androstenedione		Testosterone
3000 μg/24 h		250 μg/24 h
↓		↓
1.5%		0.15%
estrone	←	estradiol
45 μg/24 h	→	0.375 μg/24 h

Stress induced (ACTH) stimulation of androstenedione production may lead to both androgenic and estrogenic consequences of clinical significance.

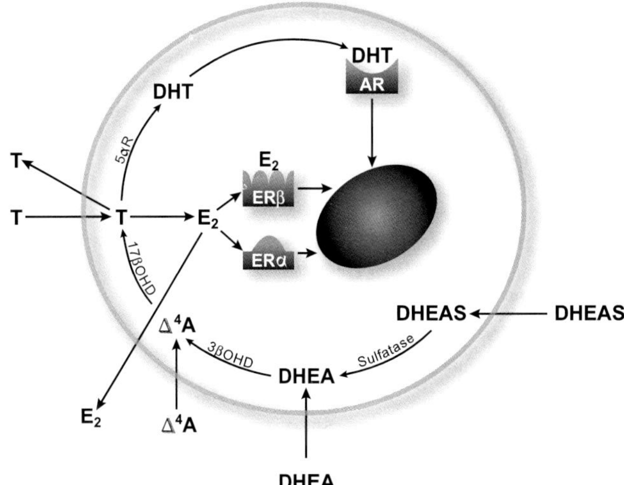

FIGURE 2A.17 The nongonadal cell production of endocrinologically active androgen and estrogen. In the process of "metabolic clearance" circulating DHA, DHAS, A, and T may be converted to "active" products (DHT, E_2) which may act locally (autocrine) or be secreted and circulated as biologically active hormones (E_2, T).

3. Androgen

By quantity, the major androgen products of the ovary are DHA and AD. Only very small amounts of T are secreted. The stroma cells and theca are the main sources of this androgen synthesis. The adrenal cortex also secretes androgens: about one-half of the daily production of DHA and AD comes from the adrenal. The production rate of testosterone in the normal female is 0.2–0.3 mg/day and of this 50% arises from peripheral conversion of androstenedione (Table 2A.6). This means roughly 50% of produced testosterone arises in equal quantities (25%) from adrenal and ovarian androstenedione. All three androgens are inactivated and excreted as ring D reduced 17 ketosteroids. DHT, a powerful androgen, is synthesized, induces activity and is metabolized entirely within its target cell and is by definition an entirely autocrine hormone.

D. Summary [92]

The complexity of extraglandular (nonovarian) synthetic and interconversion processes governing the biologic availability of estrogens and androgens is demonstrated in Fig. 2A.17.

The intracrine mechanisms whereby the synthesis in peripheral cells of estradiol (E_2) from testosterone (T) and testosterone from androstenedione (AD) and dehydroepiandrosterone (DHA) and its sulfate (DHAS) is depicted. For example, intracellular testosterone can arise from circulating androgens including testosterone which enter the cell from the blood stream. DHAS is desulfated in the cell, converted to AD by the enzyme 3β-hydroxysteroid dehydrogenase and AD converted to T by the enzyme 17β-hydroxysteroid dehydrogenase. Thereafter T can follow each of several biologically important pathways: (1) T may be secreted from the cell and re-enter the circulation in possibly augmented concentrations, (2) T may act directly on androgen receptor (AR), or (3) T may be converted to dihydrotestosterone (DHT) by the enzyme 5α reductase (isoform 1 or 2) with DHT binding to the AR. Both steps 2 and 3, depending on the "context" of the cell could yield important physiologic or pathologic androgen consequences. Finally, in step 4 T may be converted to estradiol (E_2) by the aromatase enzyme (CYP19) which in turn binds to either or both of the estrogen receptors (ERα and ERβ) to form homo or hetrodimers with resulting estrogen activity. In addition or alternatively, estradiol may be secreted from the cell and function either as a blood-borne hormone in possibly increased concentration or induce local paracrine effects on neighboring cells. Finally, in addition to endocrine, paracrine, and intracrine activities, estrogen can also act rapidly on cell surface receptors, a nongenomic action.

Steroids produced by extraglandular synthesis are a major source of circulating estrogen in the male and the postmenopausal female. They fulfill critical functions in reproductive system development and function and play an important role in the pathophysiologic manifestations of a variety of reproductive and nonreproductive system dysfunctions and diseases.

References

1. Zeleznik, A. J., and Benyo, D. F. (1994). Control of follicular development, corpus luteum function, and the recognition of pregnancy in higher primates. *In* "The Physiology of Reproduction" (E. Knobil and J. Neill, eds.), pp. 751-782. Raven Press, New York.
2. Greenwald, G., and Roy, S. Y. (1994). Follicle development and its control. *In* "The Physiology of Reproduction" (E. Knobil and J. Neill, eds), pp. 629–724. Raven Press, New York.
3. Richards, J. S., Fitzpatrick, S. L., Clemens, J. W., Morris, J. K., Alliston, T., and Sirois, J., (1995). Ovarian cell differentiation: A cascade of multiple hormones, cellular signals, and regulated genes. *Recent Prog. Horm. Res.* 50, 223–254.

4. Gougeon, A. (1996). Regulation of ovarian follicular development in primates: Facts and hypotheses. *Endocr. Rev.* 17, 121–155
5. Hirshfield, A. N. (1991). Development of follicules in the mammalian ovary. *Int. Rev. Cytol.* 124, 43–101.
6. Van Wagenen, G., and Simpson, M. E. (1965). Embryology of the ovary and testis "Homo sapiens and Macaca mulatta." Yale University Press, New Haven, CT.
7. Block, E. (1653). A quantitative morphological investigation of the follicular system in newborn female infants. *Acta Anat. (Basel)* 17, 201–206.
8. Forabosco, A., Sforza, C., De Pol, A., Vizzotto, L., Marzona, L., and Ferrario, V. F. (1991). Morphometric study of the human neonatal ovary. *Anat. Rec.* 231, 201–208.
9. De Pol, A., Vaccina, F., Forabosco, A., Cavazzuti, E., and Marzona, L. (1997). Apoptosis of germ cells during human prenatal oogenesis. *Hum. Reprod.* 12, 2235–2241.
10. Richardson, S. J., Senikas, V., and Nelson, J. F. (1987). Follicular depletion during the menopausal transition: evidence for accelerated loss and ultimate exhaustion. *J. Clin. Endocrinol. Metab.* 65, 1231–1237.
11. McGee, E.A., and Hsueh, A. J. W. (2000). Initial and cyclic recruitment of ovarian follicles. *Endocr. Rev.* 21, 200–214.
12. Makinoda, S., Uno, Y., Kikuchi, T., Tanaka, T., Ichinoe, K., and Fujimoto, S. (1988). Aging of human granulosa cells. *Program of the Satellite Symposium of the 8th International Congress of Endocrinology*, pp. 201–213. Saporo, Japan.
13. Gougeon, A. (1986). Dynamics of follicular growth in the human: a model from preliminary results. *Hum. Reprod.* 1, 81–87.
14. Harlow, C. R., Shaw, H. J., Hillier, S. G., and Hodges, J. K. (1988). Factors influencing follicle-stimulating hormone-responsive steroidogenesis in marmoset granulosa cells: Effects of adrogens and the stage of follicular maturity. *Endocrinology* 122, 2780–2787.
15. Gore, M. A., Nayudu, P. L., and Vlaisavljevic, V. (1997). Attaining dominance *in vivo*: Distinguishing dominant from challenger follicles in humans. *Hum. Reprod.* 12, 2741–2747.
16. Nahum, R., Beyth, Y., Chun, S. Y., Hsueh, A. J. W., and Tsafriri, A. (1996). Early onset of deoxyribonucleic acid fragmentation during atresia of preovulatory ovarian follicles in rats. *Biol. Reprod.* 55, 1075–1080.
17. Chun, S. Y., Eisenhauer, K. M., Minami, S., Billig, H., Perlas, E., and Hsueh, A. J. W. (1996). Hormonal regulation of apoptosis in early antral follicles: follicle-stimulating hormone as a major survival factor. *Endocrinology* 137, 1447–1456.
18. Hsueh, A .J. W., Eisenhauer, K., Chun, S. Y., Hsu, S. Y., and Billig, H. (1996). Gonadal cell apoptosis. *Recent Prog. Horm. Res.* 51, 433–455.
19. Chun, S. Y., Billig, H., Tilly, J. L., Furuta, I., Tsafriri, A., and Hsueh, A. J. W. (1994). Gonadotropin suppression of apoptosis in cultured preovulatory follicles: mediatory role of endogenous insulin-like growth factor. *I. Endocrinology* 135, 1845–1853.
20. Eisenhauer, K. M., Chun, S. Y., Billig, H., and Hsueh, A. J. W. (1995). Growth hormone suppression of apoptosis in preovulatory rat follicles and partial neutralization by insulin-like growth factor binding protein. *Biol. Reprod.* 53, 13–20.
21. Chun, S. Y., Eisenhauer, K. M., Kubo, M., and Hsueh, A. J. W. (1995). Interleukin-1β suppresses apoptosis in rat ovarian follicles by increasing nitric oxide production. *Endocrinology* 136, 3120–3127.
22. Tilly, J. L., Billing, J., Kowalski, K. I., and Hsueh, A. J. W. (1992). Epidermal growth factor and basic fibroblast growth factor suppress the spontaneous onset of apoptosis in cultured rat ovarian granulosa cells and follicles by a tyrosine kinase-dependent mechanism. *Mol. Endocrinol.* 6, 1942–1950.
23. Fauser, B. C., and Van Heusden, A. M. (1997). Manipulation of human ovarian function: Physiology concepts and clinical consequences. *Endocr. Rev.* 18, 71–106.
24. Speroff, L., Glass, R., and Kase, N. (1999). "Clinical Gynecologic Endocrinology and Infertility," pp. 201–231, 6th Edition. Williams & Wilkins, Baltimore, MD.
25. Rivier, C., Rivier, J., and Vale, W. (1986). Inhibin mediated feed-back control of FSH secretion in the female rat. *Science* 244, 205–208.
26. Bicsak, T. A., Tucker, E. M., Cappel, S., Vaughan, J., Rivier, J., Vale, W., and Hsueh, A. J. W. (1986). Hormonal regulation of granulosa cell inhibin biosynthesis. *Endocrinology* 119, 2711–2719.
27. Xiao, S., Robertson, D. M., and Findlay, J. K., (1992). Effects of activin and FSH suppressing protein/follistatin on FSH receptors and differentiation of cultured rat granulosa cells. *Endocrinology* 131, 1009–1016.
28. Matzuk, M. M., Finegold, M. J., Su, J. G., Hsueh, A. J. W., and Bradley, A. (1992). Alpha inhibin is a tumor suppressor gene with gonadal specificity in mice. *Nature* 360, 313–319.
29. Giudice, L. C. (1992). Insulin-like growth factors (IGFs) and ovarian follicle development. *Endocr. Rev.* 13, 641–669.
30. Shimasaki, S., and Ling, N. (1991). Identification and molecular characterization of IGF binding proteins (IGFBP 1–6). *Prog. Growth Factor Res.* 3, 243–266.
31. El-Roeiy, A., Chen, X., Roberts, V. J., LeRoith, D., Roberts, Jr. C. T., and Yen, S. S. C. (1993). Expression of IGF-I and IGF-II and IGF-I and IGF-II receptor genes and localization of gene products in the human ovary. *J. Clin. Endocrinol. Metab.* 77, 1411–1418.
32. Voutilainen, R., Franks, S., Mason, H. D., and Martikainen, H. (1996). Expression of (IGF, IGF receptor in RNA in normal and polycystic ovaries. *J. Clin. Endocrinol. Metab.* 81, 1003–1008.
33. Tilly, J. L., LaPolt, P. S., and Hsueh, A. J. W. (1992). Hormonal regulation of FSH receptor in RNA levels in cultured rat granulosa cells. *Endocrinology* 130, 1296–1302.
34. Dodson, W. C., and Schomberg, D. W. (1987). The effect of TGF on FSH induced differentiation of cultured rat granulosa cells. *Endocrinology* 120, 512–516.
35. Hernandez, E. R., Hurwitz, A., Payne, D. W., Dharmarajan, A. M., Purchio, A. F., and Adashi, E. Y. (1990). TGF beta inhibits ovarian androgen production gene expression cellular localization mechanisms and sites of action. *Endocrinology* 127, 2804–2811.
36. Christenson, L. K., and Stouffer, R. (1997). FSH and LH/HCG stimulation of vascular endothelial factor production by macaque granulosa cells from pre- and peri-ovulatory follicles. *J. Clin. Endocrinol. Metab.* 82, 2135–2142.
37. Lee, A., Christenson, L. K., Patton, P. E., Burry, K. A., and Stouffer, R. L. (1997). Vascular endothelial growth factor production by human luteinized granulosa cells in vitro. *Hum. Reprod.* 12, 2756–2761.
38. Kokia, E., Hurwitz, A., Ricciarelli, E., Tedeschi, D., Resknick, C. E., Mitchell, M. D., and Adashi, E. Y. (1992). IL-1 stimulated ovarian prostaglandin biosynthesis: evidence for heterologous contact-independent cell-cell interaction. *Endocrinology* 130, 3095–3097.
39. Tedeschi, C., Hagum, E., Kokia, E., Ricciarelli, E., Adashi, E. Y., and Payne, D. W. (1992). Endothelin-1 as a luteinization inhibitor: ingibition of rat granulosa cell progesterone accumulation via selective moducation of key steriodogenic steps affecting both progesterone formation and degradation. *Endocrinology* 131, 2476–2478.
40. Palter, S. F., Tavares, A. B., Hourvitz, A., Veldhuis, J. D., and Adashi, E. Y. (2001). Are estrogens of import to primate/human ovarian folliculogenesis? *Endocr. Rev.* 22, 389–424.
41. Mason, H. D., Cwyfan-Hughes, S. C., Heinrich, G., Franks, S., and Holly, J. M. P. (1996). IGF I and II, IGF-BPs and IGF binding protein proteases are produced by theca and stroma of normal and polycystic ovaries. *J. Clin. Endocrinol. Metab.* 81, 276–284.
42. Bergh, C., Carlsson, B., Olason, J. H., Selleskog, U., and Hillensjo, T. (1993). Regulation of androgen production in cultured human theca cells by IGF-I and insulin. *Fertil. Steril.* 59, 323–331.
43. Thierry-van Dessel, H. J., Chandrasekher, Y. A., Yap, O. W., Lee, P. D., Hintz, R. L., Faessel, G. H., Braat, D. D., Fauser, B. C., and Giudice, L. C. (1995). Serum and follicular fluid levels of IGF-I, IGF-II and IGF binding proteins 1 and 3 during the normal menstrual cycle. *J. Clin. Endocrinol. Metab.* 81, 1224–1231.

44. Cataldo, N. A., and Giudice, L. C. (1992). IGFBP profiles in human ovarian follicular fluid correlate with follicle functional status. *J. Clin. Endocrinol. Metab.* 74, 821–829.
45. Lockwood, G. M., Muttukrishna, S., and Ledger, W. L. (1998). Inhibins and activins in human ovulation, conception and pregnancy. *Hum. Reprod. Update* 4, 284–295.
46. Groome, N. P., Illingworth, P. G., O'Brien, M., Pai, R., Rodger, F. E., Mather, J. P., and McNeilly, A. S. (1996). Measurement of dimeric inhibin B throughout the human menstrual cycle. *J. Clin. Endocrinol. Metab.* 81, 1401–1405.
47. Sawetawan, C., Carr, B. R., McGee, E., Bird, I. M., Hong, T. L., and Rainey, W. E. (1996). Inhibin and activin differentially regulate androgen production and 17 alpha-hydroxylase expression in human ovarian thecal-like tumor cells. *J. Endocrinol.* 148, 213–221.
48. McLachlan, R. I., Cohen, N. L., Vale, W. W., Rivier, J. E., Burger, H. G., Bremner, W. J., and Soules, M. R. The importance of luteinizing hormone in the control of inhibin and progesterone secretion by the human corpus luteum. *J. Clin. Endocrinol. Metab.* 68, 1078–1085.
49. O'Shaughnessy, J., McLelland, D., and McBride, M. W. (1997). Regulation of luteinizing hormone-receptor and follicle-stimulating hormone-receptor messenger ribonucleic acid levels during development in the neonatal mouse ovary. *Biol. Reprod.* 57, 602–608.
50. Oktay, K., Briggs, D., and Gosden, R. G. (1997). Ontogeny of follicle-stimulating hormone receptor gene expression in isolated human ovarian follicles *J. Clin. Endocrinol. Metab.* 82, 3748–3751.
51. Mayerhofer, A., Dissen, G. A., Costa, M. E., and Ojeda, S. R. (1997). A role for neurotransmitters in early follicular development: induction of functional follicle-stimulating hormone receptors in newly formed follicles of the rat ovary. *Endocrinology* 138, 3320–3329.
52. Trounson, A., Anderiesz, C., Jones, G. M., Kausche, A., Lolatgis, N., and Wood, C. (1998). Oocyte maturation. *Hum. Reprod.* 3, 52–62.
53. Chun, S. Y., McGee, E. A., Hsu, S. Y., Minami, S., LaPolt, P. S., Yao, H. H., Bahr, J. M., Gougeon, A., Schomberg, D. W., and Hsueh, A. J. (1999). Restricted expression of WT1 messenger ribonucleic acid in immature ovarian follicles: Uniformity in mammalian and avian species and maintenance during reproductive senescence. *Biol. Reprod.* 60, 365–373.
54. Kotsuji, F., and Tominaga, T., (1994). The role of granulosa and theca cell interactions in ovarian structure and function. *Microsc Res. Technol.* 27, 97–107.
55. Parrott, J. A., and Skinner, M. K. (1998). Thecal cell-granulosa cell interactions involve a positive feedback loop among keratinocyte growth factor, hepatocyte growth factor, and Kit ligand during ovarian follicular development. *Endocrinology* 139, 2240–2245.
56. Li, R., Phillips, D .M., and Mather, J. P. (1995). Activin promotes ovarian follicle development in vitro. *Endocrinology* 136, 849–856.
57. Levy, M. J., Hernandez, E. R., Adashi, E. Y., Stillman, R. J., Roberts, C. T., Jr., and LeRoith, D. (1992). Expression of the insulin-like growth factor (IGF)-I and -II and the IGF-I and -II receptor genes during postnatal development of the rat ovary. *Endorcrinolgy* 131, 1202–1206.
58. Zhou, J., Kumar, T. R., Matzuk, M. M., and Bondy, C. (1997). Insulin-like growth factor I regulates gonadotropin responsiveness in the murine ovary. *Mol. Endocrinol.* 11, 1924–1933.
59. Hsueh, A. J. W., Adashi, E. Y., Jones, P. B., and Welsh, T. H., Jr. (1984). Hormonal regulation of the differentiation of cultured ovarian granulosa cells. *Endocrinol. Rev.* 5, 76–127.
60. Pauerstein, C. J., Eddy, C. A., Croxatto, H. D., Hess, R., Siler-Khodr, T. M., and Croxatto, H. B. (1978). Temporal relationships of estrogen, progesterone, and luteinizing hormone levels to ovulation in women and infrahuman primates. *Am. J. Obstet. Gynecol.* 130, 876–886.
61. Fritz, M. A., McLachlan, R. I., Cohen, N. L., Dahl, K. D., Bremner, W. J., and Soules, M. R. (1992). Onset and characteristics of the midcycle surge in bioactive and immunoactive luteinizing hormone secretion in normal women: Influence of physiological variations in periovulatory ovarian steroid hormone secretion. *J. Clin. Endocrinol. Metab.* 75, 489–493.
62. Yong, E. L., Baird, D. T., Yates, R., Reichert, L. E., Jr., and Hillier, S. G. (1992). Hormonal regulation of the growth and steroidogenic function of human granulosa cells. *J. Clin. Endocrinol. Metab.* 74, 842–849.
63. Couzinet, B., Brailly, S., Bouchard, P., and Schaison, G. (1992). Progesterone stimulates luteinizing hormone secretion by acting directly on the pituitary. *J. Clin. Endocrinol. Metab.* 74, 374–378.
64. Schneyer, A. L., Fujiwara, T., Fox, J., Welt, C. K., Adams, J., Messerlian, G. M., and Taylor, A. E. (2000). Dynamic changes in the intrafollicular inhibin/activin/follistatin axis during human follicular development: relationship to circulating hormone concentrations. *J. Clin. Endocrinol. Metab.* 85, 3319–3330.
65. Makrigiannakis, A., Amin, K., Coukos, G., Tilly, J. L., and Coutifaris, C. (2000). Regulated expression and potential roles of p53 and Wilms' tumor suppressor gene (WT1) during follicular development in the human ovary. *J .Clin. Endocrinol. Metab.* 85, 449–459.
66. Temporal relationships between ovulation and defined changes in the concentration of plasma estradiol-17 beta, luteinizing hormone, follicle-stimulating hormone, and progesterone. I. Probit analysis. World Health Organization, Task Force on Methods for the Determination of the Fertile Period, Special Programme of Research, Development and Research Training in Human Reproduction (1980). *Am. J. Obstet. Gynecol.* 138, 383-390.
67. Hoff, D., Quigley, M. E., and Yen, S. S. (1983). Hormonal dynamics at midcycle: A reevaluation. *J. Clin. Endocrinol. Metab.* 57, 792–796.
68. Zelinski-Wooten, M. B., Hutchison, J. S., Chandrasekher, Y. A., Wolf, D. P., and Stouffer, R. L. (1992). Administration of human luteinizing hormone (hLH) to macaques after follicular development: further titration of LH surge requirements for ovulatory changes in primate follicles. *J. Clin. Endocrinol. Metab.* 75, 502-507.
69. Yoshimura, Y., Santulli, R., Atlas, S. J., Fujii, S., and Wallach, E. E. (1987). The effects of proteolytic enzymes on in vitro ovulation in the rabbit. *Am. J. Obstet. Gynecol.* 157, 468–475.
70. Espey, L. L., Tanaka, N., Adams, R. F., and Okamura, H. (1191). Ovarian hydroxyeicosatetraenoic acids compared with prostanoids and steroids during ovulation in rats. *Am. J. Physiol.* 260, E163–E169.
71. Watanabe, H., Nagai, K., Yamaguchi, M., Ikenoue, T., and Mori, N. (1993). *Prostaglandins Leukot. Essent. Fatty Acids* 49, 963–967.
72. Smith, S. K., Lenton, E. A., and Cooke, I. D. (1985). Plasma gonadotrophin and ovarian steroid concentrations in women with menstrual cycles with a short luteal phase. *J. Reprod. Fertil.* 75, 363–368.
73. Fraser, H. M., Lunn, S. F., Morris, K. D., and Deghenghi, R. (1997). Initiation of high dose gonadotrophin-releasing hormone antagonist treatment during the late follicular phase in the macaque abolishes luteal function irrespective of effects upon the luteinizing hormone surge. *Hum. Reprod.* 12, 430–435.
74. Brannian, J. D., Shiigi, S. M., and Stouffer, R. L. (1992). Gonadotropin surge increases fluorescent-tagged low-density lipoprotein uptake by macaque granulosa cells from preovulatory follicles. *Biol. Reprod.* 47, 355–360.
75. McLachlan, R. I., Cohen, N. L., Vale, W. W., Rivier, J. E., Burger, H. G., Bremner, W. J., and Soules, M. R. (1989). The importance of luteinizing hormone in the control of inhibin and progesterone secretion by the human corpus luteum. *J. Clin. Endocrinol. Metab.* 68, 1078–1085.
76. Runesson, D., Ivarsson, K., Janson, P. O., and Brannstrom, M. (2000). Gonadotropin- and cytokine-regulated expression of the chemokine interleukin 8 in the human preovulatory follicle of the menstrual cycle. *J. Clin. Endocrinol. Metab.* 85, 4387–4395.
77. Sugino, N., Suzuki, T., Kashida, S., Karube, A., Takiguchi, S., and Kato, H. (2000). Expression of Bcl-2 and Bax in the human corpus luteum during the menstrual cycle and early pregnancy: Regulation by human chorionic gonadotropin. *J. Clin. Endocrinol. Metab.* 85, 4379–4386.

78. Sugino, N., Kashida, S., Takiguchi, S., Karube, A., and Kato, H. (2000). Expression of vascular endothelial growth factor and its receptors in the human corpus luteum during the menstrual cycle and in early pregancy. *J. Clin. Endocrinol. Metab.* 85, 3919–3924.
79. Wulff, C., Wilson, H., Largue, P., Duncan, W. C., Armstrong, D. G., and Fraser, H. M. (2000). Angiogenesis in the human corpus luteum: localization and changes in angiopoietins, tie-2, and vascular endothelial growth factor messenger ribonucleic acid. *J. Clin. Endocrinol. Metab.* 85, 4302–4309.
80. Retamales, I., Carrasco, I., Troncoso, J. L., Las Heras, J., Devoto, L., and Vega, M. (1994). Morpho-functional study of human luteal cell subpopulations. *Hum. Reprod.* 9, 591–596.
81. Maas, S., Jarry, H., Teichmann, A., Rath W., Kuhn, W., and Wuttke, W. (1992). Paracrine actions of exytocin, prostaglandin F2 alpha, and estradiol within the human corpus luteum. *J. Clin. Endocrinol. Metab.* 74, 306–312.
82. Khan-Dawood, F. S. (1997). Oxytocin in intercellular communication in the corpus luteum. *Sem. Reprod. Endocrinol.* 4, 395–407.
83. Girsh, E., Milvae, R. A., Wang, W., Meidan, R. (1996). Effect of endothelin-1 on bovine luteal cell function: role in prostaglandin F2alpha-induced antisteroidogenic action. *Endocrinology* 137, 1306–1312.
84. Miceli, F., Minici, F., Garcia Pardo, M., Navarra, P., Mancuso, S., Lanzone, A., and Apa, R. (2001). Endothelins enhance prostaglandin (PGE(2) and PGF(2alpha)) biosynthesis and release by human luteal cells: evidence of a new paracrine/autocrine regulation of luteal function. *J. Clin. Endocrinol. Metab.* 86, 811–817.
85. Shikone, T., Yamoto, M., Kokawa, K., Yamashita, K., Nishimori, K., and Nakano, R. (1996). Apoptosis of human corpora lutea during cyclic luteal regression and early pregnancy. *J. Clin. Endocrinol. Metab.* 81, 2376–2380.
86. Ryan, K. J., and Short, R.V. (1965). Formation of estradiol by granulosa and theca cells of the equine ovarian follicle. *Endocrinology* 76, 108–114.
87. Ryan, K. J., and Smith, O. W. (1965). Biogenesis of steriod hormones in the human ovary. *Recent Prog. Horm. Res.* 21, 367–409.
88. Erickson, G. F. (1996). Physiologic basis of ovulation induction. *Sem. Reprod. Endocrinol.* 14, 287–297.
89. Falck, B. (1959). Site of production of oestrogen in the rat ovary as studied in microtransplants. *Acta Physiol. Scand.* (Suppl. 47) 163, 1–9.
90. Speroff, L., Glass, H., and Kase, N.G. (1999). "Clinical Gynecologic Endocrinology and Fertility," 6th Ed., pp. 31–105. Lippincott Williams & Wilkins, Baltimore, MD.
91. Peiris, A. N., Sothmann, M. S., Aiman, E. J., and Kissebah, A. H. (1989). The relationship of insulin to sex hormone-binding globulin: role of adiposity. *Fertil. Steril.* 52, 69–72.
92. Grumbach, M. M., and Auchus, R. J. (1999). Estrogen: Consequences and implications of human mutations in synthesis and action. *J. Clin. Endocrinol. Metab.* 84, 4677–4694.

C H A P T E R

2B

The Normal Human Ovary Part II

How Steroid Hormones Work

NATHAN G. KASE

Department of Obstetrics, Gynecology and Reproductive Science
The Mount Sinai School of Medicine and Hospital
New York, New York 10029

I. INTRODUCTION

Estrogen (E) and progesterone (P) play a central role in both the endocrine and intracrine regulation of all aspects of female reproduction. Together they act at the level of the hypothalamus, anterior pituitary, ovary, and uterus to coordinate neuroendocrine pulsatile secretion of gonadotropin releasing hormone, cyclic release of gonadotropins FSH and LH, ovulation, and endometrial development in preparation for implantation and maintenance of fertilized embryos. In addition, both hormones are essential for pubescent and pregnancy mammary gland development (ductal morphogenesis in the case of estrogen and further ductal branding with lobulo–alveolar differentiation in the case of P). Both hormones are involved in the biology of the cardiovascular, immune, central nervous, and skeletal systems. Estrogen therapy in particular has been shown to induce salutary effects in these systems (see Chapter 27).

This chapter will focus on the mechanism of action of the principal steroid secretory products of the ovary—estradiol and progesterone. Before undertaking a detailed examination of these functions in the reproductive system as well as their involvement in other nonreproductive physiologic systems, for example, the heart and brain, the general principles of steroid hormone action will be reviewed.

II. THE "FUNCTIONAL CONTEXT" OF STEROID HORMONE–TARGET CELL INTERACTIONS

To understand how hormones produce different effects in different tissues at different times, it is necessary to consider the numerous variables which might dramatically change the final biological result of the basic steroid hormone-receptor-DNA transcription activation cascade. These include

- The structure and concentration of the steroid
- Concentration, distribution, and temporal expression of cognate receptors in various tissues

- The concentration and distribution of receptor subtypes and/or isoforms of each receptor in a specific cell
- Whether a receptor is located in the nucleus or on the plasma membrane (or both)
- The degree to which *steroid action* may proceed even *without* involvement in genomic transcriptional processes or *without* interaction with a receptor
- The degree to which *receptor activity* may be initiated in the *absence* of its classic steroid ligand
- The existence of "cross talk" between diverse receptors and signaling pathways within a cell
- Cellular and hormone specific variations in the conformational shape of the ligand–receptor complex affecting dimerization and recruitment of adaptor proteins
- Differential generation of steroid receptor co-regulators, both co-activators and co-repressors

All these variables contribute to the *functional diversity* of steroid action displayed in different organ systems. The implicit tension imposed by the various systems designed to "fine tune" cell responses, particularly the balance between positive and negative influences on the transcription mechanism has given impetus to the development of *selective receptor modulators* capable of generating tissue-specific beneficial effects (whether stimulatory or repressive) with possible clinical utility.

In summary, the modular nature of receptors allows ligand, tissue, and promoter specific interaction with selected subsets of regulators capable of elaborating distinct transcriptional and thus distinct physiological responses to a steroid signal.

III. THE MECHANISMS OF ESTRADIOL AND ESTROGEN RECEPTOR (ER) SIGNALING [1, 2]

Since the cloning of the first ER cDNA more than a decade ago, the remarkable complexity of the molecular mechanisms underlying the diverse physiologic actions of estradiol (E_2) and its many natural and synthetic ligands are now emerging. *Four* pathways for the molecular mechanisms of estrogen signaling are appreciated:

1. Classical nuclear ligand–dependent
2. Cell surface (nongenomic) ligand–dependent
3. Ligand–independent
4. DNA binding–independent

Furthermore several modifying elements such as receptor subtypes, co-regulator (stimulatory and repressive) generation, and cross talk between steroid receptor and other signaling pathways modulate these molecular mechanisms to yield tissue/cellular specificity.

A. Classical Mechanism of Estrogen Action: Ligand-Dependent [3]

The specificity of the reaction of a cell to estrogen's hormone "instruction" is due in part to the presence of initially unoccupied, inactivated, target cell intranuclear receptor proteins.

In the absence of hormone, the receptor is sequestered in a multiprotein inhibitory complex within the nucleus of target cells. The binding of estrogen (the ligand) to the receptor induces activation of the complex.

The classic pathway follows these steps (see Fig. 2B.1):

1. Free steroid enters the target cell by passive diffusion through both the plasma membrane and nuclear membrane and binds with high affinity to its cognate receptor.
2. The steroid receptor complex undergoes *activation*, a process which involves release from heat shock protein, receptor dimerization, posttranslational modification, and tertiary and quaternary conformational changes which expose high affinity DNA binding sites.
3. The activated steroid-receptor complex binds with specific DNA sequences referred to as estrogen response elements (EREs) which are enhancers located within the regulatory regions of target genes.
4. The activated steroid receptor complex functions as a general transcription factor modulating the synthesis of specific mRNAs and proteins, which are responsible in part for the cellular action of the hormone.
5. Critical to the ligand and tissue specificity of this cascade, in addition to the conformational changes in the receptors following steroid binding, the activated receptor not only binds to specific enhancer DNA elements in the promoters of specific genes but also recruits *co-regulatory* proteins which interact with the general transcriptional machinery to elaborate and/or modify hormone triggered changes.[4] The agonist (stimulatory) ligands of receptors promote binding of co-activator proteins, which promote transcription. On the other hand, binding with antagonists (inhibitory) promotes interaction with co-repressor proteins that induce transcription repression.
6. The ligand-dependent transcriptional activity of ERα is mediated by two separate activation domains, constitutive activation function-1 (AF-1) located within the N terminus (A/B domain—see Fig. 2B.2) and a hormone-dependent AF-2 located in the hormone-binding domain.[5] Both AF-2 and AF-1 activity depends on recruitment and interaction with shared as well as unique families of co-regulatory proteins.[6, 7] Co-activator proteins work in at least two ways. As noted they recruit proteins of the general transcription apparatus (which transcribes DNA into RNA). They also possess enzymatic activity such as histone acetyl transferases that unwind DNA from its histone scaffold which facilitates transcription of RNA.

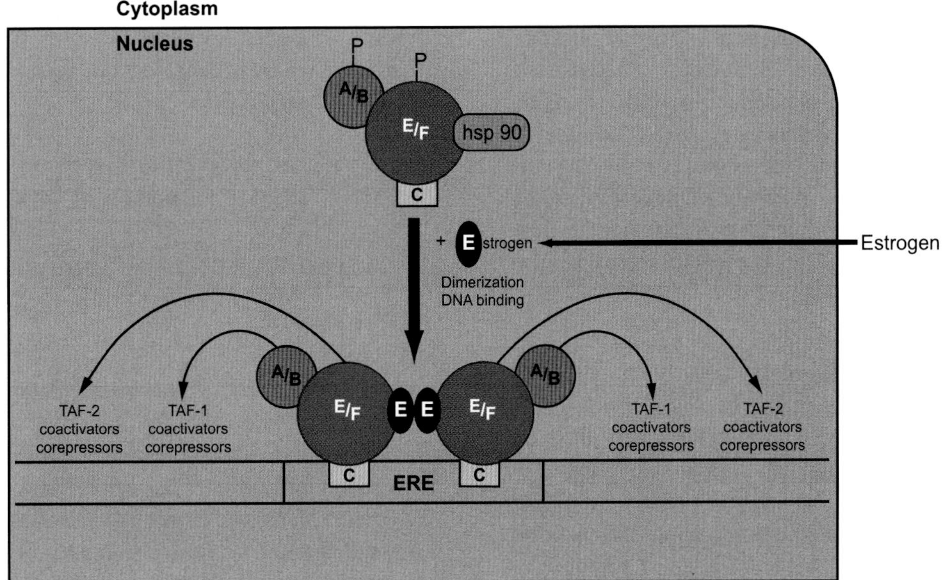

FIGURE 2B.1 The classic mechanism of estrogen action. Estrogen enters the nucleus and binds to the estrogen receptor (ER) at its ligand binding domain (E/F). Dimerization follows with DNA binding of the dimeric E-ER complex at estrogen response elements (ERE) via the DNA binding domain (C) of each ER. In addition, transcription activation factors AF-1 and AF-2 recruit and interact with a variety of co-regulatory factors, both stimulatory and inhibitory (co-activators and co-repressors) which confer ligand specific and tissue specific physiologic and pharmacologic diversity.

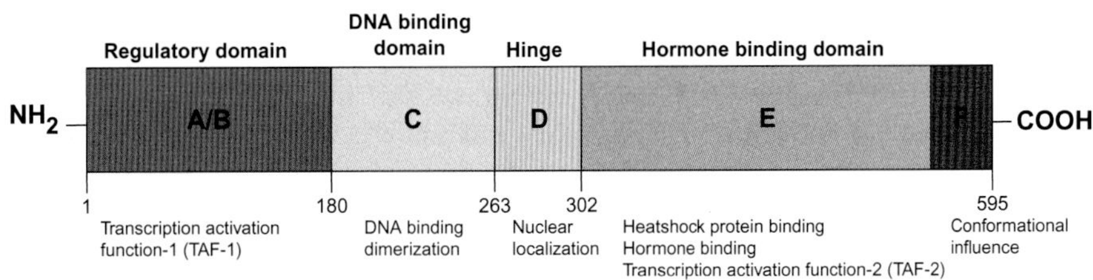

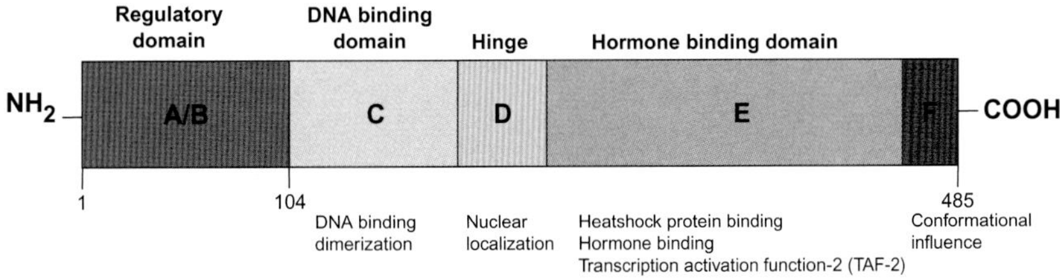

FIGURE 2B.2 The estrogen nuclear receptor subtypes, ERα and ERβ and their functional domains.

7. Transcription leads to translation; mRNA-mediated protein synthesis on the ribosomes and generation of specific biologic activity. Although activated steroid hormone receptors are thought of as primarily affecting gene transcription, they also regulate posttranslational events.

8. Biologic activity is maintained only while the nuclear site is occupied with the hormone-receptor complex. The dissociation rate of the hormone from its receptor as well as the half-life of the nuclear chromatin-bound complex are factors in the biologic response of the hormone.

Thus, *duration of exposure to a hormone is as important as concentration*. For example, only small amounts of estrogen need to be present in the circulation because the long half-life of the estradiol hormone-receptor complex. Indeed, a major factor in the potency differences among the various estrogens (estradiol, estrone, and estriol) is the length of time the estrogen-receptor complex occupies the nucleus. Cortisol and progesterone must circulate in large concentrations because their receptor complexes have short half-lives in the nucleus.

An important action of estrogen is the generation of its own and other steroid hormone activity by affecting receptor concentrations. In a process called *replenishment*, estrogen increases target tissue responsiveness to itself and to progestins and androgens by increasing the concentration of its own receptor and that of the intracellular progestin and androgen receptors. Progesterone and clomiphene, on the other hand, limit tissue response to estrogen in part by blocking the replenishment mechanism, thus decreasing the concentration of estrogen receptors over time. Replenishment, the synthesis of the sex hormone receptors, takes place in the cytoplasm, but in the case of estrogen and progestin receptors, synthesis is quickly followed by transport into the nucleus.

9. The fate of the hormone-receptor complex after gene activation is referred to as hormone-receptor *processing*. In the case of estrogen receptors, processing involves the conversion of high-affinity estrogen receptor sites to a rapidly dissociating form followed by loss of binding capacity, which is completed in about 6 h.

IV. THE GENERATION OF FUNCTIONAL DIVERSITY

A. Steroid Receptor Co-regulators and Physiologic Diversity of Hormone Response

For detailed reviews of this at once dauntingly complex but physiologically and clinically important element of steroid hormone action and the potential for pharmacologic manipulation and modification please see reviews by Robyr *et al.* [8] McKenna *et al.* [4] and Rosenfeld and Glass [9] (Table 2B.1).

Ligand-dependent implementation of receptor activity requires recruitment of a complex group of co-activators including chromatin remodeling, the unwinding nucleosome-disrupting histone acetyltransferases (SRC family members PCAF and P300), mediator proteins that bridge receptor complexes (e.g., DRIP/TRAP220/ARC), an RNA helicase p68, and elements of the ubiquitin proteosome degradation system including ubiquitin ligases (E6AP and RPF1).

Literally scores of putative co-activators have been identified. As the number of potential co-activators clearly exceeds the capacity for direct interaction with a single receptor, it is

TABLE 2B.1 Multifaceted Nature of Transcriptional Regulation by Nuclear Receptor Co-regulators: Nuclear Receptors, Through their Interactions with Co-regulators, Recruit Diverse Functional Domains and Enzyme Activities to the Promoter to Achieve Efficient Transcriptional Regulation *in vivo*

Property	Co-regulator	Target	Function
Activation domain	SRC-1, TIF2/hSRC-2, RAC3/ hSRC-3	Basal transcription factors	Stabilization of preinitiation complex
Repression domain	NcoR, SMRT, SUNCoR	Basal transcription factors	Destabilization of preinitiation complex
Acetylase	PCAF, CBP/p300, SRC-1, ACTR/hSRC-3	Core histones	Disruption of histone-DNA, histone-histone interactions
	p300	p53	Enhances p53 DNA binding
	CBP	TCF	Uncouples *Wingless* signaling in *Drosophila*
	PCAF	PR	Unknown
Deacetylase	HDAC-1/ HDAC-2	Core histones, others?	Restoration of DNA-histone, hitosne-histone interaction
Protease	Siah2/26S proteosome	NCoR	Protein degradation
Ubiquitin ligase	E6-AP	Unknown	Protein degradation
ATPase	BRG-1, Trip-1	Chromatin, others?	Domain remodeling during activation
	SNAF2 ATPase	Chromatin, others?	Domain remodeling during repression?
Kinase	TIF1α	TFIIEα, $TAF_{II}28$, $TAF_{II}35$	Stabilization/destabilization of target proteins?
	ER-associated kinase	?	
	ANPK (AR-associated Kinase)	AR coregulators?	

likely that different protein complexes can act either sequentially, combinationally, or in parallel.[10, 11] For example, a "division of labor" among co-activators would lead to the sequence of chromatin remodeling, followed by acetyltransferase activity, protein bridging, and finally complexes of co-activators that enhance RNA polymerase II recruitment to the promoter.

A number of co-repressors have also been identified including the histone deacetylases N-COR and SMRT and the estrogen receptor interacting proteins RIP140 and REA.

Studies on the comparative spatiotemporal expression of some co-regulator proteins and steroid receptors in different mammalian tissues combined with generation of knockout mouse models carrying null mutations of several co-regulatory proteins have begun to fill in the details of the essential role of these proteins in mediating selective steroid responses in health and disease.

For example, it is now clear that expression of some co-regulator proteins in steroid-responsive tissues is developmentally and hormonally controlled. The expression of co-activator SRC-1 is absent from estrogen reactive cells during postpubertal mammary gland development but can be co-localized with estrogen-receptor-positive breast cells during pregnancy. In addition, aberrant expression of co-regulator proteins has been found in breast cancer. These reports *show increased co-activator levels associated with tumorigenesis* while *the expression of co-repressors is diminished*. For example, levels of CBP, TRAP220, and a number of SRC family members—all co-activators—are elevated in breast tumors. Conversely levels of the co-repressor N-COR are decreased and even more dramatically in invasive compared to *in situ* disease. N-COR is also decreased in the mouse model of tamoxifen-resistant breast cancer. Furthermore mice carrying a null mutation of either SRC-1 or SRC-3 show that deletion of either protein results in partial hormone resistance in mammary gland developmental responses to estrogen and progesterone indicating overlapping responsibilities of the two co-activators in yielding a full hormonal response. On the other hand, SRC-1 expression is essential in eliciting full growth and differentiation of the uterus in response to E and/or P whereas deletion of SRC-3 leaves uterine function unaffected.

Validation of the essential role of co-repressors in mediating the specific transcriptional responses to ligand–ER complexes is also in hand. Studies of responses of mouse embryonic fibroblasts carrying a null mutation of the co-repressor N-COR to the estrogen receptor antagonist 4-OH tamoxifen demonstrated that the presence of this co-repressor was essential to the action of the antagonist. Ablation of N-COR converted 4-OHT to a full estrogen *agonist*.

In summary, abnormal co-regulator function may contribute to a variety of hormone-related diseases including steroid resistance syndromes, reproductive dysfunction, and steroid-responsive cell tumorigenesis. Clinicians are all too familiar with both the virtues and disadvantages of selective estrogen receptor modulators (SERM) application in their practice. The intense vasomotor reactions of some women to tamoxifen frequently limits sustained compliance. The appearance of tamoxifen-resistant breast cancer recurrences after 5 years of use is another example of the too proximal insertion of SERM action in the mechanism of estrogen action. At this point, the next generation of pharmaceutical approaches to tissue-specific steroid action modulation will emerge with identification and perturbation of tissue-specific cell co-regulatory proteins.

Of equal importance is the potential for co-regulatory "profiles" in identification of individuals at risk for steroid dysfunction, disease, or neoplasm. In the last instance, i.e., tumorigenesis, co-regulator profiles may determine degrees of aggressive invasive behavior as well as dictate individualized treatment methodologies and the sequence of their applications.[1]

B. Estrogen Nuclear Receptor Subtypes (Fig. 2B.2)

Receptors for estrogen are expressed as two structurally related subtypes designated as estrogen receptor alpha (ERα) and estrogen receptor beta (ERβ).[11, 12] ERα is translated from a 6.8-kb mRNA derived from a gene on the long arm of chromosome 6. The more recently discovered ERβ is encoded by a gene localized to chromosome 14,q22q24.

Both proteins show a high degree of amino acid conservation in their DNA-binding domains (97%) and lesser but still significant (59%) homology in the hormone-binding domain. However, substantial differences exist between α and β in their transactivation domains, as well as the hinge and the F domains which confer differential conformational "flexibility."

Two functionally distinct transactivation domains exist in both receptor proteins.[5–7] The first (AF-1) is located in the poorly conserved amino terminal domain and a second (AF-2) located in the ligand-binding domain. AF-1 and AF-2 may contribute either independently or synergistically to either agonist ligand receptor transcription activity or ligand-independent phosphorylation pathways of receptor activation. Furthermore, their relative activities vary depending on the specific cellular and promoter contexts. For example, transcriptional responses of each receptor to estradiol (a ligand with which they both bind with equal affinity) varies significantly in part due to sequence divergence in their AF-1 domains and to a differential preference of individual receptor subtypes for specific co-activator proteins.

1. Genomic Receptor Subtype Distribution: Reproductive System [13–15]

Immunocytochemical localization of ERα and β in *human* reproductive organs demonstrates a cell specific localization for each of the ER subtypes.[16] In the *ovary* ERβ immunoreactivity is found in the nuclei of granulosa cells in all stages of follicle growth (from primary to mature follicles), in the interstitial cells and germinal epithelium. ERα is seen in the theca cells as well as interstitium and germinal epithelium. Thus, each receptor can exert different functions according to their specific cellular locations. In the *uterus and vagina*, ERα is most likely the subtype involved in the action of estrogen: strong ERα immunoreactivity is detected in epithelial, stromal, and muscle cells (ERβ is seen but provides a much weaker signal). Only ERα is detected in the vagina. In the mammary gland, both ER subtypes are equally observed in epithelial cells and stromal cells. Finally, the differential distribution of ERα and ERβ mRNA in intrauterine tissues of the pregnant rhesus monkey has been studied.[17] Both subtypes are expressed in myometrium, amnion, and chorio-decidua but not in the placenta. Both ER proteins are expressed in the smooth muscle and endothelium of myometrial blood vessels.

While the functional consequences of the differential distribution of the ER subtypes in humans awaits further investigation, selective ablation of ERα (αERKO), ERβ (βERKO), and combined α and βER (αβERKO) in *mice* has provided definitive evidence that these receptor sub- types mediate distinct physiologic responses bearing on reproduction.[18]

ERα is the dominant subtype expressed throughout the female mouse reproductive tract and its ablation (αERKO) results in infertility due to defects in sexual behavior, neuroendocrine gonadotropin regulation, ovulation, uterine function, and postpubertal mammary gland development. For example, the αERKO ovary is characterized by the presence of large, hemorrhagic and cystic follicles, a sparse number of early stage follicles, and a complete absence of corpora lutea. Prolonged treatment with a GnRH agonist (resulting in normalized LH levels) leads to a resolution of the polycystic ovary phenotype in αERKO mice suggesting that it is chronic gonadotropin hyperstimulation due to a defect in anterior pituitary ERα function that causes the polycystic changes. In contrast, βERKO results in a subfertile phenotype due exclusively to intrinsic ovarian dysfunction. Fewer follicles are developed and fewer ovulate. In the gonadotropin-induced super ovulation model, βERKO display diminished capacity to conclude meiosis I as well as a high frequency of unruptured follicles.[19]

Compound knockout mice (αβERKO) exhibit phenotypes that resemble those of αERKO. However, in these animals the ovaries show progressive germ cell loss and redifferentiation of the surrounding somatic cells indicating that both ER forms are necessary in formation and maintenance of this tissue.[15]

The ERα subtype also plays an essential role in male fertility and mediates many of the nonreproductive activities of estrogen including regulation of bone resorption, bone growth, cardiovascular endothelial regeneration, adipogenesis, and sexual behavior. ERβ is detected in osteoblasts, chondrocytes, the cardiovascular system, and the central nervous system. It appears to play an essential role in cortical neuronal survival and regeneration [20] and appears to contribute, with ERα to protect against cardiovascular injury.[21]

These knockout models have contributed substantially to understanding the distributive functions of ERα and ERβ in mediating the tissue-specific physiologic responses to estrogen. In addition, they have demonstrated that embryonic *development* of the female reproductive tract proceeds normally in the *absence* of E-ER interaction. Similarly, they have validated the existence of alternate signaling pathways to function (see below) that are independent of either E-ligand or E-receptor. For example, catecholestrogen may stimulate the uterus in the absence of ER. On the other hand, ERα is an essential mediator of uterine proliferative responses stimulated by epidermal growth factor *in the absence of estrogen*—validation that a physiologic response can follow steroid hormone ligand independent activation of estrogen receptors. In this regard, ovarian nuclear receptors have been reported to be activated by different signaling pathways including those stimulated by dopamine, EGF, TGFα and IGF-I.[22–25] (See next section.)

Finally in cells in which both ERα and ERβ are expressed overall estrogen responsiveness may be determined by the ERα : ERβ *ratio*. In this fashion ERβ may compensate for a relative lack of ERα. The ability to form heterodimers suggest that both ERs share similar activation pathways. In still other respects, ERβ may attenuate the action of ERα.

Superimposed upon this distributive and receptor subtype concentration diversity are other receptor linked factors which yield unique cellular responses. These include:

1. Identification and characterization [26] of a novel human estrogen receptor (ER)β isoform called ERβcx which after heterodimer formation with ERα (not ERβ) *inhibits* ERα DNA binding and transactivation. ERαcx is expressed in the ovary, testes, thymus, prostate, and a number of human cultured cell lines.
2. Ability of different estrogen receptor agonist and antagonist ligands to induce ligand-specific conformational modification particularly in the AF domains, thereby creating a spectrum of transcriptional responses by recruitment of a variety of co-activators and co-repressors. This is the mechanism by which SERMs elicit selective tissue-specific agonist activities of estrogen. (See next section).

C. Cell-Surface, Nongenomic Signaling of Steroids

The rapid biologic effects of E_2 in bone, breast, vasculature, and nervous system suggests that estrogen may work through a nongenomic process using cell surface ER forms linked to intracellular signal transduction proteins (see Fig. 2B.3).[27, 28]

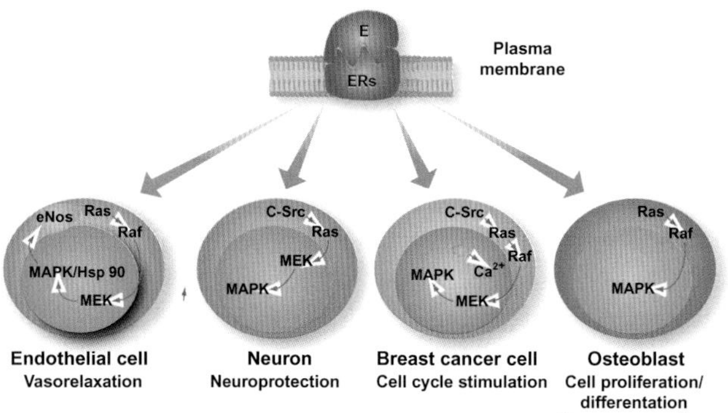

FIGURE 2B.3 Cell surface, nongenomic estrogen signaling pathways. Depending on target cell system involved, estrogen (E) links to plasma membrane estrogen receptors (ERs) and activates a variety of rapid, nongenomic signaling pathways. eNOS = nitric oxide synthase; Hsp 90 = heat shock protein 90; MAPK and MEK = steps in the mitogen activation protein kinase pathway; Ca^{2+} = calcium ion; C-Src = from cellular sarcoma gene (a tyrosine protein kinase); Ras = a member of the GTP-ase superfamily: an oncogen first isolated from *R*ats with *S*arcoma; Raf = like Ras relates to isolation from sarcoma virus: a serine/threonine kinase is part of the Src-Ras-Raf-MEK-MAPK intracellular pathway cascade that links the cytosolic face of the activated receptor to effector sites.

A large body of data supports the existence of these steroid effects which cannot be explained by the classic model of steroid-target cell nuclear interaction. These *nongenomic* processes possess the following characteristics: (1) the activity is too rapid for involvement of changes in mRNA and protein synthesis, (2) are seen in cells unable to accomplish mRNA and protein synthesis (spermatozoa) or in cells lacking steroid nuclear receptors, (3) activity can be induced even by steroids coupled with high molecular weight substances that prevent passage through the cell or nuclear membrane, (4) are not blocked by antagonists of the classic, genomic steroid receptor, and (5) are highly specific since steroids with similar but not identical structure may show various degrees of inductive potencies. In sum, these rapid effects are compatible with activation of signal transduction mechanisms similar to those activated by peptide hormones after interaction with their membrane receptors.[28, 29, 30]

ER and membrane coupled tyrosine kinase pathways are linked with E_2 activation of the MAPK signaling pathway in a variety of cells. Some of the vascular protective effects of E_2 through ERα are mediated via a nongenomic pathway involving activation of endothelial nitric oxide synthase and nitric oxide release through MAPK and phosphatidyl-inositol 3-kinase/Akt pathways.[31, 32] Similarly E_2-MAPK activation may be a mechanism for the protective effects of estrogen on bone.

The reproductive cell types in which rapid cellular responses to estrogens are prominent include transduction of the estrogen signal from the cell surface of granulosa cells, endometrial cells, and oocytes.[33, 22] In mammalian granulosa cells for example, estradiol induced a 4- to 8-fold increase in intracellular calcium (Ca^{2+}). This rise in calcium ion is likely an important regulating mechanism by modulating the function of Ca^{2+} binding signal proteins (such as calmodulin), affect the secretion of Ca^{2+} sensitive autocrine/paracrine factors (such as TGF-α), stimulate cell proliferation and modify cell to cell intraovarian communication. Because the classic nuclear ER is a substrate of the calmodulin-dependent protein kinase II, the transient rise in Ca^{2+} could mediate 'cross talk' interaction between membrane and nuclear ERs. (See Section IV.C.1).

In endometrial cells, estrogen elicits both functional and morphologic changes too rapidly to be mediated by the classic genomic pathway. Estradiol stimulates Ca^{2+} uptake by mouse endometrial cells and in a biphasic effect over 1–7 min increases the number, density, length, and clustering of microvilli on the endometrial cell's luminal surface ciliation.

Human oocytes at the germinal vesicle stage within a few seconds demonstrate a rapid influx of Ca^{2+} in response to estradiol. The presence of estradiol does not influence the nuclear progression through meiotic maturation but improves the subsequent fertilization potential of *in vitro* matured oocytes as demonstrated in better cleavage rates and development of resulting embryos. Thus, E_2 at least in these models does not appear to affect nuclear maturation but exerts a beneficial cytoplasmic effect on human oocytes.

1. 'Cross talk' between Nongenomic and Genomic Pathways in the Responses of Cells to Estrogen

Unlike oocytes, an active genomic estrogen response mechanism coexists with the nongenomic one in endometrial and mammary glands and breast cancer cells.[34, 35] Thus, the same steroid ligand can activate simultaneously or consecutively, a membrane associated receptor *and* the classic nuclear receptor. The resultant steroid effect on the cell represents a superimposition of the two distinct receptor-mediated events in which one may condition, synergize with, or modify the other. Finally, nongenomic and genomic actions may synergize causing biphasic effects that have both a rapid onset and a long-lasting persistence.

D. Ligand-Independent Activation of ER: Cross Talk with Peptide Growth Factors

ER function can be modulated by extracellular signals in the absence of E_2. The polypeptide growth factors such as EGF and IGF-I can activate ER and increase the expression of ER target genes.[36] Furthermore, multiple-site steroid membrane receptors are located in close proximity to binding sites for peptide hormones. This finding raises the probability that a complex system of cell regulation involves not only steroid and peptide hormone action on the same target cells but also utilizing the same intracellular messengers, and modulating the same signaling pathways. Biologically these hormone-independent growth factor pathways may enhance mitogenesis in ER-positive tissues or simply allow ER activation in the presence of low E_2 levels. Accordingly, each pathway may be dependent on the other for full manifestation of either response. For example, an EGF response will be diminished or obliterated by administration of a full antiestrogen or in an αERKO mouse model.

E. DNA-Independent Genomic Actions of ER [2]

E_2-ER can lead to gene activation and regulation in the absence of direct DNA binding as in the absence of an ERE site. This is seen in E_2-ERα activation of IGF-I and collagenase expression mediated through interaction with Fos and Jun at AP-I binding sites via the p160 coactivators SRC-1 and GRIP-1.[37]

V. TISSUE-SPECIFIC ACTIVATION OF ER: SERMs

SERMs are a class of synthetic compounds that stimulates a spectrum of estrogen actions and tissue specificities which exploits the existence of multiple cellular pathways of ER action in different target tissues. The classical receptor theory that agonists function to turn on inherently inactive ERs whereas antagonists competitively inhibit agonist binding and "lock" the ER in a latent state cannot explain the mixed agonist/antagonist properties of SERMs. The activity of these synthetic ER ligands are dependent on specific properties of target tissues which confer beneficial effects on bone, brain, and cardiovascular tissues but without the mitogenic and possibly carcinogenic actions on breast and endometrium. They do so by modifying ER structure producing unique conformational changes within the ER which are distinct from those seen when E_2 occupies receptors [38–41] and with consequent production of unique co-activator complexes and unique tissue-specific functional results. These synthetic ligands differ from pure estrogen antagonists in that the latter oppose estrogen activity in all tissues both *in vitro* and *in vivo*. This is accomplished by inhibition of dimerization of the ligand-bound receptor, prevention of DNA binding and disproportionate cytoplasmic metabolism of receptor without compensatory replenishment.

VI. TISSUE SELECTIVE PHYSIOLOGIC RESPONSES: NONREPRODUCTIVE SYSTEM EXAMPLES

A. Estrogen and the Cardiovascular System [42]

The atheroprotective effect of estrogen in women extends beyond the salutary influence of the hormone on serum lipid concentrations. Data now demonstrate that the direct actions of estrogen on normal blood vessels contribute substantially to the cardiovascular protective activity of estrogen. The vasculature is now recognized as an important target of estrogen action.

Estrogen induces vasodilation and inhibits the response of blood vessels to injury and the development of atherosclerosis. The former response occurs within 5–20 min after estrogen administration, is not dependent on changes in gene expression, and is therefore categorized as nongenomic. On the other hand, the hormone-induced inhibition of responses to vascular injury and the prevention of atherogenesis occur over a period of many hours or days and are dependent on the classic genomic receptor complex gene expression pathway.[21]

Vascular endothelial and smooth muscle cells bind estrogen with high affinity and both estrogen receptors α and β have been identified and functional in both types of vascular cells as well as in myocardial cells.[43, 44] However, the relative proportions of these receptors in different normal vascular beds and in diseased tissue have not been fully elucidated. That α and β not only form homodimers but heterodimers as well, that variant forms of ERα are expressed in vascular cells and that estrogen receptors can be activated by growth factors in the absence of estrogen adds further complexity to determining the influence of estrogen and the different intracellular pathways that might modulate the propagation or prevention of vascular disease. Suffice to say the presence of either of the two known estrogen receptors is sufficient to protect against vascular injury. Furthermore, the SERM tamoxifen among its other attributes appears to function as an estrogen agonist in vascular tissues but no SERM has been identified which works only on blood vessels or the heart.

1. Cardiovascular Effects of Estrogen

In addition to altering serum lipid concentrations, estrogen influences the coagulation, fibrinolytic, and antioxidant systems as well as the production of other vasoactive molecules such as nitric oxide and prostaglandins. The broad range of systemic effects of estrogen activated specific target genes in vascular smooth muscle and endothelial cells have been summarized by Mendelsohn and Karas [42] and appear in Table 2B.2. Only the major elements are reviewed here.

a. Effects on Serum Lipoproteins

The effects of estrogen therapy on serum lipid levels include a reduction in total cholesterol, LDL-C, and L_p(a) lipoprotein concentrations and an increase in serum HDL-C and triglycerides.[45] The route of administration is important since these effects are largely the result of oral "first pass" estrogen-receptor-mediated hepatic expression of apoprotein genes. Transdermal estrogen therapy avoids this

TABLE 2B.2 Estrogen-Regulated Genes of Potential Importance in Vascular Physiology and Disease

Gene product	Physiologic or pathophysiologic role[a]
Candidate estrogen-regulated genes (vascular cells)	
Prostacyclin synthase	Vasodilatation
Endothelial nitric oxide synthase	Vasodilatation
Inducible nitric oxide synthase	Vasodilatation in response to vascular injury
Endothelin-I	Vasoconstriction
Collagen	Vascular-matrix formation
Matrix metalloproteinase 2	Vascular-matrix remodeling
E-selectin	Cell adhesion
Vascular-cell adhesion molecule	Cell adhesion
Vascular endothelial growth factor	Angiogenesis and endothelial-cell proliferation
Candidate estrogen-regulated genes (nonvascular cells)	
Growth- and development-related genes	
Transforming growth factor β_1	Wound healing
Epidermal growth factor receptor	Cell growth in response to vascular injury
Platelet-derived growth factor	Cell growth in response to vascular injury
flt-4 tyrosine kinase	Angiogenesis and endothelial-cell proliferation
Coagulation- and fibrinolysis-related genes	
Tissue factor	Hemostasis in response to thrombosis
Fibrinogen	Hemostasis in response to thrombosis
Protein S	Hemostasis in response to thrombosis
Coagulation factor Vll	Hemostasis in response to thrombosis
Coagulation factor Xll	Hemostasis in response to thrombosis
Plasminogen-activator inhibitor 1	Hemostasis in response to thrombosis
Tissue plasminogen activator	Fibrinolysis
Antithrombin III	Anticoagulation
Signaling-related and miscellaneous genes	
Estrogen receptor α	Hormonal regulation and gene expression
Estrogen receptor β	Hormonal regulation and gene expression
Monocyte chemotactic protein 1	Monocyte recruitment and atherosclerosis
I_{SK} and HK2 (cardiac potassium channels)	Cardiac conduction
Connexin 43	Cardiac conduction
Leptin	Fat metabolism and obesity
Apolipoproteins A, B, D, and E and Lp(a)	Lipid metabolism and atherosclerosis
Angiotensin-converting enzyme	Vasoconstriction
Angiotensin II receptor, type 1	Vasoconstriction

[a]Data from Mendelsohn, M. E., and Karas, R. H. (1999). *N. Engl. J. Med.* 340, Table 1, p 1804.

first pass impact and has less effect on serum concentrations than the oral route. Co-administration of a progestin blunts these oral effects,[45] whereas SERMs induce less pronounced estrogen-like changes on serum lipids.

b. Systemic Effects on Coagulation, Fibrinolytic and Other Vasoactive Proteins [46–48]

The net effect of estrogen on *coagulation* depends on the form, dose, and the duration of estrogen therapy. High serum estrogen concentrations are associated with decreased plasma fibrinogen concentrations and the anticoagulant proteins antithrombin III and protein S. On the other hand, estrogen also decreases plasma levels of the antifibrinolytic protein plasminogen-activator inhibitor type I. Given the balance of these factors, whether thrombogenesis or fibrinolysis occurs may depend on flow velocity (i.e., arterial versus venous) or vasoconstriction versus vasodilation.

Vasomotor tone is directly regulated by estrogen through both its short- and long-term influences on the vasculature. In addition to an increased ratio of nitric oxide (dilation) [49] to endothelin-I (constriction) in plasma,[50] long-term effects include decreased renin and angiotensin-converting enzyme plasma concentrations, the net effect of which is vasodilation.

Finally, in postmenopausal women both short- and long-term administration of estradiol decreases the oxidation of LDL cholesterol.[51]

c. Direct Effects on Vascular Cells

Estrogens can cause short-term vasodilation by both endothelium-dependent and -independent pathways.

Membrane based, nongenomic rapid effects are achieved largely through two mechanisms: ion channel effects [52, 53] and nitric oxide generation.[50, 54] At physiologic concentrations estrogens stimulate the opening of calcium-activated potassium channels through a nitric oxide and cyclic GMP-dependent pathway. This relaxes smooth muscle and promotes vasodilatation. On the other hand, at pharmacologic concentrations, estrogen inhibits influx of extracellular calcium into vascular smooth muscle cells.

Normal endothelium secretes nitric oxide, which both relaxes vascular smooth muscle and inhibits platelet activation. In cultured endothelial cells, physiologic concentrations of estrogen cause a rapid release of nitric oxide without altering gene expression. This rapid effect appears to be mediated by the estrogen receptor α located in the plasma membrane, which activates nitric oxide synthase.[55, 56] A substantial body of pharmacologic data derived from studies in cholesterol fed ovariectomized primates [57] and postmenopausal women [58] demonstrate that estrogen acutely dilates coronary and brachial arteries and prolongs duration of treadmill exercise before the onset of ischemia.

As noted, these short-term coronary vasodilatory effects of estrogens in humans are mediated in large measure by increased production of nitric oxide. But the estrogen-estrogen receptor α complex also acts as a transcription factor to mediate the long-term effects of estrogen on gene expression. Thus, estrogen increases the expression of genes for important vasodilatory enzymes such as prostacyclin synthase and nitric oxide synthase.[58–60] The rapid effects of estrogen via membrane ERα therefore are attributable and proportional to the long-term nuclear ERα generated increases in the synthetic capacity of vascular cells to secrete vasoactive substances.

Finally, estrogen induces beneficial responses to vascular injury and contributes to long-term vascular protection against atherogenesis both directly and indirectly by inhibiting the proliferation and migration of vascular smooth muscle cells (via nitric oxide),[61] and reducing apoptosis and accelerating the growth of normal endothelial cells (in part due to local expression of vascular endothelial growth factor—VEGF).[42]

B. Central Nervous System Effects of Estrogen [62]

Estrogens act on brain areas important for learning and memory, emotions and affective state, motor coordination, and pain sensitivity.[63] However, in the CNS it cannot be overemphasized that rather than one estrogen-regulated process or action on one brain region, many types of estrogen actions on a number of neurochemical, neuroanatomical substrates, and molecular mechanisms underlie these activities.

1. Cellular and Molecular Mechanisms of Estrogen Action in the Brain

The variety of estrogen effects include classic ERα and ERβ genomic and nongenomic expression, rapid actions such as excitability of neuronal cells,[29] activation of cAMP and mitogen activated protein kinase (MAP kinase) pathways, [64] effects on calcium channel and calcium ion entry,[65] and the protective mechanisms defending neurons from damage by excitotoxins and free radicals as well as inducing repair and regeneration (Table 2B.3).[66, 67] These observations expand the action of estrogen to novel mechanisms by which estrogens can participate in cellular events also regulated by growth factors and neurotransmitters.

Even the stereospecific preference for 17β- rather than 17α- estradiol demonstrated in most other tissues does not apply in the CNS. The emergence of a broader influence for the ring A 3 hydroxyl group (as opposed to the 17-hydroxy) of the estrogen molecule as a major ligand characteristic reinforces the existence of a variety of novel estrogen signal mechanisms in the CNS.[63]

The added complexity of steroid-brain interactions is understandable given the diversity of estrogen's spatiotemporal influences on the CNS. These include prenatal brain development and organization, activation (as in pubescence), as well as estrogen influences on cognition, stress, sexuality, pregnancy and parturition, and aging. Induction of receptors, neurotransmitter activation and modulation, receptor subtype 'cross talk', neural and glial effects, oxidative metabolism, and apoptosis all must be involved in these brain functions.

Although separate mechanisms of E action will be discussed in the following paragraphs, it must be remembered that all may participate in combination or sequentially to induce or modify activity.

a. Intracellular ERs

ERα shows a characteristic distribution in the CNS with high levels in the pituitary, hypothalamus, preoptic area, amygdala, hippocampus, and cerebral cortex. The distribution of ERβ is less certain but low-level widespread localization includes the olfactory bulbs, cerebellum, and cerebral cortex.[20, 68] Co-localization (and the possibility of heterodimer formation) of ERα and ERβ has been demonstrated in

TABLE 2B.3 Actions of Estrogens Related to Excitability and Cell Membrane Events

Membrane binding sites: identified but not well characterized
Genomic effects on membrane events, e.g.: induction of the MINK potassium channel in pituitary via genomic mechanism; calcium channel expression in pituitary and hippocampus
Apparent nongenomic actions, e.g.: rapid excitation of electrical activity in cerebellum, hippocampus, striatum, and cerebral cortex; effects occur within seconds and are unlikely to involve a transcriptional activation
Second messenger activation
CREB phosphorylation: genomic versus nongenomic mechanism unclear.
MAP kinase activation: possible novel receptor pathway or involvement of classical ER in a novel signaling pathway.
Calcium homeostasis
Rapid actions: 17βE is more potent, and tamoxifen is an agonist.
Rapid actions: 17αE is as potent as 17βE on calcium entry.
Possible genomic actions: delayed and sustained increase in Ca channel activity.
Neuroprotection
Rapid actions: 17αE is as potent as 17βE versus oxidative damage.
Genomic actions: 17βE is more potent; antiestrogen blockade.

For detailed summary, see Ref. 66. Note that these estrogen actions are not mutually exclusive, but may represent different end points of interacting intracellular signaling cascades.

the hypothalamic preoptic area, portions of the stria terminals, and medial amygdaloid nucleus.[69] Estrogen actions on cholinergic, noradrenergic, serotoninergic, and hypothalamic dopaminergic pathways probably proceed via classic genomic nuclear ERα and ERβ receptors.[63]

Shughrue [70] has studied the classic genomic activity of estrogen and estrogen agonist/antagonists in the CNS. Using progesterone receptor mRNA expression as an index of estrogenic activity, as expected 17β-E_2 and DES but also 17α-E_2 increased this expression. However the SERMs tamoxifen, raloxifene, and clomiphene alone showed no effect and were *antagonists* to 17β-E_2 when combined with that steroid. An antagonist without agonist effect of SERMs has significant clinical connotations with respect to generation of vasomotor reactions; it remains to be seen if neuroprotection and other agonists benefits are also voided with the use of these nonsteroidal agents. In this regard, concerns have arisen over the failure of raloxifene to influence cognitive function in a large group of postmenopausal women (mean age of 66) when compared to placebo.[71]

b. Membrane ERs

Membrane ERs exist in the CNS as well as elsewhere in the body. Some of these receptors display a specificity for estrogens that differs from that of intracellular ER. These membrane receptors can participate (as in the vasculature) in second messenger-related effects, and appear not to discriminate between 17β- and 17α-estradiol. Noteworthy among these novel actions of estrogen is the activation of phosphorylation of the transcription regulator cAMP response element binding protein,[72] and of the MAP kinase pathway.[64] As noted these "options" would permit estrogen interaction with other cell surface receptors modulating cellular events also regulated by growth factors and neurotransmitters. Finally, while some of the neuroprotective effects of estrogen proceed via genomic mRNA expression which can be blocked by antiestrogens, estrogen also reduces the production and/or activity of cell damaging and apoptosis inducing free radicals by processes which are not blocked by estrogen antagonists.

2. Unique Properties of Estrogen Signal Transmission in the Brain

Despite the complex array of functional options for estrogen influence on the brain, a basic question must be asked. With the exception of the hypothalamus, preoptic region, and the amygdala, a relative paucity of ERs (certainly when compared to other nonbrain E_2 targets) exist in the brain. How do estrogens effect so many brain regions and neurochemical systems involved in nonreproductive brain functions? While the methodologies usually applied to determine ER presence and function may not be sufficiently sensitive for neural and glial tissue, more likely the answer lies in the fact that in the brain only a few nerve cells equipped with an estrogen reactive mechanism can have powerful transsynaptic effects on neighboring neurons. For example, estradiol can induce neurons to form new synaptic connections with other cells. Estrogen complexing with intracellular receptors in interneurons can influence thousands of pyramidal neurons in their vicinity. The brain's unique neuroanatomic circuitry and neurochemical systems extend the influence of the action in one cell to an incredible array of brain centers and their functions. *For the brain, a 'paracrine' influence is not confined to local impact. Rather it dramatically parallels the reach and range of blood-borne endocrine signals outside the CNS.*

3. Estrogen and Brain Function

Estrogens affect areas of the brain not involved in reproduction (Table 2B.4). These include affective state and mood, sleep, libido and social behavior, cognitive function (including speed of processing), neuroprotection, motor coordination, neuronal excitability, and pain and auditory thresholds. Estrogen affects attention by modulating basal forebrain dopaminergic systems, memory and learning by forebrain cholinergic up-regulation, arousal and excitation by midbrain noradrenergic systems, mood, integration and affect by midbrain 5-HT, tryptophan hydroxylase and serotonin transport regulation, and finally, reward and satisfaction by midbrain dopamine turnover. Two specific estrogen activities—influence on cognitive function and memory processes and neuroprotection in reaction to aging and dementia—will be dealt with in detail.

a. Cognition and Memory

McEwen [62] has reviewed in detail the four aspects of estrogen action on the brain relevant to memory processes and their alteration during aging and neurodegenerative diseases.

First, studies of female rats show that estrogens regulate synaptogenesis in the hippocampus, a brain region important in spatial and declarative learning and memory.[73, 74] Second, there are developmentally programmed sex differences in hippocampal structure that may explain gender differences such as in solving spatial navigation problems.[75] Third, as noted estrogens have widespread effects on the catecholaminergic neurons, midbrain serotonergic pathways, dopaminergic activity, and cholinergic systems.[76–78] These are involved in attention, arousal, mood and affect, and reward. Because of the widespread projections of these systems in the forebrain, they modulate specific actions involved in learning and remembering verbal information.[63] Fourth, clinical studies with estrogen replacement have reported specific enhancements to certain cognitive elements. These include tests of verbal memory, vigilance, reasoning, and motor speed.[79]

TABLE 2B.4 Gonadal Hormone Effects on Clinically Relevant Nonreproductive Brain Functions

Affective state and mood
- Premenstrual syndrome (cyclic symptoms)
- Depressive illness (antidepressive effects on E)

Cognitive function: positive effects of estrogen
- Short-term verbal memory
- Fine motor skills
- Spatial abilities

Dementia: positive effects of estrogen
- Improve cognitive function in Alzheimer's disease (AD)
- Improve cognitive function in nondemented women
- Reported lower prevalence of AD

Motor coordination and motion disorders:
- Dose-related influence on Parkinson's disease
  - High-dose E exacerbates symptoms
  - Low-dose E facilitates dopamine function

Excitability and epilepsy:
- Catamenial epilepsy:
  - Estrogen lowers seizure threshold
  - Progestrone decreases excitability
  - Increased clearance of antiepilepsy drugs

b. Estrogens and Neuroprotection

As noted there is growing evidence that estrogens not only improve memory, affect, and motor coordination in hypoestrogenic women but also appear to prevent, delay or modify Alzheimer's disease. Estrogen protects cells from damage and destruction by free radical and β-amyloid protein.[66, 67] McEwen [62] has suggested two ways by which estrogen is able to protect the brain from neurodegeneration. First, estrogens maintain the function of key neural structures such as the hippocampus and basal forebrain and the widely projecting dopaminergic, serotonergic, and noradrenergic systems. As estrogens decline, these systems and the cognitive and other behavioral processes that depend on them also decline. However, if estrogen is provided sufficiently early in the process, functional return and morphologic (spine density and complexity) repair is induced. Second, estrogen directly blocks the negative impact of neurotoxic agents as well as inhibits their production.[80, 81] For example, estrogen treatment interferes with the toxic effects of the β-amyloid protein and the human immunodeficiency virus coat protein, both of which act via free radical generation.[82] Estrogen also enhances glucose uptake and energy metabolism and cerebral vascular flow.[83]

Glial cells are also implicated in aspects of oxidative energy metabolism, brain plasticity, brain aging, and neuroprotection.[84] Estrogens modulate glial proteins implicated in membrane formation and structural plasticity and synaptic contiguities. The mechanism of action of estrogen on glial cell function is not entirely clear; however, it appears to be partially dependent on ERα and ERβ (primarily ERα) within astrocytes, oligodendrocytes, and microglia.

Using ERKO mice, Dubal *et al.*[85] found that the ability of 17β-E_2 to protect against CNS ischemic injury was abolished with deletion of ERα but remained completely intact despite deletion of ERβ.

TABLE 2B.5 Physiological Functions of Progesterone

Tissue	Function
Uterus/ovaries	Release of oocytes
	Facilitation of implantation
	Maintenance of pregnancy: *via myometrial inhibition*
	Stimulation of stromal regeneration: *luteal phase of cycle*
Mammary gland	Lobular alveolar development
	Suppression of milk protein synthesis during pregnancy
Brain	Mediation of sexual responsiveness
Bone	Regulation of bone mass: *prevention of bone loss*

TABLE 2B.6 Tissues and Cell Types Expressing PR

Tissue	Cell type
Uterus	Endometrium
	Myometrium
Ovary	Luteinizing granulosa
	Preovulatory granulosa
	Corpus luteum
Reproductive tissues	Testes
	Vagina
Breast	Normal and neoplastic
Brain	Pituitary
	Ventromedial
	Hypothalamus
	Preoptic area
Other	Vascular endothelium
	Thymus
	Pancreatic islets
	Osteoblast-like cells
	Lung

VII. PROGESTERONE: FUNCTIONS AND MECHANISMS OF ACTION [86, 87] (TABLE 2B.5)

The major physiologic roles of progesterone in the female mammal include:

1. Release of mature oocytes, facilitation of implantation, and maintenance of pregnancy
2. Breast lobulo-alveolar development, differentiation, and function in preparation for milk secretion and suppression of milk protein synthesis before parturition
3. Mediating signals in the brain required for sexually responsive behavior
4. Diverse nonreproductive systems such as bone (regulation of bone mass and protection against bone loss)

These physiologic effects of progesterone are mediated by interactions with specific intracellular proteins—the progesterone receptors (PRs).[88]

A. The Progesterone Receptors

The PR is induced by estrogens at the transcriptional level and decreased by progestins at both the transcriptional and translational levels. The PR has two major isoforms, designated the A and B receptors. The two forms are expressed in rodents and humans by a single gene; the two forms are a consequence of transcription from distinctly different promoters, in a complex system of transcription regulation (Table 2B.6). [89, 90] Each form is associated with additional proteins, which are important for folding of the polypeptide into a structure that allows hormone binding and receptor activity.

Progestational agents can elicit a variety of responses determined by target tissue production and activity of the two receptor forms with dimerization as AA and BB (homodimers) or AB (heterodimer). The PRs function pursuing the general mechanism shared by the superfamily of receptors: initially an unbound complex with heat shock proteins, then hormone binding, homodimerization, significant conformational changes,[91] increased receptor phosphorylation [92] and DNA binding at a progesterone response element, interaction of the receptor complex with specific co-activator proteins and general transcription factors [93] resulting in a productive transcription initiating complex on specific target tissue gene promoters.[94]

The structural features of PRs have been defined (Fig. 2B.4).[87] The amino terminal region is poorly conserved among species and contains transactivation functions (AF-1 and AF-3) that regulate the level and promoter specificity of target gene activation. A centrally located, highly conserved DNA binding domain contributes to receptor dimerization and the specificity of DNA binding. AF-2 is located downstream from the DNA binding domain and is an additional transactivation domain. The ligand binding domain serves numerous functions: in addition to progesterone binding, it contains sequences important for interaction with heat shock proteins, dimerization, and transactivation.[95]

Similar to estrogen receptors, PRs can be activated in a ligand-independent manner by cell permeable agents which increase intracellular kinase activity [96] and by stimulators of cell membrane receptors which stimulate intracellular phosphorylation pathways such as growth factors, catecholamine neurotransmitters, and dopamine.[97]

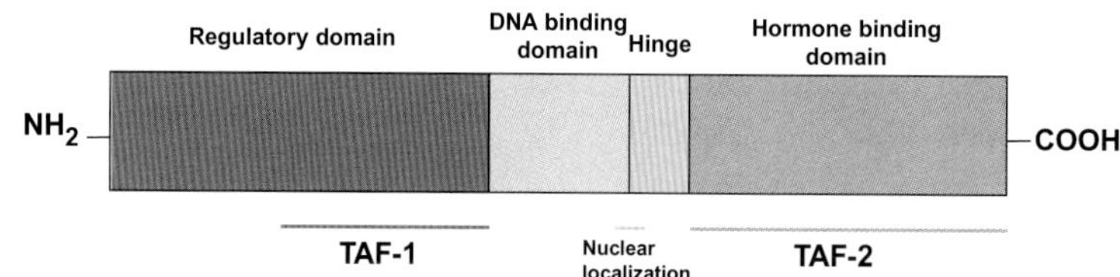

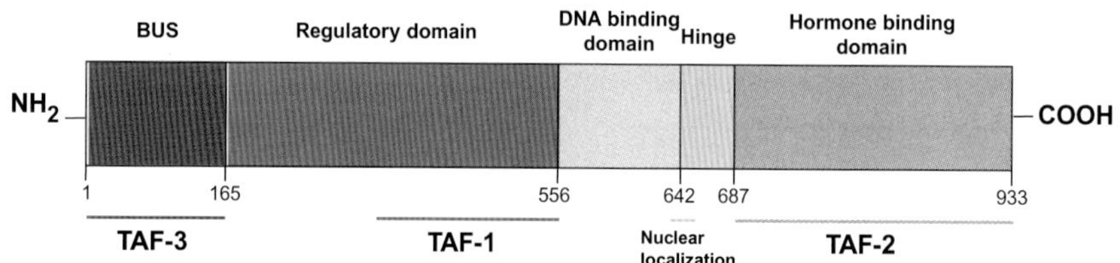

FIGURE 2B.4 The two isoforms of the progesterone receptor (PR). PRA and PRB and their functional domains. Note that PRB has three transcription activation factor components.

Studies indicate that the two receptors can be regulated independently; e.g., the relative levels differ in endometrium during the menstrual cycle.[98] However, isoforms A and B are expressed in almost equal amounts in breast and endometrial cancer cell lines. Tissue specificity of the progesterone receptor is influenced by which receptor and which dimer is active.[99] In addition the transcriptional activities of PRA and PRB depend on target cell differences, especially in the co-regulator context of the cell.[100] *However, in most cells, PRB is the positive regulator of progesterone-responsive genes, and A inhibits B activity.*[101] Repression of human estrogen receptor transcriptional activity is also dependent on the expression of PRA.[102] PRA does not form a heterodimer with the estrogen receptor nor does it prevent the estrogen receptor from binding with DNA. PRA does not change the structure of the estrogen receptor. Therefore, PRA probably competes with the estrogen receptor for a critical protein such as an essential transcription activator.[103]

PRA and PRB display different transcriptional activities and co-regulator interactions both *in vitro* and in physiologic responses to progesterone. Accordingly, the selective ability of PRA to *inhibit* transcriptional responses induced by both PRB and the estrogen receptors suggests the potential for variable progesterone induced activities in certain tissues as well as the antiestrogen effect in the endometrium.[104, 105]

B. Progesterone Isoforms and Tissue Selectivity

Female mice lacking the PR gene encoding both isoforms of PR (PRABKO) exhibit impaired sexual behavior [106] and neuroendocrine gonadotropin regulation,[107] anovulation,[108] uterine dysfunction,[109, 110] and impaired ductal and tubuloalveolar development of the breast.[88] In addition, these null mutations underscore the essential role of PRs in pregnancy, the cardiovascular system, and bone maintenance. The individual contributions of PRA and PRB have also been studied and have provided evidence that the individual isoforms do elicit distinct physiologic responses to progesterone. In PRAKO mice (expression of PRA isoform ablated), the remaining PRB isoform continues to subserve mammary development and morphogenesis but displays abnormalities in ovarian and uterine function. For example, in the absence of PRA, PRB induces a *proliferative stimulus* of P on endometrium providing proof that P bound PRA is the inhibitor of both ER and PRB stimulation of growth in this tissue. On the other hand, and of clinical importance, this inhibitory function of PRA is tissue specific. Both PRA and PRB act as growth stimulators in the breast.[111]

PRBKO (absent PRB) mice show no abnormality of either ovarian or uterine responses to P but results in reduced mammary ductal morphogenesis.[87] Thus, PRA in the mouse is both necessary and sufficient to elicit progesterone-dependent reproductive responses while PRB isoform extends progesterone effects by inducing normal mammary gland proliferation. These observations confirm the key role played by the amino terminal AF-3 domain in the tissues specific reactions to progesterone.

C. The Antiprogestin RU486 [112]

Both progesterone and the antiprogestins, RU486 (mifepristone) and ZK98299 (onapristone), form hormone-responsive element-receptor complexes that are similar, but the antiprogestin-receptor complex has a slightly different conformational change (in the hormone-binding domain) that prevents full gene activation. RU486 has some agonistic activity due to its ability to activate certain, but not all, of the transcription activation functions on the progesterone receptor.

VIII. OVERALL CONCLUSION

As has been implied throughout Part II, there is great relevance linking "how steroid hormones work" to almost all aspects of human physiology. Armed with these insights, however complex, uncertain or even barely defined—there is a legitimate basis for optimism that the mechanisms of human dysfunction and disease can also be successfully addressed. Not only does a detailed understanding of these processes have major implications for diagnosis and prevention, it also provides opportunities for development of new therapies as each of these elements become targets for manipulation by novel therapeutic interventions.

References

1. Conneely, O. M. (2001). Perspective: Female steroid hormone action. *Endocrinology* 142, 2194–2199.
2. Hall, J. M., Couse, J. F., and Korach, K. S. (2001). The multifaceted mechanisms of estradiol and estrogen receptor signaling. *J. Biol. Chem.* 276, 36869–36872.
3. Mangelsdorf, D. J., Thummel, C. J., Beato, M., Herrlich, P., Schulz, G., Umesono, K., Blumberg, B., Kastner, P., Mark, M., Chambon, P., and Evans, R. M. (1995). The nuclear receptor superfamily: The second decade. *Cell* 83, 835–883.
4. McKenna, N. J., Lanz, R. B., and O'Malley, B. W. (1999). Nuclear receptor coregulators: Cellular and molecular biology. *Endocr. Rev.* 20, 321–344.
5. Tora, L., White, J., Brow, C., Tasset, D., Webster, N., Scheer, E. and Chambon, P. (1998). The human estrogen receptor has two independent non acidic transcriptional activation functions. *Cell* 59, 477–487.
6. Heery, D. M., Kalkhoven, E., Hoare, S., and Parker, M. G. (1997). A signature motif in transcriptional coactivators mediates binding to nuclear receptors. *Nature* 387, 733–736.
7. Webb, P., Nguyen, P., Shinsako, J., Anderson, C., Feng, W., Nguyen, M. P., Chen, D., Huang, S. M., Subramanian, S., McKinerney, E., Katzenellenbogen, B. S., Stallcup, M. R., and Kushner, P. J. (1998). Estrogen receptor activator function 1 works by binding p160 coactivator proteins. *Mol. Endocrinol.* 12, 1605–1618.
8. Robyr, D., Wolffe, A. P., and Wahli, W. (2000). Nuclear hormone receptor coregulators in action: Diversity for shared tasks. *Mol. Endocrinol.* 14, 329–347.
9. Rosenfeld, M. G., and Glass, C. J. (2001). Coregulator codes of transcriptional regulation by nuclear receptors. *J. Biol. Chem.* 276, 36885–36868.
10. McNally, J. G., Muller, W. G., Walker, D., Wolford, R., Hager, G. L. (2000). The glucocorticoid receptor: rapid exchange with regulatory sites in living cells. *Science* 287, 1262–1265.
11. Shang, Y., Hu, X., DiRenzo, J., Lazar, M. A., and Brown, M. (2000). Cofactor dynamics and sufficiency in estrogen receptor-regulated transcription. *Cell* 103, 843–852.
12. Giguere, V., Tremblay, A., and Tremblay, G. B. (1998). Estrogen receptor beta: Re-evaluation of estrogen and antiestrogen signaling. *Steroids* 63, 335–339.
13. Couse, J. F., and Korach, K. S. (1999). Estrogen receptor null mice: What have we learned and where will they lead us? *Endocr. Rev.* 20, 358–417.
14. Couse, J. F., Curtis-Hewitt, S., Bunch, D. O., Sar, M., Walker, V. R., Davis, B. J., and Korach, K. S. (1999). Postnatal sex reversal of the ovaries in mice lacking ER_α and ER_β. *Science* 286, 2328–2331.
15. Dupont, S., Krust, A., Gansmuller, A., Dierich, A., Chambon, P., and Mark, M. (2000). Effect of single and compound knockouts of ER_α and ER_β on mouse reproductive phenotypes. *Development* 127, 4277–4291.
16. Pelletier, G., and El-Alfy, M. (2000). Immunocytochemical localization of estrogen receptors alpha and beta in the human reproductive organs. *J. Clin. Endocrinol. Metab.* 85, 4835–4840.
17. Wu, W. X., Ma, X. H., Smith, G. C., and Nathanielsz, P. W. (2000). Differential distribution of ER_α and ER_β mRNA in intrauterine tissues of the pregnant rhesus monkey. *Am. J. Physiol. Cell Physiol.* 278, 190–198.
18. Couse, J. F., Curtis-Hewitt, S., and Korach, K. S. (2000). Receptor null mice reveal contrasting roles for estrogen receptor alpha and beta in reproductive tissues. *J. Steroid Biochem. Mol. Biol.* 74, 287–296.
19. Couse, J. F., Lindzey, J., Grandien, K., Gustafsson, J. A., and Korach, K. S. (1997). Tissue distribution and quantitative analysis of estrogen receptor-alpha (ERalpha) and estrogen receptor-beta (ERbeta) messenger ribonucleic acid in the wild-type and ERalpha-knockout mouse. *Endocrinology* 138, 4613–4621.
20. Shughrue, P. J., Lane, M. V., and Merchenthaler, I. (1997). Comparative distribution of estrogen receptor-alpha and -beta mRNA in the rat central nervous system. *J. Comp. Neurol.* 388, 507–525.
21. Mendelsohn, M. E. (2000). Mechanisms of estrogen action in the cardiovascular system. *J. Steroid Biochem. Mol. Biol.* 74, 337–343.
22. Palter, S. F., Tavares, A. B., Hourvitz, A., Veldhuis, J. D., and Adashi, E. Y. (2001). Are estrogens of import to primate/human ovarian folliculogenesis? *Endocr. Rev.* 22, 389–424.
23. Ignar-Trowbridge, D. M., Pimentel, M., Parker, M. G., McLachlan, J. A., and Korach, K. S. (1996). Peptide growth factor cross-talk with the estrogen receptor requires the A/B domain and occurs independently of protein kinase C or estradiol. *Endocrinology* 137, 1735–1744.
24. Bunone, G., Briand, P. A., Miksicek, R. J., and Picard, D. (1996). Activation of the unliganded estrogen receptor by EGF involves the MAP kinase pathway and direct phosphorylation. *EMBO J.* 15, 2174–2183.
25. Aronica, S. M., and Katzenellenbogen, B. S. (1993). Stimulation of estrogen receptor-mediated transcription and alteration in the phosphorylation state of the rat uterine estrogen receptor by estrogen, cyclic adenosine monophosphate, and insulin-like growth factor-I. *Mol. Endocrinol.* 7, 743–752.
26. Ogawa, S., Inoue, S., Watanabe, T., Orimo, A., Hosoi, T., Ouchi, Y., and Muramatsu, M. (1998). Molecular cloning and characterization of human estrogen receptor betacx: a potential inhibitor of estrogen action in human. *Nucleic Acids Res.* 26, 3505–3512.
27. Revelli, A., Massobrio, M., and Tesarik, J. (1998). Nongenomic actions of steroid hormones in reproductive tissues. *Endocr. Rev.* 19, 3–17
28. Collins, P., and Webb, C. (1999). Estrogen hits the surface. *Nat. Med.* 5, 1130–1131.
29. Razandi, M., Pedram, A., Greene, G. L., and Levin, E. R. (1999). Cell membrane and nuclear estrogen receptors (ERs) originate from a single transcript: studies of ERalpha and ERbeta expressed in Chinese hamster ovary cells. *Mol. Endocrinol.* 13, 307–319.
30. Gu, Q., Korach, K. S., and Moss, R. L. (1999). Rapid action of 17beta-estradiol on kainate-induced currents in hippocampal neurons lacking intracellular estrogen receptors. *Endocrinology* 140, 660–666.
31. Mendelsohn, M. E. (2000). Nongenomic, ER-mediated activation of endothelial nitric oxide synthase: How does it work? What does it mean? *Circ. Res.* 87, 956–960.

32. Simoncini, T., Hafezi-Moghadam, A., Brazil, D. P., Ley, K., Chin, W. W., and Liao, J. K. (2000). Interaction of estrogen receptor with the regulatory subunit of phosphatidylinositol-3-OH kinase. *Nature* 407, 538–541.
33. Kousteni, S., Bellido, T., Plotkin, L. I., O'Brien, C. A., Bodenner, D. L., Han, L., Han, K., DiGregorio, G. B., Katzenellenbogen, J. A., Katzenellenbogen, B. S., Roberson, P. K., Weinstein, R. S., Jalka, R. L., and Manolagas, S. C. (2001). Nongenotropic, sex-nonspecific signaling through the estrogen or androgen receptors: Dissociation from transcriptional activity. *Cell* 104, 719–730.
34. Silberstein, G. B., Strickland, P., Trumpbour, V., Coleman, S., and Daniel, C. W. (1984). In vivo, cAMP stimulates growth and morphogenesis of mouse mammary ducts. *Proc. Natl. Acad. Sci. USA* 81, 4950–4954.
35. Sheffield, L. G., and Welsch, C. W. (1985). Cholera-toxin-enhanced growth of human breast cancer cell lines *in vitro* and *in vivo*: Interaction with estrogen. *Int. J. Cancer* 36, 479–483.
36. Smith, C. L. (1998). Cross-talk between peptide growth factor and estrogen receptor signaling pathways. *Biol. Reprod.* 58, 627–632.
37. Kushner, P. J., Agard, D. A., Greene, G. L., Scanlan, T. S., Shiau, A. K., Uht, R. M., and Webb, P. (2000). Estrogen receptor pathways to AP-1. *J. Steroid Biochem. Mol. Biol.* 74, 311–317.
38. Brzozowski, A. M., Pike, A. C., Dauter, Z., Hubbard, R. E., Bonn, T., Engstrom, O., Ohman, L., Greene, G. L., Gustafsson, J. A., and Carlquist, M. (1997). Molecular basis of agonism and antagonism in the estrogen receptor. *Nature* 389, 753–758.
39. Pike, A. C., Brzozowski, A. M., Walton, J., Hubbard, R. E., Thorsell, A. G., Li, Y. L., Gustafsson, J. A., and Carlquist, M. (2001). Structural insights into the mode of action of a pure antiestrogen. *Structure* (Camb) 9, 145–153.
40. Katzenellenbogen, B. S., Choi, I., Delage-Mourroux, R., Ediger, T. R., Martini, P. G., Montano, M., Sun, J., Weis, K., and Katzenellenbogen, J. A. (2000). Molecular mechanisms of estrogen action: selective ligands and receptor pharmacology. *J. Steroid Biochem. Mol. Biol.* 74, 279–285.
41. Jordan, V. C., and Morrow, M. (1999). Tamoxifen, raloxifene, and the prevention of breast cancer. *Endocr. Rev.* 20, 253–278.
42. Mendelsohn, M. E., and Karas, R.H. (1999). The protective effects of estrogen on the cardiovascular system. *N. Engl. J. Med.* 340, 1801–1811.
43. Venkov, C. D., Rankin, A. B., Vaughan, D. E. (1996). Identification of authentic estrogen receptor in cultured endothelial cells. A potential mechanism for steroid hormone regulation of endothelial function. *Circulation* 94, 727–733.
44. Grohe, C., Kahlert, S., Lobbert, K., Stimpel, M., Karas, R. H., Vetter, H., and Neyses L. (1997). Cardiac myocytes and fibroblasts contain functional estrogen receptors. *FEBS. Letts.* 416, 107–112.
45. The Writing Group for the PEPI Trial. Effects of estrogen or estrogen/progestin regimens on heart disease risk factors in postmenopausal women: The Postmenopausal Estrogen/Progestin Intervention (PEPI) Trial (1995). *JAMA* 273, 199–208.
46. Nabulsi, A. A., Folsom, A. R., White, A., Patsch, W., Heiss, G., Wu, K. K., and Szklo, M. (1993). Association of hormone-replacement therapy with various cardiovascular risk factors in postmenopausal women. *N. Engl. J. Med.* 15, 1069–1075.
47. The Writing Group for Estradiol Clotting Factors Study. Effect on hemostasis of hormone replacement therapy with transdermal and oral sequential medioxy progesterone acetate. *Thromb. Hemost.* 75, 476–480.
48. Koh, K. K., Mincemoyer, R., Bui, M. N., Csako, G., Pucino, F., Guetta, V., Waclawinw, M., and Cannon, R. O. 3rd (1997). Effects of hormone-replacement therapy on fibrinolysis in postmenopausal women. *N. Engl. J. Med.* 336, 683–690.
49. Moncada, S., and Higgs, A. (1993). The L-arginine-nitric oxide pathway. *N. Engl. J. Med.* 329, 2002–2012.
50. Best, P. J., Berger, P. B., Miller, V. M., and Lerman, A. (1998). The effect of estrogen replacement therapy on plasma nitric oxide and endothelin-1 levels in postmenopausal women. *Ann. Intern. Med.* 128, 285–288.
51. Sach, M. N., Rader, D. J., and Cannon, R. O. (1994). Estradiol and inhibition of oxidation of low density lipoprotein in postmenopausal women. *Lancet* 343, 269–270.
52. White, R. E., Darkow, D. J., and Lang, J. L. F. (1995). Estrogen relaxes coronary arteries by opening BK_{ca} channels through a cGMP dependent mechanism. *Circ. Res.* 77, 936–942.
53. Wellman, G. C., Bonev, A. D., Nelson, M. T., and Brayden, J. E. (1996). Gender differences in coronary artery diameter involve estrogen, nitric oxide, and Ca(2+)-dependent K+ channels. *Circ. Res.* 79, 1024–1030.
54. Caulin-Glaser, T., Garcia-Cardena, G., Sarrel, P., Sessa, W. C., and Bender, J. R. (1997). 17 beta-estradiol regulation of human endothelial cell basal nitric oxide release, independent of cytosolic Ca2+ mobilization. *Circ. Res.* 81, 885–892.
55. Pappas, T. C., Gametchu, B., and Watson, C. S. (1995). Membrane estrogen receptors identified by multiple antibody labeling and impeded-ligand binding. *FASEB J.* 9, 404–410.
56. Chen, Z., Yuhanna, I. S., Galcheva-Gargova, Z, Karas, R. H., Mendelsohn, M. E., and Shaul, P. W. (1999). Estrogen receptor alpha mediates the nongenomic activation of endothelial nitric oxide synthase by estrogen. *J. Clin. Invest.* 103, 401–106.
57. Williams, J. K., Adams, M. R., Herrington, D. M., and Clarkson, T. B. (1992). Short-term administration of estrogen and vascular responses of atherosclerotic coronary arteries. *J. Am. Coll. Cardiol.* 20, 452–457.
58. Reis, S. E., Gloth, S. T., Blumenthal, R. S., Resar, J. R., Zacur, H. A., Gerstenblith, G., and Brinker, J. A. (1994). Ethinyl estradiol acutely attenuates abnormal coronary vasomotor responses to acetylcholine in postmenopausal women. *Circulation* 89, 52–60.
59. Binko, J., and Majewski, H. (1998). 17 beta-estradiol reduces vasoconstriction in endothelium-denuded rat aortas through inducible NOS. *Am. J. Physiol.* 274, 853–859.
60. Weiner, C. P., Lizasoain, I., Baylis, S. A., Knowles, R. G., Charles, I. G., and Moncada, S. (1994). Induction of calcium-dependent nitric oxide synthases by sex hormones. *Proc. Natl. Acad. Sci. USA* 91, 5212–5216.
61. Cornwell, T. L., Arnold, E., Boerth, N. J., and Lincoln, T. M. (1994). Inhibition of smooth muscle cell growth by nitric oxide and activation of cAMP-dependent protein kinase by cGMP. *Am. J. Physiol.* 267, c1405–c1413.
62. McEwen, B. S. (1999). The molecular and neuroanatomic basis for estrogen effects in the central nervous system. *J. Clin. Endocrinol. Metab.* 84, 1790–1797.
63. McEwen, B. S., and Alves, S. H. (1999). Estrogen actions in the central nervous system. *Endocr. Rev.* 20, 278–306.
64. Singh, M., Setal, G. J., Guan, X., Warren, M., and Toran-Allerand, C. D. (1999). Estrogen induced activation of mitogen activated protein kinase in cerebral cortical explants: Convergence of estrogen and neurotropic signaling pathways. *J. Neurosci.* 29, 1179–1188.
65. Mermelstein, P. G., Becker, J. B., and Surmeier, D. J. (1996). Estradiol reduces calcium currents in rat neostriatal neurons via a membrane receptor. *J. Neurosci.* 16, 595–604.
66. Green, P. S., Gridley, K. E., and Simpkins, J. W. (1996). Estradiol protects against beta-amyloid (25–35)-induced toxicity in SK-N-SH human neuroblastoma cells. *Neuroscience* 218, 165–168.
67. Singer, C. A., Rogers, K. L., Strickland, T. M., and Dorsa, D. M. (1996). Estrogen protects primary cortical neurons from glutamate toxicity. *Neuroscience* 212, 13–16.
68. Kuiper, G. C., Shughrue, P. J., Merchenthaler, I., and Gustafsson, J. A. (1998). The estrogen receptor beta subtype: A novel mediator of estrogen action in neuroendocrine system. *Neuroendocrinology* 19, 253–286.

69. Hrabovszky, E., Kallo, I., Hajszan, T., Shughrue, P. J., Merchenthaler, I., and Liposits, Z. (1998). Expression of estrogen receptor-beta messenger ribonucleic acid in oxytocin and vasopressin neurons of the rat supraoptic and paraventricular nuclei. *Endocrinology* 139, 2600–2604.
70. Shughrue, P. J., Lane, M. V., and Merchenthaler, I. (1997). Regulation of progesterone receptor messenger ribonucleic acid in the rat medial preoptic nucleus by estrogenic and antiestrogenic compounds: an *in situ* hybridization study. *Endocrinology* 138, 5476–5484.
71. Yaffe, K., Krueger, K., Sarkar, S., Grady, D., Barrett-Connor, E., Cox, D. A., and Nickelsen, T. (2001). Cognitive function in postmenopausal women treated with raloxifene. *N. Engl. J. Med.* 344, 1207–1213.
72. Zhou, Y., Watters, J. J., and Dorsa, D. M. (1997). Estrogen rapidly induces the phosphorylation of cAMP response element binding protein in rat brain. *Endocrinology* 137, 2163–2166.
73. Woolley, C. S., and McEwen, B. S. (1993). Roles of estradiol and progesterone in regulation of hippocampal dendritic spine density during the estrous cycle in the rat. *J. Comp. Neurol.* 336, 293–306.
74. Woolley, C. S., and McEwen, B. S. (1994). Estradiol regulates hippocampal dendritic spine density via an *N*-methyl-D-aspartate receptor-dependent mechanism. *J. Neurosci.* 14, 7680–7687.
75. Kimura, D. (1992). Sex differences in the brain. *Sci. Am.* 267, 118–125.
76. Bethea, C. L., Pecins-Thompson, M., Schutzer, W. E., Gundlah, C., and Lu, Z. N. (1999). Ovarian steroids and serotonin neural function. *Mol. Neurobiol.* 18, 87–123.
77. Luine, V. N., Renner, K. J., and McEwen, B. S. (1986). Sex-dependent differences in estrogen regulation of choline acetyltransferase are altered by neonatal treatments. *Endocrinology* 119, 874–878.
78. Gibbs, R. B., and Aggarwal, P. (1998). Estrogen and basal forebrain cholinergic neurons: implications for brain aging and Alzheimer's disease-related cognitive decline. *Horm. Behav.* 34, 98–111.
79. LeBlanc, E. S., Janowsky, J., Chan, B. K. S., and Nelson, H. D. (2001). Hormone replacement therapy and cognition: Systematic review and meta-analysis. *JAMA* 285, 1489–1499.
80. Xu, H., Gouras, G. K., and Greenfield, J. P. (1998). Estrogen reduces neural generation of Alzheimer B amyloid peptides. *Nat. Med.* 4, 447–451.
81. Goodman, Y., Bruce, A. J., Cheng, B., and Mattson, M. P. (1996). Estrogens attenuate and corticosterone exacerbates excitotoxicity, oxidative injury, and amyloid beta-peptide toxicity in hippocampal neurons. *J. Neurochem.* 66, 1863–1844.
82. Brooke, S., Chan, R., Howard, S., and Sapolsky, R. (1997). Endocrine modulation of the neurotoxicity of gp-120: Implications for AIDS-related dementia complex. *Proc. Natl. Acad. Sci. USA* 94, 9457–9462.
83. Resnick, S. M., Maki, P. M., Golski, S., Kraut, M. A., and Zonderman, A. B. (1998). Effects of ERT on PET cerebral blood flow and neuropsychological performance. *Horm. Behav.* 34, 171–182.
84. Schipper, H. M. (1996). Astrocytes, brain aging, and neurodegeneration. *Neurobiol. Aging* 17, 467–480.
85. Dubal, D. B., Zhu, H., Yu, J., Rau, S. W., Shughrue, P. J., Merchenthaler, I., Kindy, M. S., and Wise, P. M. (2001). Estrogen receptor alpha, not beta, is critical link in estradiol-mediated protection against brain injury. *Proc. Natl. Acad. Sci. USA* 98, 1952–1957.
86. Graham, J. D., and Clarke, C. L. (1997). Physiologic action of progesterone in target tissues. *Endo. Rev.* 18, 502–519.
87. Conneely, O., and Lydon, J. P. (2000). Progesterone receptors in reproduction: Functional impact of the A and B isoforms. *Steroids* 65, 571–577.
88. Lydon, J. P., DeMayo, F. J., and Funk, C. R. (1995). Mice lacking progesterone receptor exhibit pleiotropic reproduction abnormalities. *Genes Dev.* 9, 2266–2278.
89. Kastner, P., Krust, A., and Turcotte, B. (1990). Two distinct estrogen-regulated promoters generate transcripts encoding the two functionally different human progesterone receptor forms A & B. *EMBO J.* 9, 1603–1614.
90. Kraus, W. L., Montano, M. M., and Katzenellenbogen, B. S. (1993). Cloning of the rat progesterone receptor gene 5′-region and identification of two functionally distinct promoters. *Mol. Endocrinol.* 7, 1603–1616.
91. Allan, G. F., Tsai, S. Y., Tsai, M.-J., and O'Malley, B. W. (1992). Hormonal induced conformation changes in the progesterone receptor are required for events following binding to DNA. *Proc. Natl. Acad. Sci.* USA 89, 11750–11754.
92. Weigel, N. L. (1994). Receptor phosphorylation. *In* "Mechanism of Steroid Hormone Regulation of Gene Transcription" (M.-J. Tsai, and B. W. O'Malley, eds.), pp. 93–110. R. G. Landes Co., Austin, Tx.
93. Gronemeyer, H. (1991). Transcription activation by estrogen and progesterone receptors. *Ann. Rev. Genet.* 25, 89–123.
94. Onate, S. A., Tsai, S. Y., Tsai, M.-J., and O'Malley, B. W. (1995). Sequence and characterization of a coactivator for the steroid hormone receptor superfamily. *Science* 270, 1354–1357.
95. Fawell, S. E., Lees, J. A., White, R., and Parker, M. G. (1990). Characterization and colocalization of steroid binding and dimerization activities in the mouse estrogen receptor. *Cell* 60, 953–962.
96. Denner, L. A., Weigel, N. L., Maxwell, B. L., Schrader, W. T., and O'Malley, B. W. (1990). Regulation of progesterone receptor mediated transcription by phosphorylation. *Science* 250, 1740–1743.
97. Power, R. F., Mani, S. K., Codina, J., Conneely, O. M., and O'Malley, B. W. (1991). Dopaminergic and ligand independent activation of steroid hormone receptors. *Science* 254, 1636–1639.
98. Mote, P. A., Balleine, R. L., McGowan, E. M., and Clarke, C. L. (1999). Colocalization of progesterone receptors A and B by dual immunofluorescent histochemistry in human endometrium during the menstrual cycle. *J. Clin. Endocrinol. Metab.* 84, 2963–2971.
99. Mulac-Jericevic, B., Mullinax, R. A., DeMayo, F. J., Lydon, J. P., and Conneely, O. M. (2000). Subgroup of reproductive functions of progesterone mediated by progesterone receptor-B isoform. *Science* 289, 1751–1754.
100. Giangrande, P. H., Kimbrel, E. A., Edwards, D. P., and McDonnell, D. P. (2000). The opposing transcriptional activities of the two isoforms of the human progesterone receptor are due to differential cofactor binding. *Mol. Cell Biol.* 20, 3102–3115.
101. Vegeto, E., Shahbaz, M. M., Wen, D. X., Goldman, M. E., O'Malley, B. W., and McDonnell, D. P. (1993). Human progesterone receptor A form is a cell- and promoter-specific repressor of human progesterone receptor B function. *Mol. Endocrinol.* 7, 1244–1255.
102. Chalbos, D., and Galtier, F. (1994). Differential effect of forms A and B of human progesterone receptor on estradiol dependent transcription. *J. Biol. Chem.* 269, 23007–23012.
103. Katzenellenbogen, B. S. (2000). Mechanism of action and cross-talk between estrogen receptor and progesterone receptor pathways. *J. Soc. Gynecol. Investig.* 7, 533–537.
104. Giangrande, P. H., Pollio, G., and McDonnell, D. P. (1997). Mapping and characterization of the functional domains responsible for the differential activity of the A and B isoforms of the human progesterone receptor. *J. Biol. Chem.* 272, 32889–32900.
105. McDonnell, D. P., and Goldman, M. E. (1994). RU 486 exerts antiestrogen activities through a novel progesterone receptor A mediated mechanism. *J. Biol. Chem.* 269, 11945–11949.
106. Mani, S., Allen, J. M. C., and Lydon, J. P. (1996). Dopamine requires the unoccupied progesterone receptors to induce sexual behavior in mice. *Mol. Endocrinol.* 10, 1728–1734.
107. Park-Sarge, O. K., and Mayo, K. E. (1994). Regulation of progesterone receptor gene by gonadotropins and cAMP in rat granulosa cells. *Endocrinology* 34, 709–718.
108. Natraj, U., and Richards, J. S., Hormonal regulation, localization and functional activity of the progesterone receptor in granulosa cells of rat preovulatory follicles. *Endocrinology* 133, 761–769.

109. Cullingford, T. E., and Pollard, J. W. (1988). RU 486 completely inhibits the action of progesterone on cell proliferation in the mouse uterus. *J. Reprod. Fertil.* 83, 909–914.

110. Tibbets, J. A., Conneely, O. M., and O'Malley, B. W. (1999). Progesterone via its receptor antagonizes the pro-inflammatory activities of estrogen in the mouse uterus. *Biol. Reprod.* 60, 1158–1165.

111. Inagawa, W., Yang, J., Guzman, R., and Nandi, S. (1994). Control of mammary gland development. *In* "The Physiology of Reproduction," 2nd Ed. (E. Knobil, and J. D. Null, eds.), pp. 1033–1063. Raven Press, New York.

112. Cadepond, F., Ulmann, A., and Baulieu, E. E. (1997). RU 486: Mechanism of action and clinical uses. *Annu. Rev. Med.* 48, 129–156.

CHAPTER

3

Recent Progress in Gonadal Dysgenesis

PAUL G. McDONOUGH

Departments of Obstetrics and Gynecology, Pediatrics and Physiology
Medical College of Georgia
Augusta, Georgia 30912

ABSTRACT

Conceptual, diagnostic, and therapeutic advances in the management of individuals with Gonadal Dysgenesis have been driven largely by technical advances in molecular biology, cardiac imaging, assisted reproduction, and the production of recombinant proteins. The surviving non-mosaic 45,X patient is less frequently diagnosed as DNA amplification techniques have provided rapid methods to detect mosaicism among patients previously diagnosed as 45,X using conventional cytogenetics. Flourescent *in situ* hybridization has facilitated the scoring of ever increasing numbers of interphase cells for the detection of somatic mosaicism (i.e., 45,X/46,XX), and for the clarification of X-Y structural alterations. The detection of low level mosaicism for cryptic Y DNA and tumor risk using PCR for Y specific sequences has become state of the art. Serial echocardiography for aortic diameter has enabled the clinician to identify patients who are at risk for aortic dissection. Gamete donation with ART have permitted gestational pregnancies for selected patients with Gonadal Dysgenesis. Recombinant growth hormone has effected modest improvements in final adult height for some patients with X-chromosome aneuploidy. A candidate gene, SHOX on both sex chromosomes that escapes inactivation has raised expectations that a more fundamental understanding of the mechanisms leading to the statural and gonadal deficients in the Turner Syndrome is not far away.

I. INTRODUCTION

Molecular biology is revolutionizing reproductive medicine. This is perhaps most evident in our increased understanding of the molecular biology of gonadal development. A considerable amount of basic information has been obtained relevant to somatic differentiation of the gonad, X-chromosome inactivation, and putative growth genes. In the clinical arena there have been major technologic advances in high-resolution and 3-D ultrasonography, magnetic resonance imaging (MRI), and operative laparoscopy that have provided new resources to assist in the diagnosis and management of patients with gonadal dysgenesis. In the laboratory the techniques of polymerase chain reaction (PCR) and fluorescence *in situ* hybridization (FISH) have added broader dimensions to the detection of sex chromosome mosaicism.

Finally, techniques of assisted reproduction using sibling and anonymous egg donors has made gestational motherhood a reality for carefully selected patients with gonadal dysgenesis.

II. BASIC RESEARCH

There have been some advances in our understanding of the basic mechanisms involved in the development of gonadal dysgenesis, but fundamental concepts related to germ cell migration, and the specific genes involved in gonadal failure, cardiovascular-renal anomalies, and short stature continue to elude us. There have been many efforts on the parts of different investigators to address some of these fundamental issues over the past several years.

A. Stature Genes

Investigators attempting to explain short stature in patients with gonadal dysgenesis invariably turned to Mary Lyon's hypothesis that X-linked genes in mammals are dosage compensated by X inactivation during early embryonic development. To explain why the absence of one normally inert X chromosome causes a human phenotype (gonadal dysgenesis) she purposed that Turner's syndrome (TS) is due to reduced dosage of genes that either act prior to X inactivation or due to genes that escape X inactivation.[1] Since males with normal stature require only one active X chromosome it has been hypothesized that copies of TS genes involved in stature are also present on the Y chromosome. In other words, the TS phenotype is the result of monosomy for a gene or genes common to the X and Y chromosomes. According to this hypothesis, the putative Turner gene or genes on the X chromosome must escape X inactivation and haploinsufficiency of such a gene in 45, X humans may provoke the characteristic TS phenotype.[2] With this in mind investigators searched for genes present on both X and Y that escape inactivation. The first functional genes in this category that mapped to both sex chromosomes were RPS4X and RPS4Y (human ribosomal protein S4). These genes encode isoforms of the ribosomal protein S4, which belongs to the small subunit of the ribosome. Consistent with the haploinsufficiency hypothesis the X-linked homolog RPS4X escapes X inaction.[3] RPS4X maps to *Xq13* proximal to the X-inactivation center (XIC). It is important to point out that these "candidate TS genes" (RPS4X and RPS4Y) have not been shown to cause any specific aspects of the phenotype. The strongest evidence against a causative role for RPS4X/Y in the TS phenotype is that short stature is a feature consistently seen with deletions of Xp22.3. to the Xp terminus (Xpter). In the latter situation both RPS4X genes are present and active, but short stature is still present.[4, 5] Similarly individuals with isochromosome for the long arm of X with the karyotype 46,X,i(X)(q10) have three copies of RPS4X and are still short in spite of expression levels for RPS4X that are one and a half times normal.

The tips of the X and Y short arms remain logical sites for a TS gene since genes examined thus far in this region (pseudoautosomal region) escape inactivation. A series of recent studies by Rao and colleagues have implicated a 700-kb interval in this pseudoautosomal region (PAR1) as a probable site for a gene involved in stature. Using exon trapping techniques the investigators have identified a candidate gene termed SHOX. This gene is a member of the homeobox-containing family of genes and is expressed from somatic cell hybrids containing either a human Y chromosome or an active or inactive X chromosome (Xp22/Yp11.3). Rao and colleagues did discover a SHOX nonsense mutation cosegregating with short stature in one family. However, the definition of short stature in most of these families is rather arbitrary (−2 s.d.) and some normal family members are as short as those members who carry the SHOX mutation (−1.9 versus −2 s.d.). The expression pattern of SHOX is consistent with a role for this gene in linear growth, but whether haploinsufficiency causes short stature in humans is not definitive at this time.[6] More recently a "second" homeobox-containing gene with similar properties to SHOX has been identified in the PAR1 region. This gene which has been named PHOG for pseudoautosomal homeobox-containing osteogenic gene also encodes a transcription factor. It seems to have a significantly higher level of expression in certain bone-derived cells compared to SHOX. Otherwise the expression pattern of PHOG is similar to SHOX.[7] In fact they appear to be the same gene and regardless of the final name this homeobox-containing gene constitutes a good candidate for the Turner stature gene. However, there are still many studies to be performed and questions to be answered before one can definitively say that haploinsufficiency of this gene (SHOX/PHOG) plays a role in the Turner phenotype.

B. Classification

The critical region or regions on the X chromosome that is consistently deleted in all individuals with gonadal failure is still unresolved. Gonadal failure and the TS phenotype may be seen with a variety of structural abnormalities of the X chromosome such as rings, isochromosomes, or terminal deletions. The only common denominator is that all patients with gonadal dysgenesis consistently demonstrate a privation or deletion of some portion of the X chromosome. It is helpful to propose a classification of these patients with this in mind. The variation in gonadal development, and consequently the phenotype seen in this group of individuals is facilitated by dividing them into two broad cytogenetic categories.

1. *X-chromosome aneuploidy including monosomy X.* These individuals have a wide range of cytogenetic findings including non-mosaic 45,X, mosaic 45,X/46,XX, 45,X/47,XXX, 45,X/46,X,i(Xq), 45,X/46,Xdel(X), and non-mosaic 46,X,i(Xq). These karyotypes have in common the absence of an overt Y chromosome and the apparent absence of varying degrees of X chromosome material. The common denominator in this group of patients is a deletion or privation of X chromosome material.
2. *Y-chromosome aneuploidy.* These individuals range from 45,X/46,XY to 45,X/46,X variant Y. The common denominator in this group of individuals is a monosomy X cell line and a second diploid cell line with a normal or variant Y chromosome. The gonadal development in these individuals varies and ranges from bilateral rudimentary streak gonads, unilateral streak with contralateral intra-abdominal or scrotal testis, and rarely bilateral scrotal testes. Consequently the clinical phenotype may be that of a non-masculinized phenotypic female, phenotypic female with clitoral enlargement, newborn with sexual ambiguity, masculinization at puberty in an individual with a quasi-Turner phenotype, or an azoospermic male with bilateral scrotal testes.[8, 9]

Gonadal dysgenesis is the preferred term for all patients who present with any form of gonadal agenesis. The groupings of X-chromosome aneuploidy, X monosomy, and Y-chromosome aneuploidy constitute a nomenclature system that stresses the cytogenetic findings. The gonadal phenotype is conveyed by the terms symmetrical and asymmetrical. Symmetrical implies that both gonads have a similar appearance while the asymmetrical designation indicates that one gonad has undergone differentiation (usually testis) while the other is a streak.

Pure gonadal dysgenesis refers to otherwise phenotypically normal individuals with bilateral streak gonads. These individuals are normal in stature and have a non-mosaic 46,XX or rarely a 46,XY (Swyer Syndrome) karyotype. Ullrich-Turner phenotypes invariably have short stature and may or may not have some of the other somatic anomalies associated with privations or deletions of sex chromosome material. This is the group covered by the broad spectrum of cytogenetic findings ranging from non-mosaic 45,X to mosaic 45,X/46,XX or 45,X/46,XY. The karyotype of these mosaic and non-mosaic forms are frequently accompanied by structural abnormalities of the X and Y chromosomes. The authors wish that the Ullrich-Turner or Turner eponyms could be abandoned completely because of the confusion they generate and the social stigmata they carry. Unfortunately, the term Turner's Syndrome has become so widely used and is so deeply ingrained in our lexicon that this change is unlikely to occur. Since a wide range of phenotypic variation is seen in gonadal dysgenesis, it might be less stigmatizing if we were to avoid the use of all eponyms in characterizing subjects with gonadal dysgenesis. Alternatively the eponym could be restricted to those individuals who clearly exhibit the somatic anomalies of the Turner phenotype.

C. X Inactivation

X-chromosome inactivation is the process by which a cell recognizes the presence of two copies of an X chromosome early in the development of XX embryos and chooses one to be active and one to be inactive. It appears that a critical part of the X-inactivation process is mediated by the XIC. The XIC, which maps to a 1500-kb region on the upper third of the X long arm recognizes the chromosomal number and initiates a signal that is propagated in cis. This signal silences or gags most of the genes on the spare X chromosome. The X-inactive-specific transcript gene (XIST) maps to the XIC (Xq13.3) region and does not encode a protein. It appears that the XIST mRNA unlike any other known RNA remains trapped in the nucleus and never reaches the cytoplasm. The XIST mRNA may interact with a nuclear factor and induce a conformation change in the DNA which inactivates it. XIST is expressed exclusively from the inactive X chromosome, and is an excellent candidate for the gene involved in the initiation and promulgation of an X-inactivation signal.[10] In gonadal dysgenesis an individual's structurally abnormal X chromosomes if present, tend to be inactivated preferentially in order to preserve the activity of the normal X. Certain small ring X chromosomes may lose the XIC region and be unable to initiate the inactivation process. In such cases the structurally abnormal X chromosome retains its activity. Some investigators note that these active ring X chromosomes may be associated with more severe phenotypes including mental retardation. This phenomenon would apply to those ring Xs that lack the sequences within the XIC that are essential for cis inactivation.[11, 12] At the present time it is premature to conclude that this association is a consistent one.

For students of gametogenesis it is important to note that at the onset of oogenesis the inactive X in each germ cell reactivates. In other words XIST expression is turned off temporarily. Both Xs in the germ line of females remain active until the cells of the fertilized embryo start to differentiate at about the 64 cell stage. At that time one of each pair of Xs is once more silenced in a random fashion. Consequently both X chromosomes are transcriptionally active and exchanging genetic material during oogenesis. It may be critical for the development of normal ovarian function to have both Xs active at this time. The lack of a second X at this time might be related to the consistent failure of ovarian function in 45,X individuals. In contrast during spermatogenesis the single active X chromosome is temporarily inactivated and the only exchange of genetic material is in the terminal portions of Xp and Yp.

This 2.6 megabase terminal portion of both sex chromosomes (pseudoautosomal region or PAR1) is the only region of the Y chromosome that undergoes homologous recombinaion with X during male meiosis. The implications of these observations and the role of XIST mutations in upsetting these mechanisms remains speculative at the present time.[12]

III. LABORATORY DEVELOPMENTS

A. Detection of Mosaicism for Cryptic Y

1. Y-Chromosome-Specific

Gonadal dysgenesis females carrying a mosaic Y cell line who masculinize at puberty because of unilateral intra-abdominal or labioscrotal testis will invariably be recognized and treated with gonadectomy. The real dilemma is the non-masculinized 45,X/46,XY individuals with bilateral rudimentary streak gonads, who will not masculinize at puberty and are at risk for dysgenetic tumor. Suspecting and detecting the presence of a Y chromosome in selected individuals in this group might test the clinical acumen of the physician. The exact number of 45,X individuals carrying an unrecognized normal or structurally altered Y chromosome appears to be small at this time. Prior to DNA analysis we have karyotyped an adolescent female as 45,X counting 50 cells and karyotyping 3 or 4. This subject developed a large unilateral dysgerminoma and contralateral gonadoblastoma. A repeat cytogenetic study counting 200 cells found 2 cells that were 46,XY. This pre-DNA case highlights the shortcomings of traditional metaphase karyotyping. It is obviously important to detect cryptic Y DNA in 45,X subjects who have low-level mosaicism for a 46,XY cell line and/or subjects carrying structurally abnormal sex chromosomes that are Y derived. This presence of Y DNA in any form is associated with an increased risk of gonadal tumors (dysgerminoma, gonadoblastoma). Conventional cytogenetic studies are limited by the numbers of cells that can be examined and the numbers of tissues that can be studied. PCR-based analysis for the presence of Y-chromosome sequences and the development of FISH permit the clarification of unknown fragments and the identification of covert Y DNA in 45,X subjects. This can be done most simply by amplifying centromeric repeat sequences (alphoid satellite DNA) that are present near the centromere on both the Y and X chromosome. Alternatively the amplification of ZFY and ZFX provides a similar set of homologous targets on the short arms of the Y and X chromosomes, respectively. The simultaneous amplification of the ZFX target provides an internal control for amplification failures. Another practical target sequence that is present on the both the X and the Y chromosome (Yp11.2) is the gene encoding the enamel protein amelogenin. Using a single pair of PCR primers one can generate distinct X- and Y-specific amelogenin bands (AMELY) on agarose gels. The use of FISH techniques in 45,X subjects with low-level Y mosaicism is not as sensitive as a PCR-based approach. The precise portion of the Y-chromosome involved in oncogenesis is still unknown, however, the Yq_{11} region is under suspicion at this time.[13] The portion of the Y chromosome identified by deletion mapping and shared in common among subjects who develop gonadal tumors has been called the GBY gene for the gonadoblastoma locus on the Y chromosome. It is still uncertain if there is a specific gene(s) involved in the etiology of these dysgenetic tumors or whether they arise secondarily, due to continued pituitary stimulation of a primitive, immature gonad. The Sex-Related-Y gene (SRY) does not appear to play a direct role in oncogenesis because it is not consistently present in subjects with gonadal tumors (gonadoblastoma/dysgerminoma).[14] The recent report of gonadal stromal tumors in mice that are homozygous deleted for alpha inhibin adds further speculation as to the relative role of genes versus endocrine environment in the predisposition to dysgenetic tumors.[15] The clinical importance of a low number of Y-positive cells in 45,X patients and the risk of neoplasia with/without virilization requires continued inquiry. For the present time it is important to recognize that SRY and the gene or genes conferring malignant potential are not the same. Failure to display SRY or a closely related sequence does not rule out the presence of the putative oncogenic segment of the Y chromosome.

In summary, DNA probes to detect Y DNA offer a partial solution to the difficult dilemma of a covert Y chromosome or an unknown chromosome fragment that might be Y derived. DNA diagnostics based on PCR are now widely available and should be a routine part of our armamentarium to complement cytogenetics in the laboratory detection of covert Y chromosomes. The practical utility of these molecular probes for Y depends upon their ability to detect (1) small amounts of Y-chromosome DNA in mosaic 45,X/46,XY subjects, and (2) structurally altered Y chromosomes. Both of these prerequisites are meet by utilizing DNA probes for Y-specific centromeric sequences with/without prior amplification of target DNA with PCR. This will be the approach of choice until the specific area or areas on the Y chromosome which are responsible for oncogenesis have been identified. A region of several hundred kilobase on the proximal portion of the Y short arm has been suggested to contain the "oncogenic gene(s), but no specific gene has been identified to date. At this point in time, probing for that tumor specific area may better select patients at risk for tumor development and in need of gonadal extirpation. At the present time it is clear that PCR is more effective than routine cytogenetic analysis for the detection of occult or cryptic Y DNA.

B. Detection of Mosaicism for X Chromosomes

1. Human Androgen Receptor Assay (HUMARA) Using PCR

The use of molecular techniques for the detection of low-level mosaicism involving X chromosomes is a little more complex, and usually requires the use of polymorphic DNA markers or dosimetry. However, it can be accomplished by amplifying with PCR a highly polymorphic CAG repeat that is located in the first exon of the human androgen receptor gene on Xq12. In the presence of a second X chromosome with a different HUMARA allele, the second band will be amplified by PCR. In this assay the CAG repeat is amplified together with its flanking DNAs, which fortuitously contain two methylation sensitive HpalI sites. In this procedure the genomic DNAs are digested with HpalI prior to PCR amplification. When an X chromosome is active these HpalI sites are not methylated and are susceptible to HpalI digestion, and thus PCR amplification fails to yield products. On the other hand when an X chromosome is inactive these sites are methylated, are resistant to digestion, and PCR yields products of the expected size. In the case of random X inactivation both alleles are randomly methylated and therefore will be equally digested and amplified. However, when one of the X chromosomes is selectively inactivated the allele of the inactive X chromosome will be resistant to HpalI digestion and will be selectively amplified.[16] In TS patients the second structurally abnormal X chromosome is selectively inactivated and will be selectively amplified. Even in patients with a 45,X/46,XX karyotype the allele of the second X will be more efficiently amplified since X chromosomes in 46,XX cells are randomly inactivated. In the latter situation both alleles will be equally amplified even in the presence of a large excess of 45,X cells. Secondly, since the locus is highly polymorphic the chance of the second X chromosome having a different allele is high. The percent heterozygosity at this locus is reported to be as high as 87%. Thirdly, since the locus for the androgen receptor is located at Xq12 between the centromere and the XIC at Xq13 even the second structurally abnormal X chromosome would probably retain the androgen receptor locus. In fact Xq11.2-q21 is retained in almost all structurally abnormal X chromosomes.[17]

Low-level mosaicism for X chromosomes can also be detected using different restriction fragment length polymorphisms and microsatellite polymorphisms. In those situations where an unknown chromosome, presumed to be X to Y is evident on conventional cytogenetic studies then the following technique of fluorescent *in situ* hybridization is the least complicated and the most effective approach to identify X marker chromosomes. The DXZ1 probe which hybridizes to alpha satellite DNA sequences located at the centromere of the X chromosome is ideal for this purpose. It is analogous to the DYZ3 probe for centromeric Y sequences.

C. FISH

A second technique that has extended the diagnostic capabilities for low-level sex chromosome mosaicism is FISH. In more recent years, several investigators have refined the techniques of FISH [18] so that fluorochromes attached to single pieces of DNA can be used to probe metaphase spreads of human chromosomes. This FISH technique has enabled investigators to identify copies of a given gene or anonymous sequence in dividing and nondividing interphase cells. This technique is very valuable for the rapid diagnosis of human aneuploidy. It is a valuable supplement to standard cytogenetics studies with or without subsequent DNA analysis. Specific fluorochrome probes attached to the Y and X chromosome are able to identify these specific targets in resting, interphase cells and provide a quick, easy method of scoring large numbers of cells in order to identify additional cell lines such as 45,X in someone who appears to be a normal non-mosaic 46,XX genotype on conventional metaphase chromosomes. For example, a patient may have ovarian failure and short stature, but is karyotyped as 46,XX using standard cell counts of 30 or 50 metaphase cells. If clinical suspicion of mosaicism persists FISH techniques give one the opportunity to score 600–2000 or more interphase cells for the presence of cells with a single signal consistent with a 45,X cell line and a mosaic or mixoploidic 45,X/46,XX karyotype.

In the future one controversy that may be resolved by FISH techniques concerns the incidence of ovarian failure in apparently 47,XXX individuals. When ovarian failure is present in such individuals it would seem to violate the axiom that ovarian failure and short stature is always related to some privation or deletion of X-chromosome material. It is likely that individuals with normal stature and gonadal function are non-mosaic 47,XXX and those who are short with gonadal failure are mosaics 45,X/47,XXX. Current evidence for this derives from prenatal diagnosis where chorionic sampling will reveal a 45,X/46,XX/47,XXX genotype, subsequent amniocentesis a 47,XXX karyotype, and neonatal blood 45X,/47,XXX. When the individual is ascertained later in life with ovarian failure only the 47,XXX cell line may be in evidence. Eugonadal non-mosaic 47,XXX individuals arise through paternal or maternal nondisjunction. Clinically the non-mosaic 47,XXX individuals should be of normal stature with normal menses, whereas the mosaic 45,X/47,XXX will be short with elevated serum FSH, and may have somatic anomalies consistent with the Turner phenotype.

In spite of the immense value of FISH techniques it is important to be aware of the laboratory criteria for scoring cell hybridizations and determining "noninformative." Information should always be provided on external controls and the minimum number of cells that must be "scorable" per probe set in order to consider FISH informative. Many laboratories will not provide a report unless 50 cells or more per probe (200 nuclei per specimen for the 5 standard probes—13,21,18,X,Y) are of scoring quality. This is especially important when one is trying to detect low-level mosaicism for a 45,X or 46,XY cell line. The laboratory should provide information on the percentage of cells that must generate two hybridization signals in order for the sample to be considered normal diploid, and/or the necessary percentages for the validation of aneuploidy. One laboratory might require 50 cells per probe and over 70% of the scorable cells must have 3 signals to diagnose aneuploidy (i.e.,46,XXX) and 80% with two signals for euploidy (i.e.,46,XX), etc. The laboratory should provide information on the controls and specify the exact laboratory criteria for informative results.

In general the data obtained from FISH are usually correct, however, there is a high noninformative rate and a significant risk of misdiagnosis. The laboratory should be clear about the reporting criteria for aneuploidy. They should specify in detail the criteria for aneuploidy, other than >3 standard deviations beyond that seen in diploid cells. This is important since the signal obtained in FISH is affected by the spatial arrangement of chromosomes within the nucleus, the size of the nucleus, overlapping signals, and the extent of condensation of the chromatin. Smaller nuclei such as G1 cells tend to produce small, compact, bright signals while the signals in larger G2 cells are more diffuse and less intense. Due to these variables different observers may not score signals at interphase in the same way. Two observers familiar with FISH work and with each other's interpretations may still show significantly different results on blinded analysis. Intraobserver and interobserver differences in scoring should be considered along with technical factors as a possible reason for the unreliability of interphase FISH interpretations using library probes. For this reason an observer variation study should be provided and the authors should specify as to whether all raters were blinded as to results of the final karyotyping. In other words the laboratory should provide specific details on controls, methodology, reporting criteria, and the analysis of the results.

IV. CLINICAL DEVELOPMENTS

A. Cardiac Imaging

Over the past two decades pediatricians have become increasingly concerned that the risk of fatal aortic abnormalities (aneurysm, dissection, or rupture) in patients with gonadal dysgenesis is underestimated. The continued surveillance of gonadal dysgenesis patients into adulthood and later life has helped to point out the danger of bicuspid aortic values. It has been increasingly apparent that gonadal dysgenesis patients with bicuspid aortic values are at greater risk for progressive dilatation of the aortic root in later life. The bicuspid aortic valve seems to produce a jet of greater pressure against the ascending aorta and predisposes to atherosclerotic disease. In addition a bicuspid aortic value may progress to stenosis and calcification. If a patient with gonadal dysgenesis has a bicuspid or functionally bicuspid aortic value she should have prophylactic antibiotics at the time of dental work or surgery to avoid bacterial endocarditis. A patient with gonadal dysgenesis should have echocardiography of her heart and aorta at an age when she is old enough for a clear definition of the aortic value structure (probably after 2 years of age). If a bicuspid aortic value is found yearly follow-up is recommended. The Genetics Committee of the American Academy of Pediatrics has recently recommended consistent referral to a cardiologist, and annual echocardiograms for all children and adults with gonadal dysgenesis.[19] The frequency of imaging is controversial, but the need for life time follow-up to detect changes in cardiac auscultation, and the diameter of the aortic root are indisputable. The first evidence of aortic dilation may be the sudden onset of aortic regurgitation on cardiac auscultation at 20–40 years of age. This is the reason that the limits of our thinking should not be constrained by the age of the patient. This type of specialized attention needs to extend well into adulthood. It should be a fundamental consideration prior to considering any gonadal dysgenesis patient for assisted reproduction using donor oocytes and transfer of the embryo(s) to the at risk proband. Aortic dissection may be a complication of the aortic dilatation and is an acute, but treatable event. It is clear that careful prepregnancy evaluation of all individuals with gonadal dysgenesis is critical before assisted reproductive techniques (ART) is considered. The stress of pregnancy on the cardiovascular system may augment the risks of aortic dilation, dissection, and rupture as they appear to do in Marfan's syndrome. To avoid multiple pregnancies the number of embryos transferred needs to be given careful thought. It is prophetic that these concerns were eloquently expressed by Mary Birdsall and Stephen Kennedy from the Nuffield Department of Obstetrics and Gynecology in a letter to the editor in the July 1996 issue of *Human Reproduction*. At that time there were 27 published case reports of dissecting aortic aneurysm in Turner patients, but none during pregnancy.[20] Their letter stressed the importance of a cardiac evaluation prior to oocyte donation on all patients with Turner's syndrome. According to Angela Lin who published the benchmark paper on this topic in 1986 with Barbara Lippe the majority of the aortic dissections have occurred in Turner patients who are older than 21 years.[21] That information illustrates the need for the adult physician to pick up the baton cleanly from the pediatrician, and even step up the probing for age-related cardiac changes.

Perhaps in the future we may have a better handle on the predictor variables (underlying cardiac defects, karyotype, age, etc.) that increase the likelihood of dissection during pregnancy. A known underlying cardiac defect (bicuspid valve, coarctation, aortic stenosis, etc.) and/or systemic hypertension are clearly risk factors for aortic dissection in the nonpregnant patient with Turner's syndrome. They become "red flags" when pregnancy is a consideration. However, a dissection of the abdominal aorta has been reported in one patient who had none of these risk factors.[22]

The demands of human pregnancy on the cardiovascular and other systems is considerable. Vigilance needs to be taken in the selection of gonadal dysgenesis mothers for ART otherwise complications related to their cardiovascular and renal anomalies may be reported with increasing frequency.

B. Assisted Reproduction

Two young women with Turner's syndrome who became pregnant by ovum donation have died suddenly in the third trimester due to aortic dissection. Physicians who use techniques of assisted reproduction for mothers who have genetic disorders need to be increasingly aware of these potential complications. Over the past two decades pediatricians have become increasingly concerned that the risk of fatal aortic abnormalities (aneurysm, dissection, or rupture) in patients with gonadal dysgenesis is underestimated. Consistent referral to a cardiologist and annual echocardiograms for all children with gonadal dysgenesis is recommended. The frequency of imaging is controversial, but the need for life time follow-up to detect changes in cardiac auscultation, and the diameter of the aortic root are indisputable.

Among the obvious medical risks of pregnancy in TS patients is the possibility of cesarean section and the exacerbation of underlying hypertension or carbohydrate intolerance. The future challenges include the development of a method that will consistently preserve the unfertilized oocyte. This would extend the opportunity for those patients with early evidence of gonadal integrity to undergo procedures of oocyte rescue and storage prior to the time of wanted pregnancy in a manner analogous to sperm preservation. Although there is an increased risk of chromosomal abnormalities in such pregnancies monitoring techniques are available.[23] The potential to be a gestational mother in patients with gonadal dysgenesis means that the uterus should be preserved.

Finally, the development of a registry for pregnancy in individuals with Turner's syndrome is important because it allows the different types of specialists who must manage these problems to be brought together. Perhaps this type of rapid communication is best done through online computer related communities. The Turner Syndrome Society would be the one of the logical choices to implement these on line registries.

V. THERAPY

Recombinant human growth hormone (rHGH) continues to be used for some TS patients with modest therapeutic benefits. In gonadal dysgenesis subjects started on rHGH at approximately 11 years of age the mean height increase after 4 years of therapy appeared to be about 5.4 cm. The adverse effects of growth hormone relate primarily to peripheral edema or arthralgias. These effects are caused by sodium retention and skeletal muscle growth or edema. Occasionally the edema may result in carpal tunnel symptoms. At this time growth hormone therapy is being touted for a wide range of symptoms or conditions ranging from aging to cardiovascular disease. It will be important to follow any adverse effects that occur in this group of older subjects. If treatment of gonadal dysgenesis patient with rHGH is undertaken then biochemical monitoring should be performed by following serum levels of IFG-I and IGFBP-3. At the present time a weekly dose of 0.375 mg/kg (approximately 1.125 IU/kg) of body weight divided into equal doses 3–7 times per week by subcutaneous is recommended (or 0.16–0.24 mg/kg). The heterogeneity of the sex chromosome abnormalities in gonadal dysgenesis makes ultimate height predictions uncertain for individual patients. Trying to derive normative data for gonadal dysgenesis patients remains an uncertain science and it is unlikely that it will change. For these reasons it is difficult to know if the agent you are using to increase final height is really making a difference. Nevertheless, one of the FDA's advisory committees has approved growth hormone therapy for this indication (December 1996). Market clearance has been granted by the FDA and by authorities in 27 other countries.

VI. PROGNOSIS

The overall prognosis for individuals with gonadal dysgenesis is excellent, provided they receive appropriate medical attention. The most recent data suggest that individuals with gonadal dysgenesis can live healthy, happy productive lives. Their cognitive function in general is not impaired. Their sexual function and their ability to be in a stable heterosexual relationship is also comparable to a control group of normal women. Physical and psychological problems seen in women with gonadal dysgenesis may be the result of their physical anomalies. Most of these can now be overcome with medical and surgical therapy.

Unfortunately, there are many myths which still persist about the intellectual, psychosexual, and physical potential of these individuals. This is particularly true whenever the eponym Turner syndrome is utilized and for this reason, we hope it will eventually be abandoned completely. Some of the problems associated with gonadal dysgenesis may stem from self-fulfilling prophecies proliferated by medical professionals.

We often face couples in whom a fetus has been diagnosed as having a 45,X or 45,X/46,XX karyotype who have been painted a dire prognosis for the fetus, particularly in terms of cognitive function.

Finally, we generally advise parents of a child with gonadal dysgenesis that the risk of recurrence is not increased over that in the general population. This presupposes a negative pedigree and excludes cases of Swyer's syndrome. Prenatal diagnostic modalities, as outlined above, are not routinely indicated but should be discussed with the prospective parents.

Much progress has been accomplished in our understanding of gonadal dysgenesis. The coming years hold great promise. The future is very bright for patients with these disorders of gonadal differentiation. Perhaps in the future unconventional nomenclature and traditional misconceptions about individuals with gonadal dysgenesis will fade away. Research will reveal the mechanisms underlying gonadal development and the statural determinants that are defective in subjects with gonadal dysgenesis. Molecular techniques can now identify all patients at risk for gonadal tumors. Operative laparoscopy will become the routine procedure for gonadectomy.

VII. FUTURE RESEARCH: ORIGIN AND FUNCTION OF THE GERM LINE

Advancement in our knowledge of the mechanism of ovarian failure in subjects with gonadal dysgenesis will depend on understanding more about the developmental pathways for primordial germ cells. There is a need to increase our knowledge of the common features of germ line determination and maintenance.

This information will not come easily because of the relative inaccessibility and small number of cells involved in the development of the germ line. To date the research in this area has been carried out primarily in *Caenorhabditis elegans* and *Drosophila melanogaster.*[24] This research centers on an understanding of the early expression pattern of primitive embryonic stem cells just as selected ones commit to be germ cells. A few genes that are expressed at this crucial time have been identified in *Drosophila,* but not in other higher model organisms. These studies may also help to clarify the mechanisms by which germ cells decide or select their sex. In summary it is an interesting time in the history of studies of gonadal dysgenesis because of the rapid advances being made through the use of the tools of modern molecular biology, and the remarkable advances in cardiovascular imaging.

References

1. Lyon, M. (1962). Sex chromatin and gene action in the mammalian X-chromosome. *Am. J. Hum. Gen.* 14, 135–148.
2. Ferguson-Smith, M. A. (1965). Karyotype-phenotype correlations in gonadal dysgenesis and their bearing on the pathogenesis of malformation. *J. Med. Genet.* 2, 142–155.
3. Fisher, E. M. C., Beer-Romero, P., Brown, L. G., Ridley, A., McNeil, J. A., Lawrence, J. B., Willard, H. F., Bieber, F. R., and Page, D. C. (1990) Homologous ribosomal protein genes on the human X and Y chromosome: Escape form X inactivation and possible implications for Turner syndrome. *Cell* 63, 1205–1218.
4. Geerkens, C., Just, W., Held, K. R., and Vogel, W. (1996). Ullrich-Turner syndrome is not caused by haploinsufficiency of RPS4X. *Hum. Genet.* 97, 39–44.
5. Omoe, K., and Endo, A. (1995). Relationship between the monosomy X phenotype and Y-linked ribosomal protein S4 (Rps4) in several species of mammals: A molecular evolutionary analysis of Rps4 homologs. *Genomics* 31, 44–50.
6. Rao, E., Weiss, B., Fukami, M., Rump, A., Niesler, B., Mertz, A. N., Muroya, K., Binder, G., Kirsch, S., Winkelmann, M., Nordsiek, G., Heinrich, U., Breuning, M. H., Ranke, M. B., Rosenthal, A., Ogata, T., and Rappold, G. A. (1997). Pseudoautosomal deletions encompassing a novel homeobox gene cause growth failure in idiopathic short stature and Turner syndrome. *Nat. Genet.* 16, 54–62.
7. Ellison, J. W., Wardak, Z., Young, M. F., Robey, P. G., Laig-Webster, M., and Chiong, W. (1997). PHOG, a candidate gene for involvement in the short stature of Turner syndrome. *Hum. Mol. Genet.* 6, 1341–1347.
8. Gantt, P. A., Byrd, J. R., Greenblatt, R. B., and McDonough, P. G. (1980). A clinical and cytogenetic study of fifteen patients with 45,X/46,XY gonadal dysgenesis. *Fertil. Steril.* 34, 216–221.
9. McDonough, P. G., and Tho, P. T. (1983). The spectrum of 45,X/46,XY gonadal dysgenesis and its implications, a study of 19 patients. *Pediatr. Adolesc. Gynecol.* 1, 1–17.
10. Belmont, J. W. (1996). Genetic control of the X inactivation and processes leading to X-inactivation skewing. *Am. J. Hum..Genet.* 58, 1101–1108.
11. Jani, M. M., Torchia, B. S., Pai, G. S., and Migeon, B. R. (1995). Molecular characterization of tiny ring chromosomes from females with functional X chromosome disomy and lack of cis inactivation. *Genomics* 27, 182–188.
12. Plenge, R. M., Hendrich, B. D., Schwartz, C., Arena, J. F., Naumova, A., Sapienza, C., Winter, R. M., and Willard, H. F. (1997). A promoter mutation in the XIST gene in two unrelated families with skewed X-chromosome inactivation. *Nat. Genet.* 17, 353–356.
13. Tho, S. P. T., Layman, L. C., Lanclos, K. D., Plouffe, L. Jr., Byrd, J. R., and McDonough, P. G. (1992). Absence of the testicular determining factor gene SRY in XX true hermaphrodites and presence of this locus in most subjects with gonadal dysgenesis caused by Y aneuploidy. *Am. J. Obstet. Gynecol.* 167, 1794–1802.
14. Tsuchiya, K., Reijo, R., Page, D., and Disteche, C. M. (1995). Gonadoblastoma: Molecular definition of the susceptibility region of the Y chromosome. *Am. J. Hum. Genet.* 57, 1400–1407.
15. Matzuk, M. M., Finegold, M. J., Su, J.-G. J., Hsueh, A. J. W., and Bradley, A. (1992). α-Inhibin is a tumour-suppressor gene with gonadal specificity in mice. *Nature* 360, 313–319.
16. Yorifuji, T., Muroi, J., Kawai, M., Sasaki, H., Momoi, T., and Furusho, K. (1997). PCR-based detection of mosaicism in Turner syndrome patients. *Hum. Genet.* 99, 62–65.
17. Allen, C. R., Zoghbi, H. Y., Moseley, A. B., Rosenblatt, H. M., and Belmont, J. W. (1992). Methylation of HpaII and HhaI sites near the polymorphic CAG repeat in the human androgen-receptor gene correlates with X chromosome inactivation. *Am. J. Hum. Genet.* 51, 1229–1239.
18. Delhanty, J. D., Griffin, D. K., Handyside, A. H., Harper, J., Atkinson, G. H., Pieters, M. H., and Winston, R. M. (1993). Detection of aneuploidy and chromosomal mosaicism in human embryo during pre-implantation sex determination by fluorescent in situ hybridization (FISH). *Hum. Mol. Genet.* 2, 1183–1185.

CHAPTER

4

Pathology of Non-Neoplastic Ovarian Enlargements

FRÉDÉRIQUE PENAULT-LLORCA
Service d'Anatomie et Cytologie Pathologiques
Clermont-Ferrand Cedex 01,
France

CATHERINE VAURS BARRIÈRE
Service d'Anatomie et Cytologie Pathologiques
Clermont-Ferrand Cedex 01,
France

MICHEL CANIS
Department of Obstetrics, Gynecology, and
Reproductive Medicine
Polyclinique CHU
63003 Clermont-Ferrand, France

JACQUES DAUPLAT
Department of Oncologic Surgery
Service d'Anatomie et Cytologie Pathologiques
Clermont-Ferrand Cedex 01, France

ABSTRACT

This chapter presents updated datas on clinical and pathological features of non-neoplastic ovarian enlargements, including dysfunctional cysts, disorders associated with estrogenic, and androgenic manifestations (including polycystic ovarian disease or PCOD; stromal hyperplasia and stromal hyperthecosis; massive edema and fibromatosis; hilus cell hyperplasia; pregnancy luteoma and hyperreactio luteinalis; endometriosis and, inflammatory lesions.

The authors go into detail about the newly established diagnosis criteria for PCOD. Moreover, the authors give highlights on the molecular and biological characteristics of PCOD and endometriosis, and on their respective associated increased risks.

I. CYSTIC LESIONS

A functional cyst corresponds to the formation of a non-neoplastic pathological structure containing a cavity filled with fluid. Cystic lesions correspond to solitary cysts of follicular origin. They result from expansion of the original cavity of the preovulatory follicles (follicular cysts) or corpora lutea (corpus luteum cysts). Their incidence is unknown, but they are considered to be common, frequently subclinical and spontaneously regressive in many cases. They are most common in nonpregnant women of reproductive age, particularly around times of menarche and menopause.[1]

Surface epithelium inclusion cysts will be discussed in Chapter 10. In ovarian pathology, the term cyst is also applied to cystic tumor, i.e., cystadenoma or cystadenocarcinoma (see Chapter 6). Ovaries displaying several cysts should be called "multicystic"; the term "polycystic" being reserved for the abnormal ovaries found in association with Stein-Leventhal or related syndromes.

A. Follicular Cyst

1. Etiology, Clinical Features

The etiology is usually a disordered function of the pituitary-ovarian axis:

- Unluteinized follicular cysts produce predominantly estradiol and result from excessive ovarian stimulation [Follicular stimulating hormone (FSH) stimulation or ovulation-induction agents].
- Granulosa lutein cysts produce progesterone (gonadotropins secretions).
- Theca lutein cysts produce androstenedione [prolonged exposure to Luteinizing hormone (LH) or human chorionic gonadotrophin (HCG)].

Chronic pelvic inflammatory disease may also contribute to cyst formation, probably by altering the blood flow from the ovaries.[2]

Despite secretion of steroid hormones, the vast majority of the patients with follicular cyst do not show endocrine symptoms. Nevertheless, Piver *et al.* [3] found that two-thirds of patients with surgically excised follicular cysts had menstrual irregularities, although a causal relationship could not be established. Torsion and rupture syndromes may precipitate clinical presentation.

Ovarian cysts have been described in the fetus.[4] They are usually unilateral and range in size from 2–11 cm, and torsion, rupture, or dystocia have been reported. Their exact etiology is unclear, but the development of these cysts may be related to the active folliculogenesis that occurs *in utero* as an abnormal response to maternal HCG and fetal gonadotrophins, which normally stimulate follicular development from the fourth gestational month.[5] Management is still controversial, especially of the asymptomatic lesions.[6]

Ovarian follicle cysts are uncommon in children, in whom they may cause isosexual pseudoprecocity. They are probably autonomous, as they are not associated with elevated gonadotrophin levels. The clinical symptoms regress after puncture, removal, or occasionally spontaneously. The presence of ovarian follicles cysts in children may be a feature of the McCune-Albright syndrome.[7]

2. Pathologic Features

The distinction between cystic atretic follicles and follicular cysts lacks absolute criteria. Most of the authors consider those less than 2–3 cm in diameter to be cystic follicles,[8] and above that size to be cysts. Follicular cysts do not usually exceed 8 cm in diameter except for those occurring in pregnancy, which may reach 25 cm.[9]

Follicle cysts have smooth inner surfaces, thin walls, and contain watery fluid. They are lined by several layers of granulosa cells, separated by the basement membrane from the underlying theca interna. Progressive thinning of granulosa may result in the formation of a cyst covered by morphologically indistinct low cuboidal epithelium. After the complete disappearance of the theca interna, the true nature of a cyst may be impossible to prove. In this situation, the term "simple cyst" is the most appropriate.

During pregnancy, both the granulosa and the theca layers of the follicular cyst may undergo luteinization, under the influence of gonadotropic hormones produced by the placenta. This results in the formation of a large (up to 25 cm in diameter) cyst covered by plump granulosa cells exhibiting nuclear hyperchromasia and pleomorphism, which should not be misdiagnosed as malignant. This cyst has been described under the name "large solitary luteinized follicle cyst of pregnancy and puerperium."[9] All the patients have had an uneventful postoperative course.

B. Corpus Luteum Cyst

1. Etiology, Clinical Features

This is a cyst derived from a corpus luteum of menstruation or pregnancy, which results from excessive central hemorrhage.[1] Normal corpus luteum frequently has a central cavity filled with blood or jelly-like coagulum remaining from the time of ovulation. When it attains 2 cm in diameter, it may be called a "corpus luteum cyst." It is most frequently asymptomatic, but its continuing production of progesterone may result in minor menstrual disturbances. It may cause menstrual irregularities and amenorrhea. The endometrium in such patients may show an inappropriate progesteronic effect, Arias Stella change, or the picture of irregular shedding. It may also rupture and cause hemoperitoneum.

The etiology of corpus luteum cysts is not clear. In pelvic inflammatory disease, they may increase, threefold, perhaps due to increased blood flow.[2]

2. Pathologic Features

Corpus luteum cyst is easily recognizable on gross examination, because of the complete or fragmented yellow rim along its circumference. The contour of the cyst is usually smooth and not folded like in the normal corpus luteum. The cavity is frequently filled with blood, which may be old, rusty, dark-brown creating a picture of the so-called "chocolate cyst." Endometriotic cysts may be impossible to be distinguished grossly from corpus luteum cysts but may be suspected if endometriosis is suspected clinically.

Plump granulosa lutein cells with smaller theca interna cells located at the periphery line corpus luteum cysts. With progressive involution, increasing fibrosis mixes with involuting vacuolated luteinized cells.

The corpus luteum cysts undergo involution the sameway as the normal corpora lutea. They may disappear without a trace or transform into corpora albicantia, some of which remain cystic (corpus albicans cyst). These cysts are nonfunctional and are too small to produce symptomatic adnexal masses. They rarely exceed 1 cm in diameter. They are composed of a convoluted outer ribbon of hyalinized fibrous tissue and inner zone of loose fibrous tissue.

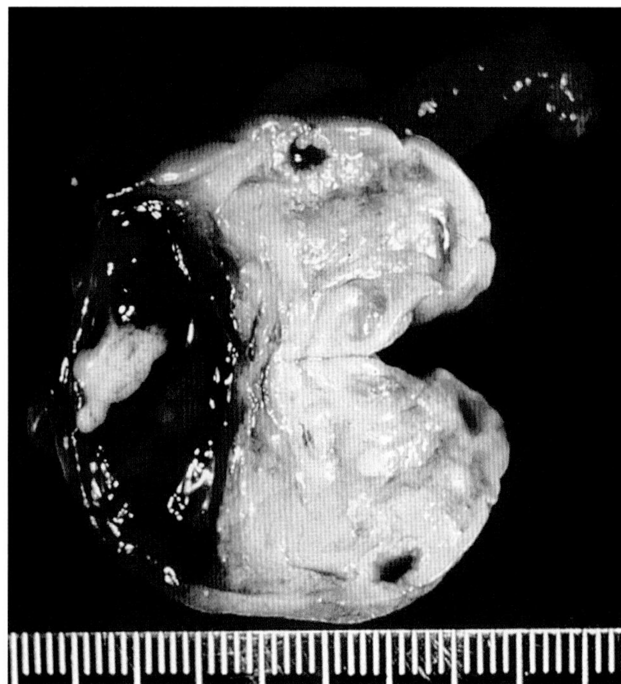

FIGURE 4.1 Sectioned surface of a hemorrhagic functional cyst. The cavity contains old blood creating a picture of the so-called "chocolate cyst".

C. Simple Cysts

This term defines ovarian cysts or cyst-like structures, which lack identifiable linings.[1] They are frequently incidental findings. The cysts are usually less than 10 cm, and show a smooth internal surface and a variable content of clear fluid or altered blood (Fig. 4.1). Some hints, like scattered involuting luteinized cells, apparent epithelial cells or granulation tissue or hematoma, suggest an origin from, respectively, the follicular apparatus, epithelial cystoma, or endometriotic cysts. All those cysts are benign and most are non-neoplastic. Their classification into different categories has probably no benefit.

D. Cytology of Simple Cysts

Aspiration of ovarian cysts is an increasingly common procedure, but its use remains controversial. Aspiration is not recommended if there is any clinical suspicion of malignancy.[10] The cytological interpretation has limitations. The diagnosis interpretation can be neoplastic versus non-neoplastic, functional versus nonfunctional,[11] serous versus functional, versus endometriotic, versus mucinous, versus borderline or malignant.[10] False-negative results may occur with variable rates.[12] False-negative results are most commonly associated with attempted aspiration of solid or semisolid lesions (inadequate sampling), or when the aspirate contains scanty cellular material or, only lymphocytes, macrophages, or a large amount of blood. Such findings may present in follicular, endometriotic, corpus luteum, atretic, or old cysts, but malignancy cannot be ruled out.

Providing that the indications have been respected, aspiration cytology is a safe, accurate, and cost-effective method of evaluating benign ovarian cysts. Increasing experience and collaboration between the cytopathologist and the clinician is of utmost importance in the proper evaluation of the ovarian cysts.[13]

II. DISORDERS ASSOCIATED WITH ESTROGENIC AND ANDROGENIC MANIFESTATIONS

Morphologic and physiologic investigations have shown that these disorders, which may be associated with evidence of androgen excess, estrogenic manifestations, or both, are part of a continuum and that sharp distinctions cannot always be made among them. In spite of this overlap, it is appropriate to describe the typical clinical and pathologic features of each separately, inasmuch as the typical cases in each category differ in several aspects.

A. Polycystic Ovarian Disease (PCOD) [14, for review]

PCOD, also called Stein-Leventhal syndrome, has been estimated to affect 3.5–7% of women of reproductive age (mainly in their third decade).

1. Diagnosis Criteria

The two criteria retained to date to diagnose PCOD is a hyperandrogenism with acne and/or hirsutism (rarely virilization) and a chronic anovulation presents as oligomenorrhea or amenorrhea of perimenarchial onset (nevertheless, a history of regular menses is also possible with a fraction of women who experienced anovulation despite reporting regular menstrual cycles).

It must be noticed that since 1990, inconstant symptoms of PCOD such as obesity, ultrasonographic characteristics, serum LH levels and LH/FSH ratio have been excluded for diagnosis.[15] Obesity is found in 40–50% of women with PCOD but normal-weight women can develop PCOD.

Ultrasonographic characteristics of PCOD correspond frequently to enlarged ovaries, usually greater than 9 mm with more than 8 mm peripherally oriented cystic structures (<10 mm) in a sonographic plane, surrounded by an increased stromal mass (>25% of the ovarian volume). However, a sonographic spectrum exists and sometimes polycystic ovaries may be absent in women with all the other classical clinical characteristics of PCOD. Conversely, ovulating women with minor evidence of hyperandrogenism, and without menstrual irregularity may also have polycystic ovaries that contain corporea lutea and albicantia, indicating lack of clear boundary between clinical PCOD and normality. Hence, ultrasonographic diagnosis alone has been estimated not to be sufficient to diagnose PCOD.

Concerning LH levels and LH/FSH ratio, they have been found elevated in 35–90% of women with PCOD. The discrepancies between the observed frequencies can be explained by pulsatile secretion of LH. In addition, LH level can be decreased by progesterone after ovulation or exogenous treatment. The serum LH level (or immunoactive LH level) does not represent the bioactive LH level, which has never been studied to our knowledge in PCOD patients. A recent study of LH levels in hyperthecosis patients suggests that the important feature in LH expression seems not to be the LH level itself, but the bioactive LH level. Hence, a single dosage of the serum LH level has been evaluated as not reliable enough to be maintained as a diagnostic criterion.[15]

2. Biological Characteristics

a. Elevated Serum Androgens

The best marker for ovarian hyperandrogenism is testosterone and particularly "free," bioactive testosterone and the best adrenal marker is dehydroepiandrosterone sulfate. However, normal levels are found in some women. The FSH level is usually low to normal and the LH level is high.

b. Mild to Severe Insulin Resistance (IR) and Hyperinsulinemia

IR is found either in obese women or in normal-weight women with PCOD from different ethnic groups. IR may be related to defective insulin receptors due to their excessive serine phosphorylation (observed in at least 50% of women with PCOD). Anovulation seems to be a major determinant of IR in women with PCOD as IR is more pronounced in women with chronic anovulation than in those who have ovulatory cycles. In addition, hyperinsulinemia might stimulate androgen synthesis and increase the free bioactive testosterone level. IR sometimes accompanied by diabetes, acanthosis nigricans, and hyperandrogenism (HAIR-AN syndrome) have been described in a small subset of women considered clinically to have PCOD or stromal hyperthecosis (see the next section).[16]

b. Altered Serum Lipid Profiles

In PCOD women, serum lipid profiles can be modified including elevated levels of cholesterol, triglycerides, low-density lipoprotein (LDL) cholesterol, and low levels of high-density lipoprotein (HDL) cholesterol and apolipoprotein A-I. The most characteristic lipid alteration in PCOD is decreased levels of HDL2. These findings vary and depend on body weight, diet, and ethnicity. Both hyperandrogenism and hyperinsulinemia probably play some role in these lipid abnormalities.

c. Impaired Fibrinolytic Activity

An impaired fibrinolytic activity is assessed by circulating levels of plasminogen activator inhibitor often found in women with PCOD.

3. Molecular Characteristics

The etiology of PCOD remains unknown but the high prevalence within families of affected cases suggests that there is a major genetic cause. The most likely mode of inheritance is autosomal dominant but recent studies suggest that PCOD may represent a complex trait involving the interaction of a small number of genes with environmental, principally nutritional, factors.[17, for review]

Among the three candidate genes tested, i.e., the 17-hydroxylase, 17/20-lyase gene, the cholesterol side chain cleavage gene (*CYP11a*), and the insulin gene (*INS*) itself, two seem to be associated with the PCOD phenotype. Hence, the most common phenotype of *CYP11a* was significantly associated with PCOD and serum testosterone levels whereas class III alleles in the variable number tandem repeat (VNTR) of *INS* were associated with anovulatory PCOD. In addition, both associations have been confirmed by linkage studies and suggest that *CYP11a* is a major susceptibility locus for hyperandrogenism in PCOD and that the *INS*-VNTR variant may have a functional role in the expression of hyperinsulinemia and/or IR in PCOD.

4. Associated Increased Risks

Patients with PCOD may have an endometrium that varies from inactive to hyperplastic. In fewer than 5% of cases, endometrial, most of them in patients under 40, and ovarian carcinomas have been reported because of the long-standing unopposed estrogen stimulation.

They may develop metabolic diseases in mid-adult life, including impaired glucose tolerance, type 2 diabetes mellitus (sixfold increased risk in later life), principally related to IR.

Finally, cardiovascular diseases in mid-adult life have been reported, including hypertension, arteriosclerosis, and a sevenfold increased risk for myocardial infarction principally related to IR but also to impaired fibrinolytic activity.

5. Pathologic Features

Grossly, the ovaries are enlarged (two to five times normal size) and rounded. Numerous small follicles are visible beneath a thickened, sclerotic, white or whitish-gray superficial cortex (Fig. 4.2). The approximately equal size of the cysts is a feature of PCOD. Occasionally, the ovaries are of normal size. The stigmata of ovulation, i.e., corpora lutea and corpora albicantia are absent or sparse, the medulla being homogenous.

The superficial layers of the cortex are hypocellular and fibrotic due to the excessive deposition of collagen. The vessels are often thick-walled. Luteinized stromal cells can be found in most cases, indicating a morphological overlap with hyperthecosis. The follicular cysts are lined by a thin layer of nonluteinized granulosa cells, which may be absent, and usually by a thick layer of luteinized theca interna cells, which may also be prominent around atretic follicles.

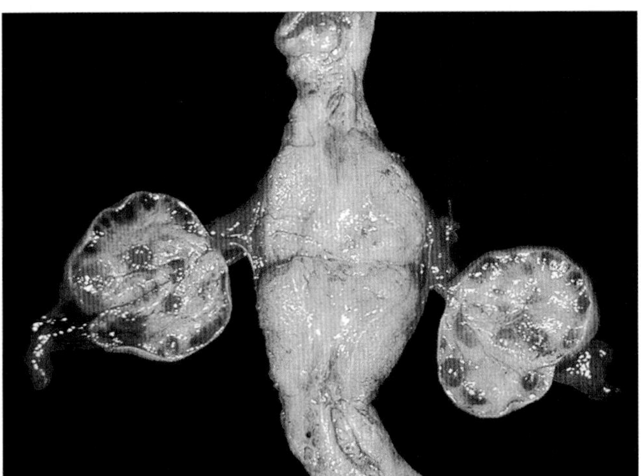

FIGURE 4.2 Polycystic ovarian disease. Sectioned surfaces of the ovaries show multiple cystic follicles.

B. Stromal Hyperplasia and Stromal Hyperthecosis

Stromal hyperplasia usually occurs in women in the sixth and seventh decades whereas clinical stromal hyperthecosis is usually encountered in patients of reproductive age, despite common findings in postmenopausal women.

Stromal hyperplasia refers to stromal proliferation from a moderate to marked degree whereas stromal hyperthecosis corresponds to the presence of large islands of luteinized thecal cells within an almost invariably hyperplastic ovarian stroma and at a distance from the follicles.

1. Diagnosis Criteria for Both Pathologies

In both pathologies, ovarian enlargements are almost always bilateral and are usually accompanied by noticeable virilization and frequent obesity (less frequent and marked in stromal hyperplasia).

2. Stromal Hyperthecosis

a. Etiology, Clinical Features

The clinical manifestations may resemble those of PCOD. But stromal hyperthecosis is seen more often as a gradual or less frequently an abrupt onset of virilization (with elevated serum testosterone level), in a premenopausal woman. Different mechanisms may be implicated in the stimulation of the ovarian androgen synthesis. First, Nagamani and Stuart have suggested that insulin may play a role trough the insulin-like growth factor [18] and recently, the same authors have shown, on three women with hyperthecosis, that stromal androgen synthesis is increased consecutively to the increased expression of the steroidogenic enzymes P450scc and P450 (17α).[19]

It must be noticed that impaired hepatic steroid metabolism (due to portal hypertension, chronic active hepatitis) has been also implicated in the development of hyperthecosis in young women (between 10 years old and middle age), which present virilization and precocious puberty in the case of the young girl.[20]

As in women with PCOD, women with hyperthecosis have insulin resistance and hyperinsulinemia. As previously reported, hyperinsulinemia may play a role in the stimulation of ovarian androgen synthesis. In addition, it has been recently shown that hyperinsulinemia induced by glucose administration has an effect, specifically in stromal hyperthecosis patients, on pituitary, increasing the bioactive LH levels (increase of the bioactive LH pulse amplitude and frequency) without changing the immunoactive LH levels.[21] The disorder is occasionally familial [22] and HAIR-AN syndrome may be associated with stromal hyperthecosis.[16]

The main diseases associated with stromal hyperthecosis are hypertension and disorders of the glucose metabolism both principally related to insulin resistance. Elevated serum estrone levels (caused by peripheral conversion of androstenedione) may cause endometrial hyperplasia or carcinoma. Estrogenic manifestations are more likely to occur in postmenopausal women, in whom the disease is usually milder.

b. Pathologic Features

Both ovaries are enlarged up to 8 cm and assume a more rounded shape. The cut surface is predominantly solid, homogenous, and yellow. Rarely, the involvement is unilateral. In premenopausal women, the tunica albuginea is thickened and few cystic follicles may be visible, but they are less numerous and large than in PCOD.

Microscopically, lipid-poor or -rich luteinized stromal cells are scattered as single cells or in small nests, throughout each ovary, within a background of stromal hyperplasia. Sometimes the luteinized cells form nodules. The distinction between nodular stromal hyperthecosis and a stromal luteoma is the size (>1 cm), and the absence of stromal hyperplasia for a diagnosis of luteoma. In premenopausal women, follicular hyperthecosis and sclerosis of the outer cortex is observed as in PCOD.

3. Stromal Hyperplasia

a. Etiology, Clinical Features

This process is a common incidental finding in the ovaries of perimenopausal or postmenopausal women. To attach clinicopathological significance to such changes, Russel and Farnsworth [23] reserve the term for definite and florid cases, and the minimum criteria are obliteration of the normal distinction between cortex and medulla or at least some nodularity of the proliferating stroma. There are androgenic or estrogenic manifestations as well as disorders of glucose metabolism, obesity, hypertension, etc., but those findings are much less common or less obtrusive than in stromal hyperthecosis.

The amount of stromal hyperplasia in postmenopausal ovaries has been related with the ovarian vein levels of androstenedione and testosterone.[24]

b. Pathologic Features

The ovaries are slightly enlarged by ill-defined, white or pale yellow, occasionally confluent nodules within the stroma of the medulla, cortex, or both. On microscopic examination, the medulla and the cortex (to a lesser extent) are replaced by nodular or diffuse, marked proliferation of small stromal cells with scanty, nonluteinized cytoplasm. Despite the absence of luteinized cells (by definition), fat stains performed on frozen sections will usually reveal widespread intracytoplasmic lipids.

The differential diagnosis includes ovarian fibroma and low-grade endometrioid stromal sarcoma (see in Chapter 8).

III. MASSIVE EDEMA AND FIBROMATOSIS

These pathologies present overlapping clinical features, indicating a probable relationship between the two entities.[25]

A. Massive Edema

1. Etiology, Clinical Features

Approximately 65 cases of this disorder have been reported so far. Patients are typically young (mean age 21, 6–33), and present with abdominal or pelvic pain, menstrual abnormalities, evidence of androgen excess or both, and abdominal swelling. The abdominal pain is sometimes so acute that it simulates appendicitis. Meig's syndrome (ascites and pleural effusion) has been described as a rare occurrence. Pelvic examination reveals a palpable adnexal mass, right-sided in most of the cases (75%), which may be due to the peculiarities of the venous drainage there. Clinical presentation simulates a malignant tumor.[26, 27]

Massive edema may be due to initial torsion or initial hyperthecosis and cortical stromal hyperplasia or fibromatosis followed by torsion. At laparotomy, ovarian enlargement is unilateral in 90% of cases, and partial or complete torsion of the ovarian pedicle is observed in over 50% of the cases.

2. Pathologic Features

The enlarged ovaries may reach up to 35 cm in size (mean 11.5 cm). They are pearly-white and on cross section, have a watery or myxoid appearance (Fig. 4.3). Usually, numerous cystic follicles are seen under the capsule and hemorrhages are quite frequent. Microscopically, edematous hypocellular stroma surrounds rather than displaces follicles and their derivatives. The peripheral cortex is spared and a sharp distinction between outer and inner cortex is obvious. Venous congestion and dilatation of lymphatics are prominent features. In one-third of the cases, there is focal hyperthecosis, which explains the occasional masculinization.

Differential diagnosis includes edematous fibroma (see Chapter 8) and Krukenberg tumor (see Chapter 9).

B. Fibromatosis

1. Etiology, Clinical Features

Patients with ovarian fibromatosis are in the same age ranges than those with massive edema (mean age 25 years 13–39). The clinical presentation is also quite similar: menstrual irregularities, abdominal pain and less commonly, hirsutism or virilization. Most of them have a palpable adnexal mass. Bilaterality is found in 20% of the cases; some involved ovaries were found twisted on their pedicles. Young and Scully [25] suggest that the massive edema is

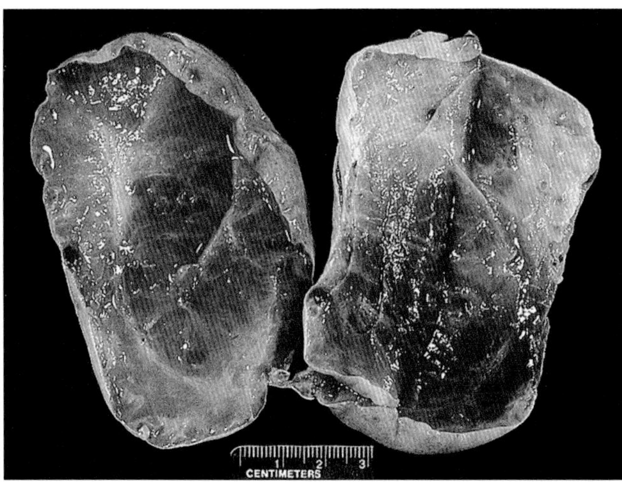

FIGURE 4.3 Massive ovarian edema.

simply ovarian fibromatosis following torsion and accumulation of edema fluid.

2. Pathologic Features

There is complete ovarian involvement by a fibromatous process. The ovaries are 8–12 cm in the maximum dimension, and have white and smooth or lobulated external surfaces. Small cysts may be visible on cut surfaces. Microscopically, follicular derivatives are surrounded by proliferating spindle cells and abundant collagen. The fibromatous proliferation is usually diffuse and thicken the superficial cortex, sometimes predominantly (i.e., cortical fibromatosis). Foci of noninvolved ovarian stroma may be present. Luteinized cells, foci of stromal edema, or focal nests of sex cord-type cells occur in rare cases.

Differential diagnosis includes fibroma, granulosa cell tumor with fibromatous component, and Brenner tumors (see Chapter 8).

IV. HILUS CELL HYPERPLASIA

In the ovarian hilus, single or grouped large epithelioid cells, with small round nuclei—hilus cells or Leydig cells—are observed in 80% of the ovaries.[28]

A. Etiology, Clinical Features

Hyperplasia of hilus cells of the ovary is rare, and generally occurs physiologically during pregnancy, or after menopause (augmentation of gonadotrophin levels). Occasionally, clinical endocrine disturbance (hirsutism) and elevated serum testosterone levels are observed.[29] In nonpregnant women, hilus cell hyperplasia is associated with stromal hyperplasia, stromal hyperthecosis, hilus cell tumor, or in the border of an epithelial ovarian tumor.

B. Pathologic Features

The hyperplasia is characterized by clusters and nodules of typical Leydig cells. Nuclear pleomorphism, hyperchromasia, multinucleation, and cellular enlargement may be observed.

Differential diagnosis with a hilus cell tumor is arbitrary with the presence of nodules over 1 cm in diameter.

V. PREGNANCY LUTEOMA AND HYPERREACTIO LUTEINALIS

Pregnancy may cause excessive luteinization of the stromal cells, resulting in one of the following conditions: pregnancy luteoma, hyperreactio luteinalis, and the large solitary luteinized follicle cyst (already described in the section follicles cyst).[30] Their recognition by pathologists and clinicians is important in order to avoid unnecessary radical surgery.[9]

A. Pregnancy Luteoma

1. Etiology, Clinical Features

HCG is necessary for the development of luteoma, but is unlikely to be the only etiological factor since the lesions are not associated with trophoblastic disease or early pregnancy when HCG levels are at their highest.

The luteoma usually presents in the third trimester, and is an incidental finding at caesarian section or postpartum tubal ligation. Rarely, a pelvic mass is palpable or obstructs the birth canal. The patients are typically multiparous and black (80%), and in their third or fourth decade. In about 25% of the cases an over-production of androgen causes hirsutism or virilization.[31] Luteomas undergo regression after termination of pregnancy, and serum androgen levels normalize within several weeks.

2. Pathologic Features

Luteomas are usually 6–12 cm in diameter but range from microscopic to larger than 20 cm. They are well-circumscribed nonencapsulated masses, which may be multinodular (50%) or bilateral (33%). On cut section, they are solid, fleshy, reddish brown, or yellow (Fig. 4.4). The nodules occasionally contain follicles filled with pale fluid or colloid like material.

Microscopically, pregnancy luteoma consists of polyhedral cells with a well-developed eosinophilic cytoplasm, large round nuclei, occasionally slightly pleomorphic, with prominent nucleoli. Mitotic figures (up to 7 mitotic figures

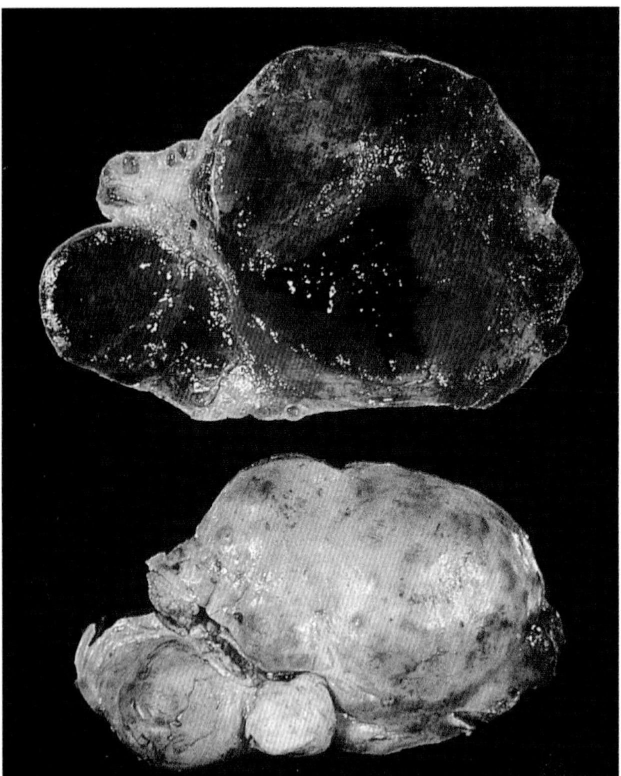

FIGURE 4.4 Pregnancy luteoma, mimicking a malignant tumor on gross examination.

per 10 hpf), are not unusual. The cytoplasm is lipid-poor and typically immunoreactive for inhibin.[32] The cells form well-circumscribed masses divided by the reticulin fibers into clusters, while in the histologically similar theca cell tumor reticulin surrounds every cell.

At postpartum regression, the lipid content of the cells increases. The luteoma is reduced to shrunken nests of degenerating cells mixed with lymphocytes and fibrosis.

Differential diagnosis includes grossly metastatic tumor, and microscopically, the different types of steroid cell tumor particularly lipid-free or lipid-poor.

B. Hyperreactio Luteinalis (Multiple Theca Lutein Cysts)

1. Etiology, Clinical Features

This condition is usually associated with molar pregnancy or choriocarcinoma (in about 25% of cases of gestational trophoblastic disease) or iatrogenic stimulation of the ovulation.[33, 34] The syndrome has also been described in women with apparently normal singleton pregnancy.[35] Virilization of the patient but not of the female infant has been described in about 15% of cases not associated with gestational trophoblastic disease. Elevated plasma testosterone levels occur in these patients as well as in other without virilization.

The hyperreactio luteinalis syndrome presents at any stage of pregnancy and even puerperium. It may be associated with marked ovarian edema, hemorrhage, torsion, rupture, hemoperitoneum, and is rarely fatal. It may cause dystocia or obstructive symptoms. The cysts may also be incidental findings at caesarian section. Regression is observed during puerperium in most of the cases. But, occasionally, cysts persist for long periods.

When the syndrome results from iatrogenic stimulation of the ovulation (by FSH and HCG or chlomiphene alone), it is more severe in patients who conceive.

2. Pathologic Features

The ovaries are both enlarged by large thin-walled cysts (up to 35 cm). They are filled with clear or hemorrhagic fluid.

Microscopically, the cysts are lined by the luteinized granulosa and theca cells, but many lose their granulosa lining and are covered only by the luteinized theca. The edematous stroma may also contain large clusters of luteinized stromal cells.

Differential diagnosis includes large solitary luteinized follicle cyst (unilateral and unilocular) and ovarian cystic tumors.

VI. ENDOMETRIOSIS

Endometriosis is one of the most common gynecological diseases that may affect more than 10% of all premenopausal women.[36] Endometriosis is a chronic disease in which tissue like the endometrium is found outside the uterine cavity. This aberrant tissue develops into growths or lesions, which respond to the menstrual cycle in the same way that the tissue of the uterine lining does: each month the tissue builds up, breaks down, and sheds. However, unlike the lining of the uterus, the tissue has no way of leaving the body. The result is internal bleeding, degeneration of blood and tissue shed, inflammation of the surrounding areas, and formation of scar tissue. In addition, adhesion to ovaries, bowel, bladder, intestines and/or other areas of the pelvic cavity can occur.

A. Diagnosis Criteria

The most common symptoms of endometriosis are painful periods, fatigue, exhaustion, diarrhea and painful bowel movements at time of period, abdominal bloating, pain at ovulation, and heavy or irregular periods. However, symptoms can vary greatly in severity, ranging from no or mild, to moderate or severe symptoms, even infertility (30–40% of cases). The amount of pain associated with the disease is not related to the extent or the size of the implants. The variety of symptoms reflects the complexity of endometriosis. It is not always a straightforward disease which is easy to detect, and many of the symptoms listed above could be caused by several other conditions.

Therefore, the only way a positive diagnosis of endometriosis can be made currently is via surgery, either a laparoscopy or the more invasive laparotomy. These techniques show the location, the size, and the extent of the growths. The difficulty in diagnosing endometriosis may explain the delay notified between the onset of pain symptoms and the surgical diagnosis (from 8–12 years).[37, 38]

B. Biological Characteristics

1. Elevated Estrogen Level

Numerous observations suggest that endometriosis is an estrogen-dependent disease. First, expression of estrogen and progesterone receptors has been demonstrated in ectopic endometrium. Secondly, the usefulness of gonadotropin-releasing hormone agonists in suppressing ovarian steroidogenesis and progestins in the management of endometriosis is well recognized. In addition, the responsiveness of endometriosis to estrogen and progesterone is also evident from hormone-dependent histological changes in this tissue similar to those in eutopic endometrium. A few years ago the delivery of estrogen to endometriotic implants had been assumed to be only via the circulating blood in an endocrine fashion. Recently, it has been demonstrated that endometriotic implants present a pattern of expression different from the eutopic endometrium, i.e., expression of aromatase and deficiency in 17β-hydroxysteroid dehydrogenase type 2 which may lead to increased local concentrations of estradiol-17β by, respectively, enhancing its production and diminishing its metabolism.[39] These findings have allowed the development of new treatment strategies with the successful use of aromatase inhibitor to treat cases of endometriosis.

C. Molecular Characteristics

1. Associated Gene Polymorphisms

Gene polymorphisms are not directly related to a certain disease but they may be implicated in an increased risk of numerous diseases. Three main classes of genes have been studied to look for a relationship between polymorphisms and endometriosis.[40]

a. Phase II Detoxification Enzymes

Three members of the phase II detoxification pathway have been studied: the glutathione S transferases M1 (GSTM1) and T1 (GSTT1) and the arylamine *N*-acetyltransferase 2 (NAT2). These enzymes are involved in the two-stage detoxification of numerous environmental toxins including dioxins. Contradictory results have been obtained between ethnic groups as some authors reported a significant excess of GSTM1 null phenotype and NAT2 slow acetylators in Russian and French patients with endometriosis,[41–44] whereas studies of the British population have not confirmed this association.[45]

Hence, in certain populations, it seems that lack of GSTM1 enzyme activity or slow acetylation activity of NAT2 could be considered a risk factor for endometriosis, as in environmentally induced cancers. These associations could explain the link between dioxin exposure and risk of endometriosis that has been reported by numerous studies.[46–49] Nevertheless, as contradictory results have been obtained between ethnic groups, further studies are necessary with more cases to definitively assess the implication of these polymorphisms in the endometriosis.

b. Galactose Metabolism

The galactose-1-phosphate uridyl transferase (GALT) catalyses the production of glucose-1-phosphate and uridyl diphosphate-galactose from galactose-1-phosphate and uridyl diphosphate-galactose-glucose and constitutes the main pathway of galactose metabolism in humans. Impairment of the GALT gene can lead to accumulation of galactose and other metabolites, which among other traits have been associated with premature ovarian failure. The most common mutation of the GALT gene is N314D, with GALT activity reduced from 75–50% for N314D heterozygotes and homozygotes, respectively. The N314D variant, which has been associated with ovarian cancer, early menopause, and Müllerian anomalies, has been found overrepresented in American women with endometriosis.[50] This result is in discrepancy with those reported in the British population.[51, 52] Hence, these last results suggest that it is more likely that this polymorphism is in linkage imbalance with a disease susceptibility locus.

c. Hormone Receptor

The estrogen receptor (ER) gene presents two types of polymorphism (one two-allele PvuII polymorphism and a multiallele (TA)n repeat) which have been used for association studies. As the ectopic endometrium expresses persistent ER with hormonal independence during the luteal phase and possibly altered biologic activity, Georgiou *et al.* [53] have looked for an association between endometriosis and the ER gene polymorphisms. They found in endometriosis patients a significant increase in the frequency of the PvuII allele (0.72 versus 0.49) and in the median repeats of the (TA)n multiallele polymorphism (15 versus 20). These results taken together with previous ones that reported an association between the PvuII allele and a low production of oocytes per follicle and fewer pregnancy [54] suggest not only an association between ER gene polymorphisms and endometriosis but also that endometriosis may be associated with genes that confer infertility.

2. Acquired Genetic Alterations

Although endometriosis is a benign condition, it shares common characteristics with malignancy including local invasion and metastases. The identification of somatic genetic events in endometriosis tissues confirms this notion. Thus, chromosomal loss or gain may play a role in the development and/or progression of endometriosis.

a. Chromosomal Gains and Oncogenes

Chromosomal gains are less frequently found than loss in endometriosis. Amplified loci have been identified on chromosomes 1q, 6q, 7q, and 17q and trisomy 11 has been reported.[55, 56] Studies of frequently altered oncogenes in tumors have shown that only c-myc is overexpressed in endometriosis (50% of cases), [57, 58] whereas cerb-B2 and K-ras seem not to be involved.[57, 59]

b. Chromosomal Loss and Tumor Suppressor Genes

TP53, a frequently tumor suppressor gene implicated in various tumor types, seems not to play an important role in endometriosis as only one mutation was found in more than 50 endometriosis cases.[59–61]

In order to identify other tumor suppressor genes that may be involved in this pathogenesis numerous loci and even the entire genome have been tested for loss of chromosomal segments in endometriosis. Losses have been observed at different loci such as 1p36.3, 5p, 6q, 9p21, 11q23.3, and 22q13 (in 15–50% of the cases). These results support the notion that tumor suppressor gene inactivation may play a role in the development of at least a subset of endometriosis cases. In addition, the observations of Jiang *et al.* [60, 61] suggest that endometrioid carcinomas may arise through malignant transformation of endometriotic lesions as identical genetic lesions are detected both in endometriosis and in adjacent endometrioid carcinoma. During the transformation of the benign lesions in carcinomas, additional loci may be lost and may correspond to those lost specifically in endometriosis adjacent to carcinomas and in carcinomas. Potential candidate genes can be suspected in some of the above-cited regions (22q12: neurofibromatose type 2 gene—*NF2*; 9p21: *GALT, CDKN2*; 6q: superoxyde dismutase gene 2—*SOD2*) but to date, none have been clearly implicated.

D. Pathologic Features

Grossly, an endometriotic cyst almost always contains old rusty blood with a brownish tinge, earning it the name chocolate cyst (Fig. 4.5).[62] The appearance of a chocolate cyst does not necessarily imply endometriosis, because there are other hemorrhagic cysts of the ovary which may look the same. They include follicular cyst, simple serous cyst, and

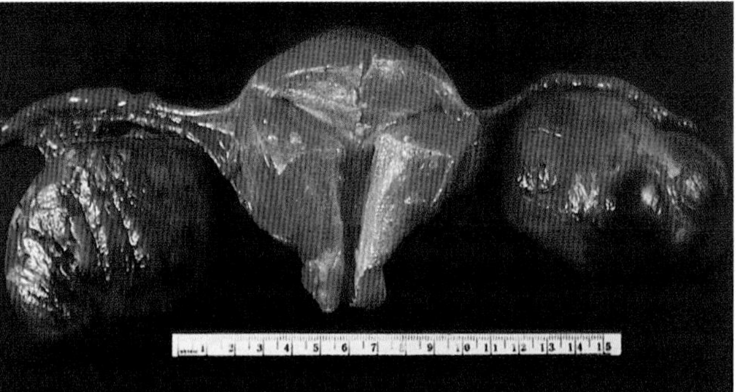

FIGURE 4.5 Bilateral ovarian endometriosis. Notice the numerous chocolate cysts.

the corpus luteum cyst. The final diagnosis must always be microscopic.

Early foci of endometriosis may not be discernible grossly, due to the absence of hemorrhage, but microscopically, they have the classical pattern of endometrium. Later, this pattern may be obscured by the degenerative changes caused by repeated menstrual discharges. As a result, only small fragments of residual endometrium remain in the lining, while most of it consists of the numerous hemosiderin-laden macrophages. Adjacent areas of the ovary usually show significant fibrosis.

In some cases, no endometrial lining can be identified, and a diagnosis of unequivocal endometriosis may be possible only if a rim of subadjacent endometrial stroma persists. When a granulation tissue has replaced the cyst lining and stroma, this appearance "strongly suggests" endometriosis. Discovery of endometriosis at other sites supports the diagnosis. Progestational changes may occur during pregnancy or progestin treatment—decidual reaction and atrophy of the glands. Atrophic changes and shrinkage of the lesions are usual after menopause or in premenopausal patients treated with danazol or oral contraceptives. The lining of the endometriotic glands may be hyperplastic or atypical. These changes may be reactive or result from estrogenic stimulus or tamoxifen therapy.[63, 64] But they may merge with neoplasm or precede it, suggesting a potential premalignant lesion.[65]

E. Associated Increased Risks

Malignant ovarian tumors have been described in up to 0.8% of cases of ovarian endometriosis. Endometrioid carcinoma and clear cell carcinoma account, respectively, for 75 and 15% of carcinoma arising within ovarian endometriosis.[65]

Different nongynecological tumors or pathologic conditions have been described in association with endometriosis, such as breast cancers, non-Hodgkin's,[66] melanoma,[67, 68] and dysplastic nevi in younger women of reproductive age.[67]

VII. INFLAMMATORY LESIONS

Involvement of the ovary by inflammation is usually secondary to pelvic inflammatory disease (PID).

A. Infectious Lesions

1. PID

PID is usually caused by the spread from salpingitis and typically takes the form of a tubo-ovarian abscess, which is usually bilateral.[69] Occasionally, the disease is a complication of an intrauterine device (IUD).[70] The disease is silent in half of the cases, the usual clinical symptoms being pelvic or abdominal pain, adnexal mass, vaginal discharge, and fever.

The appearance of the ovaries varies, depending on whether PID is acute or chronic. With acute inflammation, the surface of the ovary may be covered by an exudate. It is usually adherent to the fallopian tube, which is also inflamed. One or several abscesses may develop. The process may spread to the adherent fallopian tube with formation of the so-called "tubo-ovarian" abscess. A healed abscess may be transformed into tubo-ovarian cysts.

With resolution of acute PID, fibrous adhesions are formed around the ovary, and together with a smoldering infection of the fallopian tube, the process is known as chronic PID. There is an increase in cystic follicles and follicular and corpus luteum cysts in PID. This may be explained by altered blood supply.[2] Rarely bacterial oophoritis is observed without salpingitis resulting from direct or lymphatic spread of an intestinal infection, or postoperatively.[71] Blood-borne infections are infrequent.

2. Tuberculosis

Among granulomatous infections, the most common is tuberculosis.[72] It is almost always secondary to tubal disease, occurring in about 10–50% of the cases of genital tuberculosis. Elevation of serum CA-125 and granulomas of the adjacent peritoneum may mimic ovarian cancer. The ovaries are typically adherent to the tubal ampullae and the involvement is typically superficial (limited to the cortex).

3. Actinomycosis

The increased frequency of ovarian actinomycosis in the last three decades is associated with the use of IUDs.[73] The IUD is in place for more than 3 years. Abscesses are usually multiple and unilateral. They involve the ovary and the fallopian tube. Microscopic findings are sulfur granules admixed with a nonspecific inflammatory infiltrate composed of neutrophils and foamy histiocytes.

4. Miscellaneous Infections

Cytomegalic viral infection in the immunocompromised patients may involve ovaries and produce focal cortical necrosis.[74]

Parasitic infections affecting the ovaries include schistosomiasis and *Enterobius vermicularis*.[75, 76]

B. Noninfectious Lesions

Direct extension of Crohn's disease from the adjacent bowel may produce granulomatous inflammation in the ovary, and masquerade as ovarian tumors or tubo-ovarian abscesses.[77] Sarcoidosis and malacoplakia rarely affect the ovaries.[78]

Foreign body granulomas are related to the presence of exogenous foreign material, in ovaries and peritoneal surface, mimicking a malignant tumor at operation.[77]

References

1. Russel, P., and Farnsworth, A. (1997). Dysfunctional cysts. *In* "Surgical Pathology of the Ovaries" (P. Russel, and A. Farnsworth, eds.), pp. 115–130. Churchill Livingstone, New York.
2. Bychkov, V. (1990). Ovarian pathology in chronic pelvic inflammatory disease. *Gynecol. Obstet. Invest.* 30, 31–33.
3. Piver, M. S., Williams, L. J., and Marcuse P. M. (1970). Influence of luteal cysts on menstrual function. *Obstet. Gynecol.* 35, 740–751.
4. Sakala, E. P., Leon, Z. A., and Rouse G. A. (1991). Management of antenatally diagnosed foetal ovarian cyst. *Obstet. Gynecol. Surv.* 46, 407–414.
5. O'Hagen, D. B., Pudifin, J., and Mickel R. E. (1985). Antenatal detection of foetal ovarian cyst by real time ultrasound. A case report. *S. Afri. Med. J.* 67, 471.
6. Rizzo, N., Gabrielli, S., and Perolo A. (1989). Prenatal diagnosis and management of foetal ovarian cysts. *Prenatal Diagno.* 9, 97.
7. Danon, M., Robboy, S. J., Kim, S. *et al.* (1975). Cushing's syndrome, sexual precocity and polyostotic fibrous dysplasia (Albright Syndrome) in infancy. *J. Pediatr.* 87, 917–921.
8. Lentz, S. (1985). Ultrasonic study of follicular maturation, ovulation and development of corpus luteum during normal menstrual cycles. *Acta Obstet. Gynecol. Scand.* 64, 15–19.
9. Clement, P. B. (1993). Tumor-like lesions of the ovary associated with pregnancy. *Int. J. Gynecol. Pathol.* 12, 108–115.
10. Yee, H., Greenbaum, E., Lerner, J., Heller, D., and Timor-Trisch, I. E. (1994). Transvaginal sonographic characterization combined with cytologic evaluation in the diagnosis of ovarian and adnexal cysts. *Diagn. Cytopathol.* 10, 107–112.
11. Vacher-Lavenu, M. C., and Chapron, M. C. (1999). Ovarian puncture: Supposed functional cysts. *Ann. Pathol.* 19, 413–420.
12. Mulvany, N. J. (1996). Aspiration cytology of ovarian cysts and cystic neoplasms. A study of 325 aspirates. *Acta Cytol.* 40, 911–920.
13. Ganjiei, P., Dickinson, B., Harrison, T., Nassiri, M., and Lu, Y. (1997). Aspiration cytology of neoplastic and non neoplastic ovarian cysts: is it accurate? *Int. J. Gynecol. Pathol.* 15, 94–101.
14. Lobo R. A., and Carmina, E. (2000). The importance of diagnosing the polycystic ovary syndrome. *Ann. Intern. Med.* 132, 989–993.
15. Zawadski, J. K., and Dunaif, A. (1992). Diagnostic criteria for polycystic ovary syndrome: Towards a rational approach. *In* "Current Issue in Endocrinology and Metabolism: Polycystic Ovary Syndrome" (A. Dunaif, J. R. Givens, F. P. Haseltine, and G. R. Merriam, eds.), pp. 377–384. Blackwell Scientific Publications, Cambridge, MA.

16. Dunaif, A., Hoffman, A. R., Scully, R. E. *et al.* (1985). Clinical, biochemical and ovarian morphologic features in women with acanthosis nigricans and masculinization. *Obstet. Gynecol.* 66, 545–552.
17. Franks, S., Gharani, N., and McCarthy, M. (1999). Genetic abnormalities in polycystic ovary syndrome. *Ann. Endocrinol.* (*Paris*) 60, 131–133.
18. Nagamani, M., and Stuart, C. A. (1990). Specific binding sites for insulin-like growth factor I in the ovarian stroma of women with polycystic ovarian disease and stromal hyperthecosis. *Am. J. Obstet. Gynecol.* 163, 1992–1997.
19. Nagamani, M., and Urban, R. J. (1999). Increased expression of messenger ribonucleic acid encoding cytochrome P450 cholesterol side-chain cleavage and P450 17alpha-hydroxylase enzymes in ovarian hyperthecosis. *Fertil. Steril.* 71, 328–333.
20. Speiser, P. W., Susin, M., Sasano, H., Bohrer, S., and Markowitz, J. (2000). Ovarian hyperthecosis in the setting of portal hypertension. *J. Clin. Endocrinol. Metab.* 85, 873–877.
21. Nagamani, M., Osuampke, C., and Kelver, M. E.(1999). Increased bioactive luteinizing hormone levels and bio/immuno ratio in women with hyperthecosis of the ovaries: Possible role of hyperinsulinemia. *J. Clin. Endocrinol. Metab.* 84 ,1685–1689.
22. Judd, H. L., Scully, R. E., Herbst A. L. *et al.* (1973). Familial hyperthecosis: comparison of endocrinologic and histologic findings with polycystic ovarian disease. *Am. J. Obstet. Gynecol.* 117, 976–982.
23. Russel, P., and Farnsworth, A. (1997). Stromal Hyperplasia and hyperthecosis. *In* "Surgical Pathology of the Ovaries" (P. Russel, and A. Farnsworth, eds.), pp. 137–143. Churchill Livingstone, New York.
24. Sluijmer, A. V., Heineman, M. J., Koudstaal, J., Theunissen, P. H., de Jong F. H., and Evers, J. L. (1998). Relationship between ovarian production of estrone, estradiol, testosterone, and androstenedione and the ovarian degree of stromal hyperplasia in postmenopausal women. *Menopause* 5, 207–210.
25. Young, R. H., and Scully, R. E. (1984). Fibromatosis and massive edema of the ovary possibly related entities: A report of 14 cases of fibromatosis and 111 cases of massive edema. *Int. J. Gynecol. Pathol.* 3, 153–178.
26. Turan, C., Ugur, M., Mungan, T., Taner, D., Aydogdu, T., and Cobanoglu, O. (1996). Massive ovarian oedema: A non neoplastic adnexal mass mistaken for a neoplasm. *Aus. N. Z. J. Obstet. Gynaecol.* 36, 96–97.
27. Jacobs, S., and Prabhakar, B. R. (1996). Massive oedema of the ovary—a tumor-like condition—report of two cases. *Ind. J. Cancer* 33, 181–182.
28. Russel, P., and Farnsworth, A. (1997). Leydig cells hyperplasia. *In* "Surgical Pathology of the Ovaries" (P. Russel, and A. Farnsworth, eds.), pp. 145–146. Churchill Livingstone, New York.
29. Taylor, H. C., Pillay, I., and Setrakian, S. (2000). Diffuse stromal Leydig cell hyperplasia: A unique cause of postmenopausal hyperandrogenism and virilization. *Mayo Clin. Proc.* 75, 288–292.
30. Sternberg, W. H., and Barclay, D. L. (1996). Luteoma of pregnancy. *Am. J. Obstet. Gynecol.* 95, 165–184.
31. Manganiello, P. D., Adams, L. V., Harris, R. D., and Ornvold, K. (1995). Virilization during pregnancy with spontaneous resolution postpartum: case report and review of the English literature. *Obstet. Gynecol. Surv.* 50, 404–410.
32. Kommoss, F., Oliva, E., Bhan, A. K. *et al.* (1998). Inhibin expression in ovarian tumors and tumor-like lesions: an immunohistochemical study. *Mod. Pathol.* 11, 656–664.
33. Check, J. H., Choe, J. K., and Nazari, A. (2000). Hypereactio luteinalis despite the absence of a corpus luteum and suppressed serum follicle stimulating concentrations in a triplet pregnancy. *Hum. Reprod.* 15, 1043–1045.
34. Tanaka, Y., Yanagihara, T., Ueta, M. *et al.* (2001). Naturally conceived twin pregnancy with hypereactio luteinalis, causing hyperandrogenism and maternal virilization. *Acta Obstet. Gynecol. Scand.* 80, 277–278.
35. Csapo, Z., Szabo, I., Toth, M., Devenyi, N., and Papp, Z. (1999). Hypereactio luteinalis in a normal singleton pregnancy. A case report. *J. Reprod. Med.* 44, 53–56.
36. Mahmood, T. A., and Templeton, A. (1991). Prevalence and genesis of endometriosis. *Hum. Reprod.* 6, 544–549.
37. Kennedy, S., Mardon, H., and Barlow, D. (1995). Familial endometriosis. *J. Assist. Reprod. Genet.* 12, 32–34.
38. Hadfield, R., Mardon, H., Barlow, D., and Kennedy, S. (1996). Delay in the diagnosis of endometriosis: A survey of women from the USA and the UK. *Hum. Reprod.* 11, 878–880.
39. Bulun, S. E., Zeitoun, K. M., Takayama, K., and Sasano, H. (2000). Estrogen biosynthesis in endometriosis: Molecular basis and clinical relevance. *J. Mol. Endocrinol.* 25, 35–42.
40. Campbell, I. G., and Thomas, E. J. (2001). Endometriosis: candidate genes. *Hum. Reprod. Update* 7, 15–20.
41. Baranov, V. S., Ivaschenko, T. E., Bakay, B. *et al.* (1996). Proportion of the GSTM1 0/0 genotype in some Slavic populations and its correlation with cystic fibrosis and some multifactorial diseases. *Hum. Genet.* 97, 516–520.
42. Baranova, H., Bothorishvilli, R., Canis, M. *et al.* (1997). Glutathione S-transferase M1 gene polymorphism and susceptibility to endometriosis in a French population. *Mol. Hum. Reprod.* 3, 775–780.
43. Baranov, V. S., Ivashchenko, T. E., Shved, N.I. *et al.* (1999). Genetic factors of predisposition to endometriosis and response to its treatment *Genetika* 35, 243–248.
44. Baranova, H., Canis, M., Ivaschenko, T. *et al.* (1999). Possible involvement of arylamine *N*-acetyltransferase 2, glutathione S-transferases M1 and T1 genes in the development of endometriosis. *Mol. Hum. Reprod.* 5, 636–641.
45. Baxter, S. W., Thomas, E. J., and Campbell, I. G. (2001). GSTM1 null polymorphism and susceptibility to endometriosis and ovarian cancer. *Carcinogenesis* 22, 63–65.
46. Rier, S. E., Martin, D. C., Bowman, R. E., and Becker, J. L. (1995). Immunoresponsiveness in endometriosis: Implications of estrogenic toxicants. *Environ. Health Perspect.* 103, 151–156.
47. Mayani, A., Barel, S., Soback, S., and Almagor, M. (1997). Dioxin concentrations in women with endometriosis. *Hum. Reprod.* 12, 373–375.
48. Koninckx, P. R., Braet, P., Kennedy, S. H., and Barlow, D. H. (1994). Dioxin pollution and endometriosis in Belgium. *Hum. Reprod.* 9, 1001–1002.
49. Rier, S. E., Martin, D. C., Bowman, R. E., Dmowski, W. P., and Becker J. L. (1993). Endometriosis in rhesus monkeys (*Macaca mulatta*) following chronic exposure to 2,3,7,8-tetrachlorodibenzo-*p*-dioxin. *Fundam. Appl. Toxicol.* 21, 433–441.
50. Cramer, D. W., Hornstein, M. D., Ng, W. G., and Barbieri, R. L. (1996). Endometriosis associated with the N314D mutation of galactose-1-phosphate uridyl transferase (GALT). *Mol. Hum. Reprod.* 2, 149–152.
51. Hadfield, R. M., Manek, S., Nakago, S. *et al.* (1999). Absence of a relationship between endometriosis and the N314D polymorphism of galactose-1-phosphate uridyl transferase in a UK population. *Mol. Hum. Reprod.* 5, 990–993.
52. Morland, S. J., Jiang, X., Hitchcock, A., Thomas, E. J., and Campbell, I. G. (1998). Mutation of galactose-1-phosphate uridyl transferase and its association with ovarian cancer and endometriosis. *Int. J. Cancer* 77, 825–827.
53. Georgiou, I., Syrrou, M., Bouba, I. *et al.* (1999). Association of estrogen receptor gene polymorphisms with endometriosis. *Fertil. Steril.* 72, 164–166.
54. Georgiou, I., Konstantelli, M., Syrrou, M., Messinis, I. E., and Lolis, D. E. (1997). Oestrogen receptor gene polymorphisms and ovarian stimulation for in-vitro fertilization. *Hum. Reprod.* 12, 1430–1433.
55. Shin, J. C., Ross, H. L., Elias, S., Nguyen, D. D., Mitchell-Leef, D., Simpson, J. L., and Bischoff, F. Z. (1997). Detection of chromosomal aneuploidy in endometriosis by multi-color fluorescence in situ hybridization (FISH). *Hum. Genet.* 100, 401–406.

56. Gogusev, J., Bouquet de la Joliniere, J., Telvi, L. *et al.* (1999). Detection of DNA copy number changes in human endometriosis by comparative genomic hybridization. *Hum. Genet.* 105, 444–451.
57. Schneider, J., Jimenez, E., Rodriguez, F., and del Tanago, J. G. (1998). c-myc, c-erb-B2, nm23 and p53 expression in human endometriosis. *Oncol. Rep.* 5, 49–52.
58. Schenken, R. S., Johnson, J. V., and Riehl, R. M. (1991). C-myc protooncogene polypeptide expression in endometriosis. *Am. J. Obstet. Gynecol.* 164, 1031–1037.
59. Vercellini, P., Trecca, D., Oldani, S., Fracchiolla, N. S., Neri, A., and Crosignani, P. G. (1994). Analysis of p53 and ras gene mutations in endometriosis. *Gynecol. Obstet. Invest.* 38, 70–71
60. Jiang, X., Morland, S. J., Hitchcock, A., Thomas, E. J., and Campbell, I. G. (1998). Alletotyping of endometriosis with adjacent ovarian carcinoma reveals common lineage. *Cancer Res.* 58, 1707–1712.
61. Jiang, X., Hitchcock, A., Bryan, E. J. *et al.* (1996). Microsatellite analysis of endometriosis reveals loss of heterozygosity at ovarian tumor suppressor gene loci. *Cancer Res.* 56, 3534–3539.
62. Scurry, J., Whitehead, J., and Healey, M. (2001). Classification of ovarian endometriotic cysts. *Int. J. Gynecol. Pathol.* 20, 147–154.
63. Moutits, M. J., de Vries E. G., Willemse, P. H., Ten Hoor, K. A., Hollema, H., and Van der Zee, A. (2001). Tamoxifen treatmant and gynecologic side effects: A review. *Obstet. Gynecol.* 97, 855–866.
64. Chapman, W. B. (2001). Developments in the pathology of ovarian tumors. *Curr. Opin. Obstet. Gynecol.* 13, 53–59.
65. Stern, R. C., Dash, R., Bentley, R. C., Snyder, M. J., Haney, A. F., and Robboy, S. J. (2001). Malignancy in endometriosis: frequency and comparison of ovarian and extra ovarian types. *Int. J. Gynecol. Pathol.* 20, 133–139.
66. Brinton, L. A., Gridley, G., Persson, I., Baron, J., and Bergqvist, A. (1997). Cancer risk after a hospital discharge diagnosis of endometriosis. *Am. J. Obstet. Gynecol.* 176, 572–579.
67. Hornstein, M. D., Thomas, P. P., Sober, A. J., Wyshak, G., Albright, N. L., and Frisch, R. E. (1997). Association between endometriosis, dysplastic naevi and history of melanoma in women of reproductive age. *Hum. Reprod.* 12, 143–145.
68. Wyshak, G., Frisch, R. E., Albright, N. L., Albright, T. E., and Schiff, I. (1989). Reproductive factors and melanoma of the skin among women. *Int. J. Dermatol.* 28, 527–530.
69. Eschenbach, D. A. (1980). Epidemiology and diagnosis of acute pelvic inflammatory disease. *Obstet. Gynecol.* 55, 142S–152S.
70. Kaufman, D. W., Shapiro, S., Rosenberg, L. *et al.* (1980). Intrauterine contraceptive device use and pelvic inflammatory disease. *Am. J. Obstet. Gynecol.* 136, 159–162.
71. Mueller, B. A., Daling, J. R., Moore, D. E. *et al.* (1986). Appendectomy and the risk of tubal infertility. *N. Engl. J. Med.* 315, 1506–1508.
72. Sinha, P., Johnson, A. N., and Chidamberan-Pillai, S. (2000). Pelvic tuberculosis: An uncommon gynaecological problem presenting as ovarian mass. *BJOG* 107, 139–140.
73. Muller-Hozner, E., Ruth, N. R., Ali, V., *et al.* (1995). IUD associated pelvic actinomycosis: A report of five cases. *Int. J. Gynecol. Pathol.* 14, 70–74.
74. Subietas, A., Deppisch, L. M., and Astrloa, J. (1977). Cytomegalovirus oophoritis. *Hum. Pathol.* 8, 285–292.
75. Tiboldi, T. (1978). Involvement of human and primate ovaries in schistosomiasis. *Ann. Soc. Belge. Med. Trop.* 58, 361–373.
76. Mc Mahon, J. N., Habibi, H., Moshref, A., and Meehan, F. B. (1984). Enterobius granulomas of the uterus, ovary and pelvic peritoneum: Two cases report. *Br. J. obstet. Gynaecol.* 91, 289–290.
77. Allen, D. C., and Calvert, C. H. (1995) Crohn's ileitis and salpingo-oophoritis. *Ulster Med.* 64, 95–97.
78. McCluggage, W. G., and Allen, D. C. (1997). Ovarian granulomas: a report of 32 cases. *J. Clin. Pathol.* 50, 324–327.

CHAPTER

5

Precancerous Lesions of the Ovary

LIANE DELIGDISCH

Departments of Pathology, and Obstetrics, Gynecology and Reproductive Science
The Mount Sinai School of Medicine and Hospital
New York, New York 10029

The natural history, etiology, and histogenesis of most ovarian tumors and especially of ovarian carcinomas is still poorly understood. The late diagnosis in the vast majority of ovarian carcinomas and the high lethality due to this neoplasm are related to the paucity of symptoms and virtual absence of any screening system. With laparoscopic surgery the ovaries become more accessible. Ovarian tumors can become available for study in their early invasive or preinvasive stages. The histological identification of the precursors of epithelial cancer have contributed to a significant decrease in other gynecologic cancers, such as cervical carcinoma and endometrial carcinoma. The identification of the actual tissue changes that characterize any early neoplastic process is indispensable for any screening program.

A number of publications have reported histologic and morphometric studies aimed at the identification of precursors of ovarian cancer.[1–4] As is the case with any dysplastic changes, the biological potential to progress to invasive cancer is not predictable, and probably depends on nonmorphological factors related to host defense mechanisms, heredity, and oncogenic activity. The histologic definition of ovarian dysplasia and/or ovarian intraepithelial neoplasia (OIN) is a first step for the understanding of early ovarian neoplasia. The vast majority of ovarian malignant neoplasms arise from the surface epithelium or germinal epithelium covering the ovarian surface as an extension of the peritoneal mesothelium. This is a cuboidal to flat layer of cells, resting on a basement membrane, often displaying tall columnar cells or papillary infoldings due to inflammatory or otherwise irritating processes, such as ovulation, endometriosis, and periovarian adhesions due to a variety of causes (Fig. 5.1). This layer of cells follows the natural "crevasses" of the ovarian surface (Fig. 5.2), resulting from ovarian nodular cortical hyperplasia and often ending up as cystic cavities ranging in size from microscopic to visible with the naked eye, generally called "inclusion cysts" (Fig. 5.3). Such cysts are very common in older age groups, but were also described in infantile ovaries.[5] On the other side, the mesothelial lining of the peritoneum, which is structurally similar to the surface epithelium of the ovary is rarely the site of malignant growth. Malignant mesothelioma is uncommon in females.[6] Is this due to the fact that the underlying ovarian tissue is highly active, steroidogenic, cycling, or ovulating? The dynamic processes taking place in the ovaries during the reproductive years are associated with changes in the morphology of the epithelial layer. Neoplastic and preneoplastic processes, however, are noted in the older age group characterized by receding, i.e., shrinking, and atrophy, of the ovaries after the cessation of cyclic ovulatory changes. Carcinogenesis is a multistep, time-related process, therefore a time lag between the ovarian active period and the actual development of cancer is understandable.

Hyperplastic or metaplastic processes commonly observed in ovaries during the reproductive years have to be distinguished from neoplastic and preneoplastic changes. They are related to the microtrauma of ovulation, seen more often in women receiving ovulation stimulation therapy,[7] to endometriosis, pelvic inflammatory disease (PID), etc. In metaplastic and hyperplastic changes the cells lining the ovarian surface may show ciliated, endometrioid, clear cell, eosinophilic metaplasia. They may also form papillary structures lined by cuboidal, hyperplastic cells and form deep invaginations into the stroma. These histological features have been described as a "cancer-prone phenotype" as they were seen more often in prophylactically removed ovaries.[4]

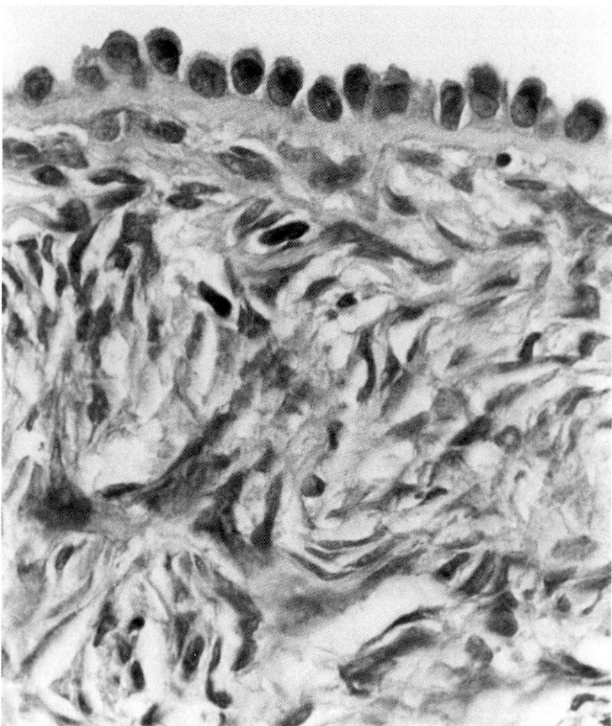

FIGURE 5.1 Ovarian surface epithelium on basement membrane overlying ovarian cortical stroma. H&E×400.

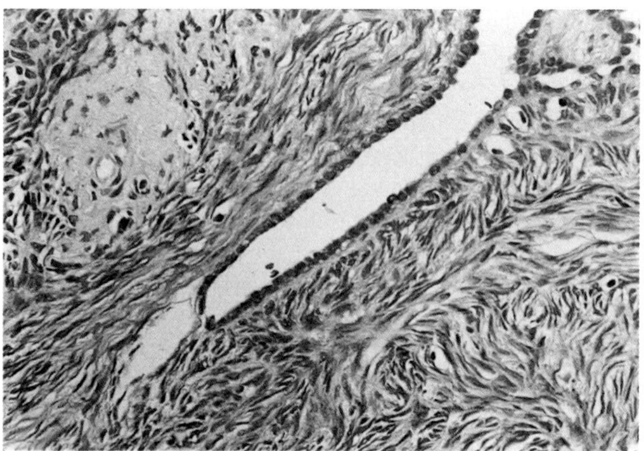

FIGURE 5.2 Papillary infolding of ovarian surface epithelium forming crevasse. H&E×100.

The criteria for dysplasia, as for any epithelial dysplastic growth, include changes in the tissue architecture such as piling-up (stratification), crowding of cells, loss of polarity, and cellular changes including increased nuclear-cytoplasmic ratio, nuclear irregularity (atypia) thickening and infolding of nuclear membranes, coarse chromatin clumping, clearing of nuclei, and prominent nucleoli. These changes can be observed by routine histologic examination. More accuracy is obtained by quantitating the individual patterns, and by a

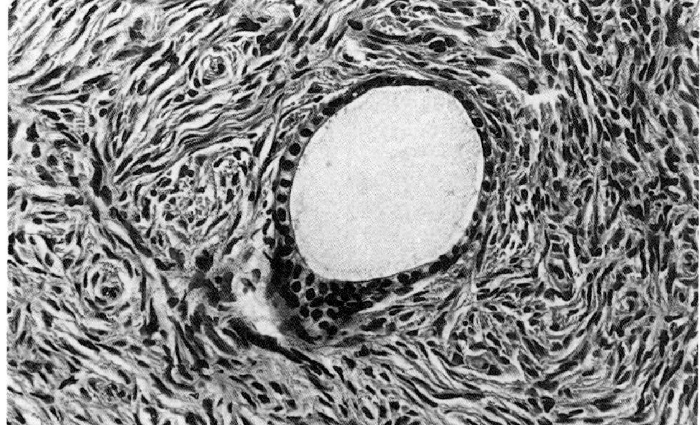

FIGURE 5.3 Ovarian epithelial inclusion cyst. H&E×100.

multivariate statistical analysis outlining the significance of the changes.

When and where should ovarian dysplasia be looked for? Of course, in patients who are at high risk to develop ovarian carcinoma, such as first-degree relatives of patients diagnosed to have ovarian cancer. A study of identical twin sisters of women with ovarian cancer [1] has revealed that their ovaries, removed prophylactically, with no gross abnormalities, display piling up of the surface epithelium, loss of polarity, and nuclear abnormalities consisting of increased nuclear-cytoplasmic ratio, chromatin clumping, prominent nucleoli, and nuclear clearing (Fig. 5.4). It is now estimated that genetic predisposition represents a strong risk factor for ovarian carcinoma.[8–11] The majority of breast and ovarian carcinoma families are linked to the BRCA1 gene and some cases of ovarian carcinoma are also apparent in breast carcinoma families linked to the BRCA2 gene.[12] It seems that >90% of familial ovarian carcinoma is due to inherited mutations in the BRCA1 breast-ovarian carcinoma susceptibility gene on chromosome 17q.[13] Familial susceptibility to cancer has been known to be transmitted with a particular allele of a genetic marker of known chromosomal location. Young women of Ashkenazi Jewish descent appear to be at particularly high risk because of the prevalence of the BRCA1 mutation 185 delAg.[14, 15] The prophylactically removed ovaries, a procedure now performed in numerous medical centers,[16, 17] have to be carefully examined in their entirety for occult neoplastic and/or dysplastic changes.[4, 18] A study of ovarian dysplasia in Ashkenazi Jewish women who tested positive for BRCA1 revealed an incidence of 77.6% ovarian dysplasia in grossly apparently normal ovaries,[18] confirming the high risk of developing ovarian carcinoma in this group.

Ovarian dysplasia can also be seen in the vicinity of ovarian neoplasms, contiguous to overt carcinoma, and to normal epithelium (Fig. 5.5), as in cervical dysplastia. Similar descriptions were made of dysplastic colonic, laryngeal, gastric, skin, etc., lesions that were identified as the periphery

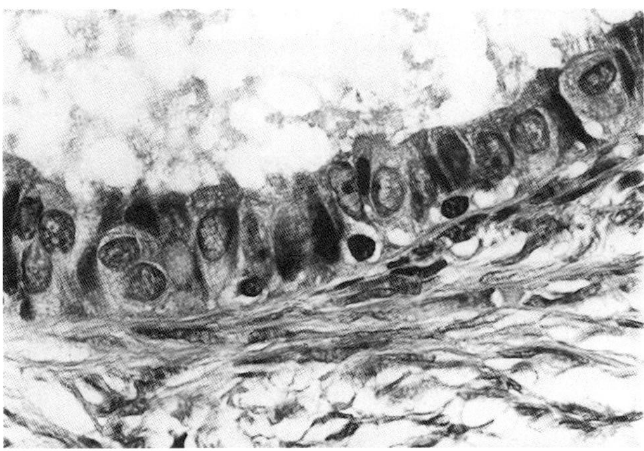

FIGURE 5.4 Ovarian dysplasia: loss of polarity, high nuclear-cytoplasmic ratio, chromatin clumping, prominent nucleoli, and nuclear clearing. H&E×1000.

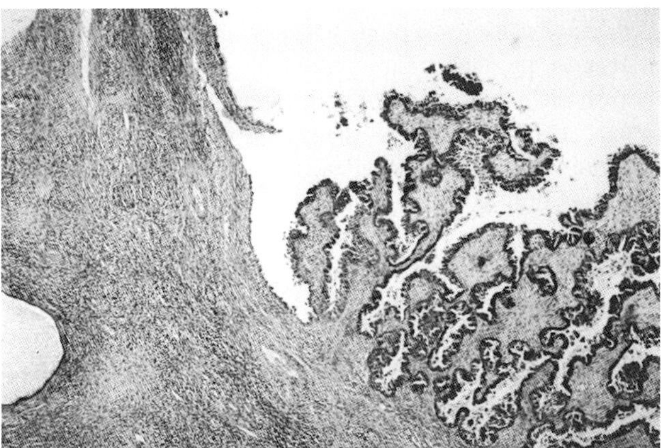

FIGURE 5.5 Ovarian dysplasia contiguous to overt carcinoma. Note also benign epithelial inclusion cyst. H&E×40.

("satellite") of overt carcinoma. Early stage ovarian carcinomas in which the neoplastic tissue is relatively confined, and adjacent noninvolved tissue is still preserved, have been suitable for the study of ovarian dysplasia.

In order to enhance the objectivity and accuracy of the diagnosis of ovarian dysplasia, or OIN, quantifiable morphologic criteria were evaluated by computerized image analysis. Interactive morphometric methods were used to assess the crowding, stratification, and loss of polarity by measuring the shortest distance between the center of nuclei and the basement membrane, and by counting the number of nuclei per unit of basement membrane (Fig. 5.6). Morphometric methods were also used to measure nuclear profiles, including perimeter, length, area, maximal chord, and circularity factor (Fig. 5.7). All these factors proved to be statistically significant, the most discriminating being the nuclear area and the distance between the nuclear center and the basement membrane.[2] A multivariate statistical analysis confirmed

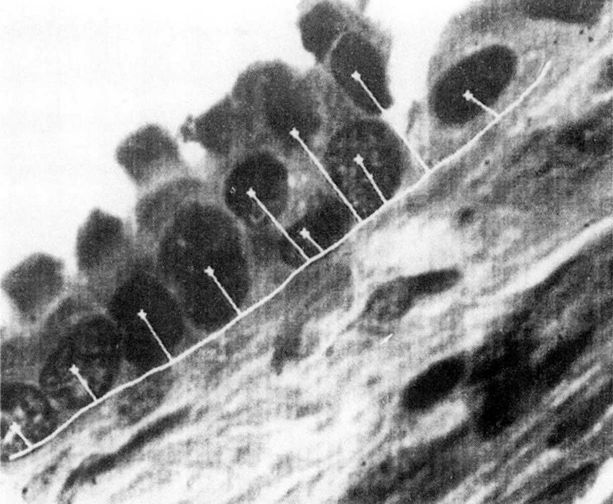

FIGURE 5.6 Morphometric analysis of crowding and stratification in dysplastic epithelium by tracing basement membrane and shortest distances from centers of nuclei to basement membrane.

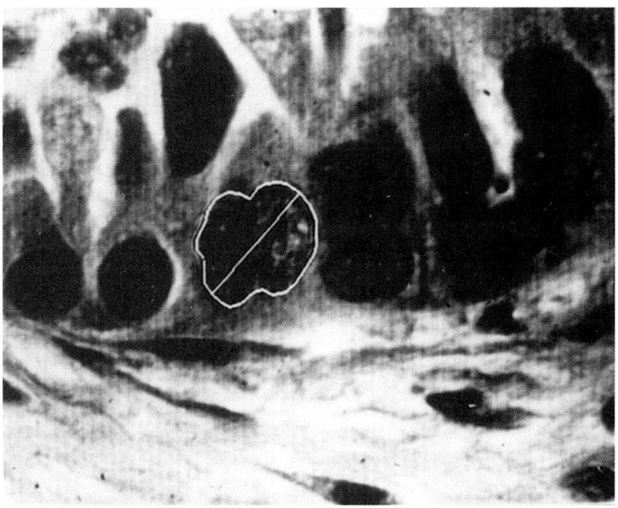

FIGURE 5.7 Morphometric analysis of nuclear profile measuring area, perimeter, and maximal chord.

the existence of dysplasia as a diagnostic category, distinct from normal and from carcinomatous epithelium. The values obtained for the dysplastic epithelium were numerically somewhat at mid-distance between normal and malignant. Nuclear area was 70 μm^2 for malignant, 44 μm^2 for dysplastic and 22 μm^2 for normal cells; on average, stratification measured by mean distances of nuclear center to basement membrane was 150 µm for malignant, 78 µm for dysplastic and 33 µm for normal tissue. Cell crowding measured by number of nuclei per unit of basement membrane were 400 in malignant, 240 in dysplastic, and 160 in normal epithelium. Subjective evaluation of histologic patterns, consistent with

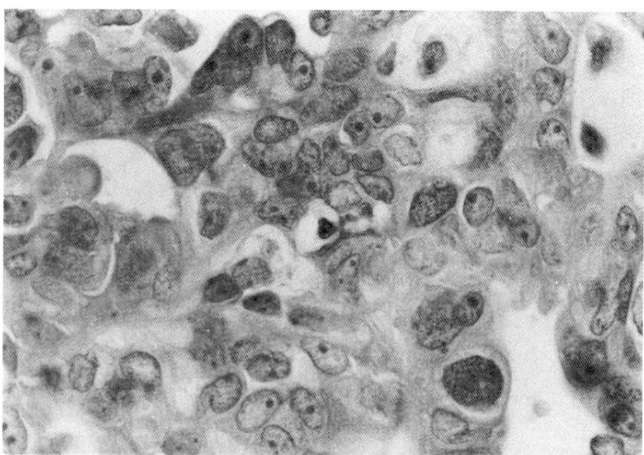

FIGURE 5.8 Malignant nuclei with coarse chromatin clumping and prominent nucleoli. H&E×1000.

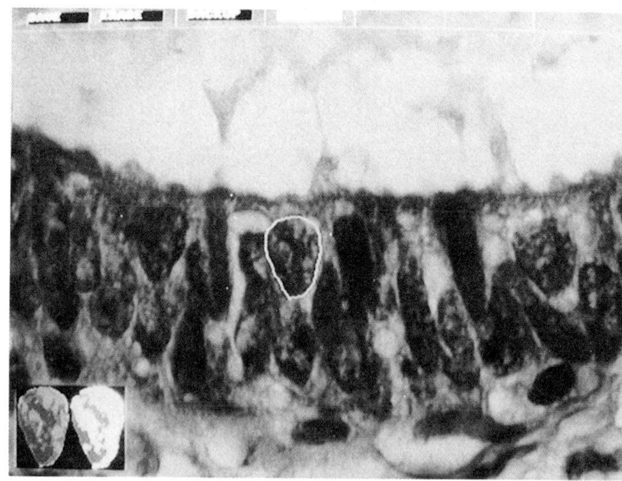

FIGURE 5.9 Histogram of dysplastic nucleus and quantitating dark, light, and gray textons.

dysplastic changes, was thus confirmed by a quantitative objective method. A database was established for the three diagnostic categories: normal, dysplasia, carcinoma, against which doubtful cases can be tested.[19]

A valuable addition to computed image analysis was the study of nuclear texture using a new method of quantification of nuclear chromatin aggregates.[20]

On routine histologic examination, the diagnosis of malignancy is often based on the characteristics of nuclear chromatin. Hyperchromatic nuclei, intranuclear clearing, coarse clumping of chromatin along with mitotic activity are characteristics of neoplastic tissue. Often there is nuclear pleomorphism consisting of an irregularity in shape, size, chromatin distribution, and staining properties of the nuclei. Obvious malignant changes are seen by simple histologic examination with routine hematoxylin-eosin stained sections (Fig. 5.8).

Subtle changes, however, as those described in ovarian dysplasia may not be as obvious to the observer and may require measurements provided by morphometric analysis.

Nuclear texture is a reflection of the chromatin structure. Histograms revealing "textons" (contiguous areas with similar levels of dark, light, or gray material) from individual nuclei were quantitated in terms of their respective areas and numbers per nucleus (Fig. 5.9).

A multivariate analysis of the findings, based on the progressive deterioration of the correlation between the size of the textons and the size of the containing nucleus as the degree of malignancy increases, confirmed again the existence of three diagnostic categories: normal, malignant, dysplastic. This morphometric study of intranuclear patterns added further accuracy to the diagnosis of ovarian dysplasia.

A number of techniques to evaluate nuclear texture had been used for fine needle aspirates of breast tissue [21, 22] and for ovarian dysplasia.[23]

A novel approach to assess the variations of intranuclear structures is by the autocorrelation procedure yielding tridimensional surface plots that show increasingly irregular images as the nuclear structure becomes less homogenous, with an increased degree of atypia from normal to dysplasia to cancer (Fig. 5.10). This method proved to be a powerful discriminant, especially when combined with the nuclear measurements used in previous studies.[18]

Ovarian dysplasia has been studied in two clinical settings: in noncancerous ovaries including those obtained by prophylactic oophorectomies for high risk or ovaries removed for reasons other than ovarian cancer (incidental dysplasia) or in areas adjacent to overt invasive ovarian cancer (adjacent dysplasia). The morphometric changes in these two groups have been compared by a highly sensitive statistical method using "neural networks."[23, 24] No significant difference was found between the two categories, thus supporting the similarity of the two conditions,[5–11] reminiscent of analogous situations seen in other dysplasias, associated or not with adjacent overt cancer, such as in the cervix, endometrium, colon, etc (Fig. 5.11).[23]

Incidental ovarian dysplasia has also been described in the contralateral ovaries of patients with unilateral ovarian carcinoma.[25] Not infrequently, ovarian epithelial inclusion cysts which are a common finding in both neoplastic and non-neoplastic ovaries, display a piled-up epithelial lining and nuclear atypia of various degrees of severity. The potential for malignant transformation of this tissue is unknown since it is surgically removed. Identification of the dysplastic ovarian lesion and the accessibility of the tissue could make a screening program possible.

At the present time, there is no implementation of a screening program for ovarian cancer. Serum tumor markers have not proven to be sensitive or specific enough for an early ovarian cancer screening.[26] As mentioned previously, in early ovarian carcinoma, the tissue adjacent to the tumor is suitable for the study of preinvasive lesions. With the advent

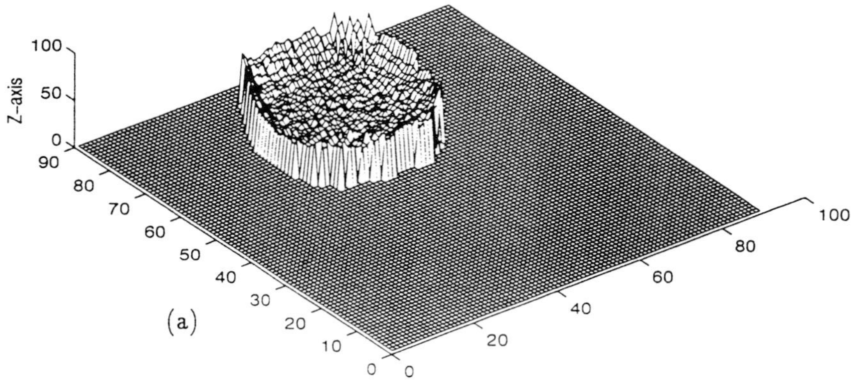

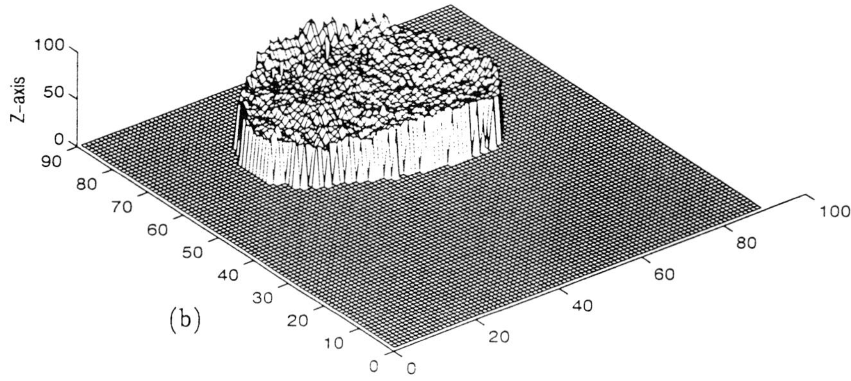

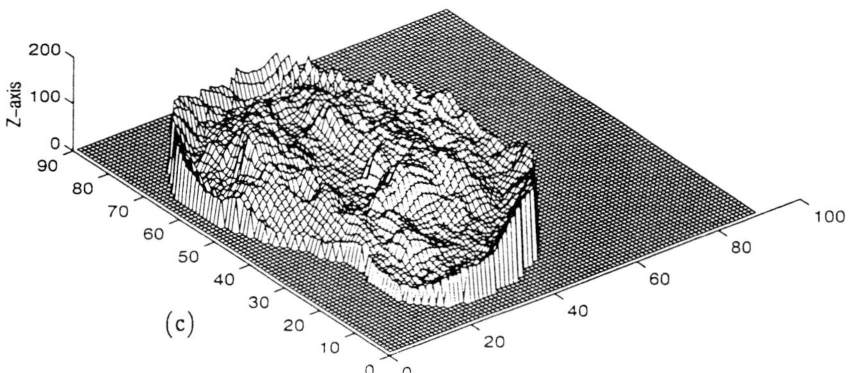

FIGURE 5.10 Three-dimensional surface plots of normal (a), dysplastic (b), and malignant (c) nuclei. Axes x and y are space conduits and the z-axis is the gray level intensity of each pixel. Note the progressive increase in nuclear size and surface complexity.

of laparoscopy, the ovary becomes more accessible and asymptomatic, low-stage ovarian cancer can be detected more readily. This may offer an opportunity for the study of changes that could precede epithelial neoplasia. The routine histologic description and the measurements performed by interactive methods of computerized image analysis on stratification, crowding, nuclear area, perimeter, and chromatin texture have revealed changes that are reproducible and recognizable by the practicing pathologist. The morphologic changes are intermediate between normal and cancerous tissue, as is the case in various other epithelial dysplasias (of the breast, larynx, uterine cervix, etc.).

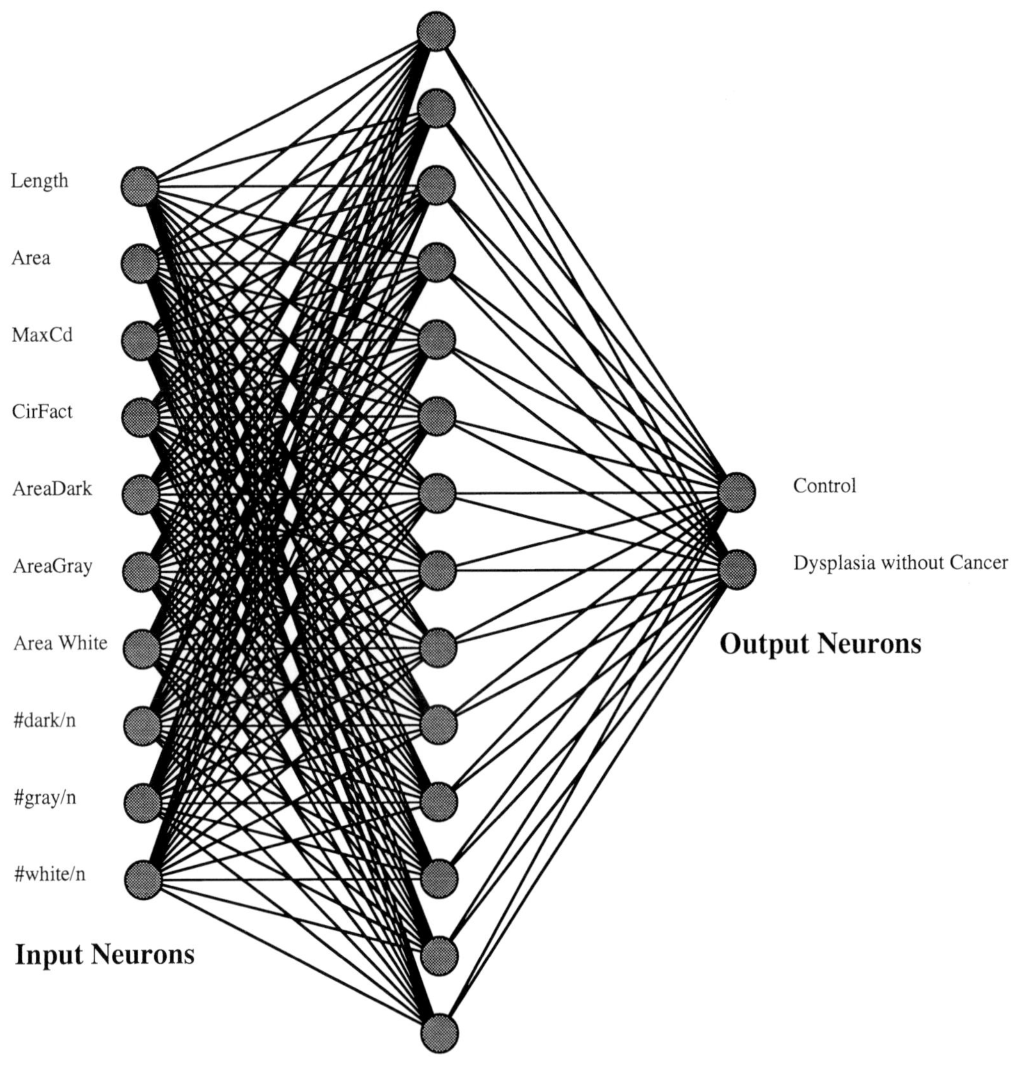

FIGURE 5.11 Neural network assessment demonstrating the difference between dysplastic (with and without cancer) and control nuclei.

Correlation with biological behavior, ploidy, and antigenic expression of oncogenes of cells diagnosed as dysplastic may shed more light on their potential to progress to overt cancer. It should be stressed again that major screening programs resulting in dramatic decrease in the morbidity and mortality due to cancer, such as those implemented a few decades ago for cervical cancer and for gastric cancer in Japan, were based on the identification of early morphologic changes. Could laparoscopy be helpful in the early detection of ovarian cancer in a similar way to colposcopy in cervical cancer? This raises the question of the possibility of detecting changes seen during laparoscopy that would suggest suspicious areas to be biopsied versus randomly performed laparoscopic biopsies. Such changes have yet to be described along with their microscopic counterparts.

It is of great interest to correlate the structural modifications of the dysplastic tissue with biological markers, DNA assessments, and oncogenic marker studies. A number of such studies are now in course (Fig. 5.12). The validation of both incidental and adjacent dysplasia by novel morphometric and statistical methods is an important step in identifying ovarian preneoplastic lesions. The diagnosis of incidental dysplasia identifies patients at risk, especially when diagnosed in women with family histories or carrying genetic mutations known to be associated with ovarian and/or breast cancer.

The increasing availability of tissue from prophylactic Oophorectomies in women at risk for ovarian cancer is promising both in terms of the discovery of occult cancer [27] and of identifying preneoplastic changes.[18, 28]

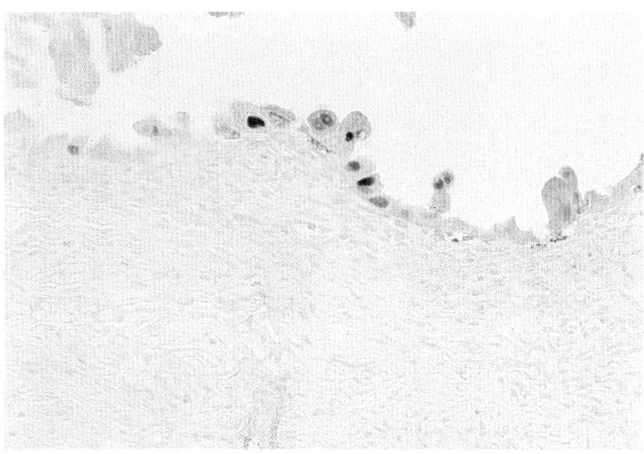

FIGURE 5.12 Immunohistologic stain for p53 showing positivity in ovarian dysplastic nuclei.

References

1. Gusberg, S. B., and Deligdisch, L. (1984). Ovarian dysplasia. A study of identical twins. *Cancer* 54, 1–4.
2. Deligdisch, L., and Gil, J. (1989). Characterization of ovarian dysplasia by interactive morphometry. *Cancer* 63, 748–755.
3. Gil, J., and Deligdisch, L. (1989). Interactive morphometric procedures and statistical analysis in the diagnosis of ovarian dysplasia and carcinoma. *Pathol. Res. Pract.* 185, 680–685.
4. Salazar, H., Godwin, A. K., Daly, M. B., Laub, P. B., Hogan, M., Rosenblum, N. *et al.* (1996). Microscopic benign and invasive malignant neoplasms in a cancer-prone phenotype in prophylactic oophorectomies. *J. Natl. Cancer. Inst.* 88, 1810–1820.
5. Blaustein, A., Kantius, M., Kaganowitz, A., Pervez, N., and Wells, J. Inclusions in ovaries of females aged day 1–30 years. *Int. J. Gynecol. Pathol.* 1, 145–153.
6. Kannerstein, M., and Churg, J. (1997). Peritoneal mesothelioma. *Hum. Pathol.* 8, 83–94.
7. Harlap, S. (1993). The epidemiology of ovarian cancer. *In* "Cancer of the Ovary" Markman M. Markman and W. J. Hoskins, (eds.), pp. 153–162. New York, Raven Press.
8. Lancaster, J. M., Wooster, R., Mangion, J., Phelan, C. M., Cochran, C., Gumbs, C. *et al.* (1996). BRCA2 mutations in primary breast and ovarian cancers. *Nat. Genet.* 13, 238–240.
9. Serova, O., Montagna, M., Torchard, D., Narod, S. A., Tonin, P., Sylla, B. *et al.* (1996). A high incidence of BRCA1 mutations in 20 breast-ovarian cancer families. *Am. J. Hum. Genet.* 58, 42–51.
10. Berman, D. B., Wagner-Costalas, J., Schultz, D. C., Lynch, H. T., Daly, M., and Godwin, A. K. (1996). Two distinct origins of a common BRCA1 mutation in breast-ovarian cancer families: A genetic study of 15 185 del AG-mutation kindreds. *Am. J. Hum. Genet.* 58, 1166–1176.
11. Gallion, H. H., and Smith, S. A. Hereditary ovarian carcinoma. (1994). *Semin. Surg. Oncol.* 10, 249–254.
12. Boyd, J., and Rubin, S. C. (1997). Hereditary ovarian cancer: Molecular genetics and clinical implications. *Gynecol. Oncol.* 64, 196–206.
13. Berchuk, A., Crisano, F., Lancaster, J. M., Schildkraut, J. M., Wiseman, R. W., Futreal, A. *et al.* (1996). Role of BRCA1 mutation screening in the management of ovarian cancer. *Am. J. Obstet. Gynecol.* 175, 738–746.
14. Friedman, L. S., Szabo, C. L., Ostermeyer, E. A., Dowd, P., Butler, I., Park, T. *et al.* (1995). Novel inherited mutations and variable expressivity of BRCA1 alleles including the founder mutation 185 delAg in Ashkenazi Jewish families. *Am. J. Hum. Genet.* 57, 1284–1297.
15. Beller, U., Halle, D., Cetane, R., Kaufman, B., Hornreich, G., Levy-Lahad, Z. (1997). High frequency of BRCA1 and BRCA2 germline mutations in Ashkenazi Jewish ovarian cancer patients, regardless of family history. *Comm. Gynecol. Oncol.* 67, 121–122.
16. Struewing, J. P., Watson, P., Easton, D. F., Ponder, B. A., Lynch, H. T., and Tucker, M. A. (1995). Prophylactic oophorectomy in inherited breast/ovarian cancer families. *Monogr. Natl. Cancer. Inst.* 17, 33–35.
17. Piver, M. S., and Wong, C. (1997). Prophylactic oophorectomy: A century-long dilemma. *Hum. Reprod.* 12, 205–206.
18. Deligdisch, L., Gil, J., Kerner, H., Wu, H., Beck, D., and Gershoni-Baruch, R. (1999). Ovarian dysplasia in prophylactic oophorectomy specimens. Cytogenetic and morphometric correlations. *Cancer* 86, 1544–1550.
19. Deligdisch, L., and Gil, J. (1989). Characterization of ovarian dysplasia by interactive morphometry. *Cancer* 67, 748–755.
20. Deligdisch, L., Miranda, C., Barba, J., and Gil, J. (1993). Ovarian dysplasia: nuclear texture analysis. *Cancer* 72, 3253–3257.
21. Einstein, A. J., Wu, H. S., Gil, J., Wallenstein, S., Bodian, C. A., Sanchez, M. *et al.* (1997). Reproductibility and accuracy of interactive segmentation procedures for image analysis in cytology. *J. Microsc.* 188, 136–148.
22. Einstein, A. J., and Gil, J. (1996). Classification procedures for diagnosis based on multiple morphometric parameters. *Acta. Stereol.* 15, 15–24.
23. Deligdisch, L., Einstein, A. B., Guera, D., and Gil, J. (1995). Ovarian dysplasia in epithelial inclusion cysts: A morphometric approach using neural networks. *Cancer* 76, 1047–1054.
24. Deligdisch, L. Ovarian dysplasia: A review. (1997). *Int. J. Gynecol. Cancer.* 7, 89–94.
25. Mittal, K. R., Zeleniuck-Jacqueot, A., Cooper, J., Demopoulos, R. I. (1993). Contralateral ovary in unilateral ovarian carcinoma—a search for pre-neoplastic lesions. *Int. J. Gynecol. Pathol.* 1003; 12, 59–63.
26. Berchuk, A., Boente, M. P., Bast, R. C., Jr. (1992). The use of tumor markers in the management of patients with gynecologic carcinomas. *Clin. Obstet. Gynecol.* 35, 45–54.
27. Weber, B. L., Punzalan, C., Eisen, A., *et al.* (2000). Ovarian cancer risk reduction after bilateral prophylactic oophorectomy in BRCA1 and BRCA2 mutation carriers. *Am. Soc. Hum. Genet.* 251.
28. Piver, M. S. (2002). Hereditary ovarian cancer, distinguished professor series. *Gynecol. Oncol.* 85, 9–17.

CHAPTER

6

Epithelial Ovarian Neoplasms

LIANE DELIGDISCH

Department of Pathology, and Obstetrics, Gynecology and Reproductive Science
The Mount Sinai School of Medicine and Hospital
New York, New York 10029

I. INTRODUCTION

This group of tumors represents about 90% of all primary malignant ovarian tumors and about 50–55% of all ovarian tumors. Their origin is in the surface or germinal epithelium that covers the ovary in continuity with the peritoneal mesothelium. Histologically, this superficial lining of the ovary is quite similar to the peritoneal mesothelial lining, consisting of a single layer of cuboidal, low columnar or flat cells. Some of these tumors include also elements from the adjacent stroma and are therefore called surface epithelial-stromal tumors.

In early embryogenesis, the coelomic mesothelium invaginates laterally to the developing gonads, forming the Mullerian ducts. The external layer of the ovary and the peritoneal and the pelvic mesothelium are thus related to the internal layer of what will become the Mullerian system (fallopian tubes, uterus, endocervix). The propensity for ovarian neoplasms to be associated with peritoneal neoplasms, and occasionally with endometrial neoplasms, can be explained by an "area response" or "field effect" to carcinogens. The "extended-Mullerian system" [1, 2] including the uterus, ovaries, and peritoneum can respond to carcinogens in a synchronous or metachronous fashion.[1, 3] The histologic patterns of these tumors show similarities regardless of their location: serous papillary tumors of the ovary are histologically identical to serous papillary tumors of the peritoneum; endometrioid tumors of ovary to endometrial carcinoma; ovarian mucinous carcinoma to endocervical carcinoma; and clear cell carcinomas are histologically identical in the endocervix, endometrium, and ovary. The concept of the multifocal response to carcinogens in the upper female genital tract is not only of academic relevance. The staging of multiple tumors in this region should discriminate between metastatic and multiple primary sites, as is the case in the concomitant occurrence of endometrial and ovarian tumors, for example.

The fact that approximately 85% of ovarian serous carcinomas are diagnosed concomitantly with peritoneal involvement by the same type of tumor, in patients who are often asymptomatic, raises the question of whether this association is due to metastatic spread or to an independent primary peritoneal neoplasm. While the general consensus is that of metastatic disease—i.e., stage III ovarian carcinoma—the fact that in about 10% of the cases, peritoneal serous papillary carcinoma is seen with no, or, in another 10% of cases,[4] minimal ovarian involvement, may support the hypothesis of independent peritoneal primary tumors. Some recent cytogenetic research, however, proposes a monoclonal nature for ovarian cancer.[5]

Another challenging aspect of ovarian epithelial neoplasms resides in the fact that, because of the late diagnosis in most cases, the tumors are usually diffusely invasive and destructive, and early histologic changes of precursor or preinvasive lesions have only recently been described. In cervical and endometrial cancers lesions adjacent to the overt cancer have been identified and studied extensively both morphologically and biologically with well-documented support for their histopathogenesis (viral for cervical cancer, hormonal for endometrial carcinoma). In the ovaries, there are only a few recent reports on precursor lesions in high-risk patients,[6] associated with early stages of invasive cancer [7] and in the contralateral ovaries [8] as well as in prophylactic oophorectomy specimens.[9]

The etiopathogenesis of ovarian epithelial tumors is poorly understood. The "trauma" of ovulation enhanced by the use of ovulation stimulation by drugs, and, conversely, the protective effect of oral contraceptives has been emphasized: strong family history for malignancy (endometrial, ovarian, colon) points toward a genetic predisposition, although only a small percentage of patients with ovarian cancer have a documented family history of cancer and/or mutational genetic abnormalities.

By and large, it has been difficult to identify a high-risk group in the general female population in order to develop a screening program for these tumors, as has been successfully accomplished for other female genital tumors.

A pre-invasive lesion such as ovarian dysplasia or ovarian intraepithelial neoplasia (OIN) in analogy with the precursor lesions in the lower female genital tract (cervical intraepithelial neoplasm [CIN], vulvar intraepithelial neoplasm [VIN], and vaginal intraepithelial neoplasm [VAIN]), or in other locations (larynx, gallbladder, colon, etc.) is a recently described entity.[10] Morphometric [11] and nuclear texture analysis [12] studies have contributed to identifying potential precursors of ovarian carcinoma.[6, 9] It should be stressed that dysplastic, or intraepithelial neoplastic changes are not borderline tumors or tumors of low malignant potential (LMP). The latter are a group of ovarian epithelial tumors with no invasive tendencies while the dysplastic ovarian epithelium is often found adjacent to an invasive ovarian neoplasm. As in any dysplastic epithelial lesion, the biological potential to progress to frankly invasive cancer is not known, and may depend on still poorly understood host factors.

Dysplastic changes can be seen in extraovarian locations, for example, in the peritoneum with endosalpingiosis. Their malignant potential is unknown.

II. CLASSIFICATION

The classification of epithelial ovarian neoplasms is based on the WHO classification.[13] This chapter will include the most common, and some of the less common tumors in this group.

A. Common Ovarian Epithelial Neoplasms

- Serous cystadenomas, serous papillary cystadenomas, and cystadenofibromas
- Serous papillary cystadenocarcinomas, tumors of low malignant potential
- Mucinous cystadenomas
- Mucinous cystadenocarcinomas
- Endometrioid tumors, benign, of LMP, endometrioid adenocarcinoma
- Clear cell carcinomas
- Brenner tumors

B. Uncommon Ovarian Epithelial Neoplasms

- Malignant mixed Mullerian tumors
- Malignant Brenner tumors
- Undifferentiated and unclassifiable tumors

III. COMMON OVARIAN EPITHELIAL NEOPLASMS

A. Serous Cystadenoma, Papillary Serous Cystadenoma, and Cystadenofibroma

The great majority of epithelial neoplasms are benign and are represented by serous and mucinous cystadenomas, which may occasionally be combined. They are often seen in the younger age group, but can occur at any age, with a peak incidence in women 40–50 years old. They are bilateral in about 10–20%, more so in older patients. These tumors originate in an invagination of the surface epithelium into the ovarian stroma which may become a component of the tumor in cystadenofibromas. The epithelium has a propensity for papillary growth somewhat reminiscent histologically of the fallopian tube mucosal folds. The external surface of the cystadenomas is smooth and shiny with a marked vascular pattern (Fig. 6.1). While many cysts have a smooth and shiny lining, others contain papillary structures that can fill part (usually less than one-third) of the cystic cavity, ranging on gross examination, between thin and friable to coarse and firm structures (Fig. 6.2). The content of the cyst is clear, yellowish ("serous") occasionally hemorrhagic or cloudy. The cysts are more often unilocular but may contain septa dividing several cavities. Histologically, the lining is

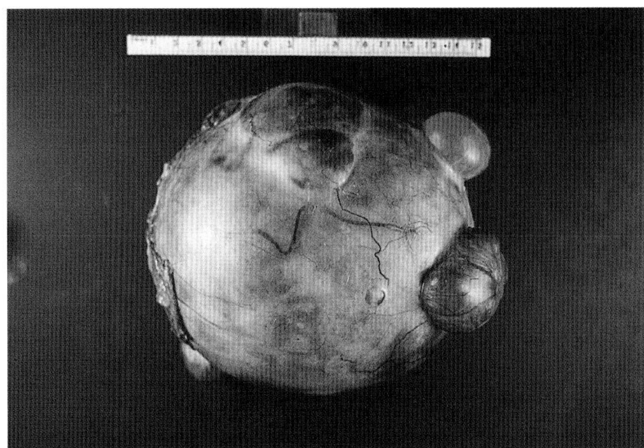

FIGURE 6.1 Ovarian serous cystadenoma. External surface is smooth, shiny, and displays a vascular pattern.

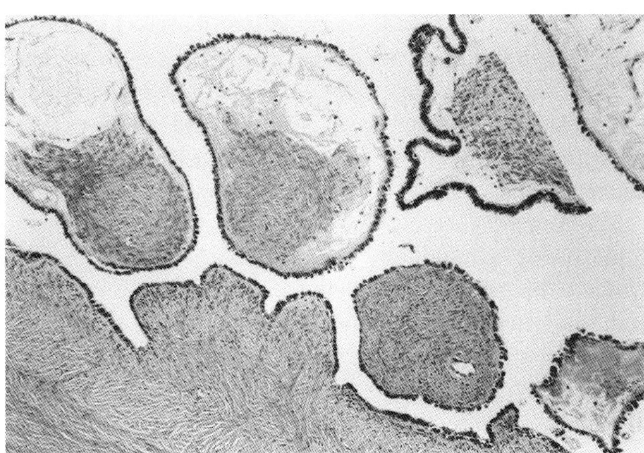

FIGURE 6.3 Ovarian papillary serous cystadenoma with fibrotic stalks lined by cuboidal epithelium. H&E×100.

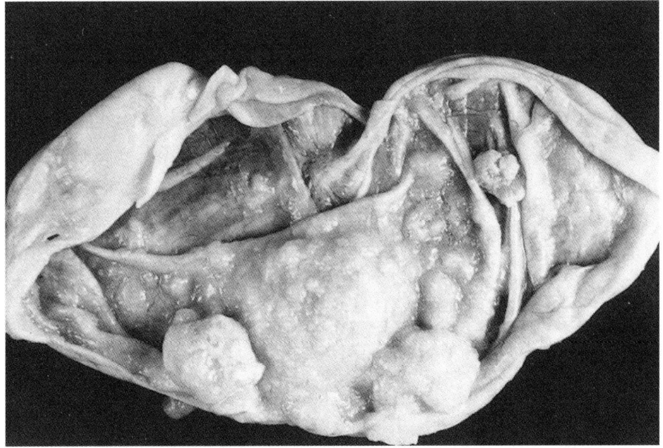

FIGURE 6.2 Ovarian papillary serous cystadenoma. Internal surface with multiple papillary projections.

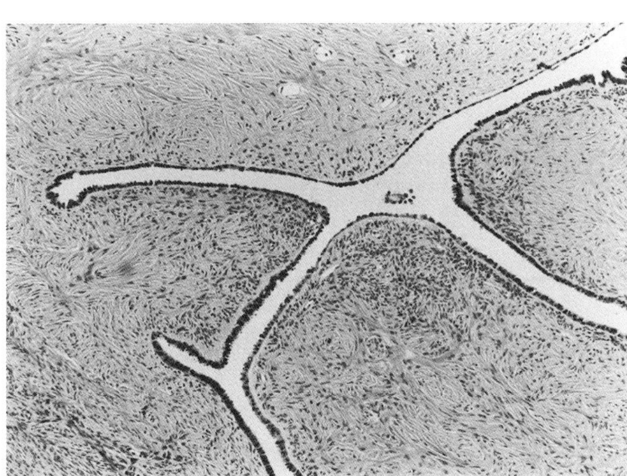

FIGURE 6.4 Ovarian cystadenofibroma. Note acellular subepithelial zone. H&E×100.

composed of cuboidal to tall columnar epithelium, occasionally flattened due to the fluid pressure (Fig. 6.3). Ciliated cells are typically seen in serous tumors, but eosinophilic and clear cells can also be found in the lining, representing metaplasias. In cystadenofibromas there is a characteristic thin acellar zone separating the epithelial lining from the underlying markedly proliferating stroma (Fig. 6.4). The solid component of the tumor has to be over 1 cm in diameter to qualify for "cystadenofibroma."[4] As in any other fibroma, there is a variable mixture of fibroblasts and collagen fibers, often with a hyalinized, and calcified matrix, therefore grossly these tumors are firm to gritty and whitish-gray. Microscopically tubular and glandular structures are seen in this dense stroma, lined by cells similar to those lining the cyst, justifying the term cystadenofibroma. The epithelial cells are generally regular, with little or no piling-up of the layers, inconspicuous mitotic activity and finely distributed nuclear chromatin. Proliferating features may be noted occasionally and have to be distinguished from the tumors of LMP or borderline which have a different biological behavior than the benign proliferating tumors.

Psammoma bodies (concentrically laminated calcific deposits) are often seen adjacent to papillary structures, or independently; their development seems to be related to a degenerative process of the papillary stalks.

B. Epithelial Ovarian Tumors of Borderline Malignancy or LMP

Despite the fact that histological criteria have been established for LMP ovarian tumors, which constitute about 15% of all malignant epithelial tumors of the ovaries, they still present a diagnostic dilemma and their management is often controversial.

Ovarian tumors of LMP or borderline are seen in younger patients than invasive carcinomas, with a peak average incidence in the fifth decade. They are more often bilateral than their benign counterparts (26–34%) [4] and are associated quite frequently (20–40%) with peritoneal, extraovarian lesions, similar histologically to the ovarian lesions.

There are no gross characteristic features for these tumors. Extensive sampling of any serous papillary tumor is recommended, especially of the more solid areas and of the more friable portions of the cyst wall. Histologically, there is an exuberant growth of epithelial cells distributed on many layers, with clusters of cells detached from the papillae. Nuclear atypia is mild to moderate and mitotic activity is occasionally present without exceeding 4 mitoses per 10 hpf. There is no invasion of the adjacent stroma (Fig. 6.5). Tangential cuts that show epithelial cells surrounded by stroma have to be distinguished from true invasion. In invasive tumors, the surrounding stroma shows edema and often a round cell infiltrate or granulation tissue representing a stromal reaction. Microinvasion of the stroma has been described in some ovarian tumors of borderline malignancy, without worsening their prognosis.[14]

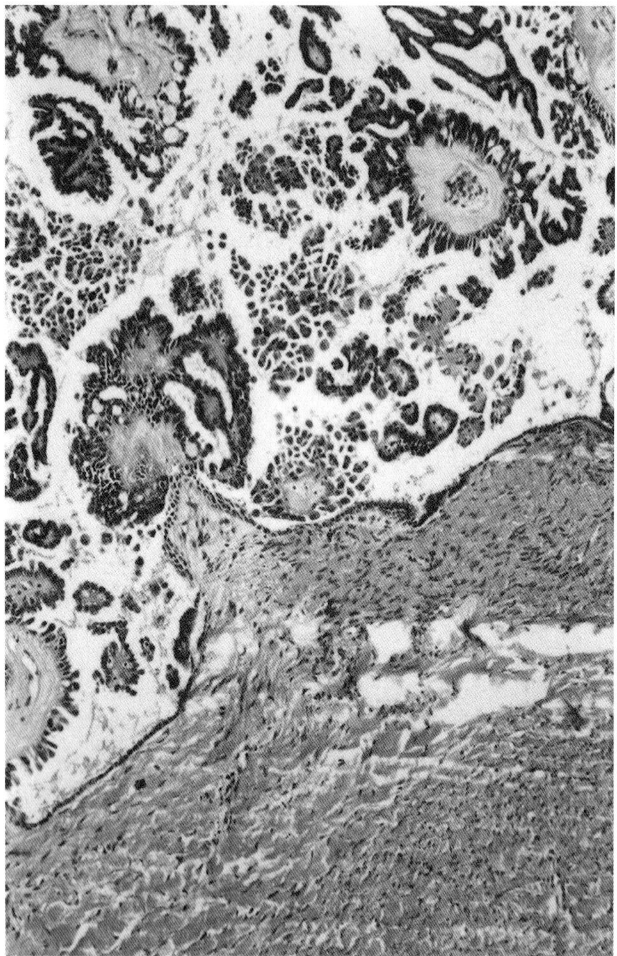

FIGURE 6.5 Ovarian serous papillary tumor of borderline malignancy. Exuberant papillary growth and detached clusters of epithelial cells, with no stromal invasion. H&E × 100.

A subset of borderline ovarian tumors has been described histologically as micropapillary or cribriform serous tumors, characterized by a highly complex papillary, filigree nonhierarchical pattern (Fig. 6.6) and a more aggressive clinical course. These tumors tend to recur and to disseminate even though the primary tumor does not invade the ovarian stroma.[15] According to other studies, the presence of a micropapillary pattern is less significant for the prognosis than the rather uncommonly encountered invasive peritoneal implants.[16] They are more often associated with peritoneal implants, representing stage II or III borderline ovarian tumors. Peritoneal implants are noninvasive or invasive, the latter being characterized by a more aggressive behavior. Noninvasive implants, epithelial or desmoplastic, resemble the papillary structures of the ovarian borderline tumor forming circumscribed lesions on the surface or in the septa of the omental adipose tissue, often surrounded by an inflammatory reaction (Fig. 6.7). Invasive implants have irregular borders with destruction of the adipose tissue, exhibiting higher degree of nuclear atypia and small rounded nests of epithelial cells. Noninvasive and invasive implants can occur in the same patient. Extensive sampling of the specimen is critical since the presence of invasive implants, more often seen with micropapillary and cribriform serous ovarian borderline tumors, is associated with a far worse prognosis. The most reliable prognostic indicator, according to Seidman and Kurman [17] is the type of peritoneal implant (95.3% survival at 7.4 years for noninvasive implants versus 66% for invasive implants).

It has also been reported that 30% of patients who have ovarian serous borderline tumors with noninvasive peritoneal implants will develop progressive or recurrent tumors.[8]

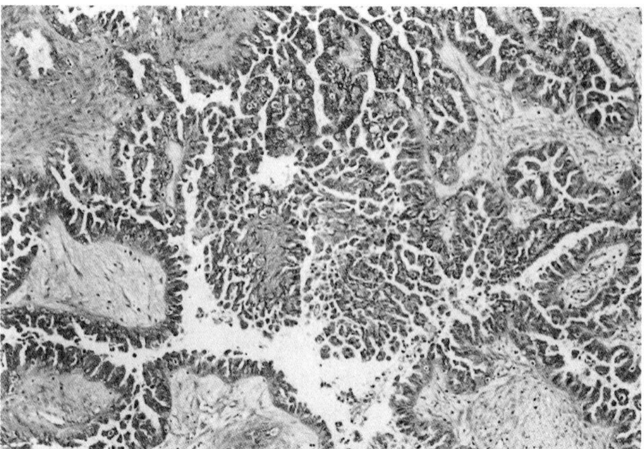

FIGURE 6.6 Borderline ovarian tumor, micropapillary type, with complex, filigree, nonhierarchical pattern. H&E × 100.

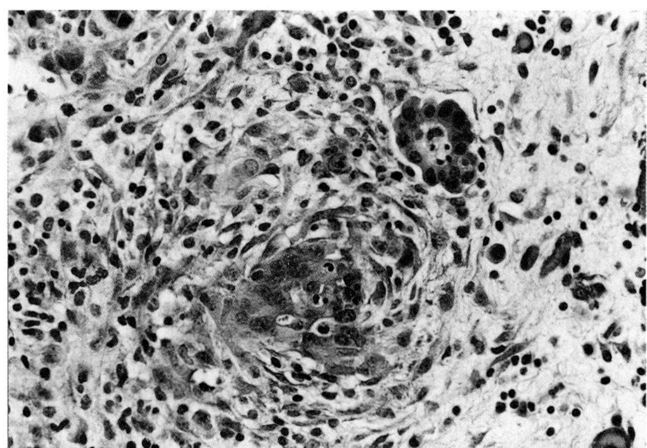

FIGURE 6.7 Peritoneal noninvasive implants of papillary tumor surrounded by inflammatory reaction. H&E×400.

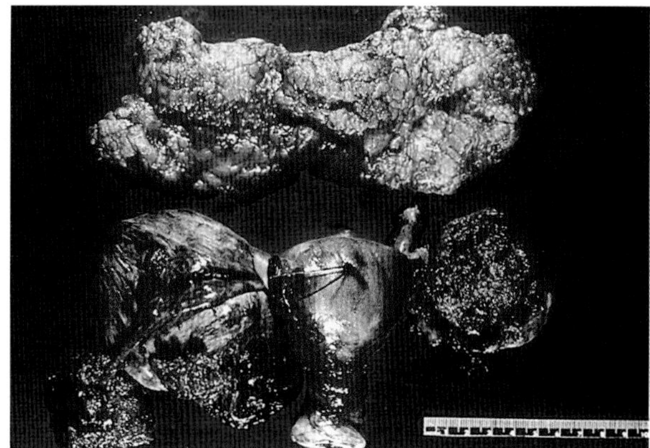

FIGURE 6.8 Ovarian serous papillary carcinoma involving both ovaries and peritoneum.

Over-expression of P53 mutations in late stage ovarian serous borderline tumors was found to be significantly associated with increased probability of progression/recurrence and decreased overall survival, along with the presence of residual tumor and of invasive implants.[19] In contrast to invasive epithelial ovarian cancer, bilateral and advanced stage serous borderline ovarian tumor may be multifocal in origin because alternate patterns of X chromosomes in activation occurred multifocally.[20]

Ovarian tumors of LMP often recur in the ovaries and/or in the peritoneal cavity. Histologically, the recurrences are usually similar to the primary tumors. If the recurrences are frankly malignant, the primary tumor might not have been an ovarian tumor of LMP. Studies by interactive morphometry combined with assessments of nucleolar organizing factors have identified further characteristics of this group of neoplasms.[21]

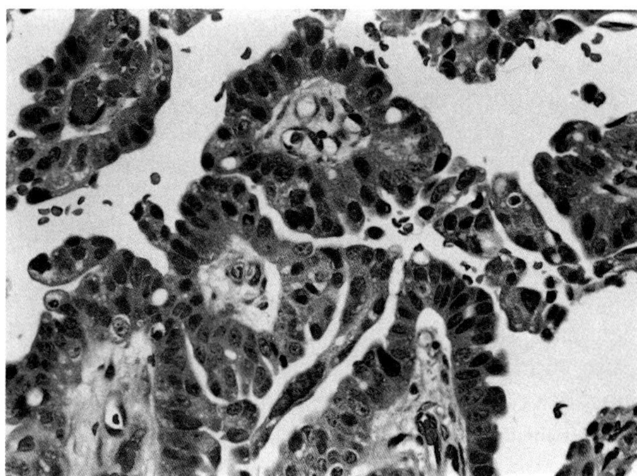

FIGURE 6.9 Serous papillary carcinoma: fibrovascular stalks are covered by malignant epithelium. H&E×1000.

C. Invasive Serous Papillary Carcinomas

These occur mostly in an older age group, with a peak at 65 years. They are the most common malignant epithelial tumors (40% of all primary ovarian malignancies) and are associated with a high mortality because of their late diagnosis. About 80% are detected in stage III, most are bilateral (about 70%) and widespread peritoneal involvement is notorious. (Fig. 6.8). The common association of peritoneal and ovarian lesions has raised some questions about the metastatic nature of the former. It has been postulated that a "field effect" of a carcinogenic agent may affect the extended Mullerian system that derives embryologically from the primitive celomic epithelium, thus involving ovarian epithelium and peritoneal mesothelium.[22] Microscopically, the serous papillary adenocarcinomas invade the ovarian stroma and show papillary structures covered by malignant epithelial cells, displaying numerous mitoses and severely atypical nuclei (Fig. 6.9). The proportion of connective tissue to epithelial tissue is related to the degree of malignancy: the more connective tissue, the better the differentiation. In well-differentiated (grade 1) tumors, the papillary structures are well represented, with broad stalks of fibroconnective tissue.

In moderately differentiated (grade 2) tumors, the epithelial proliferation partially obliterates the fibroconnective stalks, creating a lace-like pattern with micropapillary features and slits simulating glandular spaces. In poorly differentiated (grade 3) tumors, the malignant epithelium forms solid masses with only a few papillary structures (Fig. 6.10). Cellular differentiation decreases in higher grade tumors; irregular cells with large nuclei exhibiting prominent nucleoli, coarse chromatin clumps, bizarre multinucleated tumor cells with "smudged" nuclear chromatin or multinucleated tumor cells, and atypical asymmetrical mitotic figures are more numerous in the less well-differentiated tumors. Psammoma bodies are usually more frequent in the better

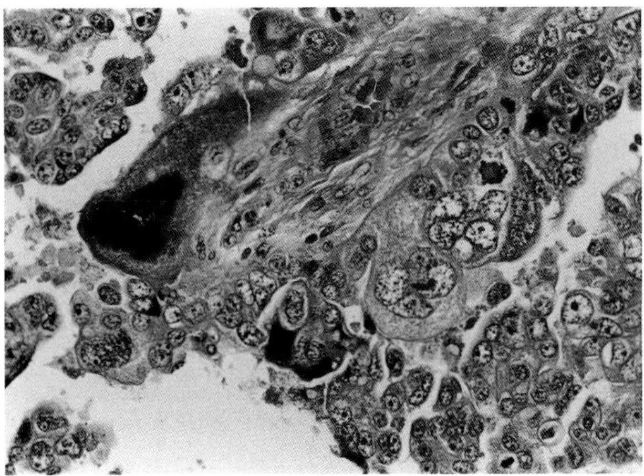

FIGURE 6.10 Poorly differentiated serous carcinoma: solid masses of tumor cells, bizarre multinucleated tumor cells with "smudged" nuclear chromatin. H&E × 1000.

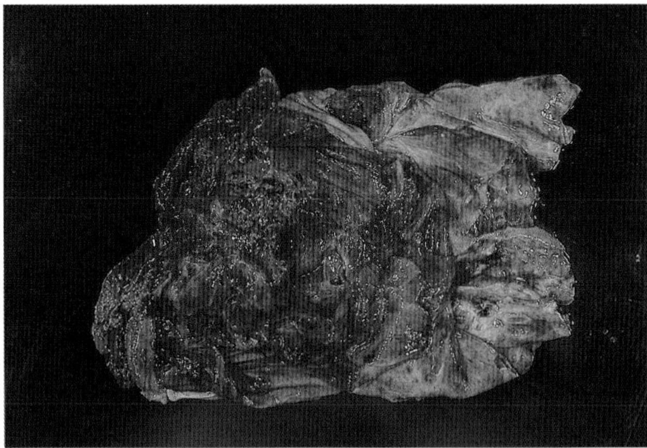

FIGURE 6.11 Ovarian mucinous cystadenocarcinoma. On frozen section it was underdiagnosed as a borderline tumor.

differentiated tumors. Large numbers of psammoma bodies seen in well-differentiated serous carcinoma are characteristic for psammocarcinoma which may be identified on x-ray films of the abdomen. They can be found in nontumoral zones, perhaps representing "burned out" papillary structures.[23] Psammoma bodies are of no prognostic value but are helpful clues in identifying a papillary tumor in an otherwise undifferentiated neoplasm, pointing to an ovarian origin in some metastatic abdominal tumors of questionable origin.[21] Often, ovarian tumors display various degrees of differentiation; it is preferable to designate the tumor with the degree of least differentiation rather than by the average, since the biological behavior and management should be that of the most virulent portion of the tumor. The chemotherapy in use is most effective in the less differentiated tumors, therefore the prognosis of ovarian tumors is not necessarily related to the degree of differentiation.[25] Along with staging and grading, the "host response" evaluated by the assessment of lymphoid cell infiltrates adjacent to the tumor has been shown to have a predictive value in ovarian serous papillary carcinomas.[26] A majority of serous carcinomas are aneuploid.[27]

D. Mucinous Tumors

Mucinous ovarian tumors represent about 15% of all ovarian tumors in the western world. Benign mucinous cystadenomas are common in women of reproductive age and are not uncommonly seen during pregnancy. They may occur at any age, with a peak during the fourth decade. They are more often unilateral than their serous counterparts and may reach large sizes. In fact, along with certain leiomyomas, they are some of the largest tumors in human gynecologic pathology. Grossly, they contain multiple cystic cavities, and may form a honeycomb structure containing small cavities divided by thin septa (Fig. 6.11). The content of the cysts is

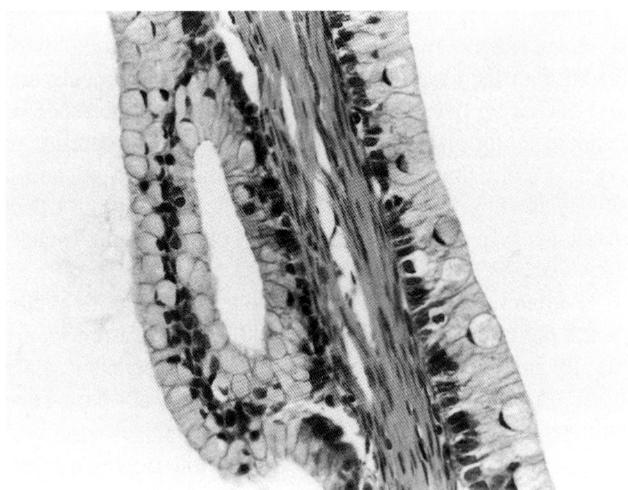

FIGURE 6.12 Mucinous cystadenoma lined by goblet cells and Paneth cells. H&E × 1000.

a jelly-like, sticky, grayish opaque material. Histologically, the cysts are lined by a single layer of tall columnar epithelium with basally located nuclei and mucin-containing vacuoles in the cytoplasm. These cells are quite similar to those lining endocervical glands. Another type of cells lining the mucinous cysts are goblet cells reminiscent of the colonic mucosa, neuroendocrine argyrophilic and Paneth cells analogous to gastric pyloric cells (Fig. 6.12). The peripheral zone of some mucinous cysts exhibits locules of "daughter cysts" in which the epithelial lining appears to be more actively growing, displaying hyperchromatic nuclei, mitoses (less than 3 per 10 hpf) and a diminished mucin content in the cytoplasm. Piling up of the epithelium is also noted, but the polarity of the cells is preserved. Extensive sampling of these areas is recommended in order to rule out an invasive tumor. Occasional leaking of the mucus content from the

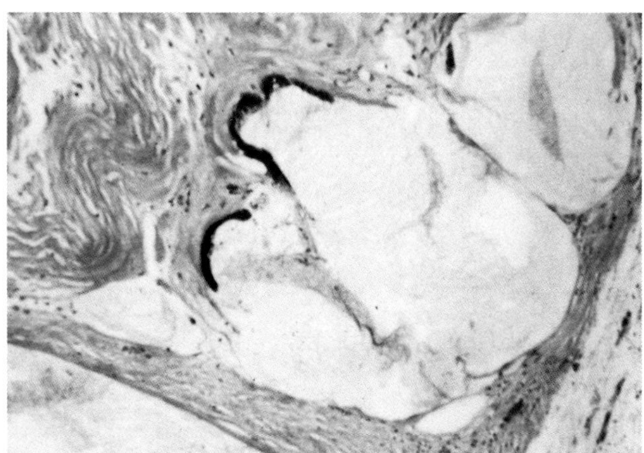

FIGURE 6.13 Pseudomyxoma peritonei: mucin pools and epithelial cells. H&E×400.

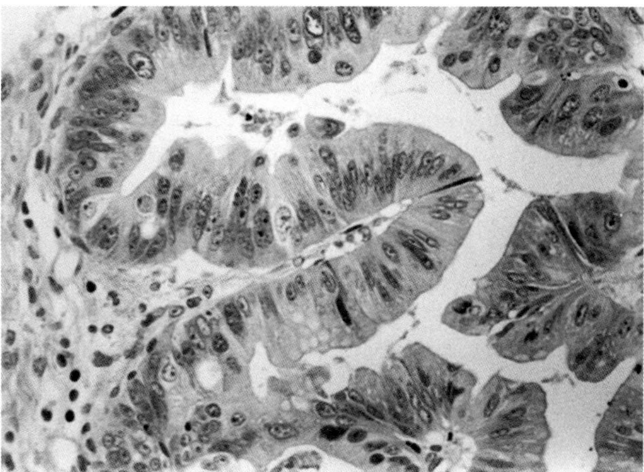

FIGURE 6.14 Mucinous ovarian tumor of borderline malignancy with diminished mucin secretion and complex proliferative pattern. H&E×1000.

cysts into the ovarian stroma can be seen in pseudomyxoma ovarii, noted more often in older patients. The finding of jelly-like masses in the peritoneal cavity, with microscopic evidence of mucin-secreting epithelium (pseudomyxoma peritonei) is associated with mucinous tumors of the ovary as well as of the appendix, or both (Fig. 6.13). Mucinous cystadenomas can be seen in association with ovarian teratomas (dermoids) and Brenner tumors.

E. Ovarian Mucinous Tumors of Borderline Malignancy (LMP) and Malignant Mucinous Tumors

These are more controversial than those of their serous counterparts. The main criterion to differentiate them from invasive tumors-stromal invasion is difficult to assess because of the fact that most histologic sections include tangentially cut mucinous glands. They have been subdivided into endocervical-like (Mullerian) and intestinal forms.[28] Histologically, the cysts are lined by multiple layers of epithelial cells (four or more) creating some complex papillary layers, and the cells are more basophilic, resembling the crypts of the colonic mucosal glands, with a large number of goblet cells and Paneth cells. Mitotic activity is higher, including atypical mitoses. Mucinous LMP tumors are difficult to distinguish from well differentiated grade 1 adenocarcinomas which show cribriform patterns (no connective tissue is seen separating the glands) and glandular structures with an irregular contour invading the stroma (Figs. 6.14 and 6.15). Like in serous tumors, the invaded stroma becomes immature, loose, and edematous, containing plump fibroblasts and inflammatory infiltrates. It has been proposed to use CA 19-9 as a serum marker for the follow-up of borderline mucinous ovarian tumors.[29]

Mucinous cystadenocarcinomas, especially the moderately differentiated mucinous adenocarcinomas (grade 2) are reminiscent of colonic carcinoma. The glandular pattern is often

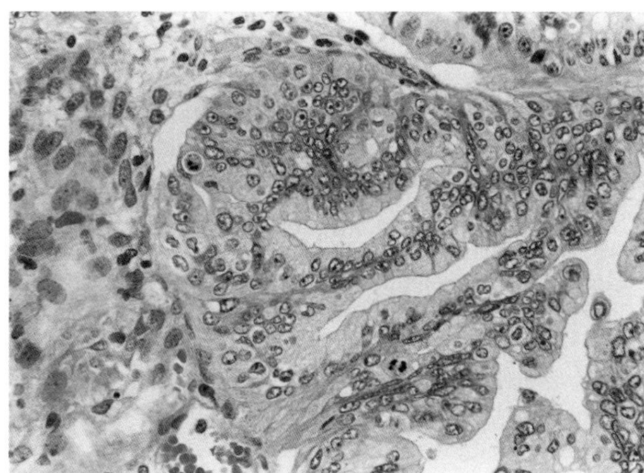

FIGURE 6.15 Well-differentiated ovarian mucinous adenocarcinoma: note cribriform pattern and mitotic activity. H&E×400.

associated with mucin pools similar to those seen in the intestinal "colloid" cancer. There is marked and atypical epithelial proliferation in the glands, with solid nests, loss of polarity, and irregular or diminished mucin secretion. Cells show marked nuclear hyperchromasia and mitotic activity. Poorly differentiated (grade 3) tumors display mostly clusters and solid sheets of tumor cells with few glandular structures and marked cellular atypia. Signet ring cells with individual cells containing mucin vacuoles and peripheral nucleus similar to Krukenberg tumors are rare in primary ovarian tumors.

Mucinous neoplasms of the ovary are often more well differentiated than their serous counterparts, and are also more often diagnosed in earlier stages of the disease. They are sometimes associated with other types of ovarian tumors, such as teratoma (most frequently dermoids) sex cord, and other mesenchymal tumors.[24] Their generally accepted histogenesis as epithelial ovarian tumors is supported by their frequent association with serous tumors. An endodermal teratomatous origin analogous to the ectodermal teratomatous origin in dermoid tumors is a less likely possibility.

Rarely, mural nodules exhibiting sarcomatous elements with bizarre nuclei and anaplastic carcinomatous elements are seen in mucinous ovarian tumors.[30] Bilateral ovarian mucinous tumors are frequently metastases from colonic primary cancer. It should be kept in mind that frozen sections of mucinous ovarian tumors are false-negative more often than other histologic entities because of sampling difficulties.

F. Endometrioid Tumors

Benign endometrioid tumors do not include endometriosis according to the WHO classification, even though the latter may present grossly as markedly enlarged tumor-like masses (endometriomas) and may histologically display an atypical epithelial lining.

Some ovarian adenofibromas show endometrial metaplasia of the epithelium lining cysts and clefts, with squamous metaplasia, but lacking an adjacent endometrial-type stroma, hemorrhage, or cyclic changes. These endometrioid cystadenofibromas are relatively uncommon tumors of mostly elderly patients. Atypical proliferative variants of endometriosis are described, more often in younger women, with associated endometriosis,[3] some presenting with infertility. Histologically, these tumors resemble endometrial hyperplasia of the uterus, including atypical hyperplasia and squamous metaplasia. Their "borderline" nature or LMP is still controversial; most of the reported cases had a rather favorable outcome.[32]

Endometrioid carcinomas of the ovary are frequent tumors, representing about 20% of all primary ovarian carcinomas. They are more often unilateral (13% are bilateral), present grossly as soft, often cystic, partly hemorrhagic, partly necrotic tumors, with a smooth capsule (Fig. 6.16). In a minority of cases (about 10–20%) there is evidence of associated endometriosis, usually in younger patients.[33] Like endometrioid endometrial carcinoma, which is concomitantly diagnosed in about 15% of the cases, this is a neoplasm of the elderly, with a peak incidence in the sixth decade.

Histologically, the tumor is identical to endometrial adenocarcinoma (Fig. 6.17). Mullerian-type glands predominate with well-formed, relatively regular glandular structures in the well-differentiated, grade 1 tumors, displaying frequently a villoglandular pattern. Solid clusters of tumor cells are admixed with glandular structures in moderately differentiated, (grade 2) adenocarcinomas, and predominate in poorly differentiated (grade 3) tumors in which there are few well-formed glands, and cellular atypia is severe. As in endometrial carcinoma, various cell types may be found in ovarian endometrioid carcinomas such as secretory, ciliated metaplastic patterns. The most common is squamous epithelium appearing as "morules," solid sheets which should not be

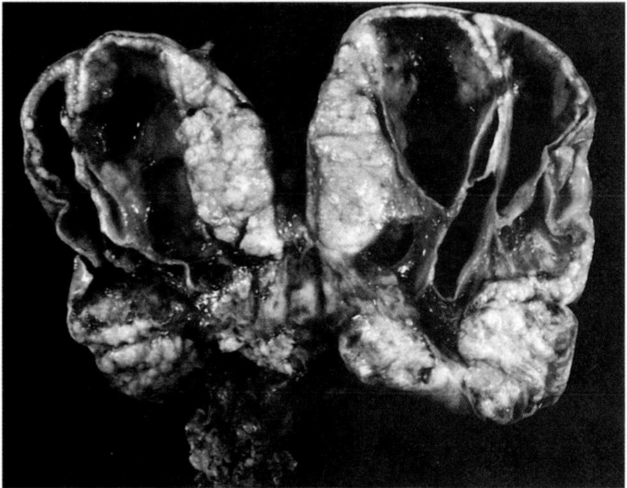

FIGURE 6.16 Endometrioid adenocarcinoma: partly cystic, partly solid tumor, with hemorrhagic and necrotic areas.

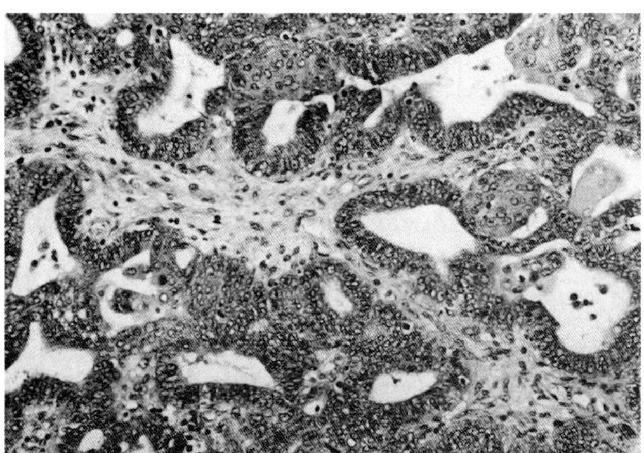

FIGURE 6.17 Endometrioid adenocarcinoma of ovary, histologically identical to endometrial adenocarcinoma, with squamoid morules. H&E×400.

mistaken for solid tumor tissue of low differentiation because of the nonglandular, solid structures. In solid tumor tissue, the cells are severely atypical, often with bizarre multinucleated tumor cells while the squamoid tissue is differentiated, displaying intercellular bridges and occasional keratin. The finding of squamoid elements in an otherwise poorly differentiated adenocarcinoma is helpful to determine the diagnosis of endometrioid carcinoma. Other commonly associated cell types are mucinous and clear cells.

The concomitant finding of uterine endometrial carcinoma and ovarian endometrioid carcinoma is probably due to the "field effect" of certain carcinogens on the upper female genital tract.[33, 34] A metastatic neoplasm from the endometrium to the ovary is more likely in the presence of deeply invasive endometrial tumor in the myometrium, and of nodular ovarian tumor masses. It may not be easy to determine if the two histologically similar malignant tumors represent separate primary tumors. More convincing evidence of their independent primary nature is the absence of myometrial invasion in the uterus and the finding of ovarian adenocarcinoma arising in an endometriotic cyst. The study of loss of heterozygosity (LOH) may be useful in determining the relationship of synchronous uterine and ovarian endometrioid neoplasms.[35, 36]

Endometrioid tumors of the ovary are diagnosed more often in lower stages than serous papillary tumors; they tend to metastasize via the blood stream. When matched for age, grade, stage, and level of cytoreduction there is no difference in 5-year survival or length of survival between endometrioid and serous carcinoma.[37]

An important differential diagnosis is that with metastatic adenocarcinoma from the gastrointestinal tract, especially from the colon, which is mostly bilateral (Fig. 6.18) and displays microscopically a more severe cytologic atypia in the glands and more necrosis and cellular debris. Another difficult differential diagnosis is that with Sertoli-Leydig cell tumors. Inhibin and Dobbs CD99 expressed by sex cord cells may be helpful markers.[38] Immunohistologic stains for Vimentin are positive and for CEA are negative in endometrioid carcinoma.

It should be mentioned that the ovarian endometrioid carcinomas are the most frequently misdiagnosed ovarian cancers. Endometrioid borderline tumors are still ill-defined entities although they were described as arising in adenofibromas and in foci of ovarian endometriosis. Criteria for their discrimination from overt endometrioid cancers have been outlined recently.[39]

G. Clear Cell Tumors

Benign clear cell tumors are very rare. Some display proliferating patterns which show atypia but no invasion and bear a favorable prognosis.[25, 26]

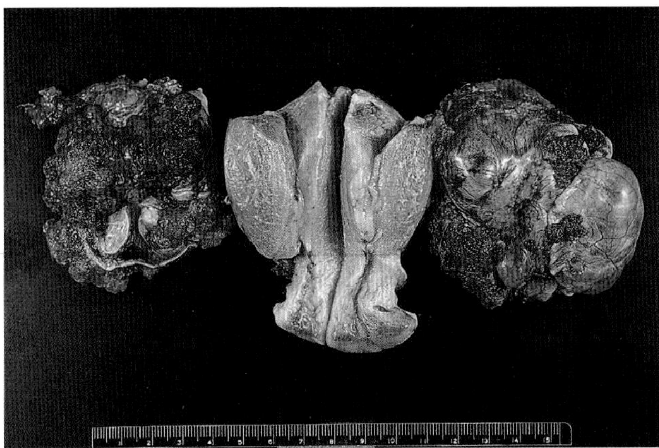

FIGURE 6.18 Metastatic ovarian carcinoma from primary colonic neoplasm, most often bilateral.

The malignant clear cell tumors, or clear cell carcinomas represent 5–10% of all primary ovarian malignancies. They are characterized by cells with clear cytoplasm resembling superficially renal cell carcinomas, and were designated in the past as mesonephroid tumors. This was a misnomer, because they originate from the extended Mullerian epithelium as proven by their frequent association with endometrioid and other epithelial ovarian tumors, and because biochemically and on ultrastructure they are similar to clear cell carcinomas of the endometrium and cervix, and different from renal cell tumors. Clear cell ovarian tumors have the highest association with ovarian and pelvic endometriosis and with paraendocrine hypercalcemia.[42]

The benign clear cell tumors have no distinctive gross features, they present as multiloculated cysts or cystadenofibromas lined by cuboidal or tall epithelium with clear glycogen-containing cytoplasm. Those with atypical proliferation display piling-up, nuclear atypia, and a low mitotic activity. They are mostly associated with adenofibromas, with or without endometrioid elements.

Clear cell carcinomas present as large tumor masses, mostly unilateral, partly cystic, partly solid with fleshy tan nodules protruding into the cystic cavities. They are often associated with endometriotic cysts. Microscopically, the tumor cells are arranged in solid sheets or form tubular-papillary structures. Their cytoplasm appears clear or finely granular and eosinophilic. It contains mostly glycogen, some fat, and no mucin. Cell borders appear distinct, and nuclei show prominent nucleoli and are irregular, sometime protruding toward the lumen ("hobnail" cells) (Fig. 6.19). Continuity with endometriotic lining and mixture with endometrioid carcinomas are not uncommon. It seems that clear cell carcinoma represents a variant of endometrioid carcinoma. The differential diagnosis in some cases can include dysgerminoma.

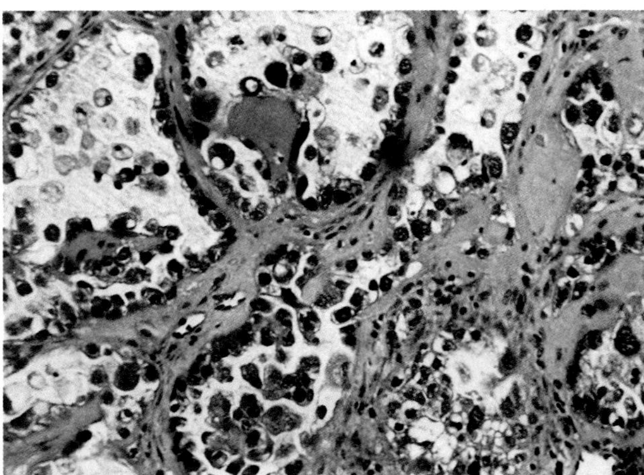

FIGURE 6.19 Ovarian clear cell carcinoma: tubular and papillary structures lined by tumor cells with clear cytoplasm and "hobnail" nuclei. H&E×400.

Epithelial membrane antigen is positive in clear cell carcinoma and negative in dysgerminoma.[42]

H. Brenner Tumors

Most Brenner tumors are benign and are incidental findings in ovaries removed for other reasons. They are usually small whitish-yellow nodules, rarely bilateral with a mean incidence in patients in their fifties. Their size rarely exceeds 6 cm and the cut surface appears firm, and whorled with occasional small cysts. Histologically, they are composed of nests of transitional type epithelium, similar to that seen in the urinary bladder, often displaying cystic cavities lined by mucin-secreting epithelium. They are identical to Walthard's nests, often seen in the adnexal region as incidental findings (Fig. 6.20). These nests are surrounded by dense hyalinized ovarian stroma, calcified areas, and occasionally by luteinized cells. Associated mucinous tumors are not uncommon. The cells are mature, with regular nuclei, but proliferating variants of Brenner tumors and Brenner tumor of borderline malignancy have been described in which nuclear atypia and mitotic activity were found. Occasionally, Brenner tumors are associated with endocrine manifestations of estrogenic or, rarely, androgenic type, probably due to steroid hormone secretion by the stromal component of the tumor.[42]

IV. UNCOMMON OVARIAN EPITHELIAL NEOPLASMS

A. Malignant Mixed Mullerian Tumors of the Ovary (MMMT)

MMMTs are less common than their uterine counterparts. They are composed of epithelial and mesenchymal elements, both derived from the primitive Mullerian and "extended Mullerian" structures. They represent a variant of endometrioid neoplasms accounting for less than 1% of all primary ovarian tumors, are seen mostly in elderly patients, and 85% present in stage III or IV. Their prognosis is generally poor.[43]

Grossly, these are large tumors, cystic and solid, with necrotic and hemorrhagic areas, and occasionally bone and cartilaginous areas, rarely within endometriotic cysts. Histologically, the epithelial components are predominantly serous papillary, but any other epithelial structures, including squamous elements can be found. The mesenchymal components, as in their uterine counterparts are homologous (carcinosarcomas) (Fig. 6.21) represented by an endometrial-type stroma, which is actually not part of the normal ovarian structure as is the case in the homologous endometrial MMMTs, and heterologous, including skeletal muscle, bone cartilage, or fat. The various components are intermixed haphazardly and extensive areas of undifferentiated tumor cells with bizarre giant cells are common as well as hyaline droplets with intra- and extracellular location (Fig. 6.22). Myxoid changes of the ground substance are characteristic for MMMT. Immunohistochemistry studies can identify their epithelial or mesenchymal nature.[44] Some MMMTs show predominantly epithelial components and their mesenchymal elements are identified only incidentally requiring extensive sampling for further confirmation. The recurrent and metastatic tumors are epithelial, occasionally mesenchymal,[45] or both. The variegated histologic composition of these tumors can be distinguished from that of malignant teratomas by the absence of neural tissues in the MMMT and the young age of the patients with teratomas. Immunostaining for P53 [46] and clonality studies [47] suggest that MMMTs are at least partly metaplastic carcinomas rather than carcinosarcomas.

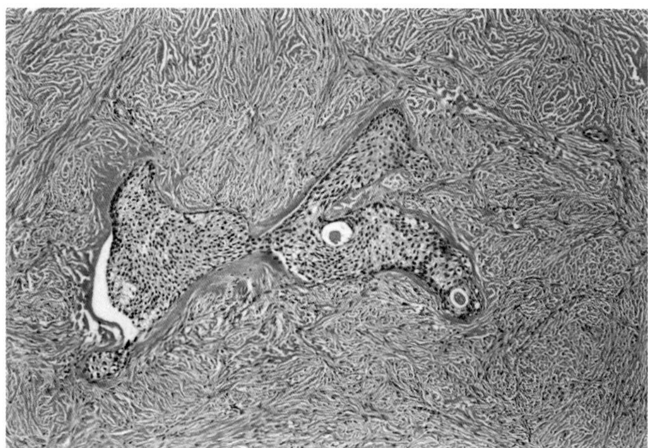

FIGURE 6.20 Ovarian Brenner tumor: nests of transitional cell carcinoma surrounded by dense ovarian stroma. H&E×100.

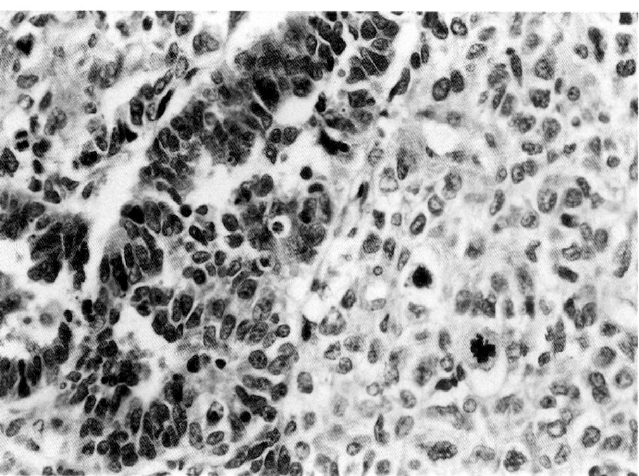

FIGURE 6.21 Ovarian carcinosarcoma (malignant mixed Mullerian tumor) composed of malignant epithelial (left) and malignant mesenchymal (right) tissue. H&E×400.

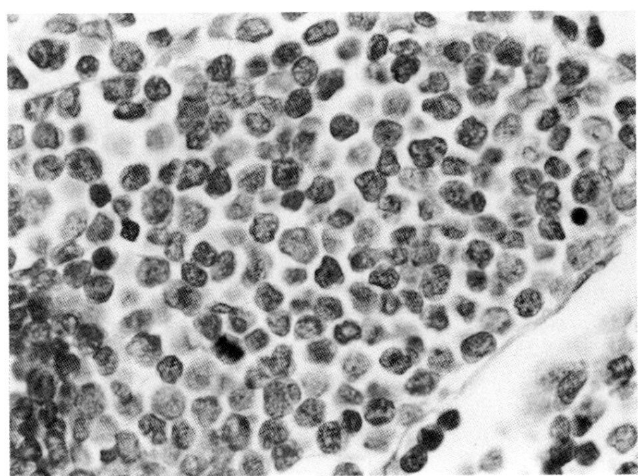

FIGURE 6.22 Small cell carcinoma of ovary. Patient was 22 years old and survived two months after diagnosis. H&E×400.

B. Malignant Brenner Tumors

Malignant Brenner tumors are very rare. They are large friable tumors, partly cystic, which show histologically a continuity between benign mesonephric-type nests and malignant epithelial tumor tissue that is of transitional, squamous, or glandular type.[48]

C. Undifferentiated and Unclassifiable Tumors

These are mostly solid tumors with necrosis and hemorrhage. Various epithelial elements may be found in tubular, glandular, or trabecular arrangements, their epithelial nature is confirmed by special immunohistochemical stains.[49] *Small cell carcinomas* of the ovary are rare neoplasms of young patients who are often hypercalcemic; the tumors are grossly solid, microscopically somewhat reminiscent of "oat cell" tumors, and have a very poor prognosis (Fig. 6.22). Their histogenesis is poorly understood and their epithelial origin is disputed, despite positive staining for some epithelial antigens.[50] Primary ovarian sarcomas are rare. Some may originate in the stromal tissue of ovarian endometriosis.[51]

References

1. Woodruff, J. D., Solomon, D., and Sullivan, H. (1985). Multifocal disease in the upper genital tract. *Obstet. Gynecol.* 65, 695–698.
2. Zaino, R. J., Under, E. R., and Whitney, C. (1984). Synchronous carcinomas of the uterine corpus and ovary. *Gynecol. Oncol.* 19, 329–335.
3. Deligdisch, L., and Szulman, A. (1975). Multifocal and multicentric carcinomas of the female genital organs. *Gynecol. Oncol.* 3, 181–190.
4. Russel, P., and Ballantyne, P. (1989). "Surgical Pathology of the Ovaries," p. 191, Churchill Livingstone, New York.
5. Griffin, C. (1993). Editorial: Is ovarian cancer a clonal disease? *Gynecol. Oncol.* 48, 1–3.
6. Gusberg, S. B., and Deligdisch, L. (1984). Ovarian dysplasia. A study of identical twins. *Cancer* 54, 1–4.
7. Plaxe, S. C., Deligdisch, L., Dottino, P. *et al.* (1990). Ovarian intraepithelial neoplasia (OIN) demonstrated in patients with stage I ovarian carcinoma. *Gynecol. Oncol.* 38, 367–372.
8. Mittal, K. P., Zelenik-Jacquot, A., Coopet, J. *et al.* (1993). Contralateral ovary in unilateral ovarian carcinoma—a search for preneoplastic lesions. *Int. J. Gynecol. Pathol.* 12, 59–63.
9. Deligdisch, L., Gil, J., Kerner, H., We, H. S., Beck, D., and Gershoni-Baruch, R. (1999). Ovarian dysplasia in prophylactic oophorectomy specimens. Cytogenetic and morphometric correlations. *Cancer* 86, 1544–1550.
10. Deligdisch, L., and Gil, J. (1989). Characterization of ovarian dysplasia by interactive morphometry. *Cancer* 4, 748–755.
11. Gil, J., and Deligdisch, L. (1989). Interactive morphometric procedures and statistical analysis in the diagnosis of ovarian dysplasia. *Pathol. Res. Pract.* 185, 680–685.
12. Aure, J. C., Hoeg, K., and Kalstad, P. (1971). Psammoma bodies in serous carcinoma of the ovary: A prognostic study. *Am. J. Obstet. Gynecol.* 109, 113.
13. Serov, S. F., Scully, R. E., and Sobin, L. H. (1973). "Histological Typing of Ovarian Tumors." Geneva, World Health Organization, a:pp. 37, b: pp. 17–18.
14. Bell, D. A., and Scully, R. E. (1990). Ovarian serous borderline tumors with stromal microinvasion: A report of 21 cases. *Hum. Pathol.* 21, 397–403.
15. Echhorn, J. H., Bell, D. A., Young, R. H., and Scully, R. E. (1999). Ovarian serous borderline tumors with micropapillary and cribriform patterns. A study of 40 cases and comparison with 44 cases without these patterns. *Am. J. Surg. Pathol.* 23, 397–409.
16. Prat, J., and de Nictolis, M. (2002). Serous borderline tumors of the ovary. A long-term follow-up study of 137 cases, including 18 with a micropapillary pattern and 20 with microinvasion. *Am. J. Surg. Pathol.* 26, 1111–1128.
17. Seidman, J. D., and Kurman, R. J. (2000). Ovarian serous borderline tumors: A critical review of the literature with emphasis on prognostic indicators. *Hum. Pathol.* 31, 539–557.
18. Gershenson, D. M., Silva, E. G., Tortolero-Luna, G., Levenback, C., Morris, M., and Tornos, C. (1998). Serous borderline tumors of the ovary with non-invasive peritoneal implants. *Cancer* 83, 2157–2163.
19. Gershenson, D. M., Deavers, M., Diaz, S., Torolero-Luna, G., Miller, B. E., Bast, R. C. Jr., Mills, G. B., and Silva, E. G. (1999). Prognostic significance of p. 53 Expression in advanced-stage ovarian serous borderline tumors. *Clin. Cancer. Res.* 5, 4053–4058.
20. Luk, H., Bell, D. A., Welch, W. R., Berkowitz, R. S., and Mok, S. K. (1998). Evidence for the mutifocal origin of bilateral and advanced human serous borderline tumors. *Cancer Res.* 58, 2328–2330.
21. Hytiroglou, P., Harpaz, N., Deligdisch, L. *et al.* (1992). Differential diagnosis of borderline and invasive serous cystadenocarcinomas of the ovary by computerized interactive morphometry of nuclear features. *Cancer* 69, 988–992.
22. Eisner, R. F., Nieberg, R. K., and Borek, J. S. (1988). Synchronous primary neoplasms of the female reproductive tract. *Gynecol. Oncol.* 33, 335–339.
23. Aure, J. C., Hoeg, K., and Kalstad, P. (1998). Psammoma bodies in serous carcinoma of the ovary: A prognostic study. *Am. J. Obstet. Gynecol.* 109, 113–118.
24. Deligdisch, L. (1994). Ovarian malignant epithelial tumors. *In* "Atlas of Ovarian Tumors." (L. Deligdisch, A. Altchek, and C. J. Cohen, eds.), pp. 87–114. Igaku-Shoin, New York.
25. Jacobs, A., Deligdisch, L., and Cohen, C. J. (1982). Histologic correlates of virulence in ovarian adenocarcinoma I. Effect of differentiation. *Am. J. Obstet. Gynecol.* 1143, 574–580.

26. Deligdisch, L., Jacobs, A., and Cohen, C. J. (1982). Prognosis of advanced ovarian carcinoma treated with cisdiaminodichloro platinum II. Morphologic correlates of host response. *Am. J. Obstet. Gynecol.* 144, 885–889.
27. Bell, D. A. (1992). Flow cytometry of ovarian neoplasms. *In*: "Current Topics in Pathology. Gynecological Tumors, Recent Progress in Diagnostic Pathology" (N. Sasano, ed.), 337–356. Springer-Verlag, Berlin.
28. Lee, K. R., and Scully, R. E. (2000). Mucinous tumors of the ovary: A clinicopathologic study of 196 borderline tumors (of intestinal type) and carcinomas, including an evaluation of 11 cases with "pseudomyxoma peritonei." *Am. J. Surg. Pathol.* 24, 1447–1464.
29. Engelen, M. J., de Bruijn, H. W., Hollema, H., ten Hoor, K. A., Willemse, P. H., Aalders, J. G., and vander Zee, A. G. (2000). Serum CA 125, carcinoembryonic antigen and CA 19-9 as tumor markers in borderline ovarian tumors. *Gynecol. Oncol.* 78, 16–20.
30. Kessler, E., Halpern, M., Koren, R., Dekel, A., and Goldman, J. (1990). Sarcoma-like mural nodules with foci of anaplastic carcinoma in ovarian mucinous tumor: Clinical, histological and immunohistochemical study of a case and review of the literature. *Surg. Pathol.* 3, 311–319.
31. McMeekin, D. S., Burger, R. A., Manetta, A., DiSaia, P., and Berman, M. L. (1995). Endometrioid adenocarcinoma of the ovary and its relationship with endometriosis. *Gynecol. Oncol.* 59, 81–86.
32. Bell, D. A., and Scully, R. E. (1985). Atypical and borderline endometrioid adenofibroma of the ovary. A report of 27 cases. *Am. J. Surg. Pathol.* 9, 205–214.
33. Tidy, J., and Mason, W. P. (1988). Endometrioid carcinoma of the ovary: A retrospective study. *Br. J. Obstet. Gynecol.* 95, 1165–1169.
34. Eisner, R. F., Nieberg, R. K., and Berek, J. S. (1988). Synchronous primary neoplasms of the female reproductive tract. *Gynecol. Oncol.* 33, 335–39.
35. Ulbright, T. M., and Roth, L. M. (1985). Metastatic and independent cancers of the endometrium and ovary: A clinico-pathologic study of 34 cases. *Hum. Pathol.* 16, 28–34.
36. Emmert-Buck, M. R., Chuaqui, R., Shuang, Z., Nogales, F., Liotta, L. A., and Merino, M. J. (1997). Molecular analysis of synchronous uterine and ovarian endometrioid tumors. *Int. J. Gynecol. Pathol.* 16, 143–148.
37. Shenson, D. L., Gallion, H. H., Powell, D. E., and Pieretti, M. (1995). Loss of heterozygosity and generic instability in synchronous endometrioid tumors of the ovary and endometrium. *Cancer* 76, 650–657.
38. Zwart, J., Geisler, J. P., and Geisler, H. E. (1998). Five-year survival in patients with endometrioid carcinoma of the ovary versus those with serous carcinoma. *Eur. J. Gynaecol. Oncol.* 19, 225–228.
39. Matias-Guiu, X., Poris, C., and Prat, J. (1998). Mullerian inhibiting substance, alpha-inhibin, and CD 99 expression in sex cord-stromal tumors and endometrioid ovarian carcinomas resembling sex cord-stromal tumors. *Hum. Pathol.* 29, 840–845.
40. Bell, D. A., and Kurman, R. J. (2000). A clinicopathologic analysis of atypical proliferative (borderline) tumors and well-differentiated endometrioid adenocarcinomas of the ovary. *Am. J. Surg. Pathol.* 24, 1465–1479.
41. Bell, D. A., and Scully, R. E. (1985). Benign and borderline clear cell adenofibroma of the ovary. *Cancer* 56, 2922.
42. Jenison, E. L., Montag, A. G., Griffiths, C. T. *et al.* (1989). Clear cell carcinoma of the ovary: A clinical analysis and comparison with serous carcinoma. *Gynecol. Oncol.* 32, 65–71.
43. Scully, R. E., Young, R. H., and Clement, P. B. (1998). Tumors of the ovary, maldeveloped gonads, fallopian tube and broad ligament. *In*: "Atlas of Tumor Pathology." Armed Forces Institute of Pathology, Washington, D.C.
44. Morrow, C. P., D'Ablaing, G., Brady, L. W. *et al.* (1984). A clinical and pathologic study of 30 cases of malignant mixed Mullerian epithelial and mesenchymal tumors: A Gynecologic Oncology Group Study. *Gynecol. Oncol.* 18, 278–292.
45. DeBrito, P. A., Silverberg, S. G., and Orenstein, J. M. (1993). Carcinosarcoma (malignant mixed mullerian [mesodermal] tumor) of the female genital tract: Immunohistochemical and ultrastructural analysis of 28 cases. *Hum. Pathol.* 24, 132–142.
46. Deligdisch, L., Plaxe, S., and Cohen, C. J. (1988). Extrauterine pelvic malignant mixed mesodermal tumors: A study of 10 cases with immunohistochemistry. *Int. J. Gynecol. Pathol.* 7, 361–372.
47. Mayall, F., Rutty, K., Campbell, F., and Coddard, H. (1994). P.53 Immunostaining suggests that uterine carcinosarcomas are monoclonal. *Histopathology* 24, 211–214.
48. Thompson, L., Chang, B., and Barsky, S. H. (1996). Monoclonal origins of malignant mixed tumors (carcinosarcomas). Evidence for a divergent histogenesis. *Am. J. Surg. Pathol.* 20, 277–285.
49. Trebeck, C. E., Friedlander, M. L., Russell, P. *et al.* (1987). Brenner tumors of the ovary: A study of the histology, immunohistochemistry and cellular DNA content in benign, borderline, and malignant ovarian tumors. *Pathology* 19, 241–246.
50. Silva, E. G., Tornos, C., Bailey, M. A. *et al.* (1991). Undifferentiated carcinoma of the ovary. *Arch. Pathol. Lab. Med.* 115, 377–381.
51. Pruett, K. M., Gordon, A. N., Estrata, R. *et al.* (1988). Small cell carcinoma of the ovary: An aggressive epithelial cancer occurring in young patients. *Gynecol. Oncol.* 29, 365–369.
52. Shakfeh, S. M., and Woodruff, J. D. (1987). Primary ovarian sarcomas; report of 46 cases and review of the literature. *Obstet. Gynecol. Surv.* 42, 331–349.

CHAPTER

7

Germ Cell Tumors of the Ovary

ALEKSANDER TALERMAN

Department of Pathology and Cell Biology
Thomas Jefferson University
Philadelphia, Pennsylvania 19107

I. GENERAL ASPECTS

Germ cell tumors are the second most common group of ovarian neoplasms after surface epithelial stromal tumors. In Europe and North America, germ cell tumors comprise approximately 20% of all ovarian neoplasms, while the incidence is relatively higher in Asian and African countries due to paucity of surface epithelial stromal tumors. The great majority of ovarian germ cell tumors are benign and consist of mature cystic teratomas. The latter make up more than 90% of ovarian germ cell tumors, while all the malignant germ cell neoplasms comprise the remaining 5–8%. Germ cell tumors are encountered at all ages, but are seen most frequently from the first to the sixth decade. It is notable that 60% of all ovarian neoplasms in children and adolescents are of germ cell origin and one-third of these are malignant. Apart from mature cystic teratoma with malignant transformation, which usually occurs in peri- and postmenopausal women, malignant germ cell tumors with rare exceptions occur from birth to menopause and the great majority are seen in patients aged less than 35 years.[1]

II. HISTOGENESIS

Germ cell tumors are ultimately derived from primitive germ cells. The most widely accepted view of the histogenesis and interrelationship of the various types of germ cell tumors, is best illustrated by a scheme proposed by Teilum [2] and depicted in Fig. 7.1. Teilum [2, 3] regarded dysgerminoma (seminoma) as a primitive germ cell neoplasm which has not acquired the potential for further differentiation. Embryonal carcinoma was considered as a morphologic as well as a conceptual entity, and as a germ cell tumor composed of multipotential cells capable of further differentiation. The view that dysgerminoma is incapable of further differentiation has been challenged by recent immunocytochemical studies which revealed the presence of occasional low molecular weight cytokeratin positive cells in some seminomas and

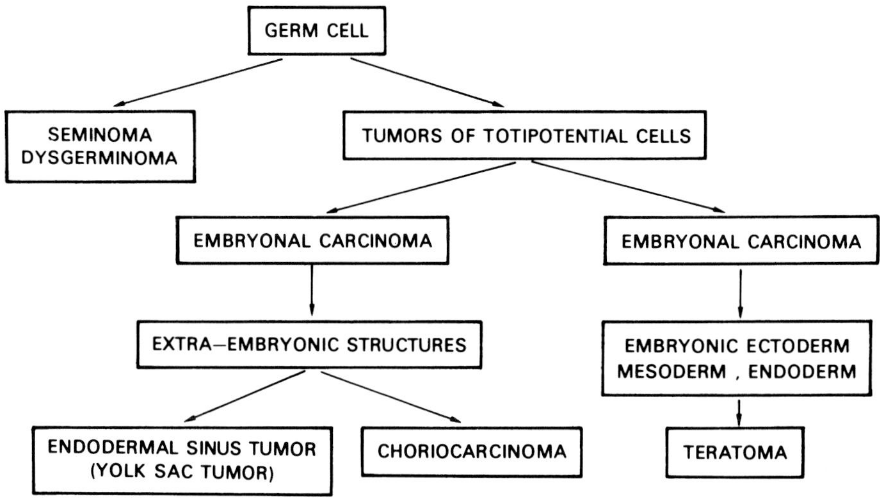

FIGURE 7.1 The histogenesis and interrelationships of germ cell neoplasms (Modified from Teilum, A. (1994). *In* "Blaustein's Pathology of the Female Genital Tract" (R. J. Kurman, ed.), 4th ed., pp. 849–914, Springer-Verlag, New York.)

dysgerminomas, suggesting that these tumors may have the capability to differentiate further.[4] This view is also supported by the intimate admixture of dysgerminoma cells with other neoplastic germ cell elements seen in a considerable number of malignant germ cell tumors.

III. CLASSIFICATION

The classification of ovarian germ cell tumors which will be followed is the widely accepted World Health Organization (WHO) classification [5] with some modifications, which are included in its updated version.[6]

Germ cell tumors
- A. Dysgerminoma
  Variant with syncytiotrophoblastic cells
- B. Yolk sac tumor (endodermal sinus tumor)
  Variants
  1. Polyvesicular vitelline tumor
  2. Hepatoid
  3. Glandular
- C. Embryonal carcinoma
- D. Polyembryoma
- E. Choriocarcinoma
- F. Teratomas
  1. Immature
  2. Mature
     a. Solid
     b. Cystic (dermoid cyst)
     c. With secondary tumor formation (specify type)
     d. Fetiform (homunculus)
  3. Monodermal and highly specialized
     a. Struma ovarii
        Variant with thyroid tumor (specify type)
     b. Carcinoid
        Insular
        Trabecular
     c. Strumal carcinoid
     d. Mucinous carcinoid
     e. Neuroectodermal tumors
     f. Sebaceous tumors
     g. Others
  4. Mixed types (tumors composed of types A through F in any combination) (specify type)

Tumors composed of germ cells and sex cord-stromal derivatives
- A. Gonadoblastoma
  Variant with dysgerminoma or other germ cell tumor
- B. Mixed germ cell-sex cord stromal tumor
  Variant with dysgerminoma or other germ cell tumor

This classification [6] differs from the original WHO classification [5] by the acceptance of the more embracing term of yolk sac tumor (YST) instead of the more specific endodermal sinus tumor, although retaining the latter as an alternative term. It also includes the more correct term mature cystic teratoma for dermoid cyst, retaining the latter as an alternative term due to its widespread use. The category of monodermal, or highly specialized teratoma includes various newly described or unusual entities. The tumors composed of germ cells and sex cord-stromal derivatives have been divided into two specific types, gonadoblastoma and mixed germ cell-sex cord stromal tumor (MGC-SCST). They will also be described and discussed in this chapter.

IV. DYSGERMINOMA

Dysgerminoma is the most common malignant ovarian germ cell neoplasm occurring in pure form.[1, 7, 8] Although at one time it was considered to be much more common than any other malignant ovarian germ cell tumor, it is now closely followed by YST. Due to more extensive sampling of the tumor, more dysgerminomas are found to be combined with other neoplastic germ cell elements than reported previously. Such tumors are included in the category of malignant mixed germ cell tumors.[9–11]

Recent studies [8, 12] support previous observations regarding the age incidence of patients with dysgerminoma. They indicate that the majority of the affected subjects are adolescent or young adult females. The peak incidence is in the second and third decades, and 80% of patients are younger than 30 years.

The great majority of patients with dysgerminoma are normally developed young females with a normal 46,XX chromosome complement.[1] Although dysgerminoma is the most common germ cell tumor observed in subjects with gonadal maldevelopment and chromosomal abnormalities, only 5–10% of dysgerminomas occur in such subjects. Abdominal enlargement is the most frequent presenting symptom.[1, 7, 8, 12] Dysgerminoma may be found incidentally, or during the investigation of patients with primary amenorrhea. In the latter case, it is usually associated with gonadoblastoma. Due to its age incidence, dysgerminoma is one of the most common ovarian neoplasms occurring during pregnancy and puerperium. Occasionally, patients present with acute abdominal emergency due to torsion of the tumor.[1]

Dysgerminoma is mainly unilateral, but bilateral involvement is observed in approximately 10% of cases.[1, 8, 12] It differs in this respect from other malignant ovarian germ cell tumors which are almost always unilateral. Bilaterality must be distinguished from metastatic involvement. The finding of multiple tumor nodules scattered throughout the ovarian tissue, either grossly or microscopically, is strongly suggestive of metastatic spread from the contralateral ovary.

Pure dysgerminomas are gray-yellow, solid, round, oval or lobulated, rapidly growing tumors, usually with a smooth glistening capsule. On cross section, pure dysgerminomas are solid and vary in consistency from soft to rubbery, depending on the amount of fibrous tissue present. Microscopically, dysgerminoma is composed of aggregates, islands, nests, or strands of large uniform cells separated by connective tissue which contains lymphocytes, other inflammatory cells (Figs. 7.2 and 7.3), and a granulomatous reaction with foreign body and Langhans giant cells (Fig. 7.4). The amount of connective tissue varies from fine fibrovascular septa to large fibrous bands and tends to determine the microscopic appearance of the tumor (Figs. 7.2–7.4). Thus dysgerminomas vary from very cellular tumors containing only imperceptible amounts of connective tissue to tumors composed mainly of dense fibrous connective tissue containing a small number of tumor cells.

The great majority of dysgerminoma cells do not react with any intermediate filament antibodies including low molecular weight cytokeratin, while cells of embryonal carcinoma, YST, and choriocarcinoma show uniformly positive staining. This provides a useful method for differentiating between dysgerminoma and the other malignant germ cell tumors mentioned above. Like its testicular counterpart, dysgerminoma cells stain positively with placental specific alkaline phosphatase (PLAP) showing fine membranous staining. Strong positive membranous staining for PLAP provides good confirmatory evidence for the diagnosis of dysgerminoma. Dysgerminoma cells contain double the amount of DNA present in normal somatic cells.[13, 14] Ultrastructurally, dysgerminoma cells are characterized by a cytoplasm showing

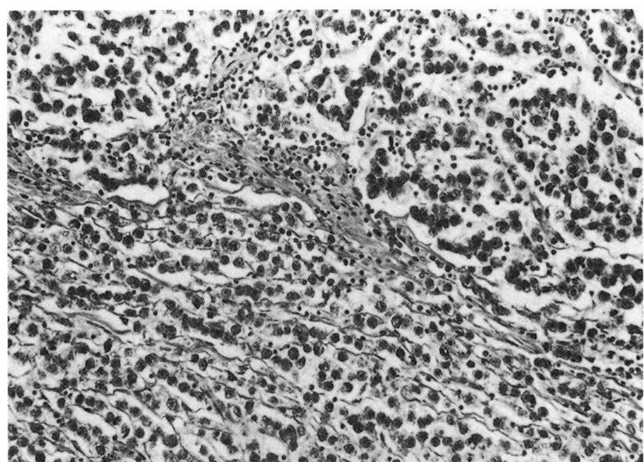

FIGURE 7.2 Dysgerminoma. The tumor is composed of aggregates of uniform cells forming strands surrounded by fine fibrovascular septa (bottom) and nests (top). Note the fibrous septum containing lymphocytes (center).

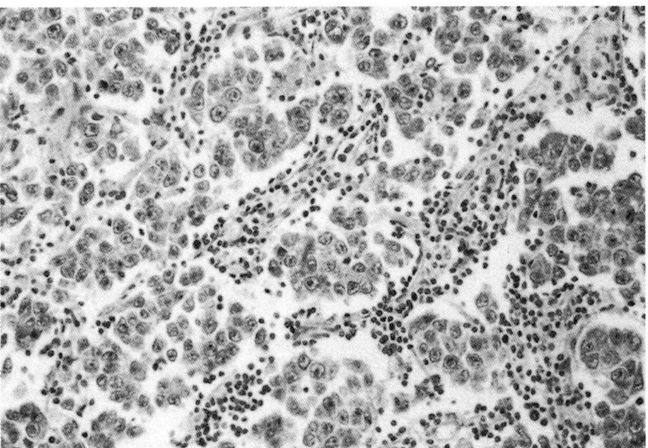

FIGURE 7.3 Dysgerminoma. Note the typical uniform appearance of the tumor cells, which are surrounded by fibrous septa containing lymphocytes.

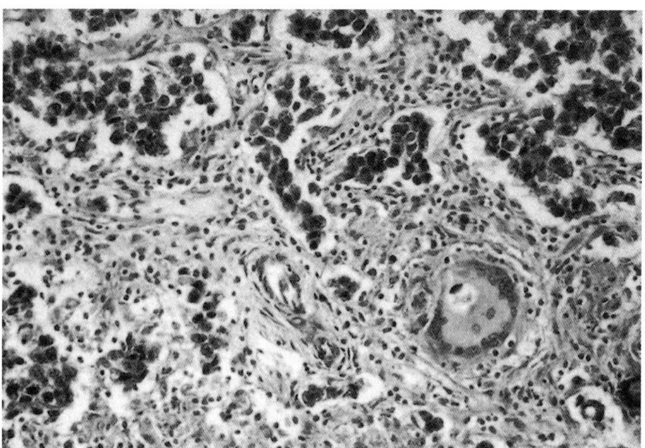

FIGURE 7.4 Dysgerminoma associated with granulomatous reaction. Note a Langhans giant cell (center) and collections of histiocytes (bottom) which surround groups of tumor cells.

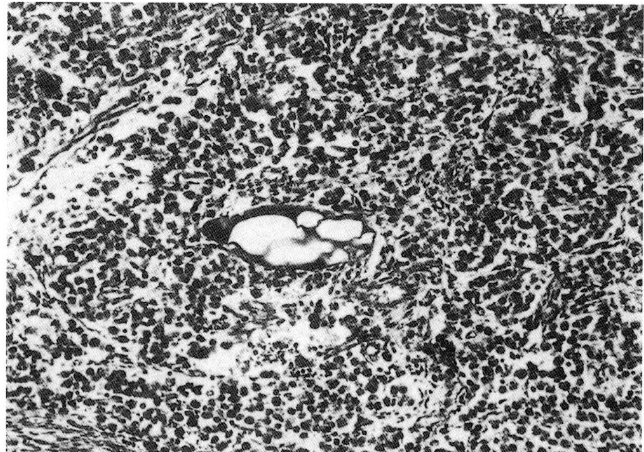

FIGURE 7.5 Dysgerminoma containing a large vacuolated syncytiotrophoblastic giant cell (center). This cell stained positively for beta-HCG.

paucity of organelles, and a large nucleus with prominent strand-like nucleolonema.

It has been suggested that dysgerminomas showing paucity of lymphocytic and granulomatous infiltration, scanty fibrous tissue, increased cellularity, and mitotic activity in common with the so-called "anaplastic" testicular classic seminoma, follow a more aggressive course and are associated with a worse prognosis. Recent studies describing therapeutic results in patients with dysgerminoma have failed to confirm these views, or to detect a group of patients with worse prognosis.[8]

Between 6 and 8% of dysgerminomas contain syncytiotrophoblastic giant cells (Fig. 7.5), which have been conclusively shown to produce HCG and beta-HCG.[1, 15] Cytotrophoblastic cells have not been observed in conjunction with the syncytiotrophoblastic giant cells. The latter must be differentiated from foreign body and Langhans giant cells (Fig. 7.4). Patients with dysgerminoma containing syncytiotrophoblastic giant cells usually show elevations of serum HCG or beta-HCG, although the levels are usually much lower than in patients with tumors composed of dysgerminoma admixed with choriocarcinoma. The serial estimation of these substances in the serum may be used for monitoring the progress of the disease in the same way as in patients with gestational or nongestational choriocarcinoma. There is no evidence that patients with dysgerminoma containing syncytiotrophoblastic giant cells have a worse prognosis. It is of utmost importance to recognize these cells correctly as syncytiotrophoblastic giant cells and not to misinterpret them as choriocarcinoma. As dysgerminoma is frequently combined with other malignant neoplastic germ cell elements, and as the presence of these elements alters the therapeutic approach, the importance of judicious and extensive sampling of the tumor and of careful histological examination are strongly emphasized.

Dysgerminoma is an aggressive neoplasm which grows rapidly invading and destroying ovarian tissue. Direct invasion of the surrounding organs and structures is seen with large tumors. Dysgerminoma first metastasizes via the lymphatics to the para-iliac and para-aortic lymph nodes. Hematogenous spread occurs later and metastases are found in the lungs, liver, bones, and other sites. Although the metastases are usually composed of dysgerminoma, in approximately 10% of cases they contain other malignant neoplastic germ cell elements.

Alpha-fetoprotein (AFP) and HCG are not elevated in the serum of patients with pure dysgerminoma.[16] Elevated levels of serum lactic dehydrogenase (LDH) have been noted in patients with dysgerminoma [17] and more recently an even better correlation was noted when isoenzymes 1 and 2 of LDH were estimated.[18, 19] There is a good correlation between the amount of tumor present and the serum enzyme levels.[17] The amount of tumor tissue needed to produce elevated levels is relatively large, thus limiting the use of these substances as tumor markers. In cases with larger tumors the estimation of LDH and especially its isoenzymes 1 and 2 is of considerable diagnostic value.[17, 19]

V. YST (YOLK SAC TUMOR)

Yolk sac tumor is the second most common ovarian malignant germ cell neoplasm occurring in pure form, and is also a frequent component of mixed germ cell tumors.[1] Originally YST was considered to be very rare, but it is now diagnosed with much greater frequency. The increase in incidence is due to the much better recognition of YST as a specific pathological entity, and to the fact that presence of perivascular formations (Schiller-Duval bodies) (Fig. 7.6) is not a prerequisite for the diagnosis of YST.[1, 3, 20]

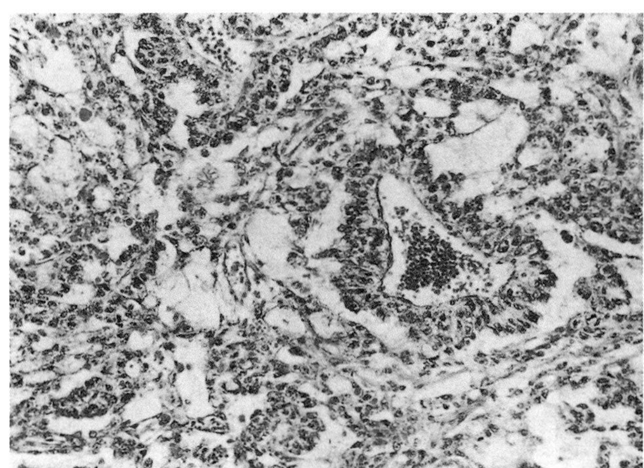

FIGURE 7.6 Yolk sac (endodermal sinus) tumor (YST). Typical perivascular formation (Schiller-Duval body) considered a hallmark of YST. Other histologic patterns of this tumor are seen in its vicinity.

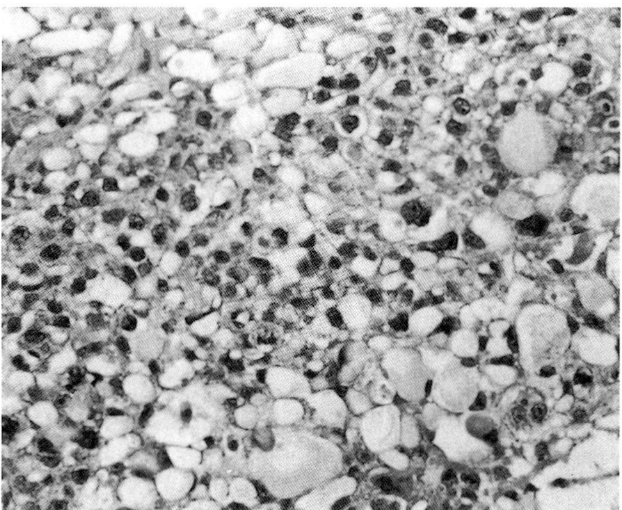

FIGURE 7.7 Yolk sac tumor showing microcystic and solid patterns. Note the typical microcysts (top and bottom) and solid aggregates of tumor cells (left).

YST is encountered most frequently in the second and third decades, followed by first and fourth, and is rare in women in the fifth decade.[1, 3, 7, 20, 21] It is very rare after menopause.[1] Most ovarian YSTs occurring in postmenopausal women are examples of metaplastic transformation of a surface epithelial stromal tumor, and not of germ cell origin. It is very important to recognize this, as these tumors behave differently from YSTs of germ cell origin and do not respond as well to the combination therapy used so successfully to treat the latter.[22–24]

Patients with ovarian YST usually present with abdominal enlargement, abdominal pain, or both. The tumors grow rapidly. Due to its age incidence, YST may be encountered during pregnancy. Occasionally, it is discovered incidentally. YST is unilateral, but metastatic involvement of the contralateral ovary may be observed and must be differentiated from bilaterality.[1] YST, like any other malignant germ cell tumor, may be associated with mature cystic teratoma in the contralateral ovary, Macroscopically the tumor is soft, round, oval, or lobulated. When large, it may invade the surrounding structures. On cross section, it is solid, gray-white, often with hemorrhagic and necrotic areas and its surface is mucoid.[1–3, 7]

Microscopically, YST usually shows a variety of histological patterns. Ten histological patterns have been described [1, 25] as follows:

1. Endodermal sinus (Fig. 7.6)
2. Microcystic (Fig. 7.7)
3. Papillary (Fig. 7.8)
4. Glandular-alveolar (Fig. 7.9)
5. Solid (Fig. 7.7)
6. Myxomatous (Figs. 7.8 and 7.9)
7. Macrocystic (Fig. 7.10)
8. Polyvesicular vitelline (Fig. 7.11)

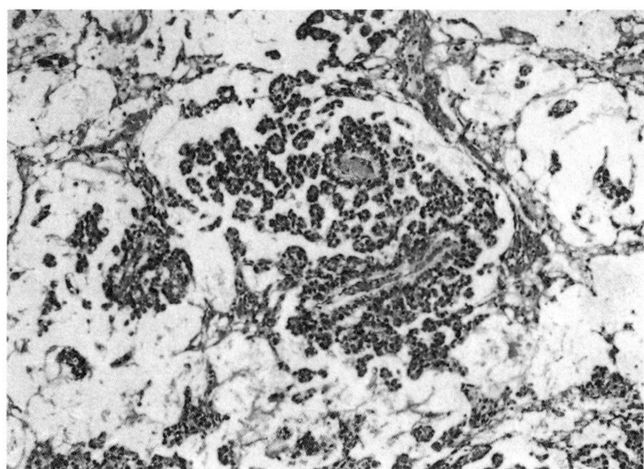

FIGURE 7.8 Yolk sac tumor showing papillary and myxomatous patterns. Two perivascular formations, one sectioned transversely, the other longitudinally are seen in the center.

9. Hepatoid (Fig. 7.12)
10. Primitive intestinal (enteric) (Fig 7.13)

While many of the histological patterns of YST may be seen in one tumor, occasionally, a tumor may exhibit a single pattern causing diagnostic difficulties. Three histological patterns of YST are most frequently seen in pure form; the polyvesicular vitelline pattern [2] (Fig. 7.11), the hepatoid pattern [26] (Fig. 7.12), and the primitive intestinal pattern [27, 28] (Fig. 7.13). The polyvesicular vitelline pattern is characterized by the presence of numerous small vesicles and cysts, usually oval, sometimes with central constriction, and lined by columnar, cuboidal, or flattened epithelial cells.

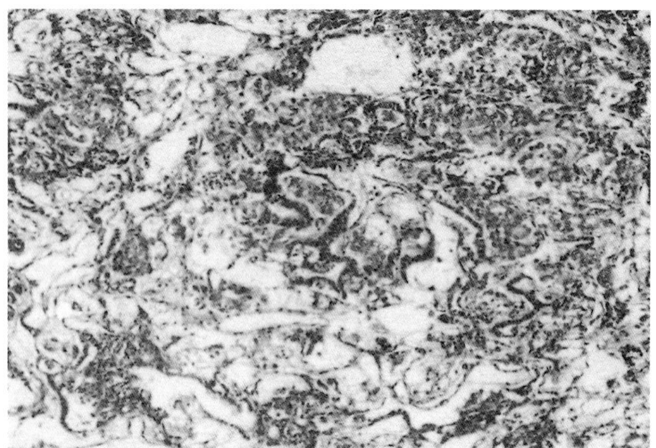

FIGURE 7.9 Yolk sac tumor showing glandular-alveolar and myxomatous patterns.

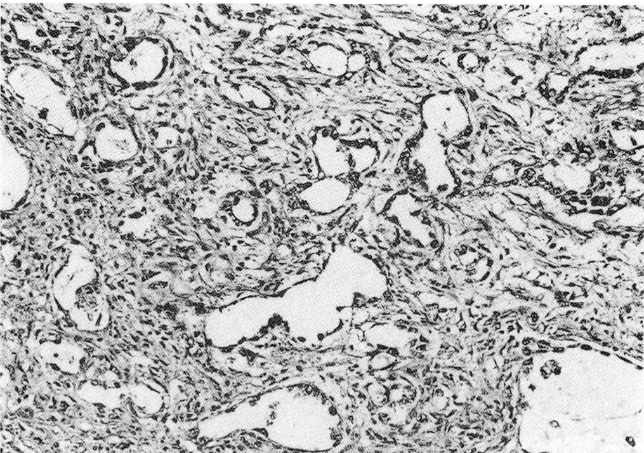

FIGURE 7.11 Yolk sac tumor showing polyvesicular vitelline pattern and composed of numerous vesicles varying in shape surrounded by loose connective tissue.

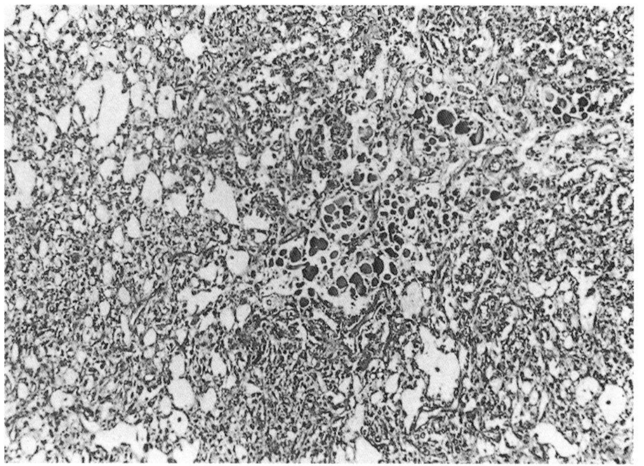

FIGURE 7.10 Yolk sac tumor showing cystic pattern. Focally papillary and solid patterns are also seen. Note the numerous hyaline bodies (center) which are not diagnostic of YST, but are frequently seen in this tumor.

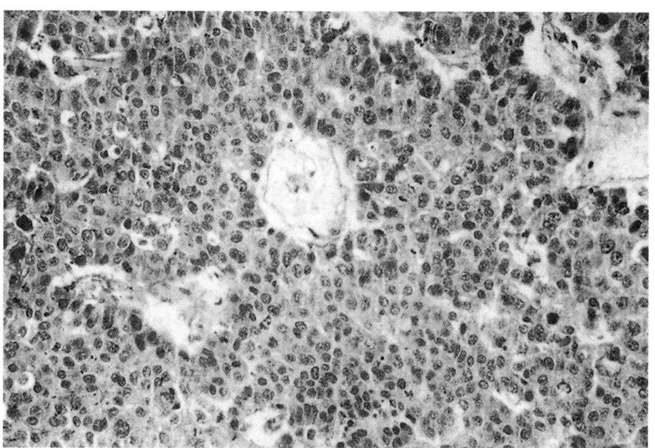

FIGURE 7.12 Yolk sac tumor showing hepatoid pattern and composed of aggregates of medium-sized cells with granular cytoplasm and large round or oval nuclei resembling hepatocytes.

They are surrounded by connective tissue which may vary from dense cellular to loose and edematous. The hepatoid pattern [26] resembles the appearance of hepatocellular carcinoma or primitive (embryonal or fetal) hepatic tissue. The tumor is composed of large polygonal cells with eosinophilic cytoplasm, which usually show a considerable degree of cellular and nuclear pleomorphism and brisk mitotic activity (Fig. 7.12). The primitive intestinal pattern [27, 28] is characterized by collections of glands lined by pleomorphic cells with large hyperchromatic nuclei and showing brisk mitotic activity (Fig. 7.13). The glands contain mucin, which may be dense and inspissated. Hyaline globules may be numerous in places. The collections of glands are surrounded by connective tissue, the amount and appearance of which may vary [27, 28]. Another variant of this pattern is characterized by primitive glands of various sizes lined by tall columnar or cuboid cells with clear cytoplasm which may resemble secretory endometrial carcinoma.[29]

The demonstration of AFP within the tumor tissue by immunocytochemistry or immunofluorescence and of elevated levels in the serum is helpful in making the diagnosis in these cases. The serum AFP levels can be correlated with the amount of YST present within the tumor, and estimation of serum AFP can be used for evaluation of the results of primary surgical treatment, for monitoring patients during chemotherapy, and for early detection of metastases and recurrences.[1, 16]

YST is a highly malignant neoplasm which grows rapidly, invades the surrounding structures, and metastasizes early to the regional lymph nodes and by hematogenous spread to the lungs, liver, and other organs.

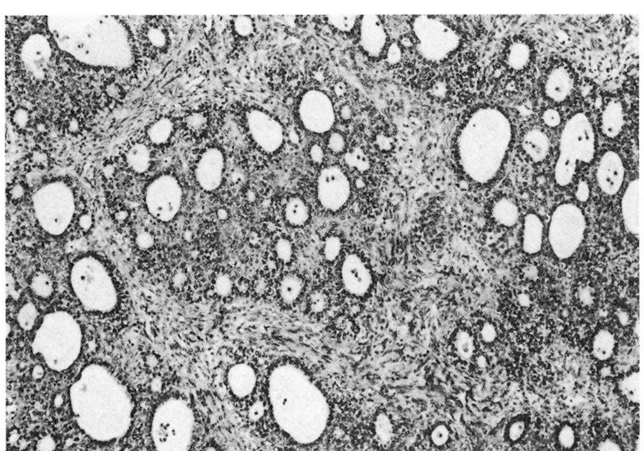

FIGURE 7.13 Yolk sac tumor showing the primitive intestinal pattern and composed of nests of primitive endodermal cells which show grandular differentiation.

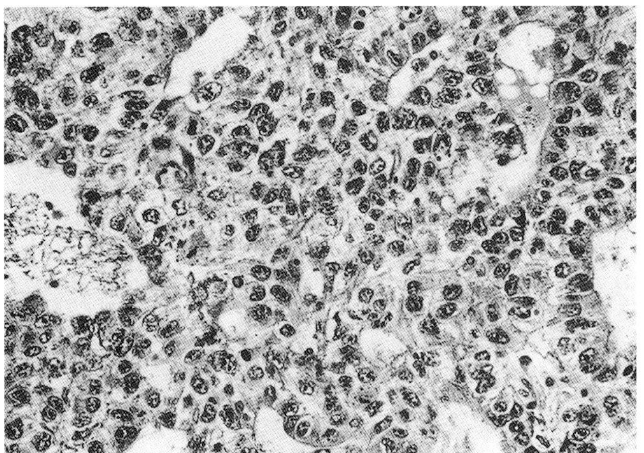

FIGURE 7.14 Embryonal carcinoma composed of aggregates of primitive epithelial-like cells forming solid pattern. Occasional clefts or spaces resembling glands are present.

VI. EMBRYONAL CARCINOMA

The term embryonal carcinoma is employed here to describe only the ovarian germ cell neoplasms showing the same histological appearance (Fig. 7.14) as their more common testicular counterparts.[25, 30] This is important, as in the past the term embryonal carcinoma was used not only to describe this entity, but the more common YST. Strict diagnostic criteria should be followed when making this diagnosis. Ovarian tumors composed entirely of embryonal carcinoma are very rare, and embryonal carcinoma is usually encountered as a component of a mixed germ cell tumor, most frequently combined with YST.[1]

Embryonal carcinoma is seen in the same age group as other malignant ovarian germ cell tumors with which it has many features in common. It frequently contains syncytiotrophoblastic giant cells, and occasionally is combined with choriocarcinoma. Elevated levels of serum HCG or beta-HCG are seen in either instance, but the levels tend to be much higher when choriocarcinoma is present. The behavior of embryonal carcinoma is similar to that of YST.

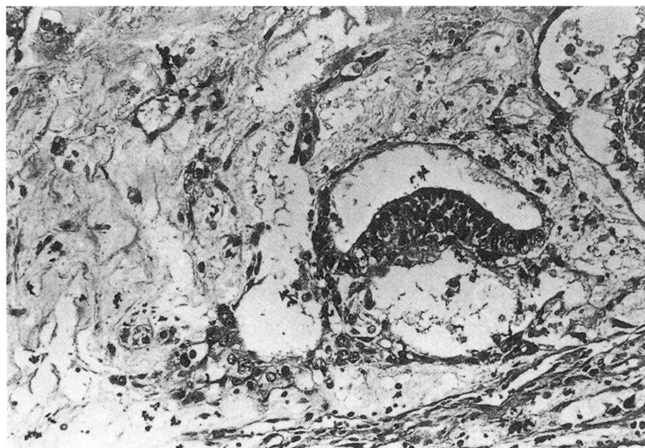

FIGURE 7.15 Embryoid body surrounded by myxomatous stroma. Tumors containing many such structures are known as polyembryomas. Note the embryonic disc (center), amniotic cavity (top), and yolk sac (bottom).

VII. POLYEMBRYOMA

Polyembryoma is a germ cell neoplasm composed entirely of embryoid bodies resembling morphologically presomite embryos, which do not develop beyond the 18-day stage. Pure polyembryoma has not been observed in the ovary, and in the few reported cases the tumor was combined with other neoplastic germ cell elements.[1] Tumors reported as polyembryoma were usually large and did not differ substantially from other malignant ovarian germ cell tumors. Microscopically, polyembryoma is composed of embryoid bodies which when well formed consist of an embryonic disc located in the center and surrounded on one side by an amniotic cavity and on the other by yolk sac (Fig. 7.15). Atypical or malformed embryoid bodies may contain an embryonic disc, which may not be well formed, and two, or more yolk sacs with a single amniotic cavity, or vice versa. The embryoid bodies are surrounded by myxomatous tissue (Fig. 7.15), or primitive mesenchymal tissue. Syncytiotrophoblastic giant cells are often seen in the vicinity of the embryoid bodies, and teratomatous elements are also often present.[1] The behavior is similar to that observed in other malignant ovarian germ cell tumors.

VIII. CHORIOCARCINOMA

The nongestational choriocarcinoma discussed here is a germ cell neoplasm, which is histologically indistinguishable from its more common gestational counterpart. It has the same age incidence as other malignant ovarian germ cell tumors, and therefore, when occurring in pure form during the reproductive years, can only be diagnosed after very careful investigations, which must exclude the presence of its gestational counterpart.[1] Nongestational choriocarcinoma is seen as a component of mixed germ cell tumors,[1] and is very rare in pure form.

Choriocarcinoma can only be diagnosed when both syncytiotrophoblast and cytotrophoblast are present within the tumor (Figs. 7.16 and 7.17). Scattered syncytiotrophoblastic giant cells, which may be present in a number of malignant germ cell neoplasms do not constitute choriocarcinoma. Choriocarcinoma produces large amounts of HCG and elevated serum levels are present. HCG, and preferably its beta-subunit (beta-HCG), which does not crossreact with lutinizing hormone (LH) is a valuable tumor marker for patients with ovarian germ cell tumors containing choriocarcinoma.[1] Tumors containing choriocarcinoma are usually large, solid, rapidly growing and are invariably hemorrhagic. They are unilateral, but may be associated with metastases or mature cystic teratoma in the contralateral ovary. Choriocarcinoma is composed of aggregates of medium-sized cytotrophoblastic cells and large uni- or multinucleated syncytiotrophoblastic cells with large hyperchromatic or pyknotic nuclei (Figs. 7.16 and 7.17). The tumor is usually associated with hemorrhage (Figs. 7.16 and 7.17). Nongestational choriocarcinoma is an aggressive component of malignant germ cell tumors, which metastasizes widely via hematogenous and lymphatic routes and invades locally.

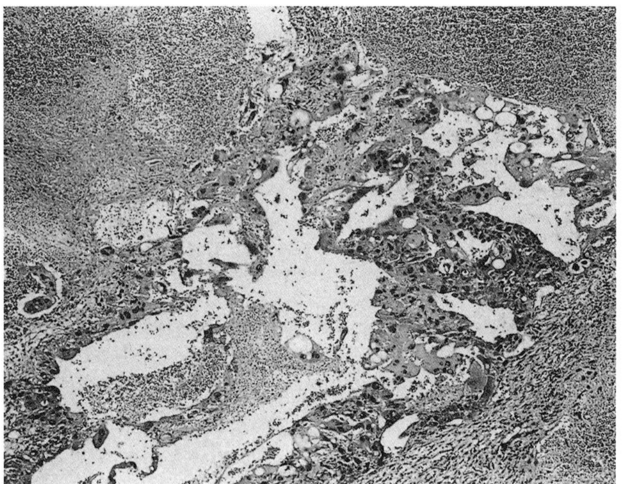

FIGURE 7.16 Choriocarcinoma. Note the numerous large vacuolated and multinucleated synctiotrophoblastic cells, small number of cytotrophoblastic cells (left), and marked hemorrhage and necrosis.

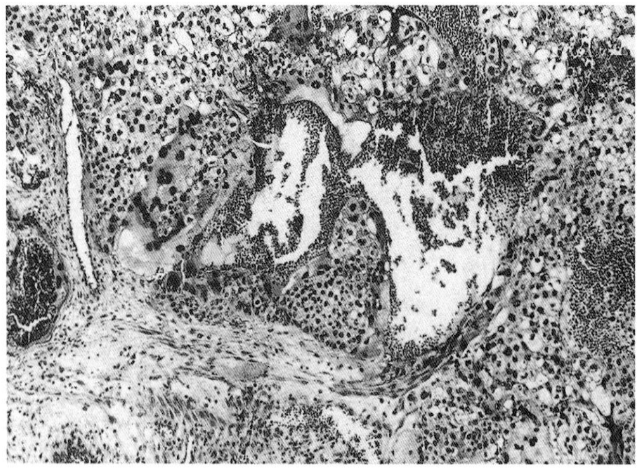

FIGURE 7.17 Choriocarcinoma. Note the smaller cytotrophoblastic cells, the large syncytiotrophoblastic cells, and hemorrhage in the center.

IX. TERATOMA

Teratomas are germ cell neoplasmas composed of derivatives of the three primitive germ layers, ectoderm, mesoderm, and endoderm. They represent the result of further differentiation of embryonal carcinoma along the somatic or embryonic pathway. As the process of differentiation of teratoma is dynamic, they exhibit varying degrees of maturity. In the ovary, the overwhelming majority (99%) of teratomas are mature and cystic. They are classified as mature cystic teratomas or dermoid cysts, and by virtue of complete maturity of the constituent tissues are benign.

A. Mature Cystic Teratoma (Dermoid Cyst)

Unlike the malignant germ cell neoplasms described above, which occur from birth to premenopause, mature cystic teratoma has a much wider age range and is encountered from birth to old age. It is more common in the first five decades of life, and therefore, has the same tendency as other germ cell tumors of the ovary to occur in younger subjects. It has been observed in fetuses and newborns.

The majority of the tumors are small, or medium-sized with a smooth surface. The wall is thin, but is thicker in places (Fig. 7.18). The tumor is usually uniloculated. Mature cystic teratomas are generally unilateral. Bilaterality is seen in approximately 10–15% of cases, and in a number of cases may be associated with a malignant germ cell tumor in the contralateral ovary. Occasionally multiple tumors may be present in the same ovary. Microscopically, the tumor is composed of a variety of tissues showing orderly arrangement with skin and its adnexa predominating (Fig. 7.19). Adipose and neural tissue (Fig. 7.20), bone, cartilage, smooth muscle, intestinal and bronchial mucosa, and thyroid tissue are frequent constituents. Well-formed teeth may be seen (Fig. 7.21). All the tissues are fully mature and the tumor is benign. Occasionally mature cystic teratoma may be associated with

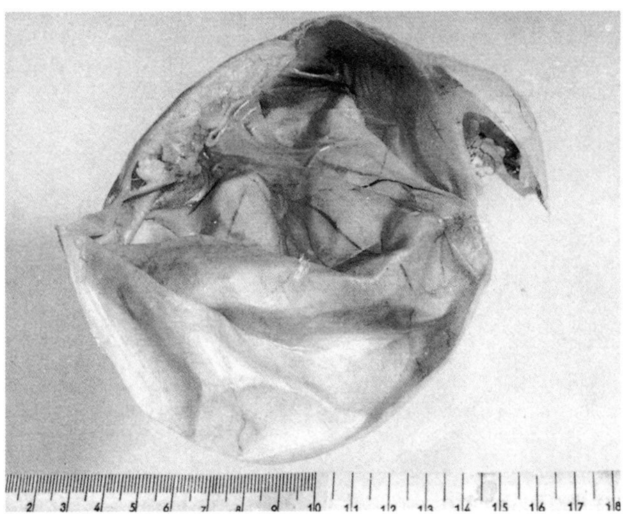

FIGURE 7.18 Mature cystic teratoma (dermoid cyst). The protuberance or mamilla which contains a variety of tissues is seen at the top where the thin and smooth wall of the cyst becomes thicker.

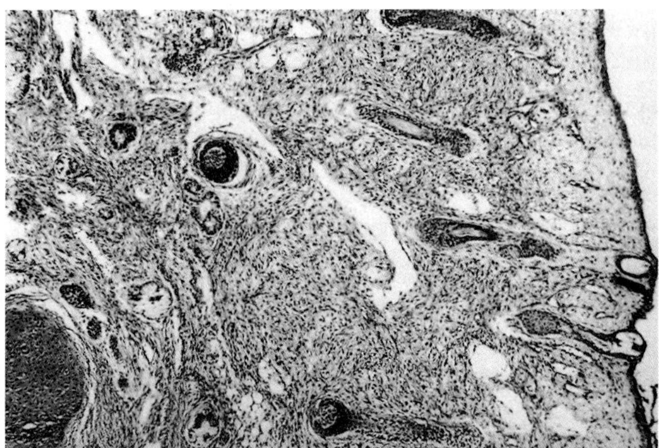

FIGURE 7.19 Mature cystic teratoma showing skin and its adnexal structures which are the most frequent constituents of the tumor. Also note a plate of cartilage (bottom left).

mature neural (glial) implants in the peritoneal cavity also known as gliomatosis peritonei.[7, 31] Because these implants are fully mature, they are benign. It is very important to recognize that gliomatosis peritonei is a benign condition and not necessitating further therapy in spite of its frequently alarming appearance with the presence of multiple peritoneal implants.

B. Mature Solid Teratoma

Mature solid teratoma is very rare.[1, 7] Since the great majority of solid teratomas contain immature elements and are malignant, the diagnosis of mature solid teratoma can only be made after extensive sampling and very careful histological examination. Mature solid teratoma occurs in young

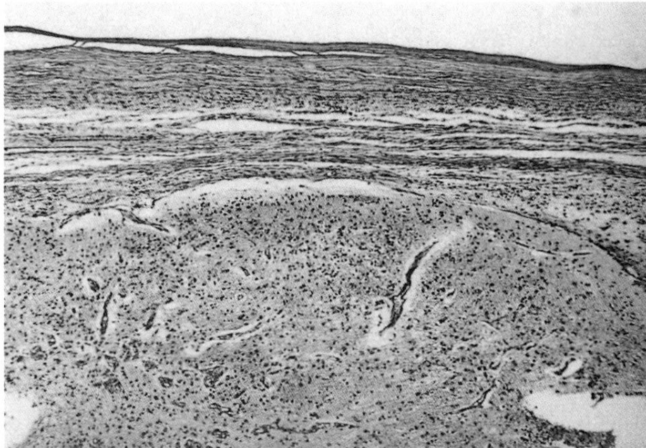

FIGURE 7.20 Mature cystic teratoma lined by squamous epithelium (top) and containing a large amount of mature neural tissue (center and bottom).

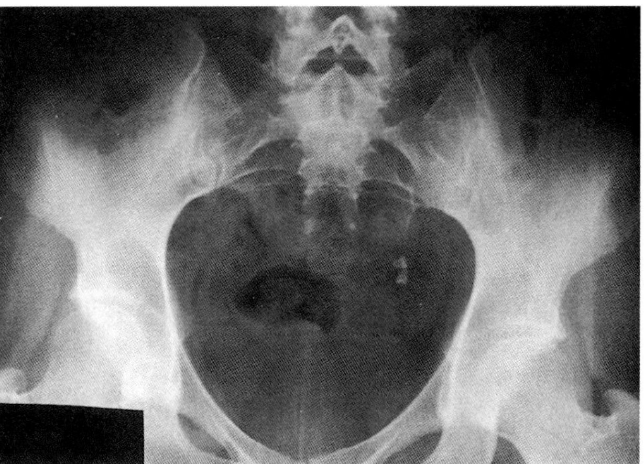

FIGURE 7.21 Mature cystic teratoma. A radiograph showing well formed teeth present within the tumor.

subjects.[1] Because all its constituent tissues are mature, the tumor is benign.

C. Immature Teratoma

Immature teratoma is uncommon and comprises less than one percent of ovarian teratomas. It is unilateral, but may be associated with mature cystic teratoma in the contralateral ovary.[1, 7] Immature teratomas tend to be larger than their mature counterparts. The tumors are usually large, round or oval, and solid. They may contain cystic areas. Microscopically, the tumors are composed of immature tissues derived from the three primitive germ layers, and show a varying degree of immaturity (Fig. 7.22). Mature elements are frequently intermingled with the immature, which usually predominate. The arrangement of the various tissues is less orderly and more haphazard than in mature teratoma.

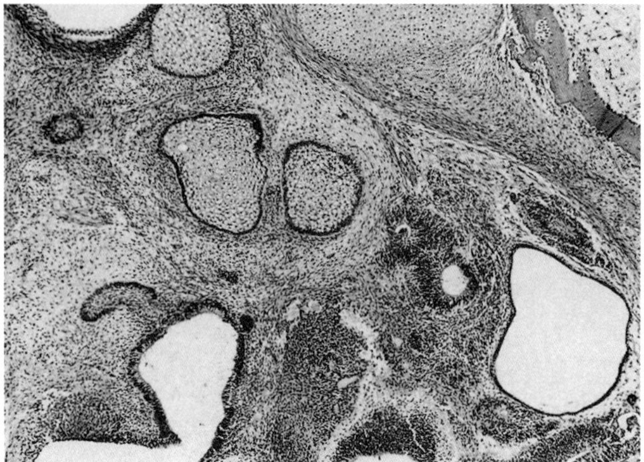

FIGURE 7.22 Immature teratoma. Note the lack of orderly arrangement seen in mature cystic teratoma, the numerous tissues present which are mostly immature, but mature bone is also present (top right).

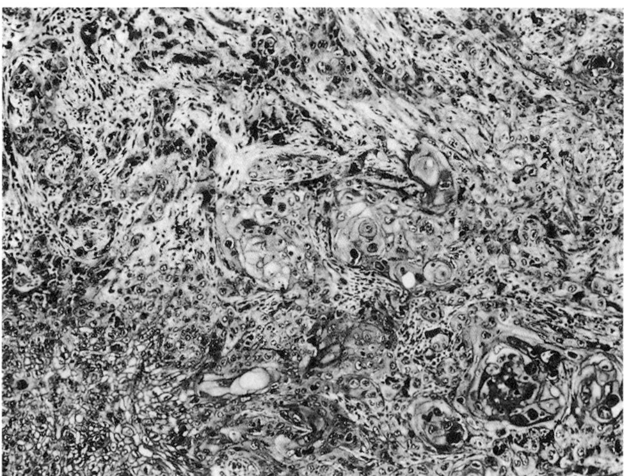

FIGURE 7.23 Mature cystic teratoma with malignant transformation and formation of invasive squamous cell carcinoma. This is the most common type.

Immature teratoma may be combined with other malignant neoplastic germ cell elements forming a malignant mixed germ cell tumor. In such cases, the levels of serum AFP and beta-HCG may be elevated reflecting the presence of YST, or choriocarcinoma. There is a strong correlation between the degree of immaturity of the tumor and its behavior. This has led to the formulation of grading systems, two of which tend to be used nowadays. One system is based on the degree of immaturity of the neural elements, which frequently tend to form the predominant component in these tumors,[32] while the other [1, 33] takes into consideration the degree of immaturity of all the elements present within the tumor. The latter system [1, 33] shown below is advocated.

Grade 0: All tissues mature; no mitotic activity

Grade 1: Minor foci of abnormally cellular or embryonal tissue mixed with mature elements; slight mitotic activity

Grade 2: Moderate quantities of embryonal tissue mixed with mature elements; moderate mitotic activity

Grade 3: Large quantities of embryonal tissue present, high mitotic activity

Immature teratoma shows many features in common with other malignant germ cell neoplasms described above and behaves in a similar manner.

D. Mature Cystic Teratoma (Dermoid Cyst) with Malignant Transformation

Malignant transformation is an uncommon complication, which occurs in approximately 2% of mature cystic teratomas.[1, 7] Unlike the vast majority of patients with malignant ovarian germ cell tumors who are premenopausal, most of the patients with this tumor are postmenopausal.[1, 7, 34] The tumors are unilateral, but may be associated with mature cystic teratoma in the contralateral ovary. The tumors are usually large and may invade the surrounding structures. They may be associated with extensive involvement of the peritoneal cavity by tumor deposits.

Microscopically, the tumor at least in some areas shows appearances of typical mature cystic teratoma, and malignant transformation of one of its components, usually squamous epithelium which forms a squamous cell carcinoma (Fig. 7.23). The latter is often well differentiated, but the degree of differentiation may vary. Any tissue within the tumor may undergo malignant change. Mature cystic teratoma with malignant transformation does not spread via the lymphatic and hematogenous routes, but spreads extensively throughout the abdominal cavity. When the tumor is composed of squamous cell carcinoma and is confined to the ovary, patients have a 63%, 5-year survival. Patients with disseminated disease have only a 15%, 5-year survival. The prognosis is even worse when the malignant element is not a squamous cell carcinoma. Early stage at diagnosis and complete excision of the tumor are at present the best prognostic features.[1, 7]

X. MONODERMAL OR HIGHLY SPECIALIZED TERATOMAS

The tumors comprising this group are composed of a single tissue and are considered to represent one-sided development of a teratoma.

XI. STRUMA OVARII

Struma ovarii is the best known member of this group of neoplasms. It is composed of thyroid tissue. Struma ovarii is uncommon comprising approximately one percent of ovarian teratomas.[1, 7] It must be distinguished from mature cystic teratoma containing thyroid tissue, which is much more common. The age incidence is the same as that of mature cystic teratoma, and patients present in the same manner. The tumors vary in size, and are usually unilateral, but in 15% of cases are associated with mature cystic teratoma in the contralateral ovary. The tumor is usually soft, smooth, round or oval, fleshy, and light tan. Microscopically, it is composed of normal thyroid tissue (Fig. 7.24), which may in parts exhibit evidence of hyperplastic, nodular, or adenomatous changes. Occasionally, such changes may be extensive, and it is important to distinguish them from malignant change.[1] Struma ovarii is treated by excision of the affected adnexa. When malignant change occurs, it manifests itself as papillary or follicular carcinoma, and the tumor is indistinguishable from its counterparts occurring within the thyroid gland. The tumors are usually well differentiated and metastasize first to the para-aortic lymph nodes.[1]

XII. CARCINOID

Ovarian carcinoid tumors comprise the second most common type of monodermal teratoma after struma ovarii. The classification of carcinoid tumors of the ovary is as follows:

1. Primary
   a. Insular (carcinoid tumors of midgut derivation)
   b. Trabecular carcinoid (carcinoid tumors of foregut and hindgut derivation)
   c. Mucinous (goblet, adenocarcinoid)
   d. Mixed (composed of two, or rarely of three of the above subtypes)
2. Metastatic

A. Insular Carcinoid

Insular carcinoid is the most common type of primary ovarian carcinoid tumor. It is usually found in association with mature cystic teratoma, but may be seen with other teratomatous tumors, and occasionally with Sertoli-Leydig cell tumor.[7] In 40% of cases, it is seen in pure form. The majority of patients are either post- or perimenopausal. They present with an ovarian mass which may be associated with abdominal pain. One-third of patients exhibit stigmata of the carcinoid syndrome.[36] Because the venous drainage of the ovary enters the systemic circulation and bypasses the liver, which is capable of detoxifying the serotonin produced by the tumor, the carcinoid syndrome is seen in the absence of metastatic disease. There is a good correlation between the size of the tumor and the presence of the syndrome, which is virtually only seen in patients with tumors larger than 10 cm.[7] Excision of the tumor results in remission of the symptoms, and the disappearance of serotonin from the blood and 5-hydroxyindole acetic acid (5-HIAA) from the urine. Serotonin and 5-HIAA can be used as tumor markers in patients with functioning ovarian insular carcinoid tumors.

Insular carcinoid forms a solid, yellow-gray tumor nodule within a mature cystic teratoma, or a similar nodule within an ovary when occurring in pure form. The tumor is nearly always unilateral, but may be associated with mature cystic teratoma in the contralateral ovary. Microscopically, it shows typical appearances of a midgut carcinoid tumor and is composed of solid nests and collections of small acini (Fig. 7.25) made up of uniform polygonal cells with ample amount of cytoplasm, and centrally located round or oval nuclei (Fig. 7.26). The cytoplasm contains orange, red, or brown granules which show the argyrophil and argentaffin reactions. The cellular nests are surrounded by connective tissue, which may be dense and hyalinized (Fig. 7.25). The amount of the connective tissue may be very large obscuring the cellular areas and posing diagnostic problems. Ultrastructural examination shows numerous neurosecretory granules which are very pleomorphic, varying in shape and size. Cytokeratin, chromogranin, serotonin, and gastrin can be demonstrated

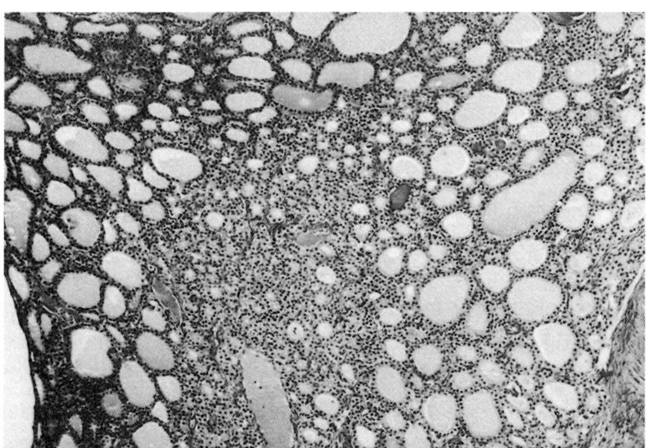

FIGURE 7.24 Struma ovarii. The tumor is composed of normal thyroid tissue.

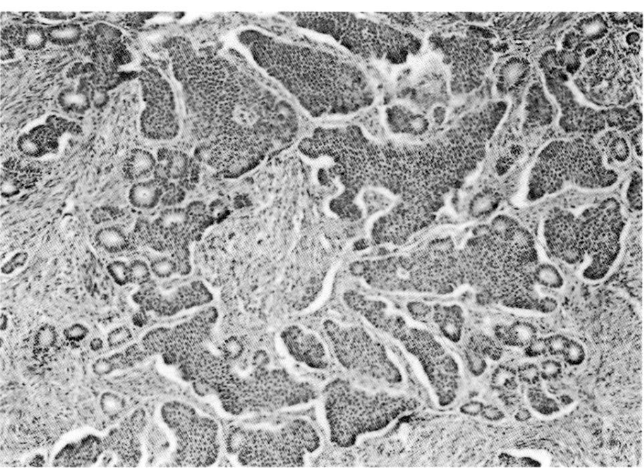

FIGURE 7.25 Insular carcinoid tumor composed of solid cellular nests and small acini surrounded by dense connective tissue.

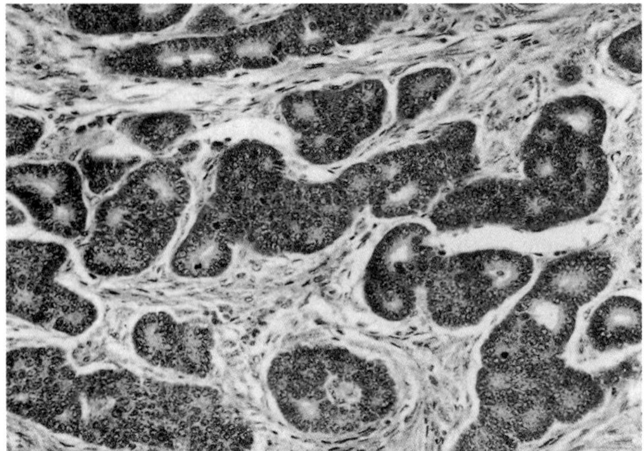

FIGURE 7.26 Insular carcinoid tumor. Note the small acini lined by uniform cells, and the dense connective tissue surrounding them.

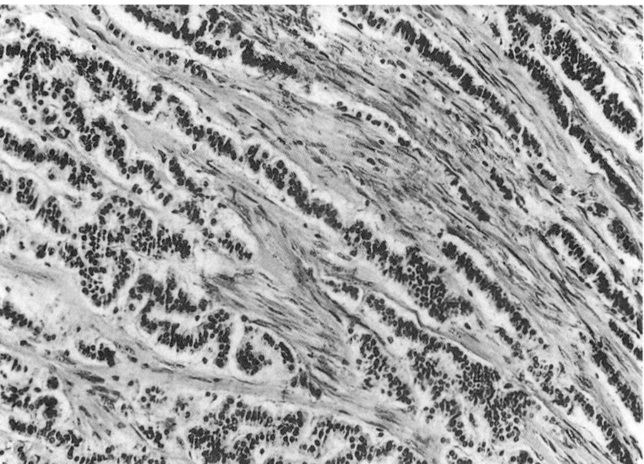

FIGURE 7.27 Trabecular carcinoid tumor composed of long wavy cords or ribbons surrounded by dense connective tissue.

within the tumor cells by immunocytochemistry, but the range of neurohormonal polypeptides, which can be demonstrated is much more limited than in the case of trabecular or strumal carcinoids.[37] Insular carcinoid behaves as a neoplasm of low-grade malignancy and only occasionally has been associated with metastases.[1, 7, 36]

B. Trabecular Carcinoid

Trabecular carcinoid is by far less common than its insular counterpart.[35, 38] It is usually seen in association with mature cystic teratoma, but may also occur in pure form. The affected patients are mainly postmenopausal.[35] The presentation is similar to insular carcinoid, except that like carcinoid tumors of foregut and hindgut derivation, trabecular carcinoid is not associated with the carcinoid syndrome.[35] The macroscopic appearance is similar to insular carcinoid. Microscopically, trabecular carcinoid is composed of long wavy cords, or ribbons, running in parallel and surrounded by narrow bands of connective tissue (Fig. 7.27). The cells are columnar, or polygonal and the cytoplasm may contain orange-red granules. Ultrastructurally, uniformly round or oval neurosecretory granules are present, differing from the pleomorphic granules seen in insular carcinoid.[39] Immunocytochemistry shows a much wider range of neurohormonal polypeptides compared with insular carcinoid.[37] Trabecular carcinoid to date has not been associated with metastases.[35]

C. Mucinous (Goblet Cell, Adenocarcinoid) Carcinoid

Mucinous carcinoid is the least common type pf primary ovarian carcinoid tumor.[35] It shows a wider age range than other types of carcinoid tumors. It is often seen in pure form, but is also observed in association with teratomatous elements.

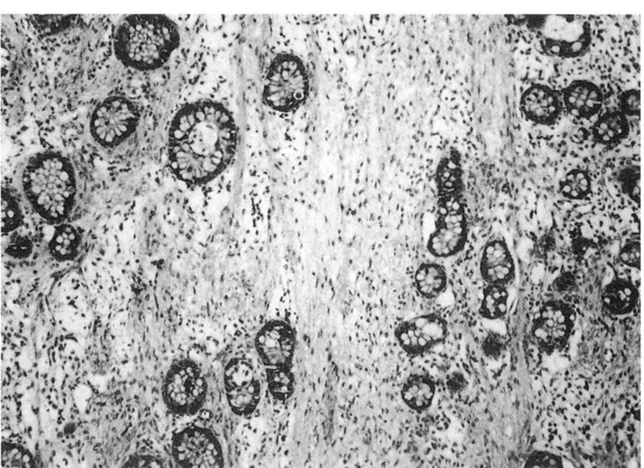

FIGURE 7.28 Mucinous carcinoid tumor composed of numerous small glands with prominent goblet cells and surrounded by loose connective tissue.

It is usually unilateral, but may be associated with mature cystic teratoma, or metastases in the contralateral ovary.[40, 41] The tumor is usually of medium to large size, gray-yellow, and solid, but may contain cystic areas. Microscopically, mucinous carcinoid is composed of numerous small glands or acini with very small lumina, surrounded by connective tissue (Fig. 7.28). The glands are lined by uniform cuboid or columnar cells with pale or clear cytoplasm, and goblet cells with clear and vacuolated cytoplasm (Fig. 7.28). The nuclei vary from small and round to large and hyperchromatic. Some cells are distended with mucin and their nuclei are compressed and may be of the signet-ring type. Other cells may be disrupted due to overdistention with mucin (Fig. 7.28). In some tumors, less well-differentiated areas are present with tumor cells forming larger aggregates with numerous signet-ring cells, larger glands lined by atypical cells, and foci of typical Krukenberg tumor.[35, 40, 41] Ultrastructurally, pleomorphic neurosecretory granules are present, similar to those seen in insular carcinoids.[35, 40] Mucinous carcinoid is more malignant than other types of ovarian carcinoids, and may metastasize widely via small lymphatics. Microscopic metastases may be present at the time of diagnosis.[1, 25, 40, 41]

D. Metastatic Carcinoid Tumors

Primary ovarian carcinoids must be distinguished from metastatic carcinoids, usually of the insular type,[35, 36, 42] but occasionally of the mucinous type.[35] Metastatic carcinoids invariably involve both ovaries and tumor deposits are diffusely scattered throughout the ovarian tissue.

E. Strumal Carcinoid (Struma Ovarii and Carcinoid)

Strumal carcinoid is composed of thyroid tissue intimately admixed with carcinoid tumor which in most cases is of the trabecular [43] type. Strumal carcinoid is the second most common type of ovarian carcinoid tumor after the insular carcinoid.[35, 43, 44] It has the same age distribution and symptomatology as other ovarian carcinoids. It may comprise a part of a mature cystic teratoma, or may occur in pure form. The former is more common. Microscopically, it is composed of thyroid tissue which is intimately admixed with carcinoid tumor most frequently of the trabecular type (Fig. 7.29). Argyrophil and argentaffin granules are present in the tumor cells.[43, 44] Metastases have only been reported in a single case.[43]

XIII. OTHER TYPES OF MONODERMAL TERATOMA

Other types of monodermal teratoma include monodermal teratomas with neuroectodermal differentiation, which comprise both malignant [45, 46] and benign [47, 48] entities, and monodermal teratomas composed of vascular tissue.[49]

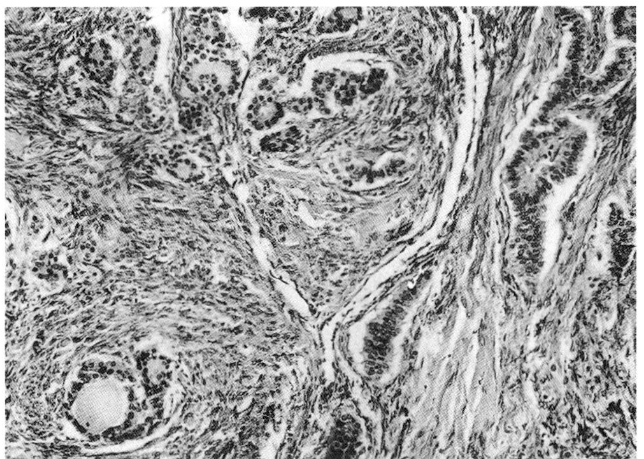

FIGURE 7.29 Strumal carcinoid tumor composed of carcinoid tumor showing trabecular pattern (right) and thyroid follicles (bottom).

At least 15–20% of mucinous tumors of the ovary show intestinal differentiation and a further 5% are associated with mature cystic teratoma or a carcinoid tumor. These tumors are considered to be of germ cell origin.

XIV. MIXED GERM CELL TUMORS

This group of ovarian germ cell neoplasms comprises all tumors composed of more than one germ cell element, and therefore, all the neoplasms included in this category are malignant. Although in the past, mixed or combined germ cell tumors were considered to be rare, more recent studies indicate that they are much more common.[9–11] The importance of recognizing the presence of different elements within a germ cell tumor needs little emphasis, as it provides the correct diagnosis and forms a basis for the appropriate therapy.

XV. TUMORS COMPOSED OF GERM CELLS AND SEX CORD-STROMAL DERIVATIVES

Tumors composed of germ cells intimately admixed with sex cord-stromal derivatives are uncommon, and consist of two distinct types:

1. Gonadoblastoma
2. Mixed germ cell—sex cord stromal tumor (MGC-SCST)

XVI. GONADOBLASTOMA

Gonadoblastoma occurs predominantly in young phenotypic females (80%), and less frequently in phenotypic male pseudohermaphrodites (20%).[50] The majority of phenotypic females with gonadoblastoma (60%) show signs of virilization. Nearly all patients (96%) are chromatin negative, and have a Y Chromosome. The most common karyotypes observed are 46,XY; 45,X/46,XY; and various other forms of mosaicism. Gonadoblastoma has been described occasionally in patients with Turner's syndrome, in ovotestes of true hermaphrodites, and in phenotypic females with normal ovaries and normal 46,XX karyotype.[1] The gonad of origin is often indeterminate, but when discernible, it is usually a testis or a streak gonad. The contralateral gonad is either a testis, a streak, or is indeterminate, and in more than 50% of cases, it also contains a gonadoblastoma.

Gonadoblastoma is usually small, gray-yellow, solid, and hard, and is frequently partly calcified. Microscopically, it is composed of small cellular nests surrounded by connective tissue which is usually dense and fibrous (Fig. 7.30), but

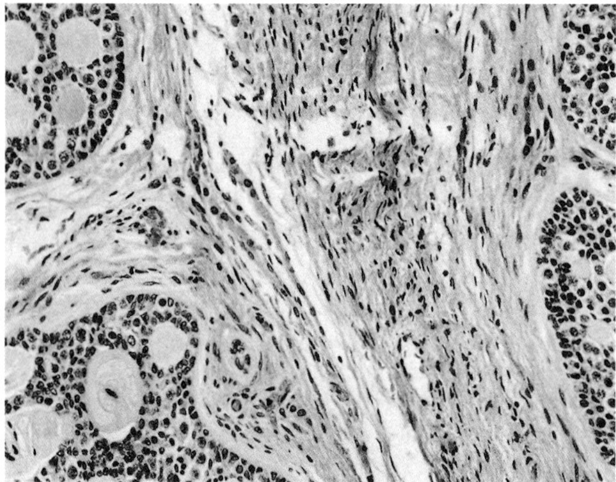

FIGURE 7.30 Gonadoblastoma composed of cellular nests surrounded by connective tissue. Note the hyaline Call-Exner-like bodies within the tumor nests and a small collection of lutein or Leydig-like cells (center).

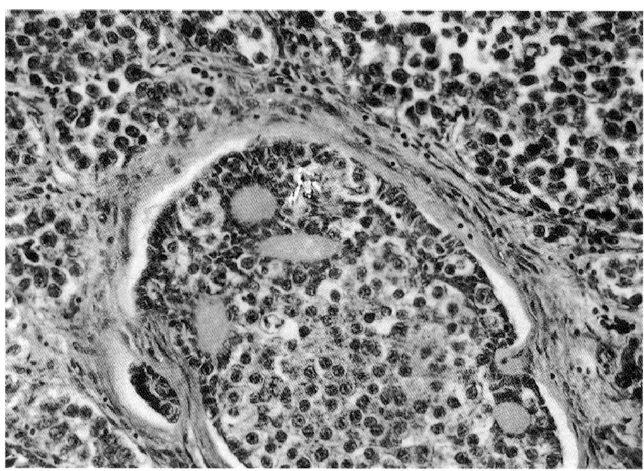

FIGURE 7.31 Gonadoblastoma overgrown by dysgerminoma. The gonadoblastoma nest contains an increased number of germ cells. Sex cord derivatives are seen mainly at the periphery of the nest, which is surrounded by dysgerminoma cells.

may be loose and edematous. The nests contain a mixture of germ cells and sex cord derivatives resembling immature Sertoli and granulosa cells [1, 7, 50, 51] (Figs. 7.30 and 7.31). The latter are arranged within the nests in three typical patterns (Figs. 7.30 and 7.31):

1. They line the periphery of the nests in a coronal pattern.
2. They surround individual or collections of germ cells.
3. They surround small spaces containing amorphous hyaline eosinophilic and PAS-positive material, resembling Call-Exner bodies.

Mitotic activity is seen in the germ cells, but not in the sex cord derivatives. The connective tissue surrounding the tumor nests may contain collections of cells resembling lutein or Leydig cells (Fig. 7.30), but Reinke crystals have never been observed within them. The basic pattern of gonadoblastoma described above may be altered by three processes: hyalinization, calcification, and overgrowth by neoplastic germ cell elements, usually dysgerminoma (Fig. 7.31). These processes may lead to the obliteration of the gonadoblastoma nests.

Gonadoblastoma is frequently admixed with dysgerminoma (Fig. 7.31). This is seen in more than 50% of cases. In another 10% it is admixed with other malignant neoplastic germ cell elements.[1, 7, 50, 51] When gonadoblastoma is associated with dysgerminoma the latter tends to metastasise less frequently and later than dysgerminoma arising *de novo*, and the prognosis is very favorable. Although it has been suggested that gonadoblastoma may be combined with mixed germ cell-sex cord stromal tumor,[52] the documentation in the case describing such association is highly unsatisfactory, and the tumor described and depicted [52] is a conventional gonadoblastoma.

XVII. MGC-SCST

The MGC-SCST is encountered most frequently in normal ovaries of phenotypic female infants and children with normal 46,XX karyotype.[1, 51] It also occurs in ovaries of genetically normal young women, some of whom had normal pregnancies, as well as in descended testes of genetically normal adult males, some of whom are known to have fathered children.[1, 51] MGC-SCST has not been associated with gonadal dysgenesis or abnormal karyotypes.[1] The female patients present with an abdominal mass, which may be associated with pain. Infants and prepubertal children may present with isosexual precocious pseudopuberty which regresses following the excision of the tumor. The tumors are usually unilateral, large, gray-white, smooth, and solid, but may contain cystic areas similar to those observed in cystic sex-cord stromal tumors.

Microscopically, MGC-SCST is composed of germ cells intimately admixed with sex cord derivatives (Figs. 7.32 and 7.33). MGC-SCST exhibits three different histological patterns showing:

1. Long, narrow, ramifying cords, or trabeculae which in places expand to form large, round or oval cellular aggregates or wide columns surrounded by connective tissue (Fig. 7.32)
2. Solid tubular structures devoid of a lumen and surrounded by connective tissue septa (Fig. 7.33)
3. Large aggregates of germ cells and sex cord derivatives devoid of any specific arrangement

All these patterns may be observed in the same tumor, although one of the patterns may predominate. The two

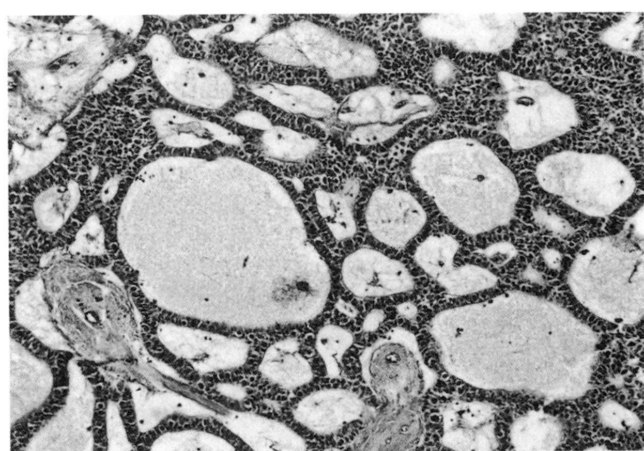

FIGURE 7.32 Mixed germ cell-sex cord stromal tumor (MGC-SCST). The tumor shows a pronounced cord-like pattern. Note the edematous connective tissue between the cords.

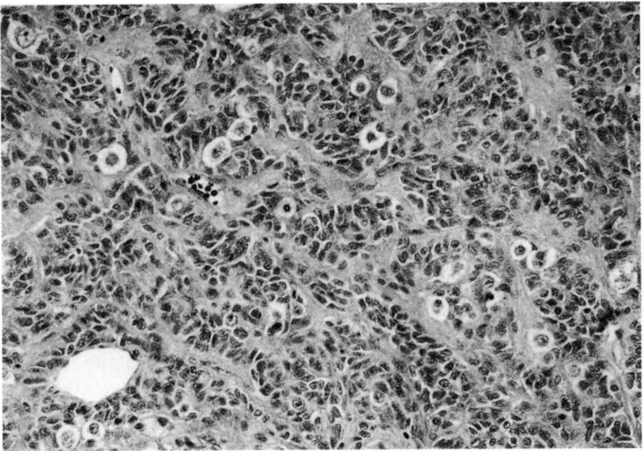

FIGURE 7.33 Mixed germ cell-sex cord stromal tumor with tubular pattern. Note the solid tubules composed of the smaller more numerous sex cord derivatives and larger germ cells with clear cytoplasm and prominent round nuclei.

components, the germ cells and sex cord derivatives are intimately admixed, although in some areas, one of them may predominate. Mitotic activity is seen in both components. Although originally MGC-SCST was observed only in pure form, occasional cases of MGC-SCST associated with dysgerminoma or other malignant neoplastic germ cell elements have been encountered.[1, 51] Although the frequency of this complication is by far lower than in patients with gonadoblastoma, it should certainly be borne in mind.

Two well-documented cases of metastasizing pure MGC-SCST occurring in anatomically and genetically normal females have been reported.[53, 54] The metastases were present in the para-aortic lymph nodes and the peritoneal cavity. Both patients were well without evidence of disease two years after surgery and combination chemotherapy. MGC-SCST is, therefore, capable of metastatic spread although this is very rare. There are cases on record where the patient was known to harbor the tumor for a number of years without developing metastases.[1, 55] The prognosis of patients with pure MGC-SCST is very favorable.[1] Even when the tumor is associated with other malignant neoplastic germ cell elements, excision of the tumor and treatment with combination chemotherapy results in a complete cure.[1]

References

1. Talerman, A. (2002). Germ cell tumors of the ovary. *In* "Blaustein's Pathology of the Female Genital Tract" (R. J. Kurman, ed.), 5th ed., pp. 967–1033. Springer-Verlag, New York.
2. Teilum, G. (1965). Classification of endodermal sinus tumour (mesoblastoma vitellinum) and so-called "embryonal carcinoma" of the ovary. *Acta Pathol. Microbiol. Scand.* 64, 407–429.
3. Teilum, G. (1976). "Special Tumors of the Ovary and Testis. Comparative Histology and Identification." 2nd ed., Munksgaard, Copenhagen.
4. Miettinen, M., Virtanen, I., and Talerman, A. (1986). Intermediate filaments in germ cell tumors. *In* "Pathology of the Testis and its Adnexa" (A. Talerman and L. M. Roth, eds.), pp. 181–191. Churchill Livingstone, New York.
5. Serov, S. F., Scully, R. E., and Sobin, L. H. (1973). "Histological Typing of Ovarian Tumours. International Histological Classification of Tumours." No. 9, pp. 19–20. World Health Organization, Geneva.
6. Scully, R. E. (1999). "Histological Typing of Ovarian Tumours. World Health Organization International Histological Classification of Tumours." 2nd ed., pp. 28–36. Springer-Verlag, Heidelberg.
7. Scully, R. E., Young, R. H., and Clement, P. B. (1998). "Tumors of the Ovary, Maldeveloped Gonads, Fallopian Tube, and Broad Ligament. Atlas of Tumor Pathology." 3rd Series, Fascicle 23, pp. 239–312. Armed Forces Institute of Pathology, Washington, D.C.
8. Bjorkholm, E., Lundell, M., Gyftodimos, A. *et al.* (1990). Dysgerminoma. The Radiumhemmet Series 1927–1984. *Cancer* 65, 38–44.
9. Talerman, A., Huyzinga, W. T., and Kuipers, T. (1973). Dysgerminoma. Clinicopathologic study of 22 cases. *Obstet. Gynecol.* 41, 137–147.
10. Kurman, R. J., and Norris, H. J. (1976). Malignant mixed germ cell tumors of the ovary. A clinical and pathologic analysis of 30 cases. *Obstet. Gynecol.* 48, 579–589.
11. Gershenson, D. M., Del-Junco, G., Copeland, L. J. *et al.* (1984). Mixed germ cell tumors of the ovary. *Obstet. Gynecol.* 64, 200–206.
12. Gordon, A., Lipton, D., and Woodruff, J. D. (1981). Dysgerminoma. A review of 158 cases from the Emil Novak Ovarian Tumor Registry. *Obstet. Gynecol.* 58, 497–504.
13. Asadourian, L. A., and Taylor, H. B. (1969). Dysgerminoma. An analysis of 105 cases. *Obstet. Gynecol.* 33, 370–379.
14. Kommoss, F., Bibbo, M., and Talerman, A. (1990). Nuclear deoxyribonucleic acid content (ploidy) of endodermal sinus (yolk sac) tumor. *Lab. Invest.* 62, 223–231.
15. Zaloudek, C. J., Tavassoli, F. A., and Norris, H. J. (1981). Dysgerminoma with syncytiotrophoblastic giant cells. A histologically and clinically distinctive subtype of dysgerminoma. *Am. J. Surg. Pathol.* 5, 361–367.
16. Talerman, A., Haije, W. G., and Baggerman, L. (1980). Serum alphafetoprotein (AFP) in patients with germ cell tumors of the gonads and extragonadal sites. Correlation between endodermal sinus (yolk sac) tumor and raised serum AFP. *Cancer* 46, 380–385.
17. Awais, G. M. (1983). Dysgerminoma and serum lactic dehydrogenase levels. *Obstet. Gynecol.* 61, 99–101.
18. Fujii, S., Konishi, I., Suzuki, A. *et al.* (1985). Analysis of serum lactic dehydrogenase levels and its isoenzymes in ovarian dysgerminoma. *Gynecol. Oncol.* 22, 65–72.

19. Schwartz, P. E., and Morris, J. M. (1988). Serum lactic dehydrogenase. A tumor marker for dysgerminoma. *Obstet. Gynecol.* 72, 511–515.
20. Langely, F. A., Govan, A. D. T., Anderson, M. C. *et al.* (1981). Yolk sac and allied tumors of the ovary. *Histopathology* 5, 389–401.
21. Kurman, R. J., and Norris, H. J. (1976). Endodermal sinus tumor of the ovary. A clinical and pathologic analysis of 71 cases. *Cancer* 38, 2404–2419.
22. Rutgers, J. L., Young, R. H., and Scully, R. E. (1987). Ovarian yolk sac tumor arising from an endometrioid adenocarcinoma. *Hum. Pathol.* 18, 1296–1299.
23. Mazur, M. T., Talbot, W. H., Jr., and Talerman, A. (1988). Endodermal sinus tumor and mucinous cystadenofibroma of the ovary. Occurrence in an 82 year old women. *Cancer* 62, 2011–2015.
24. Nogales, F. F., Bergeron, C., Carvia, R. E. *et al.* (1996). Ovarian endometrioid tumors with yolk sac component: an unusual form of ovarian neoplasm. Analysis of six cases. *Am. J. Surg. Pathol.* 20, 1056–1066.
25. Jacobsen, G. K., and Talerman, A. (1989). "Atlas of Germ Cell Tumours." Munksgaard, Copenhagen.
26. Prat, J., Bhan, A. K., Dickersin, R. G. *et al.* (1982). Hepatoid yolk sac tumor of the ovary (endodermal sinus tumor with hepatoid differentiation). A light microscopic, ultrastructural and immunohistochemical study of seven cases. *Cancer* 50, 2355–2368.
27. Cohen, M. B., Mulchahey, K. M., and Molnar, J. J. (1986). Ovarian endodermal sinus tumor with intestinal differentiation. *Cancer* 57, 1580–1583.
28. Cohen, M. B., Talerman, A., Friend, D. S. *et al.* (1987). Gonadal endodermal sinus (yolk sac) tumor with pure intestinal differentiation: A new histologic type. *Pathol. Res. Pract.* 182, 609–616.
29. Clement, P. B., Young, R. H., and Scully, R. E. (1987). Endometrioid-like variant of ovarian yolk sac tumor. A clinicopathological analysis of eight cases. *Am. J. Surg. Pathol.* 11, 767–778.
30. Mostofi, F. K., and Sesterhenn, I. A. (1998). "Histological Typing of Testis Tumours. International Histological Classification of Tumours." 2nd ed. Springer-Verlag, Heidelberg.
31. Robboy, S. J., and Scully, R. E. (1970). Ovarian teratoma with glial implants on the peritoneum. *Hum. Pathol.* 1, 643–653.
32. Norris, H. J., Zirkin, H. J., and Benson, W. L. (1976). Immature (malignant) teratoma of the ovary. A clinical and pathologic study of 58 cases. *Cancer* 37, 2359–2372.
33. Thurlbeck. W. M., and Scully, R. E. (1960). Solid teratoma of the ovary. *Cancer* 13, 804–811.
34. Stamp, G. W. H., and McConnell, E. M. (1983). Malignancy arising in cystic ovarian teratomas. *Br. J. Obstet. Gynaecol.* 90, 671–675.
35. Talerman, A. (1984). Carcinoid tumors of the ovary. *J. Cancer Res. Clin. Oncol.* 107, 125–135.
36. Robboy, S. J., Norris, H. J., and Scully, R. E. (1975). Insular carcinoid primary in the ovary. A clinicopathologic analysis of 48 cases. *Cancer* 36, 404–418.
37. Sporrong, B., Falkmer, S., Robboy, S. J. *et al.* (1982). Neurohormonal peptides in ovarian carcinoids: An immunohistochemical study of 81 primary carcinoids and of intraovarian metastases from six mid-gut carcinoids. *Cancer* 49, 68–74.
38. Talerman, A., and Evans, M. I. (1982). Primary trabecular carcinoid tumor of the ovary. *Cancer* 50, 1403–1407.
39. Talerman, A., and Okagaki, T. (1985). Ultrastructural features of primary trabecular carcinoid tumor of the ovary. *Int. J. Gynecol. Pathol.* 4, 153–160.
40. Altenghat, E., Okagaki, T., and Talerman, A. (1986). Primary mucinous carcinoid tumor of the ovary. *Cancer* 58, 777–783.
41. Baker, P. M., Oliva, E., Young, R. H. *et al.* (2001). Ovarian mucinous carcinoids, including some with a carcinomatous component: A report of 17 cases. *Am. J. Surg. Pathol.* 25, 557–568.
42. Robboy, S. J., Scully, R. E., and Norris, H. J. (1974). Carcinoid metastatic to the ovary. A clinicopathologic analysis of 35 cases. *Cancer* 33, 798–811.
43. Robboy, S. J., and Scully, R. E. (1980). Strumal carcinoid of the ovary: An analysis of 50 cases of a distinctive tumor composed of thyroid tissue and carcinoid. *Cancer* 46, 2019–2034.
44. Snyder, R., and Tavassoli, F. A. (1986). Ovarian strumal carcinoid: Immunohistochemical, ultrastructural and clinicopathologic observations. *Int. J. Gynecol. Pathol.* 5, 187–201.
45. Aguirre, P., and Scully, R. E. (1982). Malignant neuroectodermal tumor of the ovary, a distinctive form of monodermal teratoma. Report of five cases. *Am. J. Surg. Pathol.* 6, 283–292.
46. Kleinman, G. M., Young, R. H., and Scully, R. E. (1984). Ependymoma of the ovary: Report of three cases. *Hum. Pathol.* 15, 632–638.
47. Ulirsch, R. C., and Goldman, R. L. (1982). An unusual teratoma of the ovary: Neurogenic cyst with lactating breast tissue. *Obstet. Gynecol.* 60, 400–402.
48. Tiltman, A. J. (1985). Ependymal cyst of the ovary. *S. Afr. Med. J.* 68, 424–425.
49. Talerman, A. Unpublished observations.
50. Scully, R. E. (1970). Gonadoblastoma. A review of 74 cases. *Cancer* 25, 1340–1356.
51. Talerman, A. (1980). Pathology of gonadal neoplasms composed of germ cells and sex cord stroma derivatives. *Pathol. Res. Pract.* 170, 24–38.
52. Bhatena, D., Haning, R. V., Jr., Shapiro, S. *et al.* (1985). Coexistence of a gonadoblastoma and mixed germ cell-sex cord stroma tumor. *Pathol. Res. Pract.* 180, 203–206.
53. Lacson, A. G., Gillis, D. A., and Shawwa, A. (1988). Malignant mixed germ cell-sex cord stromal tumors of the ovary associated with isosexual precocious puberty. *Cancer* 61, 2122–2133.
54. Arroyo, J. G., Harris, W., and Laden, S. A. (1998). Recurrent mixed germ cell-sex cord stromal tumor of the ovary in an adult. *Int. J. Gynecol. Pathol.* 17, 281–283.
55. Talerman, A., and van der Harten, J. J. (1977). A mixed germ cell-sex cord stroma tumor of the ovary associated with isosexual precocious puberty in a normal girl. *Cancer* 40, 889–894.

CHAPTER

8

Gonadal Sex Cord-Stromal Tumors

DOROTA POPIOLEK
Department of Pathology,
Division of OB/GYN Pathology
New York University School of Medicine
Bellevue Hospital Center
New York, New York 10016

RITA DEMOPOULOS
Department of Pathology
Division of OB/GYN Pathology
New York University School of Medicine
Bellevue Hospital Center
New York, New York 10016

I. INTRODUCTION

Sex cord-stromal tumors are uncommon but fascinating neoplasms, from a clinical, morphological, and embryologic perspective. They represent the group of ovarian tumors which most often present with a wide range of endocrine manifestations due to estrogenic or androgenic hormone secretion. In addition, the morphologic features seen in these tumors are confoundingly diverse; they are usually categorized as biphasic neoplasms, composed of both stromal and sex-cord elements derived from male and female anlage.

These facts are reflected in the World Health Organization (WHO) [1] classification of ovarian tumor where the term sex cord-stromal tumor for these neoplasms has been adopted (Table 8.1). The use by the WHO of the generic term, sex cord-stromal tumor, is not intended to reflect a commitment to any one theory of gonadogenesis, but only acknowledges the presence in these tumors of two distinct categories of ovarian and testicular homologous cell types: granulosa and Sertoli cells (sex cord elements) and theca, Leydig, and non-specific stromal type cells (stromal elements).

TABLE 8.1 Classification of Sex Cord-Stromal Tumors of the Ovary [1]

1. Granulosa-stromal cell tumors
   - Granulosa cell tumor
     - Adult
     - Juvenile
   - Thecoma-fibroma group
     - Thecoma (typical, lutenized)
     - Fibroma
     - Cellular Fibroma
     - Fibrosarcoma
     - Stromal tumor with sex cord elements
     - Sclerosing stromal tumor
     - Stromal luteoma, see Steroid cell tumors
     - Unclassified/Others
2. Sertoli-stromal cell tumors, androblastomas
   - Sertoli cell tumor (tubular androblastoma)
   - Sertoli-Leydig cell tumor
     - Well differentiated
     - Intermediate differentiation
       - Variant—with heterologous elements
     - Poorly differentiated
       - Variant—with heterologous elements
     - Retiform
       - Variant—with heterologous elements
   - Leydig cell tumor, see Section 3
3. Steroid (lipid) cell tumors
   - Stromal luteoma
   - Leydig cell tumor
     - Hilar type (hilus cell tumor)
     - Nonhilar type
   - Steroid cell tumor, unclassified (not otherwise specified)
4. Others
   - Sex cord stromal tumor with annular tubules
   - Gynandroblastoma
     - Unclassified

The various terminology used for these tumors reflects the different views on the embryologic derivation/differentiation of normal ovarian components and their counterparts in neoplastic growth. Those who believe that both sex cord and stromal cells are derived from mesenchyme of the genital ridge, advocate the term gonadal stromal tumor.[2] On the other hand those who favor, along with many embryologists, the origin of sex cord elements from celomic epithelium of the gonadal ridge, prefer the term sex cord stromal tumor.[1]

A recent study of gonadogenesis in human embryos illustrates that although sex cord elements originate from mesonephros, they possess epithelial and not mesenchymal characteristics.[3]

The term sex cord-stromal tumor emphasizes the biphasic nature of these neoplasms represented by an epithelial-like component (sex cord elements: granulosa cells and Sertoli cells), although of mesodermal origin, and a mesenchymal component (fibroblasts, theca cells, and Leydig cells). The notion that granulosa and Sertoli cells are of epithelial nature is strengthened by the cytoplasmic immunoreactivity for cytokeratin in normal granulosa cells and Sertoli cells of fetal [4] and of adults testes.[5] A similar phenomenon is observed in neoplastic cells differentiating toward granulosa and Sertoli cells.[4]

The majority of sex cord-stromal tumors of the ovary display morphologic features of its normal counterpart, that is granulosa and stromal cells in granulosa-stromal cell tumors. Less frequently, the tumor cells differentiate toward testicular cell types (Sertoli-Leydig cell tumors). In some rare cases testicular and ovarian elements are present in the same tumor (gynandroblastoma). In still other cases, the sex cord elements are not mature enough and thus lack morphologic characteristics specific to either granulosa or Sertoli cells, and are therefore put into a category of sex cord-stromal tumor, unclassified.

Sex cord-stromal tumors are uncommon neoplasms and constitute approximately 8% of all ovarian tumors.[6] Granulosa-stromal cell tumors are composed of neoplastic cells resembling granulosa cells, theca cells, or stromal fibroblasts in various combination. Tumors in which granulosa cells account for more than a minor component (at least 10%) are granulosa cell tumors. Tumors in which neoplastic cells resemble fibroblasts producing collagen or theca cells belong to the fibroma-thecoma group. Tumors in the fibroma-thecoma group, which contain occasional tubules lined by Sertoli cells or nests of granulosa cells (less than 10% of the tumor) have been referred to as fibroma or thecoma with minor sex cord elements. Furthermore two subtypes of granulosa cell tumors exist—adult and juvenile types—with distinct clinical and histological features. In this chapter, we follow classification of the sex cord-stromal tumors presented in Table 8.1 which is based on WHO classification.

II. GRANULOSA CELL TUMOR (GCT)

A. Clinical Features

Adult granulosa cell tumors (AGCT) account for 95% of all granulosa cell tumors and 1–2% of all ovarian tumors.[6] They occur in middle-age and older women in over 90% of cases, and are more frequent in postmenopausal than in premonpausal women with a peak incidence at 50–55 years of age. The juvenile type of granulosa cell tumor (JGCT) is much rarer and occurs in the first three decades of life in over 90% of cases, but the patients range in age from newborn to 67 years (average 13 years).[7] Regardless of type, granulosa cell tumors are the most common ovarian tumors which present with estrogenic manifestations which vary according to the age of the patient. Thus 82% of prepubertal patients with JGCTs present with isosexual pseudoprecocity.[7] Patients in the reproductive age group develop menstrual irregularities or amenorrhea, and postmenopausal women present with vaginal bleeding. Hyperestrinism may result in endometrial hyperplasia, and less than 5% of patients develop endometrioid type adenocarcinoma, most commonly well differentiated. Rare cases with androgenic manifestation are reported, ranging from hirsutism to virilization. In one such a case ultrastructurally proven Leydig cells with crystals of Reinke were found and appeared to originate from the ovarian stroma.[8] An unexplained association exists between androgenic manifestions and predominantly cystic tumors.[6] In addition, some patients present with abdominal pain and/or swelling, or acute abdomen due the rupture of a cystic mass, or hemoperitoneum.

Inhibin, a peptide hormone, is produced by ovarian granulosa cells and granulosa cell tumors, both adult and juvenile types, and serum measurements can be used to monitor these neoplasms. Elevated serum level can indicate recurrent or metastatic disease, before it becomes clinically apparent.[9] It should be noted, however, that inhibin is not a granulosa cell specific marker. It is also produced by Sertoli cells in both normal testes and its neoplastic counterpart,[10] and ovarian luteinized stromal cells. Therefore a modest elevation in serum inhibin concentration may occur with primary and secondary ovarian epithelial tumors, especially primary mucinous adenocarcinoma,[11] which contain ovarian-type stroma.

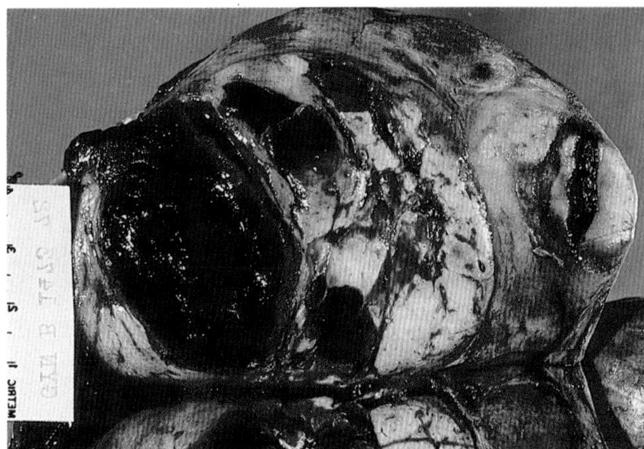

FIGURE 8.1 Adult granulosa cell tumor. Solid and cystic areas with hemorrhage.

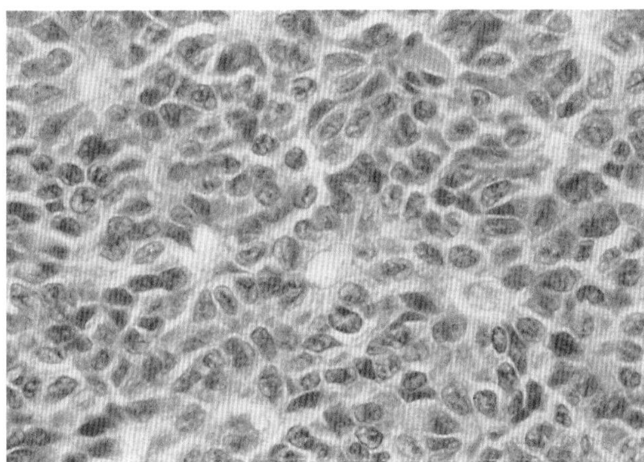

FIGURE 8.2 Adult granulosa cell tumor. Microfollicular pattern with numerous Call-Exner bodies. The granulosa cells are arranged around spaces, some containing eosinophilic fluid. The nuclei are pale, angular to oval, and occasionally grooved.

B. Gross Pathology

Adult and juvenile granulosa cell tumors share many gross characteristics. They are unilateral in over 95% of cases and vary in size from microscopic to large masses which may result in abdominal distention. The external surface is smooth. Most tumors are composed of solid and cystic areas, but purely solid or cystic masses are encountered. The cystic tumors can be multilocular or unilocular and have a smooth inner lining. The sectioned surfaces vary from soft to rubbery depending on the amount of fibrothecomatous component and from yellow to tan according to the cytoplasmic lipid content. Areas of hemorrage are common (Fig. 8.1) and occasionally necrosis is present. Seventy six to 92% of AGCT [12–14] and 97% of JGCT were stage I in one reported series.[7] Most of the remainder of AGCT were stage II, with about 5% stage III, whereas in JGCT only 2% were stage II and none stage III, in that series.

C. Microscopic Pathology

The cells of AGCT typically are characterized by uniform and pale nuclei which are angular or oval, and usually grooved. They are surrounded by scanty cytoplasm. Rare tumors, approximately 2%, are luteinized, with moderate to abundant cytoplasm. The tumor cells are arranged in a variety of patterns including follicular (microfollicular, macrofollicular) (Figs. 8.2 and 8.3), insular and trabecular, encountered in better differentiated tumors, diffuse (epithelioid and sarcomatoid), and gyriform or watered-silk (Fig. 8.4) in less differentiated tumors. Different patterns may be admixed in a single tumor. The follicular pattern, although not most frequent, is the most characteristic, in particular the microfollicular subtype. This is characterized by a small, round, and uniform in size cavity filled with pink fluid and possibly a few degenerated nuclei, closely resembling the Call-Exner body of a developing follicle, which are separated by haphazardly arranged sheets of granulosa cells (Fig. 8.2). The macrofollicular pattern is composed of regular cysts lined by granulosa cells with adjacent theca cells within its wall (Fig. 8.3).

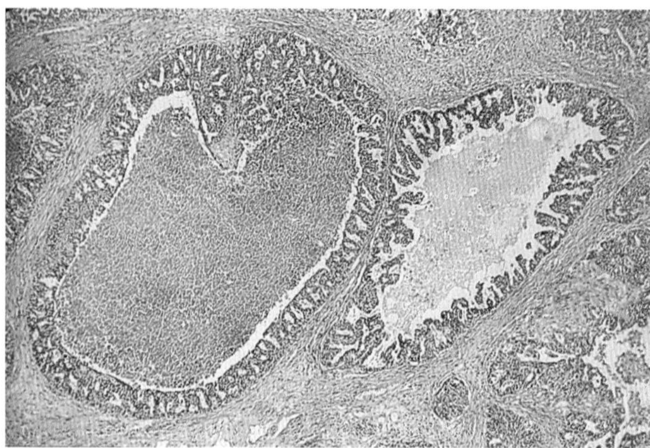

FIGURE 8.3 Adult granulosa cell tumor. Macrofollicular pattern showing large follicle-like spaces lined by multilayered granulosa cells forming Call-Exner bodies.

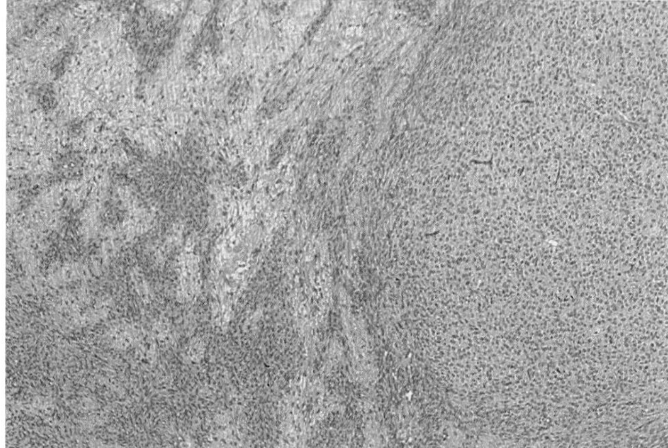

FIGURE 8.5 Adult granulosa cell tumor. Diffuse pattern on the right with prominent fibrothecomatous component on the left.

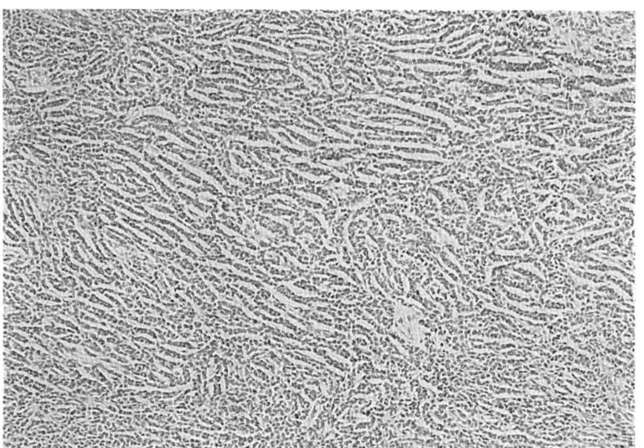

FIGURE 8.4 Adult granulosa cell tumor. Watered-silk pattern. The granulosa cells are arranged in thin, parallel cords.

The diffuse pattern was reported as the most common on low-power view, in one series [12] where the tumor cells grow in diffuse sheets, focally separated by fibrothecomatous stroma, which occasionally may be prominent and may simulate fibroma-thecoma (Fig. 8.5). In trabecular and insular patterns the granulosa cells are arranged in multilayered ribbons and well-demarcated nests, respectively, embedded in stroma. The thecomatous component of GCTs in mice has been shown to have increased numbers of gonadotropin receptors [15] and appears to represent luteinized granulosa cells as evidenced by the presence of desmosomes and other junctional complexes.[16] The gonadotropic hormone binding to human ovarian tumors of various histologic types including sex cord-stromal tumors were investigated.[17] Although no consistent association was demonstrated between histologic tumor type and the presence of gonadotropic hormone binding, two sex cord-stromal tumors and a serous cystadenocarcinoma with areas of stromal luteinization, bound FSH and HCG. Therefore it was suggested that gonadotropic hormones may play an important role in the growth of granulosa-theca cell tumors in humans.

Rare granulosa cell tumors contain solid or hollow tubules indistinguishable from well-differentiated Sertoli cell tumor; if they account for more than 10% the diagnosis of a gynandroblastoma is appropriate, otherwise the diagnosis of GCT remains unchanged. Mitotic activity in AGCT varies from less than 1 per 10 hpf (49% of cases) to more than 6 per 10 hpf (9% of cases),[13] therefore mitosis is not prominent.

The cells of JGCT are usually luteinized with a moderate to abundant amount of eosinophilic or clear (lipid-rich) cytoplasm resembling the enlarged granulosa cells of the corpus luteum. The nuclei are distinct and differ from AGCT. They are round, darker than those of the AGCT, and rarely grooved. The tumor cells have a solid pattern of growth with frequent nodular areas with scattered follicles (Fig. 8.6). The follicles can be round or oval but are more frequently irregular and of variable sizes as compared with AGCT, and Call-Exner bodies are mostly lacking. The granulosa cells lining them are multilayered and are either surrounded by a mantle of theca cells or blend into the solid areas. Rare tumor cells facing the lumen of the follicle are reminiscent of hobnail cells seen in clear cell carcinoma. The degree of nuclear atypia and mitotic rate in JGCT are greater than in AGCT and the average mitotic rate is directly proportional to the degree of nuclear atypia.[7]

D. Differential Diagnosis

Endometrioid adenocarcinoma with small, uniform glands may resemble microfollicular AGCT, but foci of squamous differentiation are encountered frequently in the former, especially with the use of antibody against "high molecular weight cytokeratin," (34βE12).[18] Undifferentiated carcinoma

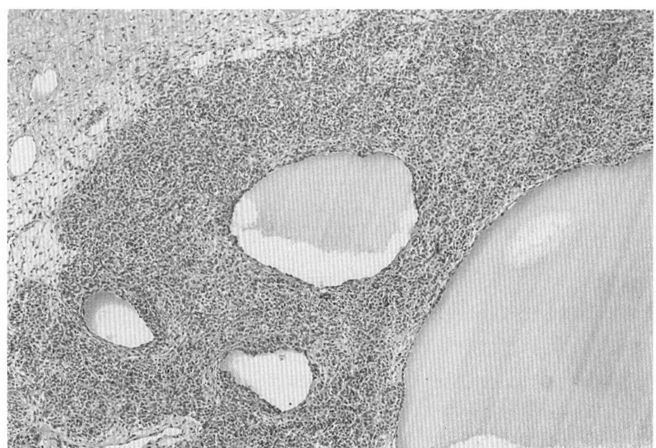

FIGURE 8.6 Juvenile granulosa cell tumor. The tumor cells have a solid pattern of growth with scattered follicles. Call-Exner bodies or nuclear grooves are lacking.

may mimic AGCT on low power. However, the nuclear characteristic of AGCT is very helpful, since instead of being pleomorphic and hyperchromatic, they are uniform, pale, and grooved, at least focally. In addition, α-inhibin expression [19] and absence of epithelial membrane antigen (EMA) in GCTs differentiates them from carcinomas.[20] Cytokeratin may be detected in GCTs, although in dot-like perinuclear distribution.[20] In addition, all GCTs were positive for vimentin, 92% reacted with smooth muscle actin, and all were negative for desmin in one series.[20] The diagnostic value of inhibin and its high sensitivity, especially the α-subunit, as a marker of ovarian sex cord-stromal tumors has been demonstrated in the published literature.[19] But caution should be exercised when using anti-inhibin antibody since 59% of adenocarcinomas of various sites, both ovarian and extraovarian, were positive for β-subunit and 26% of these tumors were also found positve for α-subunit in one study.[21] Inhibin is a dimeric peptide hormone composed of an α- and β-subunit, which in a female is produced by ovarian granulosa cells and inhibits the release of follicle stimulating hormone (FSH) from the pituitary gland and thus acts as a modulator of folliculogenesis. Inhibin is also produced by ovarian granulosa cell tumors of both adult and juvenile types, testicular Sertoli cells, trophoblasts (predominantly syncytiotrophoblasts, with little or no production in cytotrophoblasts), adrenal gland, and pituitary gland. Activin is a related hormone composed of two β-subunits (A and B forms of β-subunits are recognized) but with generally opposing actions to inhibin. Commercially available monoclonal antibodies R1 and E4 react against the α- and βA-subunits of human inhibin/activin, respectively. It has been shown that epithelial ovarian tumors usually express β-subunit, but no α-subunit, whereas GCTs stain positively with both α- and β-subunit.[21] Thus suggesting that GCTs express inhibin and ovarian carcinoma probably express activin. Therefore it is advocated to include inhibin as part of a larger panel to distinguish sex cord-stromal tumor from other neoplasms that may be close histologic mimics. This panel may include recently proposed markers of sex cord-stromal differentiation such as CD99, Mullerian inhibiting substance, and melan-A.[22–25]

Carcinoid tumors enter the differential diagnosis and again the nuclei here lack grooves, are darker with a salt and pepper distribution of chromatin, and there are cytoplasmic endocrine granules which can be detected immunohistochemically or ultrastructurally.

Pure stromal tumor of the fibroma-thecoma group may be confused with diffuse AGCTs, especially those with a prominent fibrothecomatous component. But reticulin stain can help to differentiate these two since in AGCT the reticulin fibrils surround clusters of the tumor cells, rather than investing individual cells, as in a thecoma.

Endometrial stromal sarcoma, in particular with sex-cord-like elements may share some morphologic characteristics with AGCTs but positive staining with CD10 in the former may be helpful in difficult cases.

A unilocular cystic AGCT and a large luteinized follicle cyst of pregnancy and the puerperium have the same gross appearance, but the latter is lined by diffusely luteinized cells with abundant cytoplasm and occasionally with bizarre nuclei.

JGCTs must be distinguished from small cell carcinoma of hypercalcemic type since both may occur in young patients and they are similar morphologically on low-power examination. But JGCTs are associated with estrogenic manifestations and small cell carcinoma with hypercalcemia. Microscopically, although both have diffuse growth patterns with interspersed follicles, the cells of JGCTs are large with abundant cytoplasm and thus a low nuclear-cytoplasmic (N/C) ratio, whereas the opposite is true for small cell carcinoma. In addition the latter is characterized by much higher mitotic activity.

Metastatic malignant melanoma may be confused with AGCT, but the presence of melanin pigment, intranuclear cytoplasmic inclusions, nuclear pleomorphism, and a combination of HMB-45 expression with lack of inhibin expression should confirm the diagnosis of melanoma. S-100 protein, although positive in melanoma, is also detected in half of GCTs [20] and therefore is not a helpful marker.

Another metastatic tumor which may be misleadingly similar is mammary carcinoma, especially the lobular type. The clinical history of carcinoma of the breast and positive stains for mucin (intracytoplasmic), epithelial membrane antigen, gross cystic disease, fluid protein-15, and negative stain for α-inhibin should confirm the diagnosis of secondary carcinoma from a breast primary.

E. Treatment and Prognosis

In menopausal patients the optimal treatment is total hysterectomy with bilateral salpingo-oopherectomy. For women who wish to preserve their fertility, unilateral salpingo-oopherectomy is an option, provided no evidence of spread of the tumor is present at the time of surgery.

Although AGCT tumors are malignant neoplasms, they pursue a clinical course of low malignant potential tumor characterized by local recurrence within the pelvis and lower abdomen up to three or more decades after the initial therapy; rarely distant metastases have been reported in many sites. On the other hand in a majority of JGCTs which recurred locally and as distant metastasis, they did so within three postoperative years.[7]

In AGCTs several features have been correlated with the prognosis such as: stage, size, histologic pattern, nuclear atypia, mitotic rate, and rupture. Patients with stage I disease have an 86–96% 10-year survival rate versus only 26–49% in higher stages.[13, 14] The size of AGCTs has been analyzed in relation to prognosis and when the survival rate was corrected for stage, the improvement in prognosis for smaller stage I tumors was not statistically significant. Therefore a relationship between tumor size and prognosis independent of stage has not been clearly established. The histologic pattern was shown to influence the survival rate in one series [26] but not in others [13, 14]. The mitotic rate and nuclear atypia have been shown to correlate with outcome with varying degree of success.[12–14, 27] Rupture adversely affects survival.[14]

In JGCTs analysis of the effect of these factors on prognosis in one series [7] revealed that stage was the factor of greatest prognostic significance. A correlation also existed for size, nuclear atypia, and mitotic activity when tumors of all stages were evaluated, but no such correlation was evident when only stage I tumors were considered.

III. FIBROMA-THECOMA GROUP

Tumors of fibroma-thecoma group form a spectrum composed of spindle-shaped cells resembling collagen-producing fibroblasts, and round to oval cells resembling theca cells, in various proportions; thus the terms fibroma and thecoma are used, respectively. Tumors in which a precise distinction between these two forms is impossible exist, and we believe the term fibrothecoma is acceptable.

IV. THECOMA

A. Clinical Features

The thecoma occurs at an older average age than the AGCT, 84% of patients being postmenopausal with mean age of 59 years and only 10% being younger than 30 years of age.[28] They are typically estrogenic in almost all cases. The exception is luteinized thecoma where only 50% are estrogenic and 11% are androgenic and in addition they occur in younger patients (30% in the first three decades of life).[29] Rare luteinized thecomas, some with marked mitotic activity and bilaterality, are associated with sclerosing peritonitis.[30]

B. Gross and Microscopic Pathology

Similar to GCTs they are unilateral in 97% of cases and vary in size from microscopic to large masses, which are round, oval, and solid. Sectioned surfaces are yellow and separated into nodules by fibrous bands (Fig. 8.7). Thecomas are composed of large round to oval cells with ill-defined cell borders and moderate to abundant pale cytoplasm (Fig. 8.8), which is usually lipid-rich, alternating with a variable component of spindle-shaped cells producing collagen and often forming conspicuous hyaline plaques (Fig. 8.9). The nuclei vary from round to spindle-shaped, lack atypia, and mitosis

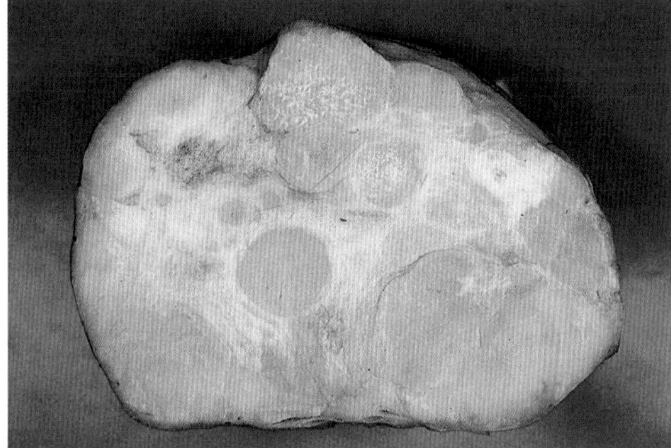

FIGURE 8.7 Thecoma. Sectioned surface is yellow and separated into nodules by fibrous septae.

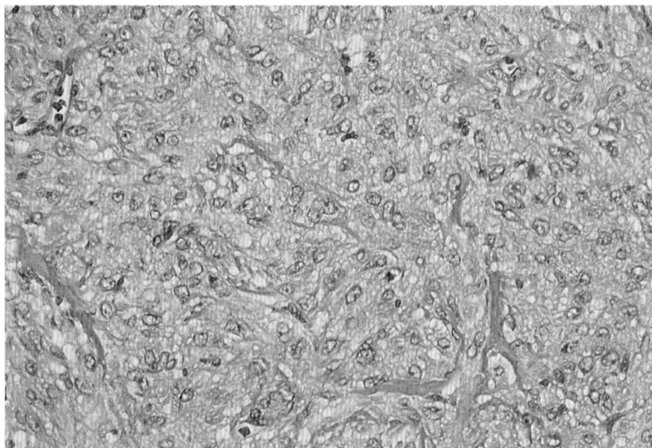

FIGURE 8.8 Thecoma composed of large cells with pale and abundant cytoplasm with ill-defined cell borders and vesicular nuclei.

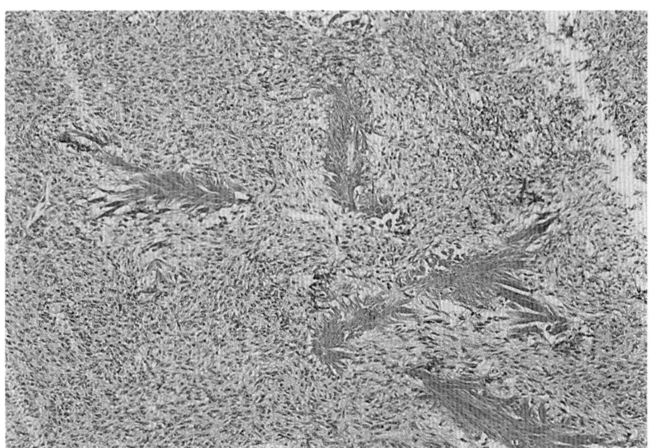

FIGURE 8.9 Thecoma with conspicuous hyaline plaques.

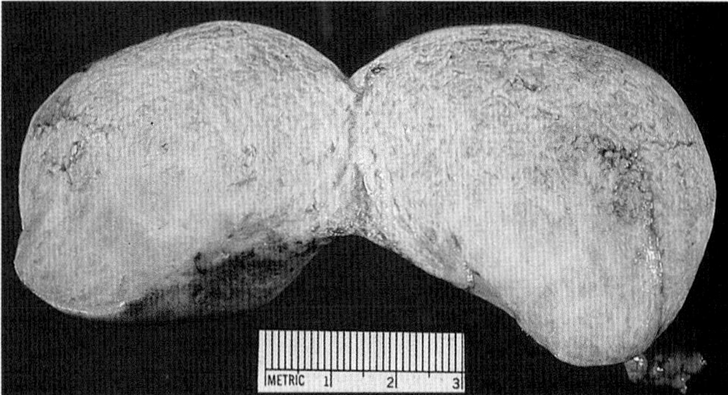

FIGURE 8.10 Fibroma. Sectioned surfaces are white and whorled.

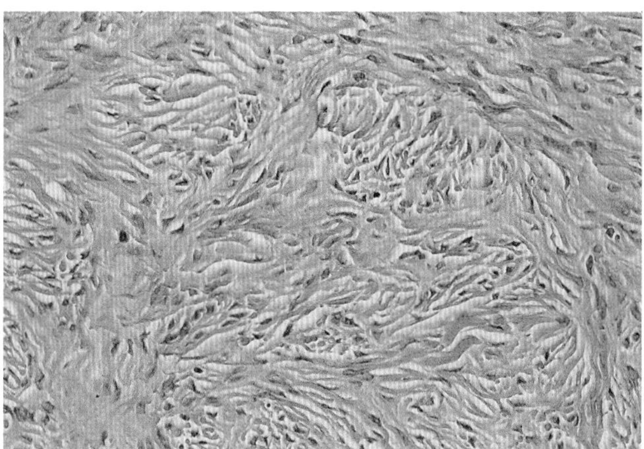

FIGURE 8.11 Fibroma. The spindle-shaped tumor cells are arranged in short interlacing fascicles.

is infrequent. The luteinized thecoma is characterized by a collection of luteinized theca or stromal cells within a fibromatous background.

Thecomas are almost always benign tumors and should be distinguished from diffuse adult granulosa cell tumors. Reticulin stain can be useful since it highlights fibrils encasing nests of granulosa cells in GCTs versus individual tumor cells as in thecoma, but sometimes the pattern is indeterminate. Although rare cases of malignant thecomas are encountered in the literature,[29, 31–33] it is not a clearly defined entity and the terms stromal sarcoma or fibrosarcoma are advocated for them.[31]

V. FIBROMA

A. Clinical Features

They account for approximately 50% of cases in the sex cord-stromal category of ovarian neoplasms and are only rarely associated with steroid hormone production. They occur in a broad age range but are most common in middle-age with an average age of 48 years and are uncommonly found in patients younger than 30 years of age.

An association exists between fibroma and two uncommon syndromes, Demons-Meig's [34] and the basal cell nevus syndrome.

Meig's syndrome is defined as the presence of a fibrous ovarian tumor accompanied by ascites and pleural effusion which disappear after the removal of the tumor. Fibromas with this clinical presentation are more likely to be edematous. The nevoid basal cell carcinoma syndrome is also referred to as the basal cell nevus syndrome and Gorlin's syndrome.[35] It is characterized by the presence of one or more of the following: basal cell carcinoma in early life, keratocysts of the jaw, calcification of the dura, mesenteric cyst, and less commonly other lesions as well as the fibroma. In this setting fibromas are usually bilateral, multinodular, and calcified.[36]

B. Gross and Microscopic Pathology

Fibromas vary in size from microscopic to large masses which are round, oval, and usually unilateral. Sectioned surfaces are firm, white, and whorled (Fig. 8.10). The tumor cells are spindle-shaped and are arranged in intersecting fascicles often forming a storiform pattern (Fig. 8.11). They produce collagen and hyalinized bands may be encountered.

Occasionally typical fibromas contain foci of sex cord elements (Fig. 8.12) and are therefore designated as fibromas with minor sex cord elements, and their clinical behavior is similar to typical fibroma.[37]

Rare fibromas composed of cells with closely packed nuclei, with absent or minimal nuclear atypia, a scant amount of collagen and with 1–3 mitoses per 10 hpf are designated as cellular fibromas (Fig. 8.13). They may recur, especially if they are ruptured or adherent to adjacent structures,

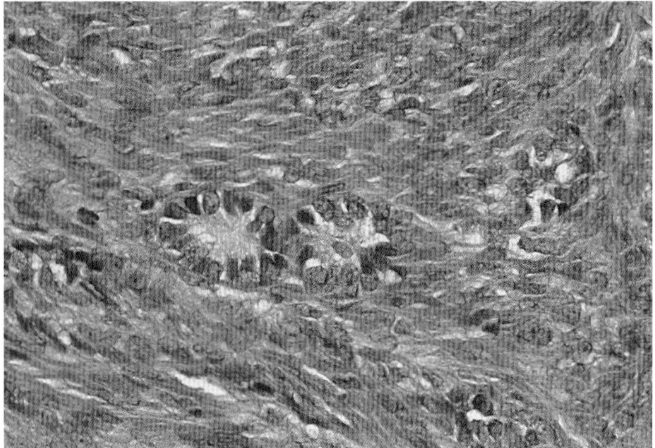

FIGURE 8.12 Fibroma with minor sex cord elements.

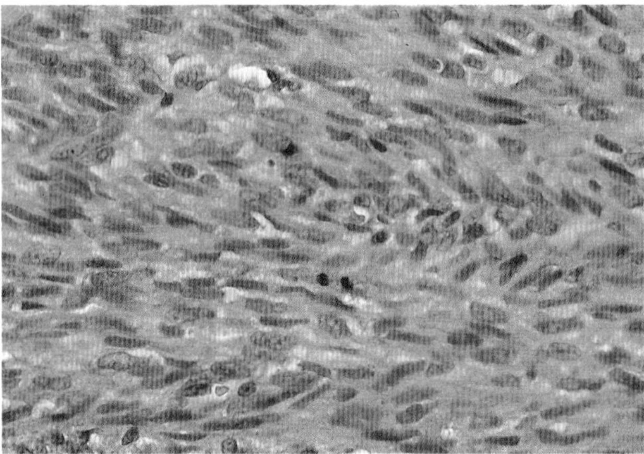

FIGURE 8.13 Cellular fibroma, devoid of significant cellular atypia, but mitotic figures are evident.

therefore they are considered by some to be a tumor of low malignant potential.[38]

Fibroblastic tumors with more than 3 mitoses per 10 hpf and at least moderate nuclear atypia often have a malignant course and are designated as fibrosarcomas.[38]

VI. SCLEROSING STROMAL TUMOR

A. Clinical Features

They are rare ovarian stromal tumors occurring in the first three decades of life in the majority of cases [39] in contrast to the fibroma-thecoma group, and endocrine manifestations are an exception rather than a rule in this tumor.[40] The most common presenting symptoms are menstrual irregularities and abdominal pain; only rarely patients develop acute abdomen due to tumor rupture with hemoperitoneum. Although ascites frequently complicates fibromas it is not a feature of sclerosing stromal tumors.

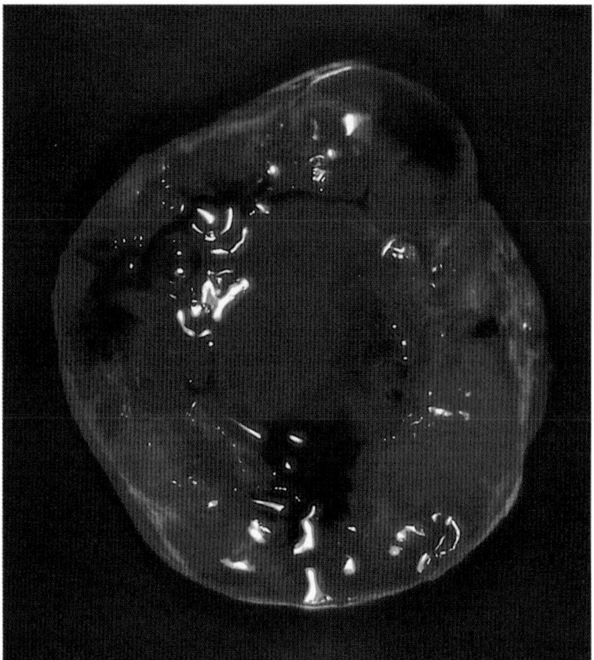

FIGURE 8.14 Sclerosing stromal tumor. Sectioned surface is solid and edematous with a central, and foci of hemorrhage.

B. Gross and Microscopic Pathology

Sclerosing stromal tumors are unilateral, with very rare exceptions,[39] round to oval masses with a smooth outer surface and predominantly solid, white, and frequently edematous sectioned surfaces. Cystic spaces of variable sizes are common which may coalesce and form a central cyst occasionally filled with blood clot (Fig. 8.14).

Microscopically they are distinct, composed of cellular areas separated by fibrous tissue which is either densely collageneous or edematous, into irregular islands imparting a pseudolobular low-power appearance (Fig. 8.15). The tumor cells in these areas have indistinct cell borders and vary in size and shape from round, oval, to spindle-shaped (Fig. 8.16). The nuclei are predominantly vesicular with occasional nucleoli, but some nuclei are pyknotic and shrunken. Mitosis is infrequent, up to 1 per 10 hpf, but cases with 3–4 mitoses per 10 hpf have been encountered. The cytoplasm is usually finely vacuolated or clear with some cells resembling signet ring cells. The cellular areas are characterized by a rich capillary vascular network, but larger dilated vessels reminiscent of hemagiopericytoma are common.

This unique constellation of microscopic features distinguishes this tumor from the fibroma-thecoma group and massive ovarian edema. Although massive ovarian edema occurs in a similar age group and may present with similar gross findings, it lacks the pseudolobular pattern and normal ovarian structures such as folllicles and corpora lutea or albicantia

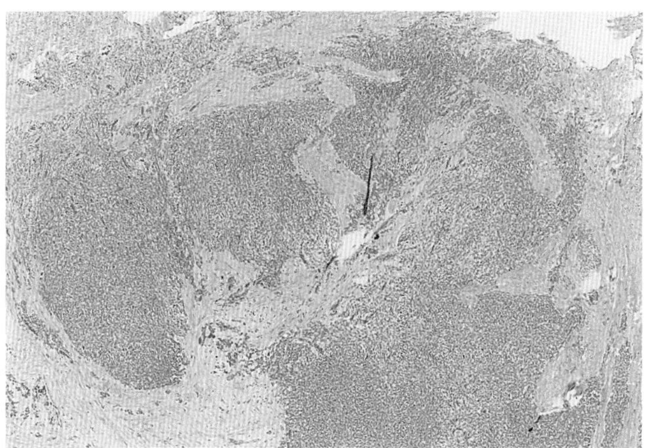

FIGURE 8.15 Sclerosing stromal tumor. Cellular areas are separated by edematous fibrous stroma imparting a pseudolobular appearance.

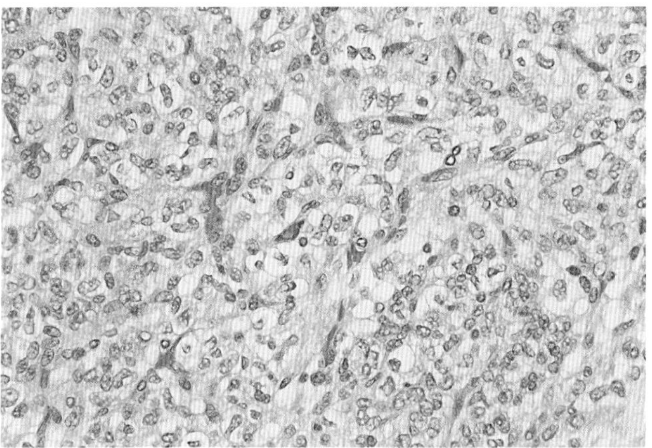

FIGURE 8.16 Sclerosing stromal tumor. The tumor cells are round to oval and spindle-shaped containing focally vacuolated cytoplasm. A rich capillary vascular network is evident.

are identified within the edematous stroma. All the cases reported in the literature behaved in a benign fashion.

VII. SERTOLI-STROMAL CELL TUMOR

This category represents a spectrum of tumors composed almost exclusively of Sertoli cells, or of Sertoli cells in various combination with cells resembling rete testis/ovary, fibroblasts, or Leydig cells at various levels of differentiation.

VIII. SERTOLI CELL TUMOR

A. Clinical Features

They occur in a broad age range with an average of 30 years.[41] They are usually nonfunctional, but may be estrogenic, especially the lipid-rich type, which has been associated with isosexual pseudoprecocity. Rare tumors may present with androgenic manifestations. All Sertoli cell tumors studied had a benign clinical course, except one which developed distant metastases.

B. Gross and Microscopic Pathology

Pure Sertoli cell tumors reported in the literature are unilateral and stage I.[41] They are lobulated firm masses with solid yellow to brown sectioned surfaces. Microscopically they are composed of hollow or solid tubules separated by fibrovascular stroma that contains only occasional or no Leydig cells (Fig. 8.17). The cells lining the tubules are cuboidal with moderate to abundant cytoplasm which is dense, eosinophilic, or vacuolated and occasionally clear with abundant lipids (lipid-rich Sertoli cell tumor). The Sertoli tumor cells may grow focally in a diffuse manner, and although nuclear atypia and mitosis are not the characteristic features, occasional tumors may contain such areas. One fatal tumor had these features focally and was classified as poorly differentiated.[41] Although a majority of the reported cases were well differentiated, rare tumors of intermediate and poor differentiation are on record, as mentioned above.

IX. SERTOLI-LEYDIG CELL TUMOR

A. General Features

Sertoli-Leydig cell tumors (SLCTs) are rare and constitute about 0.5% of all ovarian tumors. They occur in young patients, 75% in the first three decades of life, with an average age of 25 years (range 2–75).[42] Only about one-third of patients present with unequivocal evidence of androgen overproduction and many tumors are nonfunctioning and some are estrogenic. Thus terms such as "androblastoma" or "arrhenoblastoma" should be restricted to those cases with virilization. Androgenic manifestations vary from amenorrhea, atrophy of breasts, acne, hirsutism, temporal balding to deepening of the voice, and clitoromegaly. Rarely estrogenic manifestations such as menorrhagia or postmenopausal bleeding in pre- and postmenopausal women, respectively, occur. In the WHO classification they are divided into four subtypes:

1. Well differentiated
2. Intermediately differentiated
3. Poorly differentiated
4. Retiform

B. Gross Pathology

The vast majority of SLCTs are unilateral and stage I (98.5 and 97.5%, respectively) with only 2.5% being stages II and III in one of the largest series.[43] They vary from microscopic

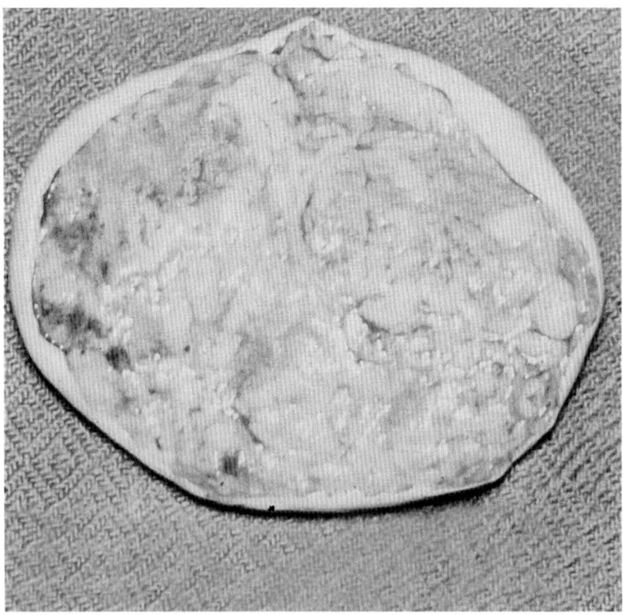

FIGURE 8.17 Sertoli-Leydig cell tumor. This tumor is round and solid with soft, brain-like consistency.

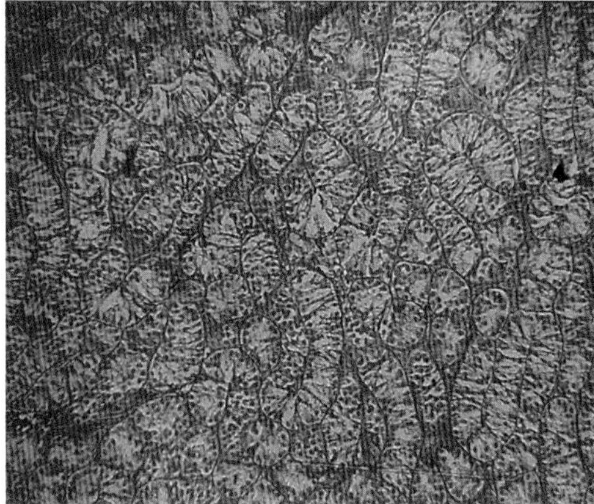

FIGURE 8.18 Sertoli cell tumor. Hollow tubules are lined by Sertoli cells with clear, lipid-rich cytoplasm.

to 51 cm in diameter (average 13.5 cm). Rupture of the tumor was reported in 15% of cases. Over half of the tumors are both solid and cystic, 38% solid, and only 4% cystic. The solid areas are tan (Fig. 8.17) to yellow and may exhibit necrosis and hemorrhage, more frequently in poorly differentiated tumors. The cystic areas are more common in the retiform variant and in tumors with heterologous elements. The retiform variant may contain intraluminal excrescences and closely simulates a papillary epithelial tumor.

C. Microscopic Pathology

Microscopic appearance reflects the degree of differentiation. SLCTs of intermediate differentiation are the most common type constituting 54% of all SLCTs, followed by poorly differentiated type 13%, and well-differentiated type 11%. *Well-differentiated SLCTs* are composed of Sertoli cells forming well-defined tubules and contain more than a small amount of Leydig cells within the intervening stroma. The tubules can be either solid or hollow. They are usually small, round to oval, but occasionally they may be more irregular, especially the hollow type and are lined by Sertoli cells with stratified nuclei and thus reminiscent of endometrial type glands. The Sertoli cells lining them are uniform in size and shape and have a moderate to abundant amount of cytoplasm which is eosinophilic, or vacuolated, and less often clear and lipid-rich. The cells are cuboidal or columnar with oval nuclei, which are stratified occasionally, and are characterized by dark, evenly distributed chromatin without discernible nucleoli. Mitotic figures are rare and nuclear atypia is mild. The stroma separating the tubules consists of mature fibrous tissue and contains clusters of polygonal Leydig cells with abundant eosinophilic or clear cytoplasm, some with lipochrome pigment and rarely crystals of Reinke.

1. SLCTs of Intermediate Differentiation

These are characterized by cellular areas separated by paucicellular or edematous connective tissue which imparts lobular appearance on low-power magnification (Fig. 8.19). The cellular lobules are composed of immature Sertoli cells with inconspicuous cytoplasm and ill-defined cell borders and with small, oval to round nuclei. These immature Sertoli cells are arranged in islands, focally solid/hollow tubules, and short one to two cell thick ribbons resembling the sex cords of the embryonic testis, and are commonly admixed with typical Leydig cells (Fig. 8.20). The Sertoli and Leydig cells are usually most apparent at the periphery of the cellular lobules. In some SLCTs the immature Sertoli cells in the cellular lobules are spindle-shaped. In addition small and large cysts with eosinophilic fluid may be observed reminiscent of thyroid follicles, and occasionally hobnail-like cells line these cysts. The connective tissue stroma may be edematous, particularly in pregnant patients and may also contain large clusters of Leydig cells. Nuclear atypia is of mild to moderate degree and the mitotic rate ranges from less than 1–28 per 10 hpf, with an average of 5.5 per 10 hpf.

2. Poorly Differentiated SLCTs

In most cases they have a diffuse growth pattern of round to oval and often spindle-shaped primitive tumor cells (Fig. 8.21)

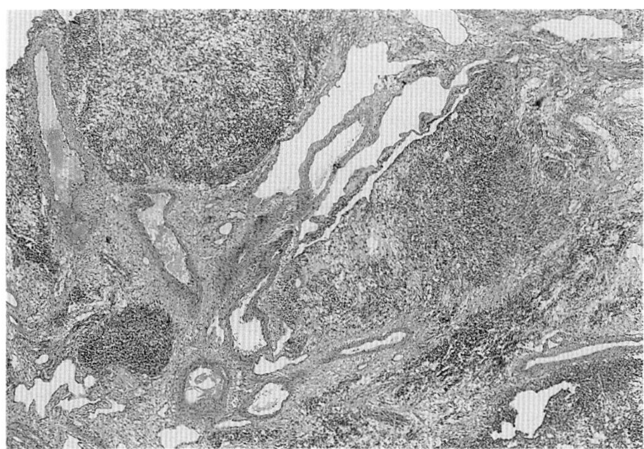

FIGURE 8.19 Sertoli-Leydig cell tumor of intermediate differentiation. The cellular areas are surrounded by edematous connective tissue imparting a lobular pattern on low power.

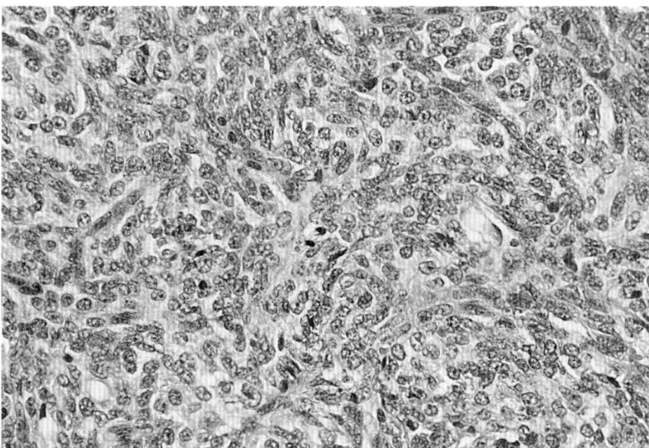

FIGURE 8.21 Sertoli-Leydig cell tumor, poorly differentiated. The tumor cells are spindle-shaped and primitive in appearance and reminiscent of fibrosarcoma.

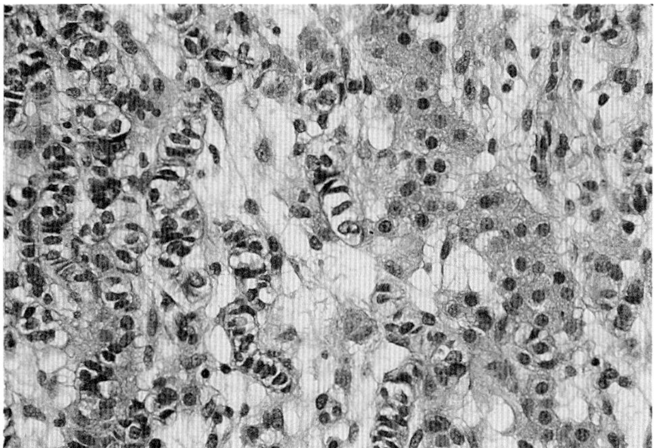

FIGURE 8.20 Sertoli-Leydig cell tumor of intermediate differentiation. The Sertoli cells are arranged in short cords on the right and are accompanied by clusters of Leydig cells on the left.

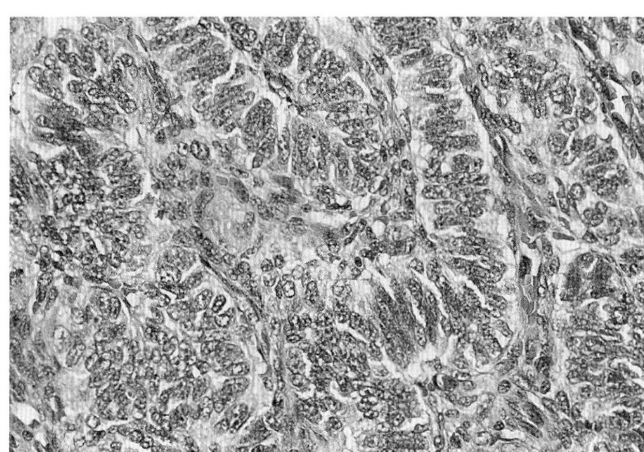

FIGURE 8.22 Sertoli-Leydig cell tumor, poorly differentiated. The primitive Sertoli cells form abortive sex cords.

which either lack or show only focal lobular arrangement. The diagnostic elements such as tubules, either solid or hollow, sex cord-like formation (Fig. 8.22), or retiform pattern are present only in minor foci in most cases. Thus they closely resemble fibrosarcoma, aside from the above-mentioned characteristic diagnostic elements. Nuclear atypia is usually moderate to severe. The mitotic rate, although ranging from 6–66 per 10 hpf, is ≥10 per 10 hpf in 85% of cases seen in the largest series.[42]

About 15–17% of SLCTs [42, 43] contain a prominent retiform pattern which resembles the normal rete testis in its architecture and cell type. Although it is recognized as a separate category in the WHO classification,[1] all of the reported cases also contain areas of SLCT of either intermediate (68% of cases) or poor (32% of cases) differentiation.[43]

Another unusual feature encountered only in approximately 20% of SLCTs of intermediate and poor differentiation is the presence of heterologous elements such as gastrointestinal epithelium or a mesenchymal component including cartilage and skeletal muscle.[44, 45] Most commonly the gastrointestinal epithelium is cytologically benign, but in rare tumors it is of borderline malignancy or frankly malignant. It is in the form of glands or cysts lined by intestinal-type epithelium including goblet, endocrine, and rarely Paneth cells; occasionally gastric-type epithelium is seen. Tumors with a mucinous component may rarely contain foci of insular or mucinous carcinoid tumor and mucin extravasation which may induce a giant cell reaction. Rarely, the tumor is largely composed of gastrointestinal elements and only small areas of SLCT and vice versa. Mesenchymal heterologous elements are observed in 5% of SLCTs and are represented most commonly by embryonal rhabdomyosarcoma and immature cartilage in a sarcomatous background. Almost all SLCTs with mesenchymal heterologous elements (91%) in one series [46] were poorly differentiated in contrast to SLCTs with a gastrointestinal component in which only 12.5% of tumors belong to this category.[44]

D. Differential Diagnosis

Although various primary and metastatic tumors must be considered in the differential diagnosis due to the broad spectrum of morphologic features seen in SLCTs, they can be put in three major categories: epithelial neoplasms, germ cell tumors, and rarely, sarcoma. All of them are negative for α-inhibin in contrast to SLCTs. In SLCTs the Sertoli and Leydig cells express α-inhibin, although more strongly in Leydig cells.[22, 46]

Endometrioid adenocarcinoma with elongated glands, nuclear stratification within cells lining them, accompanied by luteinized stroma may be a source of diagnostic confusion.

But the frequent presence of squamous differentiation, postmenopasal age, and diffuse positivity for cytokeratin and EMA and lack of α-inhibin expression should help to solve the dilemma.

Tubular Krukenberg tumor without readily apparent intracytoplasmic mucin and prominent luteinization of the stroma which may be responsible for virilization, especially during pregnancy, enters into the differential diagnosis. Again the above immunohistochemical stains, combined with a positive mucin stain and the frequent bilateral involvement of the ovaries, are useful to identify this secondary carcinoma.

The retiform variant of SLCT has areas similar to papillary serous tumors of low malignant potential or well-differentiated serous carcinoma, but the diagnostic sex cord elements should be present.

In the germ cell tumor category carcinoid tumor of trabecular and insular types may mimic ribbons and solid tubules of SLCTs, and similarly stroma ovarii may contain structures reminiscent of tubules of SLCTs. Endocrine markers and thyroglobulin immunostains are very useful, and the fact that about 70% of germ cell tumors are associated with other teratomatous elements are very useful features. Another germ cell tumor with structures similar to that observed in retiform SLCTs is endodermal sinus tumor, but alpha-fetoprotein expression in the latter is diagnostic.

SLCTs with heterologous mucinous differentiation and only focal sex cords elements may simulate pure mucinous tumor. Whereas SLCTs with heterologous mesenchymal elements in the form of rhabdomyoblastic foci or poorly differentiated SLCTs may mimic sarcoma or malignant mixed Mullerian tumor.

Endometrial stromal sarcoma, especially with sex-cord-like elements may closely mimic SLCTs of intermediate or poor differentiation and the positivity for CD10 in the former may be useful.

Immunohistochemistry of sex cord-stromal tumors is described in more detail in the Section II.D.

E. Treatment

Since 75% of SLCTs occur in the first three decades of life and approximately 97% are unilateral and stage I tumors, the most appropriate treatment is unilateral salpingo-oopherectomy for tumors involving one ovary only. In higher stage tumors and in stage I tumors of poor differentiation and ruptured tumors of intermediate differentiation more aggressive surgical therapy and chemotherapy are advocated. Recurrent tumors are rare and therefore experience is limited. Chemotherapy and radiotherapy have been reported to be helpful in some cases.[47]

F. Prognosis

The prognosis strongly correlates with the stage and differentiation of the tumor. All tumors higher than stage I are clinically malignant. None of the well-differentiated tumors, 11% of the intermediate differentiation, 59% of the poorly differentiated, and 19% of the tumors with heterologous elements were malignant in the largest series.[42] Rupture and a retiform pattern are unfavorable prognostic factors. In contrast to granulosa cell tumors which often recur late, SLCTs typically recur early. Sixty-six percent of the malignant SLCTs in the largest series [42] recurred within 1 year, whereas only 6.6% recurred after 5 years. Metastatic tumor was usually confined to the pelvis or abdomen, but lung metastases were present in two patients, scalp metastases were present in one, and supraclavicular lymph node metastases were found in one case.

X. SEX CORD TUMOR WITH ANNULAR TUBULES (SCTAT)

A. General Features

SCTAT in the WHO classification is recognized as a separate category, although some investigators consider it a subtype of Sertoli cell tumors because of the presence of Charcot-Bottcher filaments in the tumor cells in some of the cases.[48] SCTAT presents in two different clinical settings, in patients with the Peutz-Jeghers syndrome (PJS) and patients without it. In the latter group they are discovered on physical examination as palpable pelvic masses; in contrast in the former group they are usually an incidental finding during surgery for another indication. In patients with PJS the average age at presentation is 27 years and the clinical course is benign. Patients without PJS present at average age of 34 years and 20% of them follow a malignant course.[49]

B. Gross and Microscopic Pathology

The tumors in the PJS group are often microscopic with a range up to 3 cm. They are bilateral in two-thirds of the patients and frequently calcified, compared with tumors in patients without PJS which are predominantly unilateral and up to 20 cm in diameter.

Microscopically they are composed of simple or complex annular tubules (Fig. 8.23) composed of cells with abundant clear cytoplasm with indistinct cell borders containing uniform, round nuclei without nucleoli, which form rings around eosinophilic globules of basement membrane material (Fig. 8.24). The smaller rings are within larger rings imparting a complex annular pattern. In patients without PJS, foci of granulosa cell tumor, microfollicular type, and well-differentiated Sertoli-Leydig cell tumor are encountered, but not in SCTAT associated with PJS, where the tumors are small and frequently microscopic in the form of tumorlets.

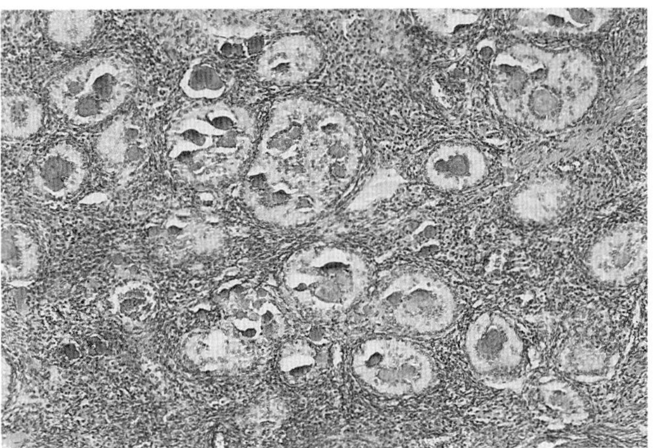

FIGURE 8.23 Sex cord tumor with annular tubules. A few simple and complex annular tubules with focal calcification, most prominent in the left upper quadrant (from a patient with PJS).

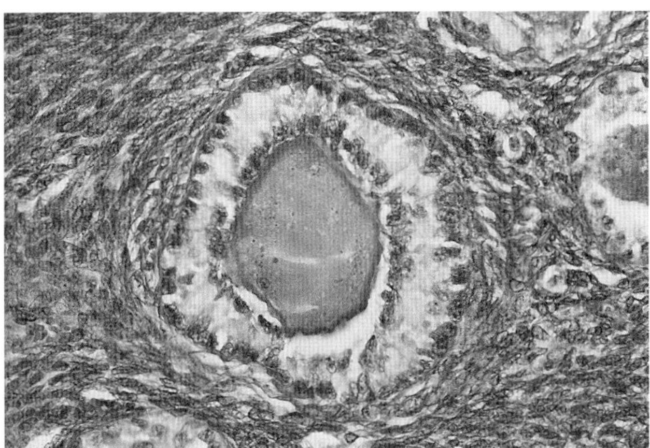

FIGURE 8.24 Sex cord tumor with annular tubules. The round nuclei form rings around the eosinophilic globules of basement membrane material.

XI. GYNANDROBLASTOMA

This is a very rare mixed tumor with two well-differentiated components including granulosa cell tumor with typical Call-Exner bodies coexisting with Sertoli cell tumor with hollow tubules, and each component should constitute at least 10% of the tumor mass. Typical Sertoli-stromal cell tumors may contain minor foci of granulosa cells with Call-Exner bodies (less than 10%) and granulosa cell tumors may show minor foci of tubules lined by Sertoli cells (less than 10%), respectively. This definition excludes cases where the sex cord elements are less well differentiated and the ovarian and testicular characteristics are not clear. This group of tumors in the WHO [1] classification is put into the category of unclassified sex cord-stromal tumor. Almost all gynandroblastomas are confined to the ovaries and follow a benign course. They may present with either estrogenic or androgenic manifestations.

XII. STEROID (LIPID) CELL TUMOR

These are tumors composed almost entirely of cells with features characteristic of steroid hormone secreting cells and thus resembling Leydig, lutein, and adrenal cortical cells.

They are rare and account for about 0.1% of all ovarian tumors and the majority produce steroid hormones and a smaller proportion contain the intracytoplasmic lipid for which they are named. In the WHO classification [1] they have been divided into three subtypes:

1. Stromal luteoma
2. Leydig cell tumor
   - Hilar type (Hilus cell tumor)
   - Nonhilar type
3. Steroid cell tumor, unclassified (not otherwise specified)

Stromal luteoma is located within the stroma of the ovary and is composed of steroid cells presumably of ovarian stromal or lutein cell origin that lack the crystals of Reinke.

The Leydig cell tumor of nonhilar type has the same location as stromal luteoma, but the steroid cells contain the crystals of Reinke and therefore are designated as such.

The Leydig cell tumor of hilar type is located in the hilus separated from the medulla and the steroid cells may or may not have crystals of Reinke. Those tumors that cannot be placed in the above categories are designated as steroid cell tumors, not otherwise specified (NOS).

XIII. STROMAL LUTEOMA

The stromal luteoma is a small tumor located within the ovarian stroma and accounts for about 20% of steroid cell tumors.[50, 51] They occur in postmenopausal women in

80% of cases who present with vaginal bleeding which is thought to be due to estrogen excess. About 12% of patients present with androgenic manifestations.[50] Stromal luteoma is accompanied by stromal hyperthecosis in the same or contralateral ovary in about 90% of cases. In nodular hyperthecosis the nodules are multiple and an arbitrary size of less than 0.5 cm is advocated by some to distinguish this entity from stromal luteoma, which is usually solitary and larger. However, it is usually less than 3 cm, since by definition it has to be confined to the ovarian stroma. Stromal luteoma defined as above has a benign course. They are unilateral with rare exceptions, solid, well-defined nodules with tan to yellow, and red or brown sectioned surface in one-third of the cases. Microscopically they are composed of cells with abundant eosinophilic cytoplasm containing single, small, uniform, and round nuclei with central, single prominent nucleoli. Lipochrome pigment may be seen. They are arranged in nests, cord, or diffusely within sparse stroma consisting of delicate connective tissue with a rich vascular network. Mitotic figures are rare.

XIV. LEYDIG CELL TUMOR

There are two subtypes in this category as defined above depending upon the location of the tumor and presence or absence of crystals of Reinke. The clinical and pathological features do not differ in these two subtypes. They are typically androgenic in 75% of cases and are detected at an average age of 58.[52] Almost all of those cases reported in the literature have been benign, except for one malignant case.[53]

They are usually small, circumscribed masses with an average diameter of 2.4 cm and unilateral (Fig. 8.25). Sectioned surfaces are tan to yellow and occasionally dark brown with bands of fibrous septa. Microscopically they are composed of lutein cells arranged diffusely and separated by eosinophilic areas devoid of nuclei (Fig. 8.26). In some tumors fibrous septa divide the tumor into lobules. Another feature seen in one-third of the cases is fibrinoid necrosis of vessel walls. Reinke crystals may be difficult to find (Fig. 8.27).

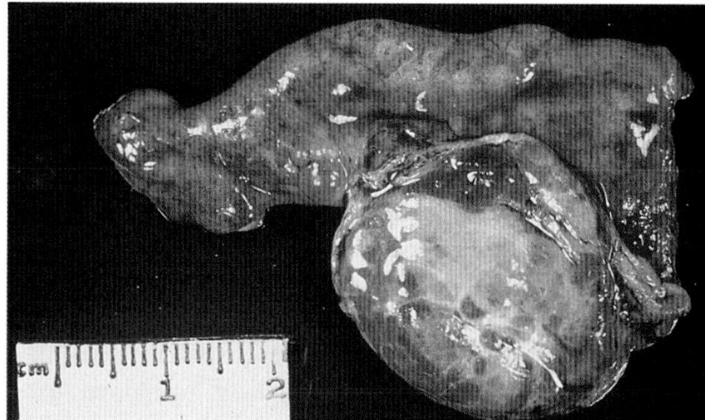

FIGURE 8.25 Leydig cell tumor. Yellow mass occupies the center of the sectioned ovary.

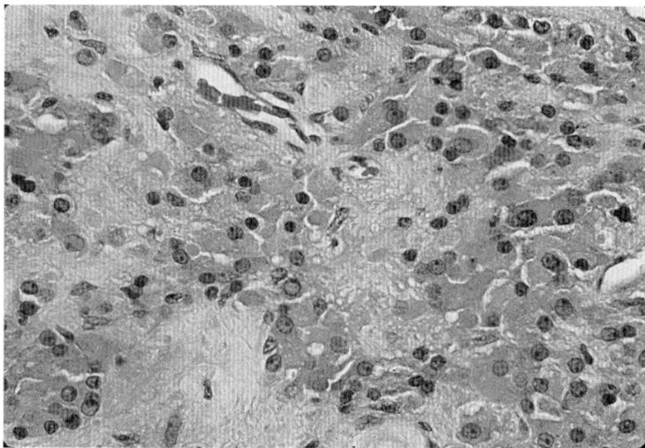

FIGURE 8.26 Leydig cell tumor. The tumor cells show abundant, finely granular eosinophilic cytoplasm and are arranged in sheets and focally, separated by pink areas which are devoid of nuclei.

XV. STEROID CELL TUMOR, NOS

A. General Features

Steroid cell tumors in this category are defined as large steroid cell tumors not confined to either cortex or medulla and lack crystals of Reinke. They account for about 60% of all steroid cell tumors. Tumors in this category represent either stromal luteoma or Leydig cell tumors lacking crystals of Reinke, but because of their large size the site of origin is obscured and thus precludes specific identification of either of the former types of tumor. The age at presentation varies from 2½ to 80 years old, with an average age of 43.[54] About 40% of patients present with virilization, rare patients have estrogenic manifestations or hypercortisolemia with Cushing's syndrome.

B. Gross and Microscopic Pathology

The tumors have a mean diameter of 8.4 cm and are solid and well circumscribed. Sectioned surfaces are yellow to dark brown depending on the lipid and lipochrome content in the cytoplasm of tumor cells. In addition necrosis and hemorrhage may be present. They are composed of steroid cells most commonly arranged diffusely, or in nests and cords. Two types of tumor cells are recognized. The more common cell type is characterized by moderate to large amount of eosinophilic, slightly granular cytoplasm (lipid-poor/free) with distinct cell borders containing small, uniform, central nuclei with single nucleoli. The less common cell type has abundant and vacuolated often spongy

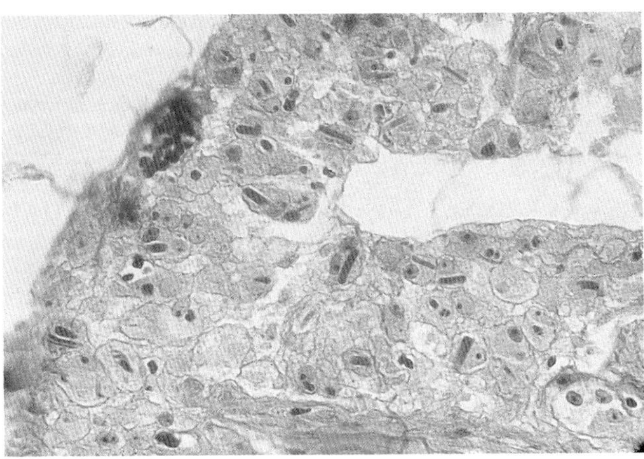

FIGURE 8.27 Hilus cell with Reinke crystals (azocarmine stain).

cytoplasm (lipid-rich) with distinct cell membranes and small but vesicular nuclei. Lipochrome pigment is present in 40% of cases and varying degrees of nuclear atypia is observed in 60% of cases.[41] The mitotic rate in cases without nuclear atypia ranges from <1–2 per 10 hpf, whereas in cases with nuclear atypia is <1–15 per 10 hpf. In the latter group necrosis and hemorrhage is more prominent.

In the largest series [54] 43% of tumors were clinically malignant and patients in this group averaged 16 years older. The best pathological correlates of malignant behavior in this series were the presence of ≥2 mitotic figures per 10 hpf, necrosis, diameter ≥7 cm, hemorrhage, and nuclear atypia.

C. Pregnancy Luteoma

Although not a neoplasic lesion, it may mimic lipid-poor/free steroid cell tumor on gross and microscopic examination. In adddition pregnancy luteoma is frequently virilizing. It is multiple in one half and bilateral in one-third of the cases.[55] Microscopically they are mitotically active but lack nuclear atypia. A solitary pregnancy luteoma may be indistinguishable from lipid-poor/free steroid cell tumor NOS.

References

1. Scully, R. E. (1999). Sex cord-stromal tumours. *In* "Histological Typing of Ovarian Tumours," 2nd ed., pp. 19–28. International Histological Classification of Tumours. World Health Organization. Springler-Verlag, Berlin.
2. Norris, H. J., and Taylor, H. B. (1968). Prognosis of granulosa-theca tumors of the ovary. *Cancer* 21, 255.
3. Satoh, M. (1991). Histogenesis and organogenesis of the gonad in human embryos. *J. Anat.* 177, 85–107.
4. Benjamin, E., Law, S., and Bobrow, L. G. (1987). Intermediate filaments cytokeratin and vimentin in ovarian sex cord-stromal tumours with correlative studies in adult and fetal ovaries. *J. Pathol.* 152, 253–263.
5. Miettinen, M., Virtanen, I., and Talerman, A. (1985). Intermediate filament proteins in human testis and testicular germ cell tumors. *Am. J. Pathol.* 120, 402–410.
6. Young, R. H., and Scully, R. E. (1994). Sex cord-stromal tumor, steroid cell, and other ovarian tumors with endocrine, paraendocrine, and paraneoplastic manifestations. *In* "Blaustein's Pathology of the Female Genital Tract," 4th ed. (R. J. Kurman., ed.), pp. 783–847. Springer-Verlag, New York.
7. Young, R. H., Dickersin, G. R., and Scully, R. E. (1984). Juvenile granulosa cell tumor of the ovary. A clinicopathological analysis of 125 cases. *Am. J. Surg. Pathol.* 8(8), 575–596.
8. Demopoulos, R. I., and Bell, D. A. (1983). The fine structure of a virilizing human granulosa-theca cell tumor: Observations on the nature of the hormone producing cell. *Cancer* 51, 1858–1865.
9. Lappohn, R. E., Burger, H. G., Bouma, J., Bangah, M., Krans, M., and de Bruijn, H. W. A. (1989). Inhibin as a marker for granulosa-cell tumor. *N. Eng. J. Med.* 321, 790–793.
10. McCluggage, W. G., Shanks, J. S., Whiteside, C., Maxwell, P., Banerjee, S. S., and Biggart, J. D. (1998). Immunohistochemical study of testicular sex cord-stromal tumors, including staining with anti-inhibin antibody. *Am. J. Surg. Pathol.* 22, 615–619.
11. Healy, D. L., Burger, H. B., and Bouna, J. (1993). Elevated serum inhibin concentration in postmenopausal women with ovarian tumors. *N. Eng. J. Med.* 329, 1539–1542.
12. Malmstrom, H., Hogberg, T., Bjorn, R., and Simonsen, E. (1994). Granulosa cell tumors of the ovary: Prognostic factors and outcome. *Gynecol. Oncol.* 52, 50–55.
13. Stenwig, J. T., Hazekamp, J. T., and Beecham, J. B. (1979). Granulosa cell tumors of the ovary. A clinicopathological study of 118 cases with long-term follow-up. *Gynecol. Oncol.* 7, 136–152.
14. Bjorkholm, E., and Silfversward, C. (1981). Prognostic factors in granulosa cell tumors. *Gynecol. Oncol.* 11, 261–274.
15. Kammerman, S., Demopoulos, R. I., and Ross, J. (1977). Gonadotropin receptors in experimentally induced ovarian tumors in mice. *Cancer Res.* 37, 2578–2582.
16. Demopoulos, R. I., and Kammerman, S. (1981). Fine structural evidence on the origin of gonadotropin-induced ovarian tumors in mice. *Cancer Res.* 41, 871–876.
17. Kammerman, S., Demopoulos, R. I., Raphael, C., and Ross, J. (1981). Gonadotropic hormone binding to human ovarian tumors. *Hum. Pathol.* 12, 886–890.
18. Yaziji, H., and Gown, A. M. (2001). Immunohistochemical analysis of gynecologic tumors. *Int. J. Gynecol. Pathol.* 20, 64–78.
19. McCluggage, W. G. (2001). Value of inhibin staining in gynecologic pathology. *Int. J. Gynecol. Pathol.* 20, 79–85.
20. Costa, M. J., DeRose, P. B., Roth, L. M., Brescia, R. J., Zaloudek, C. J., and Cohen, C. (1994). Immunohistochemical phenotype of ovarian granulosa cell tumors: Absence of epithelial membrane antigen has diagnostic value. *Hum. Pathol.* 25, 60–66.
21. McCluggage, W. G., and Maxwell, P. (1999). Adenocarcinomas of various sites may exhibit immunoreactivity with anti-inhibin antibodies. *Histopathology* 35, 216–220.
22. Matias-Guiu, X., Pons, C., and Prat, J. (1998). Mullerian inhibiting substance, alpha-inhibin, and CD99 expression in sex cord-stromal tumors and endometrioid ovarian carcinomas resembling sex cord-stromal tumors. *Hum. Pathol.* 29, 840–845.
23. Gordon, M. D., Corless, C., Renshaw, A. A., and Beckstead, J. (1998). CD99, keratin, and vimentin staining of sex cord-stromal tumors, normal ovary, and testis. *Mod. Pathol.* 11(8), 769–773.
24. Busam, K. J., Iversen, K., Coplan, K. A., Old, L. J., Stockert, E., Chen, Y. T., McGregor, D., and Jungbluth, A. (1998). Immunoreactivity for A103, an antibody to Melan-A (Mart-1), in adrenocortical and other steroid tumors. *Am. J. Surg. Pathol.* 22(1), 57–63.

25. Stewart, C. J., Nandini, C. L., and Richmond, J. A. (2000). Value of A103 (melan-A) immunostaining in the differential diagnosis of ovarian sex cord stromal tumors. *J. Clin. Pathol.* 53, 206–211.
26. Kottmeier, H. L. (1953). Carcinoma of the female genitalia. The Abraham Flexner Lectures, Series no 11. Williams & Wilkins, Baltimore, MD.
27. Fox, H., Agrawal, K., and Langley, F. A. (1975). A clinicopathological study of 92 cases of granulosa cell tumor of the ovary with special reference to the factors influencing prognosis. *Cancer* 35, 231–241.
28. Bjorkholm, E., and Silfversward, C. (1980). Theca cell tumors. Clinical features and prognosis. *Acta Radiol. Oncol. Radiat. Phys. Biol.* 19, 241.
29. Zhang, J., Young, R. H., Arseneau, J., and Scully, R. E. (1982). Ovarian stromal tumors containing lutein or Leydig cells (luteinized thecomas and stromal Leydig cell tumors). A clinicopathological analysis of fifty cases. *Int. J. Gynecol. Pathol.* 1, 270–285.
30. Clement, P. B., Young, R. H., and Scully, R. E. (1994). Sclerosing peritonitis associated with luteinized thecomas of the ovary. A clinicopathological analysis of six cases. *Am. J. Surg. Pathol.* 18(1), 1–13.
31. Waxman, M., Vuletin, J. C., Urcuyo, R., and Belling, C. G. (1979). Ovarian low-grade stromal sarcoma with thecomatous features. A critical reappraisal of the so-called "malignant thecoma." *Cancer* 44, 2206–2217.
32. Dudzinski, M., Cohen, M., and Ducatman, B. (1989). Ovarian malignant luteinized thecoma–an unusual tumor in an adolescent. *Gynecol. Oncol.* 35, 104–109.
33. McCluggage, W. G., Sloan, J. M., Boyle, D. D., and Toner, P. G. (1998). Malignant fibrothecomatous tumour of the ovary: Diagnostic value of anti-inhibin immunostaining. *J. Clin. Pathol.* 51, 868–871.
34. Meigs, J. V. (1954). Fibroma of the ovary with ascites and hydrothorax. Meigs' syndrome. *Am. J. Obstet. Gynecol.* 67, 962.
35. Gorlin, R. J. (1987). Nevoid basal cell carcinoma syndrome. *Medicine* 66, 98–113.
36. Case records of the Massachusetts General Hospital. Case 14–1976. (1976). *N. Engl. J. Med.* 294, 772–777.
37. Young, R. H., and Scully, R. E. (1983). Ovarian stromal tumors with minor sex cord elements. A report of seven cases. *Int. J. Gynecol. Pathol.* 2, 227–234.
38. Prat, J., and Scully, R. E. (1981). Cellular fibromas and fibrosarcomas of the ovary. A comparative clinicopathological analysis of seventeen cases. *Cancer* 47, 2663–2670.
39. Chalvardjian, A., and Scully, R. E. (1973). Sclerosing stromal tumors of the ovary. *Cancer* 31, 664–670.
40. Ismail, S. M., and Walker, S. M. (1990). Bilateral virilizing sclerosing stromal tumours of the ovary in a pregnant woman with Gorlin's syndrome: Implications for pathogenesis of ovarian stromal neoplasms. *Histopathology* 17, 159–163.
41. Young, R. H., and Scully, R. E. (1984). Ovarian Sertoli cell tumors. A report of ten cases. *Int. J. Gynecol. Pathol.* 2, 349–363.
42. Young, R. H., and Scully, R. E. (1985). Ovarian Sertoli-Leydig cell tumors. A clinicopathological analysis of 207 cases. *Am. J. Surg. Pathol.* 9(8), 543–569.
43. Young, R. H., and Scully, R. E. (1983). Ovarian Sertoli-Leydig cell tumors with a retiform pattern: a problem with histopathologic diagnosis. A report of 25 cases. *Am. J. Surg. Pathol.* 7(8), 755–771.
44. Young, R. H., Prat, J., and Scully, R. E. (1982). Ovarian Sertoli-Leydig cell tumors with heterologous elements. (I) Gastrointestinal epithelium and carcinoid: A clinicopathologic analysis of thirty-six cases. *Cancer* 50, 2448–2456.
45. Prat, J., Young, R. H., and Scully, R. E. (1982). Ovarian Sertoli-Leydig cell tumors with heterologous elements.(II). Cartilage and skeletal muscle: a clinicopathologic analysis of twelve cases. *Cancer* 50, 2465–2475.
46. Scully, R. E., Young, R. H., and Clement, P. B. (1998). Sex cord-stromal tumor, granulosa cell tumors. *In* "Tumors of the Ovary and Maldeveloped Gonads." Atlas of Tumor Pathology, 3rd Ser., pp. 169–188. Armed Forces Institute of Pathology, Washington, D.C.
47. Gershenson, D. M., Copeland, L. J., Kavanagh, J. J., Sringer, C. A., Saul, P. B., and Wharton, J. T. (1987). Treatment of metastatic stromal tumors of the ovary with cisplatin, doxorubicin, and cyclophosphamide. *Obstet. Gynecol.* 70, 765–769.
48. Tavassoli, F. A., and Norris, H. J. (1980). Sertoli tumors of the ovary. A clinicopathologic study of 28 cases with ultrastructural observations. *Cancer* 46, 2281–2297.
49. Young, R. H., Welch, W. R., Dickersin, G. R., and Scully, R. E. (1982). Ovarian sex cord tumors with annular tubules: Review of 74 cases including 27 with Peutz-Jeghers syndrome and 4 with adenoma malignum of the cervix. *Cancer* 50, 1384–1402.
50. Hayes, M. C., and Scully, R. E. (1987). Stromal luteoma of the ovary: A clinicopathological analysis of 25 cases. *Int. J. Gynecol. Pathol.* 6, 313–321.
51. Scully, R. E. (1964). A distinctive type of lipoid cell tumor. *Cancer* 17, 769–778.
52. Paraskevas, M., and Scully, R. E. (1989). Hilus cell tumors of the ovary. A clinicopathological analysis of 12 Reinke crystal-positive and 9 crystal negative cases. *Int. J. Gynecol. Pathol.* 8, 299–310.
53. Echt, C. R., and Hadd, H. E. (1968). Androgen excretion pattern in a patient with metastatic hilus cell tumor of the ovary. *Am. J. Obstet. Gynecol.* 100, 1055–1061.
54. Hayes, M. C., and Scully, R. E. (1987). Ovarian steroid tumors (not otherwise specified). A clinicopathological analysis of 63 cases. *Am. J. Surg. Pathol.* 11(11), 835–845.
55. Norris, H. J., and Taylor, H. B. (1967). Nodular theca-lutin hyperplasia of pregnancy (so-called "pregnancy luteoma"). A clinical and pathological study of 15 cases. *Am. J. Surg. Pathol.* 47, 557–566.

C H A P T E R

9

Metastatic Tumors of the Ovary

TAMARA KALIR

Department of Pathology
The Mount Sinai School of Medicine
New York, New York 10029

The ovaries, being richly vascular organs, may receive metastases from numerous tissues, and tend to be the most common site in the female genital tract for involvement by metastatic disease. Estimates of the frequency with which tumors metastasize to the ovaries will vary with the study design, i.e., whether autopsies or surgical pathology specimens were used, whether prophylactically removed organs were included, if patients with clinically apparent disease only were counted, or if patients with clinically silent disease were also incorporated. Additionally, the estimate will be influenced by the nationality of the patients studied, since disease prevalence varies among countries. For example, gastric cancer, which has a higher prevalence in Japan than in the U.S., tends to be a more common cause of metastasis to the ovaries in Japan than in America. Regardless, metastases to the ovaries tend to be fairly rare. One estimate states that 1% of all ovarian tumors are metastatic, and that 3% of all cancers of the ovary are metastases.[1] The organs most frequently responsible for metastasis to the ovaries include: breast, large intestine, endometrium, and stomach.

Tumors spread to the ovaries by different modes, which include direct extension (seen with tumors of the fallopian tube, uterus, colon), transtubal migration (from tumors of the endometrium), blood and lymphatic vascular invasion (employed by many cancers and sarcomas), and via dissemination through the peritoneal fluid (from intra-abdominal tumors).

Ovarian metastases may range in size from microscopic, to grossly large, bulky tumors. Cut section generally tends to be solid and white to tan, but cysts, when present, mimic some primary ovarian tumors. The majority of metastases, from 60–75%, are bilateral. Other features of metastatic tumors include a grossly multinodular distribution in the ovarian parenchyma, and focal surface deposits.

Ovarian metastases histologically may show a multinodular distribution, and sometimes lymphatic/blood vascular invasion, particularly in hilar vessels. These gross and microscopic features of metastases may be very helpful, if present, in certain histologies where primary ovarian and metastatic tumors resemble each other. For example, hepatoid endometrioid carcinoma of the ovary and hepatocellular carcinoma; mucinous ovarian and colonic cancers; endometrioid ovarian carcinoma and non-mucinous colon cancers, and carcinoids. In addition, as will be discussed later, special histochemical, or immunohistochemical stains may be performed in attempts to identify the primary site.

I. BREAST CANCER

Breast cancers metastasize to the ovaries reportedly in 6–40% of cases.[2] Most tend to involve the ovaries bilaterally. The histologic appearance bears resemblance to the primary tumor. Lobular carcinomas, which are more likely than ductal tumors to spread to the ovaries, may show characteristic "Indian-filing," or insular growth patterns.

Immunohistochemical staining for breast antigen (gross cystic disease protein 15) may be helpful. Figure 9.1 illustrates a high-power view of the histologic appearance of a metastatic lobular carcinoma in the ovary from a 47-year-old nulliparous woman, being treated with Megace for previously resected breast cancer, who presented with ascites and a pelvic mass. Both ovaries were involved by tumor, which showed a multinodular appearance, and characteristic, so-called "Indian file" pattern (cells lined up in a row) seen in the figure. Estrogen and progesterone receptor studies were positive in tumor cells, and breast antigen was negative. Patients with clinically apparent metastases tend to have a poorer prognosis.

II. COLON CANCER

Colon cancers are the most common of the intestinal primaries to metastasize to the ovaries. Approximately 4% of women with intestinal cancer have metastasis to the ovaries.[3] Such patients have a very poor prognosis. More than half the tumors tend to involve the ovaries bilaterally. The histologic appearance resembles the colonic primary, which frequently is a mucinous carcinoma with goblet cells. These tumors also resemble primary ovarian mucinous carcinomas. Characteristic findings for an intestinal metastasis are the presence of so-called "dirty" intraluminal necrosis, which describes the presence of necrotic cells, inflammatory cells, and debris within tumor gland lumina, and additionally, garland-like formation of glands at the edge of necrotic material.[4] Some colonic cancers are non-mucinous, and resemble endometrioid carcinomas of the ovary. To distinguish bilaterality, if present, is a helpful feature. Other findings in favor of an intestinal primary include the presence of extensive confluent necrosis, and discrepancy between architectural and cytologic grades. In colon cancers, well-differentiated tumors (low architectural grade), tend to have high-grade nuclear features. In contrast, gynecologic tumors with low architectural grade tend to exhibit low nuclear grade. Findings which are in favor of ovarian origin include the presence of squamous differentiation within the tumor, and, though counterintuitive, the presence of goblet cells. If the findings are not definitive, then special immunohistochemical stains may be attempted. Cytokeratin 7 and human alveolar macrophage antigens tend to be more common in primary ovarian tumors.[5] Cytokeratin 20 and carcinoembryonic antigen are more common in primary colonic cancers.[6] Figure 9.2 illustrates an ovarian metastasis removed from an 83-year-old lady who presented with severe abdominal distention and underwent exploratory laparotomy, colonic resection, bilateral salpingo-oophorectomy, and omentectomy. She had a mucinous adenocarcinoma of the colon, with bilateral ovarian tumors. Immunohistochemical staining of the ovarian tumors showed positivity for cytokeratin 20 and CEA, and negativity for cytokeratin 7. This immunophenotype is characteristic of

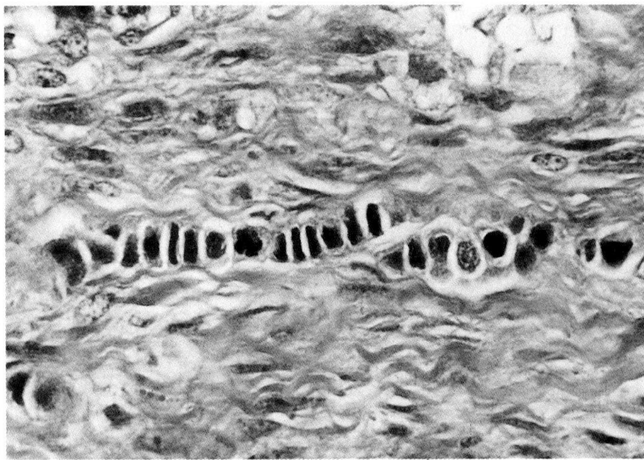

FIGURE 9.1 High-power view showing the characteristic "Indian file" pattern, or linear, single cell arrangement of metastatic lobular carcinoma of the breast, to the ovary (40×).

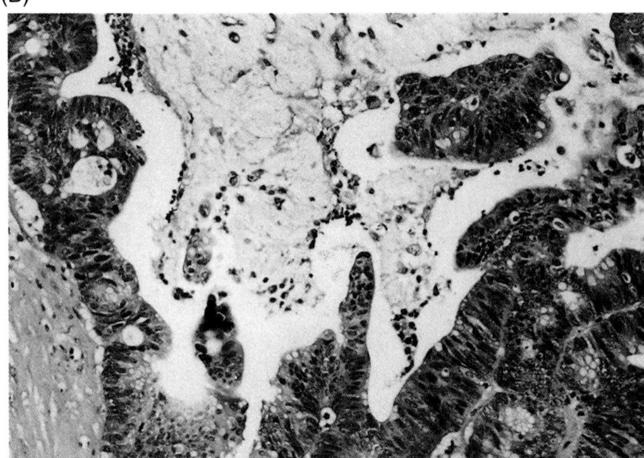

FIGURE 9.2 (A) Metastatic mucinous adenocarcinoma, from the colon, showing the usual intestinal morphology, with tall columnar (skyscraper) cells (4×). (B) Metastatic mucinous carcinoma, colonic, showing intraluminal debris, and moderate nuclear grade (10×).

colon cancer. Figure 9.2A shows a low-power view of a mucinous, intestinal-type carcinoma, with well-differentiated (grade 1) architectural grade and goblet cells. Figure 9.2B shows scanty debris within the lumens of glands and cells with moderate (grade 2) nuclear grade.

III. GASTRIC CANCER

Gastric carcinomas with a signet ring cell histology metastasize more often than gastric carcinomas of other histologic types. Such cases have a very poor prognosis. The signet ring cell resembles the familiar graduation ring and morphologically is filled with intracytoplasmic mucus, which compresses the nucleus, and pushes it off to one side. Metastatic ovarian tumors which show a predominantly signet ring cell histology are called Krukenberg tumors. The most common organs of origin of Krukenberg tumors are stomach, colon, appendix, and breast. The existence of a primary Krukenberg tumor of the ovary is controversial. Some authors believe that all Krukenberg tumors are metastases, and that in cases with signet ring cell carcinoma in the ovary(ies) and no detectable primary, that the primary tumor may have regressed, or simply was too small to be identified. Occasionally, Krukenberg tumors may incite a luteinization of surrounding stromal cells, which in turn may secrete estrogens or androgens. The differential diagnosis would then include a sex cord-stromal tumor, especially if the primary has not yet been identified. Figure 9.3A, B shows the histologic appearance of an ovarian metastasis from a 39-year-old female who presented with a pelvic mass, and history of previously resected gastric carcinoma. The cells show the signet ring morphology characteristic of a Krukenberg tumor, and are compatible with metastasis from her gastric carcinoma.

(A)

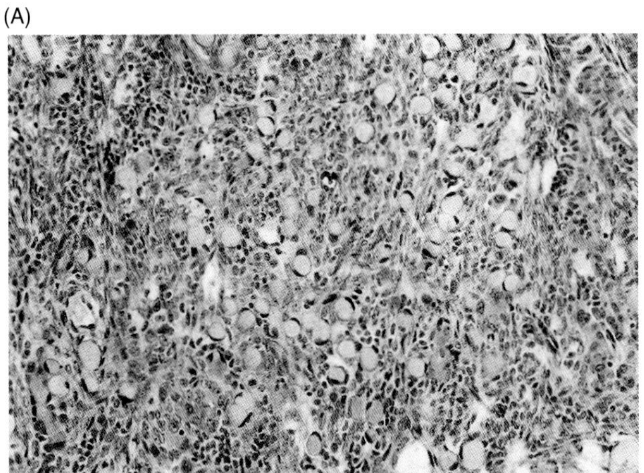

FIGURE 9.3 (A) Low-power view of a Krukenberg tumor, showing the characteristic signet ring cells within the ovarian parenchyma (10×). (B) High-power view of Krukenberg tumor, showing signet ring cells distended by intracytoplasmic mucus, and peripherally compressed nucleus (40×).

(B)

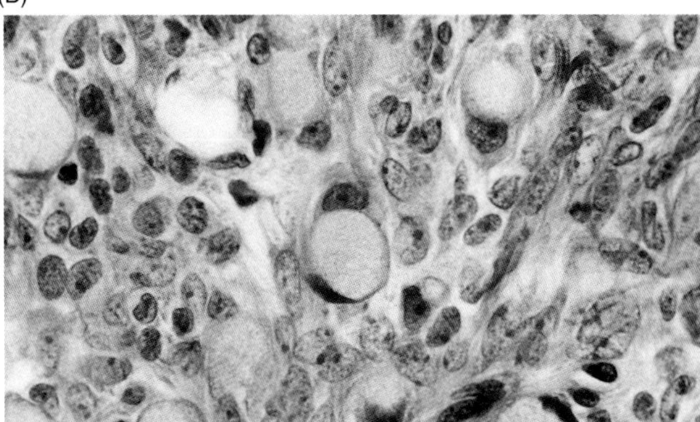

FIGURE 9.3 *(Continued)*

IV. APPENDICEAL CANCER

Ovarian metastases from the appendix range in appearance from usual intestinal type carcinomas, to carcinoids, to low-grade mucinous tumors. In some cases, patients have pseudomyxoma peritonei (Fig. 9.4), pseudomyxoma ovarii, and appendiceal pathology which ranges from overtly malignant, to benign, such as an adenoma or a mucocele. In our experience, the greater proportion of cases of pseudomyxoma peritonei have exhibited benign-appearing epithelium, so-called disseminated peritoneal adenomucinosis.[7] There is controversy in the literature about the origin of tumors that simultaneously involve the appendix and ovary. Some studies have provided evidence that the majority of such tumors arise in the appendix.[5, 8]

Carcinoid tumors account for approximately 2% of metastases to the ovary. Most are small intestinal in origin, but may also derive from elsewhere in the gastrointestinal tract or lung. Most mucinous carcinoids arise in the appendix. Again, bilateral ovarian involvement favors a metastatic process. Figure 9.5A, B shows the histologic appearance of a mucinous carcinoid metastatic to the ovaries from the appendix. The patient was a 67-year-old woman who presented with ascites and constipation. Although her tumor was debulked and she received postsurgical chemotherapy, the patient died eight months later. As shown in Fig. 9.5A, the insular pattern is the most common histologic pattern. These tumors may elicit a fibroma-like stromal proliferation, with hyalinization. The differential diagnosis then includes sex cord-stromal tumor, Brenner tumor, adenofibroma, and adenocarcinoma. Nuclear features are helpful. For example, carcinoids have a "salt and pepper" chromatin pattern, while Brenner tumors and sex cord tumors have a smooth chromatin with prominent intranuclear grooves (uncut coffee bean appearance). Special stains may be employed to help distinguish, if necessary. Histochemical stains detect argentaffin

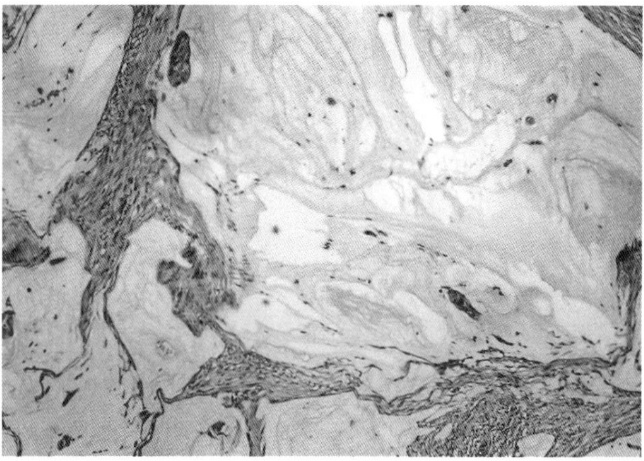

FIGURE 9.4 Pseudomyxoma peritonei, showing tissue disrupted by pools of dissecting mucus, which contains occasional inflammatory cells and is devoid of epithelial cells (2×).

(A)

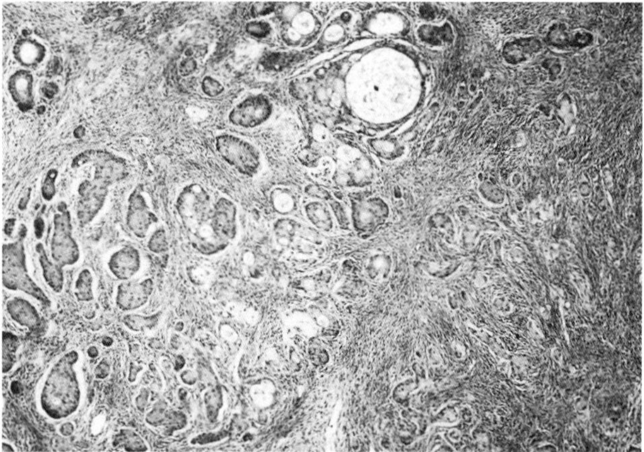

(B)

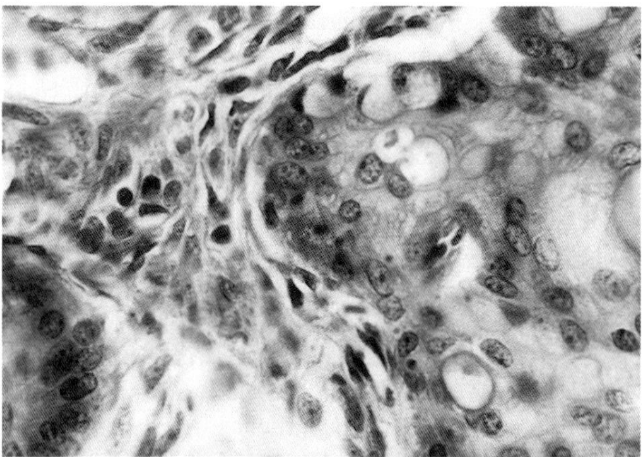

FIGURE 9.5 (A) Metastatic mucinous carcinoid from the appendix, showing insular arrangement of tumor cell nests (10×). (B) Metastatic mucinous carcinoid from the appendix, showing occasional goblet cells, and other cells with speckled (salt and pepper) chromatin pattern (40×).

and argyrophil granules, and immunohistochemical stains highlight neurosecretory granules in carcinoids. Electron microscopy may also be employed to demonstrate neurosecretory granules. Alternatively, a carcinoid amidst teratomatous elements would favor an ovarian origin, arising in a dermoid. Finally, a mucinous carcinoid will exhibit mucin-positive cells, in addition to carcinoid cells.

V. ENDOMETRIAL CANCER

At least one quarter of endometrial cancers spread to the ovaries.[9] In cases with simultaneous, histologically similar tumors in the ovary and endometrium, it may be difficult to determine whether a patient has synchronous primaries or a primary with metastasis. Features which are in favor of a primary endometrial cancer with metastases to the ovaries include [10] precancerous lesion in the endometrium (hyperplasia), deep myometrial penetration by the endometrial tumor, presence of lymphatic vascular invasion in the myometrium, freely floating intraluminal fallopian tube tumor cell clusters, tumor cells either in ovarian lymphatic or blood vessels, or involving the ovarian surface(s), and bilateral ovarian involvement. The usual tumor histology is endometrioid carcinoma. Primary ovarian endometrioid carcinoma usually is unilateral. Features in favor of synchronous primaries include a small and superficially invasive uterine corpus tumor, and the presence of endometriosis in the ovary(ies), which is felt to be a low-risk, but potentially precancerous lesion. In our experience with simultaneous ovarian and endometrial cancers of similar histologic type, distinction between the two possibilities generally can be made, and is important, because of the prognostic implications for the patient. Survival rates in cases of synchronous independent primaries tend to be higher than those with a single primary and metastasis.

VI. OTHER SITES

Metastases from other organs are rare and include sarcomas as well as carcinomas. We have had several cases of hepatic carcinoma metastatic to the ovaries. Because hepatocellular carcinoma resembles the hepatoid variant of ovarian endometrioid carcinoma, it is important to know whether the ovaries are enlarged bilaterally, and whether there is a hepatic mass, both features in favor of metastasis. Tumors from the biliary tree, gallbladder, and pancreas may metastasize to the ovaries. Again, bilateral ovarian involvement is a helpful finding. These tumors will characteristically have foci that exhibit small, sharply contoured, or comma-shaped glands, embedded in a desmoplastic stroma. In contrast, primary ovarian and Mullerian tumors tend to exhibit

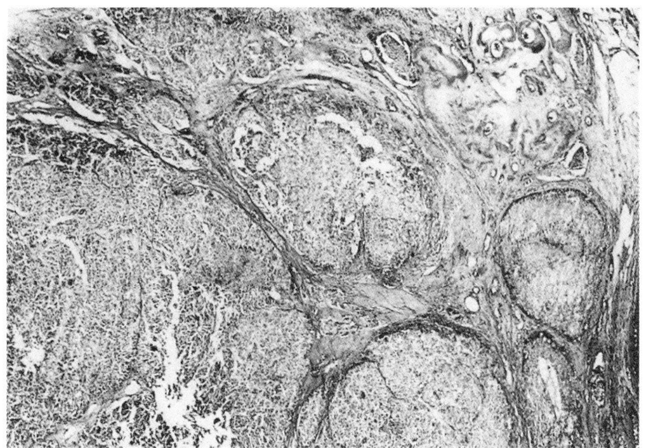

FIGURE 9.6 Adenosquamous carcinoma, metastatic to the ovary from the uterine cervix, displaying a multinodular pattern, with vascular space invasion (2×).

smoothly contoured glands, without comparable desmoplasia. One exception is clear cell carcinoma of the ovary, which tends to exhibit a hyalinized stroma, and may resemble desmoplasia. Approximately 5% of lung cancers metastasize to the ovaries.[11] Distinction from a primary ovarian endometrioid carcinoma, or undifferentiated carcinoma, may be difficult. In such cases, a special immunohistochemical stain for thyroid transcription factor (TTF1) tends to be positive in tumors of lung origin, and negative in ovarian adenocarcinomas.[12] Metastases from tumors of all histologic types from the uterine cervix are unusual. Figure 9.6 shows a recent case of a metastatic adenosquamous carcinoma from the cervix, which clinically appeared as a unilateral adnexal mass in a 40-year-old woman who presented with abnormal bleeding from the vagina. After surgery, the cervix was found to be extensively involved by tumor, with lymphatic invasion, and there was multinodular involvement of the right ovary. The patient is currently receiving chemotherapy. With the exception of malignant melanoma, metastases from skin lesions are very rare. In the past 10 years, we have had one case of a 50-year-old woman who presented with abdominal distension, and from whom bilateral blackened ovarian masses were resected. After a diagnosis of malignant melanoma, careful search revealed a primary lesion on the chest skin underlying her right pendulous breast. The patient was subsequently lost to follow-up, but her outlook was grim. Extremely rare are reports of metastasis to the ovaries from tumors of the thyroid gland, head and neck, and brain.

References

1. Robboy, S. J., Duggan, M. A., and Kurman, R. J. (1999). The female reproductive system. *In* "Pathology" (E. Rubin and J. L. Farber, eds.), p. 1015. Lippincott-Raven, New York.
2. Viadana, E., Bross, I. D. J., and Pickren, J. W. (1973). An autopsy study of some routes of dissemination of cancer of the breast. *Br. J. Cancer* 27, 336–340.
3. Burt, C. A. V. (1951). Prophylactic oophorectomy with resection of the large bowel for cancer. *Am. J. Surg.* 82, 572–577.
4. Lash, R. H., and Hart, W. R. (1987). Intestinal adenocarcinomas metastatic to the ovaries. A clinicopathologic evaluation of 22 cases. *Am. J. Surg. Pathol.* 11, 114–121.
5. Ronnett, B. M., Shmookler, B. M., Diener-West, M., Sugarbeker, P. H., and Kurman, R. J. (1997). Immunohistochemical evidence supporting the appendiceal origin of pseudomyxoma peritonei in women. *Int. J. Gynecol. Pathol.* 16, 1–9.
6. Berezowski, K., Stastny, J. F., and Kornstein, M. J. (1996). Cytokeratins 7 and 20 and carcinoembryonic antigen in ovarian and colonic carcinoma. *Mod. Pathol.* 9, 426–429.
7. Ronnett, B. M., Zahn, C. M., Kurman, R. J., Kass, M. E., Sugarbaker, P. H., and Shmookler, B. M. (1995). Disseminated peritoneal adenomucinosis and peritoneal mucinous carcinomatosis. A clinicopathologic analysis of 109 cases with emphasis on distinguishing pathologic features, site of origin, prognosis, and relationship to 'pseudomyxoma peritonei.' *Am. J. Surg. Pathol.* 19, 1390–1408.
8. Prayson, R. A., Hart, W. R., and Petras, R. E. (1994). Pseudomyxoma peritonei. A clinicopathologic study of 19 cases with emphasis on site of origin and nature of associated ovarian tumors. *Am. J. Surg. Pathol.* 18, 591–603.
9. Beck, R. P., and Latour, J. P. A. (1963). Necropsy reports on 36 cases of endometrial carcinoma. *Am. J. Obstet. Gynecol.* 85, 307–311.
10. Young, R. H., and Scully, R. E. (1994). Metastatic tumors of the ovary. *In* "Blaustein's Pathology of the Female Genital Tract" (R. J. Kurman, ed.), p. 943. Springer-Verlag, New York.
11. Mazur, M. T., Hsueh, S., and Gersell, D. J. (1984). Metastases to the female genital tract. Analysis of 325 cases. *Cancer* 53, 1978–1984.
12. Reis-Filho, J. S., Carrilho, C., Valenti, C., Leitao, D., Ribeiro, C. A., Reibeiro, S. G., and Schmitt, F. C. (2000). Is TTF1 a good immunohistochemical marker to distinguish primary from metastatic lung carcinomas? *Pathol. Res. Pract.* 196, 835–840.

C H A P T E R

10

Peritoneal Lesions Related to Ovarian Neoplasms

LIANE DELIGDISCH

Departments of Pathology, Obstetrics, Gynecology and Reproductive Science
The Mount Sinai School of Medicine and Hospital
New York, New York 10029

I. BENIGN LESIONS

A. Endometriosis

This lesion is defined as the presence of endometrial epithelium, stroma, and blood vessels in an ectopic location, outside the uterine body. Ovarian endometriosis is the most common ectopic site (85%), followed by other pelvic peritoneal locations such as the ligaments (utero-sacral, broad, round), recto-vaginal septum, cul-de-sac, and the peritoneum covering uterus, tubes, rectosigmoid, and bladder. Less commonly, endometriosis has been described in almost every organ, including bowel, cervix, vagina, urinary system, lungs, pancreas, skin, bones, and skeletal muscles.

The pathogenesis of endometriosis remains controversial. The most accepted mechanisms include metaplastic changes of the ovary and peritoneum, with its potential to differentiate into Mullerian-type structures (secondary or extended Mullerian tissue), and/or retrograde menstruation with implantation of endometrial tissue. Endometriosis is found in women of reproductive age, often presenting with infertility (30–40% of cases), or delaying pregnancy.[1] Vascular or lymphatic spread is probably responsible for distantly located endometriosis. The role of estrogen replacement therapy in postmenopausal women, in maintaining endometriosis that normally regresses after menopause, is still to be clarified. It is possible that the ectopic implantation of endometrial tissue is associated with a decreased cell-mediated immunity, as shown by the reduced apoptosis in ectopic endometrium.[2] Symptomatic endometriosis includes dysmenorrhea, pelvic pain, dyspareunia, irregular bleeding, and infertility. The intensity of the symptoms is not related to the extent of the lesions; many cases are completely asymptomatic.

Ovarian endometriosis is bilateral in less than half of the cases. The endometrial tissue present ranges in size from microscopic foci to lesions that compress and replace the ovarian parenchyma, forming cysts up to 15 cm in diameter. In the peritoneum the endometriosis is present as multiple bluish or brownish lesions, often surrounded by fibrosis and adhesions, or forming nodules or cysts similar to those in the ovaries. Laparoscopic studies have emphasized that early endometriosis may not be present as pigmented lesions and may show peritoneal defects.[3] During the reproductive years, cyclic changes often occur in the ectopic endometrial tissue, resulting in a menstrual-type shedding with hemorrhage accumulating in cystic cavities. The hemosiderin released from this menstrual blood elicits a reaction from the surrounding tissue that consists of macrophage proliferation with phagocytosis of hemosiderin pigment and fibrosis. The implantation of exfoliated endometrial tissue in the peritoneum may be related to generation and maintenance of blood supply, associated with vascular endothelial growth factor.[4]

Ovarian endometriosis is not included in the WHO classification of ovarian tumors, although some cystic lesions may reach large dimensions and are often designated as endometriomas. Grossly, ovarian endometriosis may present as cystic masses filled with a brown semi-fluid ("chocolate cysts") content, or as solid lesions with shaggy brownish irregular surfaces. Histologically, there is an epithelial lining that ranges between well-formed endometrial glands and a flat or cuboidal epithelium, surrounded by loose endometrial-type stroma and blood vessels, with fresh and/or old hemorrhage. In menopausal patients simple or cystic atrophy is often seen. In long-standing lesions, as well as in patients receiving anti-estrogenic hormone therapy, the endometrial-like characteristics may appear attenuated and be unrecognizable. Metaplastic changes are commonly seen (tubal, hobnail, clear cell, and squamous metaplasia). In patients receiving hormonal stimulation, endometriosis may flare up and reach tumoral proportions. Progesterone therapy as part of postmenopausal hormone replacement therapy may stimulate a decidual transformation of the connective tissue, resulting in solid masses that simulate tumors. In one such case, the mass compressed the ureter and produced a unilateral hydronephrosis.[5]

The epithelial lining often displays atypical features, such as the piling-up of cells, irregular nuclei with prominent nucleoli, or smudged chromatin. Mitoses are uncommon, except in the cases with cycling endometrium in premenopausal women. In rare cases, however, there is severe atypia, and high mitotic activity resembling atypical endometrial hyperplasia. Such lesions may be precancerous. An association of atypical endometriosis and ovarian cancer is seen occasionally in both ovarian and extra-ovarian (pelvic and abdominal) locations.[6, 7] When carcinoma arises in endometriosis, 75% occurs in the ovary, while 25% arises in other sites of endometriosis such as rectovaginal septum, vagina, colon, and bladder. Histologically, these are usually endometrioid or clear cell carcinomas, often with squamoid components.

A rare case of endometrioid carcinoma developing in pelvic endometriosis was seen in a patient who was 20 years postmenopausal and receiving tamoxifen for a previously diagnosed breast cancer (Fig. 10.1). Tamoxifen is known to behave as an estrogen agonist in the uterus [8] and may possibly have the same stimulating effect on endometriosis.[9]

The oncogenic potential of both ovarian and peritoneal endometriosis is low.[6, 7] Since endometriosis is associated with increased titers of serous CA125 it may preclude the early recognition of a malignant transformation. Histologic evidence of early malignant changes is presently the most reliable diagnostic method.

B. Endosalpingiosis

This consists of the presence of benign tubular structures resembling Mullerian epithelium, throughout the pelvic and abdominal cavity. As their epithelial lining often displays ciliated, secretory, and intercalate ("peg") cells, thus resembling the fallopian tube epithelium, it has been named "endosalpingiosis." The epithelium of the tubular structures is cuboidal, flat, resembling the peritoneal mesothelium, or tall columnar. The absence of endometrial-type stroma distinguishes these lesions from endometriosis. The location of endosalpingiosis is more common in the pelvic peritoneum, omentum, and periaortic tissue, including lymph nodes. These lesions may appear as whitish, granular, punctate structures, but they are usually incidental microscopic findings. Psammoma bodies are often associated with endosalpingiosis. They consist of concentrically laminated deposits of calcium appearing strongly basophilic on the routine H&E stainings (Fig. 10.2), and are considered to be the end result of a process of degeneration of the stalk of papillary excrescences. They are often encountered in papillary neoplasms.[10] In patients receiving chemotherapy for ovarian serous papillary carcinoma with peritoneal involvement, tubular or papillary structures lined by an endosalpingiosis-like epithelium or mesothelium are often seen in the proximity of psammoma bodies. They probably represent residual tumor.[11] The differential diagnosis, especially on frozen sections, between endosalpingiosis and metastatic peritoneal tumor from ovarian carcinoma is often difficult. The biological potential of these structures to revert to aggressive tumor is unknown.[11, 12] Endosalpingiosis can rarely present as a clinically evident large cystic mass.[13]

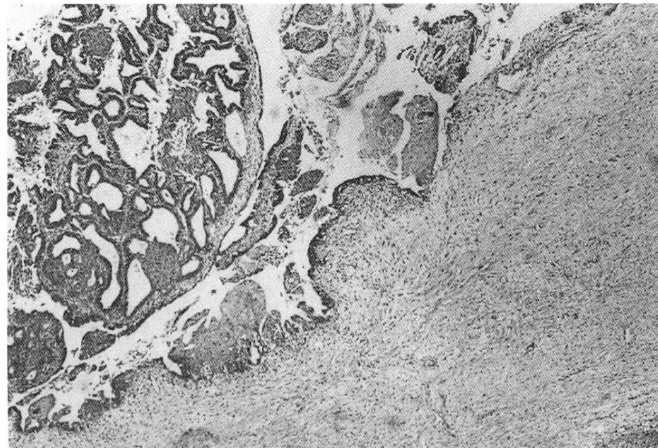

FIGURE 10.1 Pelvic endometriosis and adjacent endometrioid adenocarcinoma with squamoid areas. The patient had been treated with tamoxifen for breast cancer. H&E × 100.

Endosalpingiosis involving pelvic or abdominal lymph nodes is not uncommon and may also represent a difficult differential diagnosis with metastatic adenocarcinoma. The histologic blandness of the cells supports their benign nature. However, in patients with known ovarian malignancy, even bland-looking tubular or glandular structures in the regional lymph nodes should be viewed with caution.

Occasionally, endosalpingioisis may show hyperplastic changes consisting of stratification, cribriform pattern, atypical nuclei, and mitotic activity. This may represent, as in

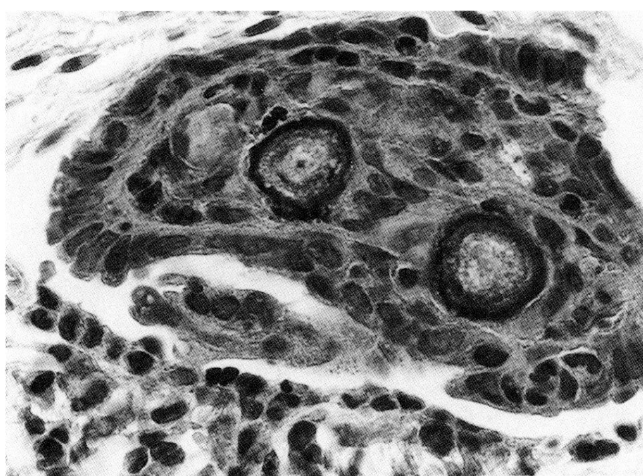

FIGURE 10.2 Psammoma bodies consisting of concentrically laminated deposits of calcium adjacent to peritoneal mesothelial hyperplasia and endosalpingiosis. H&E×400.

endometriosis, a reactive or a dysplastic, precancerous process, the former much more common than the latter. In cases of ovarian neoplasm, often in borderline serous tumors [14, 15] the proliferative activity associated with atypical changes of these inclusions may represent a "field effect" of the carcinogen that triggered the primary ovarian neoplasm. Staging may be difficult in distinguishing a metastatic lesion from a benign proliferation or from an atypical focus of endosalpingiosis.

Endosalpingiosis may represent a multifocal metaplastic process arising from the peritoneal mesothelium. When it involves the lymph nodes the endosalpingiotic glands are lined by benign Mullerian-type epithelium exhibiting the ciliated, secretory, and intercalate types of tubal epithelium. Implants from borderline ovarian tumors represent the most difficult differential diagnosis; they can be ruled out on the basis of the location, the presence of multiple cell types, and the bland aspect of the nuclei in endosalpingiosis.

C. Mesothelial Hyperplasia

This occurs very often as a result of inflammatory or otherwise irritating causes, the most common being endometriosis with the formation of adhesions, surgical scars, ascites, and foreign bodies. The mesothelium is a single cell layer composed of nonciliated, cuboidal to flat cells with eosinophilic cytoplasm, situated on a basement membrane. Histologically, the cells contain hyaluronic acid and stain negative for amylase. The peritoneal mesothelium is embryologically closely related to the ovarian surface epithelium and may respond to the same carcinogens. Mesothelial hyperplasia is often encountered on the serosal layer of the pelvic organs (uterus, fallopian tubes), of the abdominal organs, especially the bowel, and on adhesions. (Fig. 10.3).

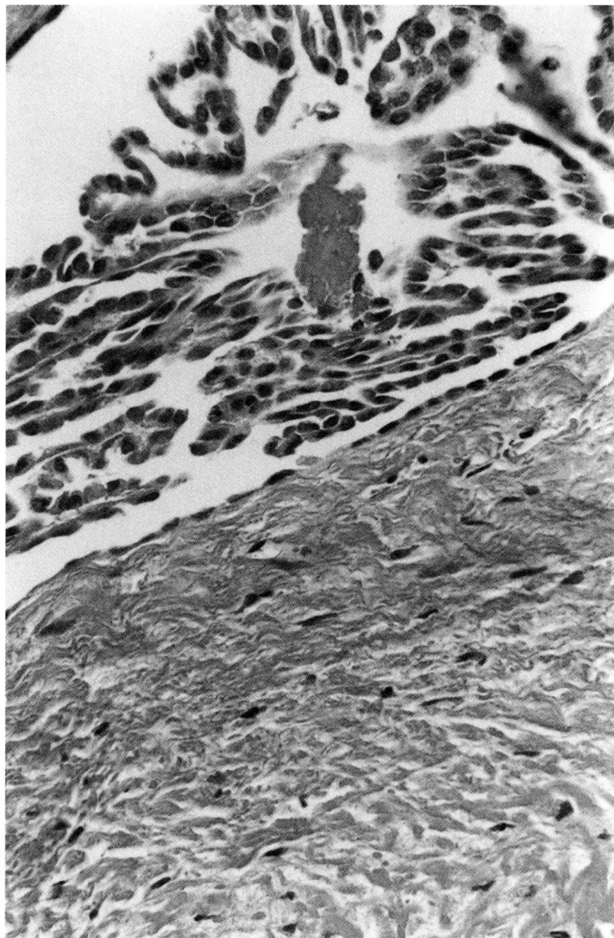

FIGURE 10.3 Periovarian adhesion with mesothelial cell hyperplasia. H&E×100.

Histologically, the hyperplastic mesothelial cells are large, with increased nuclei (Fig. 10.4). They may form trabecular or papillary structures or take a solid epithelioid appearance. In their vicinity, hemosiderin-laden macrophages, granulation tissue, and a variable amount of fibrosis can be found. The individual cells are relatively regular, uniform, and monomorphic, as opposed to the mesothelial cell atypia which is seen in neoplasms of the peritoneum (mesotheliomas). Sometimes transitional cell metaplasia (Walthard's nests) are seen on the serosal surfaces, more often of the fallopian tubes.

Morphometric studies have established a database with the size of hyperplastic mesothelial cell nuclei ranging between 22 and 27 μm^2.[12]

As with endosalpingiosis, mesothelial hyperplasia may represent a diagnostic dilemma, especially on frozen sections, with peritoneal metastatic carcinoma. The most difficult cases to differentiate from mesothelial hyperplasia are the residual peritoneal implants of ovarian carcinoma in patients treated with chemotherapy, especially those responsive, in

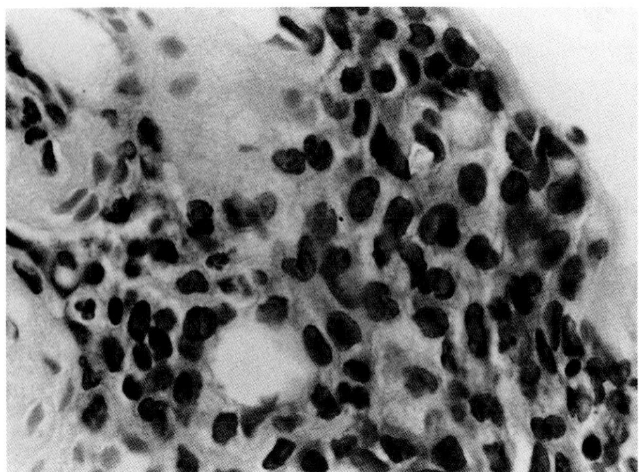

FIGURE 10.4 Hyperplastic mesothelial cells with large uniform nuclei. H&E×400.

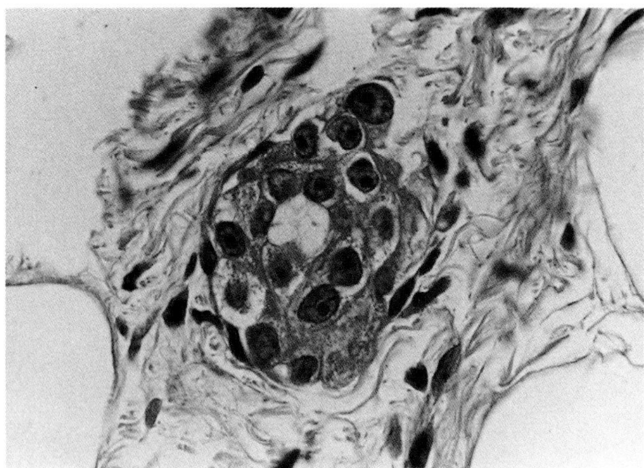

FIGURE 10.5 Peritoneal cluster of residual tumor cells from chemo therapy-treated primary ovarian carcinoma. Note prominent nucleoli. H&E×400.

which small clusters of tumor cells have a relatively bland appearance (Fig. 10.5).

II. MALIGNANT LESIONS

A. Serous Papillary Peritoneal Carcinoma

About 15% of all ovarian serous carcinomas present as tumors involving mostly the peritoneal cavity, with large omental "cakes" and peritoneal tumor masses, located in the cul-de-sac and serosal surfaces of the bowel, urinary bladder, uterus, etc., and minimal or no involvement of the ovary. Grossly, the ovary is of normal size or slightly enlarged (up to 4 cm in greatest diameter). Tumor tissue may be visible just on the surface or invading the ovarian cortex superficially (Fig. 10.6) and may be identified only by microscopic examination. Occasional serous carcinomas of the peritoneum are diagnosed in patients whose ovaries have been removed, some prophylactically, and found disease-free.[16, 17]

Grossly, the peritoneal masses are whitish, firm, and often gritty, due to calcifications. Their aspect and distribution is similar to that seen in the common form of stage III ovarian carcinoma. Histologically, the tumor is composed of papillary structures, similar to those seen in ovarian serous papillary carcinoma; an almost constant feature is the presence of abundant psammoma bodies.

Because of the location in the peritoneal cavity and the minimal or absent involvement of the ovaries, it had been postulated in the past that this tumor was a malignant mesothelioma, originating in the peritoneal mesothelium. Malignant mesothelioma is a rather uncommon neoplasm, affecting mostly male patients, with a proven etiopathogenic association with asbestos exposure, and involving the pleural and/or peritoneal cavities.

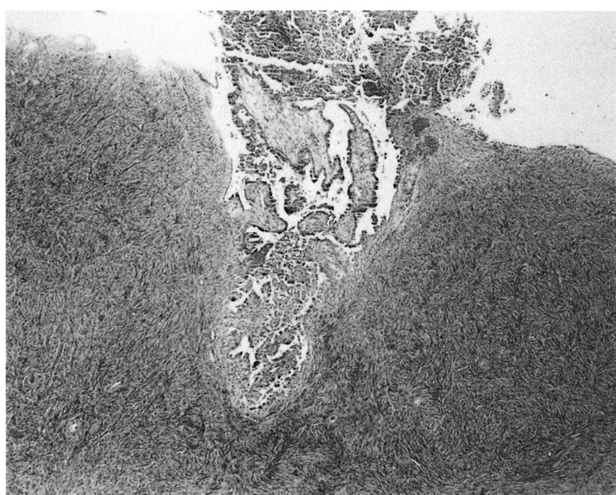

FIGURE 10.6 Serous papillary peritoneal carcinoma with focal involvement of ovarian surface and cortex. There was massive omental tumor. H&E×40.

Histologically, malignant mesotheliomas display a number of features, such as epithelioid solid, tubular, sarcomatoid, and papillary patterns, in their pure forms, or combined. They often display biphasic patterns with epithelioid and sarcomatoid elements. The papillary structures in malignant mesotheliomas are usually tubulo-papillary, with scanty connective tissue in the stalks and no psammoma bodies. The tumor cells stain positive for hyaluronic acid and express mesothelial type antigens, as opposed to the ovarian serous papillary tumor cells which are antigenically and histologically similar to Mullerian-derived epithelium, sharing only some mesothelial antigens.[13] Phenotypically, malignant mesothelioma and ovarian-type peritoneal papillary carcinoma are different tumors although both arise in the peritoneal mesothelium. The natural history and clinical behavior, including the response to chemotherapy, is also different; malignant mesotheliomas are more aggressive and respond less, or do not respond, to the currently used chemotherapy for ovarian carcinoma.[18, 19] Peritoneal tumors of low malignant potential are histologically similar to those seen in the ovary.[10, 15]

It should be mentioned that one subgroup of mesotheliomas, the benign mesotheliomas, displaying a histologic pattern dominated by papillary structures has a favorable outcome, and is usually an incidental finding in peritoneal biopsies. It should be distinguished from the two entities discussed above. The cells lining the papillary structures in benign mesothelioma are uniform and plump, with bland-appearing, round to oval nuclei. Histochemically, they are similar to normal mesothelial cells.

B. Peritoneal Neoplasms at Second-Look Operations for Ovarian Cancer

These operations are performed with the purpose of identifying minimal or microscopic disease after chemotherapy in order to re-treat those patients.

Random biopsies taken from the peritoneal surface are examined histologically. The peritoneal tumor tissue from patients who were previously "debulked" and then treated with chemotherapy, when positive, may display either characteristics similar to the original tumor, or present as clusters of relatively bland-looking cells, often adjacent to psammoma bodies.[11] The latter are not always easy to diagnose as recurrent cancer because of their quiescent appearing histology, absent mitotic activity, and resemblance to benign mesothelial hyperplasia which is often associated with repeated abdominal surgery. On frozen sections, these types of "shrinking" tumor cells may be overlooked or interpreted as mesothelial cell hyperplasia. On paraffin sections, because of the absence of well-formed papillary structures and of nuclear chromatin distribution characteristic of malignancy, and their resemblance to endosalpingiosis or mesothelial hyperplasia, they may still be difficult to interpret. Interactive morphometry and computerized image analysis have proven helpful in this difficult differential diagnosis. Measurements of nuclear profiles and multivariate statistical analyses have demonstrated that, overall, the "responsive" tumor cells are closer to hyperplastic mesothelial cells than to nonresponsive tumor cells.[12]

They are, however, different from benign hyperplastic mesothelial cells in their distribution, i.e., lack of uniformity although some overlapping of measurements in individual cells was found.

The natural history of these morphologically and morphometrically rather bland-appearing groups of tumor cells, which became different from the initial ovarian cancer due to the effect of chemotherapy, is still elusive, as is their potential to become aggressive tumor tissue again. Similar cases may elicit different morphologic responses in second-look operations for ovarian cancer. Their biological behavior at the present time is monitored by serum titers of tumor antigens of which CA125 is the most widely used.

References

1. Houston, D. E., Noller, K. I., Melton, J. *et al.* (1998). The epidemiology of pelvic endometriosis. *Clin. Obstet. Gynecol.* 31, 787–800.
2. Dmowski, W. P., Gebel, H., and Braun, D. P. (1998). Decrease of apoptosis and sensitivity to macrophage mediated cytolysis of endometrial cells in endometriosis. *Hum. Reprod. Update* 4, 696–701.
3. Redwine, D. B. (1989). Peritoneal pockets and endometriosis. Confirmation of an important relationship with further observations. *J. Reprod. Med.* 34, 270–272.
4. McLaren, J. (Update 2000). Vascular endothelial growth factor and endometriotic angiogenesis. *Hum. Reprod.* 6, 45–55.
5. Goodman, M. H., Kredentzer, D., and Deligdisch, L. (1989). Postmenopausal endometriosis associated with hormone replacement therapy. *J. Reprod. Med.* 34, 231–233.
6. Moll, U. M., Chumas, J. C., Chalas, E. *et al.* (1990). Ovarian carcinoma arising in atypical endometriosis. *Obstet. Gynecol.* 75, 537–539.
7. Heaps, J. M., Nieberg, R. K., and Berek, J. S. (1990). Malignant neoplasms arising in endometriosis. *Obstet. Gynecol.* 75, 1023–1028.
8. Deligdisch, L., Kalir, T., Cohen, C. J., deLatour, M., Le Bouedec, G., and Penault-Llorca, F. (2000). Endometrial histopathology in 700 patients treated with tamoxifen for breast cancer. *Gynecol. Oncol.* 78, 181–186.
9. Buckley, C. H. (1990). Tamoxifen and endometriosis. Case report. *Br. Obstet. Gynecol.* 97, 645–646.
10. Bell, D. A., and Scully, R. E. (1990). Serous borderline tumors of the peritoneum. *Am. J. Surg. Pathol.* 14, 230–239.
11. Deligdisch, L., Kerner, J., Dargent, D. *et al.* (1993). Morphometric differentiation between responsive tumor cells and mesothelial hyperplasia in second look operation for ovarian cancer. *Hum. Pathol.* 24, 143–147.
12. Deligdisch, L., Heller, D., and Gil, J. (1990). Interactive morphometry of normal and hyperplastic peritoneal mesothelial cells and dysplastic and malignant ovarian cells. *Hum. Pathol.* 21, 218–222.
13. Clement, P. B., and Young, R. H. (1999). Florid cystic endosalpingiosis of the uterus. *Am. J. Surg. Pathol.* 23, 166–175.
14. McCaughey, W. T. E., Kirk, M. E., Lester, W. *et al.* (1984). Peritoneal epithelial lesions associated with proliferative serous tumors of the ovary. *Histopathology* 8, 195–208.
15. Biscotti, C. V., and Hart, W. R. (1992). Peritoneal serous micropapillomatosis of low malignant potential (serous borderline tumors the peritoneum). A clinico-pathologic study of 17 cases. *Am. J. Surg. Pathol.* 16, 467–475.
16. Kemp, G. M., Hsiu, J., and Andrews, M. C. (1992). Papillary peritoneal carcinomatous after prophylactic oophorectomy. *Gynecol. Oncol.* 47, 395–397.
17. Piver, M. S., Tishi, M. F., Tsukuda, Y., and Nova, T. (1993). Primary peritoneal carcinoma after prophylactic oophorectomy in women with a family history of ovarian cancer. A report of the Gilda Radner Familial Ovarian Registry. *Cancer* 71, 2751–2755.
18. Wick, M. R., Mills, S. E., Dehner, L. P., *et al.* (1989). RE Serous papillary carcinomas arising from the peritoneum and ovaries. A clinical and immunohistochemical comparison. *Int. J. Gynecol. Pathol.* 8, 179–188.
19. Truong, L. D., Maccato, M. L., and Awalt, H. (1990). Serous surface carcinoma of the peritoneum. A clinicopathologic study of 22 cases. *Hum. Pathol.* 21, 99–110.

CHAPTER

11

The Genetic Etiology of Sporadic Ovarian Cancer

JOHNATHAN M. LANCASTER
Department of Obstetrics and Gynecology
Division of Gynecologic Oncology
Duke University Medical Center
Durham, North Carolina 27710

LAURA J. HAVRILESKY
Department of Obstetrics and Gynecology
Division of Gynecologic Oncology
Duke University Medical Center
Durham, North Carolina 27710

ANDREW BERCHUCK
Department of Obstetrics and Gynecology
Division of Gynecologic Oncology
Duke University Medical Center
Durham, North Carolina 27710

I. INTRODUCTION

Epithelial ovarian cancer is the deadliest gynecologic malignancy and a leading cause of cancer death in women. Malignant transformation of a normal ovarian epithelial cell is caused by genetic alterations that disrupt regulation of proliferation, programmed cell death, and senescence. Although approximately 10% of epithelial ovarian cancers arise in women who have inherited mutations in cancer susceptibility genes such as BRCA1 or BRCA2 (see Chapter 16), the vast majority of tumors result from the accumulation of genetic damage over the course of a lifetime and are referred to as sporadic cancers. Despite significant advances in our knowledge of the alterations that cause sporadic ovarian cancers, much remains unknown regarding their molecular etiology. The recent completion of the initial phases of the human genome project provides the framework for studies that will increase our understanding of this complex disease. Hopefully, this knowledge will lead to the development of new approaches to early diagnosis, treatment and/or prevention that will decrease ovarian cancer mortality.

A. Sporadic Ovarian Cancer is a Genetic Disease

Ovarian cancers exhibit a high degree of genetic disruption that is manifest at both the chromosomal and molecular levels. Karyotype analysis was initially used to demonstrate large chromosomal gains and losses as well as complex translocations. In one study of 23 ovarian cancers, the average number of chromosomal alterations was 7 (range 2–14).[1] More recently, studies using a technique called comparative genomic hybridization (CGH) have confirmed that most ovarian cancers have gains or losses of large segments of chromosomes. Of 44 ovarian cancers examined, 13 areas of chromosomal gain and 5 areas of chromosomal loss were seen in at least 20% of cases.[2] The most common areas of chromosomal loss were 16q and 17pter-q21, and the most frequent areas of chromosomal gain were 3q25-26 and 8q24. In another study that included 20 sporadic ovarian cancers, the average number of alterations in each cancer was 7.5, and gains were more than twice as common as losses.[3] In agreement with the studies noted above,[2] losses on 17p and gains on 8q23-24 and 3q26 were confirmed in two other studies to be among the most frequent events in ovarian cancers.[3, 4]

Differences exist in the pattern of genetic alterations observed in serous, mucinous, and endometrioid ovarian cancers.[5] Using CGH, gains at 1q have been identified frequently in endometrioid and serous tumors. Increased copy number at 10q was seen in endometrioid tumors only, whereas gains at 11q occurred mostly in serous tumors. In mucinous tumors, the most common copy number change was a gain at 17q. Although the findings of this small study, which included only 24 well or moderately differentiated cancers, cannot be considered definitive, they add weight to the theory that there are differences in the molecular pathogenesis of various histologic types of ovarian cancers.

Although when using CGH large chromosomal gains are detected more often than losses, smaller regions of allelic loss at specific genetic loci can frequently be detected using loss of heterozygosity (LOH) analysis. LOH has been demonstrated to occur at a high frequency on many chromosomal arms; including 5q,[6, 7] 6q,[8–11] 7p,[6, 12] 8p,[13] 11p,[14] 11q,[15–19] 13q,[20], 14q,[21] 16q,[19] 17p,[22] 17q,[19, 23] 22q,[24] and others.[6, 20, 25] It is unclear whether the extent of these genetic alterations reflects the need to inactivate multiple tumor-suppressor genes or is the result of generalized genomic instability. One consistent finding of various studies has been that poorly differentiated, advanced stage cancers have more genetic alterations than early stage, well-differentiated or borderline cases.[2, 20] For example, in one CGH study, the average number of alterations was 5.4 in low-grade ovarian cancers compared to 11.2 in high-grade cases.[2] This finding could be interpreted as reflective of accumulation of genetic changes with evolution of a cancer. On the other hand, it is equally plausible that advanced stage, poorly differentiated cancers are intrinsically more virulent, even early in their development, by virtue of their specific mutations and/or increased genomic instability. If this latter theory is correct, this could have significant implications for early diagnosis of ovarian cancer. Cancers that are inherently more virulent might metastasize rapidly and be less amenable to early detection.

One of the most exciting technologic advances in recent years has been the development of microarray technology, which provides the opportunity to rapidly evaluate the expression of thousands of genes in a tissue specimen. Several groups have applied this technology to the analysis of ovarian cancers.[26–28] Ono *et al.* examined the expression patterns of more than 9000 genes in 9 ovarian cancers.[26] Fifty-five genes were shown to be commonly up-regulated, and 48 genes down-regulated in cancers relative to normal cells. Differences in expression were identified between mucinous and serous tumors in 115 genes. Consequently, other groups have applied and extended the technology to describe expression patterns for larger numbers of ovarian tumors.[28] To aid interpretation of expression patterns, Welsh *et al.*[28] macrodissected normal samples into epithelial and stromal fractions, as well as hybridizing RNA from endothelial and activated B cells, in an effort to identify patterns of expression associated with infiltrating blood vessels and inflammatory cells. Cluster analysis was used to identify differences in patterns of gene expression between normal and tumor tissues, and the most informative genes included the immediate early genes *c-fos, jun-B, and EGR-1*, and estrogen responsive genes (under-expressed in tumor relative to normal tissue). Several smaller clusters of genes were under-expressed in normal relative to tumor tissue, and included *HE4* and *PRAME.* This group was able to validate their results by RT-PCR of fragments of three of the genes that exhibited differential expression patterns on microarray expression analysis.

Despite the advantages of microarray techniques, the technology is still evolving. At this time, only a subset of genes can be included in any array, and the arrays may be subject to production error and batch-to-batch variability. It is, therefore, not yet clear how accurately the expression data produced reflect true expression, such that ongoing validation using other platforms is essential. Within a cancer specimen, infiltrating normal and inflammatory cells and blood vessels can influence the expression profile considerably, necessitating careful review of tumor histology prior to analysis. Finally, one of the greatest challenges of this technique is data analysis. The interpretation of expression data from over 12,000 genes in current microarrays is daunting, and requires the highest level of expertise in biology, statistics, and computation. Future arrays may be even larger as reports from the human genome project estimate that human cells contain about 30,000 genes.

B. Etiology of Genetic Alterations

While the identification of specific genetic changes involved in ovarian carcinogenesis is an essential endeavor, an understanding of the etiology of this damage is necessary if we hope to develop effective prevention strategies. Like other sporadic cancers, most epithelial ovarian carcinomas are thought to develop due to the accumulation of genetic alterations with time. Though epidemiological and molecular studies have begun to shed some light on the etiology of ovarian cancer, the exact cause of these genetic alterations remains unclear. It is likely that genetic mutation is a multifactorial process, including effects of age and environmental exposures, on a predisposed genetic background.

Despite evidence to suggest that *sporadic* ovarian cancer generally is a monoclonal disease that originates in the ovarian surface epithelium or underlying inclusion cysts, [29, 30] there is evidence that peritoneal tumors in women who carry mutations in BRCA1 or BRCA2, may be polyclonal.[31]

It has been suggested that ovulation may be associated with the development of genetic mutations in the ovarian epithelium (Fig. 11.1), and several lines of evidence link ovulation and epithelial ovarian cancer. First, most animals—such as rats and mice—ovulate only when stimulated appropriately, and have a low incidence of epithelial ovarian cancer, whereas chickens and humans ovulate repetitively and have the highest incidence of the disease. In contrast, women with Turner's syndrome, who are anovulatory, rarely develop epithelial ovarian cancer. Additionally, the observation that pregnancy and oral contraceptive pill (OCP) use, which decrease lifetime ovulatory cycles, are strikingly protective against ovarian cancer,[32] is consistent with the theory that ovulation is the main driving force underlying the accumulation of genetic damage in the ovarian epithelium (Fig. 11.1). Molecular-epidemiological evidence supports an association between the number of ovulatory cycles and somatic DNA damage, as manifest by accumulation of mutant p53 protein.[33] Ovarian cancers that over-express mutant p53, are associated with a greater number of lifetime ovulatory cycles (mean=388) than those that do not demonstrate p53 over-expression (mean=342).[33]

It is unclear exactly why repetitive ovulation facilitates the development of ovarian cancer, and several factors including stimulation by gonadotropins, may play a role. One appealing theory is that mutations in the epithelium result from errors in DNA synthesis during the proliferative repair of ovulatory defects, as spontaneous mutations are more likely to occur in cells that are proliferating relative to those at rest.[34] Although DNA repair genes exist to maintain a high degree of fidelity in DNA synthesis, it is estimated that spontaneous errors occur—approximately once every million base pairs—that can elude repair and become fixed in the genome. In addition, the efficiency of the DNA repair systems may vary between individuals due to inherited differences in the activity of DNA repair proteins. It is also possible that mutations in the ovarian epithelium may arise due to oxidative stress as mutagenic free radicals are produced by leukocytes that infiltrate the ovulatory site in the process of corpus luteum regression and repair of the ovarian surface.

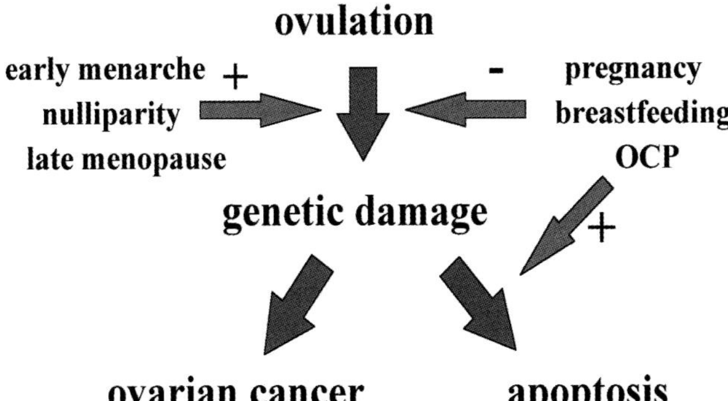

FIGURE 11.1 Schematic representation of the pathogenesis of ovarian cancer. Ovulation results in genetic damage and can lead to ovarian cancer. Factors that decrease the number of lifetime ovulatory cycles (pregnancy, breast feeding, OCP use) are protective against ovarian cancer, possibly via direct induction of apoptosis of surface epithelial cells. In contrast, early menarche, nulliparity, and late menopause are associated with an increased number of lifetime ovulatory cycles, and increased ovarian cancer risk.

Pregnancy and the OCP are protective against ovarian cancer. This effect is not simply due to a decreased rate of mutations, however. The magnitude of protection against ovarian cancer is much greater than would be predicted based simply on the number of suppressed ovulations. Five years of oral contraceptive use decreases risk by approximately 50% while decreasing lifetime ovulatory cycles by only about 10–20%.[32] Recently, however, it has been shown that administration of the progestin levonorgestrel, either alone or in combination with estrogen, stimulates apoptosis of ovarian epithelial cells in macaques.[35] This suggests that the progestagenic milieu of pregnancy and the OCP might protect against ovarian cancer by increasing apoptosis of ovarian epithelial cells, thereby cleansing the ovary of cells that have acquired genetic damage.

II. MECHANISMS OF MALIGNANT TRANSFORMATION

The number of cells in a population is dependent upon a critical balance between cellular proliferation, senescence, and apoptosis. The mutations that lead to the development of ovarian and other cancers primarily target genes involved in these processes. Development of a cancer results from disruption of these complex regulatory pathways with the net effect being an increased number of cells. Mutations that inactivate DNA repair genes accelerate the accumulation of other cancer-causing mutations. In addition to growth of a primary tumor, cancers are characterized by acquisition of a metastatic phenotype. Ovarian cancers have the ability to invade the surrounding stroma due to production of proteases that degrade connective tissue and produce angiogenic factors that stimulate the development of new blood vessels to support their growth and spread. Although these molecular pathways are integral to the process of cancer progression, there is little evidence to date to suggest that evolution of the metastatic phenotype is directly attributable to mutations in genes that encode proteases or other molecules involved in invasion and metastasis.

A. Proliferation

The rate of proliferation is a major determinant of the number of cells in a population. To prevent excessive proliferation, DNA synthesis and cell division are ordinarily restrained. When proliferation is appropriate, these inhibitory mechanisms are inactive and growth stimulatory signals are generated. Malignant tumors are characterized by alterations in genes that control proliferation. There is increased activity of genes that stimulate proliferation (oncogenes) and loss or inactivation of growth inhibitory (tumor-suppressor) genes (Table 11.1). In the past, it was thought that cancer might arise entirely because of more rapid proliferation and/or a higher fraction of cells proliferating. It is now clear that although increased proliferation is a characteristic of many cancers, the fraction of cancer cells actively dividing and the transition time of the cell cycle is not strikingly different than that seen in some normal cells. Increased proliferation is only one of several factors that contribute to cancerous growth.

The fraction of ovarian cancer cells that are actively proliferating can be measured using various techniques. One approach is to assess the DNA content of cells in a sample. This can be accomplished with flow cytometry using disaggregated nuclei or in frozen sections using image analysis. The fraction of cells with a DNA content consistent with S-phase can be distinguished from those in the G1 or G2/M phases to calculate a proliferation index. In one study, about 25% of ovarian cancers had an S-phase fraction below 5% and this correlated with early stage and favorable survival.[36] Proliferation can also be assessed using immunohistochemical techniques to identify cells that express Ki67 or PCNA, antigens that are expressed only in actively proliferating cells. In most such studies, there has been a correlation between higher proliferation indicies (>5–15%) and more advanced stage, worse grade and poor survival.[37–39]

TABLE 11.1 Classes of Genes Involved in Growth Regulatory Pathways and Malignant Transformation

Growth stimulatory (oncogenes)	
Peptide growth factors	*Corresponding receptors*
Epidermal growth factor (EGF) and transforming growth factor (TGF-α)	EGF receptor
Heregulin	erbB2 (HER-2/*neu*), erbB3, erbB4
Insulin-like growth factors (IGF-I, IGF-II)	IGF-I and II receptors
Platelet-derived growth factor (PDGF)	PDGF receptor
Fibroblast growth factors (FGFs)	FGF receptors
Macrophage-colony stimulating factor (M-CSF)	M-CSF receptor (*fms*)
Cytoplasmic factors	*Examples*
Non-receptor tyrosine kinases	*abl*, *src*, PIK3CA
G proteins	K-*ras*, H-*ras*
Serine-threonine kinases	AKT2
Nuclear factors	*Examples*
Transcription factors	*myc*, *jun*, *fos*
Cell cycle progression factors	Cyclins, E2F
Growth inhibitory (tumor-suppressor-genes)	
Extra-nuclear factors	*Examples*
Cell membrane factors	TGF-B 1–3 and their type I and II receptors
Cell adhesion factors	Cadherins, APC
Phosphatases	*PTEN*
Nuclear factors	*Examples*
Cell cycle inhibitors	Rb, p53, p16, p27
Unknown function	BRCA1, BRCA2

B. Apoptosis

Cells are capable of activating a suicide pathway of programmed cell death referred to as apoptosis. Apoptosis is an active, energy-dependent process that involves cleavage of the DNA and proteins by endonucleases and proteases. Morphologically, apoptosis is characterized by condensation of chromatin and cellular shrinkage. This is in contrast to the process of necrosis, which is characterized by loss of osmoregulation and cellular fragmentation.

Since the size of a population of cells is normally static due to a balance between the birth rate and the death rate, growth of a neoplasm theoretically could result due to either increased proliferation or decreased apoptosis. In addition to restraining the number of cells in a population, apoptosis may serve an important role in preventing malignant transformation by specifically eliminating cells that have undergone mutations. Following exposure of cells to mutagenic stimuli, including radiation and carcinogenic drugs, the cell cycle is arrested so that DNA damage may be repaired. If DNA repair is not sufficient, apoptosis occurs so cells that have undergone significant damage do not survive. This serves as an anti-cancer surveillance mechanism by which mutated cells are eliminated before they become fully transformed. The p53 tumor suppressor gene is a critical regulator of cell cycle arrest and apoptosis in response to DNA damage, but apoptosis may also be triggered via other pathways under different circumstances.

The molecular events that effect cell death in response to various stimuli have only been partially elucidated thus far, but it appears that a family of genes encoding proteins that reside in the mitochondrial membrane are directly involved.[40] The bcl-2 gene was first of these genes to be identified at a translocation breakpoint in B-cell lymphomas.

Expression of bcl-2 acts to inhibit apoptosis [41] and, paradoxically, persistence of *bcl-2* expression in ovarian cancers has been associated with favorable prognosis.[42, 43] The bcl-X_L gene, a structural and functional homolog of bcl-2, also inhibits apoptosis and has been shown to play a role in preventing apoptosis of ovarian cancer cells in response to chemotherapy.[44] Conversely, other related genes such as bax, and bcl-X_S have pro-apoptotic activity. High bax expression has been reported in 60% of newly diagnosed ovarian cancers and was associated with a favorable response to therapy.[45] The precise mechanism by which bcl-2 and these other mitochondrial proteins act to regulate apoptosis is unclear, but those that increase membrane permeability stimulate apoptosis while those that decrease permeability prevent apoptosis. Activation of a family of cytosolic proteolytic enzymes called caspases also occurs during apoptosis leading to breakdown of cellular proteins.

C. Senescence

Normal cells are only capable of undergoing division a finite number of times before becoming senescent. Recently, it has been shown that cellular senescence is due to shortening of repetitive DNA sequences (TTAGGG) called telomeres that cap the ends of each chromosome. Telomeres are thought to be involved in chromosome stabilization and in preventing recombination during mitosis. At birth chromosomes have long telomeric sequences that become progressively shorter each time a cell divides. Malignant cells appear to avoid senescence by turning on expression of telomerase activity that acts to lengthen the telomeres.[46, 47] Telomerase is a ribonucleoprotein complex and both the protein and RNA subunits have been identified. The RNA component serves as a template for telomere extension and the protein subunit acts to catalyze the synthesis of new telomeric repeats.

Because telomerase expression in most normal tissues is restricted to development, it has been suggested that telomerase might be a useful diagnostic marker in patients with cancer. Several groups have shown that telomerase activity is detectable in most ovarian cancers.[48–50] It has been suggested that persistence of telomerase activity in peritoneal washings after primary therapy for advanced ovarian cancer may predict the presence of microscopic residual disease in some cases despite negative cytologic washings and biopsies.[49] Demonstration of the utility of this approach awaits the completion of more definitive studies.

III. GROWTH STIMULATORY PATHWAYS: THE ROLE OF ONCOGENES

Oncogenes encode proteins normally involved in stimulating proliferation, but when these gene products are overactive they contribute to the process of malignant transformation (Fig. 11.2 and Table 11.2). Oncogenes can be activated via several mechanisms. In some cancers there is amplification of the number of copies of oncogenes with resultant overexpression of the corresponding protein. Some oncogenes may become overactive when affected by point mutations. Finally, oncogenes may be translocated from one chromosomal location to another and then come under the influence of promoter sequences that cause overexpression of the gene. This latter mechanism frequently occurs in leukemias and lymphomas, but has not been demonstrated in gynecologic cancers or other solid tumors.

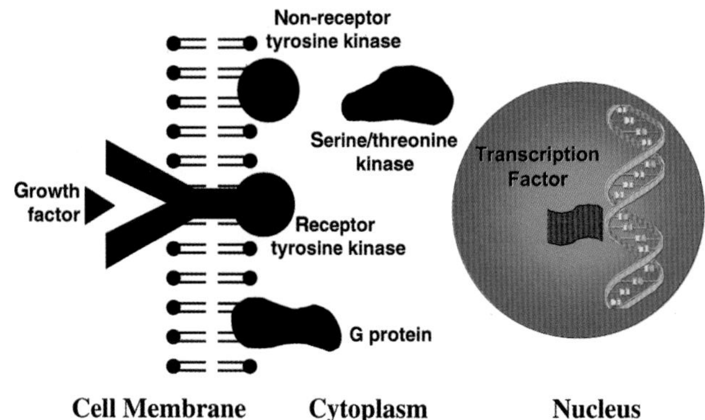

FIGURE 11.2 Classes of oncogenes.

TABLE 11.2 Molecular Alterations in Sporadic Ovarian Cancers

	Function	Alteration	Approximate Frequency
Oncogenes			
HER-2/*neu*	Tyrosine kinase	Overexpression	20%
K-*ras*	G protein	Mutation	5%
AKT2	Serine/threonine kinase	Amplification	10%
PIK3CA	Serine/threonine kinase	Amplification	?40%
c-*myc*	Transcription factor	Overexpression	20–30%
Tumor-suppressor genes			
BRCA1	?DNA repair	Mutation/deletion	5%
p53	Transcription factor	Mutation/deletion	60%
p16	cdk inhibitor	Homozygous deletion/ methylation	?15%
p27	cdk inhibitor	Decreased expression	?40%

A. Peptide Growth Factors

Peptide growth factors in the extracellular space can stimulate a cascade of molecular events that leads to proliferation by binding to cell membrane receptors. Unlike endocrine hormones, which are secreted into the blood stream to act in distant target organs, peptide growth factors usually act in the local environment where they have been secreted. The concept that autocrine growth stimulation might be a key strategy by which cancer cell proliferation becomes autonomous is intellectually appealing and has received considerable attention. In this model, it is postulated that cancers secrete stimulatory growth factors that then interact with receptors on the same cell. Although increased production of stimulatory growth factors may play a role in enhancing proliferation associated with malignant transformation, they also are involved in development, stromal-epithelial communication, tissue regeneration, and wound healing.

It has been shown that ovarian cancers produce and/or are capable of responding to various peptide growth factors. For example, epidermal growth factor (EGF) [51] and transforming growth factor-alpha (TGF-α) [52] are produced by some ovarian cancers that also express the receptor that binds these peptides (EGF receptor).[53, 54] Some cancers produce insulin-like growth factor-I (IGF-I), IGF-I binding protein, and express type 1 IGF receptor.[55] Further, growth of ovarian cancer cell lines is potently reduced by application of phosphorothioate antisense oligodeoxynucleotides (S-ODNs) to the IGF-I receptor.[56] Platelet-derived growth factor (PDGF) also is expressed by many types of epithelial cells including human ovarian cancer cell lines, but these cells usually are not responsive to PDGF.[57–59] In addition, ovarian cancers produce basic fibroblast growth factor (FGF) and its receptor, which can form a mitogenic complex in some ovarian cancers.[60] Ovarian cancers produce macrophage-colony stimulating factor (M-CSF) [61] resulting in elevated M-CSF serum levels in some patients.[62] The expression of the M-CSF receptor (*fms*) in many ovarian tumors suggests that the M-CSF autocrine pathway may be important in ovarian cancer development.[63] In addition, M-CSF could act in a paracrine fashion to stimulate recruitment and activation of macrophages. Recently, growth inhibition of three ovarian cancer cell lines by M-CSF has been demonstrated.[64] This growth inhibition was reversed by addition of anti-M-CSF monoclonal antibodies, and analysis by flow cytometry revealed that the ovarian cancer cell lines arrested in the G_0/G_1 phase of the cell cycle. Since macrophage products such as interleukin-1 (IL-1), IL-6, and tumor necrosis factor-α, (TNF-α) have been shown to stimulate proliferation of some ovarian cancer cell lines,[65–67] the potential for paracrine stimulation of the cancer by macrophages also exists. Interestingly, in the serum of patients with ovarian cancer, levels of M-CSF and IL-6 have been shown to be directly correlated, suggesting a co-regulation in production of these cytokines by tumor cells.[68] In addition to expression of peptide growth factors and their receptors, ascites of patients with ovarian cancer contain phospholipid factors that stimulate proliferation of ovarian cancer cells.[69, 70]

It has been shown that normal ovarian epithelial cells produce—and are responsive to—many of the same peptide growth factors as malignant ovarian epithelial cells.[54, 71–73] Thus, despite circumstantial evidence demonstrating the potential for autocrine and paracrine growth regulation of ovarian cancer cells by peptide growth factors, it remains unclear whether alterations in expression of growth factors are critical in the development of ovarian cancer. Peptide growth factors may function as necessary co-factors rather than as the driving force behind malignant transformation.

B. Growth Factor Receptors Including the EGF Receptor Family (EGF Receptor, HER-2/neu)

Cell membrane receptors that bind peptide growth factors are composed of an extracellular ligand binding domain, a membrane spanning region, and a cytoplasmic tyrosine kinase domain. Binding of a growth factor to the extracellular domain results in aggregation and conformational shifts in the receptor and activation of the inner tyrosine kinase.[74, 75] This kinase phosphorylates tyrosine residues on both the growth factor receptor (autophosphorylation) and targets in the cell interior leading to activation of secondary signals. For example, phosphorylation of phospholipase C leads to breakdown of cell membrane phospholipids and generation of diacylglycerol and inositol-tri-phosphate, both of which play a role in propagation of the mitogenic signal.

The role of the EGF receptor family of transmembrane receptors and their ligands in growth regulation and transformation has been a prominent focus in cancer research.[76] EGF is a peptide growth factor of 53 amino acids that maintains its secondary structure by virtue of disulfide bonds between cysteine residues. At least five other peptide growth factors, including TGF-α, also interact with and activate the EGF receptor. EFG, TGF-α, and other EGF receptor ligands are produced as pro-forms that are inserted into the cell membrane. The membrane-anchored growth factor can interact with receptors on adjacent cells, a phenomenon known as juxtacrine growth regulation. Alternatively, the active peptide then can be cleaved and released into the extracellular space. The free peptide may interact with receptors on the same (autocrine) or nearby cells (paracrine) to stimulate growth.

The EGF receptor is ubiquitously expressed in both epithelial and stromal cells and plays a role in growth stimulation of most cell types. The EGF receptor has been shown to be amplified in some squamous cancers, and the EGF receptor can be targeted therapeutically with monoclonal antibodies.[77] EGF receptor is expressed in normal ovarian epithelium and although the level of expression varies between cancers, this is not a strong predictor of clinical behavior.[78]

The EGF receptor family is often termed the *erb*B family because the first member identified was the v-*erb*B oncogene. The second member of the family (*erb*B2) initially was called *neu* because it was found to be the transforming gene responsible for the generation of neuroblastomas in rats treated with a chemical carcinogen. This Human EGF Receptor-like molecule was named both HER-2/*neu* and *erb*B2 by investigators working in the field. The transforming activity of *neu* in the animal model was due to the presence of a mutation in the transmembrane portion of the molecule that results in constitutive activation of the inner tyrosine kinase domain. Biochemical studies of HER-2/*neu* have shown that activation of this receptor is not driven by ligand binding, but rather is dependent on activation of other members of the *erb*B family (*erb*B3, *erb*B4) that heterodimerize with *erb*B2 and activate its tyrosine kinase domain.[79]

In contrast to EGF receptor, which normally is expressed in both stromal and epithelial cells, HER-2/*neu* is expressed primarily in epithelial cells. The level of HER-2/*neu* is increased in some human breast, ovarian, and other cancers due to amplification.[80, 81] The SKOV3 ovarian cancer cell line and the SKBR3 breast cancer cell line both have amplification of this gene. In human cancers, HER-2/*neu* may also be overexpressed due to alterations in regulation of transcription in the absence of gene amplification. Regardless of the underlying mechanism, it has been shown that overexpression occurs in about 20% of ovarian cancers and 30% of breast cancers and correlates with aggressive features. The level of overexpression in breast cancers generally is higher than in ovarian cancers, however, and some studies have not found overexpression of HER-2/*neu* to adversely affect prognosis in ovarian cancer.[82, 83]. It has been shown that transfection of HER-2/*neu* into normal ovarian epithelial cells can induce a malignant phenotype *in vitro* including the ability of cells to grow in an anchorage-independent fashion and to form tumors in nude mice.

As noted above, activation of the *erb*B3 and 4 transmembrane receptors is requisite for HER-2/*neu* kinase activity. At least 4 families of ligands, collectively called neuregulins (e.g., heregulin, *neu* differentiating factor), bind to e*rb*B3 and 4.[79] Interestingly, there is considerable promiscuity between *erb*B ligands and receptors. For example, amphiregulin can activate both the EGF receptor (*erb*B1) and *erb*B3. And one of the more recently described ligands (epiregulin) can activate heterodimers of any of the *erb*B family members; and these heterodimers are more potent growth stimulators than homodimers of any individual *erb*B receptor. Although their molecular signaling mechanisms have not yet been fully elucidated, the *erb*B family of receptors have also been exploited as therapeutic targets. Monoclonal antibodies that interact with HER-2/*neu* can decrease growth of breast and ovarian cancer cell lines that overexpress this receptor.[84, 85] In addition, these antibodies may enhance the sensitivity of cancers to cytotoxic chemotherapy by interfering with repair of DNA adducts.[86] Recently an anti-HER-2/*neu* antibody that induces breast cancer regression has been approved for clinical use by the FDA.[87] It is possible that this approach might also benefit some women whose ovarian cancers overexpress HER-2/*neu*.

C. Other Kinases

Following interaction of peptide growth factors and their receptors, secondary molecular signals are generated to transmit the mitogenic stimulus toward the nucleus. This function is served by a multitude of complex and overlapping signal transduction pathways that occur on the inner cell membrane and cytoplasm. Many of these signals involve phosphorylation of proteins by enzymes known as kinases.[88] Cellular processes other than growth are also regulated by kinases, but one family of kinases appears to have evolved specifically for the purpose of transmitting growth stimulatory signals. These tyrosine kinases transfer a phosphate group from ATP to tyrosine residues of target proteins. Some kinases that phosphorylate proteins on serine and/or threonine residues are also involved in stimulating proliferation. Although several families of intracellular kinases have been identified that can elicit transformation when activated *in vitro*, it remains uncertain whether structural alterations in most of these molecules play a role in the development of human cancers. The activity of kinases is regulated by phosphatases, which act in opposition to the kinases by removing phosphates from the target proteins.[89] It has been shown that a number of phosphatases are expressed by ovarian cancers and that some of these oppose the kinase activity of HER-2/*neu*.[90]

AKT2 is a gene on chromosome 19q that encodes a serine-threonine protein kinase. AKT2 was found to be amplified and overexpressed in 2 of 8 ovarian cancer cell lines and 2 of 15 primary epithelial ovarian cancers.[91] This study was confirmed by a larger series of 132 primary ovarian cancers in which 14% had AKT2 amplification or overexpression. AKT2 overexpression was found to have a statistically significant association with higher grade and worse survival.[92] More recently it has been shown that 36% (31/91) of ovarian cancers exhibit elevated AKT2 activity *in vitro*,[93] and that these tumors tend to be high grade and advanced stage. The same group demonstrated induction of apoptosis in ovarian cancer cells by inhibition of the PI3 kinase/AKT2 pathway by Wortmannin or LY294002. Further studies are needed, however, to confirm the functional significance of AKT2 overexpression in ovarian cancers.

Using CCH, the region of chromosome 3p26 that includes the regulatory subunit of phosphatidylinositol 3-kinase (PIK3CA) has been shown to be amplified in some ovarian cancer cell lines and 40% of primary ovarian cancers.[94]

Interestingly, the AKT2 gene is one of the downstream targets of PIK3CA. Thus, theoretically, amplification of either of these two genes leads to excessive activation of this mitogenic pathway.

Binding of cytokines and growth factors also activates the Janus kinase (JAK) family of protein -tyrosine kinases (PTKs). These kinases phosphorylate various signaling proteins including a unique family of transcription factors termed the signal transducers and activators of transcription, or STATs. Phosphorylation of STATs results in their transactivation, nuclear translocation, DNA binding, and dimerization, and constitutively activated STATs have been described in breast and prostate cancer cell lines and primary tumors.[95, 96] Constitutive activation of STAT 3 has been shown to be present in the ovarian cancer cell lines MDAH 2774, OV-1063, Caov-3, and O.C. 22819, but absent in normal ovarian surface epithelium.[97, 98] Further, STAT3 activation can be blocked by JAK inhibitors such as AG490 and apoptosis induced.[97] Interestingly, activation of both STATs and JAKs has also been demonstrated to be associated with enhanced expression of the breast/ovarian cancer susceptibility gene, BRCA1, in human prostate cancer cell lines.[96] Such findings underscore the critical role of the JAK/STAT system in cell signaling and provide preliminary evidence for their involvement in ovarian tumorigenesis.

D. G Proteins

G proteins represent another class of molecules involved in transmission of growth stimulatory signals toward the nucleus.[99, 100] They are located on the inner aspect of the cell membrane and have intrinsic GTPase activity that catalyzes the exchange of GTP (guanine-tri-phosphate) for GDP (guanine-di-phosphate). In their active GTP bound form, G proteins interact with kinases that are involved in relaying the mitogenic signal. Conversely, hydrolysis of GTP to GDP, which is stimulated by GTPase activating proteins (GAPs), leads to inactivation of G proteins. The *ras* family of G proteins are among the most frequently mutated oncogenes in human cancers (e.g., gastrointestinal and endometrial cancers). Activation of *ras* genes usually involves point mutations in codons 12, 13, or 61 that result in constitutively activated molecules.

Mutations in the *ras* genes do not appear to be a common feature of invasive serous epithelial ovarian cancers.[101–103] K-*ras* mutations have been noted more frequently in mucinous ovarian cancers, but these tumors comprise only a small fraction of epithelial ovarian cancers. In contrast, K-*ras* mutations are common in borderline epithelial ovarian tumors, occurring in 20–50% of cases.[104, 105] Indeed, mutations in K-*ras* have recently been found in Mullerian inclusion cysts in some patients with serous borderline tumors, suggesting that these two entities may be related.[106]

E. Nuclear Factors

If proliferation is to occur in response to signals generated in the cytoplasm, these events must lead to activation of nuclear factors responsible for DNA replication and cell division. Expression of several genes that encode nuclear proteins increases dramatically within minutes of treatment of normal cells with peptide growth factors. Once induced, the products of these genes bind to specific DNA regulatory elements and induce transcription of genes involved in DNA synthesis and cell division. When inappropriately overexpressed, however, these transcription factors can act as oncogenes. Among the nuclear transcription factors involved in stimulating proliferation, amplification and/or overexpression of members of the *myc* family has most often been implicated in the development of human cancers.[107, 108] Myc proteins are key regulators of mammalian cell proliferation and treatment of cells with myc antisense oligonucleotides inhibits proliferation. It has been shown that myc acts as part of a heterodimeric complex with the protein max to initiate transcription of other genes involved in cell cycle progression.[107]

Amplification of the c-*myc* oncogene occurs in some epithelial ovarian cancers. In five small studies, c-*myc* was reported to be amplified in a total of 24 of 77 cases (31%).[109–113] In a more recent study in which 51 epithelial ovarian cancers were analyzed, a similar incidence of c-*myc* overexpression was observed (37%).[114] c-*myc* overexpression was more frequently observed in advanced stage serous adenocarcinomas, suggesting a role in tumor progression.

IV. GROWTH INHIBITORY PATHWAYS: TUMOR-SUPPRESSOR GENES

Tumor-suppressor genes encode proteins normally involved in inhibiting proliferation and inactivation of these genes plays a role in the development of most cancers. Knudson's "two-hit" model established the paradigm that both alleles must be inactivated in order to exert a phenotypic effect on tumorigenesis.[115] The location and the type of the inactivating mutations in tumor-suppressor genes may vary from one cancer to the next. Frequently, mutations in tumor-suppressor genes alter the base sequence resulting in the production of a premature stop codon (TAG, TAA, or TGA) and truncated protein product. Such truncated protein products may result from several types of mutational events, including nonsense mutations, in which a single base substitution changes that sequence from a specific amino acid to a stop codon. In addition, microdeletions or insertions of one or several nucleotides that disrupt the reading frame of the DNA (frameshifts) also lead to the generation of stop codons downstream in the gene. In some cases, missense mutations occur which change only a single amino acid in the encoded protein. The functional significance of such a change depends upon the amino acid alteration and the location within the gene. A mutation in one allele, whether germline or somatic, is revealed following somatic inactivation of the corresponding wild-type allele, typically by deletion of part or all of the chromosome. This LOH has become recognized as the hallmark of tumor-suppressor gene inactivation.

Tumor-suppressor genes may also be inactivated by methylation of the promoter region of the gene,[116] which is proximal to the coding sequence and regulates whether or not the gene is transcribed from DNA into RNA. When the promoter is methylated it is resistant to activation and the gene is essentially silenced despite remaining structurally intact. Like oncogenes, tumor-suppressor gene products are found throughout the cell (Table 11.2). In this section the various classes of tumor-suppressor genes involved in sporadic epithelial ovarian cancers will be reviewed.

A. Extra-Nuclear Tumor-Suppressor Genes

Although most tumor-suppressor gene products are nuclear proteins, some extra-nuclear tumor suppressors have been identified. Theoretically, any protein that is normally involved in inhibition of proliferation could conceivably act as a tumor suppressor. In this regard, phosphatases that normally oppose the action of the tyrosine kinases by dephosphorylating tyrosine residues are appealing candidates.[89] Analysis of deletions on chromosome 10q23 in human cancers led to the discovery of the *PTEN* gene.[117] In addition to its phosphatase activity, *PTEN* is homologous to the cytoskeleton proteins tensin and auxin and it has been postulated that *PTEN* might act to inhibit invasion and metastasis through modulation of the cytoskeleton.[118] Interestingly, it has been shown that PIK3CA and AKT2 kinase activity can be specifically opposed by the *PTEN* phosphatase. *PTEN* mutations are rare in serous ovarian cancers, perhaps because amplification of PIK3CA or AKT2 abrogates the need for loss of *PTEN* tumor suppressor function. In contrast, *PTEN* mutations occur in about 20% of endometrioid ovarian cancers.[119]

B. TGF-β

The TGF-β family of growth factors inhibits proliferation of normal epithelial cells.[120] It is thought that TGF-β causes cell cycle arrest in G_1 by triggering pathways that result in inhibition of cyclin dependent kinases. Several closely related forms of TGF-β have been discovered which are encoded by separate genes (TGF-β1, TGF-β2, TGF-β3, and Placental TGF-β). TGF-β is secreted from cells in an inactive form bound to a portion of its precursor molecule from which it must be cleaved to release biologically active TGF-β. Active TGF-β interacts with type I and type II cell surface TGF-β receptors and initiates serine/threonine kinase activity.[121] Prominent intracellular targets include a class of molecules called Smads that translocate to the nucleus and act as transcriptional regulators.[122] Although mutations in the TGF-β receptors and Smads have been reported in some cancers, this does not appear to be a feature of ovarian cancers.

Normal ovarian epithelial cells produce, activate, and are growth inhibited by TGF-β,[123] however, most immortalized ovarian cancer cell lines have lost the ability to either produce, activate, or respond to TGF-β.[58, 123–127] This suggested that TGF-β might normally act as an autocrine growth inhibitory factor in normal ovarian epithelium, and that loss of this pathway might play a role in the development of some ovarian cancers. Although convenient to work with, immortalized cell lines frequently have undergone profound genetic alterations in tissue culture. Examination of primary ovarian cancers obtained directly from patients revealed that in almost all cases cancers were sensitive to the growth inhibitory effect of TGF-β.[128] Thus, it remains unclear whether alterations in the TGF-β pathway play a role in the development of ovarian cancers.

C. p53 Tumor-Suppressor Gene

Mutation of the p53 tumor-suppressor gene is the most frequent genetic event described thus far in human cancers (Figs. 11.3 and 11.4).[129–131] The p53 gene encodes a 393 amino acid protein that appears to play a central role in the regulation of both proliferation and apoptosis.[132–134] In normal cells, p53 protein resides in the nucleus and exerts its tumor-suppressor activity by binding to transcriptional regulatory elements of genes such as the cdk inhibitor p21 that act to arrest cells in G_1. Beyond simply inhibiting proliferation, normal p53 is thought to play a role in preventing cancer by stimulating apoptosis of cells that have undergone excessive genetic damage.[135] In this regard, p53 has been described as the "guardian of the genome" since it delays entry into S phase until the genome has been cleansed of mutations. If DNA repair is inadequate, p53 may initiate apoptosis, thereby eliminating cells with genetic damage.

Many cancers have missense mutations in one copy of the p53 gene that result in substitution of a single amino acid in exons 5 through 8, which encode the DNA binding domains (Figs. 11.4 and 11.5). Although these mutant p53 genes encode full-length proteins, they are unable to bind to DNA and regulate transcription of other genes. Mutation of one copy of the p53 gene often is accompanied by deletion of the other copy, leaving the cancer cell with only mutant p53 protein. If the cancer cell does retain one normal copy of the p53 gene, the mutant p53 protein can form a complex with wild-type p53 protein and prevent it from interacting with DNA. Because inactivation of both p53 alleles is not required for

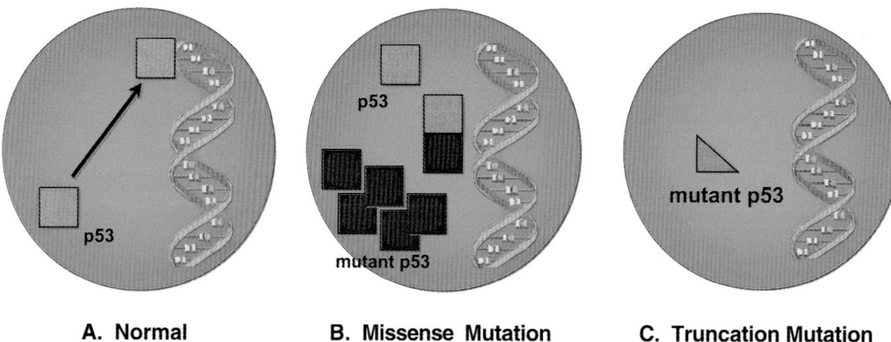

FIGURE 11.3 Inactivation of the p53 tumor suppressor gene by "dominant negative" missense mutation or by truncation mutation and deletion.

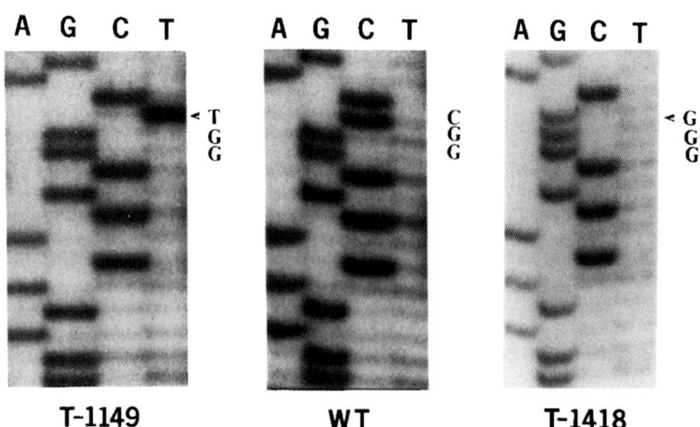

FIGURE 11.4 Transition and transversion mutations in codon 282 of the p53 gene in ovarian cancers. WT=wild type sequence CGG; T-1149=ovarian cancer with C to T transition mutation changing sequence to TGG; and T-1418=ovarian cancer with a C to G transversion mutation changing sequence to GGG.

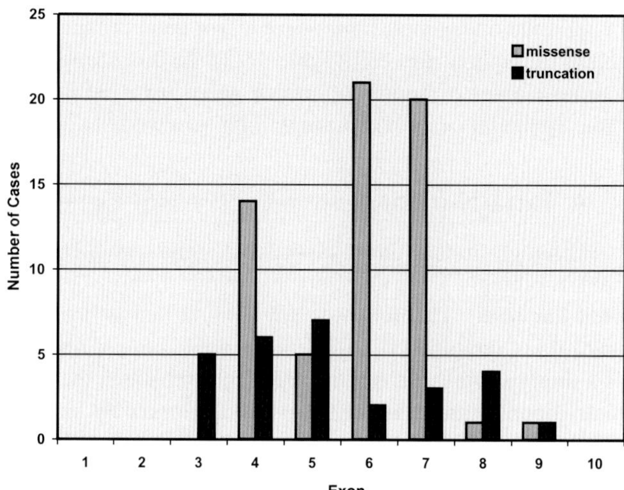

FIGURE 11.5 Spectrum of p53 mutations in advanced ovarian cancers. Missense mutations cluster in exons 5–8, whereas truncation mutations are more evenly dispersed throughout the gene.

loss of p53 function, mutant p53 is said to act in a "dominant negative" fashion. While normal cells have low levels of p53 protein because it is rapidly degraded, missense mutations encode protein products that are resistant to degradation and over-accumulate in the nucleus; and overexpression of mutant p53 protein can be detected immunohistochemically. A smaller fraction of cancers have mutations in the p53 gene that encode truncated protein products.[136] Whereas missense mutations in the p53 gene cluster in exons 5–8, truncation mutations are more evenly dispersed throughout the gene, presumably because they inactivate the p53 protein regardless of their location (Fig. 11.5). In cases of p53 truncation mutations, deletion of the other allele occurs as the second event as is seen with other tumor-suppressor genes.

Alteration of the p53 tumor-suppressor gene is the most frequent genetic event described to date in ovarian cancers.[136–143] The frequency of overexpression of mutant p53 is significantly higher in advanced stage III/IV disease (40–60%) relative to stage I cases (10–20%). In addition, p53 inactivation is uncommon in borderline tumors.[144] The higher frequency of p53 overexpression in advanced stage cases may indicate that this is a "late event" in ovarian carcinogenesis. Alternatively, the loss of p53 may confer a more aggressive metastatic phenotype. In advanced stage ovarian cancer, there is a suggestion that overexpression of p53 may be associated with somewhat worse survival.[137, 139–143, 145] The literature is not entirely consistent and most studies have not been large enough or optimally designed to yield reliable prognostic information. Finally, although there is a high concordance between p53 missense mutations and protein overexpression, about 20% of advanced ovarian cancers contain mutations that result in truncated protein products that generally are not overexpressed.[136] Overall, about 70% of advanced ovarian cancers have either missense or truncation mutations in the p53 gene.

The finding that overexpression of mutant p53 tumor suppressor genes is associated with high lifetime ovulatory cycles in women with ovarian cancer is consistent with the hypothesis that ovulation-associated proliferation may be the cause of these mutations in the ovarian epithelium.[33] In addition, most of the p53 point mutations in ovarian cancers are transitions rather than transversions,[22, 146] which also suggests that these mutations occur spontaneously, rather than due to exogenous carcinogens.

It has been suggested that loss of p53 might confer a chemoresistant phenotype, because p53 plays a role in chemotherapy-induced apoptosis. In this regard, several studies have examined the correlation between chemosensitivity and p53 mutation in ovarian cancers *in vitro*.[42, 147–150] Some have suggested a relationship between p53 mutation and loss of chemosensitivity, but in other equally valid studies such a relationship has not been observed.[151] The status of the p53 gene is probably one of a number of factors that determines sensitivity to chemotherapy.

D. BRCA1

Inherited mutations of the BRCA1 gene on chromosome 17q are the most frequent cause of hereditary ovarian cancers. Prior to the identification of BRCA1, it had been anticipated that somatic mutations in the gene would be common in ovarian cancers, since more than half of these cancers exhibit LOH in the region of BRCA1, on chromosome 17q.[23, 152, 153] Initially, two small studies reported somatic mutations in BRCA1 in about 10% of 54 ovarian cancers,[154, 155] but somatic mutations were not seen in two larger studies.[153, 156] In these initial studies, mutational screening was performed using single stranded conformation analysis.

More recently, a large study in which complete sequencing of the BRCA1 gene was performed in 103 ovarian cancers, somatic mutations were found in at least 7 cases.[157] In contrast to women with germline BRCA1 mutations whose median age at ovarian cancer diagnosis is typically in the mid 40s, the median age of women with somatic mutations was about 60. Similar to ovarian cancers with germline BRCA1 mutations, all of the ovarian cancers with somatic BRCA1 mutations were serous. In addition, loss of the wild-type BRCA1 allele invariably accompanied somatic BRCA1 mutations. These data are supportive of the hypothesis that loss of BRCA1 function occurs by way of the classic tumor-suppressor paradigm with mutation of one copy and deletion of the other. The BRCA2 gene, which is responsible for some hereditary ovarian cancer cases, also has been examined for somatic mutations, but none have been identified.[158]

E. Retinoblastoma Tumor-Suppressor Gene

Initiation of the cell cycle with resultant cell division is dependent on progression through the G_1 phase of the cycle into the DNA synthetic S phase. The retinoblastoma gene (Rb), which was the first tumor-suppressor gene discovered, plays a central role in actively regulating this process.[159,160] In the early G_1 phase of the cell cycle

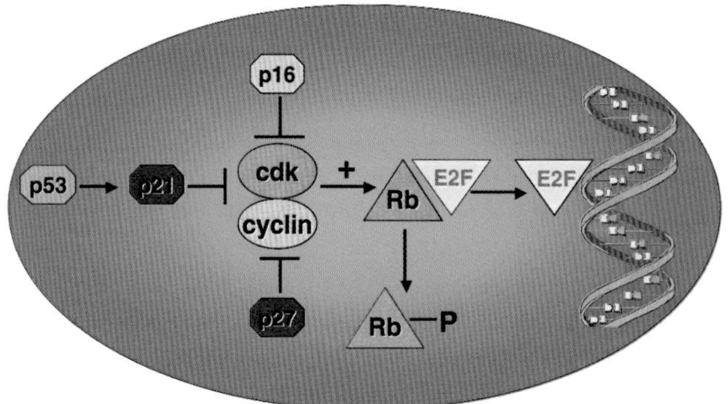

FIGURE 11.6 Regulation of cell cycle progression at G_1/S by p53 cyclins, cdks, cdk inhibitors, and Rb. In early G_1 the Rb protein binds to E2F and prevents activation of other genes involved in progression. Rb phosphorylation by a family of cdks and associated cyclins results in E2F release and stimulates entry into S phase of the cell cycle. A family of cdk inhibitors (p15, p16, p21, p27) prevent phosphorylation of Rb by cyclin-cdk complexes.

Rb protein binds to the E2F transcription factor and prevents it from activating transcription of other genes involved in cell cycle progression. When Rb is phosphorylated E2F is released and stimulates entry into the DNA synthesis phase of the cell cycle (Fig. 11.6). Mutations in the Rb gene have been noted primarily in retinoblastomas and sarcomas, but rarely in other types of cancers. LOH at the Rb locus occurs in about 30% of ovarian cancers, but mutations in the gene have not been detected [161] and functional Rb protein is present despite loss of one copy of the gene.[162]

F. Cyclins, Cyclin-Dependent Kinases (cdks), and cdk Inhibitors

Phosphorylation of Rb serves as a final common pathway with respect to initiation of proliferation; and this process is tightly controlled because of its critical importance (Fig. 11.6). Rb is phosphorylated by a family of cdks (cdk 2, 4,6) and associated cyclins (cyclin D, E), which act as regulatory subunits. Conversely, a family of cdk inhibitors (p15, p16, p21, p27) has been described that prevent phosphorylation of Rb by cyclin-cdk complexes. Although many of the intricacies of regulation of G_1 progression remain poorly understood, it is clear that inappropriately high activity of cyclins and cdks or loss of cdk inhibitors facilitates malignant transformation. Several alterations in these classes of genes have been described in human cancers including overexpression of cyclin D and loss of p16.

The p16 cdk inhibitor is the most frequently altered of the genes involved in regulating Rb phosphorylation.[116] The p16 gene on chromosome 9p21 encodes a protein that inhibits cdk4 or cdk6/cyclin D complexes from phosphorylating Rb. Initially it was noted that both copies of the p16 gene are deleted in a high fraction of immortalized cancer cell lines, including the ovarian cancer cell line, SKOV3.[163] The hypothesis that p16 loss plays a significant role in malignant transformation was strengthened by the finding that it is inactivated in some familial melanoma kindreds. Although the p16 gene also is inactivated by mutations or deletion of both alleles in some sporadic cancers, this occurs much less frequently than in immortalized cell lines. More commonly, however, the p16 gene appears to be silenced due to methylation of its promoter, which prevents transcription.

The role of the p16 gene in ovarian cancer has been studied extensively, but results are conflicting. Some studies have reported that the p16 gene is homozygously deleted or the promoter methylated in a fraction of cases,[164–166] whereas other studies have not found p16 deletions, mutations, or methylation.[167–169] The inconsistency of these various reports likely reflects the technical difficulty of assaying promoter methylation and homozygous deletions in primary tumor samples. In addition, some groups have reported that some ovarian cancers have very high levels of p16 protein,[170] but the underlying mechanism and significance of this observation has not yet been elucidated. Finally, the p14arf protein arises from an alternative reading frame of the p16 gene and has been shown to increase p53 expression by decreasing its degradation.[171] Deletions of the p16 locus would lead to loss of p14arf expression, which also could have significant consequences for regulation of G_1 progression.

There is some evidence to suggest that decreased activity of other cdk inhibitors may also play a role in the development of some cancers. The cdk inhibitor p21 binds cdk2 and the proliferating cell nuclear antigen (PCNA) during the G1/S phase of the cell cycle. Transfection of p21 into SKOV3 and OVCAR3 cell lines produced a reduction of tumor cell growth and increased susceptibility to platinum induced apoptosis, suggesting a possible role for p21 as an adjunct to platinum-based chemotherapy.[172] Reduced expression of the p27 cdk inhibitor, which is encoded by a gene on chromosome 12p, has been noted in some cancers due to increased p27 degradation. About one-third of ovarian cancers have been noted to have decreased p27 expression and this correlated with poor outcome.[173, 174] In addition, overexpression of cyclins D and/or E has been noted in some cancers. The cyclin D gene on chromosome 11q13 is translocated or amplified in some human cancers. Although the levels of cyclin D appear to be high in some ovarian cancers, overexpression has not been shown to be due to amplification or translocation.[174, 175] Likewise, cyclin E levels are high in some ovarian cancers, particularly clear cell tumors.[176]

Other cyclins, cdks, and regulatory molecules such as the chk family are involved in regulating progression from G_2 to M. Alterations in these pathways clearly play a role in the development of some cancers, but the intricacies of G_2/M transition are less well understood than those of G_1/S. Studies of G_2/M in ovarian cancers to date are preliminary and have not yielded evidence of significant alterations.

G. Other Genes

Several other known tumor-suppressor genes including *WT1* and *APC* have been examined in ovarian tumors, but do not appear to be altered frequently in these cancers. Recently, novel putative ovarian cancer tumor-suppressor genes have been described that are expressed in normal ovarian epithelial cells, but not in ovarian cancers. One of these is a *ras* homolog named *NOEY2* that was described by the group at the MD Anderson Cancer Center.[177] The *SPARC* gene, which encodes an extracellular matrix protein that is involved in adhesion,[178] and the *DOC2* gene, which is a GRB2 binding protein,[179] were described by the group at Brigham and Women's Hospital. Finally, *LOT-1*, a transcription factor [180] and the *OVCA1* and *OVCA2* genes on chromosome 17p[181] were described by the group at Fox Chase Cancer Center. The role of these and other, as yet undiscovered, tumor-suppressor genes in the development of ovarian cancers remains to be defined by future studies.

References

1. Gallion, H. H., Powell, D. E., Smith, L. W., Morrow, J. K., Martin, A. W., Van, N. J., and Donaldson, E. S. (1990): Chromosome abnormalities in human epithelial ovarian malignancies. *Gynecol. Oncol.* 38, 473–477.
2. Iwabuchi, H., Sakamoto, M., Sakunaga, H., Ma, Y. Y., Carcangiu, M. L., Pinkel, D., Yang-Feng, T. L., and Gray, J. W. (1995). Genetic analysis of benign, low-grade, and high-grade ovarian tumors. *Cancer Res.* 55, 6172–6180.
3. Elledge, R. M., and Allred, D. C. (1994). The p53 tumor suppressor gene in breast cancer. *Breast Cancer Res. Treat.* 32, 39–47.
4. Sonoda, G., Palazzo, J., du, M. S., Godwin, A. K., Feder, M., Yakushiji, M., and Testa, J. R. (1997). Comparative genomic hybridization detects frequent overrepresentation of chromosomal material from 3q26, 8q24, and 20q13 in human ovarian carcinomas. *Genes Chromos. Cancer* 20, 320–328.
5. Tapper, J., Butzow, R., Wahlstrom, T., Seppala, M., and Knuutila, S. (1997). Evidence for divergence of DNA copy number changes in serous, mucinous and endometrioid ovarian carcinomas. *Br. J. Cancer* 75, 1782–1787.
6. Cliby, W., Ritland, S., Dodson, M., Halling, K. C., Keeney, G., Podratz, K. C., and Jenkins, R. B. (1993). Human epithelial ovarian cancer allelotype. *Cancer Res.* 53, 2393–2398.
7. Tavassoli, M., Steingrimsdottir, H., Pierce, E., Jiang, X., Alagoz, M., Farzaneh, F., and Campbell, I. G. (1996). Loss of heterozygosity on chromosome 5q in ovarian cancer is frequently accompanied by TP53 mutation and identifies a tumour suppressor gene locus at 5q13.1-21. *Br. J. Cance* 74, 115–119.
8. Saito, S., Sirahama, S., Matsushima, M., Suzuki, M., Sagae, S., Kudo, R., Saito, J., Noda, K., and Nakamura, Y. (1996). Definition of a commonly deleted region in ovarian cancers to a 300-kb segment of chromosome 6q27. *Cancer Res.* 56, 5586–5589.
9. Tibiletti, M. G., Bernasconi, B., Furlan, D., Riva, C., Trubia, M., Buraggi, G., Franchi, M., Bolis, P., Mariani, A., Frigerio, L., Capella, C., and Taramelli, R. (1996). Early involvement of 6q in surface epithelial ovarian tumors. *Cancer Res.*, 56, 4493–4498.
10. Colitti, C. V., Rodabaugh, K. J., Welch, W. R., Berkowitz, R. S., and Mok, S. C. (1998). A novel 4 cM minimal deletion unit on chromosome 6q25.1-q25.2 associated with high grade invasive epithelial ovarian carcinomas. *Oncogene* 16, 555–559.

11. Shridhar, V., Staub, J., Huntley, B., Cliby, W., Jenkins, R., Pass, H. I., Hartmann, L., and Smith, D. I. (1999). A novel region of deletion on chromosome 6q23.3 spanning less than 500 Kb in high grade invasive epithelial ovarian cancer. *Oncogene* 18, 3913–3918.
12. Watson, R. H., Neville, P. J., Roy, W. J. J., Hitchcock, A., and Campbell, I. G. (1998). Loss of heterozygosity on chromosomes 7p, 7q, 9p and 11q is an early event in ovarian tumorigenesis. *Oncogene* 17, 207–212.
13. Brown, M. R., Chuaqui, R., Vocke, C. D., Berchuck, A., Middleton, L. P., Emmert-Buck, M. R., and Kohn, E. C. (1999). Allelic loss on chromosome arm 8p: analysis of sporadic epithelial ovarian tumors. *Gynecol. Oncol.* 74, 98–102.
14. Lu, K. H., Weitzel, J. N., Kodali, S., Welch, W. R., Berkowitz, R. S., and Mok, S. C. (1997). A novel 4-cM minimally deleted region on chromosome 11p15.1 associated with high grade nonmucinous epithelial ovarian carcinomas. *Cancer Res.* 57, 387–390.
15. Gabra, H., Langdon, S. P., Watson, J. E., Hawkins, R. A., Cohen, B. B., Taylor, L., Mackay, J., Steel, C. M., Leonard, R. C., and Smyth, J. F. (1995): Loss of heterozygosity at 11q22 correlates with low progesterone receptor content in epithelial ovarian cancer. *Clin. Cancer Res.* 1, 945–953.
16. Launonen, V., Stenback, F., Puistola, U., Bloigu, R., Huusko, P., Kytola, S., Kauppila, A., and Winqvist, R. (1998). Chromosome 11q22.3-q25 LOH in ovarian cancer: association with a more aggressive disease course and involved subregions. *Gynecol. Oncol.* 71, 299–304.
17. Davis, M., Hitchcock, A., Foulkes, W. D., and Campbell, I. G. (1996). Refinement of two chromosome 11q regions of loss of heterozygosity in ovarian cancer. *Cancer Res.* 56, 741–744.
18. Gabra, H., Watson, J. E., Taylor, K. J., Mackay, J., Leonard, R. C., Steel, C. M., Porteous, D. J., and Smyth, J. F. (1996). Definition and refinement of a region of loss of heterozygosity at 11q23.3-q24.3 in epithelial ovarian cancer associated with poor prognosis. *Cancer Res.* 56, 950–954.
19. Launonen, V., Mannermaa, A., Stenb, Kosma, V. M., Puistola, U., Huusko, P., Anttila, M., Bloigu, R., Saarikoski, S., Kauppila, A., and Winqvist, R. (2000). Loss of heterozygosity at chromosomes 3, 6, 8, 11, 16, and 17 in ovarian cancer: correlation to clinicopathological variables. *Cancer Genet. Cytogenet.* 122, 49–54.
20. Dodson, M. K., Hartmann, L. C., Cliby, W. A., DeLaceey, K. A., Keeney, G. L., Ritland, S. R., Su, J. Q., Podratz, K. C., and Jenkins, R. B. (1993). Comparison of loss of heterozygosity patterns in invasive low-grade and high-grade epithelial ovarian carcinomas. *Cancer Res.* 53, 4456–4460.
21. Bandera, C. A., Takahashi, H., Behbakht, K., Liu, P. C., Livolsi, V. A., Benjamin, I., Morgan, M. A., King, S. A., Rubin, S. C., and Boyd, J. (1997). Deletion mapping of two potential chromosome 14 tumor suppressor gene loci in ovarian carcinoma. *Cancer Res.* 57, 513–515.
22. Kohler, M. F., Marks, J. R., Wiseman, R. W., Jacobs, I. J., Davidoff, A. M., Clarke-Pearson, D. L., Soper, J. T., Bast, R. C., and Berchuck, A. (1993). Spectrum of mutation and frequency of allelic deletion of the p53 gene in ovarian cancer. *J. Natl. Cancer Inst.* 85, 1513–1519.
23. Jacobs, I. J., Smith, S. A., Wiseman, R. W., Futreal, P. A., Harrington, T., Osborne, R. J., Leech, V., Molyneux, A., Berchuck, A., Ponder, B. A., *et al.* (1993). A deletion unit on chromosome 17q in epithelial ovarian tumors distal to the familial breast/ovarian cancer locus. *Cancer Res.* 53, 1218–1221.
24. Bryan, E. J., Watson, R. H., Davis, M., Hitchcock, A., Foulkes, W. D., and Campbell, I. G. (1996). Localization of an ovarian cancer tumor suppressor gene to a 0.5-cM region between D22S284 and CYP2D, on chromosome 22q. *Cancer Res.* 56, 719–721.
25. Gallion, H. H., Powell, D. E., Morrow, J. K., Pieretti, M., Case, E., Turker, M. S., DePriest, P. D., Hunter, J. E., and Van Nagell, J. R. (1992). Molecular genetic changes in human epithelial ovarian malignancies. *Gynecol. Oncol.* 47, 137–142.
26. Ono, K., Tanaka, T., Tsunoda, T., Kitahara, O., Kihara, C., Okamoto, A., Ochiai, K., Takagi, T., and Nakamura, Y. (2000). Identification by cDNA microarray of genes involved in ovarian carcinogenesis. *Cancer Res.* 60, 5007–5011.
27. Wong, K. K., Cheng.R. S., and Mok, S. C. (2001). Identification of differentially expressed genes from ovarian cancer cells by MICROMAX cDNA microarray system. *Biotechniques* 30, 670–675.
28. Welsh, J. B., Zarrinkar, P. P., Sapinoso, L. M., Kern, S. G., Behling, C. A., Monk, B. J., Lockhart, D. J., Burger, R. A., and Hampton, G. M. (2001): Analysis of gene expression profiles in normal and neoplastic ovarian tissue samples identifies candidate molecular markers of epithelial ovarian cancer. *Proc. Natl. Acad. Sci. USA* 98, 1176–1181.
29. Jacobs, I. J., Kohler, M. F., Wiseman, R. W., Marks, J. R., Whitaker, R., Kerns, B. A., Humphrey, P., Berchuck, A., Ponder, B. A., and Bast, R. C., Jr. (1992). Clonal origin of epithelial ovarian carcinoma: analysis by loss of heterozygosity, p53 mutation, and X-chromosome inactivation. *J. Natl. Cancer Inst.* 84, 1793–1798.
30. Abeln, E. C., Kuipers-Dijkshoorn, N. J., Berns, E. M., Henzen-Logmans, S. C., Fleuren, G. J., and Cornelisse, C. J. (1998). Molecular genetic evidence for unifocal origin of advanced epithelial ovarian cancer and for minor clonal divergence. *Br. J. Cancer* 72, 1330–1336.
31. Schorge, J. O., Muto, M. G., Welch, W. R., Bandera, C. A., Rubin, S. C., Bell, D. A., Berkowitz, R. S., and Mok, S. C. (1998). Molecular evidence for multifocal papillary serous carcinoma of the peritoneum in patients with germline BRCA1 mutations. *J. Natl. Cancer Inst.* 90, 841–845.
32. Whittemore, A. S., Harris, R., and Itnyre, J. (1992). Characteristics relating to ovarian cancer risk. Collaborative analysis of twelve US case-control studies: IV. The pathogenesis of epithelial ovarian cancer. *Am. J. Epidemiol* 136, 1212–1220.
33. Schildkraut, J. M., Bastos, E., and Berchuck, A. (1997). Relationship between lifetime ovulatory cycles and overexpression of mutant p53 in epithelial ovarian cancer. *J. Natl. Cancer Inst.* 89, 932–938.
34. Ames, B. N. and Gold, L. S. (1990). Too many rodent carcinogens: Mitogenesis increases mutagenesis. *Science* 249, 970–971.
35. Rodriguez, G. C., Walmer, D. K., Cline, M., Krigman, H. R., Lessey, B. A., Whitaker, R. S., Dodge, R. K., and Hughes, C. L. (1998). Effect of progestin on the ovarian epithelium of macaques: Cancer prevention through apoptosis? *J. Soc. Gynecol. Invest.* 5, 271–276.
36. Reles, A. E., Gee, C., Schellschmidt, I., Schmider, A., Unger, M., Friedmann, W., Lichtenegger, W., and Press, M. F. (1998). Prognostic significance of DNA content and S-phase fraction in epithelial ovarian carcinomas analyzed by image cytometry [see comments]. *Gynecol. Oncol.* 71, 3–13.
37. Layfield, L. J., Saria, E. A., Berchuck, A., Dodge, R. K., Thompson, J. K., Conlon, D. H., and Kerns, B. J. (1997). Prognostic value of MIB-1 in advanced ovarian carcinoma as determined using automated immunohistochemistry and quantitative image analysis. *J. Surg. Oncol.* 66, 236–237.
38. Hartmann, L. C., Sebo, T. J., Kamel, N. A., Podratz, K. C., Cha, S. S., Wieand, H. S., Keeney, G. L., and Roche, P. C. (1992). Proliferating cell nuclear antigen in epithelial ovarian cancer: Relation to results at second-look laparotomy and survival. *Gynecol. Oncol.* 47, 191–195.
39. Garzetti, G. G., Ciavattini, A., Goteri, G., De Nictolis, M., Stramazzotti, D., Lucarini, G., and Biagini, G. (1995). Ki67 antigen immunostaining (MIB 1 monoclonal antibody) in serous ovarian tumors: Index of proliferative activity with prognostic significance. *Gynecol. Oncol.* 56, 169–174.
40. Green, D. R., and Reed, J. C. (1998). Mitochondria and apoptosis. *Science* 281, 1309–1312.
41. Korsmeyer, S. J. (1999). BCL-2 gene family and the regulation of programmed cell death. *Cancer Res.* 59, 1693s–1700s.
42. Herod, J. J., Eliopoulos, A. G., Warwick, J., Niedobitek, G., Young, L. S., and Kerr, D. J. (1996). The prognostic significance of Bcl-2 and p53 expression in ovarian carcinoma. *Cancer Res.* 56, 2178–2184.

43. Henriksen, R., Wilander, E., and Oberg, K. (1995). Expression and prognostic significance of Bcl-2 in ovarian tumours. *Br. J. Cancer* 72, 1324–1329.
44. Liu, J. R., Fletcher, B., Page, C., Hu, C., Nunez, G., and Baker, V. (1998). Bcl-xL is expressed in ovarian carcinoma and modulates chemotherapy-induced apoptosis. *Gynecol. Oncol.* 70, 398–403.
45. Tai, Y. T., Lee, S., Niloff, E., Weisman, C., Strobel, T., and Cannistra, S. A. (1998). BAX protein expression and clinical outcome in epithelial ovarian cancer. *J. Clin. Oncol.* 16, 2583–2590.
46. Holt, S. E., Shay, J. W., and Wright, W. E. (1996). Refining the telomere-telomerase hypothesis of aging and cancer. *Nat. Biotechnol.* 14, 836–839.
47. Shay, J. W. (1998). Telomerase in cancer: Diagnostic, prognostic, and therapeutic implications. *Cancer J. Scie. Am.* 4 Suppl. 1, S26–34.
48. Kyo, S., Takakura, M., Tanaka, M., Murakami, K., Saitoh, R., Hirano, H., and Inoue, M. (1998). Quantitative differences in telomerase activity among malignant, premalignant, and benign ovarian lesions. *Clin. Cancer Res.* 4, 399–405.
49. Duggan, B. D., Wan, M., Yu, M. C., Roman, L. D., Muderspach, L. I., Delgadillo, E., Li, W. Z., Martin, S. E., and Dubeau, L. (1998). Detection of ovarian cancer cells: Comparison of a telomerase assay and cytologic examination. *J. Natl. Cancer Inst.* 90, 238–242.
50. Wan, M., Li, W. Z., Duggan, B. D., Felix, J. C., Zhao, Y., and Dubeau, L. (1997). Telomerase activity in benign and malignant epithelial ovarian tumors. *J. Natl. Cancer Inst.* #19,89, 437–441.
51. Bauknecht, T., Kiechle, M., Bauer, G., and Siebers, J. W. (1986). Characterization of growth factors in human ovarian carcinomas. *Cancer Res.* 46, 2614–2618.
52. Kommoss, F., Wintzer, H. O., Von Kleist, S., Kohler, M., Walker, R., Langton, B., Van Tran, K., Pfleiderer, A., and Bauknecht, T. (1990). In situ distribution of transforming growth factor-α in normal human tissues and in malignant tumours of the ovary. *J. Pathol.* 162, 223–230.
53. Morishige, K., Kurachi, H., Amemiya, K., Fujita, Y., Yamamoto, T., Miyake, A., and Tanizawa, O. (1991). Evidence for the involvement of transforming growth factor-α and epidermal growth factor receptor autocrine growth mechanism in primary human ovarian cancers in vitro. *Cancer Res.* 51, 5322–5328.
54. Rodriguez, G. C., Berchuck, A., Whitaker, R. S., Schlossman, D., Clarke-Pearson, D. L., and Bast, R. C., Jr. (1991). Epidermal growth factor receptor expression in normal ovarian epithelium and ovarian cancer. II. Relationship between receptor expression and response to epidermal growth factor. *Am. J. Obstet. Gynecol.* 164, 745–750.
55. Yee, D., Morales, F. R., Hamilton, T. C., and Von Hoff, D. D. (1991). Expression of insulin-like growth factor I, its binding proteins, and its receptor in ovarian cancer. *Cancer Res.* 51, 5107–5112.
56. Muller, M., Dietel, M., Turzynski, A., and Wiechen, K. (1998). Antisense phosphorothioate oligodeoxynucleotide down-regulation of the insulin-like growth factor I receptor in ovarian cancer cells. *Int. J. Cancer* 77, 567–571.
57. Sariban, E., Sitaras, N. M., Antoniades, H. N., Kufe, D. W., and Pantazis, P. (1988). Expression of platelelt-derived growth factor (PDGF)-related transcripts and synthesis of biologically active PDGF-like proteins by human malignant epithelial cell lines. *J. Clin. Invest.* 82, 1157–1164.
58. Berchuck, A., Olt, G. J., Everitt, L., Soisson, A. P., Bast, R. C., Jr., and Boyer, C. M. (1990). The role of peptide growth factors in epithelial ovarian cancer. *Obstet. Gynecol.* 75, 255–262.
59. Henrikson, R., Funa, K., Wilander, E., Backstrom, T., Ridderheim, M., and Oberg, K. (1993). Expression and prognostic significance of platelet-derived growth factor and its receptors in epithelial ovarian neoplasms. *Cancer Res.* 53, 4550–4554.
60. Di Blasio, A. M., Cremononesi, L., Vigano, P., Ferrari, M., Gospodarowicz, D., Vignali, M., and Jaffe, R. B. (1993). Basic fibroblast growth factor and its receptor messenger ribonucleic acids are expressed in human ovarian epithelial neoplasms. *Am. J. Obstet. Gynecol.* 169, 1517–1523.
61. Ramakrishnan, S., Xu, F. J., Brandt, S. J., Niedel, J. E., Bast, R. C., Jr., and Brown, E. L. (1989). Constitutive production of macrophage colony-stimulating factor by human ovarian and breast cancer cell lines. *J. Clin. Invest.* 83, 921–926.
62. Kacinski, B. M., Stanley, E. R., Carter, D., Chambers, J. T., Chambers, S. K., Kohorn, E. I., and Schwartz, P. E. (1989). Circulating levels of CSF-1 (M-CSF) a lymphohematopoietic cytokine may be a useful marker of disease status in patients with malignant ovarian neoplasms. *Int. J. Radiat. Oncol. Biol. Phys.* 17, 159–164.
63. Kacinski, B. M., Carter, D., Mittal, K., Yee, L. D., Scata, K. A., Donofrio, L., Chambers, S. K., Wang, K., Yang-Feng, T., Rohrschneider, L. R., and Rothwell, V. M. (1990). Ovarian adenocarcinomas express *fms*-complementary transcripts and *fms* antigen, often with coexpression of CSF-1. *Am. J. Pathol.* 137:1, 135–147.
64. Kawakami, Y., Nagai, N., Ohama, K., Zeki, K., Yoshida, Y., Kuroda, E., and Yamashita, U. (2000). Macrophage-colony stimulating factor inhibits the growth of human ovarian cancer cells in vitro. *Eur. J. Cancer* 36, 1991–1997.
65. Wu, S., Rodabaugh, K., Martinez-Maza, O., Watson, J. M., Silberstein, D. S., Boyer, C. M., Peters, W. P., Weinberg, J. B., Berek, J. S., and Bast, R. C. (1992). Stimulation of ovarian tumor cell proliferation with monocyte products including interleukin-1, interleukin-6 and tumor necrosis factor-α. *Am. J. Obstet. Gynecol.* 166, 997–1007.
66. Wu, S., Boyer, C. M., Whitaker, R. S., Berchuck, A., Wiener, J. R., Weinberg, J. B., and Bast, R. C. Jr. (1993). Tumor necrosis factor-α as an autocrine and paracrine growth factor for ovarian cancer: Monokine induction of tumor cell proliferation and tumor necrosis factor-α expression. *Cancer Res.* 53, 1939–1944.
67. Naylor, S. M., Stamp, G. W. H., Foulkes, W. D., Eccles, D., and Balkwill, F. R. (1993). Tumor necrosis factor and its receptors in human ovarian cancer. *J. Clin. Invest.* 91, 2194–2206.
68. Foti, E., Ferrandina, G., Martucci, R., Romanini, M. E., Benedetti, P. P., Testa, U., Mancuso, S., and Scambia, G. (2000). IL-6, M-CSF and IAP cytokines in ovarian cancer: Simultaneous assessment of serum levels. *Oncology* 57, 211–215.
69. Fang, X., Gibson, S., Flowers, M., Furui, T., Bast, R. C. J., and Mills, G. B. (1997). Lysophosphatidylcholine stimulates activator protein 1 and the c- Jun N-terminal kinase activity. *J. Biol. Chem.* 272, 13683–13689.
70. Mills, G. B., May, C., Hill, M., Campbell, S., Shaw, P., and Marks, A. (1990). Ascitic fluid from human ovarian cancer patients contains growth factors necessary for intraperitoneal growth of human ovarian adenocarcinoma cells. *J. Clin. Invest.* 86, 851–855.
71. Siemans, C. H., and Auersperg, N. (1991). Serial propagation of human ovarian surface epithelium in culture. *J. Cell. Physiol.* 134, 347–356.
72. Lidor, Y. J., Xu, F. J., Martinez-Maza, O., Olt, G. J., Marks, J. R., Berchuck, A., Ramakrishnan, S., Berek, J. S., and Bast, R. C. (1993). Constitutive production of macrophage colony stimulating factor and interleukin-6 by human ovarian surface epithelial cells. *Exp. Cell. Res.* 207, 332–339.
73. Ziltener, H. J., Maines-Bandiera, S., Schrader, J. W., and Auersperg, N. (1993). Secretion of bioactive interleukin-1, interleukin-6 aand colony-stimulating factors by human ovarian surface epithelium. *Biol. Reprod.* 49, 635–641.
74. Pinkas-Kramarski, R., Shelly, M., Guarino, B. C., Wang, L. M., Lyass, L., Alroy, I., Alamandi, M., Kuo, A., Moyer, J. D., Lavi, S., Eisenstein, M., Ratzkin, B. J., Seger, R., Bacus, S. S., Pierce, J. H., Andrews, G. C., and Yarden, Y. (1998). ErbB tyrosine kinases and the two neuregulin families constitute a ligand-receptor network. *Mol. Cell. Biol.* 18, 6090–6101.
75. Weiss, A. and Schlessinger, J. (1998). Switching signals on or off by receptor dimerization. *Cell.* 94, 277–280.
76. Gullick, W. J. (1998). Type I growth factor receptors: current status and future work. *Biochem. Soc. Symp.* 63, 193–198.

77. Fan, Z., and Mendelsohn, J. (1998). Therapeutic application of anti-growth factor receptor antibodies. *Curr. Opin. Oncol.* 10, 67–73.
78. Berchuck, A., Rodriguez, G. C., Kamel, A., Dodge, R. K., Soper, J. T., Clarke-Pearson, D. L., and Bast, R. C., Jr. (1991). Epidermal growth factor receptor expression in normal ovarian epithelium and ovarian cancer: I. Correlation of receptor expression with prognostic factors in patients with ovarian cancer. *Am. J. Obstet. Gynecol.* 164, 669–674.
79. Alroy, I., and Yarden, Y. (1997). The ErbB signaling network in embryogenesis and oncogenesis: Signal diversification through combinatorial ligand-receptor interactions. *FEBS Lett.* 410, 83–86.
80. Slamon, D. J., Godolphin, W., Jones, L. A., Holt, J. A., Wong, S. G., Keith, D. E., Levin, L. J., Stuart, S. G., Udove, J., Ullrich, A., and Press, M. F. (1989). Studies of HER-2/*neu* proto-oncogene in human breast and ovarian cancer. *Science* 244, 707–712.
81. Berchuck, A., Kamel, A., Whitaker, R., Kerns, B., Olt, G., Kinney, R., Soper, J. T., Dodge, R., Clarke-Pearson, P., Marks, S., McKenzie, S., Yin, S., and Bast, R. C., Jr. (1990). Overexpression of HER-2/*neu* is associated with poor survival in advanced epithelial ovarian cancer. *Cancer Res.* 50, 4087–4091.
82. Rubin, S. C., Finstad, C. L., Wong, G. Y., Almadrones, L., Plante, M., and Lloyd, K. O. (1993). Prognostic significance of HER-2/*neu* expression in advanced ovarian cancer. *Am. J. Obstet. Gynecol.* 168, 162–169.
83. Kacinski, B. M., Mayer, A. G., King, B. L., Carter, D., and Chambers, S. (1992). *Neu* protein overexpression in benign, borderline, and malignant ovarian neoplasms. *Gynecol. Oncol.* 44, 245–253.
84. Rodriguez, G. C., Boente, M. P., Berchuck, A., Whitaker, R. S., O'Briant, K. C., Xu, F., and Bast, R. C., Jr. (1993). The effect of antibodies and immunotoxins reactive with HER-2/neu on growth of ovarian and breast cancer cell lines. *Am. J. Obstet. Gynecol.* 168, 228–232.
85. Pietras, R. J., Pegram, M. D., Finn, R. S., Maneval, D. A., and Slamon, D. J. (1998). Remission of human breast cancer xenografts on therapy with humanized monoclonal antibody to HER-2 receptor and DNA-reactive drugs. *Oncogene* 17, 2235–2249.
86. Pegram, M. D., Finn, R. S., Arzoo, K., Beryt, M., Pietras, R. J., and Slamon, D. J. (1997). The effect of HER-2/neu overexpression on chemotherapeutic drug sensitivity in human breast and ovarian cancer cells. *Oncogene* 15, 537–547.
87. Pegram, M. D., Lipton, A., Hayes, D. F., Weber, B. L., Baselga, J. M., Tripathy, D., Baly, D., Baughman, S. A., Twaddell, T., Glaspy, J. A., and Slamon, D. J. (1998). Phase II study of receptor-enhanced chemosensitivity using recombinant humanized anti-p185HER2/neu monoclonal antibody plus cisplatin in patients with HER2/neu-overexpressing metastatic breast cancer refractory to chemotherapy treatment. *J. Clin. Oncol.* 16, 2659–2671.
88. Schwartzberg, P. L. (1998). The many faces of Src: Multiple functions of a prototypical tyrosine kinase. *Oncogene* 17, 1463–1468.
89. Parsons, R. (1998). Phosphatases and tumorigenesis. *Curr. Opin. Oncol.* 10, 88–91.
90. Wiener, J. R., Kassim, S. K., Yu, Y., Mills, G. B., and Bast, R. C. J. (1996). Transfection of human ovarian cancer cells with the HER-2/neu receptor tyrosine kinase induces a selective increase in PTP-H1, PTP-1B, PTP-alpha expression. *Gynecol. Oncol.* 61, 233–240.
91. Cheng, J. Q., Godwin, A. K., Bellacosa, A., Taguchi, T., Frank, T. F., Hamilton, T. C., Tsischlis, P. N., and Testa, J. R. (1992). AKT2, a putative oncogene encoding a member of a subfamily of protein-serine/threonine, kinases, is amplified in human ovarian carcinomas. *Proc. Natl. Acad. Sci. USA* 89, 9267–9271.
92. Bellacosa, A., de Feo, D., Godwin, A. K., Bell, D. W., Cheng, J. Q., Altomare, D. A., Wan, M., Dubeau, L., Scambia, G., and Masciullo, V. (1995). Molecular alterations of the AKT2 oncogene in ovarian and breast carcinomas. *Int J. Cancer* 64, 280–285.
93. Yuan, Z. Q., Sun, M., Feldman, R. I., Wang, G., Ma, X., Jiang, C., Coppola, D., Nicosia, S. V., and Cheng, J. Q. (2000). Frequent activation of AKT2 and induction of apoptosis by inhibition of phosphoinositide-3-OH kinase/Akt pathway in human ovarian cancer. *Oncogene* 19, 2324–2330.
94. Shayesteh, L., Lu, Y., Kuo, W. L., Baldocchi, R., Godfrey, T., Collins, C., Pinkel, D., Powell, B., Mills, G. B., and Gray, J. W. (1999). PIK3CA is implicated as an oncogene in ovarian cancer. *Nat. Genet.* 21, 99–102.
95. Sartor, C. I., Dziubinski, M. L., Yu, C. L., Jove, R., and Ethier, S. P. (1997). Role of epidermal growth factor receptor and STAT-3 activation in autonomous proliferation of SUM-102PT human breast cancer cells. *Cancer Res.* 57, 978–987.
96. Gao, B., Shen, X., Kunos, G., Meng, Q., Goldberg, I. D., Rosen, E. M., and Fan, S. (2001). Constitutive activation of JAK-STAT3 signaling by BRCA1 in human prostate cancer cells. *FEBS Lett.* 488, 179–184.
97. Burke, W. M., Huang, M., Jin, X., Liu, J. R., Jiang, Y. B., Reynolds, K., and Lin, J. (2001). Inhibition of the constitutively active Stat3 signal pathway in human ovarian cancer cells. *Soc. Gynecol. Oncol.* (Abstract).
98. Page, H. M., Reynolds, R. K., and Lin, J. (2000). Constitutive activation of STAT3 oncogene product in human ovarian carcinoma cells. *Gynecol. Oncol.* 79, 67–73.
99. Campbell, S. L., Khosravi-Far, R., Rossman, K. L., Clark, G. J., and Der, C. J. (1998). Increasing complexity of Ras signaling. *Oncogene* 17, 1395–1413.
100. Gutkind, J. S. (1998). Cell growth control by G protein-coupled receptors: From signal transduction to signal integration. *Oncogene* 17, 1331–1342.
101. Enomoto, T., Inoue, M., Perantoni, A. O., Terakawa, N., Tanizawa, O., and Rice, J. M. (1990). K-*ras* activation in neoplasms of the human female reproductive tract. *Cancer Res.* 50, 6139–6145.
102. Feig, L. A., Bast, R. C., Jr., Knapp, R. C., and Cooper, G. M. (1984). Somatic activation of *ras*K gene in a human ovarian carcinoma. *Science* 223, 698–701.
103. Haas, M., Isakov, J., and Howell, S. B. (1987). Evidence against *ras* activation in human ovarian carcinomas. *Mol. Biol. Med.* 4, 265–275.
104. Teneriello, M. G., Ebina, M., Linnoila, R. I., Henry, M., Nash, J. D., Park, R. C., and Birrer, M. J. (1993). p53 and ki-*ras* gene mutations in epithelial ovarian neoplasms. *Cancer Res.* 53, 3103–3108.
105. Mok, S. C. H., Bell, D. A., Knapp, R. C., Fishbaugh, P. M., Welch, W. R., Muto, M. G., Berkowitz, R. S., and Tsao, S. W. (1993). Mutation of K-*ras* protooncogene in human ovarian epithelial tumors of borderline malignancy. *Cancer Res.* 53, 1489–1492.
106. Alvarez, A. A., Krigman, H. R., Whitaker, R. S., Dodge, R. K., and Rodriguez, G. C. (1999). The prognostic significance of angiogenesis in epithelial ovarian carcinoma. *Clin. Cancer Res.* 5, 587–591.
107. Facchini, L. M., and Penn, L. Z. (1998). The molecular role of Myc in growth and transformation: Recent discoveries lead to new insights. *FASEB J.* 12, 633–651.
108. Bouchard, C., Staller, P., and Eilers, M. (1998). Control of cell proliferation by Myc. *Trends. Cell. Biol.* 8, 202–206.
109. Baker, V. V., Borst, M. P., Dixon, D., Hatch, K. D., Shingleton, H. M., and Miller, D. (1990). c-*myc* amplification in ovarian cancer. *Gynecol Oncol.* 38, 340-342.
110. Zhou, D. J., Gonzalez-Cadavid, N., Ahuja, H., Battifora, H., Moore, G. E., and Cline, M. J. (1988). A unique pattern of proto-oncogene abnormalities in ovarian adenocarcinomas. *Cancer* 62, 1573–1576.
111. Serova, D. M. (1987). Amplification of c-*myc* proto-oncogene in primary tumors, metastases and blood leukocytes of patients with ovarian cancer. *Eksp. Onkol.* 9, 25–27.
112. Sasano, H., Garrett, C., Wilkinson, D., Silverberg, S., Comerford, J., and Hyde, J. (1990). Protoocogene amplification and tumor ploidy in human ovarian neoplasms. *Hum. Pathol.* 21:4, 382–391.
113. Berns, E. M. J. J., Klijn, J. G. M., Henzen-Logmans, S. C., Rodenburg, C. J., vanderBurg, M. E. L., and Foekens, J. A. (1992). Receptors for hormones and growth factors (onco)-gene amplification in human ovarian cancer. *Int. J. Cancer* 52, 218–224.

114. Tashiro, H., Niyazaki, K., Okamura, H., Iwai, A., and Fukumoto, M. (1992). c-*myc* overexpression in human primary ovarian tumors: Its relevance to tumor progression. *Int. J. Cancer* 50, 828–833.
115. Knudson, A. G. (1997). Hereditary predisposition to cancer. *Ann. N.Y. Acad. Sci.* 833, 58–67.
116. Liggett, W. H. J., and Sidransky, D. (1998). Role of the p16 tumor suppressor gene in cancer. *J. Clin. Oncol.* 16, 1197–1206.
117. Steck, P. A., Pershouse, M. A., Jasser, S. A., Yung, W. K., Lin, H., Ligon, A. H., Langford, L. A., Baumgard, M. L., Hattier, T., Davis, T., Frye, C., Hu, R., Swedlund, B., Teng, D. H., and Tavtigian, S.V. (1997). Identification of a candidate tumour suppressor gene, MMAC1, at chromosome 10q23.3 that is mutated in multiple advanced cancers. *Nat. Genet.* 15, 356–362.
118. Li, J., Yen, C., Liaw, D., Podsypanina, K., Bose, S., Wang, S. I., Puc, J., Miliaresis, C., Rodgers, L., McCombie, R., Bigner, S. H., Giovanella, B. C., Ittmann, M., Tycko, B., Hibshoosh, H., Wigler, M. H., and Parsons, R. (1997). PTEN, a putative protein tyrosine phosphatase gene mutated in human brain, breast, and prostate cancer [see comments]. *Science* 275, 1943–1947.
119. Obata, K., Morland, S. J., Watson, R. H., Hitchcock, A., Chenevix-Trench, G., Thomas, E. J., and Campbell, I. G. (1998). Frequent PTEN/MMAC mutations in endometrioid but not serous or mucinous epithelial ovarian tumors. *Cancer Res.* 58, 2095–2097.
120. Serra, R., and Moses, H. L. (1996). Tumor suppressor genes in the TGF-beta signaling pathway? *Nat. Med.* 2, 390–391.
121. Shi, Y., Wang, Y. F., Jayaraman, L., Yang, H., Massague, J., and Pavletich, N. P. (1998). Crystal structure of a Smad MH1 domain bound to DNA: Insights on DNA binding in TGF-beta signaling. *Cell* 94, 585–594.
122. Kretzschmar, M., and Massague, J. (1998). SMADs: Mediators and regulators of TGF-beta signaling. *Curr. Opin. Genet. Devel.* 8, 103–111.
123. Berchuck, A., Rodriguez, G. C., Olt, G. J., Boente, M. P., Whitaker, R. S., Arrick, B., Clarke-Pearson, D. L., and Bast, R. C., Jr. (1992). Regulation of growth of normal ovarian epithelial cells and ovarian cancer cell lines by transforming growth factor-β. *Am. J. Obstet. Gynecol.* 166, 676–684.
124. Marth, C., Lang, T., Koza, A., Mayer, I., and Daxenbichler, G. (1990). Transforming growth factor-beta and ovarian carcinoma cells: regulation of proliferation and surface antigen expression. *Cancer Lett.* 51, 221–225.
125. Bartlett, J. M. S., Rabiasz, G. J., Scott, W. N., Langdon, S. P., Smyth, J. F., and Miller, W. R. (1992). Transforming growth factor-β mRNA expression in growth control of human ovarian carcinoma cells. *Br. J. Cancer* 65, 655–660.
126. Jozan, S., Guerrin, M., Mazars, P., Dutaur, M., Monsattat, B., Cheutin, F., Bugat, R., Martel, P., and Valette, A. (1992). Transforming growth factor-β-1 (TGF- β-1) inhibits growth of a human a human ovarian cancer cell line (OVCCR-1) and is expressed in human ovarian tumors. *Int. J. Cancer* 52, 766–770.
127. Zhou, L. I., and Leung, B. S. (1992). Growth regulation of ovarian cancer cells by epidermal growth factor and transforming growth factors-α and β-1. *Biochem. Biophys. Acta.* 1080, 130–136.
128. Hurteau, J., Rodriguez, G. C., Whitaker, R. S., Shain, S., Bast, R. C., Jr., and Berchuck, A. (1994). Effect of transforming growth factor-β on on proliferation of human ovarian cancer cells obtained from ascites. *Cancer* 74, 93–99.
129. Berchuck, A., Kohler, M. F., Marks, J. R., Wiseman, R., Boyd, J., and Bast, R. C., Jr. (1994). The p53 tumor suppressor gene frequently is altered in gynecologic cancers. *Am. J. Obstet. Gynecol.* 170, 246–252.
130. Wang, X. W. and Harris, C. C. (1997). p53 tumor-suppressor gene: clues to molecular carcinogenesis. *J. Cell. Physiol.* 173, 247–255.
131. Hainaut, P., Hernandez, T., Robinson, A., Rodriguez-Tome, P., Flores, T., Hollstein, M., Harris, C. C., and Montesano, R. (1998). IARC Database of p53 gene mutations in human tumors and cell lines: Updated compilation, revised formats and new visualisation tools. *Nucleic Acids Res.* 26. 205–213.
132. Lamb, P. and Crawford, L. (1986). Characterization of the human p53 gene. *Mol. Cell. Biol.* 6, 1379–1385.
133. Braithwaite, A. W., Sturzbecher, H. W., Addison, C., Palmer, C., Rudge, K., and Jenkins, J. R. (1987). Mouse p53 inhibits SV40 origin-dependent DNA replication. *Nature* 329, 458–460.
134. Rotter, V., Abutbul, H., and Ben Zeev, A. (1983). P53 transformation-related protein accumulates in the nucleus of transformed fibroblasts in association with the chromatin and is found in the cytoplasm of non-transformed fibroblasts. *EMBO J.* 2, 1041–1047.
135. Kuerbitz, S. J., Plunkett, B. S., Walsh, W. V., and Kastan, M. B. (1992): Wild-type p53 is a cell cycle checkpoint determinant following irradiation. *Proc Natl. Acad. Sci. USA* 89, 7491–7495.
136. Casey, G., Lopez, M. E., Ramos, J. C., Plummer, S. J., Arboleda, M. J., Shaughnessy, M., Karlan, B., and Slamon, D. J. (1996). DNA sequence analysis of exons 2 through 11 and immunohistochemical staining are required to detect all known p53 alterations in human malignancies. *Oncogene* 13, 1971–1981.
137. Marks, J. R., Davidoff, A. M., Kerns, B., Humphrey, P. A., Pence, J., Dodge, R., Clarke-Pearson, D. L., Iglehart, J. D., Bast, R. C., Jr., and Berchuck, A. (1991). Overexpression and mutation of p53 in epithelial ovarian cancer. *Cancer Res.* 51, 2979–2984.
138. Kohler, M. F., Kerns, B. J., Humphrey, P. A., Marks, J. R., Bast, R. C., and Berchuck, A. (1993). Mutation and overexpression of p53 in early-stage epithelial ovarian cancer. *Obstet. Gynecol.* 81, 643–650.
139. Hartmann, L., Podratz, K., Keeney, G., Kamel, N., Edmonson, J., Grill, J., Su, J., Katzmann, J., and Roche, P. (1994). Prognostic significance of p53 immunostaining in epithelial ovarian cancer. *J. Clin. Oncol.* 12, 64–69.
140. Eltabbakh, G. H., Belinson, J. L., Kennedy, A. W., Biscotti, C. V., Casey, G., Tubbs, R. R., and Blumenson, L. E. (1997). p53 overexpression is not an independent prognostic factor for patients with primary ovarian epithelial cancer. *Cancer* 80, 892–898.
141. Henriksen, R., Strang, P., Backstrom, T., Wilander, E., Tribukait, B., and Oberg, K. (1994). Ki-67 immunostaining and DNA flow cytometry as prognostic factors in epithelial ovarian cancers. *Anticancer Res.* 14, 603–608.
142. Berns, E. M., Klijn, J. G., Van Putten, W. L., De Witte, H. H., Look, M. P., Meijer-van, Gelder, M. E., Willman, K., Portengen, H., Benraad, T. J., and Foekens, J. A. (1998). p53 protein accumulation predicts poor response to tamoxifen therapy of patients with recurrent breast cancer. *J. Clin. Oncol.* 16(1), 121–127.
143. Vander Zee, A. G., Hollema, H., Suurmeijer, A. J., Krans, M., Sluiter, W. J., Willemse, P. H., Aalders, J. G., and De Vries, E. G. (1995). Value of P-glycoprotein, glutathione S-transferase pi, c-erbB-2, and p53 as prognostic factors in ovarian carcinomas. *J. Clin. Oncol.* 13(1), 70–78.
144. Berchuck, A., Kohler, M. F., Hopkins, M. P., Clarke-Pearson, D. L., Humphrey, P. A., and Bast, R. C. (1994). Overexpression of the p53 tumor suppressor gene is not a feature of benign and early stage borderline epithelial ovarian tumors. *Gynecol. Oncol.* 52, 232–236.
145. Schildkraut, J. M., Halabi, S., Bastos, E., Marchbanks, P. A., McDonald, J. A., and Berchuck, A. (2000). Prognostic factors in early-onset epithelial ovarian cancer: A population-based study. *Obstet. Gynecol.* 95, 119–127.
146. Kupryjanczyk, J., Thor, A. D., Beauchamp, R., Merritt, V., Edgerton, S. M., Bell, D. A., and Yandell, D. W. (1993). p53 mutations and protein accumulation in human ovarian cancer. *Proc. Natl. Acad. Sci. USA* 90, 4961–4965.
147. Brown, R., Clugston, C., Burns, P., Edlin, A., Vasey, P., Vojtesek, B., and Kaye, S. B. (1993). Increased accumulation of p53 protein in cisplatin-resistant ovarian cell lines. *Int. J. Cancer* 55, 678–684.
148. Eliopoulos, A. G., Kerr, D. J., Herod, J., Hodgkins, L., Krajewski, S., Reed, J. C., and Young, L. S. (1995). The control of apoptosis and

drug resistance in ovarian cancer: Influence of p53 and Bcl-2. *Oncogene* 11, 1217–1228.

149. Righetti, S. C., Della, T. G., Pilotti, S., Menard, S., Ottone, F., Colnaghi, M. I., Pierotti, M. A., Lavarino, C., Cornarotti, M., Oriana, S., Bohm, S., Bresciani, G. L., Spatti, G., and Zunino, F. (1996). A comparative study of p53 gene mutations, protein accumulation, and response to cisplatin-based chemotherapy in advanced ovarian carcinoma. *Cancer Res.* 56, 689–693.
150. Perego, P., Giarola, M., Righetti, S. C., Supino, R., Caserini, C., Delia, D., Pierotti, M. A., Miyashita, T., Reed, J. C., and Zunino, F. (1996). Association between cisplatin resistance and mutation of p53 gene and reduced bax expression in ovarian carcinoma cell systems. *Cancer Res.* 56, 556–562.
151. Havrilesky, L. J., Elbendary, A., Hurteau, J. A., Whitaker, R. S., Rodriguez, G. C., and Berchuck, A. (1995). Chemotherapy-induced apoptosis in epithelial ovarian cancers. *Obstet. Gynecol.* 85, 1007–1010.
152. Schildkraut, J. M., Collins, N. K., Dent, G. A., Tucker, J. A., Barrett, J. C., Berchuck, A., and Boyd, J. (1995). Loss of heterozygosity on chromosome 17q11-21 in cancers of women who have both breast and ovarian cancer. *Am. J. Obstet. Gynecol.* 172, 908–913.
153. Takahashi, H., Behbakht, K., McGovern, P. E., Chiu, H. C., Couch, F. J., Weber, B. L., Friedman, L. S., King, M. C., Furusato, M., and Livolsi, V. A. (1995). Mutation analysis of the BRCA1 gene in ovarian cancers. *Cancer Res.* 55, 2998–3002.
154. Merajver, S. D., Pham, T. M., Caduff, R. F., Chen, M., Poy, E. L., Cooney, K. A., Weber, B. L., Collins, F. S., Johnston, C., and Frank, T. S. (1995). Somatic mutations in the BRCA1 gene in sporadic ovarian tumours. *Nat. Genet.* 9, 439–443.
155. Hosking, L., Trowsdale, J., Nicolai, H., Solomon, E., Foulkes, W., Stamp, G., Signer, E., and Jeffreys, A. (1995). A somatic BRCA1 mutation in an ovarian tumour. *Nat. Genet.* 9, 343–344.
156. Futreal, P. A., Liu, Q., Shattuck-Eidens, D., Cochran, C., Harshman, K., Tavtigian, S., Bennett, L. M., Haugen-Strano, A., Swensen, J., and Miki, Y. (1994): BRCA1 mutations in primary breast and ovarian carcinomas. *Science* 266, 120–122.
157. Berchuck, A., Heron, K., Carney, M. E., Lancaster, J. M., Fraser, E. G., Vinson, V.L., Deffenbaugh, A. M., Miron, A., Marks, J. R., Futreal, P. A., and Frank, T. S. (1998). Frequency of germline and somatic BRCA1 mutations in ovarian cancer. *Clin. Cancer Res.* 4, 2433–2437.
158. Lancaster, J. M., Wooster, R., Mangion, J., Phelan, C. M., Cochran, C., Gumbs, C., Seal, S., Barfoot, R., Collins, N., Bignell, G., Patel, S., Hamoudi, R., Larsson, C., Wiseman, R., Berchuck, A., Iglehart, D., Marks, J. R., Ashworth, A., Stratton, M., and Futreal, P. A. (1996). BRCA2 mutations in primary breast and ovarian cancers. *Nat. Genet.* 13, 1–5.
159. Ewen, M. E. (1998). Regulation of the cell cycle by the Rb tumor suppressor family. *Results Prob. Cell Differen.* 22, 149–179.
160. Bartek, J., Bartkova, J., and Lukas, J. (1997). The retinoblastoma protein pathway in cell cycle control and cancer. *Exp. Cell Res.* 237, 1–6.
161. Sasano, H., Comerford, J., Silverberg, S. G., and Garrett, C. T. (1990). An analysis of anormalities of the Retinoblastoma gene in human ovarian and endometrial carcinoma. *Cancer* 66, 2150–2154.
162. Dodson, M. K., Cliby, W. A., Xu, H. J., DeLacey, K. A., Hu, S. X., Keeney, G. L., Li, J., Podratz, K. C., Jenkins, R. B., and Benedict, W. F. (1994). Evidence of functional RB protein in epithelial ovarian carcinomas despite loss of heterozygosity at the RB locus. *Cancer Res.* 54, 610–613.
163. Kamb, A. (1998). Cyclin-dependent kinase inhibitors and human cancer. *Curr. Top. Microbiol. Immunol.* 227, 139–148.
164. Kanuma, T., Nishida, J., Gima, T., Barrett, J. C., and Wake, N. (1997). Alterations of the p16INK4A gene in human ovarian cancers. *Mol. Carcinog.* 18, 134–141.
165. Niederacher, D., Yan, H. Y., An, H. X., Bender, H. G., and Beckmann, M. W. (1999). CDKN2A gene inactivation in epithelial sporadic ovarian cancer. *Br. J. Cancer* 80, 1920–1926.
166. Schultz, D. C., Vanderveer, L., Buetow, K. H., Boente, M. P., Ozols, R. F., Hamilton, T. C., and Godwin, A. K. (1995). Characterization of chromosome 9 in human ovarian neoplasia identifies frequent genetic imbalance on 9q and rare alterations involving 9p, including CDKN2. *Cancer Res.* 55, 2150–2157.
167. Schuyer, M., van, S., I., Klijn, J. G., Burg, M. E., Stoter, G., Henzen-Logmans, S. C., Foekens, J. A., and Berns, E. M. (1996). Sporadic CDKN2 (MTS1/p16ink4) gene alterations in human ovarian tumours. *Br. J. Cancer* 74, 1069–1073.
168. Shih, Y. C., Kerr, J., Liu, J., Hurst, T., Khoo, S. K., Ward, B., Wainwright, B., and Chenevix-Trench, G. (1997). Rare mutations and no hypermethylation at the CDKN2A locus in epithelial ovarian tumours. *Int. J. Cancer* 70, 508–511.
169. Ryan, A., Al-Jehani, R. M., Mulligan, K. T., and Jacobs, I. J. (1998). No evidence exists for methylation inactivation of the p16 tumor suppressor gene in ovarian carcinogenesis. *Gynecol. Oncol.* 68, 14–17.
170. Shigemasa, K., Hu, C., West, C. M., Clarke, J., Parham, G. P., Parmley, T. H., Korourian, S., Baker, V. V., and O'Brien, T. J. (1997). p16 overexpression: a potential early indicator of transformation in ovarian carcinoma. *J. Soc. Gynecol. Investig.* 4, 95–102.
171. Kamijo, T., Weber, J. D., Zambetti, G., Zindy, F., Roussel, M. F., and Sherr, C. J. (1998). Functional and physical interactions of the ARF tumor suppressor with p53 and Mdm2. *Proc. Natl. Acad. Sci. USA* 95, 8292–8297.
172. Lincet, H., Poulain, L., Remy, J. S., Deslandes, E., Duigou, F., Gauduchon, P., and Staedel, C. (2000). The p21(cip1/waf1) cyclin-dependent kinase inhibitor enhances the cytotoxic effect of cisplatin in human ovarian carcinoma cells. *Cancer Lett.* 161, 17–26.
173. Masciullo, V., Sgambato, A., Pacilio, C., Pucci, B., Ferrandina, G., Palazzo, J., Carbone, A., Cittadini, A., Mancuso, S., Scambia, G., and Giordano, A. (1999). Frequent loss of expression of the cyclin-dependent kinase inhibitor p27 in epithelial ovarian cancer. *Cancer Res.* 59, 3790–3794.
174. Sui, L., Tokuda, M., Ohno, M., Hatase, O., and Hando, T. (1999). The concurrent expression of p27(kip1) and cyclin D1 in epithelial ovarian tumors. *Gynecol. Oncol.* 73, 202–209.
175. Worsley, S. D., Ponder, B. A., and Davies, B. R. (1997). Overexpression of cyclin D1 in epithelial ovarian cancers. *Gynecol. Oncol.* 64, 189–195.
176. Session, D. R., Lee, G. S., Choi, J., and Wolgemuth, D. J. (1999). Expression of cyclin E in gynecologic malignancies. *Gynecol. Oncol.* 72, 32–37.
177. Yu, Y., Xu, F., Peng, H., Fang, X., Zhao, S., Li, Y., Cuevas, B., Kuo, W. L., Gray, J. W., Siciliano, M., Mills, G. B., and Bast, R. C. J. (1999). NOEY2 (ARHI), an imprinted putative tumor suppressor gene in ovarian and breast carcinomas. *Proc. Natl. Acad. Sci. USA* 96, 214–219.
178. Mok, S. C., Chan, W. Y., Wong, K. K., Muto, M. G., and Berkowitz, R. S. (1996). SPARC, an extracellular matrix protein with tumor-suppressing activity in human ovarian epithelial cells. *Oncogene* 12, 1895–1901.
179. Mok, S. C., Chan, W. Y., Wong, K. K., Cheung, K. K., Lau, C. C., Ng, S. W., Baldini, A., Colitti, C. V., Rock, C. O., and Berkowitz, R. S. (1998). DOC-2, a candidate tumor suppressor gene in human epithelial ovarian cancer. *Oncogene* 16, 2381–2387.
180. Abdollahi, A., Godwin, A. K., Miller, P. D., Getts, L. A., Schultz, D. C., Taguchi, T., Testa, J. R., and Hamilton, T. C. (1997). Identification of a gene containing zinc-finger motifs based on lost expression in malignantly transformed rat ovarian surface epithelial cells. *Cancer Res.* 57, 2029–2034.
181. Schultz, D. C., Vanderveer, L., Berman, D. B., Hamilton, T. C., Wong, A. J., and Godwin, A. K. (1996). Identification of two candidate tumor suppressor genes on chromosome 17p13.3. *Cancer Res.* 56, 1997–2002.

PART II

DIAGNOSTIC PROCEDURES AND NEW APPROACHES

C H A P T E R

12

Diagnostic Tests for Evaluation of Ovarian Function

MICHAEL ZINGER

Department of Obstetrics and Gynecology
University of Cincinnati
Cincinnati, Ohio 45267

JAMES H. LIU

Department of Reproductive Biology
University Hospitals of Cleveland
Case Western Reserve University
Cleveland, Ohio 44106

I. INTRODUCTION

With the important exception of tumor detection, diagnosis of ovarian disorders relies on hormonal evaluation rather than ovarian imaging. Techniques of tumor detection are discussed in detail elsewhere and, thus, this chapter will primarily focus on evaluation of benign ovarian conditions. History and physical exam are important initial clues to abnormalities in ovarian function since the body serves as a bioassay for ovarian steroid hormones. The hormonal milieu can be further defined through immunoassay hormone measurements and, in some cases, response to pharmaceutical stimulation.

II. AMENORRHEA

Primary amenorrhea is the absence of menarche by age sixteen. If a lack of menarche is accompanied by a failure to develop any secondary sexual characteristics then a diagnosis of primary amenorrhea is made at age fourteen. Secondary amenorrhea is the cessation of menses for the length of at least three menstrual cycle intervals or six months. In either primary or secondary amenorrhea, investigation of potential causes is indicated. There are three possible categories for the underlying etiology: (1) a primary ovarian dysfunction, (2) inappropriate neuroendocrine regulation of the ovaries, or (3) a defect in the genital outflow tract. Figure 12.1 illustrates the diagnostic pathway for evaluation of amenorrhea.

In addition to obtaining a pregnancy test, the initial evaluation consists of completing a history and physical exam of the patient. The absence of secondary sexual characteristics should prompt measurement of serum follicle stimulating hormone (FSH). An elevated FSH in this situation suggests gonadal dysgenesis, indicating the need for karyotype analysis (see Chapter 3). A chromosomal abnormality is particularly likely when short stature is present. In contrast, if amenorrhea is first noted after age 40 then evaluation of ovarian failure may be the initial step (see Section III).

Often, the reason for amenorrhea is not initially clear and then measurement of both TSH and prolactin is indicated. If these measurements do not reveal an endocrinologic abnormality, the next step is a progestin challenge test, consisting of a 10-day course of medroxyprogesterone 10 mg orally each day. This determines whether the uterus has been sufficiently exposed to estrogen. A positive response, i.e., vaginal bleeding beginning a few days following completion of this course, is diagnostic of ovarian anovulation, a feature of polycystic ovarian syndrome (PCOS). If long-standing anovulation has been present, an endometrial biopsy is warranted due to the risk of endometrial

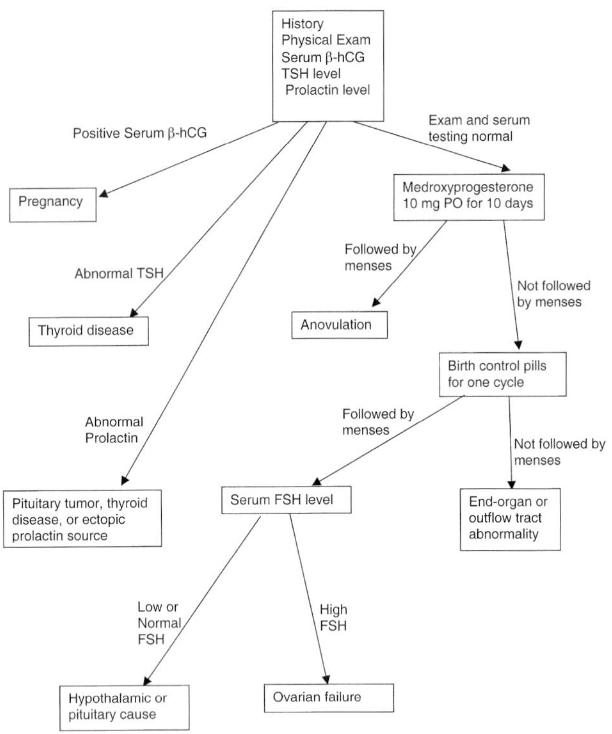

FIGURE 12.1 Evaluation of amenorrhea.

hyperplasia developing during this state of unopposed estrogen stimulation.

A negative response, i.e., failure to develop a withdrawal bleed, indicates the need for an estrogen-progestin challenge. This can be accomplished by prescribing a one-month course of oral contraceptive pills. A positive response to the estrogen-progestin challenge, following a negative response to progestin alone, indicates the absence of estrogen production. In this case, an FSH level is necessary to exclude ovarian failure (see Section III). The FSH concentration may be falsely lowered by the estrogen-progestin challenge; therefore, it is essential to wait two weeks following the last dose prior to measuring FSH. A low or normal FSH result following a negative response to the progestin challenge test is diagnostic of a hypothalamic or pituitary cause of amenorrhea.

If response to the estrogen-progestin challenge is also negative then an end-organ or outflow tract abnormality is suspected. The uterine and vaginal anatomy should be carefully evaluated for obstruction of the outflow tract or scarring of the endometrial cavity.

III. DIAGNOSIS OF OVARIAN FAILURE

Decline of ovarian function begins before birth and inevitably results in ovarian failure and menopause. When ovarian failure occurs prior to age 40, it is classified as premature and requires further investigation (see Chapter 13). At any age, a random FSH value over 40 IU/L is diagnostic of ovarian failure. Average menopausal FSH concentrations are commonly 50–100 IU/L. The elevated gonadotropin level results from a lack of ovarian hormones exerting negative feedback on the pituitary gland. Although a serum estradiol concentration is not necessary for the diagnosis, it should be below 50 pg/ml in the setting of ovarian failure. The concurrent use of oral contraceptives or hormone replacement therapy will suppress FSH levels, potentially masking the laboratory diagnosis of ovarian failure.

A random FSH level is indicated when the diagnosis of menopause is equivocal. This category includes patients that have undergone hysterectomy without oophorectomy and develop menopausal symptoms or reach an age where menopause would be likely. Additionally, ovarian failure may be suspected in younger patients that develop amenorrhea and hypoestrogenic symptoms or have a negative response to a progestin withdrawal test (see Section II).

IV. EVALUATION OF OVARIAN RESERVE

The term ovarian reserve has been used to describe the aggregate features of oocyte quantity and quality. These parameters begin to decline long before ovarian failure and menopause. The concept of ovarian reserve is important to consider in the assessment of reproductive potential and these terms are often used interchangeably.

The simplest method of assessing ovarian reserve is based on age, as it typically declines during the late 30s and more rapidly by the early 40s. However, there are significant individual variations in the onset of this decline and a more accurate assessment of ovarian reserve is needed.

Assisted reproductive technology (ART), such as *in vitro* fertilization (IVF), has spurred research in assessing ovarian reserve because this information is crucial in deciding if expense and effort should be expended in pursuing ART with the patient's own oocytes or with donor oocytes. Thus, most recent advancements in ovarian reserve assessment have been primarily studied in the setting of predicting ART success. Many studies of ovarian reserve testing have used end point measures of ovarian response to controlled ovarian hyperstimulation with exogenous gonadotropins as surrogate markers of ovarian reserve. Measures, such as peak serum estradiol concentration and number of oocytes retrieved, are expected to be positively associated with successful treatment outcome, however, difference in pregnancy rates often does not reach statistical significance. Although, it seems these methods should be applicable to predicting ovarian reserve for non-ART infertility treatments, in most cases this is unproven.

A. Basal Hormone Profile

Basal FSH level is traditionally determined on day 3 of the menstrual cycle, counting from the first day of uterine bleeding. A greater production of FSH in the anterior pituitary gland is symptomatic of inadequate production of inhibitory hormones, particularly inhibin B and estradiol, by the maturing cohort of ovarian follicles in the first few days of the follicular phase. Much of ovarian reserve testing is based on the theory that the ability of the follicles to produce these hormones is reflective of the reproductive potential of the oocytes recruited during that particular cycle.

An elevated basal FSH has been clearly shown to be prognostic of decreased likelihood of pregnancy success in IVF.[1] Furthermore, in studying almost 1500 cycles, basal FSH was shown to be a stronger predictor than age for response to ovarian stimulation as well as for the likelihood of ART resulting in an ongoing pregnancy.[2]

Unfortunately, there is not adequate standardization for FSH assays. Most assays in the U.S. today provide results in terms of the World Health Organization Second International Reference Preparation (IRP). However, these assay kits are using an estimate of the second IRP, since this preparation has not been available for years. In fact, there are significant differences in FSH results obtained for aliquots of the same serum sent to different institutions.[3] Therefore, it is crucial that each institution establish its own normative values. Typically, a sharp decrease in fertility potential will be noted with FSH levels greater than 10–17 IU/L on day 3 of the menstrual cycle.

This basal FSH measurement remains useful following unilateral oophorectomy. Although FSH concentration has been noted to be 42% higher in age-matched patients with one versus two ovaries, this FSH level accurately represents a significantly lower clinical pregnancy rate with ART.[4]

The predictive value of FSH concentration is contingent upon the timing of its measurement. Normally, the third day of the menstrual cycle represents the basal state. However, in older women the follicular phase becomes accelerated and, by cycle day three, the serum concentrations of estradiol and inhibin B have already begun to rise above their basal levels.[5] This may result in a normal-appearing day three FSH level despite a decreased ovarian reserve. This situation can be evaluated by concomitant determination of the estradiol concentration on day three. In patients with normal basal FSH, a basal serum estradiol concentration of greater than 60 pg/ml[6] to 80 pg/ml [7] is associated with significantly increased risk of poor response to ovarian stimulation. As expected, older patients with poor response are likely to have higher estradiol levels, suggesting a predisposition toward a shortened follicular phase as an early sign of decreased ovarian reserve in this group. However, it is interesting that younger patients with poor ovarian response are more likely to have lower estradiol levels.[7]

Inhibin B is a promising candidate for use in evaluation of ovarian reserve. Women with inhibin B concentrations of at least 45 pg/ml have almost seven times the likelihood of achieving pregnancy during an ART cycle compared to women with lower concentrations.[8] Additional research has suggested that inhibin B measurement may identify patients with declining ovarian reserve before they develop an elevation in basal FSH.[9] However, other investigators have disputed the usefulness of inhibin B measurement.[10] Whether inhibin B or FSH is ultimately determined to be a better marker of ovarian reserve depends on which ovarian products are best correlated to the reproductive potential of the oocyte: inhibin B or an aggregate of the other regulators of FSH secretion. The inhibin B level is not recommended as a diagnostic modality until this issue is resolved. Furthermore, inhibin B assays are expensive and should be considered investigational at this time.

There is some evidence that basal luteinizing hormone (LH) measurement is positively correlated with ovarian response to stimulation during ART.[7] However, sensitivity and specificity for this test have not been determined and are likely low as serum levels of LH are highly variable due to its pulsatile production and short serum half-life. Basal serum LH testing is not recommended as an indicator of ovarian reserve.

B. Clomiphene Citrate Challenge Test (CCCT)

Clomiphene citrate (CC), a partial estrogen receptor antagonist, blocks the negative feedback of estrogen on the hypothalamic-pituitary axis, leaving regulation of FSH release primarily to inhibin B. As noted above, inhibin B is an excellent predictor of ART outcome.[8] Thus, it follows that measuring FSH serum concentration following a course of CC during the follicular phase may improve the sensitivity of ovarian reserve testing.

The CCCT can be used to supplement day three FSH and estradiol testing. Clomiphene citrate 100 mg daily should be administered on days 5–9 of the cycle in which basal FSH was measured. Serum FSH concentration is again assessed on cycle day ten.

Unlike most ovarian reserve studies, which examine ART outcomes, two investigations have explored the value of the CCCT in predicting the pregnancy outcome of infertility patients not undergoing ART. Navot *et al.* found that among 51 unexplained infertility patients with normal day three hormone profiles, about one-third were identified by an elevated day ten FSH concentration as having a significantly decreased chance of attaining pregnancy.[11] Scott *et al.* analyzed CCCT testing in 588 infertility patients after excluding those with sperm abnormalities, moderate, or severe endometriosis, or pelvic adhesive disease.[12] An FSH concentration of greater than 10 IU/L on either day three or day ten of the CCCT cycle was considered to be an abnormal result. He found that 48.5% of patients with normal CCCT results achieved pregnancy without ART compared to 4.8% of patients with abnormal CCCT results. A comparison of the sensitivity of the CCCT to that of a simple basal FSH test was not feasible from the reported data. It is notable that an abnormal CCCT result predicted significantly lower pregnancy rates even after adjustment for age. Interestingly, age was also independently predictive of pregnancy rate among patients with a normal CCCT result.[12]

Alternate criteria for the CCCT were proposed by Loumaye *et al.*[13] The CCCT result was considered abnormal if the sum of day two and day ten FSH was above 26 IU/L. These criteria were demonstrated to be predictive of ovarian response to stimulation in ART cycles.

In amenorrheic women, once pregnancy is excluded, progestin withdrawal may be utilized to produce a menses to time drug administration for the CCCT.[14] An appropriate method of progestin withdrawal for this purpose is a 10-day, oral course of medroxyprogesterone acetate 10 mg daily. A menses would be expected two to five days following completion of this therapy and the first day of bleeding would then represent cycle day one for the purpose of the CCCT.

C. Indications for Ovarian Reserve Testing

A couple is considered to have infertility if they have not achieved pregnancy after one year of unprotected intercourse. The degree of urgency in initiation of the infertility evaluation depends primarily on the female partner's age as well as the couple's wishes. There is likely no harm in delaying fertility treatment by a few years in a 20-year-old patient. In contrast, the prognosis of fertility treatment is likely decreasing each month that treatment is delayed in a 39-year-old woman and initiation of the evaluation may be appropriate after only 6 months of unprotected intercourse.

The initial step in an infertility evaluation includes semen analysis and hysterosalpingogram. The issue of when to add ovarian reserve testing to the evaluation is not well established. In delineating appropriate candidates for ovarian reserve testing, it is important to keep in mind that the incidence of an abnormal CCCT result in infertility patients less then 34 years old is about 5 to 7%, whereas in patients 34–40 years old it is about 13–20%, and in patients greater than 40 years old it increases to 44%.[12] Some investigators have advocated screening all infertility patients older than 30 years and all unexplained infertility patients regardless of age with a CCCT,[14] while others recommend day three FSH measurement alone in infertile women over 30 years old and a CCCT in those over 37 years old.[15] Unexplained occurrence of irregular or infrequent menses associated with infertility is an indication for basal FSH testing at any age.

A day-3 estradiol measurement is most likely to be of value in women over 35 years old as an elevated basal estradiol has been demonstrated to predict decreased ovarian response in this group. However, most clinicians will order estradiol measurement whenever basal FSH is indicated because the additional information may increase the sensitivity of the testing at any age.

V. DETECTION OF OVULATION

Regular menses occurring every 25–32 days are highly suggestive of ovulation. However, during infertility evaluation, more definitive confirmation of ovulation becomes necessary. Several modalities are available to accomplish this.

A reliable method that is able to confirm ovulation with adequate warning to allow timing of intercourse during the same cycle is the assay for urinary LH. Kits for urine testing are widely available and are simple and reproducible enough for most patients to use at home. Testing should typically begin on the tenth day after initiation of menses and be repeated daily. If the result is positive on the first day that urine is tested, the patient may have a particularly shortened follicular phase. This can be confirmed by beginning urine testing a few days earlier during the next cycle. The test must be noted to change from negative to positive from one day to the next to detect an LH surge indicative of imminent ovulation.

Ovulation occurs at 34–36 h after the onset of the LH surge and 10–12 h after the LH peak.[15] Since sperm is known to remain viable within the female reproductive tract for days but the ability of the oocyte to be fertilized seems to be limited to a matter of hours after ovulation, intercourse on the day of a positive urine LH test is advisable. Repeating intercourse two days later is often recommended in case the urine LH was detected at the beginning of the LH surge.

Serum progesterone testing, although an excellent test of ovulation, is rarely necessary, given the ease and accuracy of LH urine testing. Serum progesterone should be drawn at the midluteal point, day 21 of a 28-day cycle, because this is when serum progesterone should be at its greatest concentration. A concentration of greater than 3 ng/ml indicates that ovulation has taken place. Endometrial biopsy is able to reliably demonstrate ovulation has occurred by showing progesterone's secretory effect on the endometrium. However, it is too invasive and expensive to be recommended as a routine test for ovulation.

The simplest method of confirming ovulation is to take advantage of progesterone's ability to induce an increase in the hypothalamic set point for basal body temperature.

Patients are given a graph with temperature on the Y-axis and the date along the X-axis. They are then asked to determine their temperature orally in the morning as soon as possible after waking with a special basal body temperature thermometer. A biphasic pattern of this temperature graph is confirmatory of ovulation. Specifically, an ovulatory woman should have a 0.6 °F rise in the basal body temperature beginning no more than two weeks prior to menses and lasting for at least ten days. The day of temperature rise is the approximate cycle day of ovulation. To maximize their chances of conception in future cycles, the couple can be advised to have intercourse every other day from five days before to five days after the expected rise in basal body temperature.[16]

All of the methods discussed above provide presumptive evidence of ovulation. For definitive documentation of ovulation, serial pelvic ultrasonography of the decrease in ovarian follicle size indicates follicle collapse that occurs with ovulation. In general, the developing dominant follicle that induces an LH surge to occur will ovulate, luteinize, and begin to produce an increasing amount of progesterone. An exception to this process, known as luteinized unruptured follicle, is a sporadic phenomenon that has not been found to recur consistently within any given patient.[17] Estimations of incidence range from 4[17] to 25%[18] of cycles in normal women. This phenomenon is more common in women with endometriosis[19] or infertility.[18] Since its occurrence in one cycle does not predict recurrence in future cycles, routine testing is not recommended.

VI. DIAGNOSIS OF LUTEAL PHASE DEFICIENCY (LPD)

After ovulation, the follicle is transformed into a corpus luteum. This new structure produces progesterone, the key hormone of the luteal phase. Adequate progesterone production is crucial for preparing the endometrium for implantation and the successful establishment of pregnancy. With inadequate progesterone production, the necessary secretory transformation of the endometrium will be incomplete and implantation may fail, resulting in infertility. Alternatively, insufficient transformation of the endometrium could also result from improper endometrial response to circulating progesterone. The diagnosis of LPD involves two approaches, each with their individual shortcomings: (1) analysis of the end-organ effect or (2) determination of serum progesterone concentration.

The target-tissue effects are evaluated by timed endometrial biopsy. An endometrial biopsy should be performed in the late part of the luteal phase, several days before the next menses is expected to occur. Utilizing criteria that have been described used since 1950, the endometrium is dated based on a normal 28-day cycle.[20] The actual cycle day, later determined retrospectively by setting the first day of the following menstrual period as day 28, should correspond with the histologic dating. A discordance of more than two days is considered diagnostic of LPD. Because LPD, diagnosed by these criteria, is consistently present in only about half of affected women, it is recommended that this procedure be repeated during two different cycles before a definitive diagnosis is made. If only one cycle demonstrates LPD than biopsy in a third cycle is suggested.[21]

Many clinicians are reluctant to perform two endometrial biopsies on each patient that is assessed for LPD because of the expense, delay in treatment, and discomfort to the patient. Furthermore, there are serious concerns regarding the reproducibility of histologic dating. When the same experienced observer was asked to date the same biopsy during two separate sessions the results were different by at least one day in 76% of cases and were different by greater than two days in 10% of cases.[22]

Given the disadvantages of endometrial biopsy, attention has turned toward serum progesterone measurement for the diagnosis of LPD. The rationale of this approach is that the majority of etiologies of LPD occur at or before the level of the corpus luteum and thus only impact the endometrium through decreased progesterone production. However, uterine factors, such as inadequate progesterone receptors, have also been shown to play a role in at least some cases of LPD.[23] In support of a role for uterine factors, there does not seem to be a correlation between abnormally low midluteal serum progesterone and out of phase endometrial biopsies.[24] Alternatively, this discordance may be due to the known inaccuracies of histologic dating. One study has indicated that a midluteal progesterone concentration greater than 10 ng/ml is associated with increased fecundity.[25] There has been debate regarding how many luteal phase progesterone measurements are necessary. Compared with daily testing throughout the luteal phase, a single progesterone concentration of less than 10 ng/ml, measured 4–11 days after ovulation, has a sensitivity of 82% and a specificity of 81% to detect a decrease in luteal progesterone. Changing the timing of measurement closer to the middle of the luteal phase improves the sensitivity marginally, and taking the average value of three random days during this period increases the sensitivity to 100%, while maintaining a specificity of about 80%.[26]

Determination of the length of the luteal phase, using either urine LH testing or a basal body temperature (BBT) chart, has not been found to be predictive of either endometrial biopsy results or of progesterone levels and thus is no longer recommended as a diagnostic modality for LPD.[24,26]

Testing for LPD defect should be considered in cases of unexplained infertility, or recurrent pregnancy loss, although many clinicians limit diagnostic testing to infertile women with shortened cycles or vaginal spotting of blood prior to menses. In determining which testing modality to utilize it should be kept in mind that both approaches have limitations and that a single serum progesterone measurement is approximately one-third the price of endometrial biopsy and produces much less discomfort for the patient. Given the lack of a practical test for LPD, many clinicians will opt to forgo testing and treat patients empirically with progesterone supplementation during the luteal phase if LPD is suspected.

VII. EVALUATION OF PCOS

This syndrome derived its name from the typical presence of multiple follicles in affected ovaries. Ultrasound criteria for PCOS have been arbitrarily defined as greater than ten to twelve small (<10 mm in diameter) follicles per ovary. Only 54[27] to 66%[28] of affected women have polycystic appearing ovaries on ultrasound, while 23% of normal women have polycystic ovaries on ultrasound.[29] Therefore, ultrasound may not be a useful diagnostic modality for this syndrome. The 1990 NIH-NICHD consensus conference determined that criteria for PCOS should be based on clinical features of hyperandrogenism and/or anovulation, while hormone assays should be used to exclude other conditions that may result in these features.[30] More recently, a number of researchers have evaluated the utility of hormone assays for the diagnosis of PCOS.

Increased serum LH concentration, particularly an increased ratio of serum LH to FSH, is believed to play a role in the pathophysiology of PCOS, therefore diagnostic tests based on these values have been considered. Unfortunately, much of the increased LH activity noted in PCOS is due to an increase in the bioactivity of the hormone and bioactivity is not specifically measured by routine LH assays.[31] Radiometric assays of total rather than of bioactive LH trend toward higher levels in PCOS patients, but most studies do not show a significant difference compared to controls.[27, 28, 31] The same is true of measurements of the LH/FSH ratio.[31]

In contrast, some researchers have found usefulness in measuring LH and FSH concentrations. Morales *et al.* documented a significant increase in both LH level (22.5–31.4 IU/l versus 11.3–14.3 IU/l) and the LH/FSH ratio (2.3–3.8 versus 1.0–1.1) in women with PCOS compared to controls.[32] A possible reason for this finding may have been standardization of blood draws in the fasting state and during the early follicular phase in regularly cycling controls. Koskinen *et al.* found that, out of 29 controls, none had an LH/FSH ratio greater than 1.3, while approximately 85% of the PCOS patients had results above 1.3.[33] In clinical use, the more commonly used cutoff value for the LH/FSH ratio has been 2.0.

Physical features of hyperandrogenism, such as hirsutism and acne, are among the diagnostic criteria of PCOS. A total serum testosterone concentration of greater than 72 ng/dl was found to be 97% specific although only 70% sensitive for the diagnosis of PCOS.[33] However, other researchers claim that only 36% of PCOS patients exhibit any clear laboratory evidence of hyperandrogenemia.[28] Despite the questionable efficacy of these tests in diagnosing PCOS, it is, nonetheless, important to assess serum concentrations of testosterone and possibly dehydroepiandrosterone sulfate (DHAS) in women with hirsutism, as another, pathologic source of androgen production may be revealed. This will be discussed in Section VIII.

Insulin resistance has been noted to be more prevalent in patients with PCOS. This difference has been documented on the basis of significantly higher insulin levels in response to a glucose challenge in obese PCOS patients compared to obese controls. This has led to speculation that baseline serum testing for insulin and glucose may be useful in making the diagnosis of PCOS. Unfortunately, neither the fasting insulin level nor a fasting insulin/glucose ratio is significantly different between patients with PCOS and weight-matched controls.[34, 35] Other studies from Legro *et al.* demonstrate that the fasting glucose insulin rates is a useful predictor of insulin resistance [see Reference 35a].

Metformin therapy has been adopted by many clinicians as a method of decreasing serum insulin levels. When successful, this treatment induces a decrease of hyperandrogenism and a return of regular menses. Metformin's lack of effectiveness in some patients has led to a search for a predictor of an individual patient's response to treatment. Two laboratory findings that have been shown to be predictive of response to metformin therapy are higher insulin level and lower androstenedione level.[36] Unfortunately, neither test has sufficient predictive value to recommend its use in screening candidates for metformin therapy.

VIII. EVALUATION OF HYPERANDROGENISM

The most serious cause of hyperandrogenism is an androgen-producing tumor of the ovary or the adrenal gland. A history of hirsutism, increased muscle mass, and temporal balding developing over a short time course should increase suspicion of an androgen-producing tumor. A total serum testosterone concentration greater than 200 ng/dl should prompt imaging of the ovaries and adrenal glands in search of an androgen-producing tumor. This threshold value correctly identifies 84% of patients with androgen-producing ovarian tumors and the finding of an adnexal mass on physical exam would identify a majority of the other 16%. It is interesting that tumor size does not correlate with serum testosterone level, as some of the smallest tumors produce some of the highest concentrations of testosterone.[37] Figure 12.2 illustrates the diagnostic scheme for evaluation of an androgen-producing tumor.

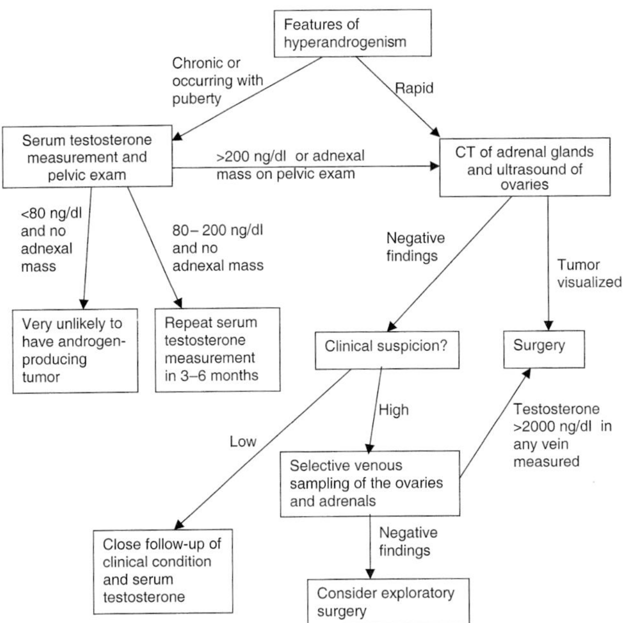

FIGURE 12.2 Screening for androgen-producing tumor.

Transvaginal ultrasonography is the preferred method for imaging the ovaries while CT scan is preferred for the adrenal glands. A strong clinical suspicion with negative imaging studies may require selective venous sampling of the ovaries and adrenal glands to determine the specific source of the excess androgens. This procedure should only be performed by a radiologist experienced in the technique. Ovarian venous testosterone concentrations greater than 2,000 ng/dl with a central to peripheral gradient will be present on the side of an androgen-producing tumor in 83% of cases.[37]

Although it has been noted that the majority of patients with a peripheral testosterone concentration >200 ng/dl will be found to have benign disease, a level of 200 ng/dl continues to be widely accepted as the threshold for implementing a search for an androgen-producing tumor.[38] Testosterone levels below this range but above 80 ng/dl should be followed with repeat testing in 3–6 months.[39] There is no added benefit to measuring free testosterone in this setting.

There is controversy regarding the need for serum DHAS levels in the evaluation of hyperandrogenic symptoms. Levels greater than twice normal may signal an adrenal tumor and should prompt imaging of the adrenal gland using CT scanning.[39] However, such elevated levels of DHAS would likely lead to high serum testosterone concentration through peripheral conversion. Thus, a testosterone level alone may be adequate to screen for both ovarian and adrenal androgen-producing tumors.[40]

Screening for late-onset 21-hydroxylase (21-OHase) deficiency, the most common form of adrenal hyperandrogenism, is also a necessary part of the evaluation of hyperandrogenism, regardless of menstrual pattern. A deficiency in this enzyme causes accumulation of its substrate, 17-hydroxyprogesterone (17-OHP). This accumulation is most notable when stimulation of the adrenal cortex by ACTH is maximal, in early morning. Sampling should be avoided during the luteal phase as the corpus luteum produces a significant amount of 17-OHP. In oligo- or amenorrheic patients, a concurrent progesterone measurement will reveal whether the patient is in the luteal phase. A follicular phase 17-OHP level, drawn between 8 and 10 a.m., of less than 200 ng/dl has been thought to exclude the diagnosis of 21-OHase deficiency,[41] although an occasional patient may be missed by this method alone.[42] A level above this threshold confers a positive predictive value of 12[43] to 80%[41]; an ACTH-stimulation test is necessary for definitive diagnosis. Concurrent use of any glucocorticoid medications could cause a false-negative result in unstimulated testing.

Pharmacological hyperstimulation of the adrenal cortex exaggerates the accumulation of 17-OHP, producing a more discriminating test. A shortened form of ACTH, the ACTH (1–24) analog (Cortrosyn, Organon, Orange, NJ), is ideal for this purpose since 0.1 mg administered intravascularly over 60 sec achieves the maximum biologic activity in normal controls without the antigenicity of natural ACTH.[44] All patients with 21-OHase deficiency will have a 17-OHP concentration greater than 1000 ng/dl 60 min following administration of 0.25 mg of synthetic ACTH.[42, 43] Results appear to be unaffected by varying the dose of ACTH from 0.1–1.0 mg, or by varying the time of day when the test is conducted.[44] Some patients that arc heterozygous for a 21-OHase mutation may have results in the lower end of the positive range and may need to be distinguished by genetic studies.[45]

IX. DIAGNOSIS OF OVARIAN REMNANT SYNDROME

Uncommonly, during bilateral oophorectomy, a small fragment of one or both ovaries may be unintentionally left behind. If the oophorectomy is technically difficult and it is suspected that ovarian tissue was not completely removed, postoperative serum FSH measurement is indicated. As with ovarian failure, an FSH concentration greater than 40 IU/l is diagnostic of absent ovaries. The FSH measurement should be delayed postoperatively for two weeks to allow FSH concentrations to reach maximal levels.[46]

If not noted intraoperatively, this complication may later be suggested by complaints of chronic pelvic pain, particularly when the oophorectomy was performed to treat endometriosis. Pelvic ultrasound may be attempted, however, ovarian remnants are often not visualized due to either their small size or to the distortion of pelvic anatomy that may result from the surgery. Measurement of serum FSH is again indicated in this situation.

When FSH levels are equivocal then a gonadotropin releasing hormone agonist stimulation test may be indicated. Leuprolide acetate, 1 mg per day, may be given subcutaneously for three days. Following this regimen, patients with functional ovarian tissue will typically exhibit an increase in serum estradiol of two- to threefold.[47] Giving CC has also been proposed. It may stimulate follicle formation and thus facilitate imaging of the ovarian remnant by ultrasound as well as localization during surgical removal of the remnant.[48] Treatment of ovarian remnant syndrome may require re-operation or low-dose pelvic radiation to eliminate viable ovarian tissue.

References

1. Scott, R. T., Toner, J. P., Muasher, S. J. *et al.* (1989). Follicle-stimulating hormone levels on cycle day 3 are predictive of in vitro fertilization outcome. *Fertil. Steril.* 51(4), 651–654.
2. Toner, J. P., Philput, C. B., Jones, G. S. *et al.* (1991). Basal follicle-stimulating hormone level is a better predictor of in vitro fertilization performance than age. *Fertil. Steril.* 55(4), 784–791.
3. Hershlag, A., Lesser, M., Montefusco, D. *et al.* (1992). Interinstitutional variability of follicle-stimulating hormone and estradiol levels. *Fertil. Steril.* 58(6), 1123–1126.
4. Khalifa, E., Toner, J. P., Muasher, S. J. *et al.* (1992). Significance of basal follicle-stimulating hormone levels in women with one ovary in a program of in vitro fertilization. *Fertil. Steril.* 57(4), 835–839.
5. Klein, N. A., Battaglia, D. E., Fujimoto, V. Y. *et al.* (1996). Reproductive aging: Accelerated ovarian follicular development associated with a monotropic follicle-stimulating hormone rise in normal older women. *J. Clin. Endocrinol. Metab.* 81(3), 1038–14045.
6. Evers, J. L., Slaats, P., Land, J. A. *et al.* (1998). Elevated levels of basal estradiol-17beta predict poor response in patients with normal basal levels of follicle-stimulating hormone undergoing in vitro fertilization. *Fertil. Steril.* 69(6), 1010–1014.
7. Frattarelli, J. L., Bergh, P. A., Drews, M. R. *et al.* (2000). Evaluation of basal estradiol levels in assisted reproductive technology cycles. *Fertil. Steril.* 74(3), 518–524.
8. Seifer, D. B., Lambert-Messerlian, G., Hogan, J. W. *et al.* (1997). Day 3 serum inhibin-B is predictive of assisted reproductive technologies outcome. *Fertil. Steril.* 67(1), 110–114.
9. Seifer, D. B., Scott, R. T., Jr., Bergh, P. A. *et al.* (1999). Women with declining ovarian reserve may demonstrate a decrease in day 3 serum inhibin B before a rise in day 3 follicle-stimulating hormone. *Fertil. Steril.* 72(1), 63–65.
10. Creus, M., Penarrubia, J., Fabregues, F. *et al.* (2000). Day 3 serum inhibin B and FSH and age as predictors of assisted reproduction treatment outcome. *Hum. Reprod.* 15(11), 2341–2346.
11. Navot, D., Rosenwaks, Z., and Margalioth, E. J. (1987). Prognostic assessment of female fecundity. *Lancet.* 2(8560), 645–647.
12. Scott, R. T., Opsahl, M. S., Leonardi, M. R. *et al.* (1995). Life table analysis of pregnancy rates in a general infertility population relative to ovarian reserve and patient age. *Hum. Reprod.* 10(7), 1706–1710.
13. Loumaye, E., Billion, J. M., Mine, J. M. *et al.* (1990). Prediction of individual response to controlled ovarian hyperstimulation by means of a clomiphene citrate challenge test. *Fertil. Steril.* 53(2), 295–301.
14. Scott, R. T., Leonardi, M. R., Hofmann, G. E. *et al.* (1993). A prospective evaluation of clomiphene citrate challenge test screening of the general infertility population. *Obstet. Gynecol.* 82(4), 539–544.
15. Barbieri, R. L. (1999). Infertility. *In* "Reproductive Endocrinology: Physiology, Pathophysiology, and Clinical Management," 4th ed. (S. S. C. Yen, R. B. Jaffe, and R. L. Barbieri eds.), pp. 562–593. W. B. Saunders Co., Philadelphia, PA.
16. Wilcox, A. J., Weinberg, C. R., and Baird, D. D. (1995). Timing of sexual intercourse in relation to ovulation. Effects on the probability of conception, survival of the pregnancy, and sex of the baby. *N. Engl. J. Med.* 333(23), 1517–1521.
17. Kerin, J. F., Kirby, C., Morris, D. *et al.* (1983). Incidence of the luteinized unruptured follicle phenomenon in cycling women. *Fertil. Steril.* 40(5), 620–626.
18. Bateman, B. G., Kolp, L. A., Nunley, W. C., Jr. *et al.* (1990). Oocyte retention after follicle luteinization. *Fertil. Steril.* 54(5), 793–798.
19. Kaya, H., and Oral, B. (1999). Effect of ovarian involvement on the frequency of luteinized unruptured follicle in endometriosis. *Gynecol. Obstet. Invest.* 48(2), 123–126.
20. Noyes, R. W., Hertig, A. T., and Rock, J. (1950). Dating the endometrial biopsy. *Fertil. Steril.* 1(1), 3–25.
21. Balasch, J., Vanrell, J. A., Creus, M. *et al.* (1985). The endometrial biopsy for diagnosis of luteal phase deficiency. *Fertil. Steril.* 44(5), 699–701.
22. Li, T. C., Dockery, P., Rogers, A. W. *et al.* (1989). How precise is histologic dating of endometrium using the standard dating criteria? *Fertil. Steril.* 51(5), 759–763.
23. Laatikainen, T., Andersson, B., Karkkainen, J. *et al.* (1983). Progestin receptor levels in endometria with delayed or incomplete secretory changes. *Obstet. Gynecol.* 62(5), 592–595.
24. Nakajima, S. T., Molloy, M. H., Oi, R. H. *et al.* (1994). Clinical evaluation of luteal function. *Obstet. Gynecol.* 84(2), 219–221.
25. Hull, M. G., Savage, P. E., Bromham, D. R. *et al.* (1982). The value of a single serum progesterone measurement in the midluteal phase as a criterion of a potentially fertile cycle "ovulation" derived form treated and untreated conception cycles. *Fertil. Steril.* 37(3), 355–360.
26. Jordan, J., Craig, K., Clifton, D. K. *et al.* (1994). Luteal phase defect: The sensitivity and specificity of diagnostic methods in common clinical use. *Fertil. Steril.* 62(1), 54–62.
27. Ehrmann, D. A., Rosenfield, R. L., Barnes, R. B. *et al.* (1992). Detection of functional ovarian hyperandrogenism in women with androgen excess. *N. Engl. J. Med.* 327(3), 157–162.
28. van Santbrink, E. J., Hop, W. C., and Fauser, B. C. (1997). Classification of normogonadotropic infertility: Polycystic ovaries diagnosed by ultrasound versus endocrine characteristics of polycystic ovary syndrome. *Fertil. Steril.* 67(3), 452–458.
29. Polson, D. W., Adams, J., Wadsworth, J. *et al.* (1988). Polycystic ovaries—a common finding in normal women. *Lancet.* 1(8590), 870–872.
30. Dewailly, D., Cortet-Rudelli, C., and Deroubaix-Allard, D. (1997). Definition, clinical manifestations, and prevalence of PCOS. *In* "Androgen Excess Disorders in Women," (R. Azziz, J. E. Nestler, and D. Dewailly, eds.), pp. 259–68. Lippincott-Raven Publishers, Philadelphia, PA.
31. Fauser, B. C., Pache, T. D., Hop, W. C. *et al.* (1992). The significance of a single serum LH measurement in women with cycle disturbances: Discrepancies between immunoreactive and bioactive hormone estimates. *Clin. Endocrinol.* 37(5), 445–452.
32. Morales, A. J., Laughlin, G. A., Butzow, T. *et al.* (1996). Insulin, somatotropic, and luteinizing hormone axes in lean and obese women with polycystic ovary syndrome: Common and distinct features. *J. Clin. Endocrinol. Metab.* 81(8), 2854–2864.
33. Koskinen, P., Penttila, T. A., Anttila, L. *et al.* (1996). Optimal use of hormone determinations in the biochemical diagnosis of the polycystic ovary syndrome. *Fertil. Steril.* 65(3), 517–522.
34. Morin-Papunen, L. C., Vauhkonen, I., Koivunen, R. M. *et al.* (2000). Insulin sensitivity, insulin secretion, and metabolic and hormonal parameters in healthy women and women with polycystic ovarian syndrome. *Hum. Reprod.* 15(6), 1266–1274.

35. Arthur, L. S., Selvakumar, R., Seshadri, M. S. *et al.* (1999). Hyperinsulinemia in polycystic ovary disease. *J. Reprod. Med.* 44(9), 783–787.
35a. Legro, R. S., Finegood, D., and Dunaif, A. (1998). A fasting glucose to insulin ratio is useful measure of insulin sensitivity in women with polycystic ovary syndrome. *J. Clin. Endocrinol. Metab.* 83, 2694–2698.
36. Moghetti, P., Castello, R., Negri, C. *et al.* (2000). Metformin effects on clinical features, endocrine and metabolic profiles, and insulin sensitivity in polycystic ovary syndrome: A randomized, double-blind, placebo-controlled 6-month trial, followed by open, long-term clinical evaluation. *J. Clin. Endocrinol. Metab.* 85(1), 139–146.
37. Meldrum, D. R., and Abraham, G. E. (1979). Peripheral and ovarian venous concentrations of various steroid hormones in virilizing ovarian tumors. *Obstet. Gynecol.* 53(1), 36–43.
38. Friedman, C. I., Schmidt, G. E., Kim, M. H. *et al.* (1985). Serum testosterone concentrations in the evaluation of androgen-producing tumors. *Am. J. Obstet. Gynecol.* 153(1), 44–49.
39. Rebar, R. W. (1999). Practical evaluation of hormonal status. *In* "Reproductive Endocrinology: Physiology, Pathophysiology, and Clinical Management," 4th ed. (S. C. C. Yen, R. B. Jaffe, and R. L. Barbieri, eds.), pp. 709–747. W.B. Saunders Co., Philadelphia, PA.
40. Speroff, L., Glass, R. H., and Kase, N. G. (1999). "Clinical Gynecologic Endocrinology and Infertility," 6th ed. Lippincott Williams & Wilkins, Baltimore, MD.
41. Azziz, R. and Zacur, H. A. (1989). 21-Hydroxylase deficiency in female hyperandrogenism: Screening and diagnosis. *J. Clin. Endocrinol. Metab.* 69(3), 577–584.
42. Fiet, J., Gueux, B., Gourmelen, M. *et al.* (1988). Comparison of basal and adrenocorticotropin-stimulated plasma 21-deoxycortisol and 17-hydroxyprogesterone values as biological markers of late-onset adrenal hyperplasia. *J. Clin. Endocrinol. Metab.* 66(4), 659–667.
43. Azziz, R., and Dewailly, D. (1997). Diagnosis, screening, and treatment of nonclassic 21-hydroxylase deficiency. *In* "Androgen Excess Disorders in Women," (R. Azziz, J. E. Nestler, and D. Dewailly, eds.), pp. 181–192. Lippincott-Raven Publishers, Philadelphia, PA.
44. Azziz, R., Bradley, E., Jr., Huth, J. *et al.* (1990). Acute adrenocorticotropin-(1-24) (ACTH) adrenal stimulation in eumenorrheic women: Reproducibility and effect of ACTH dose, subject weight, and sampling time. *J. Clin. Endocrinol. Metab.* 70(5), 1273–1279.
45. New, M. I., Lorenzen, F., Lerner, A. J. *et al.* (1983). Genotyping steroid 21-hydroxylase deficiency: Hormonal reference data. *J. Clin. Endocrinol. Metab.* 57(2), 320–326.
46. Monroe, S. E., Jaffe, R. B., and Midgley, A. R., Jr. (1972). Regulation of human gonadotropins. 13. Changes in serum gonadotropins in menstruating women in response to oophorectomy. *J. Clin. Endocrinol. Metab.* 34(2), 420–422.
47. Scott, R. T., Beatse, S. N., Illions, E. H. *et al.* (1995). Use of the GnRH agonist stimulation test in the diagnosis of ovarian remnant syndrome. A report of three cases. *J. Reprod. Med.* 40(2), 143–146.
48. Kaminski, P. F., Sorosky, J. I., Mandell, M. J. *et al.* (1990). Clomiphene citrate stimulation as an adjunct in locating ovarian tissue in ovarian remnant syndrome. *Obstet. Gynecol.* 76(5), 924–926.

CHAPTER

13

Premature Ovarian Failure

LISA KOLP

Department of Gynecology and Obstetrics
Johns Hopkins Medical Institution
Baltimore, Maryland 21287

I. INTRODUCTION

Premature ovarian failure (POF) is an ovarian disorder of diverse etiologies characterized by amenorrhea, elevated serum gonadotropins, and hypoestrogenemia in women less than 40 years of age. It affects approximately 0.1% of women by the age of 30 and 1% of women by the age of 40.[1, 2]

Historically women with amenorrhea and elevated gonadotropins have been considered to have premature *menopause* implying total depletion of their oocytes and therefore no potential for resumption of ovarian function. Goldenberg in 1973 [3] reported that virtually no follicles remained in the ovaries from women who had a serum FSH of >40 IU/l. Although there had been case reports of menstrual function and even pregnancies after the diagnosis of premature menopause, it was Rebar in 1982 [4] who first clearly documented residual ovarian function in many of these women. For that reason, the term premature ovarian *failure* is now preferred and some even recommend the term hypergonadotropic amenorrhea which carries no prognostic implications.

Although important progress has been made in the past twenty years toward a better understanding of the causes of premature ovarian failure and its long-term prognosis, many questions remain with respect to the ideal management of these women. The purpose of this review is to provide the clinician with guidance in answering the following questions:

1. How did this happen?
2. What is the appropriate work-up for these women?
3. What is their potential for fertility and pregnancy?
4. What is the appropriate long-term follow-up?

II. ETIOLOGY OF PREMATURE OVARIAN FAILURE

Series of women with secondary amenorrhea and symptoms suggestive of menopause were published in the 1950s but it required the availability of gonadotropin measurements to truly distinguish the cases of premature ovarian failure. De Moraes-Ruehsen and Jones reviewed premature ovarian failure in 1967 with the intent of helping the clinician distinguish those women with secondary amenorrhea who would respond to ovulation induction from those who had loss of oocytes, the "sine qua non" of premature ovarian failure.[5] Elevated gonadotropins were recognized as the essential diagnostic feature of premature ovarian failure.

While depletion of ovarian follicles was assumed to be present in all cases, even de Moraes-Ruehsen noted that, in one patient of 22, ovarian biopsy revealed the presence of primordial follicles. It is now clear that depletion of ovarian follicles occurs in many cases of ovarian failure but that, in a considerable number of cases, follicles remain but are, for some reason, unresponsive to stimulation by the elevated levels of circulating gonadotropins. The etiologies of premature ovarian failure are therefore generally divided into two groups: loss of ovarian function based on depletion of follicles and loss of ovarian function based on dysfunction of the follicles present in the ovaries (Table 13.1).

TABLE 13.1 Etiology of Hypergonadotropic Amenorrhea

Follicle depletion
Chromosomal Abnormalities
X chromosome
Monosomy X, mosaicism
Trisomy X, mosaicism
Mutations or deletions of Xq13–Xq26
Isochromosomes
Translocations involving X
Fragile X premutations
Trisomy 13, 18
Genetic Syndromes
Ataxia telangiectasia
Mutations of AIRE gene
BEPS syndrome
Perrault's syndrome
Iatrogenic
Ovarian surgery
Pelvic irradiation
Cancer chemotherapy
Metabolic
Mucopolysacchiridosis
Galactosemia
Infectious
Mumps
Shigella (?)
Malaria (?)
Deficient Initial Follicle Number
Thymic aplasia or hypoplasia
Idiopathic
Follicle Dysfunction
Autoimmune
Associated with other autoimmune conditions
Isolated (?)
Signal Defects
Gonadotropin or receptor abnormalities
Steroidogenic enzyme deficiencies
17α-hydroxylase
17-20 desmolase
Idiopathic

A. Causes of Follicle Depletion

During the fifth week of gestation in the human, primordial germ cells originating near the endoderm of the yolk sac migrate to the genital ridge. Mitosis of the oogonia occurs through the twenty-eighth week. At that point, meiosis begins, converting oogonia into primary oocytes. From the sixteenth week to about six months postpartum, oocytes invest themselves with coelomic epithelium-derived granulosa cells. A period of rapid atresia begins. Loss of up to 80% of the original number of germ cells occurs before birth.[6, 7] Either a reduced initial oocyte number or accelerated atresia of the oocytes can result in premature depletion of the ovarian follicles. Depletion of follicles may occur due to chromosomal abnormalities, metabolic conditions, infections, iatrogenic damage to the germ cells, or idiopathic (currently unexplained) causes.

1. Chromosomal Abnormalities Associated with POF

Numerous chromosomal abnormalities have been associated with POF. Many of these involve the X chromosome. Forty to fifty percent of girls with primary amenorrhea will have an X-chromosome anomaly.[2, 7, 8] Turner's syndrome (45X) is almost universally associated with ovarian failure prior to puberty although 3% have a short period of gonadal activity.[9] This is most likely due to accelerated atresia of oocytes during the fetal period because autopsies done on affected fetuses often show the presence of oocytes. Chromosomal mosaicism involving the X chromosome is frequently associated with POF, the most common ones being 45X/46XX, 46XX/47XXX. Other karyotypes associated with POF include 47 XXX, 46 XY, 45X/46XY as well as deletions of the short or long arms of X and balanced translocations involving the X chromosome. Low-level mosaicism not detected by standard banding techniques may be present in some "idiopathic" cases.[10]

As chromosome-banding techniques have become more sophisticated, the number of partial X-chromosome deletions or mutations recognized in cases of POF have increased. Careful review of the family history has revealed a familial syndrome of POF [11] in approximately 12% of cases of POF. A critical region of the X chromosome, Xq13–Xq26, has been identified. Mutations in this area are frequently identified in kindreds with familial POF.

While women with trisomy 21 seem to have normal ovarian function, trisomy 18 and 13 are often noted to have loss of ovarian follicles at necropsy.[12] A mutation on chromosome 3 is associated with the BEPS syndrome (blepharophimosis, epicanthus, ptosis syndrome) in which there is also absence of follicle development with resisance to gonadotropins and eventual loss of follicles. Mutations of chromosome 11 are associated with the ataxia telangietasia syndrome (cerebellar degeneration, oculomotor dysfunction, immunodeficiency, and hypoplasia of the germ cells). The autoimmune regulator (AIRE) gene, located on chromosome 21, is linked to autoimmune polyglandular failure type 1, an autosomal recessive disorder.[7] Another rare syndrome associated with POF is Perrault's syndrome: familial, autosomal recessive POF in association with deafness.[2]

There are well-documented kindreds with familial POF in whom chromosome testing appears normal and the members are otherwise phenotypically normal. POF, in this group, seems to be inherited as a dominant trait , autosomal or X-linked, with incomplete penetrance. It can be inherited through either the maternal or paternal relatives. Perhaps a subtle gene alteration will eventually be identified to explain this heritability.[11, 13, 14]

In the early 1990s, POF was recognized as an unexpected phenotype among heterozygous carriers of the fragile X premutation. The fragile X mutation involves expansion of the CGG trinucleotide repeat in the 5′ untranslated region (UTR) of the FMR1 gene located on chromosome Xq27.3. In the normal population, the CGG repeat size is highly variable with between 6–54 repeats and stably inherited. An expansion of this area to over 200 repeats is called a "full mutation." This mutation causes the fragile X syndrome which is X-linked, dominant with incomplete penetrance. Affected males have mental retardation. When the UTR of the FMR1 gene has between 60–200 repeats, the term premutation is used since premutated alleles are subject to expansion when passed from carrier to offspring. Therefore, a female carrier of the fragile X premutation is at increased risk for a male child with the fragile X syndrome.[11, 15, 16]

The incidence of fragile X premutations among women with POF is not completely clear but may be significant. In one series in which 148 women with POF were screened for the premutation, 2 of 122 with sporadic POF and 5 of 26 (19%) with familial POF showed the fragile X permutation.[15] In another large series, 760 women were studied. Of 395 premutation carriers, 16% had menopause prior to the age of 40 compared with 0 of 128 with the full mutation and 0.4% of 237 noncarriers.[17] Interestingly, the full mutation does not seem to carry the risk of POF. In another study, elevated follicular phase serum FSH concentrations were noted in women with the premutation who were still ovulating.[18] It may be especially important to recognize this etiology in women who hope to conceive or who consider using a relative for an egg donor because of the risk of a child with the full mutation.

2. Metabolic Conditions Associated with POF

There are rare conditions associated with POF including mucopolysacchiridosis in which follicle depletion is believed to be due to accumulation of some toxic substance within the ovary.[9] Similarly, galactosemia is associated with POF. Galactosemia is due to a deficiency of the enzyme galactose-1-phosphate uridyl transferase (GALT). This is a rare autosomal recessive disorder characterized by mental retardation, cataracts, hepatocellular and renal damage, and POF. [2, 4, 6, 9] While many of these girls have primary amenorrhea, most experience ovarian failure shortly after puberty.[6] The initial picture may be one of follicle dysfunction followed eventually by follicle depletion. The mechanism is not known but the excess galactose-1-phosphate, galactose, and galactriol may result in modifications of the carbohydrate moieties on the gonadotropins or have direct toxic effects on the oocytes. In an interesting rat model, it was demonstrated that high maternal serum galactose concentrations inhibited migration of embryonic germ cells to the gonadal ridge resulting in a decreased size of the initial germ cell population.[9]

3. Infectious Causes of POF

Infections are rare as a cause of POF. In a retrospective review, 3.5% of women with POF reported having had varicella, shigella, or malaria prior to the onset of ovarian failure but a cause-effect relationship has not been established.[2, 6] CMV can cause an oophoritis in immunocompromised women. During epidemics of mumps, approximately 3–7% of women who are infected will develop oophoritis, which may result in POF in some. Histologically, ovarian atrophy with fibrosis and loss of follicles has been noted after mumps oophoritis.[9]

4. Iatrogenic Causes of POF

The most common causes of iatrogenic ovarian failure include ovarian surgery, pelvic irradiation, and cancer chemotherapy. Repeated surgeries for ovarian cysts or endometriomas carry a risk of POF although the risk is difficult to quantitate. Kaaijk *et al.* reported the long-term follow-up of women with polycystic ovary syndrome who had undergone unilateral oophorectomy in an attempt to restore ovulatory cycles. At the time of follow-up the women were between 39 and 53 and there was no evidence of POF in this group.[19]

Pelvic irradiation is gonadotoxic and the effects are age- and dose-related. A dose to the ovaries of <4 Gy does not usually cause permanent ovarian failure. However, doses between 5–10 Gy in women over 40 reliably cause ovarian failure. Doses over 20 Gy may be required for POF in younger women.[20] Ovarian doses of 4–5 Gy over 4–6 weeks will cause POF in about 50% and temporary cessation of ovarian function in about 50%. Eight Gy over 3 days reliably causes POF.[4] Serious and generally irreversible ovarian damage occurs in women receiving alkylating agent chemotherapy with more than 8 Gy radiation.[21]

Radiation injury to the ovaries is age- and dose-related. Prepubertal ovaries are relatively resistant. Temporary or permanent amenorrhea may occur but return of menses does not imply that the ovaries have escaped permanent damage. These women may develop ovarian failure several years later.[9] Histologically, ovaries that have been irradiated show loss of primordial and developing follicles with fibrosis and hyalinization of the stroma and vascular sclerosis.[9]

Minimization of radiation damage is possible in some cases if the ovaries can be removed from the radiation field. For women with lymphoma or cervical cancer who will receive radiation to the para-aortic nodes, the ovaries can be transposed out of the pelvis where they may receive only about 10% of the total dose of radiation.[20]

Cancer chemotherapy is another well-recognized cause of iatrogenic ovarian failure. Again the effect is dose- and age-dependent as well as agent-dependent. Alkylating agents are particularly gonadotoxic especially in women over the age of 35 years old.[20] Younger women may experience temporary amenorrhea with resumption of menses months or even years later. Resumption of menses again does not imply that the ovaries are unscathed. Histologically, the ovaries show capsular thickening, cortical stomal fibrosis, and loss of follicles or arrest of maturation.[9] In a study of 1000 women still menstruating at the age of 21 after treatment for childhood malignancy, 42% of these women experienced ovarian failure prior to the age of 32.[20]

Conditioning regimens for bone marrow transplantation typically include high doses of chemotherapy with total body irradiation. Ovarian failure is almost universal although recovery of ovarian function in a few has occurred up to seven years later with subsequent fertility. Young girls treated for aplastic anemia with bone marrow transplantation after a conditioning regimen of thoraco-abdominal irradiation with gonadal shielding more often have normal pubertal development.[22]

Newer chemotherapeutic agents and combinations may be less gonadotoxic but limited information is available about long-term effects. Recognizing that prepubertal ovaries are more resistant to chemotherapy, attempts have been made to suppress the ovaries during chemotherapy in the hope that there will be less gonadotoxicity. Oral contraceptives have been used without convincing success. GnRH agonists have been demonstrated to have some protective effects in monkey and rat models. The depletion of the pool of primordial follicles is less profound when GnRH agonists are given 2–3 weeks prior to cyclophosphamide.[20] Whether the same will occur in humans is not clear. Small, uncontrolled series seem to demonstrate some benefit 22/id. In addition, ovarian cryopreservation is being explored as a potential means of preserving reproductive function for women facing cancer treatment. While this has exciting potential, the practical aspects have not been worked out and, to date, no pregnancies have occurred from cryopreserved ovarian tissue. It is likely that autologous reimplantation of ovarian tissue will be feasible in the near future. This will not be appropriate for many women who risk harboring some malignant cells in their cryopreserved tissue. *In vitro* maturation of cryopreserved ovarian follicles is in its infancy but may eventually address the needs of this population.[23]

5. Congenital Thymic Aplasia

Girls with congenital thymic aplasia who die before puberty have no oocytes in the ovaries at autopsy. The thymus is known to be necessary for normal gonadotropin secretion and lack of normal gonadotropin secretion results in accelerated atresia of oocytes.[4, 9] In a mouse model, thymectomy in newborn mice results in follicle depletion. However, the equivalent critical time period for action of the thymus would be *in utero* in the human and therefore, thymectomy in young girls would not be expected to cause POF.[4]

6. Idiopathic Causes of Follicle Depletion

There are many cases of premature depletion of ovarian follicles that remain unexplained at this point. While some of these may represent unrecognized chromosomal abnormalities or autoimmune dysregulation (vide infra), some may be due to an initial paucity of germ cells due, for example, to a defect in germ cell migration or a genetically regulated increased rate of atresia. Further understanding of the regulation of apoptosis will likely provide explanations for some of these cases.[9]

B. Causes of Follicle Dysfunction

While many cases of POF represent cases of depletion of essentially all ovarian follicles, there are many cases in which follicles remain but are for some reason "resistant" to stimulation with gonadotropins. This has been termed the "resistant ovary syndrome." The resistant ovary syndrome is characterized by high serum gonadotropins, numerous primordial follicles on ovarian biopsy, and insensitivity of the ovaries to exogenous gonadotropins. Forty percent will present as primary amenorrhea. Sixty percent present as secondary amenorrhea, usually in the third decade.[9]

Ovarian biopsies were once advocated as part of the evaluation of POF because it was felt that it was necessary to see if any follicles remained in order to give the patient an accurate prognosis. Even with laparotomy for biopsy, the histologic sections obtained are thought to represent <1% of an ovary of normal size.[9] Women who have been found to have no follicles on biopsy have had subsequent pregnancies indicating that the prognostic value of a biopsy is questionable.[24] By ultrasound, up to 41% of women with POF have detectable follicles,[2, 25] while only an occasional woman with menopause after the age of 50 has a detectable follicle.

Clearly there are many instances of POF in which the follicles are not depleted and in which a better understanding of the causes of this follicle dysfunction has potential for inducing a remission in these women. The best-studied causes of follicle dysfunction resulting in the "resistant ovary syndrome" include autoimmune oophoritis, gonadotropin receptor and/or postreceptor defects, and enzymatic defects.

1. Autoimmune Causes of POF

The role of autoimmunity in the pathogenesis of POF remains controversial.[9] Some consider autoimmune mechanisms to be a major cause of POF while others maintain that autoimmune mechanisms have not been established except in a few specific conditions. There are several lines of evidence implicating an autoimmune mechanism. First, there is a clear association between some forms of autoimmune endocrinopathies and POF. Second, there is a high prevalence of autoantibodies in women with POF. Third, there are changes in lymphocyte subsets in women with POF. And, finally, ovarian biopsies sometime show a lymphocyte and plasma cell infiltrate around developing follicles in women with POF.[11] The histologic finding of a mononuclear chronic inflammatory cell infiltrate is typically located around developing and atretic follicles with sparing of the primordial follicles. In early cases, the infiltrate is found primarily around the theca cells while advanced cases show infiltration of the granulosa cell layer with degeneration of some granulosa cells. The infiltrate does not extend into the stroma but may be present around hilar cells. With immunocytochemical staining, the infiltrate can be shown to be made up of polyclonal B cells, T4- and T8-positive lymphocytes, macrophages, and natural killer cells all suggestive of an antibody-dependent cell-mediated cytotoxicity.[9]

Premature ovarian failure is clearly associated with other autoimmune endocrine failure syndromes. Autoimmune polyglandular failure syndrome type I is characterized by hypoparathyroidism, adrenal failure, and mucocutaneous candidiasis and generally presents in childhood. Sixty percent of affected females have POF. Type II autoimmune polyglandular failure syndrome is characterized by adrenal failure and hypothyroidism and usually presents in the 20–40 year old age group. POF is a frequent finding in this group as well.[6] Many patients with autoimmune adrenal failure have circulating IgG antibodies directed against steroid-synthesizing cells of the adrenal. These antibodies crossreact with steroid-synthesizing cells of the ovary and can be found localizing to the hilar cells, developing follicle and theca cells of the corpus luteum.[9] These steroid-synthesizing cell antibodies (SCA) are organ-specific autoantibodies that react against a microsomal antigen common to steroid-producing cells of different tissues. They are found in 60% of women with Addison's disease and secondary amenorrhea and 95% of women with Addison's disease and primary amenorrhea. Forty percent of women with SCA and Addison's disease will develop POF in 10–15 years.[6] They are rarely found in women with POF without Addison's disease or in normal women.

The existence of an autoantibody directed against the ovary that is distinct from SCA is in doubt.[26] Autoantibodies to 3β-hydroxysteroid dehydrogenase are rare in POF.[27] While some patients with POF and adrenal failure have antibodies directed against 21-hydroxylase, 17α-hydroxylase, or P450 side chain cleavage enzyme, patients with idiopathic POF alone did not have these anti-enzyme antibodies.[6] Likewise, antibodies to the zona pellucida have been described in women with unexplained infertility and inoculation with zona pellucida proteins in some species will lead to follicle dysfunction and depletion. This antibody does not seem to play a role in human POF.[6] A specific IgG antibody that blocks the GnRH receptor has been described in two patients with POF and myasthenia gravis. In addition, IgGs from some patients with POF inhibit FSH-induced synthesis of DNA in the granulosa cells. These last two examples have used non-human gonadotropin receptors in the experimental model. Using a recombinant human gonadotropin receptor, Anasti was unable to demonstrate an IgG capable of inhibiting receptor activity in 38 women with POF.[6]

Ten percent of patients with Addison's disease will develop ovarian failure. Generally these women have SCA antibodies present. Approximately 3% of women with POF will be found to have polyglandular autoimmune failure. In type I polyglandular autoimmune failure the POF is usually diagnosed after the onset of the Addison's disease. In type II, the POF is frequently diagnosed prior to the Addison's disease.[26] This has important implications in the long-term follow-up of women with POF.

Another clear-cut autoimmune etiology of POF is associated with chronic mucocutaneous candidiasis. Anti-candida antibodies crossreact with ovarian follicular cells and can cause an autoimmune oophoritis.[9]

Some have suggested that women with multiple failed attempts at IVF because of "poor response" may have occult POF. In one study 10 of 131 such women had elevated early follicular serum FSH. Approximately 50% also had autoantibodies to adrenal, thyroid, or ovary. In the same study, 1 in 13 normal women was found to have serum antibodies that reacted with theca, thyroid, and microsomal antigens.[28]

In women with apparently idiopathic POF (no history of ovarian surgery, chemotherapy, or radiation), 10 of 24 with normal karyotypes had a positive antinuclear antibody (ANA) screen, while 0 of 8 with abnormal karyotypes had a positive ANA. Ten of 13 of the women who had POF prior to age 30 had positive ANA while none of the 11 who had POF after the age of 30 had a positive ANA. No other autoantibodies were detected in these women.[29]

Many small retrospective or observational studies have demonstrated a high prevalence of other autoimmune disorders in women with POF including especially hypothyroidism but also myasthenia gravis, Crohn's disease, vitiligo, pernicious anemia, systemic lupus, and rheumatoid arthritis. In addition, remissions of POF have been reported after treatment with corticosteroids for adrenal failure, myasthenia gravis, systemic lupus, and polyglandular autoimmune failure.[6] Plasmapheresis and thymectomy in patients with myasthenia gravis and intravenous immunoglobulin therapy in a patient with autoimmune polyglandular failure have also been associated with remissions in POF.[6]

Antiovarian antibodies have been demonstrated by a variety of methods. Some investigators have used human ovary to demonstrate antibodies by indirect immunofluorescence. In one study, serum from a variety of women was tested against normal human ovarian tissue. Fourteen of 27 women with POF showed immunofluorescence compared with 0 of 24 age-matched controls ($p<0.001$) and 1 of 22 postmenopausal women ($p<0.01$). Five of 17 women with autoimmune diseases had immunofluorescence ($p<0.01$ versus controls).[30] This method is cumbersome. More recently, ELISA assays have been used to demonstrate antibodies using ovarian antigens or proteins as substrate. Using these methods, antiovarian antibodies have been demonstrated in 10–69% of women with POF but also in a significant number of normal women.[6, 31] The correlation between the presence of the antibodies and the severity or chronology of the ovarian failure is poor. Antiovarian antibodies may be pathogenic or may represent epiphenomena secondary to antigen release after cellular damage. On the other hand, the presence of the antibodies may be transient, present early, and absent in the later stages of ovarian failure. In 215 ovarian biopsies reported over 30 years and reviewed by Anasti,[6] 11% had evidence of lymphocytic oophoritis. Seventy-eight percent of those with histologic evidence of oophoritis had SCA.

The presence of antiovarian antibodies does not prove that they are causing an autoimmune oophoritis. They can be present in Addison's disease due to tuberculosis and are also associated with neoplasia of the endometrium, kidney, bladder, or ovary. They have not been shown to be complement-binding or cytotoxic.[9]

To summarize confusing literature, there is a clear-cut relationship between the SCA frequently present in Addison's disease and POF. In addition, anti-candida antibodies have been shown to cause oophoritis. In other clinical situations, the relationship of the autoimmune condition and the ovarian failure is not as clear. Many women with POF have associated autoimmune conditions and many have circulating autoantibodies but how the apparent dysregulation of their immune systems impacts their ovarian function is not clear. The association with autoimmune conditions does have implications for the long-term follow-up of these women.

2. Abnormalities of the Gonadotropin Receptor

In theory, abnormalities of the gonadotropin receptor could produce the clinical picture of hypergonadotropic amenorrhea. Nine women with mutations in the gene for the FSH receptor have been described. The condition is inherited as an autosomal recessive and heterozygous carriers have normal fertility. Ovarian biopsies in homozygous affected women showed primordial follicles. There was variable development of secondary sexual characteristics.[2] A Finnish kindred has been described with a mutation on chromosome 2p involving the FSH receptor gene. The receptors have normal affinity but are decreased in number. This mutation has not been demonstrated in the English, French, or American populations.[7] Similarly, women with mutations in the gene for the LH receptor have amenorrhea, normal secondary sexual development, and moderately elevated serum FSH concentrations. Ovarian biopsies in these women show primordial, preantral, and antral follicles without evidence of dominant follicle formation or ovulation.[2] Other receptor or postreceptor defects could exist.[4]

In a study of 21 women with POF with normal karyotypes, attempts to demonstrate significant deletions or mutations in the FSH receptor gene did not reveal any "causative mutations."[32]

3. Abnormalities of the Gonadotropins

In theory, abnormal gonadotropins with reduced biological activity could present as hypergonadotropic amenorrhea. In addition, gonadotropins with reduced biological activity could result in accelerated atresia. There are, for example, reported cases of male pseudohermaphrodites with immunologically active but biologically inactive LH. These patients would be expected to respond normally to exogenous gonadotropins.[4]

4. Steroidogenic Enzyme Deficiencies

A deficiency in a variety of steroidogenic enzymes would be expected to produce a clinical picture of hypergonadotropic amenorrhea. Girls with a deficiency of cholesterol desmolase have no steroid hormone synthesis and rarely survive.

Deficiency of the 17α-hydroxylase enzyme impairs gonadal and adrenal function and produces a clinical picture of sexual infantilism with elevated gonadotropins as well as hypertension, hypokalemic alkalosis, and elevated serum progesterone. On ovarian biopsy, these women have large cysts and primordial follicles but no evidence of orderly follicle maturation.[2, 4] Women with 17–20 desmolase deficiency have impaired gonadal function with normal adrenal function. In both of these rare clinical syndromes, fertilizable oocytes can be obtained by assisted reproductive technologies.

Several families have been reported with an aromatase enzyme deficiency producing a clinical picture of delayed puberty, hypergonadotropic amenorrhea, and ovarian cysts.[6]

III. EVALUATION OF THE PATIENT WITH HYPERGONADOTROPIC AMENORRHEA

The differential diagnosis of hypergonadotropic amenorrhea is broad but the work-up is not complicated. It is appropriate for every woman to have a thorough evaluation on initial presentation. Being given a diagnosis of premature menopause and a prescription for hormone replacement therapy is not an adequate evaluation and does a great disservice to these women. An evaluation of hypergonadotropic amenorrhea requires a complete history and physical exam, chromosome analysis in many cases, evaluation for autoimmune disorders, and assessment of function of other endocrine organs.[2]

Table 13.2 lists the differential diagnosis and the appropriate screening or diagnostic test. In many cases, a thorough history and physical exam will provide the clinician with a diagnosis. Iatrogenic cases can be fairly easily uncovered in this way. In addition, most of the metabolic or enzymatic defects will be picked up prior to presentation with amenorrhea. It is unlikely, for example, that the practicing gynecologist will ever make the diagnosis of galactosemia based entirely on evaluation of premature ovarian failure. The important thing is to recognize the association with these syndromes with POF so that the patient and/or her family can reach some understanding of her condition.

TABLE 13.2 Differential Diagnosis of Hypergonadotropic Amenorrhea

Diagnosis	Evaluation
X chromosome abnormalities	Karyotyping
Fragile X premutation	DNA analysis for CGG repeats in FMR-1 gene
Genetic syndromes	History and physical exam
Iatrogenic	History
Metabolic	History
Infectious	History
Thymic aplasia	History
Autoimmune	
Associated with other	History, physical exam, labs: thyroid panel, B12, electrolytes, calcium, phosphorus, ACTH stimulation test, fasting glucose, rheumatoid factor
Isolated	ANA
Gonadotropin receptor defects	
Gonadotropin defects	May respond to exogenous gonadotropins
Enzyme defects	Hypertension, hypokalemia, elevated serum progesterone
17α-hydroxylase deficiency	
17-20 desmolase deficiency	

A. History

There is no typical antecedent menstrual history prior to cessation of menses in POF. Some will present with primary amenorrhea. Some will present with an abrupt cessation of menses after perfectly regular cycles and previous fertility. Some describe a more typical perimenopausal picture with oligomenorrhea prior to amenorrhea. Some will present as post-pill amenorrhea or even postpartum amenorrhea. Some will describe hot flashes but younger women frequently don't recognize hot flashes and may describe anxiety attacks or a feeling of the heart racing with sweating. A history of night sweats can often be elicited but is often not volunteered by the younger woman because she often does not realize that it is related to her presenting complaint.

The clinician should inquire carefully about a history of previous ovarian surgery, chemotherapy, or radiation. A past history of mumps or other significant infections should be sought. A past or current history of any autoimmune disease is relevant. For those with primary amenorrhea, inquire about development of secondary sexual characteristics. A family history of Addison's disease, thyroid disease, insulin-dependent diabetes mellitus, rheumatoid arthritis, Crohn's disease, vitiligo, or Sjogrens' syndrome would suggest an autoimmune etiology.

A careful review of systems should seek to elicit symptoms of hypoestrogenism as well as symptoms of other endocrine dysfunction. Symptoms suggestive of adrenal insufficiency include weight loss, anorexia, abdominal pain, weakness, increase in skin pigmentation, or salt craving. A history of premature graying can suggest hypothyroidism.[2, 4] Vitiligo is associated with autoimmune adrenal failure. Gonadotropin-producing tumors are rare in women less than 40 years but symptoms of an intracranial mass should be discussed.

B. Physical Exam

The physical exam in women with POF is most often completely normal (except for signs of hypoestrogenism).[2] The exam should include a search for signs of other associated diseases e.g., premature graying (hypothyroidism), sparse axillary and pubic hair with increased pigment in skinfolds and gums (adrenal failure), vitiligo, alopecia areata or malar rash (systemic lupus), thyroid enlargement or tenderness, and ovarian tenderness. Tanner staging should be recorded in women with primary amenorrhea.[6] Short stature might suggest Turner's syndrome which will occasionally go undiagnosed until puberty. Deafness with POF may be Perrault's syndrome.

C. Laboratory Evaluation

The diagnosis of POF should not be made until there has been at least 4 months of amenorrhea and the serum FSH has been found to be greater than 40 IU/l on at least two occasions at least one month apart. Some women will present with hot flashes and elevated serum FSH while still experiencing regular menses. This may well represent a prodromal stage of ovarian failure but in some, the symptoms will resolve and the FSH will return to normal.

A karyotype is recommended in women under thirty primarily because of the risk of gonadal tumors (gonadoblastoma and dysgerminoma) that usually present prior to the age of thirty in women with XY mosaicism. It is also appropriate to evaluate the karyotype in anyone with a family history of premature menopause or "early menopause" (prior to the age of 45).[33] Consider evaluation of the karyotype in women with younger sisters or daughters since the finding of an X-chromosome abnormality would have some prognostic significance. In addition, women who still want to try to conceive or who would consider using a relative for an egg donor should seriously consider evaluation for fragile X premutation. Fragile X premutation is now recognized with increasing prevalence in women with POF and there is a risk for a male child with fragile X syndrome and mental retardation.

The prevalence of associated autoimmune disorders is difficult to determine. It varies widely in reported series presumably due to referral patterns. In one prospective series, in 119 otherwise asymptomatic, karyotypically normal women with spontaneous POF, 22 had previously diagnosed hypothyroidism. Another 10 had abnormal thyroid function tests discovered during their evaluation for POF. Three of the 119 had previously diagnosed Addison's disease. There were no additional cases of adrenal failure discovered with ACTH stimulation tests. Two had abnormal fasting blood glucose. One had an abnormal glucose tolerance test.[34]

On the initial evaluation, a thorough search for associated autoimmune endocrine dysfunction is appropriate including: thyroid function tests, fasting blood glucose (or glucose tolerance test if there is a positive family history of diabetes), serum calcium, phosphorus, B-12, and electrolytes. Screening for evidence of systemic autoimmune dysfunction with ANA, sedimentation rate, and rheumatoid factor may be appropriate on the initial evaluation as well.[4] An MRI to look for a gonadotropin-producing tumor would only be appropriate in women with CNS symptoms.[6]

Screening for antiovarian antibodies has limited value at this time as the finding has no prognostic or therapeutic significance. The finding of steroid cell antibodies has some prognostic significance for the development of Addison's disease. Screening for SCA is not a standard part of the evaluation at this time.

Ovarian biopsy is not indicated at this time. Biopsies have proven to be unreliable for documenting the presence or absence of residual ovarian follicles. In earlier series, approximately 11–20% of women with POF were found to have follicles on biopsy. Using transvaginal ultrasound, however, up to 60% of women with POF have visible follicles.[11, 25] Weekly measurement of serum estradiol and FSH is a more practical way to document residual ovarian function and is indicated in those who wish to conceive.

IV. POTENTIAL FOR FERTILITY AND PREGNANCY

In many women with POF, the diagnosis is particularly devastating because they have not yet had children. The diagnosis of premature menopause was previously believed to be permanent and to rule out potential for future reproduction. Rebar [4] first demonstrated convincingly that many of these women have residual ovarian function. In women with spontaneous POF and normal karyotypes, approximately 40–60% will have follicles detectable on ultrasound, approximately 50% will have at least an occasional serum estradiol greater than 50 pg/ml, and nearly 20% ovulate occasionally.[35] There have been innumerable case reports of fertility and pregnancy even many years after the diagnosis of POF. It is now apparent that many cases of POF are not permanent and that, at least in some cases, the potential for reproduction exists. The difficulty is in identifying those with potential fertility and finding ways to enhance their fertility.

The most reliable and highly successful method of achieving pregnancy in women with POF is through egg donation. In many *in vitro* fertilization programs, the success rate with egg donation is around 50% per cycle. While the child is not genetically related to the mother, it is genetically related to her partner. This option is highly acceptable to many couples especially because the woman has the chance to carry the pregnancy and can breast feed if she wishes. Interestingly, when a sister of the patient is used as the egg donor, she has a higher chance of having an elevated day 3 FSH.[36]

For those women who are unable or unwilling to pursue egg donation, the clinician can accurately counsel them that there is a 20–30% chance that they will ovulate again and about a 10% chance of conception. In one study in which 46 women with various causes of amenorrhea were followed for 10 years, 10 women had no response to a progestin challenge and an elevated serum FSH. This group presumably represented women with POF. Two of the seven women had spontaneous but sporadic menses. One had regular, cyclic menses for about 6 months, but none conceived.[37] In another reported series, the likelihood of spontaneous remission of

POF varied with the etiology. Of 16 women with a surgical etiology for their POF, 3 ovulated and 1 conceived. Of three women with chemotherapy-induced POF, one ovulated again and conceived. Of 29 women with apparently idiopathic POF, 2 ovulated and 1 conceived. Of 11 women with an autoimmune etiology, 1 ovulated but did not conceive. None of the women in this series who had had radiation therapy or who had an abnormal karyotype experienced a remission.[24]

Many of the women who have had a remission of POF over the years have been on hormone replacement therapy or corticosteroid therapy. This has led to the evolution of two primary theories to explain the remissions. These theories have guided attempts to induce remissions. Based on the finding that only developing follicles have lymphocytic infiltrates on ovarian biopsies, one approach has been to suppress follicle development in order to allow an autoimmune oophoritis to subside prior to attempted ovulation induction. By using GnRH agonists to suppress follicle development followed by gonadotropin treatment or observation, some ovulatory cycles have been documented.[38] Another approach has been to use estrogen replacement either on the theory that estrogen sensitizes the granulosa cells to FSH or on the theory that suppression of gonadotropins will relieve the down-regulation of FSH receptors and restore responsivity of the follicle to FSH.[39, 40] Again some ovulations have been noted.

van Kasteren published a literature search done to address the question of efficacy of treatment for POF.[41] Fifty-two case reports of pregnancy or return of ovulation, eight observational studies, nine uncontrolled studies, and seven controlled trials were reviewed. In all, 112 pregnancies were reported resulting in 86 healthy children (including three twin pregnancies). The overall pregnancy rate for the studies was 6.3%, varying from 1.5% in the controlled studies to 18% in the uncontrolled studies. The inclusion and exclusion criteria varied widely. Some of the women in the trials were actually oligomenorrheic, not amenorrheic. The treatment protocols used were estrogen replacement to cause suppression of the FSH, GnRH agonists followed by estrogen replacement, or GnRH agonists followed by withdrawal of treatment (FSH rebound). None of the studies showed a statistically significant difference between treatment groups. Overall there was a 5–10% chance of conceiving after diagnosis and there was no evidence that these treatments altered that outcome. Most studies did not include a control group so it is not clear whether the treatments are equally effective or equally ineffective.

Treatment with corticosteroids has not proven to be efficacious either. Corenblum [42] treated 11 women with normal karyotypes and POF with prednisone 25 mg four times per day for two weeks then followed the patients with serial serum estradiol measurement and ultrasounds. Two ovulated and conceived, one on the third spontaneous cycle after the single course of corticosteroid treatment. In another study, 36 women with POF with normal karyotypes and no history of radiation or chemotherapy were treated with dexamethasone or placebo. On the fifth day of treatment, gonadotropin treatment was started. The patients were monitored by ultrasound and serial serum estradiol measurement. Eight patients had some follicle development (four in each group) but none of them ovulated. There was a slight rise in estradiol in three in the treatment group and two in the placebo group. The study was terminated due to lack of response to treatment.[41, 43]

In every study in which there was a control group, some follicle development was noted in untreated patients. This raises the question whether the best way to promote pregnancy might be by simply monitoring for signs of spontaneous follicle development. Weekly serum estradiol measurement would be adequate to detect spontaneous follicle development. If the estradiol rises significantly, ultrasound could be used to confirm and monitor follicle growth. Whether or not augmentation of follicle growth by gonadotropins would be helpful in this paradigm remains to be studied. In one study of women with regular cycles but elevated basal FSH, follicle growth was noted to be slower with smaller maximum follicle diameter. The peak serum estradiol did not differ but the peak progesterone was lower in the group with the elevated basal FSH.[44] Whether this group of women would resemble the women with POF who have some spontaneous follicle development remains to be demonstrated. In a study reported by Rosen,[38] women were treated with GnRH agonists to suppress their FSH followed by observation versus gonadotropins. Two women in each group ovulated. The women who ovulated spontaneously had lower peak serum estradiol concentrations and midluteal serum progesterones of 4.2 and 3.6 ng/ml while the women whose cycles were stimulated with gonadotropins had midluteal progesterones of 9.2 and 9.6 ng/ml. This suggests that spontaneous ovulation in women with POF might be of poor quality and that augmentation by gonadotropins may improve the chance for conception. An appropriate clinical trial is needed to answer this question.

Spontaneous remissions after chemotherapy-induced POF have been reported. The time of remission is impossible to predict and women who do not wish to conceive should be counseled to use contraception. Even after bone marrow transplant, occasional remissions are noted up to seven years after treatment. Actuarial probability of remission at 10 years after bone marrow transplantation is almost 100% if the transplant was done before the age of 18 and about 15% if the transplant was done after the age of 18.[21]

V. LONG-TERM FOLLOW-UP

Women who are diagnosed with POF require psychological support. Unless there is a family history of POF, the diagnosis usually comes as a complete shock. Because the diagnosis should not be made on the basis of a single elevated FSH, the clinician should plan to evaluate the patient over several visits. In that way, it is easier to discuss the condition in stages: the diagnosis, what caused it, what will happen next, etc., so that questions can be answered as the woman comes to understand her diagnosis. Although the condition is frequently permanent, it is not always and that can provide some hope for a young woman who has not yet started her family. It is not appropriate to hold out false hope but neither is it appropriate to tell her that there is no hope of ever conceiving.

After the initial thorough evaluation, yearly screening should focus on the most commonly diagnosed associated conditions: thyroid disorders and diabetes mellitus. An annual TSH and fasting blood glucose are appropriate. Screening for other endocrinopathies, particularly adrenal insufficiency can be done by physical exam and review of systems and does not necessarily require annual blood work. The patient should be counseled to report symptoms of adrenal insufficiency such as weight loss, anorexia, abdominal pain, weakness, pigmentation of skin creases, etc.[34]

The patient warrants the usual annual gynecologic care including pap smears and mammograms as her history warrants. In addition, consideration must be given to hormone replacement therapy. Many women with POF are quite symptomatic from hypoestrogenism. They describe night sweats, sleep interruption, hot flashes, mood swings, irritability, headaches, and symptoms of urogenital atrophy including difficulty with intercourse. Generally these symptoms respond quickly and gratifyingly to estrogen therapy.[21]

For women with primary amenorrhea, estrogen treatment is usually started with 0.3 mg of conjugated estrogens or the equivalent for about 6 months. The dose can be increased every six months or so with the addition of cyclic progestins after about a year.

For women with secondary amenorrhea for greater than 12 months, it may also be necessary to start hormone replacement therapy gradually to avoid mastalgia. The addition of androgens is sometimes used for persistent fatigue, low energy, and lack of libido. Some women prefer to use oral contraceptives because it seems more normal to them than the use of postmenopausal hormone replacement therapy. Postmenopausal doses of hormone replacement therapy will not prevent conception if ovarian function spontaneously resumes. This is a distinction that must be kept in mind when discussing options for hormone replacement.

There can be a considerable deficit in bone density in women with primary amenorrhea since a substantial portion of the eventual bone density develops in the second and third decade. Unfortunately, there is little normative data for bone density in women in their teens and twenties. A baseline bone density study may be all the clinician has for guidance but it can be followed over time for evidence of further loss of bone or improvement in bone density. Doses of estrogen higher than the usual postmenopausal doses may be required to achieve and maintain an adequate bone density in women with POF.[36] Two-thirds of women with POF have bone density Z-scores more than one standard deviation below the mean for their age groups in spite of hormone replacement therapy. Doses of 1.25 mg of conjugated estrogens or the equivalent are usually needed to maintain adequate bone density in this group.

While the metabolic effects of POF are presumed to parallel those of natural menopause, some important differences have been noted. For example, serum HDL concentrations rise in cyclophosphamide-induced ovarian failure and bone density decreases less than expected in this setting.[20] There may be some important differences between natural menopause and POF that will be delineated with time. At this time it is prudent to follow the usual clinical practices for health maintenance in postmenopausal women.

VI. SUMMARY

The diagnosis of POF almost always comes as a shock to the patient. The clinician needs to be able to discuss with the patient the issues set forth at the beginning of this chapter.

How did this happen? Once the work-up is completed, a considerable number of women will be found with an X-chromosome anomaly. With the new information about fragile X premutations, even more women will be provided with a clear reason for their ovarian failure. The next most common cause is autoimmune. A small number will have polyglandular autoimmune failure with POF. A significant number of women will carry the uncertain diagnosis of possible isolated autoimmune ovarian failure. There is no good test at this time to substantiate that diagnosis but this is probably a valid etiology in some. The vast majority of the rest of the patients will be left with "idiopathic" as their explanation. As testing becomes more and more sophisticated, etiologies will be found for more of these women, but a substantial portion will remain unexplained.

What is the appropriate work-up? Evaluation of the chromosomes especially the X chromosome is important and will often provide valuable answers. Screening for fragile X syndrome is probably appropriate in many of these women because of the implications of this familial syndrome for offspring and siblings. Screening for associated autoimmune conditions is appropriate even if the karyotype is found to be abnormal. Thorough screening at the initial diagnosis may be prudent followed by more limited and targeted screening on annual follow-up.

What is the potential for fertility? This question is difficult to answer because there is no good test to provide the answer. Clearly some of these women have reproductive potential even after many years of hypergonadotropic amenorrhea. At this point, no specific treatment has been proven beneficial to enhance the rate of ovulation and chance of conception. However, a significant portion of these women has spontaneous follicle activity. Noninvasive monitoring for signs of follicle activity (weekly serum estradiol measurement) can be undertaken if the woman is interested in trying to conceive. There is limited information about how to enhance the follicle development but augmentation with gonadotropins followed by support of the luteal phase would be logical at this point. For women who do not ovulate or conceive, *in vitro* fertilization with egg donation has a high success rate in this group. In the future, technology that is being developed to mature immature follicles from cryopreserved ovarian tissue *in vitro* may be applicable to those women with follicles present. Those who do not wish to conceive should use contraception.

What is the appropriate long-term follow-up? Long-term follow-up needs to address the risks of hypoestrogenism such as osteoporosis and increased risk of heart disease. Hormone replacement therapy is appropriate for most of these women. Those women who express concern about the need for potentially decades of hormone replacement therapy and the possible risk of breast cancer can be reassured that the hormones in replacement therapy are very weak compared to natural hormones. In their case, the hormones are not being used to artificially prolong the time interval of hormonal exposure as we do with women who experience menopause after 50 but to provide hormones during the time when the body would normally make them. A significant number of these women will develop thyroid dysfunction. Annual screening of the TSH and fasting blood glucose is appropriate. A small number will develop a polyglandular autoimmune endocrine failure. The most important condition to detect is adrenal failure. The annual exam should search for signs and symptoms of adrenal failure. An ACTH stimulation test of adrenal function should be carried out if there is suspicion of adrenal dysfunction.

It can be difficult to manage a patient with a condition as poorly understood as POF. It is important to take the time to thoroughly evaluate her, counsel her, and provide appropriate health maintenance follow-up. After the initial shock and disappointment, with the support of a caring clinician, most of these women will come to accept their diagnosis and go on to live healthy and fulfilled lives.

References

1. Coulam, C. B., Adamson, S. C., and Annegers, J. F. (1986). Incidence of premature ovarian failure. *Obstet. Gynecol.* 67, 604–606.
2. Kalantaridou, S. N., Davis, S. R., and Nelson, L. M. (1998). Premature ovarian failure. *Endocrinol. Metab. Clin. North Am.* 27, 989–1006.
3. Goldenberg, R. L., Grodin, J., Rodbard, D., and Ross, G. (1973). Gonadotropins in women with amenorrhea. *Am. J. Obstet. Gynecol.* 116, 1003–1009.
4. Rebar, R. W. (1982). Hypergonadotropic amenorrhea and premature ovarian failure: A review. *J. Reprod. Med.* 27, 179–186.
5. de Moraes-Ruehsen, M. D., and Jones, G. S. (1967). Premature ovarian failure. *Fertil. Steril.* 18, 440–461.
6. Anasti, J. N. (1998). Premature ovarian failure: An update. *Fertil. Steril.* 70, 1–15.
7. Christin-Maitre, S., Vasseur, C., Portnoi, M. F., and Bouchard, P. (1998). Genes and premature ovarian failure. *Mol. Cell. Endocrinol.* 145, 75–80.
8. Kalantaridou, S. N., and Chrousos, G. P. (2000). Molecular defects causing ovarian dysfunction. *Ann. N. Y. Acad. Sci.* 900, 40–45.
9. Fox, H. (1992). The pathology of premature ovarian failure. *J. Pathol.* 167, 357–363.
10. Devi, A. S., Metzger, D. A., Luciano, A. A., and Benn, P. A. (1998). 45,X/46,XX mosaicism in patients with idiopathic premature ovarian failure. *Fertil. Steril.* 70, 89–93.
11. van Kasteren, Y. M., Hundscheid, R. D., Smits, A. P., Cremers, F. P., van Zonneveld, P., and Braat, D. D. (1999). Familial idiopathic premature ovarian failure: An overrated and underestimated genetic disease? *Hum. Reprod.* 14, 2455–2459.
12. Simpson, J. L., and Rajkovic, A. (1999). Ovarian differentiation and gonadal failure. *Am. J. Med. Genet.* 89, 186–200.
13. Mattison, D. R., Evans, M. I., Schwimmer, W. B., White, B. J., Jensen, B., and Schulman, J. D. (1984). Familial premature ovarian failure. *Am. J. Hum. Genet.* 36, 1341–1348.
14. Tibiletti, M. G., Testa, G., Vegetti, W., Alagna, F., Taborelli, M., Dalpra, L. *et al.* (1999). The idiopathic forms of premature menopause and early menopause show the same genetic pattern. *Hum. Reprod.* 14, 2731–2734.
15. Marozzi, A., Vegetti, W., Manfredini, E., Tibiletti, M. G., Testa, G., Crosignani, P. G. *et al.* (2000). Association between idiopathic premature ovarian failure and fragile X premutation. *Hum. Reprod.* 15, 197–202.
16. Sherman, S. L. (2000). Premature ovarian failure among fragile X premutation carriers: Parent- of-origin effect? *Am. J. Hum. Genet.* 67, 11–13.
17. Allingham-Hawkins, D. J., Babul-Hirji, R., Chitayat, D., Holden, J. J., Yang, K. T., Lee, C. *et al.* (1999). Fragile X premutation is a significant risk factor for premature ovarian failure: The International Collaborative POF in Fragile X study—preliminary data. *Am. J. Med. Genet.* 83, 322–325.
18. Murray, A., Webb, J., MacSwiney, F., Shipley, E. L., Morton, N. E., and Conway, G. S. (1999). Serum concentrations of follicle stimulating hormone may predict premature ovarian failure in FRAXA premutation women. *Hum. Reprod.* 14, 1217–1218.
19. Kaaijk, E. M., Hamerlynck, J. V., Beek, J. F., and van, D. V. (1999). Clinical outcome after unilateral oophorectomy in patients with polycystic ovary syndrome. *Hum. Reprod.* 14, 889–892.
20. Howell, S., and Shalet, S. (1998). Gonadal damage from chemotherapy and radiotherapy. *Endocrinol. Metab. Clin. North Am.* 27, 927–943.
21. Spinelli, S., Chiodi, S., Bacigalupo, A., Brasca, A., Menada, M. V., Petti, A. R. *et al.* (1994). Ovarian recovery after total body irradiation and allogeneic bone marrow transplantation: Long-term follow up of 79 females. *Bone Marrow Transplant* 14, 373–380.
22. Giorgiani, G., Bozzola, M., Cisternino, M., Locatelli, F., Gambarana, D., Bonetti, F. *et al.* (1991). Gonadal function in adolescents receiving different conditioning regimens for bone marrow transplantation. *Bone Marrow Transplant* 8 Suppl. 1, 53.
23. Posada, M. N., Kolp, L., and Garcia, J. (2001). Fertility Options for women cancer patients: Fact and fiction. *Fertil. Steril.* 75, 457–463.
24. Kreiner, D., Droesch, K., Navot, D., Scott, R., and Rosenwaks, Z. (1988). Spontaneous and pharmacologically induced remissions in patients with premature ovarian failure. *Obstet. Gynecol.* 72, 926–928.
25. Mehta, A. E., Matwijiw, I., Lyons, E. A., and Faiman, C. (1992). Noninvasive diagnosis of resistant ovary syndrome by ultrasonography. *Fertil. Steril.* 57, 56–61.
26. Betterle, C., Rossi, A., Dalla, P. S., Artifoni, A., Pedini, B., Gavasso, S. *et al.* (1993). Premature ovarian failure: Autoimmunity and natural history. *Clin. Endocrinol. (Oxf)* 39, 35–43.

27. Reimand, K., Peterson, P., Hyoty, H., Uibo, R., Cooke, I., Weetman, A. P. *et al.* (2000). 3beta-hydroxysteroid dehydrogenase autoantibodies are rare in premature ovarian failure. *J. Clin. Endocrinol. Metab.* 85, 2324–2326.
28. Cameron, I. T., O'Shea, F. C., Rolland, J. M., Hughes, E. G., de Kretser, D. M., and Healy, D. L. (1988). Occult ovarian failure: A syndrome of infertility, regular menses, and elevated follicle-stimulating hormone concentrations. *J. Clin. Endocrinol. Metab.* 67, 1190–1194.
29. Ishizuka, B., Kudo, Y., Amemiya, A., Yamada, H., Matsuda, T., and Ogata, T. (1999). Anti-nuclear antibodies in patients with premature ovarian failure. *Hum. Reprod.* 14,70–75.
30. Damewood, M. D., Zacur, H. A., Hoffman, G. J., and Rock, J. A. (1986). Circulating antiovarian antibodies in premature ovarian failure. *Obstet. Gynecol.* 68, 850–854.
31. Coulam, C. B. (1983). The prevalence of autoimmune disorders among patients with primary ovarian failure. *Am. J. Reprod. Immunol.* 4, 63–66.
32. Whitney, E. A., Layman, L. C., Chan, P. J., Lee, A., Peak, D. B., and McDonough, P. G. (1995). The follicle-stimulating hormone receptor gene is polymorphic in premature ovarian failure and normal controls. *Fertil. Steril.* 64, 518–524.
33. Vegetti, W., Grazia, T. M., Testa, G., de Laurentis, Y., Alagna, F., Castoldi, E. *et al.* (1998). Inheritance in idiopathic premature ovarian failure: Analysis of 71 cases. *Hum. Reprod.* 13, 1796–1800.
34. Kim, T. J., Anasti, J. N., Flack, M. R., Kimzey, L. M., Defensor, R. A., and Nelson, L. M. (1997). Routine endocrine screening for patients with karyotypically normal spontaneous premature ovarian failure. *Obstet. Gynecol.* 89, 777–779.
35. Kalantaridou, S. N., Braddock, D. T., Patronas, N. J., and Nelson, L. M. (1999). Treatment of autoimmune premature ovarian failure. *Hum. Reprod.* 14, 1777–1782.
36. Kalantaridou, S. N., and Nelson, L. M. (2000). Premature ovarian failure is not premature menopause. *Ann. N. Y. Acad. Sci.* 900, 393–402.
37. Davajan, V., Kletzky, O., Vermesh, M., and Anderson, D. J. (1991). Ten-year follow-up of patients with secondary amenorrhea and normal prolactin. *Am. J. Obstet. Gynecol.* 164, 1666–1670.
38. Rosen, G. F., Stone, S. C., and Yee, B.(1992). Ovulation induction in women with premature ovarian failure: A prospective, crossover study. *Fertil. Steril.* 57, 448–449.
39. Nelson, L. M., Kimzey, L. M., White, B. J, and Merriam, G. R. (1992). Gonadotropin suppression for the treatment of karyotypically normal spontaneous premature ovarian failure: A controlled trial [see comments]. *Fertil. Steril.* 57, 50–55.
40. Check, J. H., Nowroozi, K., Chase, J. S., Nazari, A., Shapse, D. *et al.* (1990). Ovulation induction and pregnancies in 100 consecutive women with hypergonadotropic amenorrhea. *Fertil. Steril.* 53, 811–816.
41. van Kasteren, Y. M., and Schoemaker, J. (1999). Premature ovarian failure: A systematic review on therapeutic interventions to restore ovarian function and achieve pregnancy. *Hum. Reprod. Update.* 5, 483–492.
42. Corenblum, B., Rowe, T., and Taylor, P. J. (1993). High-dose, short-term glucocorticoids for the treatment of infertility resulting from premature ovarian failure. *Fertil. Steril.* 59, 988–991.
43. Braat, D. D., Smits, A. P., and Thomas, C. M. (1999). Menstrual disorders and endocrine profiles in fragile X carriers prior to 40 years of age: A pilot study. *Am. J. Med.Genet.* 83, 327–328.
44. Ahmed Ebbiary, N. A., Lenton, E. A., Salt, C., Ward, A. M., and Cooke, I. D. (1994). The significance of elevated basal follicle stimulating hormone in regularly menstruating infertile women. *Hum. Reprod.* 9, 245–252.

C H A P T E R

14

Ultrasound of the Ovary

KAREN JERMY
St. Georges Hospital and Medical School
London, SW1 70QT, United Kingdom

TOM BOURNE
St. Georges Hospital and Medical School
London, SW1 70QT, United Kingdom

ABSTRACT

Transvaginal ultrasound (TVS), with or without color Doppler, provides the clinician with a noninvasive, highly sensitive method of assessing ovarian morphology. The increased availability of ultrasound has led to the more frequent detection of adnexal cystic structures. The high resolution afforded by TVS allows a morphological assessment of the mass, thus facilitating appropriate management decisions. We provide an overview of normal ovarian morphology in the pre- and postmenopausal woman, with particular emphasis on the corpus luteum and the common finding of a simple cyst in the postmenopausal woman. The impact of finding an ovarian cyst during pregnancy and in the fetus is also discussed. Transvaginal ultrasound is a significant contributor to morphological scoring systems and mathematical models, and within ovarian cancer screening programs. An overview of the characterization of adnexal masses is given, including those features commonly associated with frequently encountered ovarian cysts. Particular attention is paid to endometriomas and dermoids, as they account for over one-third of persistent adnexal masses within premenopausal women. The subjective assessment of ovarian morphology based on the characteristic ultrasonographic findings in these two types of cysts is highly predictive for their diagnosis. Finally, we address the highly debated role of color Doppler in the differentiation of benign from malignant ovarian masses.

I. INTRODUCTION

Transvaginal and transabdominal (TAS) ultrasound techniques are both established imaging modalities in the examination of the pelvic organs. They are noninvasive, cost-effective, and widely available. Using a transvaginal approach means that high frequency probes can be used, in close proximity to the pelvic organs, resulting in higher resolution images. This has led to the evolution of a wide range of applications of ultrasound within gynecology. The use of TVS is well documented in infertility and for the assessment of early pregnancy complications as well as menstrual disorders and pelvic pain. TVS has an established role in the evaluation of adnexal masses, and is integral to ovarian cancer screening programs. The increased availability of gynecological ultrasound has led to the more frequent detection of adnexal cystic structures. The overwhelming advantage of TVS, when compared with TAS, is not only the identification of adnexal masses, but also their detailed morphological assessment. This lends itself to the preoperative characterization of an adnexal mass. This is paramount if we are to make correct management decisions. Absolute certainty as to the nature of an adnexal mass can only be established after histological examination of the specimen. The ability to accurately discriminate between benign and malignant disease of the ovary preoperatively allows appropriate management. This may be expectant, under the care of the gynecological oncologist or using minimal access surgical techniques. Benign ovarian cysts are common. They are frequently asymptomatic and usually resolve spontaneously. When surgery is required, the vast majority of benign adnexal masses can be treated using laparoscopic techniques. Laparoscopy, when compared to laparotomy, has been shown to reduce hospital stay, postoperative morbidity, and recovery period, without increasing the risk of spillage of the cyst contents.[1]

Knowledge of the normal ovarian anatomy and function is a prerequisite to understanding and evaluating abnormal ovarian appearances.

This chapter will aim to deal first with normal ovarian morphology and parameters, and then proceed to the issues concerning the characterization of adnexal masses.

II. THE NORMAL OVARY

Transvaginal ultrasound has high patient acceptability,[2] doesn't require a full bladder to act as an acoustic window, and has minimal interobserver variability.[3] Ovarian dimensions predicted by TVS closely correlate with surgical findings.[4] Although TVS has surpassed TAS in the assessment of ovarian morphology, the two techniques are often used in combination. The adnexa are characteristically examined after an assessment of the cervix, uterus, and endometrium has been made. Descriptions of scanning techniques and methods are widespread. A complete evaluation of the pelvic organs must include visualization of the Pouch of Douglas and the volume and character of any fluid present noted. The ovaries are measured in three planes and the volume of the ovary is calculated according to the formula of an ellipsoid:

$$\text{ovarian volume} = 0.5 \times \text{length} \times \text{width} \times \text{breadth}.$$

The distribution and size of any follicles are noted.

In the premenopausal patient the ovaries are usually located overlying the internal iliac vessels (Fig. 14.1), lateral to the uterine fundus. They are easily recognizable due to the presence of numerous echolucent follicles of varying diameters. In the postmenopausal patient, not only is the ovary a smaller structure, but these sonographic markers are also absent.

When the ovary cannot be immediately visualized, the operator can use their other hand to press on the anterior abdominal wall, as if performing a bimanual examination. This will not only bring the ovary more into the scanning field of the vaginal probe, but also offers information as to the relative mobility of the pelvic organs, and helps localize pain, if present, to a particular structure. Alternatively shifting the patient into a different position may help bring the adnexal structures into view and help displace overlying bowel.

When an ovary is not visible using the transvaginal approach, an attempt should be made to identify it transabdominally. In the presence of large uterine leiomyomas and during pregnancy the ovaries usually become abdominal structures. Also after hysterectomy the adnexal structures may be retracted out of the pelvic view.

Normal ovarian morphology and volume is dependent upon a number of factors. Paramount is the age and menopausal status (Table 14.1) of the patient. Knowledge of how ovarian volume changes with age is essential, as ovarian volume forms the basis of most ovarian cancer screening programs. Mean ovarian volumes, based on ultrasound measurements, are fairly constant at between 6.6–6.7 cm^3 until 40 years of age. After this there is a significant decrease in ovarian volume with each decade, until the mean ovarian volume in women over 70 years is 1.8 cm^3.[5] Mean ovarian volumes in postmenopausal women vary considerably between studies,

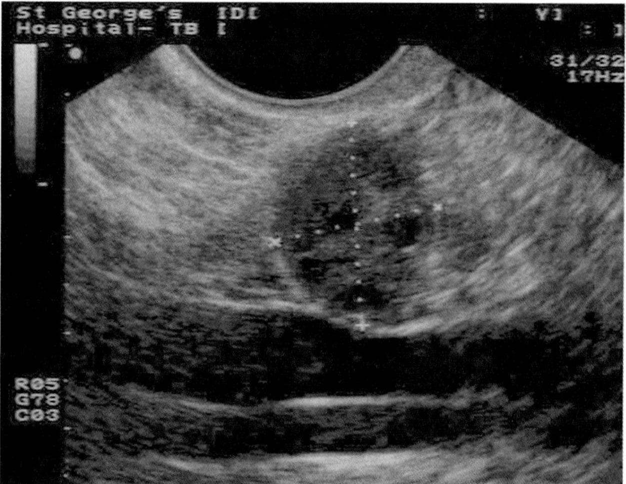

FIGURE 14.1 Normal pelvic ultrasound, demonstrating the location of the ovary overlying the internal iliac vessels.

TABLE 14.1 Ovarian Volume and Morphology Changes with Different Age Groups

Neonate	0.8 cm^3	Follicles <1 cm
2 year old	1 cm^3	Follicles <0.5 cm
Prepubertal	<2.5 cm^3	Follicles <1 cm
Postpubertal	10 $cm^3 \pm 5$ cm^3	Follicles present
Postmenopausal	↓ in size	Follicles absent[a]

[a]But up to 15% will have a simple cystic structure present.

ranging from 1.2–5.8 cm^3.[4–6, 12] No consistent relationship between weight and parity to ovarian volume has been demonstrated, although there is a statistically significant decrease in ovarian volume with exogenous estrogen use in women between 40 and 59 years (but not in older age groups).[5] This is due to the inhibition of gonadotropin production and their trophic effects on ovarian tissues by exogenous hormones, leading to a reduction in ovarian volume. Ovarian volumes persistently greater than 20 cm^3 (premenopausal) and 10 cm^3 (postmenopausal) should be a cause for concern and prompt further intervention.

A detailed history noting the day of the menstrual cycle, irregular vaginal bleeding, pelvic pain, hormonal drug use, and previous surgery will all aid the diagnosis of both ovarian normality and abnormality.

A. Premenopausal Ovarian Morphology

The premenopausal ovarian morphology is a constantly changing landscape, under the influence of the hypothalamic-pituitary axis. Knowledge of how these normal appearances vary almost each day of the ovarian cycle is important.

During the normal menstrual cycle, ovarian morphology changes on a daily basis. It is important to observe and recognize the synchrony that occurs between the ovary and endometrium. This helps us to establish the "normal" morphology we would expect at each stage during the cycle. Initial follicular growth is gonadotropin-independent, and therefore small (<5mm) follicles will be visible even in those women taking combined oral contraceptives. The dominant follicle may reach diameters of about 20 mm prior to ovulation. The follicular wall is initially well defined with a clear sharp defining edge, becoming thicker and blurred in definition as ovulation approaches. The presumed cumulus oophorus may be visualized projecting into the follicle 2–3 days prior to ovulation.

B. The Corpus Luteum

The disappearance of the dominant follicle with ovulation, results in the emergence of the corpus luteum, along with free fluid within the pouch of Douglas. The morphology of the corpus luteum will vary throughout the luteal phase, and will be predominantly cystic or solid in nature (Table 14.2). Hemorrhagic corpus lutea will demonstrate patterns of clot formation and retraction, often with fine synechiae forming a meshwork within the cyst. The internal walls of the corpus luteum may be irregular. Because of the varying morphological patterns, it can mimic a number of other pathologies, such as an ectopic gestation or an ovarian malignancy. Knowledge of the day of the menstrual cycle can aid diagnosis. If there is any doubt as to the etiology, a repeat scan in the follicular phase of a subsequent cycle will confirm resolution. Color Doppler studies of the corpus luteum (Fig. 14.2) will reflect

TABLE 14.2 The Spectrum of Corpus Luteal Morphological Characteristics

Unilocular, smooth-walled with anechoic cyst contents
Uniformly echogenic solid structure
Thick, irregular wall
Echogenic strands throughout anechoic contents
Sediment/debris present: this will move on tilting the patient

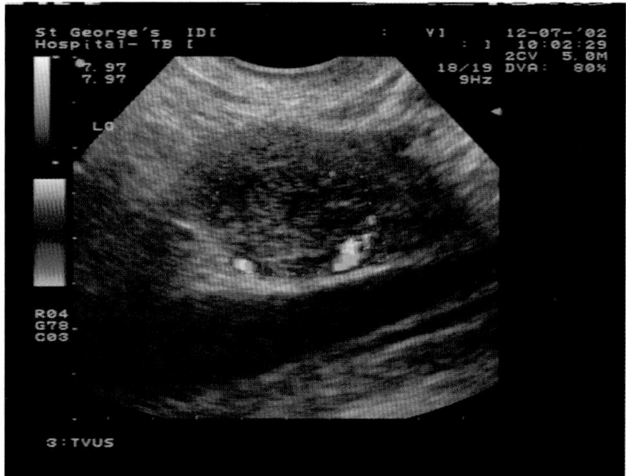

FIGURE 14.2 Color Doppler interrogation of the ovary showing the characteristic vascular pattern of the corpus luteum, a typical "ring of fire" appearance.

the neovascularization occurring as a part of normal ovarian function.[7] Detection and characterization of the corpus luteum is important in many areas of gynecology, and research into its altered morphology and vascularity in subfertility and early pregnancy complications is ongoing.

C. Polycystic Ovarian Syndrome

The polycystic ovarian syndrome (PCOS) as first described in 1935 by Stein and Leventhal, with obesity, infertility, hirsuitism, and amenorrhea, forms one extreme of the spectrum of clinical manifestations of this disorder. Up to 10% of women of reproductive age will be affected by PCOS. The diagnosis of PCOS remains the subject of much discussion and a lack of consensus remains. Originally a histological diagnosis, ultrasound currently forms the cornerstone of diagnosis, along with menstrual disturbance and hyperandrogenism or anovulation. Ovarian morphology is defined as polycystic if there are 10 or more peripheral cysts measuring 2–8 mm in diameter, typically arranged around a dense stroma ("string of pearls") (Fig. 14.3). These represent atretic subcortical follicles. The predictive value of this finding alone is not

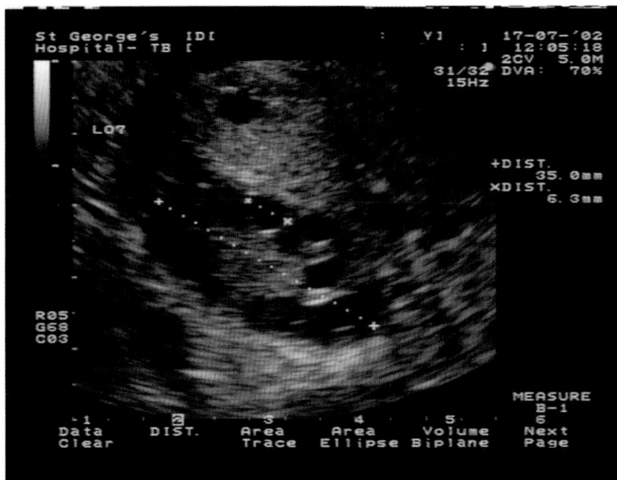

FIGURE 14.3 Polycystic ovary: Peripheral crowding of the follicles can be seen, with increased stromal density and total ovarian volume.

high; in an unselected population up to 23% of women have been shown to meet the classical ultrasound criteria historically associated with polycystic ovaries.[8] This has resulted in an attempt to refine the classification and so increase the diagnostic specificity of ultrasound in PCOS, especially in the differentiation from multifollicular ovaries. A number of studies have subjectively and objectively assessed stromal density and volumes, using TVS. These have shown that increased stromal density is frequently associated with ovarian androgenic dysfunction.[9] More applicable to routine clinical practice is the evaluation of the stromal/total area ratio taken from a standardized section. This has been shown to be significantly related to androgenic factors and is easily reproducible. Fulghesu *et al.* demonstrated 100% sensitivity and specificity in the differentiation of PCOS from multifollicular and control women based on stromal/total area ratio evaluation.[10]

D. Menopausal Ovarian Morphology

A number of ovaries will remain sonographically undetectable within the postmenopausal patient. It is widely assumed that with the use of high resolution TV probes, if an abnormality was present (in the form of a cystic lesion) then this would be detected. An inability to visualize one or both ovaries is not unusual. Studies looking at asymptomatic, healthy populations have ovarian detection rates (at least one ovary identified on TVS) of between 76 [11] and 72%.[12, 13] Two studies correlating preoperative TVS findings with pathological assessment, confirmed that sonographic nondetection of the ovary (and normal pelvic clinical examination) tends to exclude an ovarian abnormality. Fleischer *et al.* had ovarian detection rates (of at least one ovary) of 85%. The average size of ovaries not detected on TVS was 0.7×0.4 cm; most (5 out of 6) were confirmed as atrophic on pathological assessment.[14] In the study by Rodriguez *et al.*, 18% of ovaries were not visualized preoperatively and all were confirmed atrophic at histological assessment.[15]

E. The Postmenopausal Simple Ovarian Cyst

Unilocular ovarian cysts have a high prevalence within asymptomatic postmenopausal women with rates of between 3 and 17%.[16, 17] The detection of an ovarian cyst within an asymptomatic menopausal woman presents a number of dilemmas, as not only is there is an increased incidence of ovarian cancer, but the likelihood of surgery being complicated by coexistent medical conditions is also increased.

Although postmenopausal cystic activity is rarely functional in nature, the frequency of adnexal cysts in the first three years after menopause has shown to be higher than in subsequent years,[12] possibly reflecting residual ovarian activity. Spontaneous resolution will occur in up to 50% of unilocular cysts, and is unrelated to exogenous hormone use.

The risks of ovarian malignancy within a unilocular ovarian cyst, of less than 10-cm diameter, are minimal,[16, 18, 19] and the patient should be managed expectantly. Surgical intervention is warranted if the cyst wall develops irregularities or the cyst volume increases.

The most common histology of a unilocular cyst within this population is a cystadenoma. The concern is that as the natural history of ovarian cancer remains unclear, the long-term behavior of those cysts which are left *in situ* is uncertain. The degree of malignant transformation is unknown, and as such menopausal women with a simple unilocular cyst should undergo close surveillance.

F. Normal Pediatric Ovarian Morphology

The ovaries are active throughout childhood due to follicular turnover. There is continual enlargement throughout childhood, as a result of an increase in the number and size of the ovarian follicles. At approximately 8 years of age, high LH pulsatility at night results in a multifollicular appearance to the ovaries (defined on ultrasound as more than 6 follicles measuring >4 mm in diameter). Primordial follicles can be seen evenly distributed throughout the cortex by 11–12 years old. Ovulation has begun by 12–13 years old and after 14 years of age the ovary is essentially mature.

Although TVS has widespread use within gynecology it can only be used in older patients who are sexually active. A full bladder is essential for abdominal scanning and as this can be difficult in the majority of children, repeated scans throughout a session may be required.

Simple ovarian cysts are a common finding in children and adolescents. If anechoic on ultrasound, and asymptomatic in nature, expectant management in the form of serial ultrasound follow-up is recommended.

III. ABNORMAL OVARIAN PATHOLOGY

A. Characterization of Adnexal Masses

Assessment of an adnexal mass can be made using B-mode imaging alone or in conjunction with color Doppler. Although histological analysis is the only certain way of establishing the nature of a cyst, ovarian cyst characterization is central to current gynecological practice. The presence or absence of certain morphological characteristics contributes not only to the differentiation of benign from malignant, but also to the type of ovarian cyst. This latter point is important particularly when considering premenopausal women, where the background risk of malignancy is low. We will first summarize the ongoing debate of how best to discriminate between benign and malignant tumors of the ovary, and then go on to describe the morphological characteristics commonly associated with different ovarian cysts.

The subjective evaluation that any experienced ultrasonographer uses when assigning significance to particular ultrasonographic findings, such as size, echogenicity, the presence of papillary projections, and blood flow indices within an adnexal mass, has been shown to be an accurate discriminator between benign and malignant adnexal masses.[20]

Not everyone has the experience to make these decisions. Morphological scoring systems and statistical models, such as those involving multivariate logistic regression analysis and more recently artificial neural networks, have been developed, to facilitate the differentiation of benign from malignant, and in the case of mathematical models, to assign an individual "risk" of malignancy. They aim to try and mimic the processes of evaluation that occur within the mind of an experienced ultrasonographer, in assigning a risk of malignancy when presented with a number of parameters concerning a given patient or lesion.[21, 22] Considerable overlap exists between the individual ultrasonographic findings that are used to define the malignant and benign features of a mass. Initial studies set out to establish that the presence or absence of certain morphological characteristics was predictive of ovarian malignancy. Increasing complexity, in the form of locularity of the cyst, or irregularities of the cyst wall, corresponded with an increasing probability of the lesion being malignant.

1. Morphological Scoring Systems

Granberg *et al.* in 1989 demonstrated a correlation between the ultrasonographic appearance and the microscopic characteristics of a cyst.[19] Within the population studied, 296 cysts were characterized as simple and unilocular. Of these, only 1 was malignant, and this cyst was between 5–10 cm in diameter, with a macroscopically visible papillary process in a woman aged 60 years. Of the cysts with papillations 93% were malignant, and papillations were the most predictive morphological feature of malignancy, when compared to the woman's age or cyst size. There was no correlation between the size of a simple cyst and malignancy, however, increasing cyst size in complex cysts will correlate with an increased risk of malignancy.[23] It must also be remembered that a cyst size of greater than 10 cm in diameter may be difficult to characterize as a full assessment of the internal cyst wall will not always be possible due to the limited scanning field of the transvaginal probe.

An extension of initial morphological classifications was the development of scoring systems to assign a risk of malignancy to a particular mass. Sassone *et al.* developed a scoring system to allow an objective description of extrauterine pelvic disease, based on morphological characteristics.[24] In a retrospective study, they were able to differentiate benign from malignant tumors with a specificity of 83% and sensitivity of 100%. The positive and negative predictive powers were 37 and 100%, respectively. The variables studied were inner wall structure, wall thickness, septal thickness, and the echogenicity of cyst contents. Tumor size did not improve the sensitivity, and so was excluded. Benign cystic teratomas were the main cause of false-positive test results. Lerner *et al.* went onto modify this by producing a weighted scoring system including the presence or absence of acoustic shadowing, resulting in better differentiation between benign and malignant masses.[25]

Bourne *et al.* in 1993 prospectively tested the use of a morphology score as a second stage test within an ovarian cancer screening program. Its use, while significantly reducing the false-positive rate, also reduced the sensitivity to 83% from 100%.[26]

In 1990, Jacobs *et al.* proposed the risk of malignancy index (RMI) combining CA125 levels and a woman's menopausal status with sonographic morphological findings.[27] Ferazzi *et al.* went on to prospectively compare five different morphological scoring systems in order to assess the diagnostic accuracy of each system in differentiating benign from malignant adnexal masses, with a range in sensitivity of 74–88% and in specificity of 40–67%. Of note, each system maintained its diagnostic accuracy when only borderline and stage I lesions were assessed.[28]

2. Mathematical Models

More recently, mathematical models based on multivariate logistic regression analysis and artificial neural networks have been developed, with the aim of assigning an individual risk of malignancy. These are based on a statistically derived weighting system of certain ultrasonographic and demographic characteristics, rather than the arbitrary definitions of more simple morphology scores. This allows the relationship of each individual factor to be related to each other, as well as the histological diagnosis. In order to use mathematical models within routine clinical practice, a large initial data set is required.

3. Pattern Recognition

There are some lesions which can be diagnosed on the basis of "subjective impression," negating the use of complex scoring systems or models. A previous study [20] has shown that, based on subjective impression, the majority of adnexal masses are easy to characterize, with agreement between operators of varying experience in 65% of cases. Approximately 10% of cases were difficult to classify by the least experienced operators (in particular tubo-ovarian abscesses and cystadenofibromas), and it is in the classification of these cases that mathematical models should concentrate.

B. Morphological Characterization of Ovarian Cysts

The following is a summary of the salient morphological features commonly associated with the main types of ovarian cyst encountered within routine clinical practice. Classically, an adnexal mass has been described as completely cystic, mixed cystic-solid, or solid. The definitions in Table 14.3 allow clear, concise descriptions of each adnexal mass encountered to be made. This more detailed description, along with hard copy or digital image capture, allows comparisons to be made during subsequent follow-up, and to facilitate audit, research, and training. Anything other than a simple, anechoic cyst is considered complex in nature.

1. Simple Ovarian Cysts

These are thin, smoothed-walled and unilocular in nature with anechoic (sonolucent) cyst contents (Fig. 14.4). As previously mentioned, they are almost invariably benign. However, when a cyst diameter approaches and extends

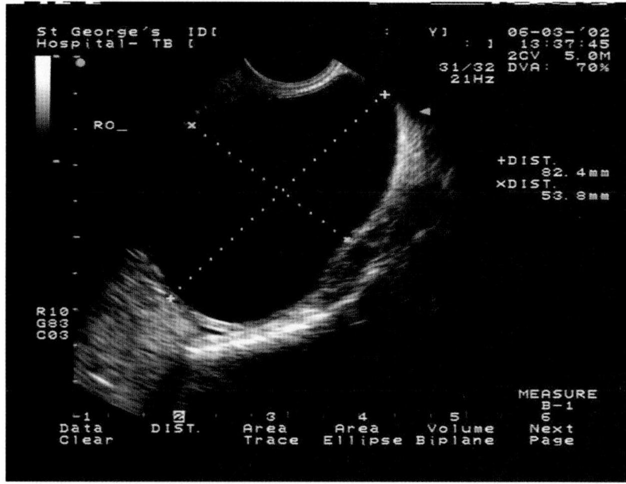

FIGURE 14.4 Transvaginal ultrasound of a simple ovarian cyst. The cyst wall is thin and regular and the cyst contents are anechoic.

beyond the range of the transvaginal probe (usually up to 8–10 cm) a complete survey of the internal wall is not possible, and "simple cyst" classification should be use with caution in these large ovarian cysts.

Physiological cysts are frequently asymptomatic and tend to resolve spontaneously. The most common within premenopausal women are follicular cysts, measuring up to 80 mm in diameter, which result from the failure of follicular fluid reabsorption. Expectant management is advised in the asymptomatic patient as a repeat ultrasound scan in the early follicular phase of a subsequent menstrual cycle should demonstrate cyst resolution. The use of hormonal manipulation to aid resolution has shown no benefit over expectant management.[29, 30] Theca lutein cysts are large, multiloculated, often bilateral cysts containing anechoic fluid. They are classically associated with ovulation induction and molar pregnancy, as a result of high circulating levels of human gonadotropin.

Persistent simple cysts tend to be serous cystadenomas. These can be large and, along with mucinous cystadenomas, form the predominant cyst type seen after menopause.

Simple adnexal cysts may also result from persistent Wolffian and Mullerian duct structures, giving rise to paratubal and paraovarian cysts. They can be large and tend to be extremely mobile, and are easily diagnosed by identifying normal adjacent ovarian morphology. Although usually an incidental finding they may predispose to ovarian or tubal torsion.

Peritoneal inclusion cysts may also mimic ovarian pathology. The patient will usually have a history of previous pelvic surgery or pelvic inflammatory disease. Morphologically the septae tend to be thin and can be seen to fluctuate within the entrapped pelvic fluid. Unusually they can be thick and vascular in nature, but will remain unchanged at subsequent examinations.

TABLE 14.3 Classification of Ovarian Cyst Morphology

Septum: strand of tissue from one wall of the cyst to the other
ocularity: defined by the presence or absence of septae
Cyst wall: thickness and regularity noted
Papillary projection: solid area of tissue projecting into the cyst cavity from the internal cyst wall
Cyst contents Anechoic Low level echogenic (mucinous tumors)

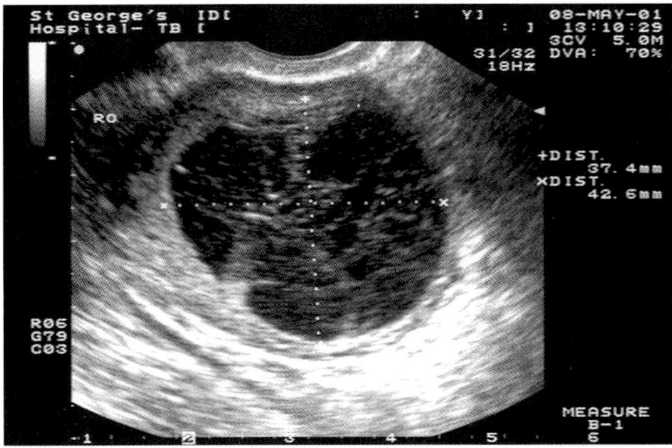

FIGURE 14.5 Transvaginal ultrasound of an ovary containing a hemorrhagic cyst. The cyst contents have a cobweb appearance as a result of fibrin deposition and clot formation.

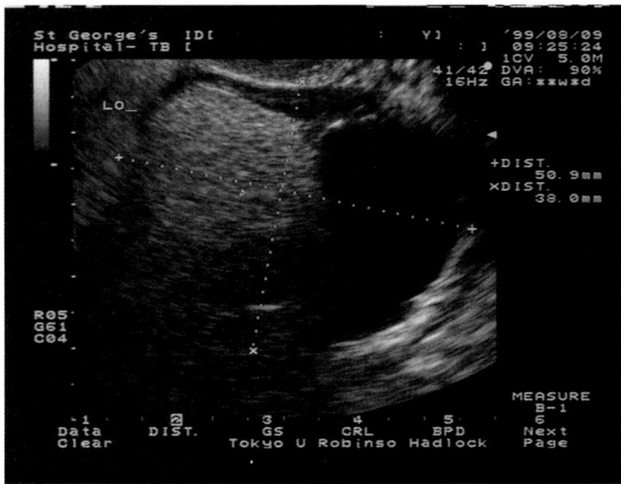

FIGURE 14.6 Transvaginal ultrasound of a dermoid ovarian cyst. The cyst contents are predominantly cystic, with posterior acoustic shadowing from the solid area; the Rokitansky protuberance.

2. Complex Ovarian Cysts

Hemorrhagic (Fig. 14.5) and corpus luteal cysts are the most common type of "complex" ovarian cyst, and their appearances have been described previously.

a. Endometriomas and Dermoids

Endometriomas and dermoid cysts account for over two-thirds of persistent adnexal masses in premenopausal women [31] and so warrant a more detailed overview. These lesions can be particularly difficult to score using morphological scoring systems and as angiogenesis is ubiquitous throughout the ovarian cycle, color Doppler is of limited value.[32] This is especially true of benign cystic teratomas and ovarian malignancy. The presence of solid components within benign cystic teratomas (Fig. 14.6) means that, in the context of morphological scoring systems, dermoids will often score as being highly suspicious of malignancy. For example, Sassone *et al.* [24] assessed the ultrasonographic characteristics of 39 histologically proven dermoids using a morphology scoring system. Of the dermoids, 32 had a score of 9 or above, representing a potentially malignant mass.

It is not only imperative to differentiate benign from malignant masses, but in a population where the background risk of ovarian malignancy is low, the characterization of benign cyst type is also important. They each have characteristic morphological patterns which aid recognition [33–35] (Tables 14.4 and 14.5) and a subjective assessment of ovarian morphology, based on characteristic ultrasonographic findings, has been shown to be highly predictive for the diagnosis of dermoids and endometriomas in a population with a low background risk of ovarian malignancy.[36]

Transvaginal ultrasonography, when used alone, can differentiate dermoids and endometriomas from other adnexal pathology with a specificity of 98 and 90%, respectively. [37, 38] The clarification of cyst type is important because the mainstay of treatment for both endometriomas and dermoids is surgical, as dermoids undergo torsion or rupture in over 10% of cases [39] and endometriomas do not respond well to medical therapy alone.[40] These rarely undergo torsion, as they are often fixed within the pelvis (Fig. 14.7), but may undergo rupture or acute hemorrhage within the cyst. Rarely they can become infected. Transvaginal ultrasonography forms the basis of the assessment of women undergoing surgery for a suspected adnexal mass. With good case selection, benign cystic teratomas can be treated laparoscopically.[41] If we can be confident in our diagnosis, patients who may

TABLE 14.4 Sonographic Characteristics of Endometriotic Ovarian Cysts

Often thick-walled
Heterogeneous, low-level echoes—"ground glass" cystic contents
May contain irregular, echogenic solid areas, representing clot (these will move on tilting the patient)
Often bilateral, may occlude pouch of Douglas if "kissing" in the midline
Other pelvic structures may be fixed

TABLE 14.5 Sonographic Characteristics of Ovarian Dermoid Cysts

Can be predominantly cystic or uniformly dense
Discrete, highly echogenic focus, with posterior acoustic shadowing (Rokitansky protuberance)
Fine, short echogenic bands within the cystic component (representing hair)
Fat-fluid level

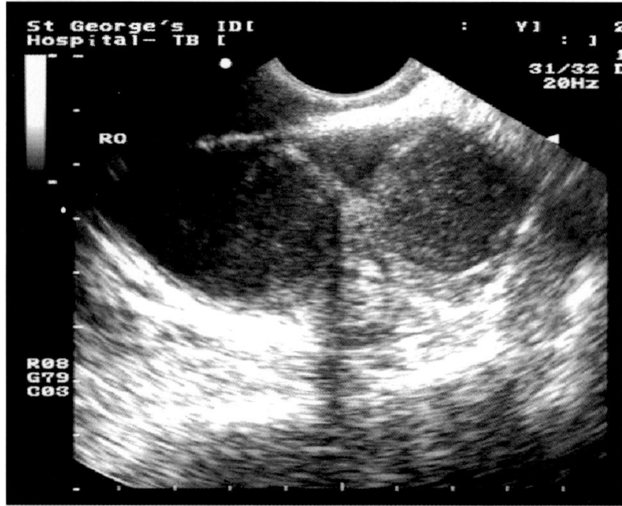

FIGURE 14.7 Transvaginal ultrasound of bilateral ovarian endometriomas. The cysts are thick walled, with homogenous low level internal echoes. They are described as "kissing" in the midline, a reflection of obliteration of the Pouch of Douglas.

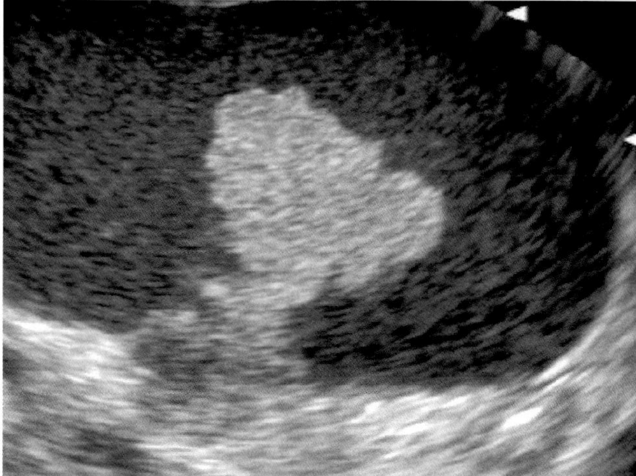

FIGURE 14.8 Papillary process. This is a magnified view of an ovarian cyst wall, demonstrating an irregular solid projection. The cyst contains are "ground glass" in appearance. The cyst histology was confirmed as a stage 1A endometroid carcinoma.

present a poor anesthetic risk can be managed conservatively and those with small dermoids managed expectantly.

b. Epithelial Tumors

Serous cystadenomas tend to be unilocular and contain anechoic fluid. They may, however, be multilocular, with smooth, internal cyst walls. The presence of irregular thickenings along the septae of a multilocular thin-walled cyst may be representative of a serous cystadenofibroma. However, the presence of multilocularity and papillary processes increases the likelihood of a serous cystadenocarcinoma. Up to 50% of these will be bilateral. Interrogation of the papillary process with color Doppler will often identify a florid, branching appearance in vascularity, likely to reflect the neovascularization associated with malignant neoplasms (Figs. 14.8 and 14.9). Occasionally, necrosis will result in absence of vascular changes despite malignant histology.

Mucinous cystadenomas (Fig 14.10) are typically multilocular, and contain low-level internal echoes, which on close inspection will appear to "fall" through the cyst contents. About 10% are bilateral. Approximately 10% will have borderline malignant characteristics. Mucinous cystadenocarcinomas can give rise to "myxoma peritonei," due to extensive intraperitoneal spread.

c. Sex Cord-Stromal Tumors

Fibromas are solid tumors, usually replacing all normal ovarian morphology. They can become very large, and can undergo cystic degeneration. Although benign, the resultant sonographic image is of a mixed cystic solid mass and ascites. Meig's syndrome rises from the association of an ovarian fibroma, ascites, and a pleural effusion.

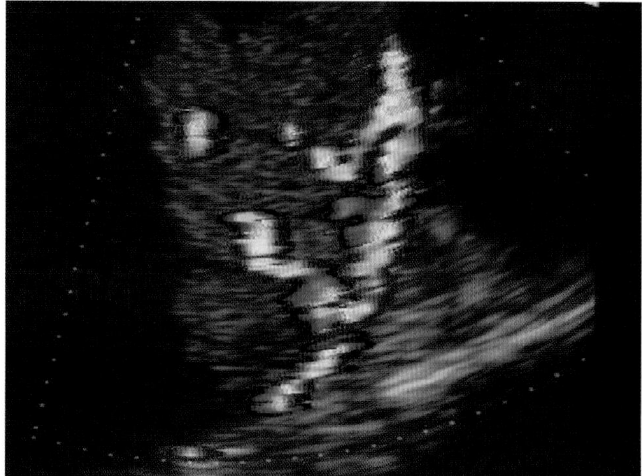

FIGURE 14.9 Color Doppler image of the same papillary process as seen in Fig. 14.8. The florid, branching pattern is highly suspicious of malignancy. This is in contrast to the pattern of blood flow seen in Figure 14.2.

C. Ovarian Cysts in Pregnancy

The increased use of ultrasound within the first trimester, either for the assessment of early pregnancy problems or first trimester screening, has led to an increased detection of coexistent adnexal pathology. The majority of ovarian cysts detected at this gestation will be corpus luteal or theca lutein in origin, and will tend to resolve by 16 weeks gestation. The incidence of ovarian cysts during pregnancy has been estimated at between 1 [42] and 4% [43], falling to 1 in 300 after 16 weeks gestation.[44, 45] This figure will vary with the degree of ultrasound surveillance performed within a unit. Those masses persisting into the second and third trimesters

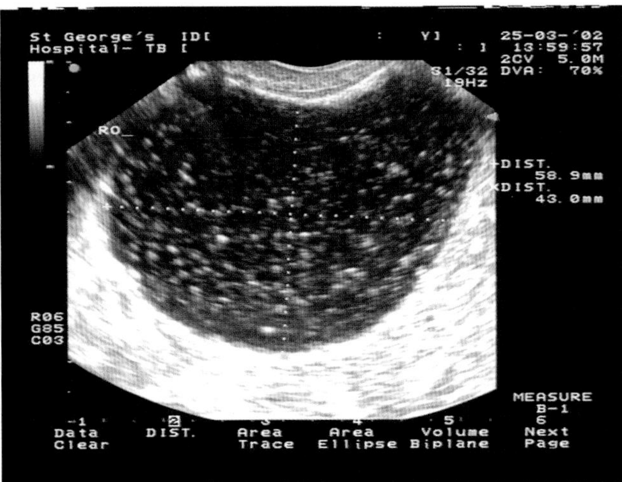

FIGURE 14.10 Transvaginal ultrasound of a mucinous cystadenoma. The cyst has a thin, smooth internal wall with characteristic low level echogenic contents.

present a number of dilemmas for the physician. The risk of malignancy within this population, although small, does exist. One series evaluated 125 persistent adnexal masses, with a 0.8% rate of ovarian malignancy, which represented 1 out of 14 complex-appearing masses.[46] A full morphological assessment of an adnexal mass using transvaginal views may be possible in early pregnancy, but in later pregnancy the ovary tends to become an abdominal organ and can be extremely difficult to visualize. Operative intervention during pregnancy will increase the risk of pregnancy complications, even if surgery is performed within the second trimester or utilizing laparoscopic techniques. So how can we adopt a conservative approach to the majority of adnexal masses during pregnancy, while ensuring that an ovarian malignancy, while rare, isn't missed? The majority of persistent ovarian cysts detected will be endometriomas, benign cystic teratomas, and simple cysts.[46] These all tend to have sonographic characteristics that permit a diagnosis to be made based on pattern recognition. Ultrasound-guided drainage of simple cysts may be useful on an individually selected basis for symptom control.

In conclusion, the majority of adnexal masses diagnosed in pregnancy will resolve by the second trimester. Those persisting can safely be managed expectantly as the rates of malignancy and ovarian torsion are both low. Ultrasonography has been shown to accurately diagnose benign cystic teratomas and endometriomas,[36] which form the largest group of histological type within this population. A repeat scan should be performed postnatally to assess the need for elective surgery. Surgical intervention should be reserved for those adnexal masses that are felt to be complex in nature, in which malignancy cannot be excluded, or the symptomatic patient where a cyst accident is suspected.

D. Fetal Ovarian Cysts

With the advent of increased ultrasound surveillance during routine pregnancy and technically advanced ultrasound equipment, more fetal ovarian cysts will be detected antenatally. The relevance of antenatally detected cysts has been addressed by a number of studies. The presence of small, follicular cysts is common throughout the neonatal period, as the ovaries, even at this early stage, are dynamic structures. Postmortem studies have shown that one-third of stillbirths and neonates have these small cysts.[47] Measuring 1–7 mm in diameter, they regress spontaneously.

Large ovarian cysts remain an uncommon finding in the antenatal and neonatal period. Antenatally, their detection should prompt ultrasound follow-up only. Intervention is rarely needed. Polyhydramnios and difficulties during vaginal delivery have been described in the presence of large ovarian cysts. These unusual circumstances may warrant *in utero* cyst decompression by needle aspiration. They are almost invariably benign and are follicular or luteal in origin. In one series, 13 neonates underwent laparotomy for antenatally detected, persistent ovarian cysts. Of these, one-third had undergone ovarian torsion and necrosis. In these cases, the cyst is often described as hypermobile, as it has either become detached completely from the adnexa, or remains attached only by a tenuous stalk.[48] A second series (17 neonates) established sonographic markers in order to differentiate between uncomplicated cysts and those complicated by torsion. An uncomplicated cyst will be anechoic in nature with a sonographically imperceptible wall. A fluid-debris level within a cyst has been shown to be a consistent feature of ovarian torsion and it also tended to have a thin echogenic wall.[49]

Most ovarian cysts persisting into the neonatal period require surgical intervention; usually in the form of laparotomy and salpingo-oophorectomy. Ovarian torsion was usually an antenatal event in the latter study and the infants were asymptomatic. Rarely, however, adnexal torsion, hemorrhage, or rupture can lead to life-threatening conditions, and as such very few ovarian cysts have been managed conservatively.

Ovarian cysts remain the most common cause of an abdominal cyst in a female fetus or neonate. Other differentials include mesenteric, bowel duplication, renal, or urachal cysts.

E. Ovarian Torsion

This is unusual with adnexal masses <5 cm.[50] However, there are no pathognomonic features specific to adnexal torsion and a high degree of clinical suspicion is essential. A clinical history of acute onset, constant pain not responding to analgesia, often with nausea and vomiting and systemic upset is typical. The central feature of ovarian torsion is the cessation of vascular supply. Color Doppler has therefore been used to interrogate the adnexal mass suspected of undergoing torsion to diagnose this gynecological emergency, as early action may allow for conservative surgery. It is likely, however, that if flow can be visualized within the mass, despite clinical symptoms and signs of ovarian torsion, that ovarian blood flow may still be compromised. This has been demonstrated by surgically proven ovarian torsion, despite normal vascularity within the mass.[51]

IV. TRANSVAGINAL COLOR DOPPLER

The degree to which color Doppler will be used to interrogate a potentially abnormal ovary will differ between individual clinicians. Angiogenesis is believed to be the integral primary step in the development of a number of malignancies.[52] These new, small blood vessels have a relative lack of intimal smooth muscle and increased arteriovenous shunting,[53] resulting in low impedance, high velocity blood flow.[54] The use of an arbitrary cut-off value of a resistance index of 0.4 will result in a number of false-positive and negative results, as the low resistance flow typically associated with malignancy can also be detected within a number of benign lesions (including the corpus luteum, tubo-ovarian abscess, and pedunculated fibroids). Vessel location and arrangement, rather than blood flow indices, can be a more accurate assessment of tumor vascularity.[20, 55]

Its use as a second-line assessment of persistent ovarian morphological abnormality will help reduce those false-positive results due to physiological lesions. The finding of persistent low impedance, high-velocity blood flow within the ovary is more likely to be significant after menopause, as the cyclical vascular characteristics reflecting normal ovarian function are no longer present. Despite its limitations, color Doppler has the potential to add a significant amount of information to initial morphological changes within the ovary.

V. OVARIAN CANCER SCREENING

Women in the western world have a 1.4% lifetime risk of developing ovarian cancer. The overall 5-year survival rates are in the region of 35–40%, although the 5-year survival rates for stage I cancers approach 90%. The majority of women still present with stage III and IV disease. In order for any screening test to be effective, the earliest form of the disease needs to be detected. B-mode ultrasound with or without color Doppler as a second stage test remains central to all ovarian cancer screening programs.

Previous screening studies for ovarian carcinoma have been criticized because of the relatively high number of false-positive test results; in one study this meant that for those women with a positive test result, approximately 51 operations were performed for each primary ovarian carcinoma detected.[56] This led to the development of second stage tests to reduce the false-positive rate. In ovarian cancer screening programs, color Doppler has been used to detect vascular indices characteristic of neovascularization within persistent morphological abnormalities [57] in an attempt to make screening more specific.

It is believed that most ovarian epithelial cancers arise *de novo* from the surface epithelium of the ovary.[58] The proportion of benign ovarian cysts which will ultimately undergo malignant transformation is unknown. Crayford *et al.* [59] have obtained long-term follow-up data from a large ovarian cancer screening study, looking at the impact of persistent ovarian cyst removal on mortality due to ovarian cancer. This demonstrated only a slight reduction in the expected mortality within the group, supporting the view that most epithelial cancers are likely to arise *de novo*, without a sonographically obvious premalignant phase.

This is evident in clinical practice with the presentation of ovarian cancer in women having had a normal screen, and also in the detection of an unsuspected cancer in women undergoing prophylactic oophorectomy. It is in this latter group of women that detailed pathological analysis of the cancer may provide important information as to ovarian cancer genesis.

VI. CONCLUSION

The assessment of ovarian morphology is paramount to many areas of gynecology. Transvaginal ultrasound, with or without color Doppler, provides the clinician with a noninvasive, highly sensitive method of achieving this, thus facilitating appropriate management decisions. It complements the routine clinical examination in the symptomatic patient and allows a diagnosis of normal ovarian morphology to be made with confidence. It is a significant contributor in the characterization of adnexal masses and within overian cancer screening programs; ongoing large multicenter trials will hopefully further define its role within these two areas.

Central to the appropriate use of TVS will be training and supervision, with up-to-date protocols and regular audit, along with an awareness of one's own limitations.

References

1. Yeun, P. M., Yu, K. M., Yip, S. K., Lau, W. C., Rogers, M. S., and Chang, A. (1997). A randomised prospective study of laparoscopy and laparotomy in the management of benign ovarian masses. *Am. J. Obstet. Gynecol.* 177, 109–114.
2. van Nagell, Jr., J. R., De Priest, P. D., Puls, L. E., Donaldson, E. S., Gallion, H. H., Pavlik, E. J., Powell, D. E., and Kryscio, P. J. (1991). Ovarian cancer screening in asymptomatic women by transvaginal ultrasonography. *Cancer* 68, 458–462.
3. Higgins, R. V., van Nagell, Jr., J. R., Woods, C. H., Thompson, E. A., and Kryscio, R. J. (1990). Interobserver variation in ovarian measurements using transvaginal sonography. *Gynecol. Oncol.* 39, 69–71.

4. DePriest, P., Gallion, H., Pavlik, E., Kryscio, R., van Nagell, Jr., J. R. (1997). Transvaginal sonography as a screening method for the detection of early ovarian cancer. *Gynecol. Oncol.* 65, 408–414.

5. Pavlik, E. J., DePriest, P. D., Gallion, H. H., Ueland, F. R., Reedy, M. B., Kryscio, R. J., van Nagell, Jr., J. R. (2000). Ovarian volume related to age. *Gynecol. Oncol.* 77(3), 410–412.

6. Cohen, H. L., Tice , H. M., and Mandel, F. S. (1990). Ovarian volumes measured by US: Bigger than we think. *Radiology* 177, 189–192.

7. Bourne, T. H., Hagstrom, H., Hahlin, M., Josefsson, B., Granberg, S., Hellberg, P., Hamberger, L., and Collins, W. P. (1996). Ultrasound studies of vascular and morphological changes in the human corpus luteum during the menstrual cycle. *Fertil. Steril.* 65, 753–758.

8. Polson, D. W., Wadsworth, J., Adams, J., and Franks, S. (1988). Polycystic ovaries-a common finding in normal women. *Lancet* 1(8590), 870–872.

9. Dewailly, D., Robert, Y., and Helin, I. (1994). Ovarian stromal hypertrophy in hyperandrogenic women. *Clin. Endocrin.* 41, 557–562.

10. Fulghesu, A. M., Ciampelli Belosi, C., Apa, R., Pavone, V., and Lanzone, A. (2001). A new ultrasound criterion for the diagnosis of polycystic ovary syndrome: The ovarian/stroma/total area ratio. *Fertil. Steril.* 76, 326–331.

11. Hata, K., Hata, T., Takamiya, O., and Kitao, M. (1989). Ultrasonographic identification and measurement of the normal ovary in postmenopausal Japanese women. *Gynecol. Obstet. Invest.* 27, 2:99–101.

12. Sladkevicius, P., Valentin, L., and Marsal, K. (1995). Transvaginal gray-scale and Doppler ultrasound examinations of the uterus and ovaries in healthy postmenopausal women. *Ultrasound Obstet. Gynecol.* 6, 81–90.

13. Hall, D. A., McCarthy, K. A., and Kopans, D. B. (1986). Sonographic visualisation of the normal postmenopausal ovary. *J. Ultrasound Med.* 5(1), 9–11.

14. Fleischer, A. C., McKee, M. S., Gordon, A. N., Page, D. L., Kepple, D. M., Worrel, J. A., Jones, H. W., Burnett, L. S., and James, Jr., A. E. (1990). Transvaginal sonography of postmenopausal ovaries with pathological correlation. *J. Ultrasound. Med.* 9(11), 637–644.

15. Rodriguez, H. M., Platt, L. D., Medearis, A. L., Lacardia, M., and Lobo, R. A. (1988). The use of transvaginal sonography for evaluation of postmenopausal ovarian size and morphology. *Am. J. Obstet. Gynecol.* 159, 810–814.

16. Auslender, R., Atlas, I., Lissak, A., Bornstein, J., Atad, J., and Abramovici, H. (1996). Follow-up of small postmenopausal ovarian cysts using vaginal ultrasound and CA-125 antigen. *J. Clin. Ultrasound* 24, 175–178.

17. Levine, D. (1994). What is the significance of the incidental discovery of a unilocular ovarian cyst in a postmenopausal woman (either with or without a family history of ovarian cancer) during a pelvic sonographic examination to exclude ovarian cancer? *AJR* 163, 215–216.

18. Bailey, C., Ueland, F., DePriest, P., Gallion, H., Kryscio, R., and van Nagell, Jr., J. R. (1988). The malignant potential of small cystic ovarian tumors in women over 50 years of age. *Gynecol. Oncol.* 69, 3–7.

19. Granberg, S., Wikland, M., and Jansson, I. (1989). Macroscopic characterisation of ovarian tumors and the relation to the histological diagnosis: Criteria to be used for ultrasound evaluation. *Gynecol. Oncol.* 35, 139–144.

20. Timmerman, D., Schwarzler, P., Collins, W. P., Claerhout, F., Coenen, M., Amant, F., Vergote., and Bourne, T. H. (1999). Subjective assessment of adnexal masses with the use of ultrasonography: An analysis of interobserver variability and experience. *Ultrasound Obstet. Gynecol.* 13, 11–16.

21. Tailor, A., Jurkovic, D., Bourne, T. H., Collins, W. P., and Campbell, S. (1998). Sonographic prediction of malignancy in adnexal masses using multivariate logistic regression analysis. *Ultrasound Obstet. Gynecol.* 10, 41–47.

22. Timmerman, D., Verrelst, H., Bourne, T. H., De Moor, B., Collins, W. P., Vergote, I., and Vandewalle, J. (1999). Artificial neural network models for the preoperative discrimination between malignant and benign adnexal masses. *Ultrasound Obstet. Gynecol.* 13,17–25.

23. Granberg, S., Norström, A., and Wikland, M. (1990). Tumors in the lower pelvis as imaged by transvaginal sonography. *Gynecol. Oncol.* 37, 224–229.

24. Sassone, A. M., Timor-Tritsch, I. E., Artner, A., Westhoff, C., and Warren, W. B. (1991). Transvaginal sonographic characterization of ovarian disease: evaluation of a new scoring system to predict ovarian malignancy. *Obstet. Gynecol.* 78, 70–76.

25. Lerner, J. P., Timor-Tritsch, I. E., Federman, A., and Abramovich, G. (1994). Transvaginal ultrasonographic characterisation of ovarian masses with an improved, weighted scoring system. *Am. J. Obstet. Gynecol.* 170, 81–85.

26. Bourne, T. H., Campbell, S., Reynolds, K. M., Whitehead, M. I., Hampson, J., Royston, P., Crayford, T. J. B., and Collins, W. P. Screening for familial ovarian cancer with transvaginal ultrasonography and colour blood flow imaging. *Br. Med. J.* 306, 1025–1029.

27. Jacobs, I., Oram, D., Fairbanks, J., Turner, J., Frost, C., and Grudzinskas, J. G. (1990). A risk of malignancy index incorporating CA 125, ultrasound and menopausal status for the accurate preoperative diagnosis of ovarian cancer. *Br. J. Obstet. Gynaecol.* 97(10), 922–929.

28. Ferrazzi, E., Zanetta, G., Dordoni, D., Berlanda, N., Mezzopane, R., and Lissoni, G. (1997). Transvaginal ultrasonographic characterization of ovarian masses: Comparison of five scoring systems in a multicenter study. *Ultrasound Obstet. Gynecol.* 10(3), 192–197.

29. Turan, C., Zorlu, C. G., Ugur, M., Ozcan, T., Kaleli, B., and Gokmen, O. (1994). Expectant management of functional ovarian cysts: An alternative to hormonal therapy. *Int. J. Gynaecol. Obstet.* 47, 257–260.

30. Nezhat, F. R., Nezhat, C. H., Borhan, S., and Nezhat, C. R. (1994). Is hormonal suppression efficacious in treating functional ovarian cysts? *J. Am. Assoc. Gynecol. Laparoscopy* 1;4:S26.

31. Koonings, P. P., Campbell, K., Mishell, D., and Grimes, D. (1989). Relative frequency of ovarian neoplasms: a 10 year review. *Obstet. Gynecol.* 74, 921–925.

32. Alcazar, J. L., Laparte, C., Jurado, M., and Lopez-Garcia, G. (1997). The role of transvaginal ultrasonography combined with color velocity imaging and pulsed Doppler in the diagnosis of endometrioma. *Fertil. Steril.* 67, 487–491.

33. Kupfer, M. C., Schwimer, S. R., and Lebovic, T. (1992). Transvaginal sonographic appearance of endometrioma: Spectrum of findings. *J. Ultrasound Med.* 11, 129–133.

34. Hertzberg, B. S., and Kliewer, M. A. (1996). Sonography of benign cystic teratoma of the ovary: Pitfalls in diagnosis. *AJR* 167, 1127–1133.

35. Cohen, L., and Sabbagha, R. (1993). Echo patterns of benign cystic teratomas by transvaginal ultrasound. *Ultrasound Obstet. Gynecol.* 3, 120–123.

36. Jermy, K., Luise, C., and Bourne, T. (2001). The characterization of common ovarian cysts in premenopausal women. *Ultrasound Obstet. Gynecol.* 17, 140–144.

37. Mais, V., Guerriero, S., Ajossa, S., Angiolucci, M., Paoletti, A. M., and Melis, G. B. (1993). The efficiency of transvaginal ultrasonography in the diagnosis of endometrioma. *Fertil. Steril.* 60, 776–780.

38. Mais, V., Guerriero, S., Ajossa, S., Angiolucci, M., Paoletti, A. M., and Melis, G. B. (1995). Transvaginal ultrasonography in the diagnosis of cystic teratoma. *Obstet. Gynecol.* 85, 48–52.

39. Ahyan, A., Aksu, T., Develioglu, O., Tuncer, Z. S., and Ayhan, A. (1991). Complications and bilaterality of mature ovarian teratomas (clinicopathological evaluation of 286 cases). *Aust. N.Z. Obstet. Gynecol.* 31, 83–85.

40. Donnez, J., Nisolle, M., Gillerot, S., Anaf, V., and Clercx-Braun, F. (1994). Ovarian endometrial cysts: The role of GnRH agonist and/or drainage. *Fertil. Steril.* 64, 63–70.

41. Shalev, E., Bustan, M., Romano, S., Goldberg, Y., and Ben-Shlomo, I. (1998). Laparoscopic resection of ovarian benign cystic teratomas: Experience with 84 cases. *Hum. Reprod.* 13(7), 1810–1812.

42. Nelson, M. J., Cavalieri, R., Graham, D., and Sanders, R. C. (1986). Cysts in pregnancy discovered by sonography. *J. Clin. Ultrasound* 14, 509–512.
43. Hill, L., Connors-Beatty, D., Nowak, A., and Tush, B. (1998). The role of ultrasonography in the detection and management of adnexal masses during the second and third trimesters of pregnancy. *Am. J. Obstet. Gynecol.* 179, 703–707.
44. Lavery, J., Koontz, W. L., Layman, L., Shaw, I., and Cumpel, U. (1986). Sonographic evaluation of the adnexa during early pregnancy. *Surg. Gynecol. Obstet.* 163, 319–923.
45. Hoyston, P., and Lilford, R. J. (1986). Ultrasound study of ovarian cysts in pregnancy: Prevalence and significance. *Br. J. Obstet. Gynaecol.* 93, 625–628.
46. Bromley, B., and Benacerraf, B. (1997). Adnexal masses during pregnancy: Accuracy of sonographic diagnosis and outcome *J. Ultrasound Med.* 16, 447–452.
47. Desa, D. J. (1975). Follicular ovarian cysts in stillbirths and neonates. *Arch. Dis. Child.* 50, 45–50.
48. Zachariou, Z., Roth, H., Boos, R., Troger, J., and Daum, R. (1989). Three years experience with large ovarian cysts diagnosed *in utero*. *J. Pediatr. Surg.* 24(5) 478–482.
49. Nussbaum, A. R., Sanders, R. C., Hartman, D. S., Dudgeon, D., and Parmley, T. H. (1988). Neonatal ovarian cysts: Sonographic-pathologic correlation. *Radiology* 168, 817–821.
50. Nichols, D., and Julian, P. (1985). Torsion of the adnexa. *Clin. Obstet. Gynecol.* 28, 375–380.
51. Rosado, W., Trambert, M., Gosink, B., and Pretorius, D. (1992). Adnexal torsion: Diagnosis by using Doppler sonography. *Am. J. Radiol.* 159, 1251–1253.
52. Folkman, J., Watson, K., Ingber, D., and Hanahan, D. (1989). Induction of angiogenesis during the transition from hyperplasia to neoplasia. *Nature* 339, 58–61.
53. Emoto, M., Iwasaki, H., Mimura, K., Kawarabayashi, T., and Kikuchi, M. (1997). Differences in the angiogenesis of benign and malignant ovarian tumors, demonstrated by analyses of colour Doppler ultr sound, immunohistochemistry and microvessel density. *Cancer* 80, 899–907.
54. Bourne, T., Campbell, S., Steer, C., Whitehead, M. I., and Collins, W. P. (1989). Transvaginal colour flow imaging: a possible new screening technique for ovarian cancer. *Br. Med. J.* 299, 1367–1370.
55. Kurjak, A., Zalud, I., Jurkovic, D., Alfirovic, Z., and Miljan, M. (1989). Transvaginal colour flow Doppler for the assessment of pelvic circulation. *Acta. Obstet. Gynecol. Scand.* 68, 131–135.
56. Campbell, S., Bhan, V., Royston, P., Whitehead, M. I., and Collins, W. P. (1989). Transabdominal ultrasound screening for early ovarian cancer. *Br. Med. J.* 299, 1363–1367.
57. Bourne, T. H. (1991). Transvaginal color Doppler in gynaecology. *Ultrasound Obstet. Gynecol.* 1, 359–373.
58. Scully, R. E. (2000). Influence of origin of ovarian cancer on efficacy of screening (commentary). *Lancet* 355, 1028–1029.
59. Crayford, T. J. B., Campbell, S., Bourne, T. H., Rawson, H., and Collins, W. P. (2000). Benign ovarian cysts and ovarian cancer: a cohort study with implications for screening. *Lancet* 255, 1060–1063.

CHAPTER

15

CA125 and Other Tumor Markers in Screening and Monitoring of Ovarian Cancer

USHA MENON

Gynecology Oncology Unit
St. Bartholomew's and The London Queen Mary's School of Medicine and Dentistry
London EC1M 6GR, United Kingdom

IAN JACOBS

Department of Obstetrics and Gynecology
Gynecology Oncology Unit
St. Bartholomew's and The London Queen Mary's School of Medicine and Dentistry
London EC1M 6GR, United Kingdom

ABSTRACT

A wide variety of serum tumor markers have been investigated in the context of screening, differential diagnosis, prognosis, and monitoring of response and recurrence in ovarian cancer. One of the oldest among them is CA125 and it still remains the tumor marker with the most well-defined and validated role in the management of this disease. The focus of this chapter is on the role of CA125 in ovarian cancer. In combination with transvaginal ultrasound, serial CA125 monitoring is undergoing evaluation in randomized controlled trials of ovarian cancer screening. It is of increasing value in the differential diagnosis of adnexal masses and changes on serial monitoring are a reliable indicator of response or progression of disease. It's clinical value as a prognostic indicator is still to be defined. New technologies including expression array and mass spectroscopy are likely to identify a wealth of new candidate markers over the next few years.

I. INTRODUCTION

A wide variety of serum tumor markers have been investigated in the context of screening, differential diagnosis, prognosis, and monitoring of response and recurrence in ovarian cancer. One of the oldest among them is CA125 and it still remains the tumor marker with the most well-defined and validated role in the management of this disease. Except in the case of specific histological subtypes of ovarian cancer, the role of other markers remains to be determined. Assays for most of these markers are not widely available and many are associated with poor specificity and/or sensitivity. Hence, the focus of this chapter will be on the role of CA125 in ovarian cancer with references to potential new markers that may contribute toward clinical care in the future.

II. CA125

CA125 was first identified by Bast, Knapp, and colleagues in 1981 using a monoclonal antibody, OC125, that had been developed from mice immunized with an ovarian cancer cell line.[1] It exists as a very large complex under natural conditions. The core CA125 subunit carries two major antigenic domains classified as A, the domain binding monoclonal antibody OC125, and B, a domain binding monoclonal antibody M11.[2] Recent studies indicate that CA125 is a typical high molecular weight mucin molecule with a high carbohydrate content.[3] Its peptide moiety has been very difficult to clone, possibly because of the mucinous nature of CA125. Using a rabbit antiserum with purified CA125 and expression cloning, a long partial cDNA sequence corresponding to a new mucin species (designated *MUC16*) has recently been cloned. It is a strong candidate for being the peptide core of the CA125 antigen.[4]

CA125 is expressed by amniotic and coelomic epithelium during fetal development. In the adult, it is found in structures derived from coelomic epithelium (the mesothelial cells of the pleura, pericardium, and peritoneum) and in tubal, endometrial, and endocervical epithelium. The surface epithelium of normal fetal and adult ovaries does not express the determinant, except in inclusion cysts, areas of metaplasia, and papillary excrescences.[5]

The currently available CA125 assays use OC125 as the capture antibody and M11 as the detection antibody. They correlate well with each other and are clinically reliable.[6] A serum value of 35 U/ml, representing 1% of healthy female donors, is often accepted as the upper limit of normal in clinical practice.[7] Overall approximately 85% of patients with epithelial ovarian cancer have CA125 levels >35 U/ml.[7] Elevated levels >35 U/ml are found in 50% of patients with stage I disease but raised levels are found in >90% of the women with more advanced stages.[8] CA125 is less often elevated in mucinous, clear cell, and borderline tumors than in serous tumors.[9, 10] While CA125 is most commonly elevated in association with ovarian malignancy, it can also be raised in some physiological situations and benign and malignant conditions (Fig. 15.1).

Physiological conditions
- Ovulation
- Pregnancy
- Retrograde menstruation

Benign gyneological conditions
- Endometriosis
- Benign Ovarian Cysts
- Uterine Leiomyomas (fibroids)

Other non-malignant disease
- Autoimmune Diseases (i.e. Sjorgrens Syndrome, Polyarteritis Nodosa, Systemic Lupus Erythematosus)
- Sarcoidosis
- Benign Gastrointestinal Diseases (i.e. Colitis, Diverticulitis)
- Chronic Active Hepatitis
- Cirrhosis
- Pericarditis
- Pancreatitis (Acute and Chronic)
- Abdominal tuberculosis
- Renal Disease with Serum Creatinine >2.0

Non ovarian malignant conditions
- Malignant Ascites
- Disseminated Malignancy (i.e. Breast, Lung)
- Disseminated Malignancies from any site involving the Pleural or Peritoneal Surfaces
- A proportion of
  - Non-Hodgkin's lymphoma
  - Pancreatic cancers
  - Cervical Cancers
  - Endometrial Cancers

FIGURE 15.1 Medical conditions known to elevate CA125 levels.

A. Screening

Serum CA125 is the most extensively evaluated tumor marker in ovarian cancer screening. Population based studies from Norway and Maryland have documented CA125 elevations up to 5 years before the diagnosis of ovarian cancer.[11, 12]

Elevation in apparently healthy postmenopausal women is a powerful predictor of increased risk of ovarian cancer.[13] This forms the basis of the multimodal ovarian cancer screening strategy proposed by Jacobs *et al.*[14, 15] Asymptomatic women are screened using serum CA125 and those with abnormal results are referred for repeat CA125 testing and an ovarian ultrasound. Using simplistic fixed cut-offs of ≥30 U/L for CA125 and ≥8.8 ml for abnormal ovarian volume, Jacobs *et al.* was able to achieve a sensitivity of 78.6% and a positive predictive value of 26.8% in the initial multimodal screening trial involving 22,000 postmenopausal women.[15] Important progress has since been made in the use of CA125 for screening. The major refinements in the multimodal strategy over the last decade have been

1. Introduction of the risk of ovarian cancer (ROC) calculation for interpretation of serum CA125 levels in place of standard cut-off levels. CA125 levels in women without ovarian cancer were noted to be static or decrease with time while levels associated with malignancy tend to rise. This has been incorporated into a computerized algorithm that uses age, rate of change of CA125 with time, and absolute levels to calculate an individual's ROC. The closer the CA125 profile to the CA125 behavior of known cases of ovarian cancer, the greater the risk of ovarian cancer.[16] This has been shown to increase the sensitivity of ovarian cancer detection from 75–85%.[17]
2. Triage of women based on the ROC algorithm (Fig. 15.2)
3. Use of ovarian morphology rather than volume to assess ovaries on transvaginal ultrasound in women with elevated CA125 levels.[18]
4. Limiting screening in the general population to postmenopausal women who are at increased risk of ovarian

cancer but have a lower incidence of benign and physiological conditions associated with CA125 elevation

There are currently underway, two large randomized control trials of ovarian cancer screening in the general population, which incorporate CA125 measurement. Both aim to assess the impact of screening on ovarian cancer mortality.

1. The Prostate, Lung, Colorectal, and Ovarian (PLCO) Cancer Screening Trial has completed enrolling 74,000 women aged 55–74 at 10 screening centers in the U.S. with balanced randomization to intervention and control arms. For ovarian cancer, women in the study arm are screened using a combined strategy (CA125 and transvaginal sonogram; TVS) for 3 years and CA125 alone for a further 2 years. Follow-up will continue for at least 13 years from randomization to assess health status and cause of death.[19, 20]
2. The United Kingdom Collaborative Trial of Ovarian Cancer Screening (UKCTOCS) started recruiting postmenopausal women from 12 centers in the UK (Fig. 15.3) in 2001. In all, 200,000 women will be randomized to control, ultrasound screening, or multimodal screening. This study also addresses the issues of target population, compliance, health economics, and physical and psychological morbidity of screening. Results are expected in 10 years. (http://www.mds.qmw.ac.uk/gynaeonc/UKCTOCS/).

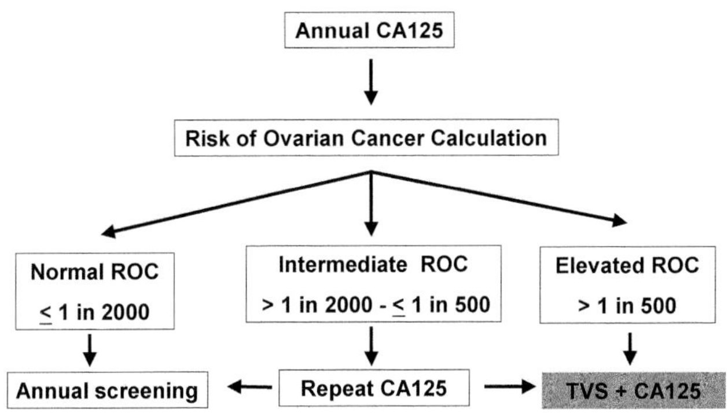

FIGURE 15.2 Risk of Ovarian Cancer Algorithm (ROCA).

In addition, trials are underway in the high-risk population where screening of women is recommended from the age of 35. There are two single arm multicentric trials aimed at developing an optimal screening strategy for the high-risk population in the U.S. and UK. The UK Familial Ovarian Cancer Screening Study (UK-FOCSS) involves 5000 "high-risk" women screened annually with CA125 measurements and transvaginal ultrasound. The U.S. trial under the auspices of the Cancer Genetics Network has a similar trial design but includes three further CA125 screens every year.

In the future, it is likely that a panel of serum markers complementary to serum CA125 maybe used in multimodal screening. Among those currently undergoing extensive testing in the U.S. is plasma lysophosphatidic acid (LPA), a bioactive phospholipid with mitogenic and growth-factor-like activities.[21]

B. Differential Diagnosis of an Adnexal Mass

Serum CA125 is of value in the differential diagnosis of benign and malignant adnexal masses, particularly in postmenopausal women. Einhorn *et al.* [22] measured CA125 preoperatively in 100 women undergoing diagnostic laparotomy for palpable adnexal masses, 23 of who were subsequently found to have a malignancy. Using an upper limit

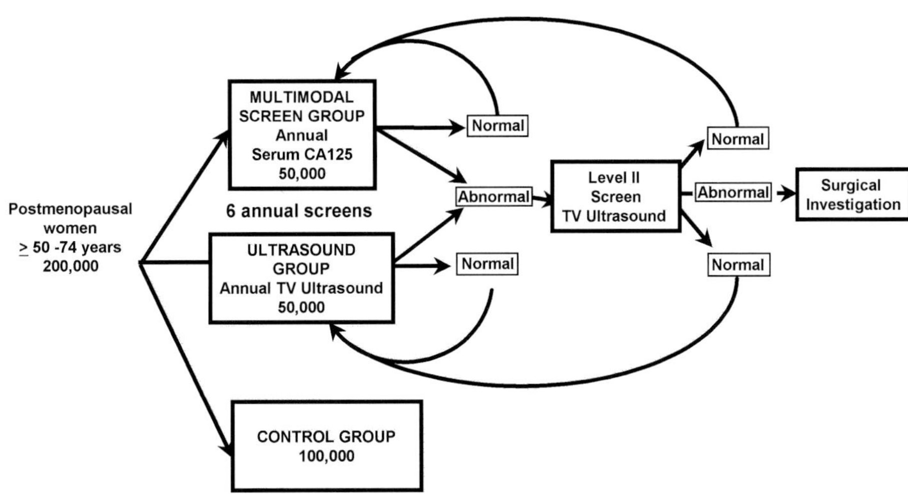

FIGURE 15.3 United Kingdom Collaborative Trial of Ovarian Cancer Screening (UKCT OCS).

of 35 U/ml, the sensitivity of serum CA125 measurements for malignant disease was 78%, specificity 95%, and positive predictive value 82%. Numerous studies have since shown that in women with a pelvic mass in addition to clinical examination and ultrasonography, determination of CA125 alone or as part of a panel of markers improves the sensitivity and specificity for detection of ovarian cancer.[23–27] Jacobs *et al.* combined serum CA125 values with ovarian ultrasound results and menopausal status to calculate a risk of malignancy index (RMI). Patients with an elevated RMI score had, on average, 42 times the background risk of cancer.[28] Tingulstad *et al.* [29] has subsequently validated the RMI prospectively in 173 women, 30 years or older, admitted for primary laparotomy of a pelvic mass. A sensitivity of 71%, specificity of 96%, and positive predictive value of 89% was achieved. For stages II, III, and IV of ovarian cancer the sensitivity increased to approximately 90% without any substantial loss in specificity. Such objective indices are useful in triaging patients with adnexal masses for referral to specialized gynecological oncology centers.

C. Prognosis

Serum CA125 levels are related to tumor stage and load in patients with CA125 positive tumors and CA125 measurements can play an important role in predicting prognosis.

1. Preoperative CA125

While some studies did not find preoperative CA125 to be an independent prognostic factor,[30–32] others have questioned this view.[33, 34] A recent retrospective study suggests that in patients with stage III ovarian cancer, the probability of performing optimal cytoreduction is approximately one in five if preoperative CA125 is >500 U/ml.[35] There is now a need for prospective studies to determine the applicability of preoperative CA125 determination in tailoring surgery and subsequent chemotherapy.[36]

2. Postoperative CA125

Levels following surgery may be a significant prognostic indicator.[31, 37] It is, however, important to note that in the immediate postoperative period, CA125 levels can be elevated as a result of tissue trauma.[38] In addition, serum levels may take some weeks to return to normal as the half-life of serum CA125 is 6 days. Residual disease should only be suspected if levels plateau or rise after 4 weeks.

3. Levels During Initial Chemotherapy

During primary chemotherapy, serum CA125 half-life, [32, 39, 40] levels prior to the third course of chemotherapy, [41–44] and the slope of the CA125 exponential regression curve [45] have all been shown to be independent prognostic factors, both for the achievement of complete remission and for survival in patients with advanced epithelial ovarian cancer. However, the prognostic information gained from CA125 alone is not sufficiently accurate to make a decision to alter the chemotherapy regime of an individual patient.[46]

4. Levels at Clinical Relapse

Serum CA125 continues to be of prognostic significance when disease recurs. Patients with normal serum CA125 levels (≤35 U/ml) at relapse have a better prognosis than those with elevated values.[31]

D. Monitoring Response to Treatment

Serum CA125 levels reflect progression or regression of disease in >90% of patients with ovarian cancer who have an elevated preoperative level.[7, 47] Several authors have explored the possibility of using serum levels to define response to treatment. The pattern of CA125 with time rather than arbitrary cut-off levels provides the most useful information. Of the several definitions proposed [48–50] the one by Rustin *et al.* [51] has been prospectively validated. In the latter study, a mathematical definition to evaluate response, using strict CA125 criteria was developed after analysis of 277 patients in the North Thames Ovary Trial 3. Response to a specific treatment was defined as a 50% decrease in CA125 after 2 samples, confirmed by a fourth sample (50% response), or a serial decrease over 3 samples of greater than 75% (75% response). The final sample had to be at least 28 days after the previous sample. The response definitions were subsequently validated in 254 patients receiving first-line chemotherapy in the North Thames Ovary 5 versus 8 Trial and 458 patients on the Gynecologic Oncology Group protocol 97.[52] In managing the individual patient, factors in addition to CA125 should be taken into account before deciding whether or not to continue therapy. It is important to note that levels can fall in response to drainage of malignant ascites or effusions. Some authors have raised concerns that in patients receiving specific drugs such as paclitaxel, CA125 changes do not correlate with response allocations according to WHO criteria.[53, 54] This question has been recently re-examined in 144 patients treated with paclitaxel in four different trials and the precise 50 or 75% CA125 response criteria were found to be as sensitive as standard response criteria.[55] The definitions proposed by Rustin *et al.* are also useful in evaluating response in patients with relapsed ovarian cancer on second-line chemotherapy.[56]

E. Detecting Recurrence

Among patients with elevated antigen levels at diagnosis, clinical detection of recurrence is often preceded by an elevation of serum CA125 levels.[52] Marker elevation predates clinical relapse by a median lead-time of 60–120 days. [52, 57] The value of marker lead-time depends ultimately on a patient's remaining therapeutic options at relapse. The influence on survival and quality of life of therapeutic intervention at preclinical diagnosis of relapse is undergoing testing in a multicenter MRC/EORTC randomized controlled trial. Patients who are in remission following treatment are randomized between treatment of relapse diagnosed on CA125 criteria versus treatment only on clinical relapse. Until the results of the trial are known, it is probably best not to routinely monitor CA125 and to use it only in the differential diagnosis of clinically suspected relapse.

F. CA125 in Combination with Other Markers

Macrophage colony-stimulating factor (M-CSF), inhibin, and LPA show promise of becoming useful supplements to CA125 in ovarian cancer. In addition, markers supplementing CA125 may play an important role in the future in monitoring disease in patients with nonepithelial ovarian cancers. In mucinous ovarian cancer, one of the gastrointestinal mucin markers, CA19-9 or CA72.4 or tumor-associated trypsin inhibitor (TATI) may prove complimentary to CA125.[58, 59] Beta-hCG,[60] TATI,[61] serum urokinase-type plasminogen activator receptor (uPAR),[62] and procollagen peptides [63] appear useful in preliminary studies as prognostic indicators.

III. OTHER TUMOR MARKERS

A. Alpha-fetoprotein

Alpha-fetoprotein (AFP) is an oncofetal glycoprotein produced by the fetal yolk sac, liver, and upper gastrointestinal tract. Elevated levels occur in pregnancy and benign liver disease. Serum levels are raised in most patients with liver tumors and in some with gastric, pancreatic, colon, and bronchogenic malignancies.[64] Elevated levels are found in endodermal sinus tumors, immature teratomas, and about 10% with dysgerminomas.[65] It accurately predicts the presence of yolk sac elements in mixed germ cell tumors. In women with elevated levels, AFP is a reliable marker for monitoring therapeutic response and detecting recurrences [66, 67] and may be useful in predicting prognosis.[68] Although AFP production is extremely rare in ovarian epithelial cancers, a case has recently been described.[69]

B. Inhibin

Inhibin was isolated from ovarian follicular fluid almost 70 years ago as a substance that selectively inhibited the secretion of FSH at the level of the pituitary gland. It is now known that inhibin is present in at least two biologically active forms (inhibin A and B) as well as in a variety of a subunit precursor forms. Interest in inhibin as a marker of ovarian malignancy was stimulated by the description of elevated levels in patients with granulosa cell tumors.[70] Several groups have since confirmed the value of serum inhibin in the differential diagnosis and follow-up of patients with ovarian sex cord-stromal tumors. Immunoreactive inhibin levels are also found to be elevated in 70–87% of mucinous tumours and 15–35% of other epithelial ovarian cancers. [71–74] Assay of sera using the specific dimeric inhibin assays has shown that ovarian tumors are able to secrete dimeric inhibin, particularly inhibin B.[75, 76] However, total inhibin measured using the less specific total inhibin immunoassays seems to be the best marker to date.[77] Used in combination with CA125 as a dual tumor marker, it appears in principle that the newly developed inhibin immunoassays may have a role in screening, differential diagnosis, and monitoring of recurrence in epithelial ovarian cancer.

C. M-CSF

Cytokines are soluble mediator substances produced by cells that exercise a specific effect on other target cells. They are becoming increasingly important in tumor biology with the demonstration that many are produced by cancer cells and can influence the malignant process both positively and negatively. Serum M-CSF or CSF-1 is the most important of the cytokines studied so far in the context of ovarian cancer. It binds to the CSF-1 receptor encoded by the *fms* proto-oncogene. Elevated levels were found in 60–70% of women with ovarian cancer.[78, 79] Recent results have indicated that serum M-CSF may be highly sensitive and specific for malignant germ cell tumors of the ovary, especially dysgerminoma.[80] The marker may be useful in combination with CA125. In two retrospective trials, use of a combination of M-CSF, OVX1, and CA125 increased sensitivity for detection of stage I ovarian cancer, but this was at the expense of specificity.[81, 82] Elevated levels were associated with poor outcome following adjustment for stage, grade, and degree of surgical clearance.[83, 84] However, serum M-CSF was not found useful in the follow-up of women with advanced ovarian cancer.[85]

D. New Markers

Multiple serum markers have been assessed in isolation and in various combinations in women with ovarian cancer, both in the context of screening and differential diagnosis as well as in assessing prognosis, monitoring response, and detecting recurrence. It is not possible in this chapter to describe the numerous studies in detail. Some of the most promising of the new markers under study are LPA,[21] kallikrien,[86–88] and prostacin.[89] In addition, novel genes have been found to be upregulated in ovarian cancer using array analysis and serum assays for markers of these genes are underway. Proteomic spectra generated by mass spectroscopy (surface-enhanced laser desorption and ionization or SELDI) is now under intense investigation as a means to identify sera from patients with ovarian cancer.[90]

IV. CONCLUSION

Numerous serum tumor markers have been investigated in the context of screening and management of ovarian cancer. No single marker or combination has, as yet emerged with a clear clinical advantage over CA125, except in specific tumor subtypes such as granulosa cell or germ cell tumors with yolk sac or chorionic elements. CA125 is of increasing value in the differential diagnosis of an adnexal mass and changes on serial monitoring is a reliable indicator of response or progression of disease according to various criteria. Its clinical value as a prognostic indicator is still to be defined. In combination with TVS, serial CA125 monitoring is undergoing evaluation in randomized controlled trials of ovarian cancer screening. New technologies including expression array and SELDI are likely to identify a wealth of new candidate markers. Development of an effective strategy to select and prioritize them is essential.

References

1. Bast, R. C., Jr., Feeney, M., Lazarus, H., Nadler, L. M., Colvin, R. B., and Knapp, R. C. (1981). Reactivity of a monoclonal antibody with human ovarian carcinoma. *J. Clin. Invest.* 68(5), 1331–1337.
2. Nustad, K., Bast, R. C., Jr., Brien, T. J., Nilsson, O., Seguin, P., Suresh, M. R. *et al.* (1996). Specificity and affinity of 26 monoclonal antibodies against the CA 125 antigen: First report from the ISOBM TD-1 workshop. International Society for Oncodevelopmental Biology and Medicine. *Tumour Biol.* 17(4), 196–219.
3. Lloyd, K. O., Yin, B. W., and Kudryashov, V. (1997). Isolation and characterization of ovarian cancer antigen CA 125 using a new monoclonal antibody (VK-8): Identification as a mucin-type molecule. *Int. J. Cancer* 71(5), 842–850.
4. Yin, B. W., and Lloyd, K. O. (2001). Molecular cloning of the CA125 ovarian cancer antigen: Identification as a new mucin, MUC16. *J. Biol. Chem.* 276(29), 27371–27375.
5. Kabawat, S. E., Bast, R. C., Jr., Bhan, A. K., Welch, W. R., Knapp, R. C., and Colvin, R. B. (1983). Tissue distribution of a coelomic-epithelium-related antigen recognized by the monoclonal antibody OC125. *Int. J. Gynecol. Pathol.* 2(3), 275–285.
6. Davelaar, E. M., van Kamp, G. J., Verstraeten, R. A., and Kenemans, P. (1998). Comparison of seven immunoassays for the quantification of CA 125 antigen in serum. *Clin. Chem.* 44(7), 1417–1422.
7. Bast, R. C., Jr., Klug, T. L., St. John, E., Jenison, E., Niloff, J. M., Lazarus, H. *et al.* (1983). A radioimmunoassay using a monoclonal antibody to monitor the course of epithelial ovarian cancer. *N. Engl. J. Med.* 309(15), 883–887.
8. Jacobs, I., and Bast, R. C., Jr. (1989). The CA 125 tumour-associated antigen: A review of the literature. *Hum. Reprod.* 4(1), 1–12.
9. Vergote, I. B., Bormer, O. P., and Abeler, V. M. (1987). Evaluation of serum CA 125 levels in the monitoring of ovarian cancer. *Am. J. Obstet. Gynecol.* 157(1), 88–92.
10. Tamakoshi, K., Kikkawa, F., Shibata, K., Tomoda, K., Obata, N. H., Wakahara, F. *et al.* (1996). Clinical value of CA125, CA19-9, CEA, CA72-4, and TPA in borderline ovarian tumor. *Gynecol. Oncol.* 62(1), 67–72.
11. Zurawski, V. R., Jr., Orjaseter, H., Andersen, A., and Jellum, E. (1988). Elevated serum CA 125 levels prior to diagnosis of ovarian neoplasia: Relevance for early detection of ovarian cancer. *Int. J. Cancer* 42(5), 677–680.
12. Helzlsouer, K. J., Bush, T. L., Alberg, A. J., Bass, K. M., Zacur, H., and Comstock, G. W. (1993). Prospective study of serum CA-125 levels as markers of ovarian cancer. *JAMA* 269(9), 1123–1126.
13. Jacobs, I. J., Skates, S., Davies, A. P., Woolas, R. P., Jeyerajah, A., Weidemann, P. *et al.* (1996). Risk of diagnosis of ovarian cancer after raised serum CA 125 concentration: A prospective cohort study. *BMJ* 313(7069), 1355–1358.
14. Jacobs, I., Stabile, I., Bridges, J., Kemsley, P., Reynolds, C., Grudzinskas, J. *et al.* (1988). Multimodal approach to screening for ovarian cancer. *Lancet* 1(8580), 268–271.
15. Jacobs, I., Davies, A. P., Bridges, J., Stabile, I., Fay, T., Lower, A. *et al.* (1993). Prevalence screening for ovarian cancer in postmenopausal women by CA 125 measurement and ultrasonography. *BMJ* 306(6884), 1030–1034.
16. Skates, S. J., Xu, F. J., Yu, Y. H., Sjovall, K., Einhorn, N., Chang, Y. *et al.* (1995). Toward an optimal algorithm for ovarian cancer screening with longitudinal tumor markers. *Cancer* 76(10 Suppl.), 2004–2010.
17. Skates, S., Pauler, D., and Jacobs, I. (2001). Screening based on the risk of cancer calculation from Bayesian hierarchical change-point and mixture models of longitudinal markers. *J. Am. Stat. Assoc.* 96(454), 429–439.
18. Menon, U., Talaat, A., Rosenthal, A. N., Macdonald, N. D., Jeyerajah, A. R., Skates, S. J. *et al.* (2000). Performance of ultrasound as a second line test to serum CA125 in ovarian cancer screening. *BJOG* 107(2), 165–169.
19. Prorok, P. C., Andriole, G. L., Bresalier, R. S., Buys, S. S., Chia, D., Crawford, E. D. *et al.* (2000). Design of the Prostate, Lung, Colorectal and Ovarian (PLCO) Cancer Screening Trial. *Control Clin. Trials* 21(6 Suppl.), 273S–309S.
20. Gohagan, J. K., Prorok, P. C., Hayes, R. B., and Kramer, B. S. (2000). The Prostate, Lung, Colorectal and Ovarian (PLCO) Cancer Screening Trial of the National Cancer Institute: History, organization, and status. *Control Clin. Trials* 21(6 Suppl.), 251S–272S.
21. Xu, Y., Shen, Z., Wiper, D. W., Wu, M., Morton, R. E., Elson, P. *et al.* (1998). Lysophosphatidic acid as a potential biomarker for ovarian and other gynecologic cancers. *JAMA* 280(8), 719–723.
22. Einhorn, N., Sjovall, K., Knapp, R. C., Hall, P., Scully, R. E,, Bast, R. C., Jr. *et al.* (1992). Prospective evaluation of serum CA 125 levels for early detection of ovarian cancer. *Obstet. Gynecol.* 80(1), 14–18.
23. Gadducci, A., Ferdeghini, M., Prontera, C., Moretti, L., Mariani, G., Bianchi, R. *et al.* (1992). The concomitant determination of different tumor markers in patients with epithelial ovarian cancer and benign ovarian masses: Relevance for differential diagnosis. *Gynecol. Oncol.* 44(2), 147–154.
24. Soper, J. T., Hunter, V. J., Daly, L., Tanner, M., Creasman, W. T., and Bast, R. C., Jr. (1990). Preoperative serum tumor-associated antigen levels in women with pelvic masses. *Obstet. Gynecol.* 75(2), 249–254.
25. Curtin, J. P. (1994). Management of the adnexal mass. *Gynecol. Oncol.* 55(3 Pt 2), S42–S46.
26. Parker, W. H., Levine, R. L., Howard, F. M., Sansone, B., and Berek, J. S. (1994). A multicenter study of laparoscopic management of selected cystic adnexal masses in postmenopausal women. *J. Am. Coll. Surg.* 179(6), 733–737.
27. Maggino, T., Gadducci, A., D'Addario, V., Pecorelli, S., Lissoni, A., Stella, M. *et al.* (1994). Prospective multicenter study on CA 125 in postmenopausal pelvic masses. *Gynecol. Oncol.* 54(2), 117–123.

28. Jacobs, I., Oram, D., Fairbanks, J., Turner, J., Frost, C., and Grudzinskas, J. G. (1990). A risk of malignancy index incorporating CA125, ultrasound and menopausal status for the accurate preoperative diagnosis of ovarian cancer. *Br. J. Obstet. Gynaecol.* 97(10), 922–929.
29. Tingulstad, S., Hagen, B., Skjeldestad, F. E., Onsrud, M., Kiserud, T., Halvorsen, T. *et al.* (1996). Evaluation of a risk of malignancy index based on serum CA125, ultrasound findings and menopausal status in the pre-operative diagnosis of pelvic masses. *Br. J. Obstet. Gynaecol.* 103(8), 826–831.
30. Venesmaa, P., Lehtovirta, P., Stenman, U. H., Leminen, A., Forss, M., and Ylikorkala, O. (1994). Tumour-associated trypsin inhibitor (TATI): Comparison with CA125 as a preoperative prognostic indicator in advanced ovarian cancer. *Br. J. Cancer* 70(6), 1188–1190.
31. Makar, A. P., Kristensen, G. B., Kaern, J., Bormer, O. P., Abeler, V. M., and Trope, C. G. (1992). Prognostic value of pre- and postoperative serum CA 125 levels in ovarian cancer: New aspects and multivariate analysis. *Obstet. Gynecol.* 79(6), 1002–1010.
32. Colakovic, S., Lukic, V., Mitrovic, L., Jelic, S., Susnjar, S., and Marinkovic, J. (2000). Prognostic value of CA125 kinetics and half-life in advanced ovarian cancer. *Int. J. Biol. Markers* 15(2), 147–152.
33. Parker, D., Bradley, C., Bogle, S. M., Lay, J., Masood, M., Hancock, A. K. *et al.* (1994). Serum albumin and CA125 are powerful predictors of survival in epithelial ovarian cancer. *Br. J. Obstet. Gynaecol.* 101(10), 888–893.
34. Nagele, F., Petru, E., Medl, M., Kainz, C., Graf, A. H., and Sevelda, P. (1995). Preoperative CA 125: An independent prognostic factor in patients with stage I epithelial ovarian cancer. *Obstet. Gynecol.* 86(2), 259–264.
35. Chi, D. S., Venkatraman, E. S., Masson, V., and Hoskins, W. J. (2000). The ability of preoperative serum CA-125 to predict optimal primary tumor cytoreduction in stage III epithelial ovarian carcinoma. *Gynecol. Oncol.* 77(2), 227–231.
36. Berek, J. S. (2000). Preoperative prediction of optimal resectability in advanced ovarian cancer using CA-125. *Gynecol. Oncol.* 77(2), 225–226.
37. Rosen, A., Sevelda, P., Klein, M., Spona, J., and Beck, A. (1990). A CA125 score as a prognostic index in patients with ovarian cancer. *Arch. Gynecol. Obstet.* 247(3), 125–129.
38. Yedema, C. A., Kenemans, P., Thomas, C. M., Massuger, L. F., Wobbes, T., Verstraeten, R. *et al.* (1993). CA 125 serum levels in the early post-operative period do not reflect tumour reduction obtained by cytoreductive surgery. *Eur. J. Cancer* 29A(7), 966–971.
39. Yedema, C. A., Kenemans, P., Voorhorst, F., Bon, G., Schijf, C., Beex, L. *et al.* (1993). CA 125 half-life in ovarian cancer: A multivariate survival analysis. *Br. J. Cancer* 67(6), 1361–1367.
40. van der Burg, M. E., Lammes, F. B., van Putten, W. L., and Stoter, G. (1988). Ovarian cancer: The prognostic value of the serum half-life of CA125 during induction chemotherapy. *Gynecol. Oncol.* 30(3), 307–312.
41. Rosman, M., Hayden, C. L., Thiel, R. P., Chambers, J. T., Kohorn, E. I., Chambers, S. K. *et al.* (1994). Prognostic indicators for poor risk epithelial ovarian carcinoma. *Cancer* 74(4), 1323–1328.
42. Gadducci, A., Zola, P., Landoni, F., Maggino, T., Sartori, E., Bergamino, T. *et al.* (1995). Serum half-life of CA 125 during early chemotherapy as an independent prognostic variable for patients with advanced epithelial ovarian cancer: Results of a multicentric Italian study. *Gynecol. Oncol.* 58(1), 42–47.
43. Makar, A. P., Kristensen, G. B., Bormer, O. P., and Trope, C. G. (1993). Serum CA 125 level allows early identification of nonresponders during induction chemotherapy. *Gynecol. Oncol.* 49(1), 73–79.
44. Redman, C. W., Blackledge, G. R., Kelly, K., Powell, J., Buxton, E. J., and Luesley, D. M. (1990). Early serum CA125 response and outcome in epithelial ovarian cancer. *Eur. J. Cancer* 26(5), 593–596.
45. Buller, R. E., Vasilev, S., and DiSaia, P. J. (1996). CA 125 kinetics: A cost-effective clinical tool to evaluate clinical trial outcomes in the 1990s. *Am. J. Obstet. Gynecol.* 174(4), 1241–1253; discussion 1253–1254.
46. Meyer, T., and Rustin, G. J. (2000). Role of tumour markers in monitoring epithelial ovarian cancer. *Br. J. Cancer* 82(9), 1535–1538.
47. Hawkins, R. E., Roberts, K., Wiltshaw, E., Mundy, J., and McCready, V. R. (1989). The clinical correlates of serum CA125 in 169 patients with epithelial ovarian carcinoma. *Br. J. Cancer* 60(4), 634–637.
48. Ng, L. W., Homesley, H. D., Barrett, R. J., Welander, C. E., and Case, L. D. (1989). CA-125 values predictive of clinical response during second-line chemotherapy for epithelial ovarian cancer. *Am. J. Clin. Oncol.* 12(2), 106–109.
49. Markman, M. (1993). A proposal to use CA-125 to evaluate activity of new antineoplastic agents in ovarian cancer. *Gynecol. Oncol.* 51(3), 297–298.
50. Rustin, G. J., van der Burg, M. E., and Berek, J. S. (1993). Advanced ovarian cancer. Tumour markers. *Ann. Oncol.* 4Suppl. 4, 71–77.
51. Rustin, G. J., Nelstrop, A. E., McClean, P., Brady, M. F., McGuire, W. P., Hoskins, W. J. *et al.* (1996). Defining response of ovarian carcinoma to initial chemotherapy according to serum CA 125. *J. Clin. Oncol.* 14(5), 1545–1551.
52. Rustin, G. J., Nelstrop, A. E., Tuxen, M. K., and Lambert, H. E. (1996). Defining progression of ovarian carcinoma during follow-up according to CA 125: A North Thames Ovary Group Study. *Ann. Oncol.* 7(4), 361–364.
53. Pearl, M. L., Yashar, C. M., Johnston, C. M., Reynolds, R. K., and Roberts, J. A. (1994). Exponential regression of CA 125 during salvage treatment of ovarian cancer with taxol. *Gynecol. Oncol.* 53(3), 339–343.
54. Davelaar, E. M., Bonfrer, J. M., Verstraeten, R. A., ten Bokkel Huinink, W. W., and Kenemans, P. (1996). CA 125: A valid marker in ovarian carcinoma patients treated with paclitaxel? *Cancer* 78(1), 118–127.
55. Bridgewater, J. A., Nelstrop, A. E., Rustin, G. J., Gore, M. E., McGuire, W. P., and Hoskins, W. J. (1999). Comparison of standard and CA-125 response criteria in patients with epithelial ovarian cancer treated with platinum or paclitaxel. *J. Clin. Oncol.* 17(2), 501–508.
56. Rustin, G. J., Nelstrop, A. E., Crawford, M., Ledermann, J., Lambert, H. E., Coleman, R. *et al.* (1997). Phase II trial of oral altretamine for relapsed ovarian carcinoma: Evaluation of defining response by serum CA125. *J. Clin. Oncol.* 15(1), 172–176.
57. Cruickshank, D. J., Terry, P. B., and Fullerton, W. T. (1991). The potential value of CA125 as a tumour marker in small volume, non-evaluable epithelial ovarian cancer. *Int. J. Biol. Markers* 6(4), 247–252.
58. Stenman, U. H., Alfthan, H., Vartiainen, J., and Lehtovirta, P. (1995). Markers supplementing CA 125 in ovarian cancer. *Ann. Med.* 27(1), 115–120.
59. Peters-Engl, C., Medl, M., Ogris, E., and Leodolter, S. (1995). Tumor-associated trypsin inhibitor (TATI) and cancer antigen 125 (CA125) in patients with epithelial ovarian cancer. *Anticancer Res.* 15(6B), 2727–2730.
60. Vartiainen, J., Lehtovirta, P., Finne, P., Stenman, U. H., and Alfthan, H. (2001). Preoperative serum concentration of hCGbeta as a prognostic factor in ovarian cancer. *Int. J. Cancer* 95(5), 313–316.
61. Venesmaa, P., Stenman, U. H., Forss, M., Leminen, A., Lehtovirta, P., Vartiainen, J. *et al.* (1998). Pre-operative serum level of tumour-associated trypsin inhibitor and residual tumour size as prognostic indicators in Stage III epithelial ovarian cancer. *Br. J. Obstet. Gynaecol.* 105(5), 508–511.
62. Sier, C. F., Stephens, R., Bizik, J., Mariani, A., Bassan, M., Pedersen, N. *et al.* (1998). The level of urokinase-type plasminogen activator receptor is increased in serum of ovarian cancer patients. *Cancer Res.* 58(9), 1843–1849.
63. Simojoki, M., Santala, M., Risteli, J., Risteli, L., and Kauppila, A. (2000). Serial determinations of aminoterminal propeptide of type III procollagen (PIIINP) and prognosis in ovarian cancer; Comparison to CA125. *Anticancer Res.* 20(6C), 4655–4660.
64. Onsrud, M. (1991). Tumour markers in gynaecologic oncology. *Scand. J. Clin. Lab. Invest. Suppl.* 206, 60–70.

65. Kawai, M., Kano, T., Kikkawa, F., Morikawa, Y., Oguchi, H., Nakashima, N. *et al.* (1992). Seven tumor markers in benign and malignant germ cell tumors of the ovary. *Gynecol. Oncol.* 45(3), 248–253.
66. Chow, S. N., Yang, J. H., Lin, Y. H., Chen, Y. P., Lai, J. I., Chen, R. J. *et al.* (1996). Malignant ovarian germ cell tumors. *Int. J. Gynaecol. Obstet.* 53(2), 151–158.
67. Zalel, Y., Piura, B., Elchalal, U., Czernobilsky, B., Antebi, S., and Dgani, R. (1996). Diagnosis and management of malignant germ cell ovarian tumors in young females. *Int. J. Gynaecol. Obstet.* 55(1), 1–10.
68. Mayordomo, J. I., Paz-Ares, L., Rivera, F., Lopez-Brea, M., Lopez Martin, E., Mendiola, C. *et al.* (1994). Ovarian and extragonadal malignant germ-cell tumors in females: A single-institution experience with 43 patients. *Ann. Oncol.* 5(3), 225–231.
69. Maida, Y., Kyo, S., Takakura, M., Kanaya, T., and Inoue, M. (1998). Ovarian endometrioid adenocarcinoma with ectopic production of alpha-fetoprotein. *Gynecol. Oncol.* 71(1), 133–136.
70. Lappohn, R. E., Burger, H. G., Bouma, J., Bangah, M., Krans, M., and de Bruijn, H. W. (1989). Inhibin as a marker for granulosa-cell tumors. *N. Engl. J. Med.* 321(12), 790–793.
71. Healy, D. L., Burger, H. G., Mamers, P., Jobling, T., Bangah, M., Quinn, M. *et al.* (1993). Elevated serum inhibin concentrations in postmenopausal women with ovarian tumors. *N. Engl. J. Med.* 329(21), 1539–1542.
72. Burger, H. G., Baillie, A., Drummond, A. E., Healy, D. L., Jobling, T., Mamers, P. *et al.* (1998). Inhibin and ovarian cancer. *J. Reprod. Immunol.* 39(1–2), 77–87.
73. Burger, H. G., Robertson, D. M., Cahir, N., Mamers, P., Healy, D. L., Jobling, T. *et al.* (1996). Characterization of inhibin immunoreactivity in post-menopausal women with ovarian tumours. *Clin. Endocrinol. (Oxf.)*;44(4), 413–418.
74. Robertson, D. M., Cahir, N., Burger, H. G., Mamers, P., McCloud, P. I., Pettersson, K. *et al.* (1999). Combined inhibin and CA125 assays in the detection of ovarian cancer. *Clin. Chem.* 45(5), 651–658.
75. Lambert-Messerlian, G. M., Steinhoff, M., Zheng, W., Canick, J. A., Gajewski, W. H., Seifer, D. B. *et al.* (1997). Multiple immunoreactive inhibin proteins in serum from postmenopausal women with epithelial ovarian cancer. *Gynecol. Oncol.* 65(3), 512–516.
76. Menon, U., Riley, S. C., Thomas, J., Bose, C., Dawnay, A., Evans, L. W. *et al.* (2000). Serum inhibin, activin and follistatin in postmenopausal women with epithelial ovarian carcinoma. *BJOG.* 107(9), 1069–1074.
77. Robertson, D. M., Stephenson, T., Pruysers, E., McCloud, P., Tsigos, A., Groome, N. *et al.* (2002). Characterization of inhibin forms and their measurement by an inhibin alpha-subunit ELISA in serum from postmenopausal women with ovarian cancer. *J. Clin. Endocrinol. Metab.* 87(2), 816–824.
78. Xu, F. J., Ramakrishnan, S., Daly, L., Soper, J. T., Berchuck, A., Clarke-Pearson, D. *et al.* (1991). Increased serum levels of macrophage colony-stimulating factor in ovarian cancer. *Am. J. Obstet. Gynecol.* 165(5 Pt 1), 1356–1362.
79. Suzuki, M., Ohwada, M., Aida, I., Tamada, T., Hanamura, T., and Nagatomo, M. (1993). Macrophage colony-stimulating factor as a tumor marker for epithelial ovarian cancer. *Obstet. Gynecol.* 82(6), 946–950.
80. Suzuki, M., Kobayashi, H., Ohwada, M., Terao, T., and Sato, I. (1998). Macrophage colony-stimulating factor as a marker for malignant germ cell tumors of the ovary. *Gynecol. Oncol.* 68(1), 35–37.
81. van Haaften-Day, C., Shen, Y., Xu, F., Yu, Y., Berchuck, A., Havrilesky, L. J. *et al.* (2001). OVX1, macrophage-colony stimulating factor, and CA-125-II as tumor markers for epithelial ovarian carcinoma: A critical appraisal. *Cancer* 92(11), 2837–2844.
82. Woolas, R. P., Xu, F. J., Jacobs, I. J., Yu, Y. H., Daly, L., Berchuck, A. *et al.* (1993). Elevation of multiple serum markers in patients with stage I ovarian cancer. *J. Natl. Cancer Inst.* 85(21), 1748–1751.
83. Scholl, S. M., Bascou, C. H., Mosseri, V., Olivares, R., Magdelenat, H., Dorval, T. *et al.* (1994). Circulating levels of colony-stimulating factor 1 as a prognostic indicator in 82 patients with epithelial ovarian cancer. *Br. J. Cancer* 69(2), 342–346.
84. Price, F. V., Chambers, S. K., Chambers, J. T., Carcangiu, M. L., Schwartz, P. E., Kohorn, E. I. *et al.* (1993). Colony-stimulating factor-1 in primary ascites of ovarian cancer is a significant predictor of survival. *Am. J. Obstet. Gynecol.* 168(2), 520–527.
85. Gadducci, A., Ferdeghini, M., Castellani, C., Annicchiarico, C., Prontera, C., Facchini, V. *et al.* (1998). Serum macrophage colony-stimulating factor (M-CSF) levels in patients with epithelial ovarian cancer. *Gynecol. Oncol.* 70(1), 111–114.
86. Diamandis, E. P., Yousef, G. M., Soosaipillai, A. R., and Bunting, P. (2000). Human kallikrein 6 (zyme/protease M/neurosin): A new serum biomarker of ovarian carcinoma. *Clin. Biochem.* 33(7), 579–583.
87. Diamandis, E. P., Okui, A., Mitsui, S., Luo, L. Y., Soosaipillai, A., Grass, L. *et al.* (2002). Human kallikrein 11: A new biomarker of prostate and ovarian carcinoma. *Cancer Res.* 62(1), 295–300.
88. Luo, L. Y., Bunting, P., Scorilas, A., and Diamandis, E. P. (2001). Human kallikrein 10: A novel tumor marker for ovarian carcinoma? *Clin. Chim. Acta* 306(1–2), 111–118.
89. Mok, S. C., Chao, J., Skates, S., Wong, K., Yiu, G. K., Muto, M. G. *et al.* (2001). Prostasin, a potential serum marker for ovarian cancer: Identification through microarray technology. *J. Natl. Cancer Inst.* 93(19), 1458–1464.
90. Petricoin, E. F., Ardekani, A. M., Hitt, B. A., Levine, P. J., Fusaro, V. A., Steinberg, S. M. *et al.* (2002). Use of proteomic patterns in serum to identify ovarian cancer. *Lancet* 359(9306), 572–577.

CHAPTER

16

BRCA1 and BRCA2 Mutations in Ovarian Carcinoma

GEORGE COUKOS
Division of Gynecologic Oncology
University of Pennsylvania Medical Center
Philadelphia, Pennsylvania 19104

STEPHEN C. RUBIN
Division of Gynecologic Oncology
University of Pennsylvania Medical Center
Philadelphia, Pennsylvania 19104

In the U.S., epithelial ovarian carcinoma causes the highest mortality of all gynecologic cancers; there are 26,700 new cases estimated and 14,800 deaths associated with this malignancy annually. The current Surveillance, Epidemiology, and End Results (SEER) estimation of lifetime risk for ovarian cancer is 1:55 (1.8%) over a woman's lifetime in the U.S., up from the 1970 figures of 1:70 (1.4%).[1,2] In African-American women such risk is approximately 1%.

Of all women who present with ovarian cancer, 20% have a family history of ovarian cancer and 8% carry a germline mutation. The term "hereditary" ovarian cancer was defined by the Breast Cancer Linkage Consortium as clustering of three or more cases of ovarian cancer or a total of four or more early-onset (younger than 60) breast or ovarian cancers at any age. Population studies and detailed analyses of familial ovarian cancer pedigrees have indicated the existence of the breast and ovarian cancer syndrome, in which multiple members of the family are affected by breast or ovarian cancer or both. Typically, family pedigrees contain five or more breast or ovarian cancers in first- or second-degree relatives [3] or at least three cases of early-onset (before age 60 years) breast or ovarian cancer.[4] This group also contains a small proportion of families with site-specific ovarian cancer.

Efforts to identify the genetic basis of familial ovarian cancer culminated in the identification of the breast/ovarian cancer susceptibility genes BRCA1 and BRCA2 through positional cloning approximately five years ago. Germline mutations in either of these genes account for the vast majority of hereditary ovarian cancers.[5] By contrast, approximately up to 60% of hereditary breast cancer cases are attributed to germline BRCA1 and BRCA2 mutations.[6] Genetic linkage analysis indicates that approximately 10–15% of hereditary ovarian cancers present as site-specific. These cases are invariably linked to BRCA1 mutations. Another 65–75% of cases belong to the far more common breast and ovarian cancer syndrome. This syndrome exhibits more genetic heterogeneity, with the majority of cases being related to mutations in BRCA1, while virtually all remaining cases are related to mutations in the BRCA2 gene.

I. FUNCTION OF BRCA1 AND BRCA2

Significant efforts have been made to characterize the functions of BRCA1 and BRCA2. Although there is apparent dissimilarity in protein sequence and structure, BRCA1 and BRCA2 likely exert similar biological functions. Their protein products exhibit similar patterns of expression and subcellular localization and are both expressed in many tissues in a cell-cycle-dependent manner.[7–11] Their levels are highest during S phase, suggesting functions during DNA replication. In fact, the C terminus of BRCA1 contains two 95-residue BRCT (BRCA1 C-terminal) domains, which are also found in many other proteins involved in DNA repair and cell cycle regulation.[12]

Both BRCA1 and BRCA2 are tumor suppressor genes. Although the exact function has not been elucidated, indirect evidence suggests that the normal protein products of BRCA1 and BRCA2 are involved in the fundamental cellular processes of maintaining genomic integrity and transcriptional regulation. BRCA1 and BRCA2 proteins participate in the control of homologous recombination and double-strand break repair during cellular response to DNA damage. Both proteins have been reported to bind to RAD51, a protein essential for DNA repair and genetic recombination.[13, 14] BRCA1 is rapidly recruited to break sites of DNA damage, where the histone H2A family member H2AX becomes extensively phosphorylated. BRCA1-deficient and BRCA2-deficient murine cells exhibit hypersensitivity to genotoxins such as x-rays.[7, 15] Cells that contain truncated BRCA1 or BRCA2 progressively accumulate aberrations in chromosome structure during passage in culture; these typically include multiradial chromosomes as well as chromosome breaks.[15] BRCA1 is involved at multiple levels in the DNA damage response, while it is possible that BRCA2 only controls the intracellular transport and function of RAD51 and through it DNA repair by homologous recombination.[16] An additional mechanism by which BRCA1 may control the response to DNA damage may be through the transcriptional regulation of genes downstream of p53, such as p21 CIP1 cyclin-dependent kinase inhibitor[17] and the GADD45 tumor suppressor,[18, 19] both of which are activated in response to DNA damage. BRCA1 co-purifies with the RNA polymerase II holoenzyme through an interaction with a helicase component.[20] These findings suggest that BRCA1 may participate in transcription-coupled DNA repair, a process entailing preferential removal of base lesions from the transcribed DNA strand following X irradiation or oxidative damage.

II. BRCA1 AND BRCA2 MUTATIONS IN OVARIAN CANCER

Together, germline mutations in BRCA1 and BRCA2 account for the great majority of families with hereditary susceptibility to breast and ovarian cancer. The breast and ovarian cancer phenotypes associated with mutations in BRCA1 and BRCA2 are similar, confirming that the two proteins exert common functions. BRCA1 and BRCA2 mutations are highly penetrant, with variation related to genetic background.[6] The majority of germline mutations are small insertions or deletions distributed throughout the genes, which result in protein truncation. Missense and nonsense alterations have also been described. A list of known mutations can be found in http://www.nhgri.nih.gov/Intramural_research/Lab transfer/Bic. Breast and ovarian tumors almost invariably exhibit loss of heterozygosity while retaining the mutant allele.[5]

The BRCA1 is localized to chromosome 17q21 locus and accounts for more than 80% of hereditary ovarian cancers and approximately 45% of breast cancers occurring within the context of breast and ovarian cancer syndrome.[21] Overall, approximately 5% of ovarian cancers have been attributed to germline BRCA1 mutations,[22, 23] but in Israel, BRCA1 mutations have been identified in 40% of ovarian cancer cases with a family history and 13% of those without such a history. Germline BRCA1 mutations are also responsible for fallopian tube and primary peritoneal carcinomas.[24] Among 45 Canadian women diagnosed with fallopian tube cancer, 11% were positive for a germline mutation in BRCA1. The incidence increased significantly (28%) when only women diagnosed at or before age 55 were considered.[25] Germline BRCA1 mutations were also detected in 26% of 43 patients with papillary serous carcinoma of the peritoneum. BRCA1 mutation carriers had a higher overall incidence of p53 mutations (89%), were more likely to exhibit multifocal or null p53 mutations and were less likely to exhibit erbB-2 overexpression than wild-type BRCA1 case subjects.[26]

The BRCA2 breast-ovarian cancer susceptibility gene is localized to chromosome 13q12. BRCA2 consists of 26 coding exons spanning over 70 kb of genomic DNA. It is also expressed in thymus, testis, breast, and ovary, but its role in normal breast and ovarian epithelium remains unclear. BRCA2 may account for as much as 10–35% of hereditary ovarian cancers. Both male and female BRCA2 carriers have a high risk of early-onset breast cancer.[5] Similarly to BRCA1, mutations of BRCA2 also occur throughout the gene and are for the most part loss-of-function or frameshift mutations. Germline BRCA2 mutations predispose to breast and ovarian carcinoma as well as fallopian tube and primary peritoneal carcinoma. Among 45 patients with fallopian tube cancers, 5% were positive for a mutation in BRCA2.[25]

How does loss of BRCA1 or BRCA2 function lead to breast or ovarian cancer? Malignant transformation in breast and ovaries of individuals with germline BRCA mutations requires somatic inactivation of the remaining wild-type allele. The inherited inactivating allele and the subsequent somatic genomic loss of the wild-type allele results in complete BRCA deficiency in ovarian epithelial cells. Cells that lack BRCA1 or BRCA2 accumulate chromosomal abnormalities including chromosomal breaks, severe aneuploidy and centrosome amplification. Chromosomal instability as a result of BRCA1 or BRCA2 deficiency may be the pathogenic basis for tumor formation. Most cells that have BRCA function loss will be unable to repair DNA damage and will die. However, if cells are subjected to stimuli promoting rapid proliferation, some repair-deficient cells may escape death and eventually undergo malignant transformation. In breast epithelium, estrogens may represent an obvious stimulus promoting proliferation, but in ovarian surface epithelium such factors to date remain elusive.

Among sporadic breast or ovarian tumors, 50–70% has lost an allele of BRCA1 and 30–50% has lost an allele of BRCA2.

These observations suggest that somatic loss of BRCA genes may be associated with sporadic breast and ovarian tumorigenesis. In addition, reduction or complete loss of BRCA1and BRCA2 protein has been documented in a large number of sporadic breast and ovarian tumors. The exact role of somatic BRCA mutations in somatic ovarian cancer, however, is unclear. Possibly, BRCA1 and BRCA2 mutations may be a late event in somatic ovarian carcinomas.

A. Risk Assessment

Thanks to the discovery of BRCA1 and BRCA2, genetic testing is today available to patients seeking estimation and reduction of cancer risk. Based on the American Society of Clinical Oncology 1996 recommendations, genetic testing for breast or ovarian cancer should be performed when the *a priori* probability of finding a germline mutation is equal to or more than 10%. The risk estimation is usually based on clinical history data including a significant familial background and/or early-onset breast cancer and/or ethnicity. Family history, especially when it reveals clustering of breast and/or ovarian carcinomas, has the best positive predictive value, ranging from 33–67%. However, the power of family history is potentially limited by anamnestic bias or lack of medically confirmed diagnoses. The number of kindred clearly influences the predictive power of pedigrees. In fact, a significant proportion of patients that tested positive for BRCA mutations only exhibit a mildly suggestive family history.[27, 28] In an earlier study from our institution, 10 BRCA1 germline mutations were identified among 116 unselected ovarian cancer patients: more than half the patients had family histories that would generally be considered unremarkable. Furthermore, the majority of ovarian cancer patients with maternal family history of breast or ovarian cancer or maternal family history of any cancer tested negative for mutations.[29]

Initial studies in families selected on the basis of strong family history and early age of onset suggested that the lifetime risk of developing ovarian cancer in women who carry a BRCA1 mutation was as high as 63% and in women who carry a BRCA2 mutation was 27%.[30, 31] More recently, the lifetime risk of ovarian cancer was reduced to 27.8% in BRCA1 carriers based on segregation analysis of reported ovarian cancer occurrence in first-degree relatives of participants in three case-control studies in the U.S.[23] Similarly, the lifetime penetrance of breast cancer at age 70 years was initially reported as high as 87% [31] and more recently as 56%.[32] In a recent study on Ashkenazi Jews, BRCA1 carriers had a lifetime risk of ovarian cancer as low as 16%,[32] but cancer cases beyond the proband were identified through questionnaires, which may underestimate the true incidence of ovarian cancer. These disparities highlight the uncertainty in our estimates, due in part to the low prevalence of specific BRCA1 or BRCA2 mutations, which limits the data set from which genotype/phenotype correlations can be derived. Additionally, different types of BRCA mutation penetrance or different genetic or environmental covariants among the different groups of women may play a role. In studies of BRCA2 founder mutations in the Icelandic population,[33, 34] the risk of cancer associated with BRCA2 *999del5* mutation was shown to vary considerably among families, resulting in differences in the age of cancer onset, the degree of penetrance, and even the type of tumor to which individuals are predisposed, suggesting that other genetic factors or tumor-host interactions may play an important role.

The relative difference in penetrance among different mutations within the same gene remains a controversial issue. Although one study from the U.K. reported that mutations in the carboxy terminus end of the BRCA1 gene favor breast cancer over ovarian cancer, while mutations in the proximal amino end of the gene resulted in a higher likelihood of developing ovarian cancer,[35] another study from the U.S. at the Myriad Genetic Laboratories performed on 798 high-risk families did not confirm this association.[36] Furthermore, differences in ovarian cancer penetrance have been observed among different families with identical BRCA1 mutations.

B. Risk Reduction Options

The medical and surgical options offered to high-risk women remain conventional. Women with proven disease-associated mutation in BRCA1 or BRCA2 have relatively few clinical management options available to reduce their risk of developing ovarian (and breast) cancer. Preventive strategies include (1) screening, (2) chemoprevention, and (3) prophylactic surgery.

Screening procedures have proven highly ineffective in the general population and the consensus is that the current screening methodologies do not perform any better in the setting of hereditary ovarian cancer. The positive predictive value of an abnormal pelvic ultrasound is 2% in women with one relative affected, while that of serum CA125 is barely 10%.

Chemoprevention of ovarian cancer is still at its infancy. Oral contraceptives have been shown to significantly reduce the risk of ovarian carcinoma in the general population and their protective effect is applicable also to women with germline BRCA1 or BRCA2 mutations. In the general population, the risk reduction depends on the length of use; multiparous and nulliparous women achieve a 40–50% risk reduction after five years of use, including low-dose formulations.[37] In a case-control study in carriers of BRCA1 or BRCA2 mutations, use of oral contraceptives conferred a risk reduction of 50%, [38] which is similar to that observed in the general population.[39] However, the effects of oral contraceptive use on breast cancer risk in patients with germline BRCA mutations are unknown. Data from a small study of young breast cancer patients suggest that long-term oral contraceptive use before first full-term pregnancy increases breast cancer risk more in BRCA mutation carriers than in noncarriers.[40] In a cohort of 87 Ashkenazi patients with breast and/or ovarian cancer and *185delAG* and *5382insC* mutations in the BRCA1 gene and *6174delT* in the BRCA2 gene, oral contraceptive use was documented in 61.3% of breast cancer patients as compared to 11.8% of ovarian cancer patients.[41] Clearly, these results need replication with larger numbers. If this notion is confirmed, the beneficial effects of oral contraceptives on life expectancy would be negated.

Progestational agents may offer superior chemoprotection of ovarian cancer compared to oral contraceptives, based on a nonhuman primate study.[42] However, progestins exert a mitogenic effect on breast tissue and may also increase the risk of breast cancer in patients with germline BRCA mutations. Finally, the synthetic retinoid 4-HPR (fenretinide) may offer protective effects. A trial designed to prevent primary cancers in the contralateral breasts of patients with localized breast cancer showed a reduction of second breast malignancies in premenopausal women. In addition, a significant decrease of circulating insulin-like growth factor (IGF)-I, a known risk factor for premenopausal breast cancer, was observed after one year of fenretinide administration in premenopausal women with breast cancer.[43, 44] Furthermore, the same study suggests fenretinide treatment may be associated with a lower incidence of ovarian carcinoma during the intervention period but such a protective effect may be lost once treatment is discontinued.[45]

Because current conservative options for ovarian cancer prevention are not effective, many high-risk women consider the option of bilateral prophylactic oophorectomy, in the hope that removal of healthy ovarian tissue will reduce their risk of developing invasive malignancy. Studies from U.S., Canadian, and European centers have shown that women carrying a BRCA mutation are more prone to undergo prophylactic oophorectomy than prophylactic mastectomy, with more than 50% of carriers opting for oophorectomy and 8–28% undergoing mastectomy.[46, 47] The recent evidence that BRCA mutation carriers are also predisposed to fallopian tube cancers raises the issue of whether oophorectomy alone is enough. Removal of the fallopian tubes appears advisable based on these observations. Because bilateral salpingo-oophorectomy does not remove the interstitial and isthmic portion of the fallopian tubes, some advocate inclusion of hysterectomy in the routine management of patients.[48] But how significant is the protection offered by prophylactic oophorectomy? The response will depend on the parameters used to monitor the beneficial effects of prophylactic oophorectomy.

At least three end points may be considered: quality of life, cancer-free survival, and overall life expectancy. Most studies have shown that quality of life improves following prophylactic oophorectomy. Among 60 women who underwent prophylactic oophorectomy or ovarian cancer surveillance at Washington University, only 7% of women undergoing surgery expressed regret about their decision, while 50% of patients undergoing surveillance expressed some regret, and 10% were frankly dissatisfied with their management.[49] In-depth interviews conducted with 14 women between 4 months and 7 years after prophylactic oophorectomy indicated a high degree of satisfaction with their decision to undergo oophorectomy. Women emphasized that the procedure had decreased their anxiety about developing ovarian cancer.[50]

Cancer-free survival following oophorectomy depends on the relative lifetime risk of developing ovarian, breast, fallopian, or peritoneal carcinoma. Currently, information is not sufficient to discriminate between highly penetrant and scarcely penetrant BRCA mutations or site-specific mutations (breast versus ovarian versus other carcinoma). As the estimated penetrance of BRCA1 or BRCA2 mutations for ovarian cancer have declined, the impact of prophylactic oophorectomy appears less significant. A woman with hereditary breast and ovarian syndrome undergoing prophylactic oophorectomy may still develop breast carcinoma, but a number of studies have suggested that prophylactic oophorectomy may reduce the risk of subsequent breast cancer. Most studies have been conducted in women with elevated but undefined breast or ovarian cancer risk.[51] In a cohort of women with disease-associated germline BRCA1 mutations from 5 North American institutions, including 43 women with BRCA1 mutations who underwent bilateral prophylactic oophorectomy but not a prophylactic mastectomy and 79 control subjects with BRCA1 mutations who had no history of oophorectomy, a statistically significant reduction in breast cancer risk was found after bilateral prophylactic oophorectomy, with an adjusted hazard ratio of 0.53 up to 5 years and 0.33 after 10 years of follow-up after surgery.[52]

The risk of developing peritoneal carcinoma after prophylactic oophorectomy has been markedly emphasized by several investigators. Among 324 women who had undergone prophylactic oophorectomy from the Gilda Radner Familial Ovarian Cancer Registry, 1.8% developed primary peritoneal carcinoma indistinguishable from ovarian cancer 1–27 years after prophylactic oophorectomy. The incidence of primary peritoneal carcinoma after prophylactic oophorectomy has been higher in other reports. The National Cancer Institute's (NCI) registry of cancer-prone families. indicated a 10.7% incidence.[53] It is important to critically analyze these data under the light provided by thorough retrospective or prospective examination of prophylactic oophorectomy specimens. In a recent study from the University of Toronto, 5 out of 60 (8.3%) consecutive prophylactic oophorectomy specimens (all from patients with known BRCA1 mutations), which appeared normal at the time of surgery, showed occult carcinoma of the ovaries and/or *in situ* or invasive carcinoma of a fallopian tube.[54] In another study, among 50 women undergoing prophylactic oophorectomy, 33 patients had a calculated risk of carrying a germline BRCA1 or BRCA2 mutation greater than 25%. Four incidental tumors were found (12%) in this group of women. All patients had germline BRCA1 or BRCA2 mutations.[55] This suggest that perhaps some of the peritoneal cancers diagnosed following prophylactic oophorectomy might have represented peritoneal spread of an undiagnosed primary ovarian cancer due to sampling error. Careful retrospective examination of the ovaries in some of these patients revealed the presence of microscopic foci of cancer that were not appreciated at the time of the initial pathologic examination.[56] An analysis of women with a first-degree relative with ovarian cancer from the same NCI registry, among whom 44 did while 346 did not undergo oophorectomy, indicated that oophorectomy reduced the risk not only of subsequent serous carcinoma of the ovary but also of the peritoneum by about half.[57] Some cases of presumed peritoneal cancer following prophylactic oophorectomy could also result from incomplete removal of ovarian tissue at the time of surgery, as may occur in the presence of extensive adhesions or scarring.

Outcome analyses vis-à-vis life expectancy are confounded by the relative impact of cancers at different sites and the consequences of surgical menopause. For example, as compared with sporadic ovarian cancers, cancers associated with BRCA1 mutation appear to have a significantly more favorable clinical course.[58] Assuming a lifetime risk of ovarian cancer to be 30% and breast cancer 80%, and a risk reduction of 75% for ovarian cancer and 47% for breast cancer, in a decision analysis concerning 30-year-old women who carry mutations in the BRCA1 gene, prophylactic oophorectomy offered a life expectancy increase of 6 years, while the addition of HRT or raloxifene did not significantly modify the gain.(Randall and Rubin, unpublished observations.) The benefit of oophorectomy, however, may become less after age 60.[59]

Women with BRCA1- or BRCA2-associated breast cancer are at increased risk for contralateral breast cancer and ovarian cancer. In a prospective study of 845 Norwegian women from breast/ovarian and ovarian cancer kindred, seven ovarian cancers were detected in 49 women with previous breast cancer (14%), while nine were detected among 754 unaffected women (1.2%); 25% of ovarian tumors were of low malignant potential.[60] Because of the excellent outcome of select breast cancers, some of these patients may have otherwise a long life expectancy and might benefit from prophylactic oophorectomy. Using a Markov model for decision analysis, total and incremental life expectancy benefit was reported in a recent study for hypothetical breast cancer patients with BRCA1 or BRCA2 mutations facing decisions about secondary cancer prevention strategies. Depending on the assumed penetrance of the BRCA mutation, compared with surveillance alone, 30-year-old early-stage breast cancer patients with BRCA mutations were found to gain in life expectancy 0.4–1.3 years from tamoxifen therapy, 0.2–1.8 years from prophylactic oophorectomy, and 0.6–2.1 years from prophylactic mastectomy. The magnitude of these gains was less for women with low-penetrance mutations (assuming a contralateral breast cancer risk of 24% and ovarian cancer risk of 6%) compared to those with high-penetrance mutations (assuming a contralateral breast cancer risk of 65% and ovarian cancer risk of 40%).[61]

Although much emphasis has been placed on observations that hereditary ovarian cancers tend to occur earlier than sporadic ones, a recent study indicates that germline mutations in BRCA1 or BRCA2 genes contribute to only a minority of cases of very early-onset epithelial ovarian cancer (occurring before age 35), suggesting that very early-onset ovarian cancer is not associated with a greatly increased risk of cancer in close relatives.[62] The incidence of ovarian cancer in BRCA1 and BRCA2 carriers does not begin to rise dramatically until about age 40. Prophylactic oophorectomy may therefore be performed in women in their late 30s or 40s. The symptoms of early surgical menopause may be quite severe and occasionally difficult to manage even with HRT. To minimize subjective side effects and metabolic effects on bone and the cardiovascular system, most patients are placed on HRT. Although concerns have been raised on the potentially adverse effect of HRT on breast cancer risk in patients with BRCA mutations, a recent report indicated that this was not the case in a cohort of 43 women with disease-associated germline BRCA1 mutations from 5 North American institutions who underwent bilateral prophylactic oophorectomy but not a prophylactic mastectomy. When compared to 79 control subjects with BRCA1 mutations who had no history of oophorectomy, prophylactic oophorectomy followed by HRT afforded a statistically significant reduction in breast cancer risk with an adjusted hazard ratio of 0.53 up to 5 years and 0.33 after 10 years of follow-up after surgery.[52]

III. CONCLUSIONS

BRCA1 and BRCA2 mutations are responsible for the vast majority of hereditary ovarian cancers, which represent up to 8–10% of all ovarian cancers. Although the exact function of these genes has not been characterized, evidence suggests that they function as tumor suppressor genes and are implicated in mechanisms of DNA repair through multiple mechanisms. Loss of BRCA1 or BRCA2 function in patients with germline mutations requires loss of the wild-type allele and confers a variable lifetime risk of ovarian carcinoma. Population-based studies are still needed to better define the risk associated to individual mutations or the genetic/environmental covariants that modify such risk. Chemoprevention of hereditary ovarian cancer is at its infancy and awaits additional preclinical evidence and/or the completion of large trials. At this time, prophylactic surgery remains the most efficient preventive measure. Removal of the fallopian tubes and careful exploration of the surgical specimen and the peritoneum should be carried out in an effort to identify occult carcinomas at the time of prophylactic surgery.

References

1. Devesa, S. S. (1995). Cancer patterns among women in the United States. *Semin. Oncol. Nurs.* 11, 78–87.
2. Kosary, C. L. (1994). FIGO stage, histology, histologic grade, age and race as prognostic factors in determining survival for cancers of the female gynecological system: An analysis of 1973-87 SEER cases of cancers of the endometrium, cervix, ovary, vulva, and vagina. *Semin. Surg. Oncol.* 10, 31–46.
3. Easton, D. F., Bishop, D. T., Ford, D., and Crockford, G. P. (1993). Genetic linkage analysis in familial breast and ovarian cancer: Results from 214 families. The Breast Cancer Linkage Consortium. *Am. J. Hum. Genet.* 52, 678–701.
4. Narod, S. A., Ford, D., Devilee, P., Barkardottir, R. B., Lynch, H. T., Smith, S. A., Ponder, B. A., Weber, B. L., Garber, J. E., Birch, J. M. *et al.* (1995). An evaluation of genetic heterogeneity in 145 breast-ovarian cancer families. Breast Cancer Linkage Consortium. *Am. J. Hum. Genet.* 56, 254–264.
5. Boyd, J., and Rubin, S. C. (1997). Hereditary ovarian cancer: Molecular genetics and clinical implications. *Gynecol. Oncol.* 64, 196–206.
6. Nathanson, K. L., and Weber, B. L. (2001). "Other" breast cancer susceptibility genes: Searching for more holy grail. *Hum. Mol. Genet.* 10, 715–720.
7. Sharan, S. K., and Bradley, A. (1998). Functional characterization of BRCA1 and BRCA2: clues from their interacting proteins. *J. Mammary Gland Biol. Neoplasia* 3, 413–421.
8. Rajan, J. V., Marquis, S. T., Gardner, H. P., and Chodosh, L. A. (1997). Developmental expression of BRCA2 colocalizes with BRCA1 and is associated with proliferation and differentiation in multiple tissues. *Dev. Biol.* 184, 385–401.
9. Connor, F., Smith, A., Wooster, R., Stratton, M., Dixon, A., Campbell, E., Tait, T. M., Freeman, T., and Ashworth, A. (1997). Cloning, chromosomal mapping and expression pattern of the mouse BRCA2 gene. *Hum. Mol. Genet.* 6, 291–300.
10. Blackshear, P. E., Goldsworthy, S. M., Foley, J. F., McAllister, K. A., Bennett, L. M., Collins, N. K., Bunch, D. O., Brown, P., Wiseman, R. W., and Davis, B. J. (1998). BRCA1 and BRCA2 expression patterns in mitotic and meiotic cells of mice. *Oncogene* 16, 61–68.
11. Bertwistle, D., Swift, S., Marston, N. J., Jackson, L. E., Crossland, S., Crompton, M. R., Marshall, C. J., and Ashworth, A. (1997). Nuclear location and cell cycle regulation of the BRCA2 protein. *Cancer Res.* 57, 5485–5488.
12. Koonin, E. V., Altschul, S. F., and Bork, P. (1996). BRCA1 protein products ... Functional motifs. *Nat. Genet.* 13, 266–268.
13. Wong, A. K., Ormonde, P. A., Pero, R., Chen, Y., Lian, L., Salada, G., Berry, S., Lawrence, Q., Dayananth, P., Ha, P., Tavtigian, S. V., Teng, D. H., and Bartel, P. L. (1998). Characterization of a carboxy-terminal BRCA1 interacting protein. *Oncogene* 17, 2279–2285.
14. Chen, J., Silver, D. P., Walpita, D., Cantor, S. B., Gazdar, A. F., Tomlinson, G., Couch, F. J., Weber, B. L., Ashley, T., Livingston, D. M., and Scully, R. (1998). Stable interaction between the products of the BRCA1 and BRCA2 tumor suppressor genes in mitotic and meiotic cells. *Mol. Cell* 2, 317–328.
15. Xu, X., Wagner, K. U., Larson, D., Weaver, Z., Li, C., Ried, T., Hennighausen, L., Wynshaw-Boris, A., and Deng, C. X. (1999). Conditional mutation of BRCA1 in mammary epithelial cells results in blunted ductal morphogenesis and tumour formation. *Nat. Genet.* 22, 37–43.
16. Davies, A. A., Masson, J. Y., McIlwraith, M. J., Stasiak, A. Z., Stasiak, A., Venkitaraman, A. R., and West, S. C. (2001). Role of BRCA2 in control of the RAD51 recombination and DNA repair protein. *Mol. Cell* 7, 273–282.
17. Somasundaram, K., Zhang, H., Zeng, Y. X., Houvras, Y., Peng, Y., Wu, G. S., Licht, J. D., Weber, B. L., and El-Deiry, W. S. (1997). Arrest of the cell cycle by the tumour-suppressor BRCA1 requires the CDK-inhibitor p21WAF1/CiP1. *Nature* 389, 187–190.
18. Zheng, L., Pan, H., Li, S., Flesken-Nikitin, A., Chen, P. L., Boyer, T. G., and Lee, W. H. (2000). Sequence-specific transcriptional corepressor function for BRCA1 through a novel zinc finger protein, ZBRK1. *Mol. Cell* 6, 757–768.
19. Harkin, D. P., Bean, J. M., Miklos, D., Song, Y. H., Truong, V. B., Englert, C., Christians, F. C., Ellisen, L. W., Maheswaran, S., Oliner, J. D., and Haber, D. A. (1999). Induction of GADD45 and JNK/SAPK-dependent apoptosis following inducible expression of BRCA1. *Cell* 97, 575–586.
20. Anderson, S. F., Schlegel, B. P., Nakajima, T., Wolpin, E. S., and Parvin, J. D. (1998). BRCA1 protein is linked to the RNA polymerase II holoenzyme complex via RNA helicase A. *Nat. Genet.* 19, 254–256.
21. Miki, Y., Swensen, J., Shattuck-Eidens, D., Futreal, P. A., Harshman, K., Tavtigian, S., Liu, Q., Cochran, C., Bennett, L. M., Ding, W. *et al.* (1994). A strong candidate for the breast and ovarian cancer susceptibility gene BRCA1. *Science* 266, 66–71.
22. Stratton, J. F., Gayther, S. A., Russell, P., Dearden, J., Gore, M., Blake, P., Easton, D., and Ponder, B. A. (1997). Contribution of BRCA1 mutations to ovarian cancer. *N. Engl. J. Med.* 336, 1125–1130.
23. Whittemore, A. S., Gong, G., and Itnyre, J. (1997). Prevalence and contribution of BRCA1 mutations in breast cancer and ovarian cancer: Results from three U.S. population-based case-control studies of ovarian cancer. *Am. J. Hum. Genet.* 60, 496–504.
24. Bandera, C. A., Muto, M. G., Welch, W. R., Berkowitz, R. S., and Mok, S. C. (1998). Genetic imbalance on chromosome 17 in papillary serous carcinoma of the peritoneum. *Oncogene* 16, 3455–3459.
25. Aziz, S., Kuperstein, G., Rosen, B., Cole, D., Nedelcu, R., McLaughlin, J., and Narod, S. A. (2001). A genetic epidemiological study of carcinoma of the fallopian tube. *Gynecol. Oncol.* 80, 341–345.
26. Schorge, J. O., Muto, M. G., Lee, S. J., Huang, L. W., Welch, W. R., Bell, D. A., Keung, E. Z., Berkowitz, R. S., and Mok, S. C. (2000). BRCA1-related papillary serous carcinoma of the peritoneum has a unique molecular pathogenesis. *Cancer Res.* 60, 1361–1364.
27. FitzGerald, M. G., MacDonald, D. J., Krainer, M., Hoover, I., O'Neil, E., Unsal, H., Silva-Arrieto, S., Finkelstein, D. M., Beer-Romero, P., Englert, C., Sgroi, D. C., Smith, B. L., Younger, J. W., Garber, J. E., Duda, R. B., Mayzel, K. A., Isselbacher, K. J., Friend, S. H., and Haber, D. A. (1996). Germ-line BRCA1 mutations in Jewish and non-Jewish women with early-onset breast cancer. *N. Engl. J. Med.* 334, 143–149.
28. Abeliovich, D., Kaduri, L., Lerer, I., Weinberg, N., Amir, G., Sagi, M., Zlotogora, J., Heching, N., and Peretz, T. (1997). The founder mutations 185delAG and 5382insC in BRCA1 and 6174delT in BRCA2 appear in 60% of ovarian cancer and 30% of early-onset breast cancer patients among Ashkenazi women. *Am. J. Hum. Genet.* 60, 505–514.
29. Rubin, S. C., Blackwood, M. A., Bandera, C., Behbakht, K., Benjamin, I., Rebbeck, T. R., and Boyd, J. (1998). BRCA1, BRCA2, and hereditary nonpolyposis colorectal cancer gene mutations in an unselected ovarian cancer population: Relationship to family history and implications for genetic testing. *Am. J. Obstet. Gynecol.* 178, 670–677.

30. Rebbeck, T. R., Couch, F. J., Kant, J., Calzone, K., DeShano, M., Peng, Y., Chen, K., Garber, J. E., and Weber, B. L. (1995). Genetic heterogeneity in hereditary breast cancer: role of BRCA1 and BRCA2. *Am. J. Hum. Genet.* 59, 547–553.
31. Easton, D. F., Ford, D., and Bishop, D. T. (1995). Breast and ovarian cancer incidence in BRCA1-mutation carriers. Breast Cancer Linkage Consortium. *Am. J. Hum. Genet.* 56, 265–271.
32. Struewing, J. P., Hartge, P., Wacholder, S., Baker, S. M., Berlin, M., McAdams, M., Timmerman, M. M., Brody, L. C., and Tucker, M. A. (1997). The risk of cancer associated with specific mutations of BRCA1 and BRCA2 among Ashkenazi Jews. *N. Engl. J. Med.* 336, 1401–1408.
33. Thorlacius, S., Olafsdottir, G., Tryggvadottir, L., Neuhausen, S., Jonasson, J. G., Tavtigian, S. V., Tulinius, H., Ogmundsdottir, H. M., and Eyfjord, J. E. (1996). A single BRCA2 mutation in male and female breast cancer families from Iceland with varied cancer phenotypes. *Nat. Genet.* 13, 117–119.
34. Tavtigian, S. V., Simard, J., Rommens, J., Couch, F., Shattuck-Eidens, D., Neuhausen, S., Merajver, S., Thorlacius, S., Offit, K., Stoppa-Lyonnet, D., Belanger, C., Bell, R., Berry, S., Bogden, R., Chen, Q., Davis, T., Dumont, M., Frye, C., Hattier, T., Jammulapati, S., Janecki, T., Jiang, P., Kehrer, R., Leblanc, J. F., Goldgar, D. E. *et al.* (1996). The complete BRCA2 gene and mutations in chromosome 13q-linked kindreds. *Nat. Genet.* 12, 333–337.
35. Gayther, S. A., Warren, W., Mazoyer, S., Russell, P. A., Harrington, P. A., Chiano, M., Seal, S., Hamoudi, R., van Rensburg, E. J., Dunning, A. M. *et al.* (1995). Germline mutations of the BRCA1 gene in breast and ovarian cancer families provide evidence for a genotype-phenotype correlation. *Nat. Genet.* 11, 428–433.
36. Shattuck-Eidens, D., Oliphant, A., McClure, M., McBride, C., Gupte, J., Rubano, T., Pruss, D., Tavtigian, S. V., Teng, D. H., Adey, N., Staebell, M., Gumpper, K., Lundstrom, R., Hulick, M., Kelly, M., Holmen, J., Lingenfelter, B., Manley, S., Fujimura, F., Luce, M., Ward, B., Cannon-Albright, L., Steele, L., Offit, K., Thomas, A. *et al.* (1997). BRCA1 sequence analysis in women at high risk for susceptibility mutations. Risk factor analysis and implications for genetic testing. *JAMA* 278, 1242–1250.
37. Rosenblatt, K. A., Thomas, D. B., and Noonan, E. A. (1992). High-dose and low-dose combined oral contraceptives: Protection against epithelial ovarian cancer and the length of the protective effect. The WHO Collaborative Study of Neoplasia and Steroid Contraceptives. *Eur. J. Cancer* 28A, 1872–1876.
38. Narod, S. A., Risch, H., Moslehi, R., Dorum, A., Neuhausen, S., Olsson, H., Provencher, D., Radice, P., Evans, G., Bishop, S., Brunet, J. S., and Ponder, B. A. (1998). Oral contraceptives and the risk of hereditary ovarian cancer. Hereditary Ovarian Cancer Clinical Study Group. *N. Engl. J. Med.* 339, 424–428.
39. Whittemore, A. S., Harris, R., and Itnyre, J. (1992). Characteristics relating to ovarian cancer risk: Collaborative analysis of 12 US case-control studies. II. Invasive epithelial ovarian cancers in white women. Collaborative Ovarian Cancer Group. *Am. J. Epidemiol.* 136, 1184–1203.
40. Ursin, G., Henderson, B. E., Haile, R. W., Pike, M. C., Zhou, N., Diep, A., and Bernstein, L. (1997). Does oral contraceptive use increase the risk of breast cancer in women with BRCA1/BRCA2 mutations more than in other women? *Cancer Res.* 57, 3678–3681.
41. Kaduri, L., Gibs, M., Hubert, A., Sagi, M., Heching, N., Lerer, I., Uziely, B., Weinberg, N., Abeliovich, D., and Peretz, T. (1999). Genetic testing of breast and ovarian cancer patients: clinical characteristics and hormonal risk modifiers. *Eur. J. Obstet. Gynecol. Reprod. Biol.* 85, 75–80.
42. Rodriguez, G. C., Walmer, D. K., Cline, M., Krigman, H., Lessey, B. A., Whitaker, R. S., Dodge, R., and Hughes, C. L. (1998). Effect of progestin on the ovarian epithelium of macaques: Cancer prevention through apoptosis? *J. Soc. Gynecol. Invest.* 5, 271–276.
43. Torrisi, R., and Decensi, A. (2000). Fenretinide and cancer prevention. *Curr. Oncol. Rep.* 2, 263–270.
44. Decensi, A., Bonanni, B., Guerrieri-Gonzaga, A., Torrisi, R., Manetti, L., Robertson, C., De Palo, G., Formelli, F., Costa, A., and Veronesi, U. (2000). Chemoprevention of breast cancer: The Italian experience. *J. Cell. Biochem. Suppl.* 34, 84–96.
45. De Palo, G., Mariani, L., Camerini, T., Marubini, E., Formelli, F., Pasini, B., Decensi, A., and Veronesi, U. (2002). Effect of fenretinide on ovarian carcinoma occurrence. *Gynecol. Oncol.* 86, 24–27.
46. Wagner, T. M., Moslinger, R., Langbauer, G., Ahner, R., Fleischmann, E., Auterith, A., Friedmann, A., Helbich, T., Zielinski, C., Pittermann, E., Seifert, M., and Oefner, P. (2000). Attitude towards prophylactic surgery and effects of genetic counselling in families with BRCA mutations. Austrian Hereditary Breast and Ovarian Cancer Group. *Br. J. Cancer* 82, 1249–1253.
47. Meijers-Heijboer, E. J., Verhoog, L. C., Brekelmans, C. T., Seynaeve, C., Tilanus-Linthorst, M. M., Wagner, A., Dukel, L., Devilee, P., van den Ouweland, A. M., van Geel, A. N., and Klijn, J. G. (2000). Presymptomatic DNA testing and prophylactic surgery in families with a BRCA1 or BRCA2 mutation. *Lancet* 355, 2015–2020.
48. Paley, P. J., Swisher, E. M., Garcia, R. L., Agoff, S. N., Greer, B. E., Peters, K. L., and Goff, B. A. (2001). Occult cancer of the fallopian tube in BRCA1 germline mutation carriers at prophylactic oophorectomy: A case for recommending hysterectomy at surgical prophylaxis. *Gynecol. Oncol.* 80, 176–180.
49. Swisher, E. (2001). Hereditary cancers in obstetrics and gynecology. *Clin. Obstet. Gynecol.* 44, 450–463.
50. Meiser, B., Tiller, K., Gleeson, M. A., Andrews, L., Robertson, G., and Tucker, K. M. (2000). Psychological impact of prophylactic oophorectomy in women at increased risk for ovarian cancer. *Psychooncology* 9, 496–503.
51. Rebbeck, T. R. (2000). Prophylactic oophorectomy in BRCA1 and BRCA2 mutation carriers. *J .Clin. Oncol.* 18, 100S–103S.
52. Rebbeck, T. R., Levin, A. M., Eisen, A., Snyder, C., Watson, P., Cannon-Albright, L., Isaacs, C., Olopade, O., Garber, J. E., Godwin, A. K., Daly, M. B., Narod, S. A., Neuhausen, S. L., Lynch, H. T., and Weber, B. L. (1999). Breast cancer risk after bilateral prophylactic oophorectomy in BRCA1 mutation carriers. *J. Natl. Cancer Inst.* 91, 1475–1479.
53. Tobacman, J. K., Greene, M. H., Tucker, M. A., Costa, J., Kase, R., and Fraumeni, J. F., Jr. (1982). Intra-abdominal carcinomatosis after prophylactic oophorectomy in ovarian-cancer-prone families. *Lancet* 2, 795–797.
54. Colgan, T. J., Murphy, J., Cole, D. E., Narod, S., and Rosen, B. (2001). Occult carcinoma in prophylactic oophorectomy specimens: prevalence and association with BRCA germline mutation status. *Am. J. Surg. Pathol.* 25, 1283–1289.
55. Lu, K. H., Garber, J. E., Cramer, D. W., Welch, W. R., Niloff, J., Schrag, D., Berkowitz, R. S., and Muto, M. G. (2000). Occult ovarian tumors in women with BRCA1 or BRCA2 mutations undergoing prophylactic oophorectomy. *J. Clin. Oncol.* 18, 2728–2732.
56. Chen, K. T., Schooley, J. L., and Flam, M. S. (1985). Peritoneal carcinomatosis after prophylactic oophorectomy in familial ovarian cancer syndrome. *Obstet. Gynecol.* 66, 93S–94S.
57. Struewing, J. P., Watson, P., Easton, D. F., Ponder, B. A., Lynch, H. T., and Tucker, M. A. (1995). Prophylactic oophorectomy in inherited breast/ovarian cancer families. *J. Natl. Cancer Inst. Monogr.* 33–35.
58. Rubin, S. C., Benjamin, I., Behbakht, K., Takahashi, H., Morgan, M. A., LiVolsi, V. A., Berchuck, A., Muto, M. G., Garber, J. E., Weber, B. L., Lynch, H. T., and Boyd, J. (1996). Clinical and pathological features of ovarian cancer in women with germ-line mutations of BRCA1. *N. Engl. J. Med.* 335, 1413–1416.
59. Schrag, D., Kuntz, K. M., Garber, J. E., and Weeks, J. C. (1997). Decision analysis—effects of prophylactic mastectomy and oophorectomy on life expectancy among women with BRCA1 or BRCA2 mutations. *N. Engl. J. Med.* 336, 1465–1471.

60. Dorum, A., Heimdal, K., Lovslett, K., Kristensen, G., Hansen, L. J., Sandvei, R., Schiefloe, A., Hagen, B., Himmelmann, A., Jerve, F., Shetelig, K., Fjaerestad, I., Trope, C., and Moller, P. (1999). Prospectively detected cancer in familial breast/ovarian cancer screening. *Acta Obstet. Gynecol. Scand.* 78, 906–911.
61. Schrag, D., Kuntz, K. M., Garber, J. E., and Weeks, J. C. (2000). Life expectancy gains from cancer prevention strategies for women with breast cancer and BRCA1 or BRCA2 mutations. *JAMA* 283, 617–624.
62. Stratton, J. F., Thompson, D., Bobrow, L., Dalal, N., Gore, M., Bishop, D. T., Scott, I., Evans, G., Daly, P., Easton, D. F., and Ponder, B. A. (1999). The genetic epidemiology of early-onset epithelial ovarian cancer: A population-based study. *Am. J. Hum. Genet.* 65, 1725–1732.

CHAPTER

17

Epidemiology of Ovarian Cancer

M. STEVEN PIVER

Sisters of Charity Hospital
Buffalo, New York 14214
Gilda Radner Familial Ovarian Cancer Registry
Roswell Park Cancer Institute
Buffalo, New York 14263

TOM S. FRANK*

Myriad Genetics Laboratories
Salt Lake City, Utah 84108

I. INTRODUCTION

Ovarian cancer remains a major public health problem, not only for the 23,100 cases that occur annually in the U.S., especially in comparison to the 182,800 annual cases of breast cancer, but because there are no accurate methods for early diagnosis. This major failing results in a disease with an insidious onset and more than 70% of cases being diagnosed in advanced stages, with a generally very poor long-term prognosis. Although significant advances have been made in cytoreductive radical surgery and platinum-based chemotherapy for women with epithelial ovarian cancer, with some improvement in the median survival and progression free survival by the end of the last millennium, the majority of women with ovarian cancer will eventually succumb to this sinister disease. One method for improving the bleak image of the gynecologic cancer with the highest fatality to case ratio is to better understand its causes and prevention.

Worldwide ovarian cancer ranks in the top 10 of cancers in women with some 165,000 cases annually. In the U.S., ovarian cancer is the sixth most common cancer in women, the fifth most common cause of cancer mortality in women, and the most common cause of gynecologic cancer mortality, essentially resulting in more deaths than all other gynecologic cancers combined. The only known etiologic factor in epithelial ovarian cancer is that some 5–10% are caused by a mutated gene inherited from the mother or the father. Notwithstanding the fact that the etiology of the remaining 90–95% of sporadic cases remains unknown, certain parts of the enigma are starting to coalesce. First, ovarian cancer occurs most often among middle and upper class women from the most highly industrialized countries with the highest incidence in Sweden, Norway, U.S. white, and England; a lower incidence in U.S. blacks and Latinos and a very low incidence in Africa, India, and Japan. However, as women from a country such as Japan with a low risk incidence of ovarian cancer migrate to a high incidence country, such as the U.S., they and their daughters develop ovarian cancer at rates that approach those of native born North Americans. This suggests some dietary, behavioral or environmental factor differences occurring in the higher incidence countries.

*Deceased.

There are hundreds upon hundreds of epidemiology studies related to the causation of ovarian cancer. With the one exception that a small percentage of cases are known to be the result of an inherited mutated gene, all of the myriad of other possible causes or risk factors for ovarian cancer remain speculative. Even for inherited ovarian cancer in which a female can be born with one mutated or abnormal allele and one wild or normal allele, it is important to establish the risk factors that result in mutation of the normal allele. Finally, it is important to know if the risk factor profile for sporadic and inherited ovarian cancer differ. Therefore, the purpose of this chapter is to review: (1) diet as related to epithelial ovarian cancer (lactose and fat); (2) ovarian epithelial injury as related to epithelial ovarian cancer (talc, asbestos, ovulation, fertility drugs); (3) infertility; (4) inherited ovarian cancer; and (5) the possible protective mechanisms against epithelial ovarian cancer (parity, lactation, oral contraceptives, tubal ligation, and hysterectomy).

Since most of the data, with the exception of mutated genes and inherited ovarian cancer, are based on statistics derived from case control studies, it is important to keep in perspective the words of Dimitrios Trichopoulos then head of the Department of Epidemiology, Harvard School of Public Health. "We, epidemiologists, are fast becoming a nuisance to society. People don't take us seriously anymore and when they do take us seriously, we may unintentionally do more harm than good."

II. INCREASE RISK FACTORS

A. Diet

One of the major dietary customs differentiating women from industrialized countries is their higher consumption of animal fat in the "western" diet. In theory, this could partly explain why women from highly industrialized Japan with a low fat "Asian" diet have higher rates of ovarian cancer when they migrate to the United States and are exposed to the western diet. Although historically Japan had one of the lowest worldwide rates of ovarian cancer, mortality from ovarian cancer in Japanese females has risen significantly since 1955 paralleling the increase in fat content in the Japanese diet, again lending support to the role of dietary fat and ovarian cancer.[1] This is also consistent with the hypothesis that a higher dietary fat content may be associated with increased risk of ovarian cancer is a report by Mettlin and Piver.[2] The authors' studied the milk drinking habits of ovarian cancer cases. The relative risk for ovarian cancer was 3.1 for women who drank more than one glass of whole milk daily as compared to control women who never drank whole milk (Table 17.1). Moreover, women who drank only whole milk were at significantly increased risk for ovarian cancer as opposed to those women who drank

TABLE 17.1 Ovarian Cancer and Whole Milk Consumption

Frequency (total)	Ovarian cancer (297 total)	Controls (587 total)	Relative risk
Never	174	410	1
Less than one glass daily	62	109	1.3
One glass daily	25	41	1.4
More than one glass daily	36	27	3.1
$P<0.001$			

Adapted from Mettlin, C. and Piver, M.S. (1990). *Am. J. Epidemiol.* 132, 873.

2% or skim milk, suggesting that it is the increased amount of animal fat in whole milk as the origin of the increased risk. In support of this hypothesis, Webb *et al.* in a report of 800 cases, found that ovarian cancer risk was positively associated with increasing consumption of whole milk and inversely associated with consumption of low fat milk.[3]

In 1989 Cramer and co-authors reported that women who consume significantly larger amounts of cottage cheese and yogurt (foods high in lactose) had significant increased risk for developing ovarian cancer than did controls.[4] The authors' study was based on the theory that the mammalian ovary is very susceptible to damage from the effects of galactose and galactose metabolites. Dairy products are the most frequent source of dietary galactose. The main source of dietary galactose in humans is cow milk. Lactose in milk is hydrolyzed to glucose and galactose. Since it is frequently recommended that women consume significant amounts of dairy products to reduce their risk for osteoporosis, linking lactose intake in dairy products to increased risk for ovarian cancer could have significant public health implications. In the 1989 study Cramer reported that women who consumed increased dietary galactose (lactose) from dairy products also had low levels of galactose I phosphate uridyltransferase (GALT), an enzyme important in the metabolism of galactose (Table 17.2). The authors posited that women who inherited abnormally low levels of GALT would have their ovaries exposed to the accumulated damage by galactose thus resulting in their increased risk for the development of ovarian cancer. However, 11 years later (2000) Cramer and co–authors reported in a case control study of 563 women with epithelial ovarian cancer and 523 control women that there was no significant difference between ovarian cancer cases and controls in consumption of dairy products or daily lactose, the principle source of dietary galactose.[5] Moreover, the RBC activity of GALT did not differ between cases and controls and the authors concluded that "adult consumption of galactose carries no clear risk for the disease (ovarian cancer)."

TABLE 17.2 Risks for Ovarian Cancer by Lactose Consumption and Transferase Activity

Combination		No. of subjects (%)		
Lactose consumption (g/d)	Transferase activity (μmol/h per g Hb)	Cases (n=145)	Controls (n=127)	RR (95% CI)
≤11	≥22.9	29 (20)	36 (28)	1.0
≤11	<22.9	30 (21)	35 (28)	1.1 (0.5–2.2)
>11	≥22.9	33 (23)	29 (23)	1.3 (0.6–2.7)
>11	<22.9	53 (36)	27 (21)	2.2 (1.1–4.5)

CI=confidence interval; RR=relative risk. From Cramer, D. W., Harlow, B. L., Willett, W. C. *et al.* (1989). Lancet, 2, 66.

The most recent report on lactose consumption from dairy products and the risk of ovarian cancer is a report by Fairfield and co-authors of a prospective study of dietary lactose in ovarian cancer.[6] The authors prospectively evaluated consumption of lactose, milk, and milk products in relation to ovarian cancer among 80,326 women in the Nurses Health Study who completed questionnaires in 1980, 1984, 1986, and 1990. There were 301 cases of invasive epithelial ovarian cancer documented during the 16 years of dietary follow-up. The authors reported a 44% greater risk for women with the highest consumption of lactose compared to the lowest (RR 1.44; 95% CI 1.01–207; *p* for trend 0.07). Skim and low fat milk were the largest contributors to dietary lactose. The authors observed an increased risk for serous tumors in women consuming five or more servings of yogurt per week (RR 2.35; 95% CI 109–507; *p* for trend 0.04) but no association with all subtypes of tumor together.

Recommending a diet low in yogurt, skim milk, and cottage cheese could have significant long-term health implications for women. It is clear that the role of dietary fat and dietary lactose in relation to ovarian cancer risk remains unsettled.

B. Ovarian Epithelial Injury

Any hypothesis relating ovarian epithelial injury secondary to retrograde transmission of possible toxins via the vagina needs to have a counterbalancing mechanism explaining the possible protective effects against ovarian cancer by tubal ligation and hysterectomy.

1. Hygienic Perineal Talc

Asbestos is a known carcinogen. Because there are chemical similarities between talc and asbestos, talc has been implicated as a possible ovarian carcinogen. The mineral talc consists of pulverized hydrus magnesium silicate. Prior to 1976, cosmetic talc powder was contaminated by significant amounts of asbestos: tremolite, chrysolite, and crocidolet. Subsequently, manufacturers of talc voluntarily tried to limit asbestos particles from cosmetic talc. As early as 1979, Henderson demonstrated talc particles in normal ovarian tissue.[7] Recently, Heller demonstrated by electron microscopy that asbestos chrysotile and asbestos crocidolite fibers were present in the majority of tissue blocks from fallopian tube and ovaries in women with no known exposure to asbestos.[8] The authors concluded that asbestos chrysotile is ubiquitous in the environment and that there is background exposure in everyone. Theoretically, talc powders (or asbestos) placed on the perineum can reach the ovaries via retrograde flow through the cervix and fallopian tubes. The possible link between perineal talc use in genital hygiene and ovarian cancer was initially reported by Cramer and co-authors in 1982.[9] The authors reported a relative risk of 1.9 ($p<0.03$) for ovarian cancer among talc users. The relative risk was 3.28 for women who used talcum powder on perineal napkins and dusting powder on the perineum (Table 17.3). In a follow-up study reported 19 years later, Cramer *et al.* reported a population-based case control study involving 563 women with epithelial ovarian cancer and 523 control women.[10] The authors again reported an elevated odds ratio for women who directly powdered the perineal area (OR 1.45); powdered sanitary napkins (OR 1.45); or powdered underwear (OR 1.21). The authors reviewed data from 14 case control studies, including their own, on the risk of ovarian cancer and any use of genital talc. They reported a combined odds ratio of 1.36 (95% CI 1.24–1.49) which was statistically significant and concluded that the "odds ratio of 1.36 suggests that between 10–11% of ovarian cancers in these populations are attributable to the genital use of talc." In contrast Wong and co-authors in a case control study reported no increased risk for ovarian cancer and the use of perineal talc.[11] In addition, there was no increased risk with duration of use (Table 17.4).

Although there are conflicting reports on the possible link between cosmetic perineal talc use and ovarian cancer, most of the positive studies show a weak association with no biological mechanism or no dose response association. However, the carcinogenic potential of talc remains unsettled as evidenced by the fact in the year 2000, the National Toxicology Program, a branch of the National Institute of Health, that meets every two years to update the federal list of proven and suspected cancer causing substances, refused to add talc powder to the list stating that there was not enough evidence linking its use in feminine hygiene products to ovarian cancer.

C. Ovulation and Fertility Drugs

One of the most prominent theories related to ovarian carcinogenesis is the incessant ovulation hypothesis. This hypothesis posits that women who incessantly ovulate, uninterrupted by resting the ovarian epithelium by pregnancy,

TABLE 17.3 Ovarian Cancer and Talc Exposure

Exposure	Ovarian cancer (215 total)	Controls (215 total)	Relative risk
No exposure	57%	72%	
Any exposure	43%	28%	1.92 (p <0.003)

Adapted from Cramer, D. W., Welch, W. R., Scully, R. E. *et al.* (1982). *Cancer* 50, 372.

TABLE 17.4 Perineal Talc Exposure and Ovarian Cancer

Years	Controls	Ovarian cancer	Odds ratio
None	382	241	1.0
1–9	61	39	0.9
10–19	50	49	1.4
≥20	161	101	0.9

Adapted from Wong, C., Hempling, R. E., Piver, M. S. *et al.* (1998). *Obstet. Gynecol.* 93, 372.

oral contraceptive use, or breastfeeding are at increased risk for the development of ovarian cancer. It is theorized that excessive ovulation damages the ovarian epithelium. Damaged ovarian epithelial cells at the point of follicular rupture are characterized by marked inflammatory process. This inflammatory process produces oxidants that damage DNA. Therefore, the more frequent proliferative process resulting from incessant ovulation with or without exposure to environmental toxins such as talc or asbestos, the higher the likelihood of defective DNA repair at the site of follicular damage with resultant mutagenesis leading to ovarian cancer.

If ovulation results primarily in once a month disruption of the ovarian epithelium, then the use of fertility drugs in infertile women would result in hyperovulation with multiple follicular disruptions more prone to errors in DNA replication and repair. The most commonly used fertility drugs are clomiphene citrate (Clomid) and human menopausal gonadotropin (Pergonal).

In 1992, Whittemore reported the combined analysis of 12 U.S. case control studies on the possible association of fertility drugs in women with physician diagnosed infertility.[12] The odds ratio was 2.8 (95% CI 1.3–6) for women who took fertility drugs as compared to infertile women who did not (Table 17.5). Although there were many limitations and much criticism of this study, the study was reported widely by the national television and print media resulting in significant anxiety for many thousands of infertile women who had or were taking fertility drugs. In 1994 Rossing and co-authors reported an increased ovarian cancer risk (RR 2.3; 95% CI 0.5–11.4) for women attending an infertility clinic in

TABLE 17.5 Fertility Drugs and Ovarian Cancers

Fertility drug	Ovarian cancer	Controls	Odds ratio
No	76	124	0.91
Yes	20	11	2.80
Total	96	135	

Adapted from whittemore, A. S., Harris, R., Intyre, J., and the Collaborative Ovarian Cancer Group (1992). *Am. J. Epidemiol.* 136, 1184.

Seattle, WA, treated with Clomid.[13] For those women who took ≥12 monthly courses of Clomid, the RR was 11.1 (95% CI 1.5–82.3) but there was no increase risk for those women who took only 1–11 courses. Notwithstanding the fact that this study was reported in the prestigious *New England Journal of Medicine*, the criticisms were myriad, not the least of which the authors only had 11 cases of ovarian tumors, 4 invasive epithelial ovarian cancers, 5 borderline epithelial ovarian cancers, and 2 granulosa cell tumors. The latter two may not have any true malignant potential leaving a study based on nine ovarian cancers. Two years later in 1996, Shushan *et al.* reported an odds ratio of 3.19 (95% CI 0.86–11.82) for women treated with human menopausal gonadotropin alone for infertility in a nationwide case control study from Israel.[14] These conflicting results have lead to numerous editorials denouncing the reported possible relationship between fertility drugs and ovarian cancer. However, conceptually the effects of fertility drugs is consistent with the hypothesis of repeated DNA turnover with possible defects in DNA repair. Also, lending some credence to the possibility that superovulation leads to ovarian cancer is the animal model whereby hyperovulatory hens have an increased risk for developing ovarian cancer. Although surveys document that most physicians do not believe that ovulation induction increases the risk for ovarian cancer, most physicians have now limited the length of treatment with fertility drugs and many are now doing surveillance for ovarian cancer in infertile women who have taken fertility drugs.

D. Infertility

If conception decreases risk for ovarian cancer, then infertility should have the opposite effect. Whittemore reporting on 12 U.S. case control studies reported that ovulatory women who had sexual intercourse unprotected by any type of contraception had a nearly double risk for developing ovarian cancer (Table 17.6).[15] At present there is no explanation relating reproductive dysfunction (infertility) and increased risk of ovarian cancer. However, it has been suggested that there may be a genetic mutation not only responsible for the development of ovarian cancer but also as a causation of infertility. Nieto and co-workers retrospectively reviewed

TABLE 17.6 Ovarian Cancer Risk of Unprotected Intercourse

Years of unprotected intercourse	Ovarian cancer	Controls	Relative risk	*p* Value
<2	91 (50%)	323 (62%)	1	
2–9	48 (26%)	117 (22%)	1.5	0.08
>10	43 (24%)	82 (16%)	1.8	0.01

Adapted from Whittemore, A. S., Wu, M. L., Paffenbarger, R. S. *et al.* (1989). *Cancer Res.* 49, 4047.

TABLE 17.7 Parity and Risk of Ovarian Cancer Nurses Health Study 1976–1988

Parity	Cases	Person years	Age adjusted relative risk
0	30	78,382	1.0
1	29	88,337	0.93
2	72	329,091	0.68
3	61	320,098	0.53
4	34	192,026	0.44
5	16	89,891	0.41
≥6	13	77,504	0.35

Adapted from Hankinson, S. E., Colditz, G. A., Hunter, D. J. *et al.* (1995). *Cancer* 76, 284.

the prevalence of ovarian cancer in first-degree relatives of infertile women.[16] The prevalence of ovarian cancer in first-degree relatives of ovarian cancer women was 1.45% compared to 0.74% in relatives of fertile women (RR 1.95; CI 0.36–10–55). This difference was only in relatives of women who did not conceive in spite of treatment for infertility. The authors suggested that there may be a common abnormality between infertility and ovarian cancer, but that this anomaly only occurs in women who are childless in spite of infertility treatment.

III. PROTECTIVE MECHANISMS

A. Parity

Consistent with the incessant ovulation hypothesis is the protection against ovarian cancer of parity. Pregnancy results in high levels of estrogen and progesterone which inhibit follicular stimulating and luteinizing hormone thus preventing ovulation. In the Nurses Health Study 121,700 married female registered nurses were 30–55 at the beginning of the 1976 prospective study.[17] By 1988 there was follow-up of 107,865 who were evaluable for parity (number of pregnancies lasting six months or more). From this population, 260 cases of ovarian cancer were confirmed. The highly protective effect of parity was evident by the 45% decrease in ovarian cancer risk relative to nulliparous women (age adjusted risk=0.55; 95% CI 0.3–0.80). Although there was only a very slight decrease in risk with only one child (RR 0.93), there was a 16% decreased risk for each subsequent birth (Table 17.7). Results from the analysis of 12 U.S. case control studies also observed a similar 15% reduction in risk for ovarian cancer for each subsequent pregnancy after the first.[12]

B. Lactation

To a lesser degree, breastfeeding lowers the risk for ovarian cancer. Lactation would theoretically reduce the risk for ovarian cancer by inhibiting pituitary luteinizing hormone and thus suppressing ovulation. There does not appear to be a relation, however, between duration of lactation and decrease in ovarian cancer risk.

C. Tubal Ligation and Hysterectomy

It has been demonstrated that carbon particles placed in the vagina immediately prior to hysterectomy can be recovered from fallopian tubes.[18] In addition, talc particles and asbestos fibers have been found to be present in normal ovarian tissue. Therefore, since environmental toxins such as talc particles and asbestos fibers can gain egress to the ovarian epithelium via retrograde transmission from the vagina, then theoretically tubal ligation or hysterectomy should result in a decreased risk for ovarian cancer.

In the largest study to date, The Nurses Health Study, 121,700 registered nurses were prospectively studied after 12 years of follow-up.[19] There was nearly a 70% (RR 0.33; CI 95% 0.16–0.64) decrease in the risk of ovarian in the nurses who underwent tubal ligation (Table 17.8). Cornelison and co-authors in a case control study (300 cases of epithelial ovarian cancer and 606 nonmalignant controls) reported a near 50% decrease in the risk of developing ovarian cancer (RR 0.52).[20] Also of importance in this latter study was the fact that the greatest protection against the development of ovarian cancer was associated with the youngest patient ages at the time of tubal ligation. This is consistent with the concept that the longer the prevention of ascending migration by toxins or carcinogens, the greater the protection.

Although the mechanism of the protective effects of tubal ligation are unknown, speculative theories include: (1) impairment of blood supply to the ovaries; (2) prevention of retrograde toxins from the vagina; (3) altered levels of estradiol and progesterone suppressing ovulation; and (4) induction of inflammatory changes in the ovarian epithelium.

TABLE 17.8 Tubal Ligation and Ovarian Cancer Risk Nurses Health Study 1976–1988

Tubal ligation	Premenopausal ovarian cancer cases	Person years	Age adjusted RR (95% CI)
No	149	690,508	1.0
Yes	9	169,283	0.29 (0.15–0.55)

RR=relative risk; CI=confidence interval. Adapted from Hankinson, S. E., Hunter, D. J., Colditz, G. A. *et al.* (1993). *JAMA* 270, 2813.

In the Nurses Health Study, hysterectomy reduced the risk of ovarian cancer by 33% (RR 0.67; 95% CI 0.45–0.099). Confounding this observation is a report that hysterectomy provided no protective effects in women who had undergone tubal ligation prior to hysterectomy.[15]

Although one would not advocate tubal ligation or hysterectomy (with preservation of the ovaries) as a method for reducing the risk for the development of ovarian cancer, the reports that there may be a decreased risk for ovarian cancer associated with these procedures necessitates further study into the role of exogenous toxins and this disease.

D. Oral Contraceptives

In 1987 the Cancer and Steroid Hormone (CASH) of the Centers for Disease Control and the National Institute of Health and Human Development reported a case control study of oral contraceptive use in ovarian cancer cases and controls.[21] Even with as little as 3–6 months of use, there was a 40% decrease for the development of ovarian cancer and this increased with duration of use to 80% with ≥10 years of use (Table 17.9).

In a 1994 study using updated data from the CASH study combined with data from Surveillance Epidemiology and End Results (SEER), the authors concluded that five or more years of oral contraceptive use by nulliparous women can reduce their risk for ovarian cancer to that of parous women who never used oral contraceptives.[22] In addition, ten years of oral contraceptive use by women with a family history of ovarian cancer can decrease their risk to below that for women without a family history of ovarian cancer and never used oral contraceptives.

Oral contraceptives probably reduced the risk of developing ovarian cancer by suppressing ovulation and pituitary gonadotropin secretion. However, they may also have a direct effect on ovarian epithelium. Rodriguez and co-authors using a monkey model reported that progestins induce cell death (apoptoses) in ovarian epithelium.[23]

In a 1993 study from the Gilda Radner Familial Ovarian Cancer Registry for those women on which data on oral contraceptive use was available, the use of oral contraceptives

TABLE 17.9 Cumulative Duration of Oral Contraceptive Use and Ovarian Cancer

Duration	Ovarian cancer	Controls	Relative risk
Never	242	1532	1.0
3–6 months	26	280	0.6
7–11 months	14	134	0.7
1–2 years	65	602	0.7
3–4 years	40	397	0.6
5–9 years	39	594	0.4
7–10 years	13	328	0.2

Adapted from The Cancer and Steroid Hormone Study for Disease Control and the National Institute of Child Health and Human Development (1987). *N. Engl. J. Med.* 316, 650.

was much less common in the group of index cases who had developed ovarian cancer than the group of index cases who had not developed ovarian cancer (p<0.01) suggesting a possible protective role for oral contraceptives even in women who might carry a deleterious gene.[24] This study was prior to the discovery of the genes BRCA1 and BRCA2 responsible for most cases of inherited ovarian and breast cancer.

Narod *et al.* reported a case control study of 207 women with hereditary ovarian cancer all of whom carried a pathogenic mutation of BRCA1 (179) or BRCA2 (28).[25] The cases were matched to 161 sisters as controls. There was a 50% (OR 0.5; 95% CI 0.3–0.8) decrease in ovarian cancer risk associated with any past use of oral contraceptives. The protective effect of oral contraceptives was increased with increased duration of use with a 60% reduction for 6 or more years of use. If this study is verified by other groups, oral contraceptive use could be added to the armamentarium for preventing ovarian cancer, now limited to prophylactic oophorectomy in women at high risk (Table 17.10).

Given the significant protective effects of oral contraceptives, the discovery of oral contraceptives by John Rock and Gregory Pincus and the FDA approval in 1960 for the use of oral contraceptives may be the most important discovery to date in lowering the incidence and thus mortality from ovarian cancer. Support for this statement comes from the study by Gnagy *et al.* of the decline in observed U.S. rates of ovarian cancer incidence and mortality in the years 1970–1995 [26] and the more recent American Cancer Society's statistics from 1996–2000.[27]

Using a statistical model, Gnagy and co-authors predicted that the decrease in incidence and mortality was secondary to the decrease in parity and the increase in oral contraceptive use over that time period. In women up to age 50 (30–49), the decrease in rates were consistent with the data of decreased parity and increased oral contraceptive use during that time, but in postmenopausal women 50–64 the model predicted a greater reduction than was observed suggesting the protective effect of oral contraceptive use declines with age. However, adding support to their thesis is the 1996–2000 data on U.S. cancer incidence and mortality.[27] For the first time there was a significant decrease in the number of ovarian cancer cases occurring between 1996 (26,700) and 2000 (23,100) and a significant decrease in the death rate from 1996 of 14,800 to 2000 of 14,000 deaths (Table 17.11).

IV. HEREDITARY RISKS OF OVARIAN CANCER

A. Biological Basis

While a myriad of genetic factors undoubtedly influence a woman's lifetime risk of any cancer, approximately 10% of ovarian carcinomas are the direct consequence of mutations in specific genes inherited from one parent or the other.[28] Such mutations confer greatly increased risk of ovarian cancer as an autosomal dominant trait. Most hereditary ovarian carcinomas are the result of mutations in two genes, BRCA1 and BRCA2.[29] These genes are also responsible for greatly increasing the risk of early-onset breast cancer, and in fact most hereditary ovarian cancer occurs in association with familial breast cancer. Some families with mutations in BRCA1 and BRCA2 nonetheless exhibit clustering of site-specific ovarian cancer. A minority (probably fewer than 10%) of hereditary ovarian cancers result from germline mutations in the genes responsible for hereditary nonpolyposis colorectal cancer (HNPCC, or "Lynch syndrome"). Two genes in particular, MLH1 and MSH2, account by far for most of HNPCC. Mutations in these genes are primarily associated with familial clusters of early-onset colorectal and endometrial carcinoma, with ovarian carcinoma reported in a minority of families. It appears that some HNPCC families exhibit more clustering of gynecologic malignancies than others, and many of these may be due to mutations in a third gene, MSH6,[30] for which no test is currently available.

The genes BRCA1, BRCA2, MLH1, and MSH2 encode proteins that repair mutations in other genes. The BRCA1 and BRCA2 proteins are responsible for repairing double-stranded breaks in DNA,[31] whereas the protein products of MLH1 and MSH2 are responsible for repair of mismatches that occur between aligned bases of the double-stranded DNA molecule.[32] By repairing damage in other genes, the protein products of these genes prevent the accumulation of mutations and thus suppress the development of cancer. Thus, such genes are generally considered to be tumor suppressor genes. When an inherited mutation in a critical tumor suppressor gene is inherited from a parent, each cell is approximately one million times more likely than a normal cell to undergo malignant transformation.

TABLE 17.10 Oral Contraceptives and Ovarian Cancer

Years	Controls sisters (Odds ratio)	BRCA1 or BRCA2 mutations
0	1.0	1.0
<3	0.8	0.4
3–<6	0.4	0.4
≥6	0.4	0.3

Adapted from Narod, S. A., Rish, H., Moslehi, R. *et al.* (1998). *N. Engl. J. Med.* 339, 424.

TABLE 17.11 U.S. Ovarian Cancer Cases and Deaths 1996–2000

Year	Cases	Deaths
1996	26,700	14,800
1997	26,800	14,200
1998	25,400	14,500
1999	25,200	14,500
2000	23,100	14,000

Adapted from Greenlee, R. T., Murray, T., Bolden, S. *et al.* (2000). *CA* 50, 7.

B. Hereditary Cancer Risk

The risk of ovarian carcinoma conferred by mutations in BRCA1 and BRCA2 appears to be higher than for the HNPCC genes (Table 17.12). Mutations in BRCA1 are associated with a risk of ovarian carcinoma between 28% [33] and 44% [34, 35] by age 70. The risks of ovarian carcinoma conferred by mutations in BRCA2 appear to be somewhat lower than for BRCA1, or about 27% by age 70.[29] Women already diagnosed with breast cancer due to a mutation in BRCA1 and BRCA2 have a tenfold increase in their risk of ovarian cancer compared to other women with early-onset breast cancer.[36] This risk is at least 16%.[37]

The risk of ovarian cancer associated with mutations in the HNPCC genes (Table 17.13) is approximately 12%.[38] Although lower than the risk associated with mutations in BRCA1 and BRCA2, this nonetheless represents a nearly tenfold increase above the general population risk.

Mutations in these genes appear to confer higher ovarian cancer risk in some families than in others. There is some evidence that this is related to the location of the mutation within a particular gene,[39, 40] although other studies do not support such an association.[36] What is becoming increasingly evident is that other genes modify the risk of ovarian cancer conferred by inherited mutations in BRCA1, BRCA2, MLH1, and MSH2. For example, genes on chromosome 11

TABLE 17.12 Cancer Risks for BRCA1–BRCA2 Mutation Carriers

Site	Population risk	Risk associated with inherited mutation in BRCA1–BRCA2
Breast	2% by age 50	33–50% by age 50
	7% by age 70	56–87% by age 70
Ovary	1% by age 70	28–44% by age 70 (BRCA1)
		27% by age 70 (BRCA2)
		(16% risk by age 70 following breast cancer)

TABLE 17.13 Cancer Risks for MLH1–MSH2 Mutation Carriers

Site	Population risk	Risk associated with inherited mutation in MLH1–MSH2
Colon	0.2% by age 50	>25% by age 50
	2.0% by age 70	82% by age 70
Endometrium	0.2% by age 50	20% by age 50
	1.5% by age 70	60% by age 70
Ovary	1% by age 70	12% by age 70

and the X chromosome have been specifically implicated as modifiers of ovarian cancer risk in women who carry mutations in BRCA1.[41, 42] These so-called "modifier genes" have not yet been fully characterized and so clinical tests for them are not currently available.

It is important to note that men and women who carry a mutation in genes such as BRCA1, BRCA2, MLH1, and MSH2 still have one normal copy of each gene, which means that each of their children has the same chance of inheriting the normal copy as the mutated copy. Only those offspring who inherit the mutated gene from their father or mother are at a greatly increased risk of ovarian cancer, whereas those who inherit the normal copy from that parent are not at increased risk of ovarian cancer despite having a family history that would suggest otherwise. Thus, mutations in BRCA1, BRCA2, MLH1, and MSH2 confer cancer risk in an autosomal dominant fashion, with offspring having an equal chance each of either being at greatly increased risk of cancer or of being at the general population risk.

C. Features of Hereditary Cancer

Hereditary ovarian cancers, whether due to BRCA1, BRCA2, MLH1, or MSH2, are epithelial. Malignancies of germ cell and sex cord-stromal origin are not generally seen in association with mutations in these genes. Most hereditary ovarian carcinomas are invasive, although tumors of low malignant potential ("borderline tumors") have also been reported in affected families. The majority of the carcinomas reported in women with inherited mutations in BRCA1 and BRCA2 are papillary serous,[43, 44] although other histologic subtypes have also been observed. In contrast to hereditary breast cancer, which largely occurs prior to age 50, hereditary ovarian cancer is most commonly diagnosed after age 50 years.[29, 45] There is some evidence that inherited mutations in BRCA1 and BRCA2 are associated with improved survival compared to sporadic ovarian cancer.[45] The features of HNPCC-associated ovarian cancer are not as well-defined as those due to mutations in BRCA1 and BRCA2, but the histologic spectrum appears to be similar to that of sporadic ovarian carcinoma.[38]

Mutations in BRCA1 and BRCA2 have been identified in 5–10% of presumed sporadic ovarian carcinomas [46, 47] in which the mutation is present in the cancer, but not in the woman's germline. This is in contrast to breast cancer, where only inherited mutations in these genes have been reported are inherited. The prevalence of somatic MLH1 and MSH2 mutations in sporadic ovarian cancer has not yet been characterized.

D. Identification of Hereditary Risk of Ovarian Cancer

Family history is an important way to assess whether a woman's ovarian cancer is likely the result of an inherited mutation in a tumor suppressor gene. Since most hereditary ovarian cancer occurs in association with a family history of tumors of other sites, a family history of such other cancers can indicate the possibility of hereditary risk of ovarian cancer. An inherited mutation in BRCA1 or BRCA2, for example, is suggested by one or more relatives with breast cancer diagnosed before age 50, often in the absence of a known family history of ovarian cancer. Even a single first- or second-degree relative with breast cancer under 50 indicates an approximately 40% chance that a woman's ovarian cancer is due to a mutation in BRCA1 or BRCA2.[36] When hereditary ovarian cancer is due to HNPCC the family history usually includes at least one first- or second-degree relative with colorectal and/or endometrial cancer diagnosed before age 50.

In assessing a family history it is important to keep in mind that mutations in BRCA1, BRCA2, MLH2, or MSH2 can be inherited from either a woman's father or mother. Fully half of women with hereditary risk of ovarian cancer inherited the causative mutation from their father's side of the family. Women who inherit such mutations from their fathers have the same increased risk of ovarian cancer as if they inherited it from their mother.

Assessment of family history can identify the possibility of hereditary risk of ovarian cancer but cannot confirm whether an individual woman is herself at risk. This is because increased cancer susceptibility due to BRCA1, BRCA2, MLH1, and MSH2 is inherited as an autosomal dominant trait, so that each offspring of a mutation carrier has an equal chance of being at greatly increased risk of cancer, or not, depending upon whether she inherited the abnormal copy of the gene. Direct analysis of these genes can provide a "tissue diagnosis" of hereditary cancer risk, which is useful because risk assessment based on family history alone will likely underestimate a woman's risk of cancer if she actually carries the mutation in her family and overestimate that risk if in fact she does not. Specific interventions are available for women found to carry mutations that increase the risk of ovarian cancer,[25, 48, 49] while those found not to carry the mutation in their family can avoid unnecessary interventions that might otherwise have been recommended on the basis of their family history.

Genetic testing for hereditary risk of ovarian cancer is not a general population screen but is appropriate only for women with a greatly increased chance of carrying a mutation compared to the general population. Such tests can be obtained only by a healthcare professional. Appropriate counseling for the individual being tested is strongly recommended, and documentation of informed consent is required. The most sensitive test for hereditary ovarian cancer risk is gene sequence analysis in which the genes are "proofread" in their entirety.

V. CONCLUSION

In the past quarter of a century scientists have studied and written a great deal about the possible etiology(s) of epithelial ovarian cancer. As this chapter discusses, these theories cover the entire gamut of diet (high fat versus high lactose), perineal talc powder, physician diagnosed infertility, fertility stimulating drugs (Clomid, Pergonal), mutations in the "wounded" ovarian surface epithelium caused by "incessant" ovulation and an abnormal ovarian (and breast) cancer gene inherited from one's mother or father. However, the latter (an inherited gene) is the only known cause of epithelial ovarian cancer. It has been posited that inheritance of an abnormal gene might be a possibility when in two successive years (1978 and 1979) two families each with five members with epithelial ovarian cancer spanning three generations came under the author's care. A review of the English medical literature at that time demonstrated that this was a rarely reported occurrence as evidenced by the fact that over a 40-year span (1929–1969) there were only 5 reported families with multiple cases of epithelial ovarian cancer.[50]

In 1981 the Familial Ovarian Cancer Registry was established to study the occurrence of such families in the U.S. The registry was subsequently renamed in honor of the memory of the great comedian Gilda Radner, the Gilda Radner Familial Ovarian Cancer Registry. Through the year 2000, 1606 families with two or more first- or first- and second-degree relatives (range 2–10) had been accessioned into the Gilda Radner Familial Ovarian Cancer Registry (Fig. 17.1) documenting that this is not the extremely rare event as suggested by the 5 families reported from 1929–1969. The challenge for the future is to discover what environmental factors may increase (for example, diet, talc, fertility drugs, infertility) or decrease (for example, oral contraceptives, tubal ligation, pregnancy) the chance of mutation in the normal allele that was inherited along with the mutated (BRCA1, 2, ?BRCA3, 4, 5) ovarian cancer allele that eventually causes inherited epithelial ovarian cancer. Since only 5–10% of epithelial ovarian cancer is caused by an inherited gene, the bigger challenge for the future is the discovery of the etiology of sporadic or noninherited epithelial ovarian cancer. Then and only then will the mortality from the leading cause of death from gynecologic cancer in the U.S. truly decline.

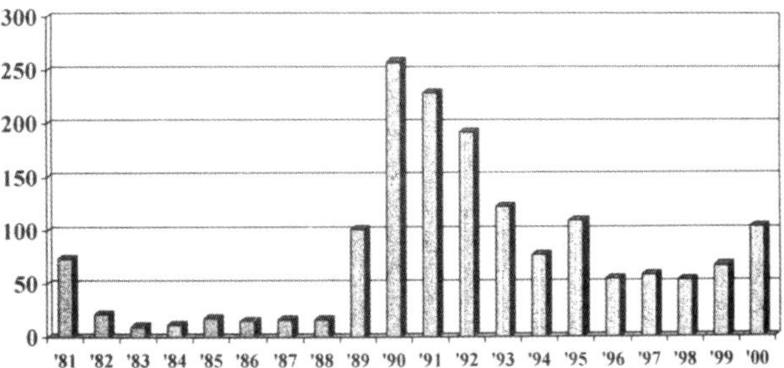

FIGURE 17.1 The Gilda Radner Familial Ovarian Cancer Registry. From 1981–1999 the Registry, renamed in Gilda Radner's honor in 1989, has enrolled 1606 families with two or more close relatives with ovarian cancer.

References

1. Rose, D. P., Boyar, A. P., and Wynder, E. L.(1986). International comparison of mortality rates for cancer of the breast, ovary, and colon and per capita food consumption. *Cancer* 58, 2363–2371.
2. Mettlin, C. J., and Piver, M. S. (1990). A case control study of milk drinking and ovarian cancer risk. *Am. J. Epidemiol.* 132, 871–876.
3. Webb, P. M., Bain, C. J., Purdie, D. M., Harvey, P. W., and Green, A. (1988). Milk consumption, galactose metabolism and ovarian cancer (Australia). *Cancer Causes Control* 9, 637–644.
4. Cramer, D. W., Harlow, B. L., and Willett, W. C. *et al.* (1988). Galactose consumption and metabolism in relation to the risk of ovarian cancer. *Lancet* 2, 66–71.
5. Cramer, D. W., Greenberg, E. R., Titus-Ernstoff, L., Liberman, R. F., Welch, W. R., Li, E., and Ng, W. G. (2000). A case-control study of galactose consumption and metabolism in relation to ovarian cancer. *Cancer Epidemio. Biomarkers Prevent.* 9, 95–101.
6. Fairfield, K. M., Hunter, D. J., Colditz, G. A., Fuchs, C. S., Speizer, F. E., Willett, W. C., and Hankinson, S. E. (2000). A prospective study of dietary lactose and ovarian cancer. *J. Gen. Int. Med.* 15, 205–206.
7. Henderson, W., Hamilton, T., and Griffin, K. (1979). Talc in normal and malignant ovarian tissue. *Lancet* 5, 449.
8. Heller, D. S., Gordon, R. E., and Katz, N. (1999). Correlation of asbestos fiber burdens in fallopian tubes and ovarian tissue. *Am. J. Obstet. Gynecol.* 181, 346–347.
9. Cramer, D. W., Welch, W. R., and Scully, R. E. *et al.* (1982). Ovarian cancer and talc: A case-control study. *Cancer* 50, 372–376.

10. Cramer, D. W., Liberman, R. F., Titus-Ernstoff, L., Welch, W. R., Greenberg, E. R., Baron, J. A., and Harlow, B. L. (1999). Genital talc exposure and risk of ovarian cancer. *Int. J. Cancer* 81, 351–356.
11. Wong, C., Hempling, R. E., Piver, M. S., Natarajan, N., and Mettlin, C. J. (1999). Perineal talc exposure and subsequent epithelial ovarian cancer: A case-control study. *Obstet. Gynecol.* 93, 372–376.
12. Whittemore, A. S., Harris, R., Itnyre, J., and the Collaborative Ovarian Cancer Group (1992). Characteristics relating to ovarian cancer risk: Collaborative analysis of 12 U.S. case-control studies: Part II. Invasive epithelial ovarian cancers in white women. *Am. J. Epidemiol.* 136, 1184–1203.
13. Rossing, M. A., Daling, J. R., and Weiss, N. S. *et al.* (1994). Ovarian tumors in a cohort of infertile women. *N. Engl. J. Med.* 331, 771–776.
14. Shushan, A., Paltiel, O., and Iscovich, J. *et al.* (1996). Human menopausal gonadotropin and the risk of epithelial ovarian cancer. *Fertil. Steril.* 65, 13–18.
15. Whittemore, A. S., Wu, M. L., Paffenbarger, R. S., Sarles, D. L., Kampert, J. B., Grosser, S., Jung, D. L., Ballon, S., Hendrickson, M., and Mohle-Boetani, J. (1989). Epithelial ovarian cancer and the ability to conceive. *Cancer Res.* 49, 4047–4052.
16. Nieto, J. J., Rolfe, K. J., MacLean, A. B., and Hardiman, P. (1999). Ovarian cancer and infertility: A genetic link? *Lancet* 354, 649.
17. Hankinson, S. E., Colditz, G. A., and Hunter, D. J. *et al.* (1995). A prospective study of reproductive factors and risk of epithelial ovarian cancer. *Cancer* 76, 284–290.
18. Egli, G. E., and Newton, M. (1961). The transport of carbon particles in the human female reproductive tract. *Fertil. Steril.* 12, 151–155.
19. Hankinson, S. E., Hunter, D. J., and Colditz, G. A. *et al.* (1993). Tubal ligation, hysterectomy and risk of ovarian cancer: A prospective study. *JAMA* 270, 2813–2818.
20. Cornelison, T. L., Natarajan, N., and Piver, M. S. *et al.* (1997). Tubal ligation and risk of ovarian cancer. *Cancer Detect. Prevent.* 21, 1–6.
21. The Cancer and Steroid Hormone Study of the Centers for Disease Control and the National Institute of Child Health and Human Development (1987). The reduction in risk of ovarian cancer associated with oral contraceptive use. *N. Engl. J. Med.* 316, 650–655.
22. Gross, T. P., and Schlesselman, J. J. (1994). The estimated effect of oral contraceptive use in the cumulative risk of epithelial ovarian cancer. *Obste. Gynecol.* 83, 419–424.
23. Rodriguez, G. C., Walmer, D. K., Cline, M., Krigman, H., Lessey, B. A., Whitaker, R. S., Dodge, R., and Hughes, C.L. (1998). Effect of progestin on the ovarian epithelium of macaques: Cancer prevention through apoprosis. *J. Soc. Gynecol. Invest.* 5, 271–276.
24. Piver, M. S., Baker, T. R., Jishi, M. F., Sandecki, A. M., Tsukada, Y., Natarajan, N., Mettlin, C. J., and Blake, C. (1993). Familial ovarian cancer: A report of 658 families from the Gilda Radner Familial Ovarian Cancer Registry 1981–1991. *Cancer* 71, 582–588.
25. Narod, S. A., Risch, H., Moslehi, R., Dorum, A., Neuhausen, S., Olsson, H., Provencher, D., Radice, P., Evans, G., Bishop, S., Brunet, J. S., Ponder, B. A. J., and the Hereditary Ovarian Cancer Clinical Study Group (1998). Oral contraceptives and the risk of hereditary ovarian cancer. *N. Engl. J. Med.* 339, 424–428.
26. Gnagy, S., Ming, E. E., Devesa, S. S., Hartge, P., and Whittemore, A. S. (2000). Declining ovarian cancer rates in U.S. women in relation to parity and oral contraceptive use. *Epidemiology* 11, 102–105.
27. Greenlee, R. T., Murray, T., Bolden, S., and Wingo, P. A. (2000). Cancer statistics 2000. *CA* 1.
28. Claus, E. B., Schildkraut, J. M., Thompson, W. D., and Risch, N. J. (1996). The genetic attributable risk of breast and ovarian cancer. *Cancer* 77, 2318–2324.
29. Ford, D., Easton, D. F., and Stratton, M. *et al.* (1998). Genetic heterogeneity and penetrance analysis of the BRCA1 and BRCA2 genes in breast cancer families. *Am. J. Hum. Genet.* 62, 676–689.
30. Wijnen, J., de Leeuw, W., and Vasen, H. *et al.* (1999). Familial endometrial cancer in female carriers of MSH6 germline mutations. *Nat. Genet.* 23, 142–144.
31. Welcsh, P. L., Owens, K. N., and King, M. C. (2000). Insights into the functions of BRCA1 and BRCA2. *Trends Genet.* 16, 69–74.
32. Marra, G., and Boland, C. R. (1995). Hereditary nonpolyposis colorectal cancer. The syndrome, the genes, and historical perspectives. *J. Natl. Inst.* 87, 1114–1125.
33. Whittemore, A. S., Gong, G., and Itnyre, J. (1997). Prevalence and contribution of BRCA1 mutations in breast cancer and ovarian cancer: Results from three U.S. population-based case-control studies of ovarian cancer. *Am. J. Hum. Genet.* 60, 496–504.
34. Ford, D., Easton, D. F., Bishop, D. T., Narod, S. A., and Goldgar, D. E. (1994). Breast Cancer Linkage Consortium: Risks of cancer in BRCA1-mutation carriers. *Lancet* 343, 692–695.
35. Easton, D. F., Ford, D., Bishop, D. T., and Breast Cancer Linkage Consortium (1995). Breast and ovarian cancer incidence in BRCA1-mutation carriers. *Am. J. Hum. Genet.* 56, 265–271.
36. Frank, T. S., Manley, S. A., Olopade, O. I. *et al.* (1998). Sequence analysis of BRCA1 and BRCA2: Correlation of mutations with family history and ovarian cancer risk. *J. Clin. Oncol.* 16, 2417–2425.
37. The Breast Cancer Linkage Consortium (1999). Cancer Risks in BRCA2 Mutation Carriers. *J. Natl. Cancer Inst.* 91, 1310–1316.
38. Aarnio, M., Sankila, R., and Pukkala, E. *et al.* (1999). Cancer Risk in mutation carriers of DNA-mismatch-repair genes. *Int. J. Cancer* 81, 214–218.
39. Gayther, S. A., Warren, W., Mazoyer, S. *et al.* (1995). Germline mutations of the BRCA1 gene in breast and ovarian cancer families provide evidence for a genotype-phenotype correlation. *Nat. Genet.* 11, 428–433.
40. Gayther, S. A., Mangion, J., Russell, P. *et al.* (1997). Variation of risks of breast and ovarian cancer associated with different germline mutations of the BRCA2 gene. *Nat. Genet.* 15, 103–105.
41. Phelan, C. M., Rebbeck, T. R., Weber, B. L. *et al.* (1996). Ovarian cancer risk in BRCA1 carriers is modified by the HRAS1 variable number of tandem repeat (VNTR) locus. *Nat. Genet.* 12, 309–433.
42. Buller, R. E., Sood, A. K., Lallas, T., Buekers, T., and Skilling, J. S. (1999). Association between nonrandom X-chromosome inactivation and BRCA1 mutation in germline DNA of patients with ovarian cancer. *J. Natl. Cancer. Inst.* 91, 339–346.
43. Rubin, S. C., Benjamin, I., Behbakht, K. *et al.* (1996). Clinical and pathological features of ovarian cancer in women with germ-line mutations of BRCA1. *N. Eng. J. Med.* 335, 1413–1416.
44. Stratton, J. F., Gayther, S. A., Russell, P. *et al.* (1997). Contribution of BRCA1 mutations to ovarian cancer. *N. Eng. J. Med.* 336, 1125–1130.
45. Boyd, J., Sonoda, Y., and Federici, M. G. *et al.* (2000). Clinicopathologic Features of BRCA-Linked and Sporadic Ovarian Cancer. *JAMA* 283, 2260–2265.
46. Merajver, S. D., Pham, T. M., Caduff, R. F. *et al.* (1995). Somatic mutations in the BRCA1 in sporadic ovarian tumors. *Nat. Genet.* 9, 439–443.
47. Berchuck, A., Heron, K. A., Carney, M. E. *et al.* (1998). Frequency of germline and somatic BRCA1 mutations in ovarian cancer. *Clin. Cancer. Res.* 4, 2433–2437.
48. Burke, W., Daly, M., Garber, J. *et al.* (1997). Recommendations for follow-up care of individuals with an inherited predisposition to cancer. II. BRCA1 and BRCA2. Cancer Genetics Studies Consortium. *JAMA* 277, 997–1003.
49. Weber, B. L., Punzalan, C., Eisen, A. *et al.* (2000). Ovarian cancer risk reduction after bilateral prophylactic oophorectomy (BPO) in BRCA1 and BRCA2 mutation carriers. *Am. J. Hum. Genet.* 67(S2), 59.
50. Piver, M. S., Barlow, J. J., and Sawyer, D. M. (1982). Familial ovarian cancer: Increase in ferquency? *Obstet. Gynecol.* 60, 397–399.

CHAPTER

18

Early Diagnosis and Screening for Ovarian Cancer

MARK H. EINSTEIN

Division of Gynecologic Oncology
Department of Obstetrics, Gynecology, and Women's Health
Albert Einstein College of Medicine and Montefiore Medical Center
Bronx, New York 10461

CAROLYN D. RUNOWICZ

Department of Obstetrics and Gynecology
St. Luke's-Roosevelt Hospital Center
New York, New York 10019

I. INTRODUCTION

Making a diagnosis of early stage ovarian cancer is a difficult task. Currently there are no acceptable screening methods for the general population for this disease. This chapter discusses some of the cellular and pathologic models that support a multistep oncogenic process from a single ovarian epithelial cell that provides a rationale for screening. Since the survival is better in early-stage ovarian cancer, attempts at early detection through tumor markers and screening strategies have been studied. Some tumor markers have been shown to have some usefulness in the detection of ovarian cancer, especially CA125. Most of the tumor markers, however, have poor specificity and positive predictive values when used alone for screening. Ultrasonography can detect cystic and solid processes of the ovary and has been used for cancer screening. Morphology scoring indices have been used for cancer screening. Morphology scoring indices have been used to quantify real-time ultrasound findings, and have been correlated with histopathologic diagnosis. Screening strategies utilizing transvaginal ultrasonography, serum CA125 measurements, and other indices have been performed in clinical trials with some promising data. No current screening strategies have been found to reduce the mortality rate from ovarian cancer, but some have been shown to have a shift to an earlier stage at time of diagnosis. Risk factors and current screening guidelines are also presented in this chapter. BRCA1/2 mutation carriers are at high risk for developing ovarian cancer. Screening guidelines are different for those patients than for the rest of the population. For those patients at risk, there are surgical and chemopreventative measures that can be taken to reduce this risk.

Presently, the early diagnosis of ovarian cancer is a serendipitous finding, rather than a triumph of medicine.[1] Most early ovarian cancer cases are found incidentally at the time of laparoscopy or laparotomy, or as a result of endocrine activity from functional stromal cell tumors.

The goal of early detection is to improve treatment outcome, as measured by a reduction in morbidity and mortality, in a group of individuals at risk for developing this disease. Ovarian cancer eludes this goal. Abdominal discomfort, dyspepsia, flatulence, bloating, mild digestive disturbances, and pelvic pain have all been described as early symptoms of ovarian cancer.[2] The time required to develop an invasive cancer, or the interval for progression from stage I to stage III is unknown. Limited literature exists regarding the possibility of a precursor lesion for ovarian carcinoma. Observational studies have led to the hypothesis that dysplasia or hyperplasia arising within epithelial inclusion cysts may represent a histologic precursor to ovarian carcinoma [3–10] (Table 18.1). Molecular analysis suggests a multistep molecular oncogenesis from a single ovarian epithelial cell.[11] Thus, there

TABLE 18.1 Ovarian Cancer Precursors

Study	N	Pathology
Plaxe (1990) [4]	50 patients stage I 50 patients incidental oophorectomy	Ovarian intraepithelial neoplasia (OIN)
Deligdish (1993) [5]	12 patients ovarian cancer 12 patients ovarian dysplasia 11 patients control	Computerized image analysis of OIN
Salazar (1996) [6]	20 patients "high-risk" 20 patients incidental oophorectomy	1. Surface epithelial pseudo-stratification 2. Cortical invagination 3. Inclusion cysts
Stratton (1999) [8]	11 patients BRCA1/2 26 patients "high-risk"	No difference in groups
Barakat (2000) [7]	18 patients BRCA1 20 controls	No difference in groups
Werness (2000) [9]	Case-study BRCA	1. Laser capture microdissection 2. p53 mutations 3. LOH prior to stromal invasion
Pothuri (2001) [10]	39 prophylactic oophorectomies in BRCA mutation carriers 8 stage I	1. TP53 mutation in 31% of prophylactic oophorectomies (laser capture microdissection) 2. All cases had inclusion cysts 3. Dysplasia preceded carcinoma

may be a biologic rationale to justify screening efforts directed at finding "precancerous" or early-stage cancers of the ovary. However, the more laudable long-term goal is to prevent the onset of the disease by risk reduction interventions, including chemoprevention and prophylactic surgery.

II. SCREENING

Currently, there are no screening guidelines for the general population to detect ovarian cancer in an earlier stage. The most serious obstacle is the low incidence of the disease. The minimum positive predictive value for consideration of a screening program for ovarian cancer suggested in the literature is 10%.[12] For ovarian cancer, this requires a high sensitivity [13], a high specificity [14], reproducibility, accessibility, and affordability. The screening test must also result in the reduction in mortality.

Based on known risk factors, one cannot easily identify or pinpoint a group of women at increased risk for ovarian cancer, except for those with a strong family history of ovarian cancer (Table 18.2). Of the hormonal, genetic, and environmental risk factors, genetics plays the largest role. However, women with inherited familial syndromes account for only 10% of all of the patients with ovarian cancer cancers.[15] The majority of women with a family history of ovarian cancer are not from families with hereditary ovarian cancer syndromes. Of the women with inherited syndromes, the majority of genetic mutations (85%) are in the tumor suppressor genes, BRCA1, located on chromosome 17q21, and BRCA2, on chromosome 13q. These genes are inherited in an autosomal dominant pattern, with variable or incomplete penetrance and have been associated with breast, ovarian, and prostate cancers. The hereditary nonpolyposis colon cancer (HNPCC) syndrome accounts for a small percentage of patients with inherited ovarian cancer. With the completion of the Human Genome Project, as well as the use of microarray technology, other genes will be identified.

For the general population, the lifetime risk is 1.8%. The risk increases to 5% with one affected first-degree relative and 7% with two or more first-degree relatives.[16] In the Ashkenazi Jewish population, the most recent studies estimate that BRCA1/2 mutation carriers have a 16.5% lifetime risk by the age of 70 of developing ovarian cancer.[17] Depending on the population studied, the lifetime risk will vary (Table 18.3). In women with breast cancer, mutations in BRCA1 and BRCA2 have been associated with a tenfold increased risk of subsequent ovarian carcinoma.[18]

Screening guidelines for genetic testing include patients with a >10% risk of having a mutation, the ability to interpret the results, and a willingness of the patient to act on the result.[19] Patients with a >10% risk for a mutation include:

1. Breast and ovarian cancer (any age) within the same family, particularly, if within the same woman
2. Cases of male breast cancer

TABLE 18.2 Risk Factors for Developing Ovarian Cancer

Risk factor	RR
Late menopause (age ≥52 or later vs. <49)	2.4
Early menarche	1.5–2
Nulliparity	
(versus 1 child)	2.0
(versus 5 children)	5.0
Infertility	2–5
Older age	3
Caucasian race	1.5
Higher Education or income	1.5–2
History of breast, endometrial, or colon cancer	3–50

Adapted from Runowicz, C. D., and Fields, A. L. (1999). *Surg. Oncol. Clin. N. Am.* 8(4), 703–723.

TABLE 18.3 Estimates of BRCA1 Penetrance for Ovarian Cancer

Study	Gene	Lifetime risk
Easton (1995) [82]	BRCA1	63%
Easton (1997) [83]	BRCA2	27%
Struewing (1997) [17]	BRCA1/2	16%
Ford (1998) [84]	BRCA2	27%
Moslehi (2000) [85]	BRCA1	51%
	BRCA2	20%
General population		1.8%

3. Multiple cases of early onset breast cancer disease (<age 50)
4. Bilateral breast cancers

Currently, a federal law (through HIPAA) protects patients, identified with mutations, against discrimination with respect to health insurance.

Once a high-risk family has been identified and counseled, a living affected member should be offered testing for the most commonly identified mutations:

185delAG } BRCA1
5382insC }
6174delT–BRCA2

If these mutations are not identified, full gene sequencing may be offered. If the affected member tests positive for one of the mutations, the unaffected members may be offered testing. If the unaffected member tests positive for the identified mutation, that person is at increased risk for developing a malignancy. Preventative strategies should be discussed. If the unaffected member tests negative, she is at the same risk as the general population for developing a breast and/or ovarian cancer.

III. TUMOR MARKERS

CA125 is an antigenic determinant on a high molecular weight glycoprotein recognized by the murine monoclonal antibody OC125.[20] In the adult, it is found in structures derived from coelomic epithelium and in tubal, endometrial, and endocervical epithelium. Overall, approximately 85% of patients with epithelial ovarian cancer have CA125 levels >35 U/ml.[21, 22] CA125 is not in and of itself, a good screening test for ovarian cancer because it has a low specificity and positive predictive value. Most premenopausal patients with elevated CA125 levels will have benign or physiologic conditions such as: pregnancy, menstruation, pelvic inflammatory disease, and endometriosis. Other conditions that elevate CA125 levels include malignancies of the colon, pancreas, breast, and lung.[22] Liver and renal failure will also elevate CA125. Less than half of patients with stage I ovarian cancer will have an elevated CA125.[23] Newer CA125 assays have been developed. The second generation CA125 assay utilizes a new high-affinity antibody (M11) in combination with OC125. The enhanced affinity diminishes the variability by 50%.[24]

Other tumor markers have been utilized in screening protocols for the early detection of ovarian cancer. None have yet been shown to have more than a minor additional discriminative value over CA125 as a tumor marker. Table 18.4 lists of some of the tumor markers that have been used alone, or in combination for screening.

Multiple biomarker profiles have been utilized in ovarian cancer screening. Berek reports that serial measurements of complementary serum markers can improve the sensitivity, specificity, and positive predictive value of serum markers CA125 and OVX1.[25] Woolas and colleagues reported that a serum panel of 5 separate markers had a sensitivity of 83.3% and specificity of 84% when 2 or more markers were elevated.[26] CA125, menopausal status, and ultrasonography have been found to be superior to a panel of three tumor markers (CA125, CA15-3 and TAG72-3) in the preoperative differential diagnosis of a pelvic mass.[27] In asymptomatic healthy women, five separate tumor markers behaved independently and the false-positive rate could be estimated by the sum of the individual false positive rates.[28] Thus, a drawback to ordering too many markers is the high probability that the false-positive results may lead to further testing, including surgery for a benign process.[28, 29]

Some investigators have focused on the biologic behavior of CA125. An algorithm proposed by Skates shows that not only a rise, but the rate in rise of CA125 may be significant. This risk of ovarian cancer (ROC) algorithm may be a better indicator for early detection.[30]

Traditional technologies and laboratory testing has yet been able to detect early state ovarian cancer. Utilizing proleomics and bioinformatics, Petricoin *et al.* [30a] produced an algorithm that identifies a cluster pattern in ovarian cancer.

TABLE 18.4 Tumor Markers

Tumor marker	Comment
Lysophospatidic acid (LPA)	More sensitive than CA125 in early-stage disease, but also in 10% of the population [86]
Lipid-associated sialic acid (LASA)	Is elevated in leukemia, sarcoma, melanoma, Hodgkin's disease, oropharyngeal tumors, and ovarian cancer [87–89]
OVX1	The antibody recognizes a unique antigenic determinant present in ovarian and breast cancer cells, it does not bind to normal ovarian tissues [90]
Macrophage colony-stimulating factor (M-CSF)	Has been found to be measurable in 68% of patients with clinically detectable ovarian carcinoma residual disease [91, 92]
CA19-9	An antigen that is part of the Lewis Blood Group antigens, elevated in pancreatic, ovarian, GI, lung, and endometrial cancer [93]

Importantly, the discriminatory pattern correctly identified all 18 stage I cases. Although far from routine clinical use, the use of this new technology yielded a sensitivity of 100% and specificity of 95% with a positive predictive value of 94% as compared to the positive predictive value of 4% using CA125 alone. The use of proleomics and bioinformatics may be used as a screening tool for ovarian cancer as well as detection of other cancers in the near future.

IV. ULTRASONOGRAPHY

Real-time ultrasonography has been used to visualize the ovaries. The transvaginal route improves the definition of ovarian imaging and may achieve a small increase in specificity, when used in the screening setting.[31–33] Morphology scoring indices have been used to quantify the real-time ultrasound findings, and have been correlated with the histopathologic diagnosis.[31, 34–36] These scoring indices include:

1. Ovarian volume
2. Cyst wall structure
   - Thickness
3. Papillary vegetations
4. Septations
5. Echogenicity
6. Color Doppler imaging (CDI)
   - Resistance
   - Impedance

No scoring system has been universally agreed upon. However, all agree that papillary vegetations are the most ominous finding associated with the diagnosis of ovarian carcinoma. The specificity of ultrasound for ovarian cancer is limited by the detection of cystic and solid benign processes.[37]

Even in patients at increased risk for ovarian cancer, only one in three women with a family history of ovarian cancer and a "positive" screen will have histologic evidence of ovarian cancer.[38] Due to the time required to perform the test and associated expense, ultrasonography will most likely be used as a second-level screening modality.[39]

CDI characterizes blood flow. The biologic rationale for evaluating of blood flow is based on the observation that neovascularization is an obligate early event in tumor growth and neoplasia.[40] Early changes in angiogenesis may be detectable prior to morphologic changes in ovarian architecture.[41] With CDI, "malignant" vascular patterns may theoretically be differentiated from "benign" vascular patterns. Using CDI, the blood flow, vessel location and arrangement, impedance values, and the presence or absence of a diastolic flow can be assessed.[42] Using CDI, clinical studies have reported that normal physiologic changes in the premenopausal ovary near ovulation have impedence flow patterns that mimic "malignant" flow patterns,[43, 44] thus, limiting its usefulness in the premenopausal woman.

Patients, however, do have an interest in participating in such ultrasound-based screening studies. In a study performed by Pavlik *et al.*, 13,963 women continued to participate in an ovarian cancer screening program even at 5 and 7.5 years after starting the trial.[45]

Multimodal screening with serial CA125 and ultrasonography has been investigated.[46–50] Investigators from the Royal Hospital in London randomized 22,000 women aged 45 or older to a control group and screened group (Fig. 18.1). Of the 468 women in the screened group that had an elevated CA125, 29 were referred to a gynecologist. Six index cancers were detected by the screen and an additional 10 women in the screening group developed an index cancer during the follow-up of 8 years. Twenty women in the control group developed cancer. The positive predictive value of this screening protocol was 20.7%. There was a survival benefit in the screened group (median survival 72.9 months versus 41.8 months in the control group). However, this did not reach statistical significance.[13] There was a trend to an earlier stage distribution of cancers in the screened cohort.

The European randomized clinical trial (RCT) of ovarian cancer screening will recruit 200,000 postmenopausal women for a screening trial (Table 18.5). More than 20 centers will be employed to perform this trial over an approximate period of 6 years to screen. Study end points include mortality, quality of life, and cost. As part of the trial, the patient's ROC will be calculated. This formula is based on the intercept, slope, and assay variability (Figs. 18.2 and 18.3). The ROC algorithm using the CA125II assay has an estimated positive predictive value of 16%, substantially greater than the positive predictive value based on a single assay.[30] Figure 18.2 displays the increasing slope of CA125II levels over time in a patient with ovarian cancer. Figure 18.3 displays

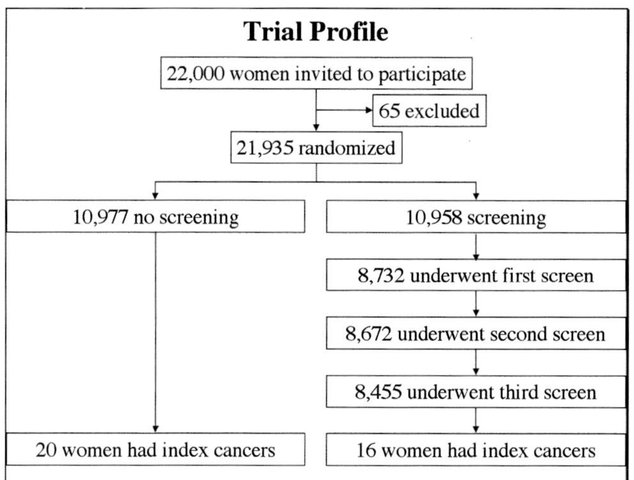

FIGURE 18.1 Trial profile for Royal Hospital in London ovarian cancer screening study. (Adapted from Jacobs, I. J. *et al. Lancet* 1999; 353; 1207.)

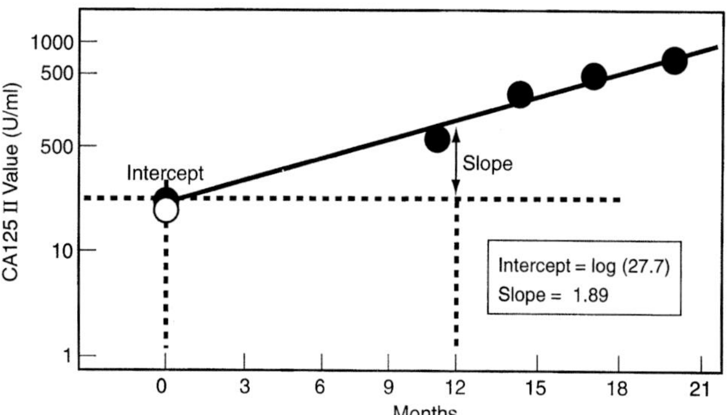

FIGURE 18.2 Log-transformed increasing slope of CA125II value in an ovarian cancer patient.

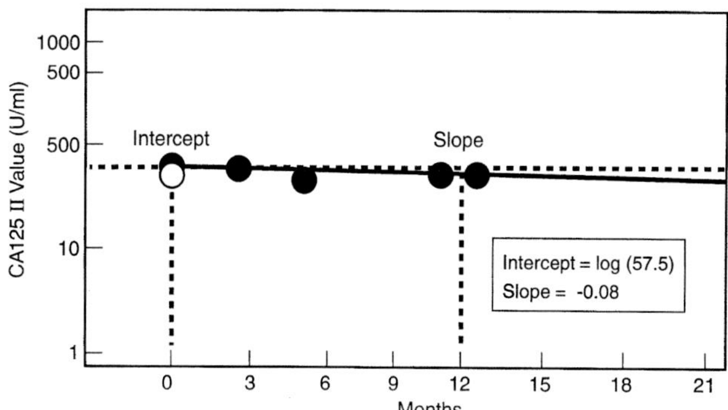

FIGURE 18.3 Log-transformed unchanged slope of CA125II value in a patient who does not have ovarian cancer.

TABLE 18.5 European RCT of Ovarian Cancer Screening (EURCTOCS)

200,000 Postmenopausal >50 years old; no family history
50,000 multimodal:annual CA125 (ROC), TVS
50,000: annual TVS
Time period: 3-year recruitment, >20 centers
6 years screening
Endpoints
Mortality
Quality of Life
Cost

an ROC curve of a patient without ovarian cancer. Although the CA125 is markedly elevated, the straight line over time is consistent with a benign process.

A smaller study of approximately 5000 women used a similar multimodal screening protocol. Patients with elevated CA125 levels had a transabdominal ultrasound. Six cases of ovarian cancer occurred in women >50 years who had an elevated CA125 level. The diagnosed cases were stage IA(2), IIB(2), and IIIC(2). Three patients, all under age 50, with normal range CA125 levels were subsequently found to have ovarian cancer. The positive predictive value of this screening protocol proved to be 50%.[14]

A larger trial in the U.S., the National Institutes of Health (NIH) PLCO (prostate, lung, colon, and ovary) cancer screening trial, is testing a multimodal screening protocol utilizing pelvic examinations, ultrasonography, and CA125 to detect ovarian cancer in women 60–74 years old.[51] If the patient has any abnormal results, she will be referred for gynecologic evaluation. PLCO is a larger randomized trial with a control arm to determine the impact of the screening interventions on ovarian cancer mortality. Based on a power of 80%, it will take 16 years to demonstrate a 30% reduction in mortality in this study.

A large Japanese screening study identified a shift in stage in women undergoing transvaginal sonogram (TVS) as a screening procedure (Table 18.6).[52] A total of 183,034 women participated in primary screening and participants who underwent the primary screening repeatedly were included in the analysis. Of those women, 51,500 took part in screening for the first time with follow-up screening required in 5309 patients. Of the participants, 324 underwent surgery. There were 17/22 stage I tumors identified, with elevated tumor markers in only 5/17 (29.4%). As compared to historical controls, the authors have demonstrated a shift in stage with 29.7% of the patients diagnosed with stage I disease from 1981–1987, as compared to 59% in the screened interval. Whether this results in improved survival was not demonstrated in this study.

A similar shift in stage was reported by van Nagell *et al.* in a large screening trial consisting of 14,469 asymptomatic women.[53] The women were either ≥50 years of age or ≥25 years of age with a family history of ovarian cancer. Women with persistently abnormal TVS had a repeat sonogram in

TABLE 18.6 Stage of Ovarian Cancer Before and After Induction of Screening (N = 51,550)

Stage	1981–1987 # of patients (%)	1988–1998 # of patients (%)
I	11 (29.7)	50 (58.8)
II	5 (13.5)	8 (9.4)
III	16 (43.3)	19 (22.4)
IV	5 (13.5)	8 (9.4)
Total	37	85

Adapted from Sato, S. *et al.* (2000). *Cancer* 89, 582–588.

TABLE 18.7 Case-Specific Ovarian Cancer Survival in Screened Population

Annually screened	N	2 years	5 years
All cases	21	95%	88%
Invasive cases	15	93%	84%
FIGO (1998)			47%

Adapted from van Nagell, J. R., *et al.* (2000). *Gynecol. Oncol.* 77(3), 350–356.

4–6 weeks and those with two repeat abnormal sonograms had a serum CA125 determination as well as tumor morphology indexing, Doppler flow sonography, and were advised to have the mass removed. In 180 patients with persistently abnormal TVS 17 ovarian cancers were detected (11 stage I, 3 stage II, 3 stage III). Survival is shown in Table 18.7. The authors conclude that annual TVS screening is associated with a shift in stage resulting in a decrease in case-specific ovarian cancer mortality as compared to PIGO data.[53]

Morgante *et al.* described two malignancy risk indices incorporating ultrasound, CA125, and menopausal status to aid in the identification of women with ovarian cancer.[54] Statistically significant differences were found between the groups with benign and malignant pathology. This type of index may be helpful for diagnosing early ovarian cancer in the future.

The cost of multimodal screening has been analyzed. The cost per screen is highest during the first year of screening. At the lowest, the cost per ultrasound screen is $39 as reported by DePriest and colleagues.[55] However, the cost of the ultrasound for their studies is underwritten by a research grant. In the U.S., the cost of a nonobstetrical sonogram is approximately $275 and the cost of a CA125 is approximately $45. If every woman aged 45 years or older had these two diagnostic procedures, there would be an increase in healthcare costs of about $13,760,000,000 per year without any guarantee of lowering the death rate of ovarian cancer.[56]

V. RISK-FACTOR-BASED SCREENING TRIALS

In order to improve the yield in screening for ovarian cancer, screening trials based on risk factors have been evaluated. A family history of ovarian cancer and advanced age are the two most significant risk factors for ovarian cancer.[1, 41] However, relying on family history means that we are only screening up to 10% of the population.

Bourne and co-workers evaluated patients with a family history of ovarian cancer.[38] Of the 1601 women screened, 61 (3.8%) were found to have a positive screen. Six ovarian cancers (5 stage I, 3 of which were low-malignant potential, and 1 stage III) and 48 benign neoplasms were found. In seven women, no abnormality could be found. In the subsequent 2–4 years of follow-up, three more stage III ovarian cancers were detected. Because of these late-stage patients, the authors concluded that ovarian cancer screening should be performed more often than annually. Karlan and colleagues have been following a cohort of 1079 "high-risk" women with CDI, ultrasonography, and five different serum tumor biomarkers. Thirty-four women underwent bilateral oophorectomies for persistently abnormal test results. Another 37 women underwent elective prophylactic oophorectomy, following genetic counseling and testing. In the group with abnormal results, one stage IA and one stage IB low-malignant potential ovarian cancers were found as well as one stage IA grade 3 endometrial cancer. Disappointingly, one patient presented with abdominal symptoms, 4 months after normal screening results and prophylactic oophorectomy, and was found to have a stage IIIC primary peritoneal cancer. A consistent pattern of ovarian pathology or precursor lesions were not identified in the surgical specimens.[41]

VI. OVARIAN CANCER SCREENING RECOMMENDATIONS FOR INDIVIDUALS AT RISK

Screening recommendations for patients with one or two affected family members cannot be made at this time. The benefits of screening a woman who has one or no first-degree relatives with ovarian cancer are unproven.[57] In fact, the risks of unnecessary screening may outweigh the benefits, particularly in women with no family history or other high risk factors. The NIH consensus statement states that despite the absence of prospective data, a woman with one first-degree relative with ovarian cancer may choose to be screened. This opportunity should be made available to the woman by her physician. Women with two or more family members affected by ovarian cancer should have counseling by a gynecologic oncologist or other qualified specialist about her individual risk and screening.[57] In patients with a hereditary ovarian cancer syndrome, the experts in the NIH consensus conference recommended an annual pelvic examination, CA125 level, and TVS.[57] However, they also comment that there is no data demonstrating that screening reduces mortality of ovarian cancer.

The Cancer Genetics Studies Consortium made recommendations for individuals carrying mutations in the BRCA1 or BRCA2 genes.[58] Although these recommendations are based on expert opinion only and not prospective trials, the consortium recommends:

1. Transvaginal ultrasonography with color doppler and serum CA125 levels
2. Begin at age 25–35
3. Annual or semi-annual screen

Transvaginal ultrasound should be timed to avoid ovulation and reduce false-positive results. BRCA2 mutation carriers should consider surveillance, but their lower risk reduces the likelihood of any benefit.[58] This screening strategy has not been shown to reduce mortality.

Based on a survey of 16 European family cancer clinics, the European Familial Breast Cancer Collaborative Group recommends an annual gynecologic examination, TVS, and CA125 level in all BRCA1 and BRCA2-mutation carriers and in members from breast/ovarian cancer families starting from age 30–35.[59] Some European centers even recommend testing in "breast cancer only" families also, but this is the recommendation of only a few institutions based on expert opinion only.[59]

VII. SURGICAL PREVENTION OF OVARIAN CANCER

Data collected from the Centers for Disease Control reveal that only about 40–50% of patients undergoing hysterectomy at 40 years of age or older had a prophylactic oophorectomy.[60] Approximately 1000 ovarian cancer cases could be prevented if prophylactic oophorectomy were performed in all women older than 40 who undergo a hysterectomy.[61] If the woman at risk for ovarian cancer is having abdominal surgery for other indications, a prophylactic oophorectomy should be considered, especially in the peri- and postmenopausal patient.[37] The added surgical morbidity of oophorectomy at the time of other surgery is minimal.[60] However, the benefits of prophylactic oophorectomy must be weighed against the consequences of early estrogen loss:

1. Physiologic adjustments to a premature surgical menopause, especially vasomotor symptoms; the prevention of cardiovascular disease and osteoporosis remains a critical issue.
2. Psychosocial adjustments to premature menopause
3. Hormone replacement therapy, especially in these women with a high risk of breast cancer

Prophylactic oophorectomy should be encouraged in women with inherited ovarian cancer syndromes (BRCA1/2). Based on expert opinion, the NIH Consensus Conference recommended a bilateral prophylactic oophorectomy when childbearing is complete or by the age of 35 in high-risk women.[57] An ovarian cancer risk reduction of 50% has been reported with a bilateral prophylactic oophorectomy in high-risk families.[62] However, this did not reach statistical significance. The Cancer Genetics Studies Consortium, organized by the National Human Genome Research Institute, felt there was insufficient evidence to recommend for or against bilateral prophylactic oophorectomy.[58] Soon after the consortium statement, Rebbeck *et al.* published multi-institutional data regarding the efforts of prophylatic oophorectomy incarriers of BRCA1 or BRCA2 mutation carriers. Patients were carefully screened to fall into categories of mutation carriers who had a prophylactic oophorectomy and mutation carriers who were alive with both ovaries intact at the time the woman with whom she was matched with underwent prophylactic oophorectomy. Using these criteria, 259 eligible subjects and 292 controls were identified.

Of the 259 subjects who underwent prophylactic oophorectomy, 8 (3.1%) received a diagnosis of ovarian or primary peritoneal cancer at or after oophorectomy as compared with 58 or 292 controls (19.9%). Of the 8 cases in prophylactic oophorectomy patients, 6 were stage I cases that were diagnosed at the time of surgery. Neither breast nor ovarian cancer developed in 185 of the 259 prophylatic oophorectomy patients (71.4%) as compared with 153 of 292 controls (52.4%), $p<0.001$). When the upper bound of the 95% confidence interval of the hazard ration was taken as a conservative estimate, prophylactic oophorectomy reduced the risk of ovarian cancer in mutation carriers by approximately 85% and the risk of breast cancer by approximately 25%.[63] Although only 55% of the patients in this study were followed prospectively,[64] this is convincing data to perform a prophylactic oophorectomy in BRCA1 or 2 mutation carriers.

In a small study, foci of malignant tumors were detected in prophylactic oophorectomy specimens, in women at high risk for ovarian cancer.[65] Frozen section should be performed on all prophylactic oophorectomy specimens, with appropriate surgical staging, if microscopic disease is present.

Tubal sterilization procedures have also been shown to be protective against ovarian cancer. In a prospective assessment of the relationship of tubal ligation and hysterectomy, the risk of ovarian cancer during the 12 years of follow-up in the Nurses Health Study was analyzed. When adjusted for age, parity, oral contraception (OC) use, and other ovarian cancer risk factors, there was a strong inverse association between tubal ligation and ovarian cancer.[66] There was also an association between hysterectomy and ovarian cancer risk reduction.[66]

VIII. CHEMOPREVENTION

Multiple studies consistently report that OCs significantly decrease the incidence of ovarian cancer.[67] The Cancer and Steroid Hormone Study of the CDC and NIH showed that women who used OCs had a risk reduction of epithelial cancer of 0.6% for ovarian cancer, as compared with those who never used them. More importantly, the protective effect continued for 15 years after OC use ended, even in women who used them for only 3–6 months.[68] Use of OCs for 6 or more years in patients with a risk of hereditary ovarian cancer has also been associated with a 60% reduction in ovarian cancer risk. The risk decreased with increasing duration of use.[69, 70] Newer, low-dose OCs may have slightly weaker protection.[71]

The biologic basis for this protection is unknown. Prevention of unnecessary ovulation may be one of the mechanisms. The number of lifetime ovulatory cycles has been correlated with p53-positive ovarian cancers, suggesting that proliferation-associated DNA damage may cause a p53 mutation.[72] The progesterone component of the OCs may be the most important component resulting in protection. In monkey studies, progesterone induces apoptosis in the ovarian epithelium significantly more than estrogen.[73]

Retinoids have been shown to have anti-tumor activity *in vivo* and antiovarian cancer activity *in vitro*. Retinoids refer to a class of compounds which includes vitamin A, its natural derivatives, and thousands of analogs.[74] Retinoic acid receptors (RARs) belong to the superfamily of steroid and thyroid receptors. RARs act as transcription factors, binding as dimers to retinoid response elements in the promoter regions of target genes to enhance or repress transcription.[74] 4HPR or fenretinamide has been shown to reduce oncogenicity of ovarian cancer cell lines A2780 and IGROV-1 clones which overexpress RAR.[75] Cell cycle kinetics of ovarian carcinoma cell growth was inhibited in two ovarian cancer cell lines, CA-OV3 and SK-OV3, by retinoids.[74] OVCAR-3, CAOV-3, and SK-OV3 treated with a variety of retinoids had growth inhibition and increased apoptosis.[76] A phase I trial of 9-cis retinoic acid in adults with solid tumors showed human dosing was feasible with adequate plasma levels achieved with oral administration.[77] In a randomized clinical trial for patients with T1 or T2 breast cancer in an adjurant, women were assigned to receive either 4-HPR or no treatment. During the 5 years of intervention, 6 patients in the control group developed an ovarian carcinoma whereas no case of ovarian carcinoma occurred during the same period in the 4-HPR group. This difference in the incidence rate of ovarian carcinoma was significant ($p = 0.0162$).[78]

Anti-inflammatory drugs have recently been shown to have an effect on ovarian cancer risk reduction (Table 18.8).[79] Although most of the confidence intervals cross one, the data is intriguing. The anti-tumorigenic effects of aspirin have been proven in colon cancer. In a preliminary report, prospective questionnaires in 12,329 women suggested that at least six months of regular aspirin use was associated with a reduced risk of ovarian cancer.[80] However, the results of this study were not statistically significant and are limited by the sampling bias of the questionnaires. An inverse association between paracetamol use and ovarian cancer risk has been reported.[81] However, the confidence intervals cross one (Table 18.8). Rodent studies show that high-dose paracetamol causes ovarian atrophy, thus suggesting a biologic mechanism for such a finding in humans.

TABLE 18.8 Role NSAID and Other Anti-Inflammatory Agents in Ovarian Cancer Risk Prevention 5 Case-Control Studies

Study	#OC cases	Odds ratio	95% Conf. interval
Tzonou (1993) [94]	189	0.51	0.26–1.02
Cramer (1998) [81]	563	0.75	0.52–1.10
Tavani (2000) [79]	749	0.93	0.53–1.62
Rosenberg (2000) [95]	780	0.50	0.2–1.0
Akhmedkhanov (2001) [80]	68	0.60	0.26–1.36

IX. SUMMARY

All women should have a comprehensive family history taken by a physician knowledgeable in the risks associated with ovarian cancer and should continue to undergo annual pelvic examination as part of routine medical care. There are no suitable means to screen for ovarian cancer in the general population at this time. Large prospective trials may provide better insight as to the best screening protocol for those individuals at increased risk for developing ovarian cancer. Participation in these clinical trials should be encouraged for all patients at risk. Lastly, medical and surgical methods that reduce ovarian cancer risk should be discussed with all patients who are found to be at an increased risk of ovarian cancer.

References

1. Barber, H. (1993). "Ovarian Carcinoma: Etiology, Diagnosis and Treatment." Springer-Verlag, New York.
2. Goff, B. A., Mandel, L., Muntz, H. G., and Melancon, C. H. (2000). Ovarian carcinoma diagnosis. *Cancer* 89, 2068–2075.
3. Deligdisch, L., Gil, J., Kerner, H., Wu, H. S., Beck, D., and Gershoni-Baruch, R. (1999). Ovarian dysplasia in prophylactic oophorectomy specimens: Cytogenetic and morphometric correlations. *Cancer* 86, 1544–1550.
4. Plaxe, S. C., Deligdisch, L., Dottino, P. R., and Cohen, C. J. (1990). Ovarian intraepithelial neoplasia demonstrated in patients with stage I ovarian carcinoma. *Gynecol. Oncol.* 38, 367–372.
5. Deligdisch, L., Miranda, C., Barba, J., and Gil, J. (1993). Ovarian dysplasia: Nuclear texture analysis. *Cancer* 72, 3253–3257.

6. Salazar, H., Godwin, A. K., Daly, M. B. *et al.* (1996). Microscopic benign and invasive malignant neoplasms and a cancer-prone phenotype in prophylactic oophorectomies. *J. Natl. Cancer Inst.* 88, 1810–1820.
7. Barakat, R. R., Federici, M. G., Saigo, P. E., Robson, M. E., Offit, K., and Boyd, J. (2000). Absence of premalignant histologic, molecular, or cell biologic alterations in prophylactic oophorectomy specimens from BRCA1 heterozygotes. *Cancer* 89, 383–390.
8. Stratton, J. F, Buckley, C. H., Lowe, D., and Ponder, B. A. (1999). Comparison of prophylactic oophorectomy specimens from carriers and noncarriers of a BRCA1 or BRCA2 gene mutation. United Kingdom Coordinating Committee on Cancer Research (UKCCCR) Familial Ovarian Cancer Study Group. *J. Natl. Cancer Inst.* 91, 626–628.
9. Werness, B. A., Parvatiyar, P., Ramus, S. J. *et al.* (2000). Ovarian carcinoma in situ with germline BRCA1 mutation and loss of heterozygosity at BRCA1 and TP53. *J. Natl. Cancer Inst.* 92, 1088–1091.
10. Pothuri, B., Leitao, M., Barakat, R. *et al.* (2001). Genetic Analysis of Ovarian Carcinoma Histogenesis. *Proc. Soc. Gynecol. Oncol.* Nashville, TN, 43.
11. Gusberg, S. B., and Deligdisch, L. (1984). Ovarian dysplasia. A study of identical twins. *Cancer* 54, 1–4.
12. Jacobs, I., and Bast, R. C., Jr. (1989). The CA 125 tumour-associated antigen: A review of the literature. *Hum. Reprod.* 4, 1–12.
13. Jacobs, I. J., Skates, S. J., MacDonald, N. *et al.* (1999). Screening for ovarian cancer: A pilot randomised controlled trial. *Lancet* 353, 1207–1210.
14. Einhorn, N., Sjovall, K., Knapp, R. C. *et al.* (1992). Prospective evaluation of serum CA 125 levels for early detection of ovarian cancer. *Obstet. Gynecol.* 80, 14–18.
15. Claus, E. B., Schildkraut, J. M., Thompson, W. D., and Risch, N. J. (1996). The genetic attributable risk of breast and ovarian cancer. *Cancer* 77, 2318–2324.
16. Kerlikowske, K., Brown, J. S., and Grady, D. G. (1992). Should women with familial ovarian cancer undergo prophylactic oophorectomy? *Obstet. Gynecol.* 80, 700–707.
17. Struewing, J. P., Hartge, P, Wacholder, S. *et al.* (1997). The risk of cancer associated with specific mutations of BRCA1 and BRCA2 among Ashkenazi Jews. *N. Engl. J. Med.* 336, 1401–1408.
18. Frank, T. S., Manley, S. A., Olopade, O. I. *et al.* (1998). Sequence analysis of BRCA1 and BRCA2: Correlation of mutations with family history and ovarian cancer risk. *J. Clin. Oncol.* 16, 2417–2425.
19. Statement of the American Society of Clinical Oncology (1996). Genetic testing for cancer susceptibility, adopted on February 20, 1996. *J. Clin. Oncol.* 14, 1730–1736; discussion 1737–1740.
20. Bast, R. C., Feeney, M, Lazarus, H., Nadler, L. M., Colvin, R. B., and Knapp, R. C. (1981). Reactivity of a monoclonal antibody with human ovarian carcinoma. *J. Clin. Invest.* 68, 1331–1337.
21. Bast, R. C., Klug, T. L., St. John, E. *et al.* (1983). A radioimmunoassay using a monoclonal antibody to monitor the course of epithelial ovarian cancer. *N. Engl. J. Med.* 309, 883–887.
22. Canney, P. A., Moore, M., Wilkinson, P. M., and James, R. D. (1984). Ovarian cancer antigen CA125: A prospective clinical assessment of its role as a tumour marker. *Br. J. Cancer* 50, 765–769.
23. Woolas, R. P., Xu, F. J., Jacobs, I. J. *et al.* (1993). Elevation of multiple serum markers in patients with stage I ovarian cancer. *J. Natl. Cancer Inst.* 85, 1748–1751.
24. Bast, R. C., Boyer, C. M., Xu, F. J. *et al.* (1995). Molecular approaches to prevention and detection of epithelial ovarian cancer. *J. Cell Biochem. Suppl.* 23, 219–222.
25. Berek, J. S., and Bast, R. C. (1995). Ovarian cancer screening. The use of serial complementary tumor markers to improve sensitivity and specificity for early detection. *Cancer* 76, 2092–2096.
26. Woolas, R. P., Conaway, M. R., Xu, F. *et al.* (1995). Combinations of multiple serum markers are superior to individual assays for discriminating malignant from benign pelvic masses. *Gynecol. Oncol.* 59, 111–116.
27. Jacobs, I. J., Rivera, H., Oram, D. H., and Bast, R. C. (1993). Differential diagnosis of ovarian cancer with tumour markers CA 125, CA 15-3 and TAG 72.3. *Br. J. Obstet. Gynaecol.* 100, 1120–1124.
28. Crump, C., McIntosh, M. W., Urban, N., Anderson, G., and Karlan, B. Y. (2000). Ovarian cancer tumor marker behavior in asymptomatic healthy women: Implications for screening. *Cancer Epidemiol. Biomarkers Prevent.* 9, 1107–1111.
29. Jeyarajah, A. R., Ind, T. E., Skates, S, Oram, D. H., and Jacobs, I. J. (1999). Serum CA125 elevation and risk of clinical detection of cancer in asymptomatic postmenopausal women. *Cancer* 85, 2068–2072.
30. Skates, S. J., Xu, F. J., Yu, Y. H. *et al.* (1995). Toward an optimal algorithm for ovarian cancer screening with longitudinal tumor markers. *Cancer* 76, 2004–2010.
30a. Petricoin, E. F., Ardekani, A. M., Hitt, B. A. *et al.* (2002). Use of proleomic patterns in serum to identify ovarian cancer. *Lancet* 359, 572–577.
31. Bourne, T. H., Campbell, S., Reynolds, K. M. *et al.* (1993). Screening for early familial ovarian cancer with transvaginal ultrasonography and colour blood flow imaging. *BMJ* 306, 1025–1029.
32. van Nagell, J. R., DePriest, P. D., Gallion, H. H., and Pavlik, E. J. (1993). Ovarian cancer screening. *Cancer* 71, 1523–1528.
33. Fishman, D. A., and Cohen, L. S. (2000). Is transvaginal ultrasound effective for screening asymptomatic women for the detection of early-stage epithelial ovarian carcinoma? *Gynecol. Oncol.* 77, 347–349.
34. DePriest, P. D., Shenson, D., Fried, A. *et al.* (1993). A morphology index based on sonographic findings in ovarian cancer. *Gynecol. Oncol.* 51, 7–11.
35. Lerner, J. P., Timor-Tritsch, I. E., Federman, A., and Abramovich, G. (1994). Transvaginal ultrasonographic characterization of ovarian masses with an improved, weighted scoring system. *Am. J. Obstet. Gynecol.* 170, 81–85.
36. Bohm-Velez, M., Mendelson, E., Bree, R. *et al.* (2000). Ovarian cancer screening. American College of Radiology. ACR Appropriateness Criteria. *Radiology* 215 Suppl, 861–871.
37. Runowicz, C. D., and Fields, A. L. (1999). Screening for gynecologic malignancies: A continuing responsibility. *Surg. Oncol. Clin. N. Am.* 8, 703–723, vii.
38. Bourne, T. H., Whitehead, M. I., Campbell, S., Royston, P., Bhan, V., and Collins, W. P. (1991). Ultrasound screening for familial ovarian cancer. *Gynecol. Oncol.* 43, 92–97.
39. Menon, U., Talaat, A., Rosenthal, A. N. *et al.* (2000). Performance of ultrasound as a second line test to serum CA125 in ovarian cancer screening. *BJOG* 107, 165–169.
40. Folkman, J., Watson, K., Ingber, D., and Hanahan, D. (1989). Induction of angiogenesis during the transition from hyperplasia to neoplasia. *Nature* 339, 58–61.
41. Karlan, B. Y. (1997). The status of ultrasound and color Doppler imaging for the early detection of ovarian carcinoma. *Cancer Invest.* 15, 265–269.
42. Karlan, B. Y., and Platt, L. D. (1995). Ovarian cancer screening. The role of ultrasound in early detection. *Cancer* 76, 2011–2015.
43. Karlan, B. Y., Raffel, L. J., Crvenkovic, G. *et al.* (1993). A multidisciplinary approach to the early detection of ovarian carcinoma: Rationale, protocol design, and early results. *Am. J. Obstet. Gynecol.* 169, 494–501.
44. Karlan, B. Y., and Platt, L. D. (1994). The current status of ultrasound and color Doppler imaging in screening for ovarian cancer. *Gynecol. Oncol.* 55, S28–33.
45. Pavlik, E. J., Johnson, T. L., 2nd, Depriest, P. D., Andrykowski, M. A., Kryscio, R. J., and van Nagell, J. R., Jr. (2000). Continuing participation supports ultrasound screening for ovarian cancer. *Ultrasound Obstet. Gynecol.* 15, 354–364.

46. Jacobs, I. (1994). Genetic, biochemical, and multimodal approaches to screening for ovarian cancer. *Gynecol. Oncol.* 55, S22–S27.
47. Jacobs, I. J., Skates, S., Davies, A. P. *et al.* (1996). Risk of diagnosis of ovarian cancer after raised serum CA 125 concentration: A prospective cohort study. *BMJ* 313, 1355–1358.
48. Menon, U., and Jacobs, I. J. (2000). Recent developments in ovarian cancer screening. *Curr. Opin. Obstet. Gynecol.* 12, 39–42.
49. Menon, U., and Jacobs, I. J. (2001). Ovarian cancer screening in the general population. *Curr. Opin. Obstet. Gynecol.* 13, 61–64.
50. Brewer, M. A., Mitchell, M. F., and Bast, R. C. (1999). Prevention of ovarian cancer. *In Vivo* 13, 99–106.
51. Kramer, B. S., Gohagan, J., Prorok, P. C., and Smart, C. (1993). A National Cancer Institute sponsored screening trial for prostatic, lung, colorectal, and ovarian cancers. *Cancer* 71, 589–593.
52. Sato, S., Yokoyama, Y., Sakamoto, T., Futagami, M., and Saito, Y. (2000). Usefulness of mass screening for ovarian carcinoma using transvaginal ultrasonography. *Cancer* 89, 582–588.
53. van Nagell, J. R., Jr., and DePriest, P. D., Reedy, M. B. *et al.* (2000). The efficacy of transvaginal sonographic screening in asymptomatic women at risk for ovarian cancer. *Gynecol. Oncol.* 77, 350–356.
54. Morgante, G., la Marca, A., Ditto, A., and De Leo, V. (1999). Comparison of two malignancy risk indices based on serum CA125, ultrasound score and menopausal status in the diagnosis of ovarian masses. *Br. J. Obstet. Gynaecol.* 106, 524–527.
55. DePriest, P. D., Gallion, H. H., Pavlik, E. J., Kryscio, R. J., and van Nagell, J. R. (1997). Transvaginal sonography as a screening method for the detection of early ovarian cancer. *Gynecol. Oncol.* 65, 408–414.
56. Creasman, W. T., and DiSaia, P. J. (1991). Screening in ovarian cancer. *Am. J. Obstet. Gynecol.* 165, 7–10.
57. NIH Consensus Conference. (1995). Ovarian cancer. Screening, treatment, and follow–up. NIH Consensus Development Panel on Ovarian Cancer. *JAMA* 273, 491–497.
58. Burke, W., Daly, M., Garber, J. *et al.* (1997). Recommendations for follow-up care of individuals with an inherited predisposition to cancer. II. BRCA1 and BRCA2. Cancer Genetics Studies Consortium. *JAMA* 277, 997–1003.
59. Vasen, H. F., Haites, N. E., Evans, D. G. *et al.* (1998). Current policies for surveillance and management in women at risk of breast and ovarian cancer: A survey among 16 European family cancer clinics. European Familial Breast Cancer Collaborative Group. *Eur. J. Cancer* 34, 1922–1926.
60. ACOG Practice Bulletin. Prophylactic Oophorectomy. Number 7, September 1999. Clinical management guidelines for obstetrician-gynecologists. American College of Obstetricians and Gynecologists. *Int. J. Gynaecol. Obstet.* 67, 193–199.
61. Sightler, S. E., Boike, G. M., Estape, R. E., and Averette, H. E. (1991). Ovarian cancer in women with prior hysterectomy: A 14-year experience at the University of Miami. *Obstet. Gynecol.* 78, 681–684.
62. Struewing, J. P., Watson, P., Easton, D. F., Ponder, B. A., Lynch, H. T., and Tucker, M. A. (1995). Prophylactic oophorectomy in inherited breast/ovarian cancer families. *J. Natl. Cancer Inst. Monogr.* 33–35.
63. Rebbeck, T. R., Lynch, H. T., Neuhausen, S. L. *et al.* (2002). Prophylactic oophorectomy in carriers of BRCA1 or BRCA2 mutations. *N. Engl. J. Med.* 346, 1616–1622.
64. Rebbeck, T. R., and Webber, B. L. (2002). Correspondence. *N. Engl. J. Med.* 347, 1039–1040.
65. Lu, K. H., Garber, J. E., Cramer, D. W. *et al.* (2000). Occult ovarian tumors in women with BRCA1 or BRCA2 mutations undergoing prophylactic oophorectomy. *J. Clin. Oncol.* 18, 2728–2732.
66. Hankinson, S. E., Hunter, D. J., Colditz, G. A. *et al.* (1993). Tubal ligation, hysterectomy, and risk of ovarian cancer. A prospective study. *JAMA* 270, 2813–2818.
67. Rubin, S. C. (1998). Chemoprevention of hereditary ovarian cancer. *N. Engl. J. Med.* 339, 469–471.
68. The reduction in risk of ovarian cancer associated with oral-contraceptive use. The Cancer and Steroid Hormone Study of the Centers for Disease Control and the National Institute of Child Health and Human Development. (1987). *N. Engl. J. Med.* 316, 650–655.
69. Narod, S. A., Risch, H., Moslehi, R. *et al.* (1998). Oral contraceptives and the risk of hereditary ovarian cancer. Hereditary Ovarian Cancer Clinical Study Group. *N. Engl. J. Med.* 339, 424–428.
70. Gross, T. P., and Schlesselman, J. J. (1994). The estimated effect of oral contraceptive use on the cumulative risk of epithelial ovarian cancer. *Obstet. Gynecol.* 83, 419–424.
71. Rosenblatt, K. A., Thomas, D. B., and Noonan, E. A. (1992). High-dose and low-dose combined oral contraceptives: Protection against epithelial ovarian cancer and the length of the protective effect. The WHO Collaborative Study of Neoplasia and Steroid Contraceptives. *Eur. J. Cancer* 28A, 1872–1876.
72. Schildkraut, J. M., Bastos, E., and Berchuck, A. (1997). Relationship between lifetime ovulatory cycles and overexpression of mutant p53 in epithelial ovarian cancer. *J. Natl. Cancer Inst.* 89, 932–938.
73 Rodriguez, G. C., Walmer, D. K., Cline, M. *et al.* (1998). Effect of progestin on the ovarian epithelium of macaques: Cancer prevention through apoptosis? *J. Soc. Gynecol. Invest.* 5, 271–276.
74. Zhang, D., Holmes, W. F., Wu, S., Soprano, D. R., and Soprano, K. J. (2000). Retinoids and ovarian cancer. *J. Cell Physiol.* 185, 1–20.
75. Pergolizzi, R., Appierto, V., Crosti, M. *et al.* (1999). Role of retinoic acid receptor overexpression in sensitivity to fenretinide and tumorigenicity of human ovarian carcinoma cells. *Int. J. Cancer* 81, 829–834.
76. Spencer, C. C. (2000). Effects of retinoids on ovarian cancer cells. *Obstet. Gynecol.* 95, S5.
77. Kurie, J. M., Lee, J. S., Griffin, T. *et al.* (1996). Phase I trial of 9-cis retinoic acid in adults with solid tumors. *Clin. Cancer Res.* 2, 287–293.
78. De Palo, G., Veronesi, U., Camerini, T. *et al.* (1995). Can fenretinide protect women against ovarian cancer? *J. Natl. Cancer Inst.* 87, 146–147.
79. Tavani, A., Gallus, S., La Vecchia, C., Conti, E., Montella, M., and Franceschi, S. (2000). Aspirin and ovarian cancer: An Italian case-control study. *Ann. Oncol.* 11, 1171–1173.
80. Akmedkhanov, A., Toniolo, P., Zeleniuch-Jacquotte, A., Kato, I., Koenig, K., and Shore, R. (2001). Aspirin and risk of epithelial ovarian cancer. *Proc. Soc. Gynecol. Oncol.* Nashville, TN, 68.
81. Cramer, D. W., Harlow, B. L., Titus-Ernstoff, L., Bohlke, K., Welch, W. R., and Greenberg, E. R. (1998). Over-the-counter analgesics and risk of ovarian cancer. *Lancet* 351, 104–107.
82. Easton, D. F., Ford, D., and Bishop, D. T. (1995). Breast and ovarian cancer incidence in BRCA1-mutation carriers. Breast Cancer Linkage Consortium. *Am. J. Hum. Genet.* 56, 265–271.
83 Easton, D. F., Steele, L., Fields, P. *et al.* (1997). Cancer risks in two large breast cancer families linked to BRCA2 on chromosome 13q12-13. *Am. J. Hum. Genet.* 61, 120–128.
84. Ford, D., Easton, D. F., Stratton, M. *et al.* (1998). Genetic heterogeneity and penetrance analysis of the BRCA1 and BRCA2 genes in breast cancer families. The Breast Cancer Linkage Consortium. *Am. J. Hum. Genet.* 62, 676–689.
85. Moslehi, R., Chu, W., Karlan, B. *et al.* (2000). BRCA1 and BRCA2 mutation analysis of 208 Ashkenazi Jewish women with ovarian cancer. *Am. J. Hum. Genet.* 66, 1259–1272.
86. Xu, Y., Shen, Z., Wiper, D. W. *et al.* (1998). Lysophosphatidic acid as a potential biomarker for ovarian and other gynecologic cancers. *JAMA* 280, 719–723.
87. Schutter, E. M., Visser, J. J., van Kamp, G. J. *et al.* (1992). The utility of lipid-associated sialic acid (LASA or LSA) as a serum marker for malignancy. A review of the literature. *Tumour Biol.* 13, 121–132.
88. Patsner, B., Mann, W. J., Vissicchio, M., and Loesch, M. (1988). Comparison of serum CA-125 and lipid-associated sialic acid (LASA-P)

in monitoring patients with invasive ovarian adenocarcinoma. *Gynecol. Oncol.* 30, 98–103.

89. Petru, E., Sevin, B. U., Averette, H. E., Koechli, O. R., Perras, J. P., and Hilsenbeck, S. (1990). Comparison of three tumor markers—CA-125, lipid-associated sialic acid (LSA), and NB/70K—in monitoring ovarian cancer. *Gynecol. Oncol.* 38, 181–186.
90. Xu, F. J., Yu, Y. H., Li, B. Y. *et al.* (1991). Development of two new monoclonal antibodies reactive to a surface antigen present on human ovarian epithelial cancer cells. *Cancer Res.* 51, 4012–4019.
91. Ramakrishnan, S., Xu, F. J., Brandt, S. J., Niedel, J. E., Bast, R. C., and Brown, E. L. (1989). Constitutive production of macrophage colony-stimulating factor by human ovarian and breast cancer cell lines. *J. Clin. Invest.* 83, 921–926.
92. Xu, F. J., Ramakrishnan, S., Daly, L. *et al.* (1991). Increased serum levels of macrophage colony-stimulating factor in ovarian cancer. *Am. J. Obstet. Gynecol.* 165, 1356–1362.
93. Tamakoshi, K., Kikkawa, F., Shibata, K. *et al.* (1996). Clinical value of CA125, CA19-9, CEA, CA72-4, and TPA in borderline ovarian tumor. *Gynecol. Oncol.* 62, 67–72.
94. Tzonou, A., Polychronopoulou, A., Hsieh, C. C., Rebelakos, A., and Karakatsani, A., and Trichopoulos, D. (1993). Hair dyes, analgesics, tranquilizers and perineal talc application as risk factors for ovarian cancer. *Int. J. Cancer* 55, 408–410.
95. Rosenberg, L., Palmer, J. R., Rao, R. S. *et al.* (2000). A case-control study of analgesic use and ovarian cancer. *Cancer Epidemiol. Biomarkers Prevent.* 9, 933–937.

CHAPTER

19

Clues to Tumors: New Concepts of Symptoms, Signs, Syndromes, Paraneoplastic Syndromes, and Predisposition to Ovarian Cancer

ALBERT ALTCHEK

Department of Obstetrics, Gynecology and Reproductive Science
The Mount Sinai School of Medicine and Hospital
New York, New York 10128

ABSTRACT

There are no early symptoms and/or no unique symptoms of ovarian tumors except possibly those which are hormonally active or sudden, new symptoms. There is a possible new paraneoplastic syndrome for early diagnosis of the common "dyspepsia."

Physical examination for ovarian epithelial cancer is unreliable, especially early. Transvaginal ultrasound and serum tumor markers (CA125) are helpful but not completely reliable.

It is often unappreciated that the recognition of a syndrome may alert the physician to the increased chance of a tumor. For those with high risk, prophylactic surgery is an option after childbearing.

An even more important potentially overlooked diagnostic opportunity is the recognition of a paraneoplastic syndrome which may appear early in (or even infrequently before) tumor formation. Although considered to be rare, it maybe more common than expected and subclinical cases possibly might be detected by serum tests.

Although hereditary genetic ovarian cancer is associated with autosomal dominant, highly penetrant gene mutations of BRCA1 and BRCA2 as well as with certain paraneoplastic syndromes, there may be a larger number of hereditary ovarian cancer cases associated with combinations of less penetrant recessive gene mutations, which are difficult to identify by pedigree.

I. INTRODUCTION

The goal of early diagnosis of ovarian cancer is to improve the cure rate since there is about a 90% cure rate in early cases. However, there are unknown biologic factors suggesting that perhaps early-stage diagnosed tumors are less virulent, slower growing, more responsive to chemotherapy, and more resectable.

Nevertheless, continuous efforts are made to improve our clinical skills which determine the entrance of the patient to the medical care system.

About 70–85% of ovarian cancer derives from the surface epithelium and is referred to as "common epithelial tumors."

About 75–85% of epithelial cancer is diagnosed in an advanced stage of spread (stage III or IV). Despite surgical resection (debulking, cytoreduction, reducing tumor burden) and platinum combination chemotherapy with subsequent no sign of tumor, there is a high recurrence rate close 50%. Thus, the 5-year cure rate remains relatively low, perhaps about 40%, and the 10-year cure rate even lower. Early diagnosis has not been achieved in the majority of cases.

II. SYMPTOMS—IS "DYSPEPSIA" A PARANEOPLASTIC SYNDROME?

Early symptoms are vague and nonspecific. Normal humans often have similar symptoms. On the other hand, sometimes when symptoms are first present the tumor is already widespread. The symptoms appear often after the ovary is already enlarged, when there is abdominal or pelvic pain or discomfort due to pressure, when there is abdominal distention, and nonspecific gastrointestinal symptoms. There may also be urinary frequency, dysuria, and vaginal bleeding. The most frequent symptoms of epithelial ovarian cancer are abdominal swelling, pain, dyspepsia, urinary frequency, and weight change.[1]

Despite this discouraging outlook, there is continuing hope for improving symptom recognition. "It is time, however, to change the generally accepted notion that there are no early symptoms of ovarian cancer. Symptoms often include vague abdominal discomfort, dyspepsia, and other mild digestive disturbances, which may be present for several months before the diagnosis." Women between 40 and 70 years of age with "...persistent gastrointestinal symptoms that cannot be diagnosed" are suspect.[1, Chap. 11, p. 297]

Barber established a triad index of suspicion for ovarian epithelial cancer: over age 40, history of ovarian dysfunction and infertility, and vague abdominal discomfort and mild digestive symptoms which persist (dyspepsia, flatulence, and distention after eating).[2]

A recent study by a novel in-person interview with a structured questionnaire by trained interviewers rather than the usual retrospective record review found that 92% of 166 women with invasive ovarian tumors had 4 months of symptoms prior to discovery.[3] The symptoms were 71% pelvic discomfort, 47% bowel irregularity, 37% urinary frequency and/or urgency, and 53% with other symptoms. Each "other" symptom was "reported by less than 10%," and included bowel pain, menstrual irregularities, vaginal bleeding or discharge, weight change, dyspareunia, fatigue, respiratory difficulties, back pain, anorexia, leg pain or swelling, lump or mass, night sweats or hot flashes, and fever. "The relatively short median duration of symptoms among women with invasive (mostly late-stage) cancers suggests that the disease progresses rapidly."[3] Another possibility is rapid increase after the development of asymptomatic advanced disease.

The median number of months from the first consultation to diagnosis of invasive cancer was one month, with 75% diagnosed within 3 months. Women who were young, non-white and with lower household income took a longer time to diagnose. "Symptom duration (onset to diagnosis) reflects patient, physician, and system-related delays in diagnosis."[3] A separate control group (unpublished data) found 14% with pelvic discomfort, 13% with bowel irregularity, and 18% with urinary frequency. These symptoms are often found in the normal population.[3]

Unfortunately, as attractive as the concept of symptom recognition pattern is, it does not work. Normal women often have nonspecific, suggestive symptoms while 8% of invasive cancer cases are asymptomatic. To immediately investigate all women of the general population with nonspecific symptoms would not be feasible because of the high incidence of false-positive symptoms, especially with apprehensive women and those with problems known to cause symptoms such as irritable bowel syndrome and cholecystitis and lack of cost effectiveness.

Although borderline and invasive cases had similar symptoms, the former had no symptoms in 16% (versus 8%), had longer prediagnostic symptom duration of 6 months (versus 4 months), and 28% were diagnosed by routine examination (versus 16%). Invasive cases were diagnosed because of symptoms in 62% whereas, versus 48% of borderline cases.[3]

A smaller study found that the majority (78%) of women with early-stage ovarian cancer have nonspecific symptoms including abdominal or pelvic pain, bloatedness, and vaginal bleeding. These symptoms were also present in 68% of women with borderline ovarian tumors. The time from onset of symptoms to diagnosis was 3–4 months for invasive cases and 8 months for borderline tumor.[4]

The above symptom analysis applies to the general public with a low incidence of ovarian cancer. In high risk cases, women are alerted to report symptoms promptly. There should be increased concern in women over age 40, nulliparous, who did not take oral contraceptives, who had ovarian dysfunction, infertility, and who have syndromes or paraneoplastic syndromes or family histories related to ovarian tumors.

Long duration of symptoms before diagnosis (13-month patient delay, 1- to 6-month physician delay) had a worse prognosis compared to women with a short delay (2–4 and 0 months).[5]

In a retrospective review from the Mayo Clinic Gastroenterology Research Unit, of 12 patients with paraneoplastic gastrointestinal (GI) motor dysfunction with malignant tumors there were nine with small cell lung carcinoma, one with anaplastic lung adenocarcinoma, one with retroperitoneal lymphoma, and one with ovarian papillary serous adenocarcinoma who also had cerebellar degeneration, another paraneoplastic syndrome. Six of the patients were women.[6]

Even though there was only one ovarian cancer, it is not unreasonable to consider that this new paraneoplastic syndrome may be extremely significant.

This overlooked report might be the breakthrough in explaining the common "dyspepsia" symptom of early ovarian epithelial cancer before tumor enlargement or ascites. If so, it opens the possibility of early diagnosis based on the usual earliest but vague symptom of "dyspepsia"—in fact a previously unrecognized paraneoplastic gastrointestinal motor dysfunction syndrome due to autoantibodies.

The symptoms of paraneoplastic GI motor dysfunction included weight loss, nausea and vomiting, pain, dysphagia, constipation, and acute distention. (These symptoms are the same as the vague symptoms several months before the diagnosis of ovarian cancer.) The symptoms were relatively acute in onset, and progressed rapidly in this group mainly of aggressive lung cancer. The findings included delayed gastric emptying, esophageal dysmotility, and abnormal autonomic reflex tests. The ovarian cancer patients had type 1 Purkinje cell cytoplasmic antibody (PCA-1 or anti-Yo) (the only case and in high titer) and N-type calcium channel antibodies.[6]

The authors recommended a panel of serological tests for paraneoplastic autoantibodies, scintigraphic gastric emptying, and esophageal manometry for screening tests. "Seropositivity for ANNA-1, PCA-1, or N-type calcium channel-binding antibodies should prompt further evaluation for an underlying malignancy even when routine imaging studies are negative."[6, p. 373]

III. SIGNS

The patient with advanced ovarian cancer present for a certain time may be detected from afar because of fatigue, cachexia, distended abdomen, and spindly extremities.

At the other extreme is stage III (advanced) cancer without signs (or symptoms) despite examination by experienced gynecologists.

To make the situation worse, nongynecologists are usually not trained in and often do not do routine clinical pelvic examinations. Most ovarian cancer is sporadic without high risk background (90%), and routine screening of the general population by transvaginal ultrasound and serum CA125 is not done. Nevertheless, it is the clinical visit which is the entrance to the medical care system. Unfortunately, medical students are only given minimal instruction in physical examination. It requires an empty bladder and bowel and a relaxed patient. Pelvic examination begins with abdominal examination.

Usually signs and symptoms are related to the peritoneal cavity.

Most cases of epithelial cancer are discovered with advanced cancer in stage III. About 40–75% have a palpable abdominal mass and about 20–30% have clinical ascites. However, even with symptomatic ovarian cancer there may be a negative pelvic examination. Abdominal distention may be due to ascites or a large tumor. Ascites gives a fluid wave, shifting dullness, umbilical hernia enlargement, and bowel tympany in the anterior midline in the supine position. There may be umbilical lymph node involvement (Sister Mary Joseph's node). A large ovarian cyst may give a fluid wave (especially if mucinous), no shifting dullness or umbilical enlargement, and bowel tympany laterally. Upper abdominal omental metastases ("omental cake") may have a solid irregular feel. There may also be a partial bowel obstruction or ileus. There may be a pleural effusion if ascites is present.

Pelvic examination includes bimanual palpation with the vaginal fingers as sensing structures while the abdominal hand gently presses downward. Following this bimanual rectovaginal examination is done and the stool is tested for occult blood.

A frequent error is considering an ovarian tumor to be a uterine fibroid. With the latter, abdominal pressing is transmitted directly to the rigidly attached cervix, while pressing on ovarian tumors usually does not move the cervix.

Benign ovarian tumors tend to be mobile, smooth, cystic, unilateral, and under 10 cm. There may be a huge, unilateral, benign mucinous cystadenoma. Malignant tumors tend to be solid, fixed, irregular, nodular, of shoddy consistency with soft rubbery areas, bilateral, large, and with cul-de-sac nodularity (like a "handful of knuckles").[2] The earliest sign usually in the asymptomatic woman with localized tumor found by routine pelvic examination is an ovarian mass,[2] however, most are not carcinoma.

Infrequent signs include inguinal and supraclavicular adenopathy, pleural effusion, skin and lung metastases.

There may be an ovarian metastatic enlarged axillary node with the histology of adenocarcinoma, and misdiagnosed as consistent with primary breast cancer. Immunohistochemistry may be helpful.[7] Following later recurrent epithelial ovarian cancer, there may be unusual metastatic presentations including bleeding intramural gastric metastasis, central nervous system, and bone.

Less common clinical signs relate to functional (hormone-producing) neoplasms which may secrete mainly estrogen, androgen, and progesterone, alone or in combination. This may result in primary or secondary amenorrhea, masculinization, precocious puberty, menometrorrhagia, and postmenopausal bleeding. The endometrium may show hyperplasia or decidual change.

Ovarian carcinoma may be secondary from gastrointestinal or pancreatic primary cancers. Multilocularity with ultrasound or magnetic resonance favors primary rather than secondary ovarian malignancy, however, it is difficult to accurately distinguish between them. Neither a solid appearance nor bilaterality is significant.[8]

Colorectal cancer may simulate ovarian cancer because of proximity, adhesions, and constitutional symptoms.

A. Malignant Germ Cell Tumors

Although malignant germ cell tumors (MGCTs) make up less than 5% of all ovarian neoplasms and are therefore rare, when they do occur it is usually in adolescents and young women. The age range is from 6–46 with a median range of 16–20. About 15–20% of dysgerminomas are found during pregnancy or postpartum.[9] Whereas epithelial malignancies are relatively slow in growth and tend not to cause acute symptoms, germ cell malignancies grow relatively rapidly and are associated with relatively acute or subacute symptoms. With tumor hemorrhage, necrosis, stretching, torsion, and rupture there may be sudden abdominal pain, nausea, bladder and rectal pressure, abdominal distention, and abnormal vaginal bleeding.

"One of the classic initial signs of a dysgerminoma is hematoperitoneum from rupture of the capsule of the lesion as it rapidly enlarges."[1, p. 352, Chap. 12] It may be confused with pregnancy complications or acute appendicitis. The usual symptom is abdominal pain present in 87%, of which 10% have acute pain. About 35% have abdominal distention, 10% have fever, and 10% have vaginal bleeding. Isosexual precocious puberty due to human chorionic gonadotropin (hCG) secretion occurs rarely. There may be elevated serum tumor markers.

A palpable mass is present 85% of the time. A large tumor may rise out of the pelvis and present as an abdominal mass. The size varies from 7–40 cm with a median size of 16 cm. Although dysgerminomas may be bilateral in 10–15%, other MGCTs are almost never bilateral. About 30% have ascites. Rupture occurs in 20%. For 5–10% of the cases of MGCTs, there may be an associated benign mature cystic teratoma and sometimes with gonadal dysgenesis and gonadoblastoma. MGCTs might metastasize more to nodes, liver, or lung more than epithelial cell tumors. About 60–70% are found in stage I and 25–30% in stage III.[9–10] In the prepubertal child, the ovaries are abdominal rather than pelvic in location.

If feasible, before surgery for an ovarian neoplasm in premenarchal girls, because of the high incidence of germ cell tumors, consider[10]:

1. Quantitative serum tumor markers of alpha-fetoprotein (AFP), hCG, lactic dehydrogenase (LDH), and CA125, as well as a stored frozen serum sample for unexpected hormone associated neoplasms
2. Chest X-ray for pulmonary metastases.
3. Blood karyotype to rule out a tumor developing from a dysgenetic gonad
4. Computed tomography (CT) scan or magnetic resonance imaging (MRI) for retroperitoneal lymphadenopathy, hepatic metastases, and tumor

B. Other Signs

In premenarchal girls an adnexal mass of 2 cm is viewed with suspicion, and a solid 2-cm mass associated with symptoms usually requires surgery.[10] With recent extensive use of ultrasound, physiological simple unilocular asymptomatic cysts of the ovary in premenarchal girls are found to be not unusual and generally spontaneously disappear. They may be associated with a transient spurt of precocious puberty.

Sudden severe abdominopelvic pain may be due to a biologic accident such as torsion of an ovarian mass and/or fallopian tube. The child/adolescent is at increased risk because of a long pedicle from the infundibulopelvic ligament. Such torsion can occur even from a benign hemorraghic corpus luteum or dermoid cyst. Prompt diagnosis and surgical detorsion may salvage the ovary. This might require resection of the cyst to reduce the ovarian size and attaching the ovarian ligament to the back of the uterus to prevent repeat torsion. Another acute surgical problem is spontaneous rupture of a malignant ovarian tumor with bleeding.

For the young adult postmenarchal woman, a simple asymptomatic ovarian cyst up to 8 cm in diameter with negative tumor markers, may be observed with a repeat transvaginal ultrasound in 6–8 weeks or may be given a 2-month trial of hormonal (oral contraceptive) suppression for two cycles. With decreasing tumor size, the patient may be continued to be observed. This may occur with a hemorrhagic corpus luteum cyst which may show a high-volume, low-pressure flow erroneously suggestive of malignancy with color Doppler flow study. Such physiological angiogenesis means that such a study is best done in the proliferative phase. Ectopic pregnancy or endometrioma may also give a false-positive study. If after two cycles, there is an increase or persistence in size, surgery is considered. If the cyst is over 8 cm or is solid, has a suspicious ultrasound appearance, is symptomatic, or has positive tumor markers, then prompt surgery is advised.

With ovulation induction in fertility cases, there may be an ovarian hyperstimulation syndrome with huge tender ovaries and ascites. This usually responds with time and support.

A recent concern is the question of persistent ovulation induction inducing carcinoma. This is complicated by the fact that with carcinoma or a predisposition to it, there is reduced fertility and with hereditary ovarian carcinoma each generation tends to have an earlier onset of carcinoma. Reported cases have neglected pedigree history. A reasonable number of ovulation induction cycles is still standard practice.

In former years, it was thought that the postmenopausal ovary was always small, quiescent, and nonpalpable. The palpable firm ovary of the size of a menstruating ovary in a postmenopausal woman might be a sign of early cancer, but it is usually benign.

In recent years, it has been found that about 14% of normal asymptomatic postmenopausal women have small, unilocular ovarian cysts, many of which spontaneously disappear or recur after a few months. These cysts have not been reported generally in the pathology literature. Many are not palpable. Most are benign. More study is required to determine whether and how many are neoplastic versus physiologic.

Surgery for a postmenopausal cyst is considered if the cyst is suspicious on ultrasound, the cyst enlarges progressively, there is pain, there is an elevated serum CA125, or if the cyst is over 5 cm in diameter.

The discovery of, or suspicion of, a pelvic and/or abdominal mass requires an ultrasound (sonogram). The traditional abdominopelvic sonogram is appropriate for abdominal masses and for the upper pole of a large mass rising out of the true pelvis. The transvaginal ultrasound gives better definition of ovarian masses but has a relatively short range. Many use morphology indices based on gross anatomical structures to separate benign and malignant ovarian masses. Color flow with Doppler waveform analysis is based on the concept that because of an angiogenesis factor in a malignant ovarian tumor, its blood vessels are thin-walled, dilated, irregular, endothelial-lined structures with a high flow and little resistance. This is in contrast to the normal arteriole with a regular pattern and thick muscular wall with a slower flow and more resistance. Despite these theoretical considerations, preoperative ultrasound diagnosis, while helpful, is not always correct.

While ultrasound is the ideal imaging for intraperitoneal masses, the CT or MRI scan may be better for retroperitoneal nodes and masses. The general consensus is that annual screening of the general population for ovarian cancer by transvaginal ultrasound and serum tumor marker CA125 is not feasible because of the low incidence of the disease and the high cost of screening. However, when a tumor is discovered these are standard care for differential diagnosis.

About 8% of primary ovarian tumors are sex cord-stromal which includes granulosa cell, Sertoli cell, Leydig cell, and stromal fibroblasts. Most (about 87%) sex cord-stromal tumors are the thecoma-fibroma group which are benign. The most common malignant tumor of the group is granulosa (12% of the total) with 0.05% Sertoli-Leydig cell tumors. The adult granulosa cell tumor numbers 95% of all granulosa cell tumors and occurs with a peak age of 50–55, but may be seen at any age. They are the usual ovarian tumor that secretes estrogen causing endometrial hyperplasia and postmenopausal bleeding and in 5% cause endometrial cancer, and possible breast cancer. In the reproductive years there may be amenorrhea for months or years followed by irregular excessive bleeding. In the rare case of adult granulosa cell tumor in a child there is isosexual pseudoprecocious puberty. Occasionally there is progesterone or androgen secretion. There is usually an ovarian mass and 10% present with pain and hematoperitoneum due to rupture. Even if not palpable it can be imaged by ultrasound. About 85% are in stage I, unilateral, average diameter of 12 cm, with 10–15% having ruptured, and composed of solid, multicystic, all solid, or thin-walled with uni- or multiloculated cysts.[11]

Juvenile granulosa cell tumors (JGCTs) number about 5% of all granulosa cell tumors. JGCTs are found in prepubertal children usually with isosexual pseudoprecocity and occasionally also with enlargement of the clitoris. Almost all occur within the first three decades and when after puberty there may be abdominal pain, distention, menstrual irregularity, and amenorrhea. There is an association of JGCT with Ollier's disease (enchondromatosis) and Maffucci's syndrome (enchondromatosis and hemangiomatosis). In about 10% JGCT rupture during surgery. About 10% have ascites. JGCT is usually unilateral, ranging from 3–32 cm (average 12.5 cm) with a similar gross appearance as adult granulosa cell tumor. About 98% are confined to the pelvis. JGCT has a different histology than adult GCT.

Sertoli-Leydig cell tumors number less than 0.5% of all ovarian neoplasms and occur at an average age of 25 with 75% at age 30 or less. About one-third of cases have virilization with oligomenorrhea, amenorrhea, breast atrophy, loss of body contour, then masculinization with acne, hirsutism, temporal balding, deep voice, and enlargement of the clitoris. The difficult differential diagnosis is adrenal virilizing tumors. Infrequently, they may be estrogenic or associated with cervix sarcoma botryoides, thyroid adenomas, and rare familial occurrence (autosomal dominant).[11, p. 203]

In clinical practice there is a 6–7% chance that an ovarian cancer is metastatic, often intestinal, gastric, and mammary, and 70% are bilateral.[11, p. 335; 38]

IV. SYNDROMES

Syndromes have potential value: (1) remembering the syndrome facilitates recognition; (2) identifying those as increased risk for ovarian tumors; (3) the possibility of discovering overlapping or associated gene mutations with the predisposition to ovarian tumors; (4) the possibility of discovering metabolic pathways leading to tumors and of chemoprevention. "…it is likely to be worth the effort, because new information concerning tumorigenic mechanisms in man is likely to be uncovered."[12]

A. Residual Ovarian Syndrome

The residual ovarian syndrome consists of pelvic pain, pelvic mass, dyspareunia, and pressure symptoms following hysterectomy without removal of ovaries. There may be periovarian adhesions and dysfunction due to compromised blood flow. There is a 0.33–4.30% incidence of second operations for non-malignant conditions of retained ovaries, but it is probably 4–5% with lifetime followup.[13]

A 20-year study of 2561 hysterectomies not for malignancy with one or both ovaries left in resulted in a residual ovary syndrome of 2.85%. Of those who required re-exploration, 71.3% (52 cases) was due to chronic pelvic pain and an asymptomatic pelvic mass was the reason for 24.6%. Of all the explorations, by 5 years 46.6% had been done and within 10 years 75.4% had been done. Functional cysts were found in 50.7%, benign neoplasms in 42.6%, and ovarian carcinoma in 12.3%. The authors recommended routine oophorectomy in premenopausal women over 45 years of age with hysterectomy with individualization and patient participation in the decision.[14]

Of 8 women with chronic pelvic pain with residual ovarian syndrome, GnRH analog resolved the pain in 6 who later had permanent pain relief with re-operation. Thus, it might be a test of whether the chronic pelvic pain was due to the residual ovary syndrome. This would avoid potentially difficult surgery in those who would not be helped.[15]

An "acute" residual ovary syndrome developed in a 41-year-old woman who 11 weeks after hysterectomy and right salpingo-oophorectomy developed an abdominopelvic mass the size of a 24-week pregnancy. It was a huge cyst measuring $11.5 \times 11.0 \times 14.1$ cm with benign, thick-walled follicular cysts.[16]

To prevent one case of ovarian cancer in the general population, bilateral prophylactic oophorectomy would have to be done in 50 women at the time of hysterectomy in women aged 40–50.[13]

B. Ovarian Remnant Syndrome

The concept of residual ovarian syndrome has been expanded to include symptoms from incompletely removed ovaries which tends to happen with pelvic inflammatory disease and endometriosis, and is referred to as ovarian remnant syndrome. The ovarian remnant syndrome usually presents as a pelvic mass and chronic pain following a bilateral oophorectomy.[17]

A report of 19 cases of laporoscopic oophorectomy leaving ovarian remnants found the risk factors were improper tissue extraction or misapplication or improper use of pretied surgical loops, linear staples, or bipolor electrodessication on the infundibulopelvic ligament, especially with prior multiple pelvic surgeries, adhesions, or endometriosis.[18]

With prophylactic laparoscopic salpingo-oophorectomy to prevent ovarian cancer there is the possibility of incomplete removal of the ovary by transection close to the ovary to avoid the ureter as it goes through the base of the infundibulopelvic ligament containing the ovarian blood vessels. Since the patient has an hereditary ovarian cancer predisposition, the ovarian remnant can form an ovarian cancer.[19]

The ovarian remnant may develop a benign corpus luteum and follicular cyst which may mimic a malignancy.[20]

Both residual ovaries and ovarian remnants are recognized causes of pelvic pain and pelvic tenderness. Of 7 with residual ovaries and 10 with ovarian remnants, following re-operation, 6 of the first and 9 of the second group had relief of pain and pelvic tenderness and improved quality of life. Diagnosis and re-operation are "frequently difficult."[21]

A report of 10 cases of ovarian remnant syndrome reported a high incidence of ureteral and bowel injury in corrective surgery and one case of ovarian cancer.[22] Most series do not sufficiently emphasize the risks of re-exploration.

There was a case reported of ovarian remnant syndrome following bilateral salpingo-oophorectomy with recurrent ureteral obstruction after corrective surgery. It was managed successfully by GnRH analog treatment. Recurrence of residual ovarian tissue after corrective surgery was considered "common."[23]

C. Meigs' Syndrome

Meigs' syndrome is a benign solid ovarian tumor with the gross appearance of a fibroma with ascites and hydrothorax. Removal of the tumor promptly cures the ascites and hydrothorax. The histology would be a fibroma, thecoma, or granulosa cell tumor.[24] When other benign ovarian teratomas or cysts are present rather than a fibrous tumor it is called pseudo-Meigs' syndrome. Struma ovarii, an ovarian teratoma with predominant mature thyroid tissue, may also cause pseudo-Meigs' syndrome. One-third of cases may have ascites. Despite the histology, only about 5% have clinical hyperthyroidism.[25, 26] Psuedo-Meigs' syndrome has been found with bilateral polycystic ovarian cortical stromal hyperplasia [27] and uterine leiomyoma including broad ligament leiomyomas [28] and paraovarian fibroma [29] without ovarian tumor causing ascites and hydrothorax.[30]

There are several theories to explain the ascites including tumor lymphatic leakage possibly from slight torsion as well as mechanical peritoneal inflammation from the tumor. The pleural fluid is thought to originate from rapid passage through minute diaphragmatic openings and possibly via lymphatics.[26, 30]

There are markedly elevated levels of vasoactive factors in ascitic and pleuritic fluid (vascular endothelial and fibroblast growth factors and interleukin 6) which decrease with clinical improvement after removal of the ovarian tumors.[31]

Subsequent to Meigs' description, serum CA125 measurement was developed and has been found to be elevated in some cases of Meigs' and psuedo-Meigs' syndrome. Serum CA125 is a marker of benign, nonspecific peritoneal irritation [32] and not directly due to the ovarian fibroma.[26] Apparently this is in accordance with the peritoneum being a more efficient producer of CA125 than ovarian epithelial carcinoma. Elevated serum CA125 may be found including the classic ovarian fibromas,[33] and thecoma,[34] as well as with pseudo-Meigs' syndrome due to uterine leiomyoma,[35] with degenerating leiomyoma,[30, 36] and as a variety of benign "false-positives."[37] With benign conditions pleural and ascitic fluid have negative cytology and there are no peritoneal implants with CT scan.[38]

The exact chance of Meigs' syndrome having an elevated serum CA125 is unknown but may well be an integral part of the syndrome since it is associated with peritoneal irritation. Thus, the patient with Meigs' syndrome may mimic the patient with advanced ovarian epithelial cancer. The diagnostic dilemma is made more difficult since rarely pseudo-Meigs' syndrome may result from ovarian malignancies including malignant stroma ovarii, adenocarcinoma of the ovary and fallopian tube,[39] bilateral ovarian endometrioid carcinoma, seminoma (dysgerminoma) endodermal sinus tumor,[40] proliferative and malignant Brenner tumors of the ovary,[41, 42] and ovarian borderline mucinous tumor.[43] Psuedo-Meigs' syndrome may be caused by metastatic ovarian gastrointestinal origin tumors form the colon, rectum, or stomach.[44]

When benign leiomyoma is the cause, myomectomy is curative.[45] A case report described cure by resection of a benign ovarian fibrothecoma, and 30 years later it recurred with elevated CA125 and was again cured by resection of a peritoneal recurrence.[46] The differential diagnosis includes ovarian hyperstimulation syndrome due to exogeneous gonadotropin and genital tuberculosis with peritonitis.[47] In 1937, Joe Vincent Meigs, Professor of Gynecology at Harvard, described ovarian fibromas associated with ascites and hydrothorax [48] which were promptly cured by removal of the tumor.[49] The syndrome was named in his honor. A letter to the editor [50] cites a report [40] concerning a Bordeaux surgeon Demons, who in 1887, described cystic ovarian neoplasms with ascites and pleural effusion and indicates that in France the syndrome has the eponym Demons-Meigs.

D. Polycystic Ovary Syndrome

Polycystic ovarian syndrome (PCOS) is also called polycystic ovarian disease (PCOD), hyperandrogenic chronic anovulation syndrome, Stein-Leventhal syndrome, and sclerotic ovaries. It is characterized by (1) chronic anovulation; (2) hyperandrogenism (increased testosterone, free testosterone, androstenedione); (3) continuous elevation of serum LH, low serum FSH, increased LH/FSH ratio of 3:1 or greater; (4) polycystic ovaries on ultrasound (bilateral, slightly enlarged with many follicular cysts up to 1 cm size close to the surface "like a string of pearls"); and (5) occurrence only during menstrual life. Clinically there may be amenorrhea, oligomenorrhea, dysfunctional intensive uterine bleeding of adolescence, infertility, hirsutism, acne, acanthosis nigricans, and insulin resistance. The possible unappreciated long-term consequences include an increased chance of type 2 diabetes mellitus, elevated cholesterol, endometrial hyperplasia and carcinoma, and hypertension. PCOS may present in adolescence with heavy irregular bleeding and oligomenorrhea in young adulthood. About 20% of normal women have polycystic ovaries on ultrasound, while only about 60% of those with PCOS have polycystic ovaries. PCOS may be the most common female endocrinopathy affecting about 10%, and PCOS may wax and wane. Some believe that any cause of ovulation will result in PCOS. Others feel that PCOS is a primary ovarian syndrome, but that adrenal and pituitary disease has to be ruled out. About 5% of PCOS may be due to atypical congenital adrenal hyperplasia which can be ruled out by elevated serum 17-hydroxyprogesterone in the early proliferative phase and/or ACTH stimulation test. Another possible problem is a faulty anterior pituitary and/or hypothalamus which does not cycle. PCOS has been associated with a variety of syndromes which include familial impaired insulin receptor binding and insulin resistant diabetes. The ovarian hyperthecosis syndrome may be a variant of polycystic ovarian syndrome.[51]

About one-third of women in the United Kingdom have polycystic ovaries on ultrasound, defined as 10 or more follicles per ovary. However, only one-third are actually PCOS, defined as polycystic ovaries together with one or more of hirsutism, male-pattern baldness, acne, oligomenorrhea or amenorrhea, obesity or increased serum testosterone and/or luteinizing hormone. The frequently associated insulin resistance and abnormal serum lipids increase the risk of later diabetes mellitus.[52]

In obese adolescents with PCOS, glucose intolerance is associated with metabolic abnormalities which are precursors of type 2 diabetes and are present early in the course of PCOS. The absence of nocturnal blood pressure dipping may be a sign of later risk of cardiovascular disease.[53] The recent epidemic of adolescent obesity in the United States has caused the usual late adult-onset of type 2 diabetes mellitus to develop in the adolescent.

E. Metabolic Syndrome

Some believe that at this population level, PCOS is a distinct subgroup of a wider problem referred to as metabolic syndrome. The latter is defined if 3 of the 8 criteria are present: (1) first-degree relative with type 2 diabetes; (2) body mass index greater or equal to 30 kg/m^2; (3) waist/hip ratio greater or equal to 0.88; (4) blood pressure greater than or equal to 160/95; (5) fasting serum triglyceride level greater than or equal to 1.70 mmol/L; (6) high-density lipoprotein cholesterol value 1.20 mmol/L; (7) abnormal glucose metabolism; (8) fasting insulin value greater than or equal to 13.0 mU/L. Oligomenorrhea is more common in metabolic syndrome (46.2%) than in otherwise normal obese (25.4%) and lean (15.1%) women. Polycystic-like ovaries were found by vaginal ultrasonography with the same frequency in all (about 14%). "Surprisingly, few women with metabolic syndrome had symptoms suggestive of PCOS, in comparison with obese and lean women."[54]

HAIR-AN syndrome is a variety of the insulin-resistant subset of PCOS. It is often associated with PCOS and ovarian stromal hypoplasia. HAIR-AN syndrome consists of hyperandrogenism, insulin resistance, elevated insulin if there is adequate pancreatic beta-islet cell reserve, and acanthosis nigricans. The latter is an epiphenomenon. The hyperinsulinemia stimulates ovarian androgen secretion which in turn causes further insulin resistance and hyperinsulinemia. The severity of insulin resistance correlates with the severity of hyperandrogenism. The syndrome is overlooked because hyperandrogenic women are not screened for insulin resistance, or acanthosis nigricans. The association of insulin resistance and hyperandrogenism explains the hyperandrogenemia in obesity, acromegaly, lipoatrophic diabetes, leprechaunism, and Kahn types A and B insulin resistance.[51]

A possible mechanism for insulin resistance and hyperinsulinism is insulin receptor antibodies.[55]

Oral insulin-sensitizing agents and weight loss can reduce hyperinsulinemia and hyperandrogenism and increase fertility.

Rare nonobese, insulin-resistant acanthosis nigricans syndrome has X-linked dominant inheritance.[56]

There is a familial insulin-resistant diabetes associated with anathosis nigricans, polycystic ovaries, hypogonadism, pigmentary retinopathy, labyrinthine deafness, and mental retardation.[57]

Werner's syndrome may be associated with early-onset hyperandrogenism caused by ovarian hyperthecosis, acanthosis nigricans, and peripheral neuropathy.[58]

Berardinelli-Seip syndrome (congential generalized lipodystrophy) is an hereditary autosomal recessive generalized deficiency of adipose tissue, muscular hypertrophy, tall stature, acromegaly, encephalopathy, hyperpigmentation, acanthosis nigricans, generalized hypertrichosis, clitoris hypertrophy, polycystic ovaries, extreme insulin resistance due to insulin receptor defect, hyperlipemia, and nonketonic diabetes mellitus in second decade.[59]

Miescher syndrome (Bloch-Miescher syndrome, Mendenhall syndrome, Ralson-Mendenhall syndrome) is autosomal recessive, consists of insulin receptor defect, congential acanthosis nigricans (neck, axillary, inguinal, genital), hypertrichosis, failure to thrive, short stature, dysmorphism of the jaw and mouth, severe insulin-resistant diabetes mellitus due to impaired insulin binding and a characteristic appearance. It resembles congenital generalized lipodystrophy. There may be clitoromegaly, goiter, and nodular hyperplasia of the pineal body [59, p. 362, #177; 56, p. 396].

The *Mendenhall syndrome* of insulin resistance and pineal hyperplasia is autosomal recessive. There is clitoromegaly, hypertrichosis, and acanthosis nigricans.[56, p. 396]

F. Malignant Acanthosis Nigricans Syndrome

Acanthosis nigricans may also be found with ovarian carcinoma ("malignant acanthosis nigricans") typically "…in older women in association with a malignant tumor, usually an adenocarcinoma, which in most cases has metastasized by the time of its discovery. The cutaneous lesions may precede, coincide with, or follow the detection of the neoplasm."[11, p. 386]

G. Ovarian Hyperstimulation Syndrome

Ovarian hyperstimulation syndrome (OHSS) is a serious, iatrogenic, somewhat unpredictable complication of assisted reproduction. There is marked ovarian enlargement with luteinization, hemoconcentration, increased capillary permeability, ascites, hydrothorax, pericardial effusion, and in severe cases thromboembolic phenomena, respiratory distress, and renal failure. It might be associated with inflammatory cytokines and vascular endothelial growth factors. Management is supportive with correction of fluid imbalance and maintaining renal perfusion. Ultrasound and serum estradiol are guides to prevention.[60–63] Follicular fluid interleukin IL-6 concentrations at oocyte retrieval and serum IL concentrations at embryo transfer were higher in OHSS and may be an early predictor.[62]

Early OHSS is due to "excessive" preovulatory response to stimulation with higher serum estradiol (E2) levels and lower gonadotropin requirements. Early or late OHSS had more oocytes collected than those without OHSS. With late OHSS serum E2 and oocyte numbers could not predict risk, clinical pregnancies occurred in all cycles with late OHSS, and there were more multiple pregnancies, and late OHSS was more likely to be severe. Thus, late OHSS is only poorly related to preovulatory events.[64]

Most cases of thrombosis present in pregnancy are late complications of OHSS.[65] There may be thrombosis in the internal jugular vein,[65, 66] subclavian vein,[67] superior vena cava,[68] and ileofemoral deep vein.[69] There may also be abdominal compartment syndrome.[69]

OHSS risk is not prevented even with empty follicle syndrome (following salvage),[70] or even with the sole administration of a gonadotropin-releasing hormone agonist.[71]

The MR scans of OHSS show bilateral symmetric enlargement with multiple cystic changes giving a "wheel-spoke" appearance with internal hemorrhage in some cysts. The differential diagnosis is cystic neoplasm.[72] Severe OHSS occurred in 3 cases of 1000 oocyte donors.[73]

The stress of OHSS may cause a perforation of a preexisting duodenal ulcer.[74]

Aside from careful observation of serum E2 levels and ultrasound to prevent OHSS there have been several other approaches. Postponing human chorionic gonadotropin while continuing daily gonadotropin-releasing hormone agonist therapy ("coasting") prevented recurrent OHSS in women with PCOS.[75] High doses of intramuscular progesterone were effective in preventing OHSS in high-risk women.[76] Another approach is a single administration of gonadotropin-releasing hormone agonist to trigger ovulation while avoiding OHSS.[77]

H. Other Syndromes

Luteinized unruptured follicle syndrome (LUF) is the absence of oocyte expulsion from a primary follicle persisting more than 48 h after luteinizing hormone (LH) blood peak. The Doppler blood flow of perifollicular ovarian arteries shows a follicular phase of low diastolic velocities and high resistance.[78] The LUF syndrome is the explanation for failures of pregnancy with ovulation stimulation despite a rise in progesterone. Thus there may be "biochemical ovulation" without true ovulation. There may be two types of LUF syndrome: (1) the mature follicle; and (2) the premature luteinized follicle.

The *Resistant ovary syndrome* is amenorrhea, elevated gonadotropins, and ovarian failure, but with ovarian follicles present. It may be associated with autoimmune endocrinopathy and a benign thymoma.

Empty follicle syndrome (EFS) had been diagnosed originally by transvaginal ultrasound and had been thought to cause a high percent of infertility (43.4%) and recurrent miscarriage.[79] At present it is diagnosed by failure to retrieve oocytes during *in vitro* fertilization. It occurs only in 1.8%. The chance of EFS increases with age, being 24% in the 35–39 year age group and 57% for those over 40. Thus it is assumed that ovarian aging is a major factor in folliculogenesis.[80] A question was raised of the possibility of a borderline form of EFS.[80a]

Primary empty sella syndrome is a neuroanatomical-radiological entity with variable endocrine implications. There may be multiple endocrine abnormalities due to panhypopituitarism including lack of response to gonadotropin-releasing hormone and posterior pituitary deficiency (diabetes insipidus). It may result from trauma, tumor, or meningoencephalitis.

In *Bardet-Biedl syndrome* CT scanning shows empty sella associated with obesity and primary hypogonadism.[81]

McCune-Albright syndrome (Albright syndrome, Weil-Albright syndrome, osteitis fibrous dysplasia) refers to polyostatic fibrous dysplasia (especially long bones and pelvis), irregular, sharp, café au lait skin pigmentation (usually unilateral, over sacrum, buttocks, and upper spine), and an unusual type of precocious puberty with premature menarche first followed by premature breast and pubic hair development. It is due to a gonadotropin-independent autonomous estrogen-secreting ovarian cyst. The mechanism is a somatic mosaic-activating mutation in early embryogenesis of the gene encoding the α-subunit of the G protein which affects signal transduction of cyclic adenosive monophosphate (cAMP). This stimulates growth and function of gonads, adrenal cortex, pituitary, osteoblasts, and melanocytes.

There may also be hyperthyroidism, hyperparathyroidism, pituitary adenoma-secreting growth hormone, acromegaly, Cushing's syndrome, and hyperprolactinemia. The syndrome is sporadic and not transmitted.[59, #176, p. 360; 82] The endocrinologic abnormalities result from autonomous multi-endocrine hyperfunction rather than from pituitary stimulation.

In girls with polycystic ovaries and gonadotropin-independent isosexual precocious puberty without clinical or molecular features of McCune-Albright syndrome there were no germline activating mutations in exon 10 of the follicle stimulating hormone receptor (FSHR) gene somatic activation of the FSHR.[83]

A possible diagnostic tool for evaluating an ovarian cyst is percutaneous aspiration to detect McCune-Albright syndrome molecular Arg 201 His mutation of the Gs alpha gene.[84]

In differential diagnosis gonadotropin-independent precocious puberty has to be distinguished from ovarian JGCT.

The ovarian vein syndrome is a clinical concept of pain in the right lower quadrant or lumbar area or renal colic which is often first noticed in pregnancy and later recurs with menstruation and urinary tract infection. The theory is that it is due to a dilatation of the normally larger right ovarian vein, with a thickened wall and adherence to and pressure on the ureter with the external iliac artery. It has been reported on the left side due to compression of the ureter between the dilated vein and the psoas muscle.[85]

Pelvic congestion syndrome refers to pelvic pain and fullness made worse by prolonged standing, coitus, and in the premenstrual period in multiparous women. There are vulvar varices which communicate with the saphenous vein in the groin with thigh and buttock varices. The original diagnostic approach was ovarian venography showing reflux to the ovaries and thigh. The original surgical treatment was ligation by bilateral retroperitoneal incisions. The first use of laparoscopic transperitoneal ligation was in 1995.[86]

Recently transcatheter ovarian vein embolization has been used to treat symptomatic cases and/or women with extremity,[87] vulvar, or tubo-ovarian varicosities with ovarian and iliac vein coils or embolization.[88]

The existence of the syndrome has always been controversial since incompetent and dilated ovarian veins are frequently seen on CT scanning in asymptomatic parous women.[89] This has also been observed generally at surgery for other conditions.

Acute pelvic pain syndrome is a common emergency syndrome in women and is usually due to gynecologic problems such as ectopic pregnancy, miscarriage, and pelvic inflammatory disease. It may also be due to appendicitis, sigmoid diverticulitis, urinary tract infection, and renal colic.[90]

Munchausen's syndrome is a chronic factitious psychologic disorder of hospitalizations, self-inflicted injuries, and pretending illness, including operative placement of a Port-A-Cath and chemotherapy for "advanced ovarian cancer."[91]

Sotos syndrome (Cerebral Gigantism) "is a pleiotropic syndrome of multiple congenital anomalies, developmental delay, and overgrowth characterized by macrocephaly, prominent forehead, variable mental deficiency, hypotonia, hyperreflexia, prenatal onset of excessive size, large hands and feet, advanced bone age, downslanting palpebral fissures, a high hairline, a prominent jaw, a high narrow palate, generalized overgrowth, and psychomotor developmental delay."

"Sotos syndrome belongs to overgrowth syndromes, which have an increased risk of neoplasms, including Wilms tumor, adrenal carcinoma, gonadoblastoma, hepatoblastoma in Beckwith-Wiedemann syndrome, mesodermal hamartomas in Ruvalcaba-Myhre-Smith syndrome, neuroblastoma in Weaver syndrome, neurofibromas, astrocytomas, cutaneous angiomas, subcutaneous leiomyomas, carcinoid tumors, xanthogranulomas, acoustic neuromas in neurofibromatosis, subcutaneous hamartomas and fibroadenomas in Proteus syndrome, and cavernous hemangiomas in Klippel-Trenaunay-Weber syndrome." Neoplasms found with Sotos syndrome include: Wilms tumor, hepatocarcinoma, vaginal epidermoid carcinoma, osteochondroma, neuroectodermal tumor, giant cell granuloma of mandible, neuroblastoma, multiple hemangiomas, non-Hodgkin lymphoma, acute lymphocytic leukemia, small cell lung carcinoma, testicular yolk sac tumor, sacrococcygeal teratoma, mixed parotid tumor, and cardiac fibroma of the left ventricle. A 26-year-old woman with Sotos syndrome had a left 8-cm and a right 3-cm ovarian fibroma with extensive foci of calcification and occasional ossification. This is similar to young women with basal cell nevus syndrome. Since Sotos syndrome and bilateral calcified ovarian fibromas in young women are rare it "...suggests the effect of overgrowth in Sotos syndrome on ovarian tumorigenesis."[92]

There was one report of four successive generations with ovarian fibromas, diagnosed at an early age (as young as 3), sometimes bilateral multinodular or multiple and calcified. These were similar to ovarian fibromas of nevoid basal cell carcinoma syndrome (NBCS) but there were no other signs of NBCS.[11, p. 388; 93]

I. Nevoid Basel Carcinoma Syndrome

Nevoid Basal Cell Carcinoma syndrome (NBCS) (Basal Cell Nevus syndrome, Gorlin's syndrome) is an autosomal dominant inherited disorder with high penetrance but variable presentations which increase with age. They include multiple nevoid basal cell carcinomas, multiple jaw keratocysts, skeletal developmental defects (rib, vertebral, craniofacial), palmar and plantar skin pits, epidermal inclusion cysts, milia, ectopic calcification (falx cerebri diaphragma sellae), and a variety of extracutaneous neoplasms especially of the ovary, brain (meduloblastoma, meningioma), and fibroma of the heart.

About 75% of women with NBCS have ovarian fibromas, usually bilateral and multinodular or multifocal and calcified. They are usually found in young adults, adolescents, and even children and may recur after excision.[94] Rarely an ovarian fibrosarcoma may develop secondarily. Gestational hypertension may develop from renin secretion from the ovarian tumor. One case of NBCS had a bilateral sclerosing stromal tumor found during pregnancy.[11, p. 387, 388]

In the general population, ovarian fibromyomas cause 4% of ovarian neoplasms, develop at an average age of 48, are usually unilateral, not calcified, are single, and unusual under age 30.[11, p. 194]

In a population-based study from Manchester, England, the major complications of basal cell carcinomas and jaw cysts occurred in over 90% by age 40, but some even before age 10. Ovarian fibroma with calcification were found in 24%, ophthalmic abnormalities (squint, cataract) in 26%, and 5% with meduloblastoma, cleft palate, and cardiac fibroma.[95]

Despite the risk of recurrence in young women, the ovarian fibroma should be removed but the normal ovary should be preserved.[94]

A 37-year-old woman with NBCS with a unilateral ovarian fibroma was found to have an endometrial adenocarcinoma.[96]

The molecular defect is considered to be a mutation of the human homolog of *Drosophilia* patched gene (PTC) which permits easy identification of allelic loss in lesions.[97] The gene mutation is in chromosome 9 q23.1–q31 and acts as a tumor-suppressor gene.[98]

J. Other Syndromes

Proteus syndrome is a rare, sporadic complex disorder causing malformations, and postnatal overgrowth of multiple tissues in mosaic patterns involving hypertrophy of limbs, digits, connective tissue, and epidermal nevus and hyperostoses. There may be various hamartomas and benign and malignant tumors. "Bilateral ovarian cystadenomas are regarded as having diagnostic value in Proteus syndrome when occurring within the first two decades of life." Bilateral cystic paraovarian cystadenomas of the broad ligament were found in a 3-year-old-girl. The usual tumors are hemangiomas, lympangiomas, and lipomas.[99] A unilateral JGCT causing precocious puberty was found in a 7-month-old-girl.[100]

The *Townes syndrome* (Townes-Brocks syndrome) of anomalies of the ears, thumbs, anus, kidneys, and cystic ovaries is an autosomal dominant.[98]

The *Rudiger syndrome* of developmental failure of limbs and diaphragm with coarse facial features and autosomal recessive inheritance has ovarian cysts.[56]

Fraser and associated syndromes include autosomal recessive cryptophthalmos, fused eye lids, anomalies of the head, ears, and nose, and syndactyly.[101]

In females, 54% have genital anomalies including large clitoris, bicornuate uterus, vaginal atresia, rudimentary uterus, and cystic ovaries. About one-third have urinary tract anomalies including renal agenesis.[102]

Von Hippel-Lindau syndrome is a serious, autosomal dominant disease with varying expression of a tumor-suppressor gene of the short arm of chromosome 3 p25–26. The association of angiomatous retina (von Hippel disease) and angiomatous tumors of the cerebellum and central nervous system was recognized by Lindau in 1926 and over 500 cases have been reported. It may be underestimated because only half of those with the gene mutation have only one symptomatic lesion. There may also be diffuse hemangiomata as well as pheochromocytoma, polycythema, and ovarian papillary cystadenoma.[98, p. 511]

Weaver syndrome of macrosomia, accelerated skeleton maturation, camptodactyly, and unusual facies has been found to have cardiovascular anomalies and neoplasia with an ovarian endodermal sinus tumor reported.[103]

Sclerosing peritonitis syndrome may be associated with ovarian luteinized thecomas. There is fibrotic thickening of the peritoneum, especially of the omentum and small bowel with small bowel obstruction and ascites.[104–107] The reason for the sclerosing is unknown. There may be ascites, abdominal swelling, and pain with omental and peritoneal nodules. It has also been found with a benign cystic teratoma,[108] florid mesothelial hyperplasia, ovarian fibromatosis, and endometriosis.[109] It may present as an acute abdomen due to hemorrhagic necrosis secondary to infarction.[110] One paper reported a fatality from extensive sclerosing peritonitis associated with high mitotic activity of the ovarian luteinized thecoma implying peritoneal dissemination of an ovarian cancer as the mechanism of sclerosis.[111]

Lymphangioleiomyomatosis syndrome is a rare disorder of menstrual life with hamartomatous proliferation of smooth muscle around pulmonary airways, vessels, and lymphatics similar to the tuberous sclerosis complex. There may be extrapulmonary involvement of the uterus and ovaries which may improve with progestin therapy.[11, p. 389]

K. Peutz-Jeghers and Related Syndrome

Peutz-Jeghers syndrome (PJS) is a rare autosomal dominant inherited condition clinically diagnosed by perioral dark mucocutaneous melanin pigmentation (which may fade with age). There may also be persistent pigmentation of buccal mucosa, genital mucosa, hands and feet,[112] and bridge of the nose; and by diffuse gastrointestinal hamartomatous polyps.[11, p. 387; 113]

The pigmentation–hamartoma relationship was first recognized by Peutz in 1921 [114] with the definitive description published in 1949.[115] The eponym was established in 1954.[113]

Most polyps are in the upper jejunum. They have characteristic hyperplasia of the smooth muscle that extends into the superficial epithelial layer in a treelike fashion.[112] It usually presents with abdominal pain due to polyp intussusception or gastrointestinal blood loss causing anemia. The average age of females diagnosed with GI polyps is 26.

In children there may be rectal prolapse or extrusion of polyps even before perioral pigmentation develops.[116]

PJS is an unappreciated general cancer susceptibility syndrome with early-age onset.[113] Aside from colorectal, gastric, and small bowel malignancies there may be malignancies of the pancreas, breast, and gynecologic, as well as thyroid, multiple myeloma, skin, and gallbladder.[11, p. 387] There may also be bronchial adenomas, biliary hamartomas, and bile duct cysts.[113]

There is a "very high relative and absolute risk for gastrointestinal and nongastrointestinal cancers," with the cumulative risk for all cancer being 93% from age 15–64.[117] The relative risk (RR) for esophagus is 57, stomach 213, small intestine 520, colon 84, pancreas 132, lung 17.0, breast 15.2, uterus 16.0, and for ovary 27.[117] Another study found the RR for cancer in women with PJS was 18.5, and the risk for breast and gynecologic cancer was 20.3. This risk for men with PJS was 6.2.[118]

There is a diversity of individual family risk patterns of extraintestinal manifestation which may be suggested by detailed pedigree analysis [113] such as simultaneous bilateral ovarian sex cord tumor with annual tubules (SCTATs), adenoma malignum of the cervix, and bilateral ovarian mucinous tumors.[119, 120] Another variant is bilateral ovarian SCTATs with mucinous neoplasm and cervical mucinous neoplasm but apparently without these classic stigmata of PJS.[121]

The gynecologic neoplasms include ovary and adenoma malignum of the cervix. There has been confusion about ovarian tumors in PJS. The usual ovarian tumor of PJS found in one-third of cases at the average age of 27 is the SCTATs. SCTAT may have focal differentiation into Sertoli cell or GCTs. They are usually discovered by coincidence.[11, p. 387] Others maintain that "the lesion has been found in almost all female patients with PJS in whom the ovaries have been examined," usually in young adults.[113] When present in about two-thirds of cases SCTATs are bilateral, usually not visible grossly, but sometimes form small yellow nodules. They are multifocal with ovaries not or minimally enlarged to less than 3 cm.

Scully indicates that all PJS tumorlets are benign.[11, p. 223] Although there is general agreement about this, the apparent "...first documented example of bilateral, malignant SCTAT rising in a patient who had PJS..." was in 2000.[122] Occasionally, SCTATs are estrogenic with manifestation of isosexual precocity, menstrual irregularities, and hyperestrogenism due to local increase in aromatase which increases estrogen production.[113]

Of 74 women with SCTATs, 27 had PJS with benign, multifocal, bilateral, very small or microscopic and calcified tumors. Of these, 12 had hyperestrogenism (menstrual irregularity in 11 and postmenopausal bleeding in 1). Of the 27, 4 had cervical adenoma malignum from which 2 died.[123]

It is not generally appreciated that ovarian SCTATs in women without PJS are completely different than in women with PJS. These tumors are usually unilateral, large (forming palpable masses), solid and yellow, and are usually discovered at an average age of 34. About 40% have estrogenic manifestations and there may also be a progesterone effect. At least 20% are clinically malignant with late multiple local and distant node recurrences. Mullerian-inhibiting substance, progesterone, and inhibin may be useful serum markers.[11, p. 221] Of 47 women with SCTATs without PJS, the tumors were unilateral and large. There was hyperestrogenism in 25 (menstrual irregularity, postmenopausal bleeding, sexual precocity), 7 were malignant, and 4 were fatal.[123]

There is an increased risk for nonepithelial ovarian cancer with ovarian SCTATs tumors, ovarian dysgenesis, precocious puberty, and paraneoplastic symptoms.

With PJS but without ovarian SCTATs, there may occur ovarian Sertoli cell tumor discovered at average age of 30 which may be nonfunctional, estrogenic, or androgenic. [11, p. 387, 124, 125] There may also occur an ovarian sex cord-stromal tumor, unclassified, which can cause isosexual precocity.[11, p. 203, 206] Two rare variants of ovarian sex cord-stromal tumor causing sexual precocity in PJS were described.[126]

Subsequently with PJS, but without SCTATs, there may be an ovarian unilateral or bilateral, benign, borderline or malignant mucinous cystic tumor.[11, p. 387]

With PJS the fallopian tube may have mucinous metaplasia and mucinous benign and malignant tumors and these may be markers for multifocal mucinous metaplasia elsewhere.[127]

Adenoma malignum, a mucinous well-differentiated carcinoma (also know as minmal deviation adenocarcinoma; MDA), of the cervix is part of PJS and especially associated with mucinous ovarian tumors. "Because of the high degree of differentiation of the tumors at both sites in such cases it may be very difficult or impossible to determine whether the ovarian tumor is an independent primary tumor or a highly differentiated metastatic tumor of cervical origin."[11, p. 83]

Adenoma malignum usually presents at age 40 with bleeding and/or a mucoid watery discharge.[113] Despite the deceptively benign histology, it has a clinical malignant behavior.

There may be an independent association of mucinous adenocarcinoma of the cervix and large cystic unilateral or bilateral ovarian (benign mixed with malignant areas) mucinous neoplasms. The average age was 44. Among 16 cases with cervical and ovarian lesions, 10 had cervical adenoma malignum, but apparently only 2 had PJS. Most of the cervical tumors were deeply invasive.[128]

Cervical adenoma malignum on ultrasound shows a hyperechoic mass with multiple cysts, while a CT scan shows a low attenuated endocervical mass.[120]

A case of intra-abdominal paraovarian desmoplastic small cell tumor with peritoneal metastases was reported in a 23-year-old woman with PJS. It might be an association or fortuitous.[129]

Males with PJS in the first decade may have gynecomastia, rapid growth, advanced bone age, and small bilateral multinodular testacles. Upward of 20% of the latter may be malignant.[113] Testicular ultrasound is done periodically.

Women with PJS should be carefully observed. Aside from history and clinical examination there might be an annual blood count and periodic pelvic and pancreatic ultrasound (or CT), and serum CA19-9. Careful endocervical cytology and possible endocervical curettage are done, and perhaps additional four-quadrant microendocervical punch biopsies (personal series unpublished). "All children in a family with PJS should be properly investigated" for intestinal polyposis.[130]

In more than half of the cases with PJS, the SCTATs had histologic calcification of the tubules. Since it is "...occasionally extensive,"[11, p. 221] personal speculation is that it might be possible to visualize microcalcific spots analogous to mammography.

Sex cord-stromal tumors may be hormonally active (estrogenic and virilization). Ultrasound of a fibrous tumor suggests fibrothecoma, a large hemorrhage multicystic mass in a child with precocious puberty suggests JGCT, PJS, Ollier disease, and Maffucci syndrome.[131]

The main clinical problem with PJS is the multiple small bowel polyposes.[113] There should be surgical removal of symptomatic polyps, those over 1.5 cm or with suspicion of malignancy by laparotomy (with intraoperative enteroscopy of the small bowel) or enteroscopic polypectomy. Extensive small bowel removal should be avoided to avoid short bowel syndrome.[111, 132, 133]

In differential diagnosis, juvenile polyposis syndrome (JPS) is the most common hamartomatous syndrome, inherited as an autosomal dominant and associated with congenital birth defects including midgut malrotation as well as in genitourinary and cardiac systems. The polyps are in the rectosigmoid with a dense inflammatory response and pathognomonic cystic dilatation of epithelial line spaces.[112] The genetic mechanism is different from PJS.

In addition to PJS there are other autosomal dominant mucocutaneous lentginosis syndromes with multiple tumors (thyroid, breast, ovarian, testicular, etc.) and endocrine manifestations including Carney complex, Cowden disease, and Bannayan-Riley-Ruvalcaba-Zonana syndrome,[113] but they have different genetic loci.[134]

Most, but not all cases with PJS have a novel germline mutation in chromosome 19p13.3 (of gene LKB1 and also known as STK11) that uncodes a multifunctional serine threonine kinase epithelial tumor suppressor with an unexpected loss in kinase activity. Other cancer susceptibility syndromes have an increased kinase activity.[112, 113, 135]

PJS-related tumors have a distinct pathway of carcinogenesis in contrast to the colorectal adenocarcinoma sequence.[136]

Gastrointestinal hamartomatous polyps in PJS cases result from germline mutation inactivation of the LKB1 gene plus somatic mutation or loss of heterozygosity (LOH) of the unaffected allele, and additional mutations of the beta-catenin gene and p53 gene which change the polyps into adenomatous and carcinomatous lesions.[137] LKB1 associates with p53 to regulate specific p53-dependent apoptosis cell death. PJS polyps lack LKB1 staining and have reduced apoptotic cells.[138] LKB1 mutation requires phosphoylation to suppress cell growth.[139] Like BRCA1 and BRCA2, LKB1 mutations can cause ovarian tumors when inheritied as a germline mutation, but only rarely is it a somatic or acquired mutation.[140, 141]

In sporadic (non-PJS) cases of ovarian SCTATs and uterine cervix MDA there were no somatic mutations of region 19p13.3 gene STK11 although there was LOH. "...a yet-to-be defined tumor-suppressor gene in the 19p13.3 region may be the specific target of inactivation in these tumors.[141]

The second unidentified putative gene causing PJS might be on chromosome 19q13.4.[142]

Cowden's syndrome (multiple hamartoma syndrome) is a rare, autosomal dominant heritable syndrome of pink or brown warty facial papules (tricholemmomas) and of the oral mucous membrane, flat keratotic papules of the dorsal hands, palms, and soles, and gastrointestinal polyps. About 20% are associated with breast cancer and 8% with thyroid cancer and variable internal hamartomas, including ovarian cysts and tumors with menstrual irregularities.[143, 56, p. 134] Cowden's disease (CD) has germ-line mutations of the PTEN gene. (10q22–23) Ruvalcaba-Myhre-Smith syndrome may be a variant of Cowden's syndrome. [112, 56, p. 542]

Bannayan-Riley-Ruvalcaba syndrome (Ruvalcaba-Myhre syndrome, Riley-Smith syndrome, Bannayan syndrome) is a grouping of three previously described autosomal dominant syndromes which are variations of a theme of macrocephaly, hamartomatous ileal and colon polyps, mucocutaneous and genital lentiginosis, and multiple tumors. There may be cutaneous angiolipomas encapsulated or infiltrating, diabetes, acanthosis nigricans, hemangiomas, lymphangiomyomas, mental deficiency, and pseudopapilledema.[98, p. 528] There is a carnitine-deficient lipid storage skeletal muscle myopathy.

Carney complex (CNC) syndrome is an inherited familial autosomal dominant complex of spotty skin pigmentation, myxomas, and endocrine overactivity. It is a lentiginosis and multiple neoplasia syndrome. It may present to the endocrinologist because of Cushing's syndrome, acromegaly, and male precocious puberty.[12] There is a predisposition to colon polyps and carcinoma, and gastrointestinal, thyroid, and breast cancers.

Some features overlap with PJS with hamartoses and multiple endocrine neoplasias (MEN) with pigmented nodular adrenocortical disease, Gonadotropin hormone (GH) producing pituitary adenomas, testicular tumors, and thyroid lesions. Large cell calcifying Sertoli cell tumors of the testes occur frequently in males and occasionally in PJS.

Strangely, this tumor does not appear in the ovary in CNC.[144] CNC, PJS, CD, and Bannayan-Zonana syndrome (BZS) have similar features of mucocutaneous lentigines, multiple tumors (thyroid, breast, ovarian, and testicular), and autosomal dominance. Nevertheless, they have different genetic loci.[134]

Contrary to the traditional and expected viewpoint, women with CNC are not predisposed to the ovarian tumors associated with PJS. Nevertheless, women with CNC are predisposed to ovarian tumors and cysts and may be at risk for ovarian carcinoma. These tumors have copy number gain of chromosome 2p16 characteristic of CNC, suggesting molecular involvement of the CNC gene(s). "...although CNC and PJS have some clinical similaries, they do not share LOH of the STK11/LKB1 locus." Although ovarian tumors are not a major part of CNC, they are increased above the general population.

"...ovarian ultrasound may be part of the initial evaluation of patients with CNC; followup of any unidentified lesion is recommended, because of the possible risk for malignancy."[145]

Isolated mucocutaneous melanotic pigmentation syndrome (IMMP) is a recently described related PJS syndrome without intestinal polyposis. Of 26 cases reviewed at the Mayo Clinic, 10 developed malignancies, with an RR increase of breast and gynecologic cancers of 7.8. Additional malignancies were in the cervix, endometrium, kidney, lung, colon, and lymphatics. Of interest is that there were no LKB1 mutation found which is common with PJS. Thus, IMMP is another lentiginosis with cancer predisposition.[146]

L. Ollier's and Maffucci's Syndromes

Juvenile granulosa cell tumor (JGCT) and Sertoli-Leydig tumor of the ovary occur with Ollier's or Maffucci's syndromes in the first or second decades as part of a generalized mesodermal dysplasia.[147] JGCT can cause isosexual precocious puberty, and sometimes presents with acute symptoms due to hemorrhage and necrosis.[11, p. 180] For the usually unilateral stage I JGCT unilateral salpingo-oophorectomy "...is almost always curative."[11, p. 186] Recurrences, if they develop, usually appear within 3 years, unlike the adult

GCT with late recurrences.[11, p. 186] In a series of 125 ovarian JGCTs, the average age was 13, 44% were age 10 or younger, 34% were between 11 and 20, 18% were between 21 and 30, and only 3% were over 30. Almost 82% of prepubertal children presented with isosexual pseudoprecocity, whereas the older ones had abdominal pain or swelling, menstrual irregularities, or amenorrhea. Two each had Ollier's disease and Maffucci's syndrome. The JGCT was unilateral in 122 cases and stage I. With an average 5 years, follow up, 92% were free of disease, while 7 died within 3 years. One died later of chrondosarcoma.[148]

Bilateral JGCT may occur with other congenital syndromes or abnormalities such as Goldenhar's syndrome of craniofacial and skeletal abnormalities, and Potter's syndrome.[11, p. 388] Phenotypically normal females with unilateral JGCT may have bone or soft tissue tumors.[11, p. 388] Ovarian granulosa cell tumor has been associated with tamoxifen therapy and leprechaunism.

Ollier's syndrome or disease is a rare congenital but nonhereditary sporadic disorder of asymmetric, multiple sporadic enchondromas and association with enchonrosarcomas. There may be a rare ovarian fibroma or fibrosarcoma. There is also an association with ovarian JGCT [147] with isosexual precocious puberty in the first or second decade. Enchondrosarcomas usually occur after the second decade.[11, p. 388; 98, p. 519]

Maffucci's syndrome is enchondromal (like Ollier's syndrome) but with soft tissue hemangiomatosis. Ovarian JGCT may occur and there have been single cases with ovarian fibroma and fibrosarcoma.[11, p. 388]

Association of sertoli-leydig cell tumors (SLCTs) and thyroid adenomas, an unnamed syndrome, is a familial inherited autosomal dominant with a variable degree of expressivity. Occasionally there is an additional ovarian mucinous cystadenoma or cystadenocarcinoma. Even those under 30 with sporadic SLCTs have an increase in thyroid masses. The usual thyroid masses in familial and sporadic SLCTs are solitary or multiple adenomas or nodular goiter, but also there has been hyperthyroidism and carcinoma.[11, p. 388]

M. Ovarian Size Syndromes

Normal-sized ovary carcinoma syndrome (NOCS) "...is characterized by diffuse metastatic malignant disease of the abdominal cavity in females with normal-sized ovaries...."[149] A series of four cases from Japan indicated that the clinical stage of NOCS was higher than the non-NOCS which was attributed to intraperitoneal rapid spread of ovarian serous surface papillary adenocarcinoma.[149] A retrospective review of 11 cases indicated that 7 or 11 were extraovarian peritoneal serous papillary carcinoma, one was metastatic, and only two were primary ovarian serous adenocarcinoma.[150] (*Editorial comment*: NOCS is probably primary peritoneal carcinoma with ovarian carcinoma histology.)

The postmenopausal palpable ovary syndrome (PPOS) is the palpation of what is a normal sized ovary for the premenopausal woman, but is indicative of an enlargement in the postmenopausal woman. It refers to size and consistence. It does not refer to small cysts reported on ultrasound.[151] Of 20 women who had surgical exploration for PPOS, 13 (60%) had a malignant or borderline malignant ovarian neoplasm.[152] Current clinical management is conservation using transvaginal ultrasound, serum CA125, and possible laparoscopy to reduce unnecessary surgery since other series usually found no malignancies.(153) In clinical practice about 15% of normal women may have a small asymptomatic, thin-walled, unilocular cyst on transvaginal ultrasound which may persist or disappear, and may or may not occur. It is usually not palpable, apparently benign, and the general population patient it usually observed by repeated ultrasound. In high-risk cases for ovarian cancer, especially in postmenopause, there is concern for malignancy.

The *growing teratoma syndrome* is the maturation of malignant immature teratoma (or nonseminomatous GCT or its metastasis with normalization of tumor markers) of the ovary following partial surgical removal and chemotherapy.[154] Clinically, it presents as a tumor which continues to grow but it is histologically a mature teratoma without malignant cells. The differential diagnosis includes a mass due to tumor necrosis or tumor resistance to chemotherapy. It should be removed to confirm the diagnosis, to avoid pressure symptoms, and to avoid possible later malignant degeneration. However, even without chemotherapy, pure ovarian immature teratomas may mature. Most reported cases refer to males (testes) and mediastinal location.[155]

Tumor lysis syndrome develops after aggressive chemotherapy for rapidly growing ovarian cancer with increased levels of serum lactate dehydrogenase, uric acid, phosphate, and creatinine with a decrease of calcium. It is managed with hydration, bicarbonate, furosemide, and allopurinol.[156]

N. Pseudomyxoma Peritoni Syndrome

Pseudomyxoma peritoni syndrome is a clinical designation for large intraperitoneal masses of jelly-like mucus of the lower abdomen and considered to be stage II or III ovarian borderline tumor or carcinoma.[11, p. 99] It has been a surgical problem because of the inability to scoop out all the material and its recurrence. Examination of the abdomen reveals a pronounced fluid wave. Recently, there has been disagreement whether the jelly-like mucus originates from a primary (or secondary ovarian metastasis from the appendix) ovarian mucinous neoplasm or from a perforated appendiceal mucinous adenoma.

General surgeons consider it to be a syndrome. Whereas for men the most comment presentation was suspected acute appendicitis (27%), for women the diagnosis was usually made while being evaluated for an ovarian mass (39%).

This suggests an ovarian origin for women. Increasing abdominal girth presented in 23 and 14% had new-onset inguinal hernia.[157] Rarely pseudomyxoma peritonei may result from displaced malignant colonic epithelial cells from a recurrent enteric fistula, and intraperitoneal seeding of a mucinous urachal adenocarcinoma.[158]

O. Other Syndromes

Cancer anorexia-cachexia syndrome (CACS) is a common problem in advanced cancer and especially in ovarian cancer. "Cachexia is among the most diebilitating and life-threatening aspects of cancer." It is associated with anorexia and wasting of muscle tissue and fat, and arises from an interaction of tumor and host cytokine response. There is a weight loss of more than 5% within 6 months.[159] Weight loss reduces survival time. Cachexia is increased in the elderly and in children, and in more than 20% it is the main cause of death. With ovarian tumors there are special problems of gastrointestinal obstruction, malabsorption, surgery, chemotherapy, and depression. With simple starvation, there is an increase of appetite, decrease in metabolism, and relative sparing of lean body mass. With cachexia, the appetite is reduced, the metabolic rate is increased, and there is a wasting of lean body mass resulting in reduced tolerance to therapy and increase of surgical complications.[159] Sometimes correction of possible reversible factors may bring some relief such as anemia (with erythropoietin), dehydration, infection, pain, and depression. Megestrol acetate and glucocorticoids short term have been used.

Ataxia-telangiectasia syndrome (A-T); (Louis Bar syndrome) is an autosomal recessive of cerebellar ataxia, oculocutaneous telangiectasias, and immune deficiency. The latter results in sinopulmonary infections and malignant tumors, mainly leukemias and lymphomas. A variety of other malignancies occur including thyroid and pancreas. Ovarian malignancies include dysgerminoma, yolk sac (endodermal sinus) tumor, gonadoblastoma, and carcinoma.[11, p. 389] Ovarian hypoplasia and insulin resistance may also occur.[160] A-T and yolk sac tumor produce serum alpha-fetoprotein.[98, p. 196]

A recent finding that carriers of ATM mutations, the cause of A-T, are prevalent in hereditary breast and ovarian cancer (HBOC) suggests that the ATM gene mutations of itself have an HBOC risk comparable to the risk of BRCA1 or BRCA2 mutation.[161] This could be the explanation for the rare HBOC without BRCA1 or BRCA2 mutations.

Rendu-Osler-Weber syndrome (hereditary hemorrhagic telangiectasia, HHT) is an autosomal dominant inherited disorder of aberrant vascular development complicated by gastrointestinal bleeding and pulmonary and cerebral arteriovenous malformations. It is often overlooked because of a disparity of clinical presentations. A report from northern Japan was that there was a weak yet suggestive linkage to the HHT 1 locus encoding endoglin (ENG), a homodimeric integral membrane protein expressed mainly in vascular endothelial cells. More than 30 different mutations have been reported which lead to frameshifts. Importantly there is a relatively high mutation rate and "...most mutations have risen in recent generations." The prevalence is 1:8000 to about 1:5000.[162]

Is it possible that new variation mutations of HHT are developing?

A report suggested an association with polyarthritis [163] and ovarian cancer.[164]

Bloom syndrome, characterized by short stature, malar hypoplasia, and telangiectatic erythema of the face, may have mixed microcephaly, mild mental deficiency, high-pitched voice, absence of upper lateral incisors, prominent ears, digital abnormalities, café au lait spots, and noninsulin dependent diabetes. There is immunoglobulin deficiency with impaired lymphocytic proliferation response to mitogens, and *in vitro* increased chromosomal breakage. About 25% develop malignancies, usually leukemia and various solid tumors of various sites of origin and histologic types. The mean age of malignancy is 24.8 years (range 4–40).[98, p. 104]

Li-Fraumeni syndrome (LFS) results from dominant inherited germ-line p53 mutations associated with early-onset sarcomas of bone and soft tissues, carcinomas of the breast and adrenal cortex, brain tumors, and acute leukemias. Nevertheless p53 carriers are at increased risk of other cancers. Among 738 cancer cases 77% were common type while 23% included a wide range of neoplasms.

Previous analyses of the p53 binding domain were limited to exons 5–8. "Therefore, our data likely underestimate the mutation frequency outside this domain." There is a suggestion "...that carcinomas of the stomach, colon, rectum, pancreas, and ovary and lymphomas may represent uncommon manifestations of germ-line p53 mutations." Since somatic p53 mutations are found in almost all sporadic cancer, "...it is reasonable that germ-line p53 mutations would also predispose to a wide spectrum of tumors."[165]

The p53 mutations are associated with increased vascularity of ovarian cancers and may be a factor in promoting metastases. "Cancer-risk in mutation carriers has been estimated to be 75% in males and nearly 100% in females, the difference almost entirely explained by breast cancer."[166]

Torre-Muir syndrome (Muir-Torre Syndrome or paraneoplastic syndrome) is an inherited autosomal dominant condition of solitary or multiple skin sebaceous tumors in association with internal malignancy. The skin tumors may be sebaceous adenomas, epitheliomas, carcinomas, and keratoacanthomas. The internal malignancies may be gastrointestinal and genitourinary and include ovarian carcinomas. In about 40% of cases, the skin lesions appear before or with the internal cancers, and in almost half of the cases, the internal cancers are multiple.[11, p. 386; 160] Most humans with hereditary nonpolyposis colorectal cancer have a germline mutation in the DNA mismatch repair genes MSH2 or MLH1. In Torre-Muir syndrome most germline mutations are in MSH2. Contrary to what would be expected, only one of nine skin tumors exhibited an LOH at the MSH2 locus as a "second hit" microsatellite instability. Thus LOH is not the preferred mode of inactivation of the second MSH2 allele.[167] Eruptive keratoacanthomas without sebaceous tumors have been reported with ovarian carcinomas.[11, p. 386]

Sweet's syndrome is acute neutrophilic dermatosis with tender erythematous plaques with a characteristic biopsy, fever, and leukemia. It may occur with underlying occult cancer, especially leukemia but also with ovarian carcinoma and internal malignancy.[160; 11, p. 386]

Leser-Trelat sign syndrome or sign (or paraneoplastic syndrome) is the sudden onset and rapid enlargement of seborrheic keratosis in association with an occult cancer. It has been found months before discovery of ovarian adenocarcinoma. It is considered a variant of "malignant" acanthosis nigricans.[11, p. 386]

Malignant acanthosis nigricans is a velvety or verrucous hyperpigmented epidermal hyperplasia in flexura areas associated with malignancy. In 277 cases, gastric carcinoma occurred in 55.5%, other abdominal carcinoma 17.7%, and other site malignancy 26%.[168]

Trousseau's syndrome (or paraneoplastic syndrome) is migratory thrombophlebitis which is associated with chronic disseminated intravascular coagulation (DIC). The latter may be due to tissue factors on tumor cell surfaces which set off intrinsic and extrinsic pathways [169] (see Section V).

Whereas clinical manifestations of DIC with ovarian tumors are unusual, it may be that the majority of ovarian cancer cases show serum fibrin degradation products, suggesting subclinical DIC. This suggests the possibility of a screening test for malignancy.

The nephrotic syndrome with membranous glomerulopathy may be associated in 5–15% of all neoplasms, and rarely with ovarian carcinoma. It might be related to immune complexes of DIC, but sometimes precedes ovarian serous carcinoma.[160] Although previously it was not certain that there was an association with neoplasms, it is now considered a paraneoplastic phenomenon ovarian malignancy.

Blepharophimosis syndrome is a rare, autosomal dominant eye disorder associated with ovarian dysfunction and premature menopause. A case was reported of an associated bilateral GCT. The pathogenesis was hypothesized to be the long-term hypergonadotropism reacting to the oocyte depletion associated with the syndrome. "In female patients with blepharophimosis syndrome close gynecologic surveillance should be instituted."[170]

Clostridium septicum syndrome "is highly associated with the presence of a malignancy, either known or occult at the time infection occurs." Occult tumors are usually in the cecal area. Predisposing conditions include hematologic malignancies, colon carcinoma, neutropenia, diabetes mellitus, and bowel mucosal disruption. A case was reported of a necrotic ovarian carcinoma in the wall of the ceum which resulted in distant myonecrosis with gas gangrene.[171] Rarely fever of unknown origin is the presenting symptom of ovarian cancer.[11, p. 390; 172]

P. Possible Unnamed Syndromes

The autosomal dominant with variable expressivity hereditary association of ovarian *Sertoli-Leydig cell tumors* with *thyroid adenomas*, nodular goiter, Graves disease and carcinoma.[11, p. 388]

There is an unappreciated association of *Down syndrome (trisomy 21)* and *ovarian dysgerminoma*. There is a "...relative increase in germ cell neoplasms in female patients...." Although the increased frequency of seminoma in males has been recognized the counterpart is now being recognized in females.[173] "The occurrence of cancer in Down Syndrome is unique with a high risk of leukaemia in children and a decreased risk of solid tumors in all age groups. The distinct pattern of malignancies may provide clues in the search for leukaemogenic genes and tumour suppressor genes in chromosome 21."[174]

Bilateral uveal melanocytic lesions with loss of vision are associated with abdominal cancers, including ovarian, and might be listed as a syndrome.[11, p. 390] The pathology is diffuse proliferation of melanocytes, but 1 case of 3 was malignant. Thus it might be a syndrome, a paraneoplastic syndrome, or an association with uveal malignant melanoma.[160]

Cutaneous melanosis has been found with a stromal carcinoid tumor.(11, p. 386)

Melanosis peritonei is pigmentation of the ovary and peritoneum due to melanin laden histiocytes and is associated with dermoid cysts or microscopic gastric mucosal-lined cysts. It is benign but may be confused with disseminated malignant melanoma.[11, p. 277]

1. *Ovarian Non-Hodgkin Lymphoma* (of which 20% are Burkitt Lymphoma) and Human *Immunodeficiency Virus (HIV)*

With improved HIV therapy increasing survival rates there will be an increase in cases with ovarian involvement. Previously it was rare and usually present in children, especially with infection with Epstein-Barr virus. It should be considered in women with AIDS who have abdominal or pelvic symptoms from slightly englarged, friable, hemorrhagic ovaries. The common lymphoma locations are central nervous system, bone marrow, gastrointestinal tract, and mucocutaneous tissue.[175, 176]

2. *Suppressed Immune Syndrome* and *Neoplasia*

Immunosuppressive therapy used for organ transplantation increases the risk for epithelial ovarian cancer, as well as other malignancies. With increasing transplantation there will be a continuous increase. Such observations indicate that an intact immune system is a tumor-suppressor agent and that potential neoplasms are constantly developing.

Chronic tamoxifen therapy for breast cancer has been associated with endometrial hyperplasia and malignancy and stimulation of endometriosis.[177] A case report of papillary serous ovarian adenocarcinoma after 13 years of tamoxifen [178] may now be explained by the recent report of chronic use of estrogen hormone replacement therapy predisposing to ovarian cancer [179, 180] since tamoxifen is proestrogen regarding the genital tract but antiestrogen for the breast.[179]

V. PARANEOPLASTIC SYNDROMES

Paraneoplastic syndromes are often overlooked. Although considered rare, they may be more frequent than generally appreciated, and may be (or their antibody mechanism) a clue to early diagnosis of asymptomatic localized ovarian cancer.

A. Neurologic

"Ovarian cancer is one of the malignant tumors that is most often associated with paraneoplastic disorders of the nervous system," occurring in as many as 16%.[11, p. 383]

There is a strong association with only one disorder—subacute cerebellar degeneration (SCD). About one-third of cases of paraneoplastic SCD (PCD) are due to ovarian cancer, usually poorly differentiated serous epithelial adenocarcinomas. The rest are from the heart or lung adenocarcinomas.[160, 181]

In patients with subacute cerebellar degeneration and anti-Yo antibody without ovarian or breast cancer (the usual causes), the bladder should be investigated since bladder transitional cell carcinoma can also be the cause.[182]

The pathology is a severe loss of or severe inflammatory reaction of cerebellar Purkinje cells. The pathogenesis is circulating antibodies to the tumor antigen which also by coincidence attack the host's Purkinje cells.[11, p. 383]

The symptoms of PCD include unsteady gait ataxia; dysarthria; mystagmus; truncal, limb, and appendicular ataxia; dysphagia; vertigo; headache, and diplopia.[183] Treatment results of PCD generally are not good.[184]

"The cerebellar manifestation antedated, sometimes by several years, or coincided with the initial recognition of the cancer is over 75%...." They may also precede the diagnosis of recurrent cancer.[11, p. 385; 181, 183–185]

Paraneoplastic encephalitis with neuropsychiatric symptoms "...usually predate the diagnosis of cancer by 3 months to 6 years." It may be "...the first manifestation of a very small malignant ovarian tumor."[186]

Although imaging may be negative, there may be positive anti-Yo antibodies, positive CA125, and stage IIIC adenocarcinoma of the ovary.[181]

Autoantibody screening for paraneoplastic serum antibodies has been suggested for patients with SCD.[187]

This suggests that microscopic cancer or histologic cancer precursor or possibly even molecular precursor can provoke an antibody response.

PCD symptoms have appeared 7 months after treatment with no clinical evidence of disease, suggesting an impending recurrence.[185]

PCD degeneration develops when ovarian (or breast) tumors release an onconeural antigen, cdr 2 cystoplasmic protein, which is normally expressed in cerebellar Purkinje neurons. The immune response to cdr 2 causes an autoimmune cerebellar degeneration by blocking its interaction with c-Myc.[188]

These anti-Punkinje cell antibodies (anti-Yo) are present in the serum and cerebrospinal fluid.[181]

Circulating anti-Punkinje cell antibodies are present more frequently in ovarian cancer cases without PCD than with PCD.[189] Personal speculation is that it may be related to antibody specificity, resistance of normal Punkinje cells, antibody concentration, individual variation, and a robust immune system.

The clinical speculation implications are: (1) testing all women with ovarian cancer for serum anti-Purkinje antibodies (for investigation); (2) testing for serum anti-Purkinje antibodies in women at increased risk for ovarian cancer, for patient care and screening; and (3) stimulation of antibody production against cancer antigen (without causing SCD) as a dynamic test for early detection of ovarian cancer for research.

The presence of several antibodies in some cases suggests multimodal antibody production and mechanisms.[190] Antiamphiphysin antibodies which react with a 128-kd protein found in synaptic vesicles are not specific for one type of tumor or one neurological syndrome and can be associated with other neural and non-neural antibodies.[190]

Aside from serum autoimmune cdr2 antigen neuronal degeneration in PCD, there is evidence for a specific cellular immune response by MHC class I-restricted car2-specific cytotoxic T lympoctyes.[191]

Although paraneoplastic neurologic syndromes have been classified anatomically, they are now being classified by specific antibodies. Specific autoantibodies are highly predictive for a neoplasm for sensible and autonomic neuropathy, cerebellitis, limbic encephalitis, opsoclonus-myoclonus syndrome, Stiff-man syndrome, neuromyotonia, and subacute amaurosis. Pathogenic relevance of these antibodies has been demonstrated only against Lambert-Eaton myasthenic syndrome, neuromyotonia, and retinopathy.[192]

PCD may occur during paraneoplastic encephalomyelitis and may be associated with the opsoclonus-myoclonus syndrome and Lambert-Eaton syndrome.[193]

A teenage girl with small cell ovarian carcinoma after several months developed paraneoplastic limbic encephalitis.[194]

Paraneoplastic limbic encephalitis may have neuropsychiatric symptoms which usually predate the discovery of cancer by 3 months to 6 years, and very rarely symptoms develop after cancer diagnosis. A case was reported with the simultaneous discovery of stage Ia immature ovary teratoma and the development of acute neuropsychiatric symptoms.[186]

Paraneoplastic motor neuron disease with type 1 Purkinje cell antibodies (anti-Yo) was reported with ovarian carcinoma causing progressive weakness.[195] Ovarian duct cancer has been found causing anti-Ri opsoclonus-myoclonus ataxia.[196]

A reversible severe paraneoplastic encephalomyelitis in a 24-year-old woman was caused by a benign mature ovarian teratoma (dermoid cyst) presumably by an immune response directed against neural teratoma contents which cross-reacted with normal brain, brainstem, and spinal cord antigens.[197]

A reversible severe limbic encephalitis and brainstem encephalitis in a 19-year-old woman was caused by an immature ovarian teratoma with a neuronal component. There was no identifiable immunologic cross reaction and a cell- rather than a globulin-mediated immunity was suggested.[198]

Cerebral and extracerebral vessel occlusions have been the initial manifestations of ovarian and peritoneal epithelial low malignant potential (borderline) tumors. "In stroke of unknown etiology a paraneoplastic process should be kept in mind," especially with recurrent thromboembolism in different areas and with ineffective warfarin therapy.[199a]

A 24-year-old woman was reported with disseminated intravascular coagulation, menometrorrhagia, and galactorrhea was considered to have a paraneoplastic manifestation of a borderline ovarian fibromyxoma whose removal cured the symptoms.[199]

Upper motor neuron disease may be caused by type 1 Purkinje cell antibodies (anti-Yo antibody) in serum in high dilution.[(195]

An occult asymptomatic ovarian cancer presented with two paraneoplastic syndromes—nephrotic syndrome and later PCD. The former resolved with treatment.[185]

A rare case was reported of subacute PCD being followed later by cerebellar metastasis of ovarian origin.[200]

Four percent of hospitalized ovarian carcinoma cases require neurologic consultation, generally. Of 83 consultations 4 were paraneoplastic, while iatrogenic complications were the majority.[201] Neuropathy may be due to cisplatinum therapy as well as paraneoplasia.[202] Spinal cord metastasis is unusual in ovarian carcinoma.

Although central nervous system metastases from epithelial ovarian cancer in the past was 1%, recent reports indicate a rise to 5–12%. This increase might be the result of: (1) improved primary control with longer survival thereby permitting proliferation of metastases in distant sites; and (2) minimal passage of chemotherapy across blood-brain barrier. "...in patients with ovarian cancer who present with neurologic symptoms, the possibility of brain metastases should be considered even in those who had negative second-look surgeries."[203]

B. Dermatomyositis

Dermatomyositis is one of the idiopathic inflammatory myopathies. There is a typical heliotrope skin rash and symmetrical proximal muscle weakness. The frequency increases with age especially after 40. It is a systemic disorder. Although the skin and muscles are the usual involved areas, there may also be arthralgias, arthritis, esophageal disease, and cardiopulmonary dysfunction. There are myositis-specific antibodies suggesting that it is different from all other collagen-vascular diseases.[204]

There may be characteristic skin signs of heliotrope rash, Gottron's papules, periungual telangectasia and other cuticular changes, photodistributed erythema, or poikiloderma and a scaly alopecia.[205]

"The risk of ovarian as well as other types of cancer appears to be increased in patients with dermatomyositis or polymyositis."[11, p. 385] Most ovarian tumors were high-grade serous carcinoma. Dermatomyositis usually precedes the discovery of the tumor within 2 years. Dermatomyositis may be the presenting symptom of ovarian cancer. The signs usually regress after excision of the tumor but also return with tumor recurrence.[11, p. 385; 206]

Ovarian cancer is the leading malignancy found in women with dermatomyositis. Among 14 women with dermatomyositis, 4 subsequently developed ovarian cancer (and of these 2 had elevated serum CA125) 5 and 13 months before the diagnosis of cancer was made. None of the controls without evidence of ovarian cancer had elevated CA125. The sensitivity was 50% and specificity was 100%. "Serum CA125 screening for ovarian cancer in patients having dermatomyositis may be useful...," however, more studies are needed.[207, 208]

Polymyositis (PM) (proximal neuropathic muscle weakness) with systemic involvement is similar to acute dermatomyositis (DM) except for the absence of skin lesions. Perhaps mild or transient skin lesions may not have been recorded in retrospective reviews.

Dermatomyositis is "...strongly associated with malignant disease," particularly ovarian. The national cancer rates of Sweden, Denmark, and Finland identified 618 cases of dermatomyositis (both sexes) of whom 198 had cancer, and of these 115 developed cancer after the diagnosis of DM. Aside from ovarian, other cancers included lung, pancreatic, stomach, colorectal, and non-Hodgkin lymphoma. Of 914 cases of PM, 137 had cancer, of which in 95 cases the cancer followed the PM. There was an increased risk of non-Hodgkin lymphoma, lung, and bladder cancer. The overall risk or malignant disease was only modestly increased with PM.[209]

A Mayo Clinic report found 10 cases treated of DM and PM associated with gynecologic cancer. All but two had typical skin changes of acute DM. In all cases the DM/PM preceded the cancer in from 3 months to 6 years, usually within 2 years. There were 5 ovarian, 3 cervical, 1 endometrial, and 1 vaginal cancers. The ages ranged from 40–46 (mean 53). In most cases the symptoms of DM-PM regressed markedly after treatment of the carcinoma but recurred with tumor recurrence.[210]

A report from Baylor Hospital in Texas found 25 women with DM-PM of whom 5 had a malignant tumor (3 ovarian carcinoma, 1 cervical intraepithelial carcinoma, and 1 colon carcinoma).[211]

An 11-year analysis of a medical center in Israel found 35 adult inpatients with DM/PM, 15 men and 20 women with a mean age at diagnosis of 53 ± 18. DM numbered 20 and PM were 15. There were 9 malignancies with DM (45%) and 4 with PM (27%), which is 12.6 times higher than in the general population. In 4 cases, malignancy appeared after the appearance or DM/PM, and in 6 it was simultaneous. In the mixed group (sex, DM, PM) there were a variety of malignancies aside from ovary. Eight died during the study period. "...DM/PM is associated with high rates of malignancy and mortality."[212]

A Mayo Clinic study described 14 women with DM and PM with an underlying ovarian malignancy. The mean age at diagnosis of DM and PM was 59. The 12 with DM had distinctive skin lesions. Thirteen had proximal muscle weakness confirmed by electromyographic testing and elevated creatine kinase. Five had dysphagia. DM and PM preceded ovarian cancer in 9, concomitant with it in 4 and followed it in 1. "Physical examination and imaging techniques failed to detect early ovarian cancer in our patients with dermatomyositis and polymyositis." Ovarian cancer was advanced when discovered and "...survival was poor."[213]

A report from Johns Hopkins indicated that 5 of 15 women with DM were subsequently diagnosed with metastatic ovarian papillary adenocarcinoma. "These diagnoses of advanced cancer were unexpected, as all women had undergone repeated cancer screenings beyond what is normally recommended for patients with DMM dermatomyositis."[207]

Initially all the cases of DM were misdiagnosed as photo-induced or contact dermatitis and had severe recalcitrant skin disease. It took 2–10 months to make the correct diagnosis of DMM. The ovarian cancer is usually diagnosed months or up to 6 years from the onset of DMM symptoms.[208]

A woman with DM had extensive searching for underlying malignancy unsuccessfully for 2-1/2 years. She then presented with pleural effusion and ascites due to primary papillary serous carcinoma (PPSC). After treatment, the muscle strength and enzymes remained normal but the skin manifestation persisted. Although less frequent than ovarian cancer, PPSC may occur in the female with DM. Like ovarian cancer intense surveillance failed early detection.[214]

Of 6 women with breast cancer who developed DM (before or after breast cancer) 2 developed a second primary ovarian cancer and 2 had recurrent breast cancer.[215]

Malignancy may occasionally occur in the young patient. A 16-year-old girl with DM had a dysgerminoma.[216]

All reports indicate: (1) an increase of ovarian cancer, "...especially in older women" with DM; (2) the apparent inability to detect early ovarian cancer by surveillance; and (3) the only clue is the presence of DM when it develops before (or presents at the same time as) the malignancy.

The significant increased incidence of ovarian epithelial high-grade cancer discovered in an advanced stage despite surveillance with poor prognosis creates concern regarding preventive management. It may be with greater identification of DM and with more information regarding the association with ovarian malignancy that in the future prophylactic salpingo-oophorectomy might be considered in select cases (personal opinion).

Rheumatoid-like polyarthritis and palmar fasciitis may present 1–25 months before a high-stage ovarian carcinoma. Rare associations with ovarian malignancies include hypertrophic pulmonary osteoarthropathy, rheumatoid or rheumatoid-like arthitis, scleroderma, and the shoulder-hand syndrome.[11, p. 385]

Occult advanced epithelial ovarian cancer can cause sudden severe digital ischemia and distal necrosis of all the fingers, and over 40 cases have been reported.[217, 218]

1. Multicentric Reticulohistiocytosis—A Possible Paraneoplastic Syndrome

Multicentric reticulohistiocytosis is a systemic disease with symmetric polyarthritis and papulonodular skin lesions. In a case reported characteristic biopsy lesions were present in cutaneous biopsy and synovial biopsy. Synovial fluid analysis is helpful for early diagnosis. This suggested an underlying tumor which was discovered to be an ovarian adenocarcinoma, "...especially when arthritis is the presenting symptom."[219]

Rendu-Osler disease has been associated with polyarthritis and ovarian cancer.[164]

Antiphospholipid antibody syndrome was present in a 41-year-old woman with widespread and worsening thromboembolism which did not respond to conventional anticoagulant treatment. Subsequently an ovarian endometrioid adenocarcinoma was discovered and when removed both the thromboembolism and antiphospholipid antibodies disappeared. The authors suggest that this may be a new paraneoplastic syndrome.[220]

C. Skin

"The skin markers of internal cancer are manifold. They include metastases to the skin, syndromes produced by humoral secretions from nonendrocrine tumors, a variety of proliferative and inflammatory dermatoses, and disorders indicative of a systemic or organ-related carcinogenic process."[221, p. 1]

Skin metastases may originate from the breast, stomach, lung, uterus, kidney, ovary, colon, and urinary bladder. There is usually a poor prognosis. In rare cases cutaneous metastases appeared several years before the primary carcinoma was discovered.[221, p. 1]

Cutaneous metastases from the ovary have a predisposition for the abdominal wall and periumbilical area. Breast cancer metastasizes to the anterior chest wall.[221, p. 2]

Clubbing of the fingers and toes may occur with primary ovarian cancer metastatic to the thorax.[221, p. 24]

Tripe palms refers to a form of keratoderma with exaggerated dermatoglyphics resulting in a rugose appearance. It appears to be part of a spectrum related to acanthosis nigricans associated with malignancy. A case was reported of tripe palms, acanthosis nigricans, and ovarian carcinoma. Excision of the carcinoma was followed by a complete regression of the cutaneous lesions.[222]

With Cowden disease the most common lesion is flesh-colored, flat-topped lichenoid papules ranging from less than 1–4 mm. These may be hyperkeratotic papules with central delling or umbilication on the soles and sides of the feet and on the palms and fingers.[221, p. 62]

Paraneoplastic urticaria [223] or leukocytoclastic vasculitis of palpable pruritic papules on all extremities may be the presenting signs of occult ovarian cancer.[224]

D. Hematologic

An unappreciated and overlooked high percent of women with ovarian (and other) malignancies have coagulation abnormalities which may be a clue to underlying malignancy. "The relationship between cancer and abnormalities of blood coagulation has been recognized for well over a century."[225]

The most common cause of thromboembolic disease (TE) is deep thrombosis of the lower extremities. Other events include pulmonary embolism (especially in the elderly), upper extremity vein thrombosis, and disseminated intravascular coagulation.

The underlying malignancies include ovarian, gastrointestinal, and pancreatic.[225]

Postoperative deep venous thrombosis with gynecologic malignancy was 37.9% (in contrast to the expected 10–15% in general gynecology) using fibrinogen tagged I-125 scanning. Twenty percent of the total group had isotopic evidence of bilateral venous thrombosis post-operatively. Thus, there is a need to investigate both limbs if thrombosis is suspected. Clinical diagnosis is inaccurate.[226]

A paraneoplastic superior vena cava thrombosis led to the discovery of an ovarian papillary carcinoma with pleural metastasis and effusion. With chemotherapy there was a "...disappearance" of the thrombosis.[227, 228]

"Paradoxical embolism should be considered in the differential diagnosis of ovarian cancer patients with embolic stroke and it may be appropriate to include a cardiac echo as part of the diagnostic evaluation." The mechanism was patent foramen ovale with femoral vein thrombosis occurring postoperatively.[229]

DIC probably occurs from tumor cell surface tissue factors which initiate intrinsic and extrinsic paths. Other putative mechanisms include increased serum viscosity, erythrocyte aggregation, fibrinogen, beta-thromboglobulin, and platelet factor 4.[11, p. 386]

Personal speculation is that a test for subclinical DIC might be added to other procedures for surveillance for ovarian (or other) malignancies.

Occasionally, ovarian tumors are associated with non-thrombocytopenic purpura, granulocytosis, thrombocytopenia, pancytopenia, systemic mastocytosis, and especially thrombocytosis.[11, p. 386]

Erythrocytosis occurs with androgenic ovarian tumors, and also by secretion of erythropoietin by some dermoid cysts and steroid cell tumor.[11, p. 385]

A Coombs-positive autoimmune hemolytic anemia may occur with ovarian dermoid cysts and occasionally carcinomas. Removal of the tumor gives a rapid remission perhaps because the tumor secretes an antibody to red blood cells.[11, p. 385]

E. Ocular

Bilateral diffuse uveal melanocytic proliferation with monocular cancer causing rapid blindness occurs with ovarian carcinoma, and new lesions develop with recurrence of the ovarian cancer. It mimics metastatic disease to the eye.[230] Five of 18 cases with this eye problem had ovarian carcinoma.[231]

The mechanism is a serum cancer-associated retinopathy antibody [232] such as retinal 45-kd protein.[233] "Patients with unexplained ophthalmologic symptoms may harbor an underlying gynecologic cancer."[232]

A literature review in 2001 of 18 cases of the paraneoplastic syndrome of bilateral diffuse melanocyrtic proliferation associated with extraocular cancers added 2 more cases from the Massachusetts Eye and Ear Infirmary. The average age at diagnosis was 63 years (34–89) including 13 women and 7 men. In half the cases the ocular symptoms antedated the tumors which were mainly poorly differentiated carcinomas. The most common in women were in the ovary and uterus, and in men the lung. The tumors expressed neuron-specific enolase. This report was "...the first to document a statistically significant association between this syndrome and gynecologic cancers." "...many general pathologists are not aware of this unique paraneoplastic syndrome."[234]

Another variety of unusual bilateral retinopathy and blindness as a paraneoplastic event is retinal pigmentary mottling with leaking and serous elevation in the posterior pole.[233]

VI. PARAENDOCRINE SYNDROMES

A. Hypercalcemia

Small cell carcinoma of the ovary is infrequent, however two-thirds of the cases have paraendrocrine hypercalcemia. The neoplasms are large, solid, aggressive, and occur in women of an average age of 24 (varies from 2–46).[11, p. 379] The young case was 14 months.[235] It is rarely familial. The hypercalcemia has been used to monitor therapy. Clinical signs of hypercalcemia are unusual.

Other ovarian carcinomas which rarely exhibit hypercalcemia include dysgerminoma (the second most common in the young patient); clear cell in the older age group; and serous or squamous cell arising in a dermoid cyst and mucinous.

In those tumors with hypercalcemia the pathology is not different from the non-hypercalcemic tumors.

There was a case report of a 25-year-old phenotype female, with karyotype 46,XY, with female external and internal genitalia who had a gonadoblastoma originating from dysgenetic gonads and severe hypercalcemia. The gonads were calcified.[236]

"Paraneoplastic hypercalcemia due to ovarian carcinoma may be more common than generally recognized and present as a life threatening condition requiring urgent treatment."[237]

In general, ovarian neoplasms with hypercalcemia are malignant. The mechanism might be secretion of parathyroid hormone-related protein (PTHrP).[11, p. 380]

Severe hypercalcemia resistant to medical management may occur with dysgerminomas in children. "Serum calcium levels should be checked in all children with solid ovarian tumors."[238]

1. Humoral Hypercalcemia of Malignancy Syndrome (HHM)

HHM by definition is a malignancy which produces excessive PTHrP so that the serum level increases serum calcium. The presence of elevated serum PTHrP and serum calcium has been considered pathognomonic of malignancy.

2. Benign Humoral Hypercalcemia—A Newly Appreciated Syndrome

Although increased production of PTHrP by cancer is regarded as pathognomonic of malignancy, there was a case report of a 16-cm benign ovarian dermoid cyst in a 29-year-old woman with autoimmune hepatitis and Hashimoto thyroiditis in which PTHrP was being produced in squamous epithelium, neural elements, and colonic-type mucosa. The authors point out that normal ovary produces PTHrP but it does not elevate serum levels or cause hypercalcemia. They indicate that a variety of other normal tissues synthesize PTHrP, which has a wide distribution of receptors aside from bone and kidneys. Although the exact role of PTHrP is not known it has activity in calcium hemostasis and fetal development and growth. Hypercalcemia has been found with benign conditions such as pheochromocytoma and lymphedema (lymphedema/hypercalcemia syndrome).[239]

3. Intriguing PTHrP Physiology in Pregnancy

An editorial comment suggests a molecular heterogenicity of PTHrP. It also indicates as a clinical guide that "pheochromocytoma may be the most common single diagnosis for an HHM-like syndrome that accompanies a benign tumor." The editorial points out the intriguing unknown roles of PTHrP. It is an endothelium-derived vascular smooth muscle relaxing factor. Its synthesis increases with distention of hollow organs to relax the smooth muscle walls in the rat urinary bladder and uterus. "It is present in human amniotic fluid at high concentrations; and is important for maintaining the placental calcium gradient in experimental animal models." In addition, there are "mild increases of PTHrP associated with normal pregnancy and lactation…."[240] Obviously this is a fascinating unexplored aspect of pregnancy physiology.

B. Renin

Rarely ovarian tumors, especially sex cord-stromal tumors, may cause hypertension by secretion of renin and secondary hyperaldosteronism. There may be an overlap with Gorlin's syndrome with ovarian fibroma. Sometimes there may be an aldosterone-secreting tumor with low or normal plasm renin. Rarely there may also be isosexual pseudo-precocious puberty with elevated extradiol and testosterone. There may also be an overlap with Peutz-Jeghers syndrome. Many are malignant.

Although clinical signs of hypereninism are rare with ovarian tumors, "…subclinical secretion of renin by some ovarian tumors may be relatively common." Possibly 50% of sex cord-stromal tumors may be immunocreactive for renin without hypertension of hypokalemia.[11, p. 383]

"The occurrence of renin-secreting ovarian tumors is consistent with recent observations that a complete renin-angiotension system exists in the follicular apparatus of the normal ovary."[11, p. 383]

C. Testosterone, Renin, and Erythropoietin—A Possible New Syndrome (HHP)

Although this has not been described as a syndrome, I found two case reports which to me suggest this possibility. Additional case reports have pieces of a puzzle. One was a 67-year-old woman with facial hair, hoarse voice, weight gain, elevated blood testosterone of 44 nmol/L, secondary polycythemia with hemoglobin of 19 g/L, hypertension with blood pressure 168/96 mmHg, and immunochemistry evidence of renin synthesis. She had a left, solid 6-cm ovarian steroid cell tumor which caused virilization with testosterone, probably erythropoietin production causing polycythemia and renin synthesis possibly causing hypertension.[241]

A second report was a 62-year-old woman with hirsutism, male-type temporal baldness, receding hairline, and hypertension which developed over the past year. There was plethoric facies, clitoromegaly and a 6 cm left ovarian mass. The plasma testosterone was elevated to 28.5 nmol/L, and hemoglobin elevated to 17.5 g/dl. The ultrasound showed a mixed echogenicity of the tumor. Histology showed a borderline epithelial endometriod tumor with the stroma having extensive hyalinization with prominent groups of luteinized cells and a strong positive reaction for oc-inhibin. Six months postoperatively the testosterone and blood pressure were normal, the hirsutism had regressed and the temporal hair regrew. It was assumed that the stromal hyperplasia and luteinization caused the increased testosterone. The possibility of increased erythropoietin was not mentioned as the cause of polycythemia.[242]

A 70-year-old para 7 had a firm nodular suprapubic mass and a hemoglobin of 19.0 g/dl. There was a 15-cm yellow, multinodular, solid left ovarian mass. Although the right ovary appeared normal there was a bilateral Brenner tumor. The secondary polycythemia disappeared shortly after surgery. Most Brenner tumors are small, unilateral, and hormonally inactive. Large tumors occur in an older age group. "Secondary polycythemia has been observed in association with other large ovarian tumors. This has been explained on the basis of increased erythropoietin production either by the tumor or as a result of pressure in the renal vessels. The latter mechanism was probably operational in this case." The authors did not measure erythropoietin or testosterone or report blood pressure.[243]

Other case reports describe large tumors with secondary polycythemia, without measurement of blood pressure, erythropoietin, or testosterone; virilization with borderline high hematocrit, increased testosterone, one normal blood pressure; and a malignant tumor with masculinization, elevated testosterone and erythropoietin, and mild diabetes mellitus but no report of blood pressure.

A case was reported of a 6-cm steroid cell tumor (not otherwise specified) of the right ovary removed at age 21 who at age 4 had rapid linear growth, and at age 8 virilization. She had been placed on glucocorticoids for 8 years. The only blood pressure reported was 110/80 mmHg with a hematocrit of 0.464 (borderline high) prior to surgery. Testosterone was elevated and could not be suppressed.[244]

A 61-year-old gravida 7 para 3224 with diet-controlled, type 2 diabetes mellitus had progressive masculinization for 3 years. The hemoglobin was 23.3, hematocrit was 70.8, serum testosterone 3546 mg/dl (normal less than 75 mg/dl), and serum erythropoietin 55 ng/ml (normal 7–36 ng/ml). The blood pressure was not reported. Preoperative phlebotomy was done to reduce the hematocrit to 45%. There was a 10-cm right ovarian lobular tumor, two large liver nodules, and enlarged paraaortic nodes. The tumor was a malignant lipid cell tumor. The patient died from thromboembolic complications 8 months postoperatively with a massive thrombosis in the lower abdominal aorta. Mild erythrocytosis had been reported with benign virilizing lipid cell tumors presumably because of adrogenic steroids. "The marked erythrocytosis in this patient was likely secondary to tumor production of erythropoietin." There were no previous reports found regarding erythropoietin-producing lipid cell tumors. The authors advised repeated phlebotomies to reduce the polycythemic state before surgery to prevent hemorrhagic and thromboembolic perioperative complications.[245]

A 10-year history of androgenic alopecia in an 80-year-old woman was found to be associated with a large ovarian cystic tumor. Pathology showed bilateral Leydig cell hyperplasia within the wall of the cyst and in the opposite ovarian hilus. Leydig hilus cell tumors are the most frequent postmenopausal virilizing tumors.[246]

D. Carcinoid

Carcinoid syndrome refers to bright red cutaneous flushing in the face, neck, and upper chest lasting 10–30 minutes associated with feelings of heat and swelling. With repeated episodes there develops facial telangiectasis and edema. There may also be dyspnea, asthma, abdominal cramps, severe diarrhea, hypotension, and pulmonary stenosis and tricuspid insufficiency due to right heart connective tissue thickening. Most carcinoid tumors develop in the appendix and intestine.[221] The extrarintestinal carcinoid tumors arise from the bile ducts, pancreas, ovaries, and bronchi.

The carcinoid syndrome is caused by tumors of germ cell origin which secrete 5-hydroxytryptamine and other vasoactive amines. The tumors usually are in the gastrointestinal tract and also in the lungs or ovaries. The usual symptoms are flushing, diarrhea, abdominal pain, wheezing, and shortness of breath. The flushing may be confused with menopausal hot flashes. An unappreciated symptom of trabecular carcinoid tumor of the ovary is severe constipation due to a peptide hormone (PYY) with a strong inhibitory effect on intestinal mobility. It is present in endocrine cells of the distal intestine, and in normal colon mucosal cells. PYY is the peptide having an N-terminal tyrosine and a C-terminal tyrosine.[247]

The signs include heart murmur and peripheral edema. There is an increase of urinary 5-hydroxyindole acetic acid (5-HIAA). There may be hyperinsulinemic hypoglycemia or cutaneous melanosis (with stromal ovarian carcinoid tumor).[11, p. 295]

Flushing and carcinoid heart disease are the most specific clinical manifestations of the syndrome.[248] The latter may be the first sign of carcinoid tumor, presenting as unexplained right heart failure and diagnosed by echocardiography.[249] About two-thirds of cases with carcinoid syndrome have carcinoid heart disease.[250] Tumor resection may improve prognosis.[251]

With the initial small bowel tumor there may not be any symptoms because of hepatic detoxification. Symptoms will develop after liver metastases.

With the primary tumor in the bronchus or ovary the secreted hormones enter the systemic circulation and symptoms present without metastases. The syndrome is present usually over age 50 and with tumors of 7 cm.

Primary ovarian carcinoid tumors have other teratomatous components in 85–90% of cases, usually dermoid cyst, stromal carcinoid, mature solid teratoma or a cystic mucinous tumor. Thus the tumors may have developed from a teratoma.[252] The most common type of primary ovarian carcinoid is the insular type, one of four varieties. One-third have carcinoid syndrome which may be the presenting manifestation.

Strumal carcinoid tumor is composed of a mixture of thyroid tissue and carcinoid. A literature review of 329 reported cases of carcinoid tumors of the ovary compared those with accompanying cystic dermoid teratoma (group A) and those without it (group B). There were statistically significant differences with tumor size, group A 44.7 mm versus group B 89.9 mm, rate of metastases 5.8% versus 22.1%, rate of hepatic involvement 2.1% versus 15.0%, associated carcinoid syndrome 13.8% versus 22.9%, and 5-year survival rate 93.7% versus 84%. Insular and trabecular type carcinoids were about the same one-fourth in each group. Carcinoid syndrome was present in 38.9% of insular and 7.8% of trabecular type carcinoids.[253]

Of 35 cases of carcinoid tumors metastatic to the ovary there was a median age of 57, with a range from 21 to 82. Forty percent had carcinoid syndrome. Usually the primary was in the small intestine. Metastataic carcinoid tumors are usually bilateral, solid, and large.[11, p. 345]

Carcinoid tumors may be associated with the carcinoid spectrum, ectopic ACTA syndrome, or other polypeptide hormone secreting syndromes, including MSH-like peptide, glucagons, gastrin, vasoactive intestinal peptide, insulin calcitonin, and antiduretic hormone.

E. Cushing's Syndrome

The clinical features of Cushing's syndrome include proximal muscle weakness, peripheral edema, hypertension, hirsutism, unexplained hyperglycemia, hypoleukemia, and metabolic alkalosis. It may be caused by cortisol secretion of an ovarian steroid cell tumor, which may also cause isosexual precosity. Malignant forms may be aggressive with focal necrosis, nuclear atypia, and many mitoses.

Rarely, other tumors may produce Cushing's syndrome due to ectopic secretion of adrenocorticotrophic hormone (ACTH) or corticotropin-releasing factor. Such tumors include endometroid or undifferentiated adenocarcinoma, Sertoli-Leydig cell tumor, carcinoid and pituitary tissue in a dermoid cyst [11, p. 381] as well as small cell lung cancer.

The ectopic ACTH-producing syndrome (Cushing's syndrome with hyperpigmentation) is one of the most common nonendocrine tumor syndromes causing a humoral syndrome. When due to a malignant tumor it is the most common unrecognized type of Cushing's syndrome.

Ectopic ACTH-syndrome may be due to primary ovarian carcinoma [254–256] or due to recurrent endometrioid ovarian adenocarcinoma.[257] "Cushing's syndrome is more common in patients with Zollinger-Ellison syndrome than was previously reported, occurring in 8% of all cases." "All patients with the Zollinger-Ellison syndrome and all patients with multiple endocrine neoplasia type 1 should be screened for Cushing's syndrome."[258]

F. Zollinger-Ellison Syndrome

Zollinger-Ellison Syndrome can occur with large ovarian mucinous cystadenomas, borderline tumors, and cystadenocarcinomas which have neuroendocrine intestinal-type gastrin-containing cells and clinically active elevated plasma gastrin. These argyrophil, argentaffin hormone immunoreactive cells also produce serotonin and a variety of polypeptide hormones (including corticotropin, gastrin, somatostatin, glucagon, and pancreatic polypeptide) which apparently are clinically not obvious.[160; 11, p. 381]

A case was reported of a 60-year-old woman with epigastric pain and diarrhea. There was a large multifocal ovarian cyst and also multiple ulcerations of the stomach and duodenum and a plasma level of gastrin of 1500 pg/ml. The tumor was a borderline malignant potential mucinous neoplasm with many gastrin-producing cells in the epithelium.[259]

G. Multiple Polyendocrine Neoplasia Type I

A case was reported of an ovarian gastrinoma containing somatostatin as part of multiple endocrine neoplasia type I, with primary hyperparathyroidism and Zollinger-Ellison syndrome. Oophorectomy gave the diagnosis and complete healing.[260]

A Norwegian report of 20 cases of autoimmune polyendocrine syndrome type I (APS I) found 4 different mutations of the AIRE gene. Five of eight women had premature ovarian failure. In two-thirds of the cases the patients had been hospitalized for acute adrenal insufficiency or hypocalcemic crisis. "The diagnosis APS I must be considered in children and adolescents with chronic mucocutaneous candidiasis, autoimmune adrenenocortical failure of hypoparathyroidism in order to avoid fatal complications."

Diagnostic aids include autoantibody analyses and AIRE gene mutations.[260a]

H. Hyperthyroidism

Struma ovarii is a teratoma with predominant thyroid tissue, usually recognized grossly in less than 5% of dermoid cysts with a peak frequency in the fifth decade. Although careful histology reveals thyroid tissue in 20% of dermoids, clinical hyperthyroidism occurs in only 5% of struma ovarii. There may be a high uptake of I-131 in the pelvis and a low uptake in the neck. Struma ovarii torsion or surgery may provoke thyrotoxicosis. After resection there may be an enlargement of the thyroid gland.

In pure form, the thyroid tissue in the ovary appears as a brownish, solid gelatinous tissue, occasionally mixed with a dermoid cyst or with a solid carcinoid tumor (strumal carcinoid). Infrequently the opposite ovary has a dermoid cyst or another struma.

About 5–10% of strumas are malignant, and less than half of these have spread beyond the ovary. Occasionally cases show extraovarian peritoneal spread with a histologically benign appearance ("strumosis") and an indolent course.[11, p. 285]

Most cases of struma ovarii and the strumal component of ovarian strumal carcinoids produce subclinical thyroid hormones.

Hyperthyroidism may result from hydatidiform mole or choriocarcinoma because of the thyrotropic stimulation of human chorionic gonadotropin.

I. Tumors with Functioning Stroma

These are separate from sex cord-stromal and steroid cell tumors. "Almost all types of ovarian tumors, both benign and malignant, primary and metastatic, have been reported to be associated with endocrine abnormalities of estrogenic, androgenic, or rarely, progestagenic type, or combinations thereof."[11 p. 373]

Clues to ovarian tumors with functioning stroma (OTFS) include estrogenic vaginal cytology and endometrial hyperplasia. About half of postmenopausal women with benign and malignant surface epithelial-stromal tumors or metastatic carcinoma have elevated urinary estrogen. This may explain postmenopausal women with tumors who experience bleeding from proliferative or hyperplastic endometrium or have breast tenderness. There may also be progestational change with decidual reaction or an Arias-Stella endometrium.

Virilizing ovarian tumors may have functioning stroma and since a one-third occur in pregnancy they may have virilized female children. Rarely dysgerminoma may have functioning stroma with syncytiotrophoblastic cells causing isosexual precocity. Presumably the secretion of hCG stimulates luteinization and hormone production by stromal cells.

Stromal cells of OTFS resemble steroid hormone-secreting cells. The high hCG level in pregnancy stimulates virilizing OTFS.

In general ovarian carcinoma cells have aromatase ability to convert androgens to estrogens. This also occurs more rapidly in ovarian cancer metastases where there is a larger mass of tumor cells.

The functioning stroma may be tumor intrinsic and/or adjacent stroma and histologically is stromal hyperthecosis made of plump spindle cells which is also present normally and which produces steroid hormones. Infrequently the stromal cells become Leydig cells with Reinke crystals. Possibly OTFS produces androgens which may undergo peripheral conversion to androgens.

OTFS tends to occur in malignant tumors, especially mucinous and endometrioid surface epithelial-stromal carcinomas, and large intestine metastatic tumors.

Among androgenic OTFS about one-third are gastric metastatic Krukenberg tumors but also there may be primary benign mucinous cystic tumors, rete cystadenomas, large intestine metastatic carcinomas, dermoid cysts, and strumal carcinoid tumors. In histological differential diagnosis tubular Krukenberg tumors and surface epithelial-stromal tumors with luteinized stroma may be confused with sex cord-stromal tumor.[(11, p. 373]

J. Sex Cord-Stromal Tumors

Most sex cord-stromal tumors are ovarian type granulosa-stromal cells which secrete estrogen while Sertoli-stromal cell tumors secrete androgens. Mixtures of both are gynandroblastomas. The adult granulosa cell tumor occurs mainly in middle-aged or older women. The juvenile form occurs in children and young adults.

1. Juvenile Granulosa Cell Tumor (JGCT)

This differs histologically from adult granulosa cell tumors and 97% occur under age 30. About 80% of JGCT in prepubertal children cause isosexual precocious puberty (also called pseudoprecocious because it is not due to central or true precocious puberty).

Clinically precocious puberty appears in the normal sequence starting with breast development and then sex hair. Occasionally there is also clitoromegaly. When it occurs after puberty it may have the same presentation as GCT with amenorrhea and/or menstrual irregularity. About 6% present acutely with rupture and hematoperitoneum. Rarely Ollier's disease (enchondromatosis) and Maffucci's syndrome (enchondromatosis and hemangiomatosis) may also occur. About 10% have ascites and 10% rupture in surgery. It is unilateral in 98% with an average diameter of 12.5 cm. It is a solid and cystic neoplasm with hemorrhagic fluid. The prognosis is good in stage I and "...removal of the involved ovary is almost always curative."[11, p. 186] Whereas the GCT has late recurrences, JGCT has early recurrences.

2. Adult Granulosa Cell Tumor (GCT)

This has a peak incidence between 50 and 55 years and is the most common estrogen-producing tumor. It causes endometrial cystic hyperplasia and about 5% cause well-differentiated carcinoma.

Postmenopausal women experience uterine bleeding. Menstruating women often first have amenorrhea followed later with excessive regular bleeding. With the rare case of occurrence in childhood it causes isosexual precocious puberty. Most cases have abdominal pain, swelling, a mass, and 10% present acutely with rupture and hematoperitoneum. Although 12% may not be palpable it may be visualized by ultrasound. Most are discovered in stage I and are unilateral in 95%.

The average diameter is 12.5 cm and it may be cystic and/or solid. The serum inhibin level is increased and may indicate recurrences. Recurrences are late. In the young patient, a unilateral salpingo-oophorectomy may be done if there is no spread. Tumor rupture and large size reduce survival rate.

3. Stromal Tumors

This include thecoma, luteinized thecoma with sclerosing peritonitis, fibroma, cellular fibroma, fibrosarcoma, and sclerosing stromal tumor.[11, p. 189]

The usual thecoma contains sheets of theca-like cells in a fibromatous mass. They are generally estrogenic, have a mean age of 59, and only 10% were under age 30. Most cases present with postmenopausal bleeding and 21% have endometrial carcinoma.

Luteinized thecomas also contain lutein cells. Half are estrogenic, 11% are androgenic, and 39% are nonfunctional. Clinical masculinization is unusual because of aromatization of androgen to estrogen. About 30% occur under age 30. Rare cases with Reinke crystals ("stromal Leydig cell tumor") may be virilizing. About 95% of thecomas are unilateral, mostly 5–10 cm, and solid. Extensive calcification may occur in young women. Rarely with luteinized thecomas there may be sclerosing peritonitis, usually presenting under age 30. They present with intestinal obstruction and sometimes with ascites. Both ovaries are involved ranging from normal size up to 31 cm with a nodular surface.

Fibromas appear at an average age of 48 and are rare in children. Usually there is no steroid hormone secretion. It represents 4% of all ovarian tumors. It may be associated with Meigs' syndrome in 1% of fibromas, and nevoid basal cell carcinoma syndrome (Gorlin's syndrome). When fibromas are over 10 cm there is a 10–15% chance of ascites. Fibromas are bilateral in 8%, ranging in size from microscopic to very large with an average size of 6 cm. Less than 10% have calcification; however, bilateral calcification "...is almost always present with the nevoid basal cell carcinoma syndrome."[11, p. 195] In general fibroids are benign.

4. Sertoli-Stromal Cell Tumors

There include tumors of Sertoli cells and those of Leydig cells either together or separate.[11, p. 203]

Sertoli cell tumors are rare, presenting at an average age of 30, and are occasionally estrogenic or androgenic. They may also produce progesterone and renin. There may be an association with Peutz-Jeghers syndrome. "All the Sertoli cell tumors reported to date have been unilateral and stage I," with an average size of 9 cm forming lobulated solid masses.[11, p. 203]

Sertoli-Leydig cell tumors number only 0.5% of all ovarian neoplasms. The average size is 25 cm. About one-third of cases have prominent virilization with amenorrhea, breast atrophy, and masculinization with acne, hirsutism, temporal balding, deep voice, and clitoromegaly. There may also be androgen-induced erythrocytosis. There is an increase of plasma testosterone and androstenedione. Nevertheless hormone testing to separate the ovarian Sertoli-Leydig cell tumor from a virilizing adrenal tumor may not be reliable.

Rarely Sertoli-Leydig cell tumors may be estrogenic, and have an association with cervix sarcoma botryoides or thyroid disease or have a rare familial occurrence.

Over 98% are unilateral and stage Ia in 80%, although rupture may occur in 12%. The size varies from microscopic to very large, averaging 13.5 cm. They are solid, lobulated, and yellow. If confined to one ovary in the young patient a unilateral salpingo-oophorectomy is done. Recurrences occur early.

a. Sex Cord Tumor with Annular Tubules (SCTATs)

These may have areas of Sertoli cell tumor or granulosa cell tumor. In women without PJS the tumor is palpable. About 40% are estrogenic and sometimes secrete progesterone. The average age is 27. The tumors are unilateral, solid, moderately large, and yellow. About one-fifth are malignant with late recurrences. Malignant tumors may produce large amounts of Mullerian-inhibiting substance, and progesterone and inhibin, which are clinically useful markers.

In women with PJS, the tumors are bilateral, usually not visible grossly, but occasionally yellow nodules up to 3 cm are present. The tumorlets of themselves are benign. With PJS there are gastrointestinal hamartomatosis polyps, mucocutaneous pigmentation, and sometimes adenoma malignum of the cervix, and gastrointestinal pancreatic or breast cancer.

5. Steroid Cell Tumors

These are rare, being only 0.1% of all ovarian neoplasms. They are divided into two types of known origin, the stromal luteoma and the Leydig cell tumor. These are benign.

The third type is of unknown origin (not otherwise specified, NOS).[11, p. 232]

The stromal luteoma tumor is a small solitary tumor over 0.5 cm within the ovarian stroma. In 90% of cases there is stromal hyperthecosis in the same or other ovary. About 80% occur in postmenopausal women, usually presenting as bleeding due to hyperestrogenism. It is not known whether estrogen is secreted directly or whether there is androgen secretion with peripheral conversion to estrogen.

About 12% have androgenic symptoms. Other steroid cell tumors are usually androgenic. There is a possible association with hyperandrogenism-insulin resistance-acanthosis nigricans syndrome found with polycystic ovaries. The tumors are less than 3 cm, unilateral, well circumscribed, solid and gray-white or yellow.

Leydig cell tumor is diagnosed by Reinke crystals in the neoplastic cytoplasm and may be hilar or nonhilar. The average age is 58, with three-fourth of cases causing hirsutism or virilization, and are rarely estrogenic. The androgenic change is milder and slower (up to many years) than with Sertoli-Leydig cell tumor. They produce testosterone.

The steroid cell tumor NOS represent 60% of steroid cell tumors and are probably large stromal luteomas or Leydig cell tumors but lack Reinke crystals. The average age is 43 and occasionally present before puberty. Half of the cases have slow androgenic changes over years, 10% have estrogenic change and isosexual pseudoprecocious puberty, and occasionally there are progestagenic changes, or cortisol secretion with Cushing's syndrome. Rarely there has been increased cortisol without Cushing's syndrome, hypercalcemia, erythrocytosis, or ascites. There is increased testosterone, androstenedione, and increased urinary 17-ketosteroids and 17-hydroxycorticosteroids. About 95% are unilateral, solid, and circumscribed with a mean diameter of 8.4 cm. There is a typical yellow or orange appearance on sectioning. In young patients with stage Ia unilateral oophorectomy has been done. About 20% have extraovarian spread. The chance of malignancy is 25–43% but there may be rare late recurrences. "...no malignant tumors have been reported in patients in the first two decades."[11, p. 237]

The cases with Cushing syndrome had advanced tumor. Tumors of 7-cm size were 78% malignant. "Occasionally tumors that appear cytologically benign, however, may be clinically malignant."[11, p. 237]

a. Autoimmune Hemolytic Anemia Syndrome

Rarely dermoid cysts may cause a Coombs positive autoimmune hemolytic anemia.[11, p. 385]

b. Melanosis Peritonei

Melanosis or pigmentation of the peritoneum and ovary is associated with dermoid cysts or microscopic gastric mucosal lined cysts. It may be focal or diffuse, tan to black staining nodules, and may include the peritoneum.[11] It is due to melanin-laden histiocytes. It is benign but may be confused with disseminated malignant melanoma.

c. Chronic Gonadotropin (hCG) Secretion

Clinical signs of hCG production are usually due to germ cell tumors containing syncytiotrophoblastic cells. Steroid hormones may be stimulated by luteinized tumor, stromal cells, or in the adjacent ovarian stroma.

Subclinical serum hCG has been reported with various ovarian tumors, and in 10–40% of surface epithelial benign and malignant tumors associated with "active stroma." This has also been found in metastatic gastrointestinal adenocarcinomas.[11, p. 379] hCG may activate the stroma of primary and secondary ovarian tumors.

d. Inappropriate Antidiuresis Syndrome

There was a case report of ovarian serous carcinoma with a component of small cell carcinoma of pulmonary type with neuroendocrine granules containing antidiuretic hormone. Such tumors are usually large, solid, bilateral, and aggressive.[11, p. 381]

e. Hyperprolactinemia

Rarely dermoid cysts may contain a small prolactinoma which may cause amenorrhea, galactorrhea, and hyperprolactinemia. In one case Sertoli-type cells of a gonadoblastoma stained for prolactin.[11, p. 383]

f. Hypoglycemia

Hypoglycemia is rare and may occur with various malignant and benign neoplasms because of insulin and proinsulin secretions. Carcinoid ovarian tumors may in addition cause cutaneous melanosis due to secretion of alpha-melanocytic-stimulating hormone, and rarely there is an association with parathyroid adenoma and pituitary hyperplasia as part of the type I multiple endocrine neoplasia syndrome.[11, p. 381–382]

g. Amylase Secretion

High-stage serous surface epithelial carcinomas may contain amylase and secrete it into cystic, ascitic, and pleural fluid, as well as serum and urine. Thus, aspiration of an ovarian cystic tumor may be misinterpreted as ascitic fluid, or it might mimic a pancreatic pseudocyst or acute pancreatitis. Ovarian neoplasm amylase is similar to salivary amylase and has a different electrophoretic pattern than pancreatic amylase. "The serum amylase level may be a useful marker of tumor progression and therapeutic response in such patients."[11, p. 390]

VII. CHROMOSOMAL ABNORMALITIES

Chromosome XO syndrome or Turner syndrome has also been referred to as Turner-Albright, Morgagni-Turner,

Shereshevskii-Turner, Bonnevie-Ullrich, Ullrich-Turmer, genital dwarfism, gonadal dysgenesis, ovarian dwarfism, and ovarian short stature syndrome. The classic XO due to a loss of one X chromosome is thought to be a relatively lethal condition and therefore may be unsuspected mosaicism. There is a classic XO Turner phenotype with short stature. It is the most common chromosomal abnormality in females occurring in 1 : 2500 live phenotypic female births. The classic clinical syndrome was described by Turner in 1938 as small stature, sexual infantilism, webbed neck, and cubitus valgus. The essential criteria are small stature (less than 150 cm in height) and gonadal dysgenesis. The mechanism is a sporadic absence of an X chromosome, usually from the father resulting in a total of 45 chromosomes.

The ovaries are fibrous streaks ("streak ovaries") without ovulation and do not produce estrogen resulting in primary amenorrhea due to ovarian failure.

Most XO conceptuses are lethal with early spontaneous abortions. Although the ovaries are normal in early fetal life, primary follicles do not usually develop and there is rapid degeneration of the ovaries.

Clinical clues include hypoplasia or absence of ovarian primary follicles, neonatal congenital lymphedema or dorsum of fingers and toes, broad shield shaped chest with widely spaced nipples, webbed neck, prominent auricles, prognathous, narrow palate, low posterior hairline suggesting a short neck, elbow cubitus valgus, renal and cardiac anomalies, coarctation of the aorta, and fifth short metacarpal bones.

For diagnosis karyotype is recommended for short stature in childhood, pubertal arrest, primary and secondary amenorrhea, and elevated follicle-stimulating hormone (FSH). FSH level may be helpful before age 5 and after age 10. Usually estrogen replacement therapy is used to mimic puberty and later progestin is added to give cyclic withdrawal bleeding.

Adults with Turner's syndrome (TS) have an increased chance of osteoporosis, hyperthyroidism, renal and gastrointestinal diseases, aortic dissection, ischemic heart disease, and reduced life expectancy. They should have a multidisciplinary team care.[260b]

Mosaicism 45X/47XXX may cause premature menopause and the development of streak ovaries in adult life.[260c]

Probably even more common than the monosomic XO syndrome are cases with only some cells XO and others mosaic or all mosaic. This would include XX/XO, XY/XO with varying degrees of masculine genitalia, or those with part of one X missing. In these mosaic cases there may be some ovarian function with 10–20% having spontaneous puberty and 2–5% transient spontaneous menses and rarely pregnancy. Even with this there is usually premature menopause.

Although bilateral streak gonads occur in "pure gonadal dysgenesis" (often 46,XX karyotype) and Turner's syndrome (45,X or mosaic karyotype) together with failure of puberty development there are two distinct phenotypic presentations. With the former there is normal height and no congenital abnormalities.

Swyer's syndrome is 46XY gonadal dysgenesis with a female phenotype. These cases usually do not have the Turner phenotype. There is normal height. There are streak gonads, primary amenorrhea due to ovarian failure, and atrophic but otherwise normal genitalia. There is a 25–80% chance of malignant change of the streak gonads by the age of 30 into single or multiple gonadoblastoma, dysgerminoma, or other germ cell tumors.[260d]

These cases usually have "mixed gonadal dysgenesis," a combination of streak gonads and testis. The patient is usually phenotypic female but may have some masculinization of the external genitalia and presents with primary amenorrhea. The phenotype may resemble Turner syndrome in about one-third of the cases.[260e, f]

There is a wide variability in clinical, histopathologic, and cytogenic findings including mosaicisms of 45,X/46,XY; 46,XY; 46XX; 46,XX/46XY; and 45X/46,Xi (Xq).[260e, 261a]

Most pure gonadal dysgenesis and Turner's syndrome patients do not have Y chromosomes and therefore do not have a predisposition to gonadoblastomas or germ cell tumors (dysgerminomas). "...Y mosaicism could theoretically be present in 35–40% of cases with Turner's syndrome."[261b] When a rare ovarian tumor forms (without a Y chromosome) it may be a surface epithelial stromal or hilus cell tumor.[260f]

If there is a 46,XY karyotype with pure gonadal dysgenesis or a 45,X/46,XY or mosaic karyotype in mixed gonadal dysgenesis there is an increased risk of gonadoblastoma and dysgerminoma (which is malignant). The malignancy risk by age 20 is 28% with gonadal dysgenesis and 19% with mixed gonadal dysgenesis (with Y chromosome). "...prophylactic removal of the gonads is advisable in both groups of patients at an early age."[11, p. 400]

Rarely JGCT is found in infants with gonadal dysgenesis, Y chromosome, and ambiguous genitalia.

There are differences between prenatally and postnatally diagnosed cases of 45,X/46,XY mosaicisms. Most prenatally diagnosed cases show a normal male phenotype, whereas the postnatally diagnosed cases show a wide spectrum of phenotypes. Some cases with streak gonads show homogenous 45,X suggesting selective invasion of the primitive genital ridge which induces abnormal gonad development. Some males normal at birth develop late-onset abnormalities of Turner syndrome including dysgenetic testes, infertility, and dysmorphic features.[260f]

Using polymerase chain reaction (PCR) testing of Turner's syndrome patients, 3% of Austrians [261c] and 12% of Mexicans [261d] were discovered to have unsuspected Y chromosomes or sequences.

Gonadectomy has been recommended if a Y chromosome (or Y fragments) is present because 20–40% develop gonadoblastomas.[261b] Gonadectomy has also been recommended if there are clinical signs of hyperandrogenism and/or virilization. For the latter this policy has been recently questioned because excess androgen may originate in the dysgenetic gonad with normal Y-negative chromosomes without predisposition to neoplasia, and gonadectomy for that purpose is not required. Such examples include ovarian hilus cell hyperplasia, stroma luteoma, and nodular hyperthecosis and cystadenofibroma. Nodular hyperthecosis results from prolonged high gonadotrophin.[261e]

PCR is useful to identify patients with Turner's syndrome who have Y markers in their genomic DNA corresponding to Yp region or centromere and therefore should have gonadectomy.[261e]

Using PCR peripheral blood lymphocyte testing in Turner's syndrome without Y chromosome with standard testing, might reveal Y material in as much as 9%.[261e]

The commentary points out that because of mosaicism more than one tissue should be examined in cases with virilization. Noninvasive testing could be done using buccal cells or urine cell sediment. There have been cases with virilization and Y material present in gonads but not in blood. To make it more confusing, in virilized cases "…tumors have been described in TS with no molecular evidence of Y sequences in blood or gonads." The commentary recommends considering testing for Y chromosome mosaicism in all cases with a 45,X karyotype as well as those with virilization using multiplex PCR molecular testing investigating the centromeric and proximal long arm regions of the Y chromosome (the sites of the putative gonadoblastoma gene CGBY).[261b]

A report from Denmark showed that of 114 patients with Turner's syndrome 14 or 12.2% (testing by PCR) had Y chromosome material. The karyotype in 7 did not suggest the presence of Y chromosome material. One of the 10 ovariectomized patients had a gonadoblastoma. The authors concluded that although the frequency of Y material is high the occurrence of gonadoblastoma in such cases is low (1 or 14) or 7–10%. "Gonadectomy is generally recommended; however, this consensus is questioned by the present study."[261f]

Personal opinion follows the consensus.

If there is XY/XO mosaicism, or a Y chromosome in a different location then prophylactic surgical removal of the gonads in childhood is advised to prevent malignant tumor (gonadoblastoma) formation. The uterus is preserved, contrary to previous practice, because with ovum donation and assisted reproductive technology pregnancy is still possible. There may be a variable phenotype with streak ovaries and testes.

"Because of the possible inheritance of XY gonad dysgenesia all family members should undergo a thorough screening."[261g]

With the rare true hermaphroditism with ovarian and testicular tissue, the karyotype is usually 46,XX, and there is often sexual ambiguity. Malignant gonadal tumors develop in less than 3%, usually dysgerminoma-seminoma. "Eight phenotypically female true hermaphrodites with a 46,XX or mosaic karyotype have borne children."[11, p. 401; 261h]

A. Androgen-Insensitivity Syndrome (AIS)

AIS refers to a female phenotype, 46,XY karyotype, bilateral testes, and end-organ insensitivity to androgen. The testes are usually retroperitoneal intra-abdominal (sometimes in the inguinal canal). Male internal and external development does not occur. There is no or little sex hair. Breasts develop. The testes secrete Mullerian-inhibiting substance which prevents development of the uterus and fallopian tubes. The usual mechanism is an abnormality of the androgen receptor gene in the long arm of the X chromosome. It may be sporadic or familial. The testes produce androgens and estrogens. There is puberty development. There is primary amenorrhea, a short vagina, no cervix, and possibly inguinal gonads and a family history of affected aunts. The diagnosis is readily overlooked. The patients have a normal feminine psyche and are reared as females.

After puberty there is a tendency to benign and malignant hamartomas and neoplasms. The most common are benign hamartomas and often bilateral. Sertoli cell adenomas may develop and may be confused with the malignant Sertoli cell tumor which infrequently forms.[261i] About 8% of adults develop GCTs, usually seminomas.

It is generally agreed that the testes should be removed, but there are differences of opinion regarding timing. Pediatric surgeons advise surgery in childhood for the small chance of early development of tumors and to avoid emotional trauma. Gynecologists often wait until after puberty to allow spontaneous puberty development. Psychologic aspects are important with the testes being referred to as "abnormal gonads."

AIS covers a broad spectrum with numerous infrequent varieties ranging from failure to produce androgen to failure to metabolize it.

With partial androgen insensitivity and an enlarged clitoris the gonads are removed in childhood because of a possible androgenic effect at puberty.

Pituitary hemorrhage ("apoplexy") has occurred in an LH-producing adenoma which may have developed from hyperplasia due to feedback because of lack of gonadal steroid.[(261j] Most cases of AIS are treated with hormone replacement therapy after gonadectomy.

1. Germ Cell Tumors

Under age 21 about 60% of ovarian tumors are germ cell. Most are benign dermoid cysts (mature cystic teratomas). When malignant tumors occur about two-thirds of them are germ cell tumors.

B. Tumors Associated with Abnormal Sexual Development

1. Gonadoblastoma

Gonadoblastomas are the most common tumors associated with abnormal gonadal development, usually gonadal dysgenesis with a Y or Y fragment chromosome. About two-thirds of these tumors are gonadoblastomas (sometimes mixed with germ cell tumors). Clinically the cases of gonadoblastoma are children or young adults, about one-third under age 15, and usually phenotypic females often with virilization. Pure gonadoblastomas are small to moderate size, less than 8 cm, 25% are microscopic, and one-third of cases have tumor in the opposite ovary. About 96% of gonadoblastomas develop in dysgenetic gonads with Y chromosome or fragments.

Pure gonadoblastomas do not metastasize and can regress spontaneously. They may secrete estrogen or testosterone. Because of nests of mixed germ cells, 50% may develop into dysgerminomas and 10% into other malignant germ cell neoplasm.

Karyotyping should be done for unexplained short stature even without any other Turner stigmata because there could be a female phenotype with 45,X/46,X, isodicentric (Yp) mosaicism, and a gonadoblastoma.[261k]

Rarely a dysgerminoma has formed in a 45,X Turner patient without molecular evidence of Y material in blood or tumor.[261l] Rarely with dysgerminomas (which may be hormonally active) there may be an elevated serum beta-hCG sufficient to cause a positive pregnancy test.[261m]

Gonadoblastomas themselves are benign but have a high frequency of developing into a malignant germ cell tumor. Thus bilateral gonadectomy is done except in the very rare case with an otherwise normal ovary with a normal karyotype and no underlying gonadal disorder.[11, p. 400]

Dysgerminomas are malignant and may develop from benign gonadoblastomas in phenotypic females with gonadal dysgenesis with 46,XY pure gonadal dysgenesis or with mixed gonadal dysgenesis with 45,X/46,XY mosaicism. Rarely dysgerminomas occur with ataxia-telangiectasia. In phenotypic females with androgen insensitivity syndrome (testicular feminization) and 46,XY karyotype the testes may form seminomas.

Most dysgerminomas occur in the second and third decades with an average age of late teens to early twenties. Almost all have an elevated serum lactic dehydrogenase which is helpful in diagnosis, monitoring, and detecting recurrence. Some also have elevation of serum alkaline phosphatase, CA125, neuron-specific enolase, and chorionic gonadotrophin.

Dysgerminomas average 15 cm and are solid with 10% gross laterality and 10% microscopic bilaterality. About 65% are in stage Ia. About 10% contain more than one cell type. For the young patient with stage Ia, unilateral salpingo-oophorectomy is usually done with careful follow-up since 20% may recur. "The 5-year survival rate approachs 100% for patients with stage I tumors, and 80–90% for those with higher stage reccurent tumor."[11, p. 245]

Yolk sac tumor (endometrial sinus tumor) is a very malignant germ cell tumor, with average size of 15 cm, having a 25% chance of rupture with friable and hemorrhagic necrotic tissue. They are almost always unilateral. In recent years due to new chemotherapy the prognosis has reversed from the previous poor outlook. Usual therapy is unilateral salpingo-oophorectomy, cytoreduction of extraovarian tumor, and combination chemotherapy.

Germ cell sex cord-stromal tumors, unclassified, occur with normal karyotype, normal gonads, in infants or girls under age 10, and occasionally with isosexual precocity. They are very rare and may be benign or malignant.

Combining new chemotherapy with conservative surgery for malignant germ cell tumors irrespective of subtype and stage, the survival rate was 90–100% with only slight decrease in fertility and probably no difference in congenital malformations.[261n, o]

2. Heritability of Germ Cell Malignancies

The early age of onset of malignant ovarian germ tumors suggests an inherited genetic factor. Among 78 cases up to the age of 20 with normal chromosomes, there was no increase of tumors in relatives. Dysgerminomas, the most common ovarian germ cell malignancy, and gonadoblastomas, were excluded because of their association with Y chromosomes, or germ-line cytogenetic abnormality. A larger number of cases would be required if there was a risk factor of up to 5%.[262] Familial malignant germ cell tumors with normal chromosomes have been reported in siblings [262a–c] and fathers and daughters.[262d] Both myelodysplasia and a malignant germ cell tumor in an adolescent were found to have similar abnormal chromosomes and presumably a common clonal origin.[262e]

A study of a large series from the Nordic countries of relatives of children with childhood cancers concluded that "...apart from rare cancer syndromes, paediatric cancer is not an indicator or increased risk in siblings."[262f]

VIII. SUSCEPTIBILITY TO OVARIAN CANCER

A. Sporadic, Hereditary, Breast Ovarian Cancer (HBOC) Syndrome, and Hereditary Nonpolyposis Colorectal Cancer (HNPCC) Syndrome

Most ovarian cancer is epithelial serous papillary. About 90% is considered "sporadic" due to progressive accumulated acquired genetic changes, and apparently occurring without any hereditary predisposition. The lifetime risk for the general population is about 1.8% or 1:55 with a median age of 63. The main risk factors are family history (suggesting a hereditary factor) and age of 45. Other factors include nulliparity, ovarian infertility, residence in industrialized North American and Northern Europe, and being white.

There is a reduced incidence with multiparity, the use of oral contraceptives, tubal ligation, hysterectomy, and in black and Asian populations.[262g]

About 10% of epithelial cancer is hereditary and of these about 85–90% are due to HBOC. Of these, most (about 70%) are due to mutations of BRCA1 gene. A few (about 20%) are due to mutations of BRCA2 gene which has later onset cancer and lower penetrance. An even smaller percent (about 5%) are due to another mechanism associated with HNPCC syndrome.

Despite the above with the assumption that they account for all hereditary ovarian cancer there are patients with cancer and a suggestive family history but without the above identification. They might be accounted for by other unidentified HBOC gene mutations. Other rare syndromes are associated with ovarian cancer.

There is speculation that without a family history there may be combinations of low penetrance genes which could cause hereditary cancer.

The lifetime risk with BRCA1 mutation is 16–63%, with BRCA2 mutation is 16–40%, and with HNPCC is 5%. The risk of breast cancer is higher. There is a 1/400 occurrence of BRCA1 and BRCA2 mutations in the general population. Askenazi Jewish women have a 2.6% incidence.[262g]

The HBOC and HNPCC syndrome mutated genes are autosomal dominant and highly penetrant. First-degree relatives have a 50% chance of being carriers. This explains the high rates of familial ovarian cancer which was noted prior to the discovery of the BRCA mutations.

HBOC syndrome causes 85–90% of all familial ovarian cancer cases. BRCA1 gene causes 45% of early-onset hereditary breast cancer and more than 80% of hereditary ovarian cancers.

BRCA2 causes fewer cases of ovarian cancer and there also may be a negative history. There is late-onset disease due to lower penetrance and "...the fraction of all ovarian cancers resulting from hereditary predisposition may be higher than previously suspected on the basis of estimates derived from highly penetrant genetic loci."[263, p. 114]

As patients throughout the world are studied for BRCA1 and BRCA2 mutations for breast and ovarian cancer new regional mutations are being discovered with different patterns.[264–266, 266a]

Since it is not feasible to test every patient completely it is customary to test for only the common mutations. Ideally the geographic origin should be considered, otherwise an unusual mutation will not be tested for and there will be an erroneous conclusion that the patient was in the lucky 50% noncarrier group despite a positive family history. Discovery of the unusual mutation will increase the incidence of hereditary cancer.

Unique regional mutations and frequencies of BRCA1 and BRCA2 have been reported from Switzerland, western Sweden,[267] Holland,[268] and northeastern France.[264]

With complete coding of the BRCA1 region of Norwegian women and the discovery of 11 distinct mutations because of family history, more than half had 2 founder mutations and they had significantly older age of onset of cancer. "...BRCA mutation penetrance estimates from populations with strong founder effects may be biased."[265]

The entire coding sequences of BRCA1 and BRCA2 genes were investigated in 989 unrelated patients from German breast/ovarian cancer families. There were 77 BRCA1 and 63 BRCA2 distinct deleterious mutations found in 302 cases. "More than one-third of these mutations are novel and might be specific for the German population." In addition there were 50 different rare sequence variations of unknown significance in 72 families. There were 18 common mutations in 68% of BRCA1 mutations and 13 recurrent mutations in 44% of BRCA2 mutations. This might expedite mass screening.[269]

Complete coding sequence of both genes was done in Belgium based on family history and "sporadic" early-onset disease cases of 49 families and 19 "sporadic" patients. In 15 families there were 12 BRCA1 mutations and 3 BRCA2 mutations. There was a common haplotype immediately flanking the mutation in all families suggesting that the disease alleles are identical by descent.[266]

Major genometric rearrangements of the BRCA1 gene might account for some apparently mutation negative cases. Investigation of 60 such probands found a recombination between two very similar Alu repeats. "This type of mutation is not identified by the conventional methods of mutation detection which are based on PCR amplification of single exons."[270]

B. Possible Unrecognized Genetic Factors

The highest risk of cancer (high risk genes) occurs with germ-line mutations of BRCA1, BRCA2, and TP53.[271]

Moderate-risk genes for breast and ovarian cancer may be associated with autosomal dominant inherited syndromes including Cowden disease, HNPCC, Muir-Torre syndrome, and PJS. These genes have lower penetrance than BRCA1, BRCA2, or TP53 mutations and thus have less risk of breast and/or ovarian cancer. "Low-risk genes likely require significant environmental exposure, and although they are associated with the lowest risk of cancer, they account for more cancer than high–and moderate-risk genes."[272]

Other than the high penetrance genes BRCA1 and BRCA2 involved with breast cancer, there is a 5% significance level for 13 polymorphisms in 10 genes with breast cancer. Thus, polymorphism combinations may have a risk role in breast cancer. It might be possible that rare genetic syndromes with increased breast cancer risks may play a role as with the Li-Fraumeni syndrome, the ATM gene of ataxia-telangiectasia

(A-T) the LKB1 gene and PJS. There may be a role of low penetrance breast cancer susceptibility genes. Several genes may interact. "Finally, it is not unlikely that other genes exist that give rise to variation in breast cancer susceptibility, but have not yet been identified and/or tested."[273]

Logically, if the above is valid for breast cancer, it might also apply to ovarian cancer since they are both part of the HBOC syndrome.

"It should be stressed that there are likely to exist many other gene variants that confer predisposition to one another cancer type with lower penetrance, in a recessive fashion, or through interactions with other susceptibility loci, but much less is currently known regarding these types of genes. Thus, it is likely that a much large fraction of all cancers will eventually be regarded as 'hereditary' in nature, but for the purposes of this discussion, the term 'hereditary cancer' will refer to those associated with dominant highly penitrant loci."[263, p. 111]

C. Hereditary Nonpolyposis Colorectal Cancer (HNPC) Syndrome

Hereditary nonpolyposis colorectal cancer (HNPCC), previously referred to as Lynch syndrome, affects about 1/1000. It is due to a defect in DNA mismatch repair gene, usually a germ-line mutation in hMLH1 or hMSH2. It is associated with an increased risk of cancer of the right colon as well as stomach, small bowel, hepatobiliary, ureter, brain, and skin. There is also a lifetime risk of 40–60% of endometrial cancer and of 10–12% of ovarian cancer. Most ovarian cancers are serous and endometriod, but there is wide variety.[(274] These gynecologic cancers occur 15 years earlier than with sporadic cancer.

Although HNPCC-associated endometrial cancer is only 5–10% of all endometrial cancer the cases should be investigated. "In a study that is currently in progress, a consortium of HNPCC registries in the United States and Canada found that among women with HNPCC who had more than one cancer in their lifetime, over 50% had an endometrial or ovarian cancer as their 'sentinel' cancer." They went on to develop a colon or other cancer.[274]

With HNPCC syndrome the mean age of ovarian cancer is 43, versus at least 60 for the general population. The cancer is usually discovered in an early stage and is well to moderately differentiated, and is more likely to have synchronous endometrial cancer (20%). About one-third of ovarian cancers appear before age 40.[275]

Sporadic and BRCA ovarian cancers are usually late stage and high grade.[274]

Microsatellite instability is characteristic and caused by a deficiency of DNA mismatch-repair function. It is a hallmark or HNPCC, but also occurs in 15% of sporadic cancer.

The MSH2-associated DNA mismatch-repair gene of HNCC was found to explain gynecologic malignancy susceptibility in three consecutive generations.[276]

"...The prevalence of HNPCC in the general population is likely to be closer to 1% than to 5%."[277] Prophylactic total abdominal hysterectomy and bilateral salpingo-oophorectomy is a suggested option for HNPCC syndrome patients after childbearing.[278]

D. Ataxia-Telangiectasia (A-T) and p53

The gene responsible for the inherited disease ataxia-telangiectasia (A-T) is the ATM gene. Germline ATM mutations occur in at least 8.7% of Austrian women with breast cancer. There were 11 different detrimental mutations. The penetrance is 85% at age 60. The risk of breast cancer in A-T is similar to other breast cancer genes. "The prevalence of ATM mutations in the Austrian HBOC families was similar to that of BRCA2 and about half of that for BRCA1." None of the patients with ATM mutations had BRCA mutations.[279]

The abstract did not make clear the number of patients with ovarian cancer.

The most common somatic genetic event in ovarian cancer is a mutation of the p53 gene.

"In addition to germline BRCA1 and BRCA2 mutations, somatic p53 alterations leading to p53 accumulation are an important event in hereditary ovarian cancer and are as frequent as in non-BRCA-related ovarian cancer." The range was 60–69%.[271]

References

1. Di Saia, P. J., and Creasman, W. T. (2002). "Clinical Gynecologic Oncology" 6th Edition, Chap. 11, pp. 289–350. Mosby, Inc, St. Louis, MD.
2. Barber, H. R. K. (1993). "Ovarian Carcinoma, Etiology, Diagnosis and Treatment," 3rd Edition, p. 87. Springer-Verlag, New York.
3. Vine, M. F., Ness, R. B., Calingaert, B., and Schildkraut, J. M. (2001). Types and duration of symptoms prior to diagnosis of invasive or borderline ovarian tumor. *Gynecol. Oncol.* 83, 466–471.
4. Eltabbakh, G. H., Yadev, P. R., and Morgan, A. (1999). Clinical picture of women with early stage ovarian cancer. *Gynecol. Oncol.* 75, 476–479.
5. Ranney, B., and Ahmad, M. I. (1979). Early identification, differentiation and treatment of ovarian neoplasia. *Brit. J. Gynaecol. Obstet.* 17, 209–218.
6. Lee, H.-R., Lennon, V. A., Camilleri, M., and Prather, C. M. (2001). Paraneoplastic gastrointestinal motor dysfunction: clinical and laboratory characteristics. *Am. J. Gastroenterol.* 96, 373–379.
7. Hockstein, S., Keh, P., Lurain, J. R., and Fishman, D. A. (1997). Ovarian carcinoma initially presenting as metastatic axillary lymphadenopathy. *Gynecol. Oncol.* 65, 543–547.
8. Brown, D. L., Zou, K. H., Tempany, C. M., Frates, M. C., Silverman, S. G., McNeil, B. J., and Kurtz, A. B. (2001). Primary versus secondary ovarian malignancy: imaging findings of adnexal mass in the Radiology Diagnostic Oncology Group Study. *Radiology* 219, 213–218.
9. Williams, S. D., Gershenson, D. M., Horowitz, C. J., and Silva, E. (2000). Ovarian germ-cell tumors *In* "Principles and Practice of Gynecologic Oncology," 3rd Edition. (W. J. Hoskins, C. A. Perry, and R. C. Young, eds.), Chap. 35, pp, 1059–1074. Lippincott, Williams & Wilkins, New York.
10. Berek, J. S., and Hacker, N. F. (2000). "Practical Clinical Gynecology," 3rd Edition, Chap. 12, 523, Lippincott, Williams, & Wilkins, New York.

11. Scully, R. E., Young, R. H., and Clement, P. B. (1998). "Atlas of Tumor Pathology. Third Series Fascicle 23. Tumors of the Ovary, Maldeveloped Gonads, Fallopian Tube and Broad Ligament." Chap. 9, p. 169. Armed Forces Institute of Pathology, Washington D.C.
12. Malchoff, C. D. (2000). Editorial: Carney complex—clarity and complexity. *J. Clin. Endocrinol. Metab.* 85, 4010–4012.
13. Madsen, E., Lidegaard, O., and Tabor, A. (1993). Oophorectomy in the prevention of ovarian cancer. *Acta. Obstet. Gynecol. Scand.* 72, 599–600.
14. Dekel, A., Efrat, Z., Orvieto, R., Levy, T., Dicker, D., Gal, R., and Ben-Rafael, Z. (1996). The residual ovary syndrome: A 20-year experience. *Eur. J. Obstet. Gynecol. Reprod. Biol.* 68, 159–164.
15. Carey, M. P., and Slack, M. C. (1996). GnRH analogue in assessing chronic pelvic pain in women with residual ovaries. *Brit. J. Obstet. Gynaecol.* 103, 150–153.
16. Rane, A., and Ohizua, O. (1998). "Acute" residual ovary syndrome. *Aust. NZ. J. Obstet. Gynaecol.* 38, 447–448.
17. Vavilis, D., Loufopoulos, A., Agorastos, T., Vakiani, M., Intzesiloglou, K., Kravida, A., and Brontis, J. N. (2000). Ovarian remnant syndrome: A case report and review of the literature. *Clin. Exp. Obstet. Gynecol.* 27, 121–122.
18. Nezhat, C. H., Seidman, D. S., Nezhat, F. R., Mirmalek, S. A., and Nezhat, C. R. (2000). Ovarian remnant syndrome after laparoscopic oophorectomy. *Fertil. Steril.* 74, 1024–1028.
19. Narayansingh, G., Cumming, G., Parkin, D., and Miller, I. (2000). Ovarian cancer developing in the ovarian remnant syndrome: A case report and literature review. *Aust. NZ. J. Obstet. Gynaecol.* 40, 221–223.
20. Burke, M., Talerman, A., Carlson, J. A., and Bibbo, M. (1997). Residual ovarian tissue mimicking malignancy in a patient with mucinous carcinoid tumor of the ovary. A case report. *Acta. Cytol.* 41, (4 Suppl.) 1377–1380.
21. Siddall-Allum, J., Rae, T., Rogers, V., Witherow, R., Flanagan, A., and Beard, R. W. (1994). Chronic pelvic pain caused by residual ovaries and ovarian remnants. *Br. J. Obstet. Gynaecol.* 101, 979–985.
22. Elkins, T. E., Stocker, R. J., Key, D., McGuire, E. J., and Roberts, J. A. (1994). Surgery for ovarian remnant syndrome. *J. Reprod. Med.* 39, 446–448.
23. Koch, M. O., Coussens, D., and Burnett, L. (1994). The ovarian remnant syndrome and ureteral obstruction: medical management. *J. Urol.* 152, 158–160.
24. Papathanasiou, K., Papageorgiou, C., and Tsonoglou, D. (1998). A case of Meigs' syndrome with a gigantic granulosa ovarian tumor. *Clin. Exp. Obstet. Gynecol.* 25, 61–63.
25. Long, C. Y., Chen, Y. H., Chen, S. C., Lee, J. N., Su, J.H., and Hsu, S. C. (2001). Pseudo-Meigs' syndrome and elevated levels of tumor markers associated with benign ovarian tumors. Two case reports. *Kaohsiung J. Med. Sci.* 17, 582–585.
26. Huh, J. J., Montz, F. J., and Bristow, R. E. (2002). Struma ovarii associated with pseudo-Meigs' syndrome and elevated serum CA125. *Gynecol. Oncol.* 86, 231–234.
27. Ramondetta, L. M., Carlson, J. A., and Schwarting, R. (1997). Atypical Meigs' syndrome and bilateral ovarian stromal hyperplasia. A case report. *J. Reprod. Med.* 42, 603–605.
28. Brown, R. S., Marley, J. L., and Cassoni, A. M. (1998). Pseudo-Meigs' syndrome due to broad ligament leiomyoma: A mimic of metastatic ovarian carcinoma. *Clin. Oncol. (R. Coll. Radiol.)* 10, 198–201.
29. Giannacopoulos, K., Giannacopoulou, C., Matalliotakis, I., Neonaki, M., Papanicolaou, N., and Koumatakis, E. (1998). Pseudo-Meigs' syndrome caused by paraovarian fibroma. *Eur. J. Gynaecol. Oncol.* 19, 389–390.
30. Amant, F., Gabriel, C., and Timmerman, D. (2001). Pseudo-Meigs' syndrome caused by a hydropic degenerating uterine leiomyoma with elevated CA 125. *Gynecol. Oncol.* 83, 153–157.
31. Abramov, Y., Anteby, S. O., Fasouliotis, S. J., and Barak, V. (2001). Markedly elevated levels of vascular endothelial growth factor, fibroblastic growth factor, and interleukin 6 in Meigs syndrome. *Am. J. Obstet. Gynecol.* 184, 354–355.
32. Meden, H., and Fattahi-Meibodi, A. (1998). CA 125 in benign gynecological conditions. *Int. J. Biol. Markers* 13, 231–237.
33. Abad, A., Cazorla, E., Ruiz, F., Aznar, I., Asins, E., and Llixiona, J. (1999). Meigs' syndrome with elevated CA 125: Case report and review of the literature. *Eur. J. Obstet. Gynecol. Reprod. Biol.* 82, 97–99.
34. Bognoni, V., Quartuccio, A., Jr., and Quartuccio, A. (1999). [Meigs' syndrome with high blood levels of CA 125. Clinical case and review of the literature.] [Italian]. *Minerva Ginecol.* 51, 509–512.
35. Migishima, F., Jobo, T., Hata, H., Sato, R., Ikeda, Y., Arai, M., and Kuramoto, H. (2000). Uterine leiomyoma causing massive ascites and left pleural effusion with elevated CA 125: A case report. *J. Obstet. Gynaecol. Res.* 26, 283–287.
36. Dunn, J. S., Jr., Anderson, C. D., Method, M. W., and Brost, B. C. (1998). Hydropic degenerating leiomyoma presenting as Pseudo-Meigs syndrome with elevated CA 125. *Obstet. Gynecol.* 92, (4 Pt. 2) 648–649.
37. Patsner, B. (2000). Meigs syndrome and "false positive" preoperative serum CA-125 levels: Analysis of ten cases. *Eur. J. Gynaecol. Oncol.* 21, 362–363.
38. Rouzier, R., Berger, A., and Cugenc, P. H. (1998). [Meigs' syndrome: is it possible to make a preoperative diagnosis?] [French]. *J. Gynecol. Biol. Reprod.* (Paris) 27, 517–522.
39. Chen, F. C., Fink, R. L., and Jolly, H. (1995). Meigs' syndrome in association with a locally invasive adenocarcinoma of the fallopian tube. *Aust. N.Z. J. Surg.* 65, 761–762.
40. Bridgewater, J. A., and Rustin, G. J. S. (1997). Case Report. Pseudo-Meigs' syndrome secondary to an ovarian germ cell tumor. *Gynecol. Oncol.* 66, 539–541.
41. Pratt-Thomas, H. R., Kreutner, A., Jr., Underwood, P. B., and Dondeswell, R. H. (1976). Proliferative and malignant Brenner tumors of ovary. Report of two cases, one with Meigs' syndrome, review of literature, and ultrastructural comparisons. *Gynecol. Oncol.* 42, 176–193.
42. Aoshima, M., Tanaka, H., Takahashi, M., Nakamura, K., and Makino, I. (1995). Meigs' syndrome due to Brenner tumor mimicking lupus peritonitis in a patient with systemic lupus erythematosus. *Am. J. Gastroenterol.* 90, 657–658.
43. Wiatrowska, B., Krajci, B., and Berner, A. (2000). [Pseudo-Meigs' syndrome] [Norwegian]. *Tidsskr. Nor. Laegeforen.* 120, 364–366.
44. Nagakura, S., Shirai, Y., and Hatakeyama, K. (2000). Pseudo-Meigs' syndrome caused by secondary ovarian tumors from gastrointestinal cancer. A case report and review of the literature. *Dig. Surg.* 17, 418–419.
45. Ollendorff, A. T., Keh, P., Hoff, F., Lurain, J. R., and Fishman, D. A. (1997). Leiomyoma causing massive ascites, right pleural effusion, and respiratory distress. A case report. *J. Reprod. Med.* 42, 609–612.
46. Bretella, F., Portier, M. P., Boubli, L., and Houvenaeghel, G. (2000). [Recurrence of Demons-Meigs' syndrome. A case report.] [French]. *Ann. Chir.* 125, 269–272.
47. Yang, Y. Y., Fung, C. P., and Chiang, J. H. (1999). Genital tuberculosis with peritonitis mimicking Meigs' syndrome: A case report. *J. Microbiol. Immunol. Infect.* 32, 217–221.
48. Meigs, J. V., and Cass, J. W. (1937). Fibroma of the ovary with ascites and hydrothorax, with a report of seven cases. *Am. J. Obstet. Gynecol.* 33, 249–267.
49. Lurie, S. (2000). Meigs' syndrome: The history of the eponym. *Eur. J. Obstet. Gynecol. Reprod. Biol.* 92, 199–204.
50. Menzin, A. W. (1998). Letter to the editor. A Case of pseudo-Meigs' syndrome secondary to an ovarian germ cell tumor. *Gynecol. Oncol.* 70, 441.
51. Barbieri, R. L., and Ryan, K. J. (1983). Hyperandrogenism, insulin resistance, and acanthosis nigricans syndrome: A common endocrinopathy with distinct pathophysiologic features. *Am. J. Obstet. Gynecol.* 147, 90–101.
52. Tackling polycystic ovary syndrome. (2001). *Drug Ther. Bull.* 29, 1–5.
53. Arslanian, S. A., Lewy, V. D., and Danadian, K. (2001). Glucose intolerance in obese adolescents with polycystic ovary syndrome: Roles of

insulin resistance and beta-cell dysfunction and risk of cardiovascular disease. *J. Clin. Endocrinol. Metab.* 86, 66–71.

54. Korhonen, S., Hippelainen, M., Niskanen, L., Vanhala, M., and Saarikoski, S. Relationship of the metabolic syndrome and obesity to polycystic ovary syndrome: A controlled, population-based study. *Am. J. Obstet. Gynecol.* 184, 289–296.
55. Esperanza, L. E., and Fenske, N. A. (1996). Hyperandogenism, insulin resistance, and acanthosis nigricans syndrome: Spontaneous remission in a 15-year-old girl. *J. Am. Acad. Dermatol.* 34, 892–897 (5 Pt 2).
56. Winter, R. M., and Baraitser, M. (1991). "Multiple Congenital Anomalies: A Diagnostic Compendium," p. 539. Chapman and Hall Medical, New York.
57. Boor, R., Herwig, J., Schrezenmeir, J. *et. al.* (1993). Familial insulin resistant diabetes associated with acanthosis nigricans, polycystic ovaries, hypogonadism, pigmentary retinopathy, labyrinthine deafness, and mental retardation. *Am. J. Med. Genet.* 45, 649–653.
58. Blanc, F., Hillion, B., Rass, B., Vexiau, P., Lazrak, R., and Civatt, J. (1990). [Werner's syndrome with early onset with hyperandrogenism caused by ovarian hyperthecosis, acanthosis nigricans and peripheral neuropathy.] [French]. *Ann. Dermatol. Venereol.* 117, 785–786.
59. Wiedemann, H. R., Kunze, J., and Grosse, F. R. (1997). "Clinical Syndrome," 3rd Edition, p. 318, #155.
60. McElhinney, B., and McClure, N. (2000). Ovarian hyperstimulation syndrome. *Baillieres Best Pract. Res. Clin. Obstet. Gynaecol.* 14, 103–122.
61. Whelan, J. G., 3rd, and Vlahos, N. F. (2000). The ovarian hyperstimulation syndrome. *Fertil. Steril.* 73, 883–896.
62. Chen, C. D., Chen, H. F., Lu, H. F., Chen, S. U., Ho, H. N., and Yang, Y. S. (2000). Value of serum and follicular fluid cytokine profile in the prediction of moderate to severe ovarian hyperstimulation syndrome. *Hum. Reprod.* 15, 1037–1042.
63. Barbieri, R. L. (2000). Induction of ovulation in infertile women with hyperandrogenism and insulin resistance. *Am. J. Obstet. Gynecol.* 183, 1412–1418.
64. Mathur, R. S., Akande, A. V., Keay, S. D., Hunter, L. P., and Jenkins, J. M. (2000). Distinction between early and late ovarian hyperstimulation syndrome. *Fertil. Steril.* 73, 901–907.
65. Belaen, B., Geerinckx, K., Vergauwe, P., and Thys, J. (2001). Internal jugular vein thrombosis after ovarian stimulation: Case report. *Hum. Reprod.* 16, 510–512.
66. Schanzer, A., Rockman, C. B., Jacobowitz, G. R., and Riles, T. S. (2000). Internal jugular vein thrombosis in association with the ovarian hyperstimulation syndrome. *J. Vasc. Surg.* 31, 815–818.
67. Loret de Mola, J. R., Kiwi, R., Austin, C., and Goldfarb, J. M. (2000). Subclavian deep vein thrombosis associated with the use of recombinant follicle-stimulating hormone (Gonal-F) complicating mild ovarian hyperstimulation syndrome. *Fertil. Steril.* 73, 1253–1256.
68. Lamon, D., Chang, C. K., Hruska, L., Kerlakian, G., and Smith, J. M. (2000). Superior vena cava thrombosis after *in vitro* fertilization: Case report and review of the literature. *Ann. Vasc. Surg.* 14, 2883–2885.
69. Cil, T., Tummon, I. S., House, A. A., Taylor, B., Hooker, G., Franklin, J., Rankin, R., and Carey, M. A tale of two syndromes: Ovarian hyperstimulation and abdominal compartment. *Hum. Reprod.* 15, 1058–1060.
70. Evbuomwan, I. O., Fenwick, J. D., Shiels, R., Herbert, M., and Murdoch, A. P. (1999). Severe ovarian hyperstimulation syndrome following salvage of empty follicle syndrome. *Hum. Reprod.* 14, 1707–1709.
71. Khalaf, Y., Anderson, H., Tayor, A., and Braude, P. (2000). Two rare events in one patient undergoing assisted conception: empty follicle syndrome and ovarian hyperstimulation with the sole administration of a gonadotropin-releasing hormone agonist. *Fertil. Steril.* 73, 171–172.
72. Jung, B. G., and Kim, H. (2001). Severe spontaneous ovarian hyperstimulation syndrome with MR findings. *J. Comput. Assist. Tomogr.* 25, 215–217.
73. Sauer, M. V. (2001). Defining the incidence of serious complications experienced by oocyte donors: A review of 1000 cases. *Am. J. Obstet. Gynecol.* 184, 277–278.
74. Uhler, M. L., Budinger, G. R., Gabram, S. G., and Zinaman, M. J. Perforated duodenal ulcer associated with ovarian hyperstimulation syndrome: case report. *Hum. Reprod.* 16, 174–176.
75. Ohata, Y., Harada, T., Ito, M., Yoshida, S., Iwabe, T., and Terakawa, N. (2000). Coasting may reduce the severity of the ovarian hyperstimulation syndrome in patients with polycystic ovary syndrome. *Gynecol. Obstet. Invest.* 50, 186–188.
76. Costabile, L., Unfer, V., Manna, C., Gerli, S., Rossetti, D., and Di Renzo, G. C. (2000). Use of intramuscular progesterone versus albumin for the prevention of ovarian hyperstimulation syndrome. *Gynecol. Obstet. Invest.* 50, 182–185.
77. Kol, S., and Itskovitz-Eldor, J. (2000). Severe OHSS: Yes, there is a strategy to prevent it! *Hum. Reprod.* 15, 2266–2267.
78. Summaria, V., Speca, S., and Mirk, P. (1998). Ovarian factor infertility. *Rays* 23, 709–726.
79. Hilgers, T. W., Kimball, C. R., Keck, S. J., *et al.* (1992). Assessment of the empty follicle syndrome by transvaginal sonography. *J. Ultrasound Med.* 11, 313–316.
80. Zreik, T. G., Garcia-Velasco, J. A., Vergara, T. M., Arici, A., Olive, D., and Jones, E. E. (2000). Empty follicle syndrome: Evidence for recurrence. *Hum. Reprod.* 15, 999–1002.

80a. Isik, A. Z., and Vicdan, K. (2000). Borderline form of empty follice syndrome: Is it really an entity? *Eur. J. Obstet. Gynecol. Reprod. Biol.* 88, 213–215.

81. Soliman, A. T., Rajab, A., AlSalmi, I., and Asfour, M. G. (1996). Empty sellae, impaired testosterone secretion, and defective hypothalamic-pituitary growth and gonadal axes in children with Bardet-Biedl syndrome. *Metabolism* 45, 1230–1234.
82. Jones, K. L. (1997). "Smith's Recognizable Patterns of Human Malformation," 5th Edition, p. 510. W.B. Saunders Co., Philadelphia.
83. Batista, M. C., Kohek, M. B., Frazzatto, E. S., Fragoso, M. C., Mendonca, B. B., and Latronico, A. C. (2000). Mutation analysis of the follicle-stimulating hormone receptor gene in girls with gonadotropin-independent precocious puberty resulting from autonomous cystic ovaries. *Fertil. Steril.* 73, 280–283.
84. Pienkowski, C., Lumbroso, S., Bieth, E., Sultan, C., Rochiccioli, P., and Tauber, M. (1997). Recurrent ovarian cyst and mutation of the Gs alpha gene in ovarian cyst fluid cells: What is the link with McCune-Albright syndrome? *Acta. Paediatr.* 86, 1019–1021.
85. Maubon, A., Ferru, J. M., Thiebaut, C., Berger, V., Hoche, N., and Rouanet, J. P. (1997). [Left ovarian syndrome] [French]. *J. Radiol.* 78, 223–225.
86. Mathis, B. V., Miller, J. S., Lukens, M. L., and Paluzzi, M. W. (1995). Pelvic congestion syndrome: A new approach to an unusual problem. *Am. Surg.* 61, 1016–1018.
87. Maleux, G., Stockx, L., Wilms, G., and Marchal, G. (2000). Ovarian vein embolization for the treatment of pelvic congestion syndrome: Long-term technical and clinical results. *J. Vasc. Interv. Radiol.* 11, 859–864.
88. Cordts, P. R., Eclavea, A., Buckley, P. J., DeMaioribus, C. A., Cockerill, M. L., and Yeager, T. D. (1988). Pelvic congestion syndrome: Early clinical results after transcatheter ovarian vein embolization. *J. Vasc. Surg.* 28, 862–868.
89. Rozenblit, A. M., Ricci, Z. J., Tuvia, J., and Amis, E. S., Jr. (2001). Incompetent and dilated ovarian veins: A common CT finding in asymptomatic parous women. *A.J.R. Am. J. Roentgenol.* 176, 119–122.
90. Burlet, G., and Judlin, P. (1994). [Acute pelvic pain syndrome. Diagnostic and therapeutic approach in women.] [French]. *Rev. Fr. Gynecol. Obstet.* 89, 537–542.
91. Bruns, A. D., Fishkin, P. A., Johnson, E. A., and Lee, Y. T. (1994). Munchausen's syndrome and cancer. *J. Surg. Oncol.* 56, 136–138.

92. Chen, C. P., Yang, Y. C., Lin, S. P., Wang, W., Chang, C. L., and Chang, K. M. (2002). Bilateral calcified ovarian fibromas in a patient with Sotos syndrome. *Fertil. Steril.* 77, 1285–1287.
93. Dumont-Herskowitz, R. A., Safaii, H. S., and Senior, B. (1978). Ovarian fibromata in four successive generations. *Am. J. Obstet. Gynecol.* 93, 621–624.
94. Seracchioli, R., Bagnoli, A., Colombo, F. M., Missiroli, S., and Venturoli, S. (2001). Conservative treatment of recurrent ovarian fibromas in a young patient affected by Gorlin syndrome. *Hum. Reprod.* 16, 1261–1263.
95. Evans, D. G., Ladusans, E. J., Rimmer, S., Burnell, L. D., Thakker, N., and Farndon, P. A. (1993). Complications of the naveoid basal cell carcinoma syndrome: Results of a population based study. *J. Med. Genet.* 30, 460–464.
96. Khalifa, M. A., Patterson-Cobbs, G., Hansen, C. H., Hines, J. F., and Johnson, J. C. (1997). The occurrence of endometrial adenocarcinoma in a patient with basal cell nevus syndrome. *J. Natl. Med. Assoc.* 89, 549–552.
97. Zedan, W., Robinson, P. A., and High, A. S. (2001). A novel polymorphism in the PTC gene allows easy identification of allelic loss in basal cell nevus syndrome lesions. *Diag. Mol. Pathol.* 10, 41–45.
98. Jones, K. L. (1997). "Smith's Recognizable Patterns of Malformation," 5th Ed. p. 260. W.B. Saunders, Philadelphia.
99. Raju, R. R., Hart, W. R., Magnuson, D. K., Reid, J. R., and Rogers, D. G. (2002). Genital tract tumors in Proteus syndrome: Report of a case of bilateral paraovarian endometroid cystic tumors of borderline malignancy and review of the literature. *Mod. Pathol.* 15, 172–180.
100. Ezzeldin, K. M., Ezzeldin, A. A., Zahrani, A. J., and Al-Zaiem, M. M. (2002). Precocious puberty in a female with Proteus syndrome. *Saudi Med. J.* 23, 332–334.
101. Mena, W., Krassikoff, N., and Philips, J. B. (1991). Fused eyelids, airway anomalies, ovarian cysts, and digital abnormalities in siblings: A new autosomal recessive syndrome or a variant of Fraser syndrome? *Am. J. Med. Genet.* 40, 377–381.
102. Gattuso, J., Patton, M. A., and Baraitser, M. (1995). The clinical spectrum of the Fraser syndrome: Report of three new cases and review. *In* "Congenital Malformation Syndromes," (D. Donaii and R. M. Winter, Eds.), p. 521, Chap. 65. Chapman and Hall Medical, London.
103. Huffman, C., McCandless, D., Jasty, R., Matloub, J., Robinson, H. B., Weaver, D. D., and Cohen, M. M., Jr. Weaver syndrome with neuroblastoma and cardiovascular anomalies. *Am. J. Med. Genet.* 99, 252–255.
104. Clement, P. B., Young, R. H., Hanna, W., and Scully, R. E. (1994). Sclerosing peritonitis associated with luteinized thecomas of the ovary. A clinicopathological analysis of six cases. *Am. J. Surg. Pathol.* 18, 1–13.
105. Reginella, R. F., and Sumkin, J. H. (1996). Sclerosing peritonitis associated with luteinized thecomas. *A. J. R. Am. J. Roentgenol.* 167, 512–513.
106. Iwasa, Y., Minamiguchi, S., Konishi, I., Onodera, H., Zhou, J., and Yamabe, H. (1996). Sclerosing peritonitis associated with luteinized thecoma of the ovary. *Pathol. Int.* 46, 510–514.
107. Nishida, T., Ushijima, K., Watanabe, J., Kage, M., and Nagaoka, S. (1999). Letter: Sclerosing peritonitis associated with luteinized thecoma of the ovary. *Gynecol. Oncol.* 73, 167–169.
108. Stenram, U. (1997). Sclerosing peritonitis in a case of benign cystic ovarian teratoma: A case report. *APMIS* 105, 414–416.
109. Frigerio, L., Taccagni, G. L., Mariani, A., Mangili, G., and Ferrari, A. Idiopathic sclerosing peritonitis associated with florid mesothelial hyperplasia, ovarian fibromatosis, and endometriosis : A new disorder of abdominal mass. *Am. J. Obstet. Gynecol.* 176, 721–722.
110. Spiegel, G. W., and Swiger, F. K. (1996). Luteinized thecoma with sclerosing peritonitis presenting as an acute abdomen. *Gynecol. Oncol.* 61, 275–281.
111. Werness, B. A. (1996). Luteinized thecoma with sclerosing peritonitis. *Arch. Pathol. Lab. Med.* 120, 303–306.
112. Wirtzfeld, D. A., Petrelli, N. J., and Rodriguez-Bigas, M. A. (2001). Hamartomas polyposis syndromes: Molecular genetics, neoplastic risk, and surveillance recommendations. *Ann. Surg. Oncol.* 8, 321–327.
113. McGarrity, T. J., Kulin, H. E., and Zaino, R. J. (2000). Clinical reviews. Peutz-Jeghers syndrome. *Am. J. Gastroenterol.* 95, 596–604.
114. Peutz, J. L. A. (1921). Very remarkable case of familial polyposis of mucous membrane of intestinal tract and nasopharynx accompanied by peculiar pigmentations of skin and mucous membrane. *Ned. Mandschr. Geneesk.* 10, 134–136.
115. Jeghers, H., McKusick, V. A., and Katz, K. H. (1949). Generalized intestinal polyposis and melanin spots of the oral mucosa, lips and digits: A syndrome of diagnostic significance. *N. Engl. J. Med.* 241, 993–1005.
116. Tovar, J. A., Eizaguirre, I., Albert, A., and Jeminez, J. (1983). Peutz-Jeghers syndrome in children: Report of 2 cases and review of the literature. *J. Pediatr. Surg.* 18, 1–6.
117. Giardello, F. M., Brensinger, J. D., Tersmette, A. C., Goodman, S. N., Peterson, G. M., Booker, S. V., Cruz-Correa, M., and Offerhaus, J. A. (2000). Very high risk in familial Peutz-Jeghers syndrome. *Gastroenterology* 119, 1447–1453.
118. Boardman, L. A., Pittelkow, M. R., Couch, F. J., Schaid, D. J., McDonnel, S. K., Burgart, J. A., Schwartz, D. I., Thibodeau, S. N., and Hartman, L. C. (2000). Association of Peutz-Jeghers-like mucocutaneous pigmentation with breast and gynecologic carcinomas in women. *Medicine (Baltimore)* 79, 293–298.
119. Chen, K. T. (1986). Female genital tract tumors in Peutz-Jeghers syndrome. *Hum. Pathol.* 17, 858–861.
120. Choi, C. G., Kim, S. H., Kim, J. S., Chi, J. G., Song, E. S., and Han, M. C. (1993). Adenoma malignum of uterine cervix in Peutz-Jeghers syndrome: CT and US features. *J. Comput. Assist. Tomogr.* 17, 819–821.
121. Matseoane, S., Moscovic, E., Williams, S., and Huang, J. C. (1991). Mucinous neoplasm in the cervix associated with a mucinous neoplasm in the ovary and concurrent bilateral sex cord tumors with annular tubules: Immunohistochemical study. *Gynecol. Oncol.* 43, 300–304.
122. Lele, S. M., Sawh, R. N., Zaharopoulos, P., Adesokan, A., Smith, M., Linhart, J. M., Arrastia, C. D., and Krigman, H. R. (2000). Malignant ovarian sex cord tumor with annular tubules in a patient with Peutz-Jeghers syndrome: A case report. *Mod. Pathol.* 13, 466–470.
123. Young, R. H., Welch, W. R., Dickerson, G. R., and Scully, R. E. (1982). Ovarian sex cord tumor with annular tubules: Review of 74 cases including 27 with Peutz-Jeghers syndrome and four with adenoma malignum of the cervix. *Cancer* 50, 1384–1402.
124. Ferry, J. A., Young, R. H., Engel, G., and Scully, R. E. (1994). Oxyphilic Sertoli cell tumor of the ovary: A report of three cases, two in patients with the Peutz-Jeghers syndrome. *Int. J. Gynecol. Pathol.* 3, 259–260.
125. Zung, A., Shohan, Z., Open, M., Altman, Y., Dgani, R., and Zadik, Z. (1998). Sertoli cell tumor causing precocious puberty in a girl with Peutz-Jeghers syndrome. *Gynecol. Oncol.* 70, 421–424.
126. Young, R. H., Dickerson, G. R., and Scully, R. E. (1983). A distinctive ovarian sex cord-stromal tumor causing sexual precocity in the Peutz-Jeghers syndrome. *Am. J. Surg. Pathol.* 7, 233–243.
127. Seidman, J. D. (1994). Mucinous lesions of the fallopian tube. A report of seven cases. *Am. J. Surg. Pathol.* 12, 1205–1212.
128. Young, R. H., and Scully, R. E. (1988). Mucinous ovarian tumors associated with mucinous adenocarcinomas of the cervix. A clinicopathological analysis of 16 cases. *Int. J. Gynecol. Pathol.* 7, 99–111.
129. Shintaku, M., Baba, Y., and Fujiwara, T. (1994). Intra-abdominal desmoplastic small cell tumor in a patient with Peutz-Jeghers syndrome. *Virchow Arch.* 425, 211–215.
130. Baumgartner, G., Neuweiler, J., and Herzog, D. (2000). Peutz-Jeghers syndrome: Is family screening needed? *Pediatr. Surg. Int.* 16, 437–439.
131. Outwater, E. K., Wagner, B. J., Mannion, C., McLarney, J. K., and Kim, B. (1998). Sex cord-stromal and steroid cell tumors of the ovary. *Radiographics* 18, 1523–1546.

132. Lin, B. C., Lien, J. M., Chen, R. J., Fang, J. F., and Wong, Y. C. (2000). Combined endoscopic and surgical treatment for the polyposis of Peutz-Jeghers syndrome. *Surg. Endos.* 14, 1185–1187.
133. Amaro, R., Diaz, G., Schneider, M. D., and Stollman, N. H. (2000). Peutz-Jeghers syndrome managed with a complete intraoperative endoscopy and intenstive polypectomy. *Gastrointest. Endos.* 52, 552–554.
134. Stratakis, C. A., Kirschner, L. S., Taymans, S. E., Tomlinson, I. P., Marsh, D. J., Torpy, D. J., Giatzakis, C., Eccles, D. M., Theaker, J., Houlston, R. S., Blouin, J. L., Antonarakis, S. E., Basson, C. T., Eng, C., and Carney, J. A. (1998). Carney complex, Peutz-Jeghers syndrome, Cowden disease and Bannayan-Zonana syndrome share cutaneous and endocrine manifestations but not genetic loci. *J. Clin. Endocrinol. Metab.* 83, 2972–2976.
135. Makagawa, H., Koyama, K., Tanaka, T., Miyoshi, Y., Ando, H., Baba, S., Watatanim, M., Yasutomi, M., Monden, M., and Nakamura, Y. (1998). Localization of the gene responsible for Peutz-Jeghers syndrome within a 6-c M region of chromosome 19 p 13.3. *Hum. Genet.* 102, 203–206.
136. Entius, M. M., Keller, J. J., Westerman, A. M., van Reese, B. P., van Velthuysen, M. L., de Goeij, A. F., Wilson, J. H., Giardello, F. M., and Offerhaus, G. J. (2001). Molecular genetic alterations in hamartomatous polyps and carcinomas of patients with Peutz-Jeghers syndrome. *J. Clin. Pathol.* 54, 126–131.
137. Mi Ya Ki, M., Iijima, T., Hosono, K., Ishii, R., Yasuno, M., Mori, T., Toi, M., Hishima, T., Shitara, N., Tamura, K., Utsunomiya, J., Kobayashi, N., Kuroki, T., and Iwama, T. (2000). Somatic mutations of LKB1 and beta-catenin genes in gastrointestinal polyps from patients with Peutz-Jeghers syndrome. *Cancer Res.* 60, 6311–6313.
138. Karuman, P., Gozani, O., Odze, R. D., Zhou, X. C., Zhu, H., Shaw, R., Brian, T. P., Bozzuto, C. D., Ooi, D., Cantley, L. C., and Yuan, J. (2001). The Peutz-Jeghers gene product LKB1 is a mediation of p53-dependent cell death. *Mol. Cell.* 7, 1307–1319.
139. Sapkota, G. P., Kieloch, A., Lizcano, J. M., Lain, S., Arthur, J. S., Williams, M. R., Morrice, N., Deak, M., and Alessi, D. R. (2001). Phosphorylation of the protein kinase mutated in Peutz-Jeghers cancer syndrome, LKB1/STK11, at Ser 431 by p90 (RSK) and cAMP-dependent protein kinase, but not its farnesylation at Cys (433), is essential for LKB1 to suppress cell growth. *J. Biol. Chem.* 276, 19469–19482.
140. Wang, Z. J., Churchman, M., Campbell, I. G., Xu, W. H., Yan, Z. Y., McCluggage, W. G., Foulkes, W. D., and Tomlinson, I. P. (1999). Allele loss and mutation screen at the Peutz-Jeghers (LKB1) locus (19p13.3) in sporadic ovarian tumors. *Br. J. Cancer* 80, 70–72.
141. Connoly, D. C., Katabuchi, H., Cliby, W. A., and Cho, K. R. (2000). Somatic mutations in the STK11/LKB1 gene are uncommon in rare gynecological tumor types associated with Peutz-Jeghers syndrome. *Am. J. Pathol.* 156, 339–345.
142. Marneros, A. G., Mehenni, H., Reichenberger, E., Antonarakis, S. E., Kreig, T., and Olsen, B. R. (2001). Gene for the human transmembrane-type protein tyrosine phosphatase H (PTPRH): Genomic structure, fine-mapping and its exclusion as a candidate for Peutz-Jeghers syndrome. *Cytogenet. Cell Genet.* 92, 203–210.
143. Box, J. C., and Watne, A. L. (1995). Inherited syndromes of colon polyps. *Semin. Surg. Oncol.* 11, 394–398.
144. Stratakis, C. A., Papageorgiou, T., Premkumar, A., Pack, S., Kirschner, L. S., Taymans, S. E., Zhuang, Z., Oelkers, W. H., and Carney, J. A. (2000). Ovarian lesions in Carney complex: Clinical genetics and possible predisposition to malignancy. *J. Clin. Endocrinol. Metab.* 85, 4359–4366.
145. Stratakis, C. A., Kirschner, L. S., Taymans, S. E., Tomlinson, I. P., Marsh, D. J., Torpy, D. J., Giatzakis, C., Eccles, D. M., Theaker, J., Houlston, R. S., Blouin, J. L., Antonarakis, S. E., Basson, C. T., Eng, C., and Carney, J. A. (1998). Carney complex, Peutz-Jeghers syndrome, Cowden disease and Bannayan-Zonana syndrome share cutaneous and endocrine manifestations but not genetic loci. *J. Clin. Endocrinol. Metab.* 83, 2972–2976.
146. Boardman, L. A., Pittelkow, M. R., Couch, F. J., Schaid, D. J., McDonnell, S. K., Burgart, L. J., Ahlquist, D. A., Carney, J. A., Schwartz, D. I., Thibodeau, S. N., and Hartmann, L. C. (2000). Association of Peutz-Jeghers-like mucocutaneous pigmentation with breast and gynecologic carcinomas in women. *Medicine (Baltimore)* 79, 293–298.
147. Gell, J. S., Stannard, M. W., Ramnani, D. M., and Bradshaw, K. D. (1998). Juvenile granulosa cell tumor in a 13-year-old girl with enchondromatosis (Ollier's disease): A case report. *J. Pediatr. Adoles. Gynecol.* 11, 147–150.
148. Young, R. H., Dickerson, G. R., and Scully, R. E. (1984). Juvenile granulosa cell tumor of the ovary. A clinicopathologic analysis of 125 cases. *Am. J. Surg. Pathol.* 8, 575–596.
149. Takekawa, Y., Kimura, M., Sakakibara, M., Yoshii, R., and Shikata, T. (2001). [Pathological, cytological and immunohistochemical study of normal-sized ovary carcinoma syndrome] [Japanese]. *Rinsho Byori* 49, 66–70.
150. Yao, Z., Li, L., and Yang, H. (1998). [Normal-sized ovary carcinoma syndrome–clinical and pathological analysis of 11 cases] [Chinese]. *Zhonghua Zhong Liu Za Zhi* 20, 383–386.
151. Barber, H. R. K., and Graber, E. A. (1971). The PMPO syndrome (post-menopausal palpable ovary syndrome). *Obstet. Gynecol.* 38, 921–923.
152. Miller, R. D., Nash, J. D., Weiser, E. B., and Hoskins, W. J. (1991). The postmenopausal palpable ovary syndrome. A retrospective review with histopathologic correlates. *J. Reprod. Med.* 36, 568–571.
153. Goldstein, S. R. (1996). Postmenopausal adnexal cysts: How clinical management has evolved. *Am. J. Obstet. Gynecol.* 175, 1498–1501.
154. Geisler, J. P., Goulet, R., Foster, R. S., and Sutton, G. P. (1994). Growing teratoma syndrome after chemotherapy for germ cell tumors of the ovary. *Obstet. Gynecol.* 84, 719–721 (4 Pt 2).
155. Andre, F., Fizazi, K., Culine, S., Droz, J., Taupin, P., Lhomme, C., Terrier-Lacombe, M., and Theodore, C. (2000). The growing teratoma syndrome: Results of therapy and long-term follow-up of 33 patients. *Eur. J. Cancer* 36, 1389–1394.
156. Bilgrami, S. F., and Fallon, B. G., (1993). Tumor lysis syndrome after combination chemotherapy for ovarian cancer. *Med. Pediatr. Oncol.* 21, 521–524.
157. Esquivel, J., and Sugarbaker, P. H. (2000). Clinical presentation of the *Pseudomyxoma peritonei* syndrome. *Br. J. Surg.* 87, 1414–1418.
158. Bree, E. D., Witkamp, A., Van De Vijver, M., and Zoetmulde, F. (2000). Unusual origins of *Pseudomyxoma peritonei*. *J. Surg. Oncol.* 75, 270–274.
159. Akio, I. (2002). Cancer anorexia-cachexia syndrome: Current issues in research and management. *CA cancer j. clin.* 52, 72–91.
160. Clement, P. B., Young, R. H., and Scully, R. E. (1991). Clinical syndromes associated with tumors of the female genital tract. *Semin. Diag. Pathol.* 8, 204–233.
161. Thorstenson, Y. R., Roxas, A., Kroiss, R., Wagner, T., and Oefner, P. J. (2001). Germline carriers of ATM mutations are prevalent among Austrian hereditary breast and ovarian cancer (HBOC) patients. *Am. J. Hum. Genet.* 69 (Supplement), 205, Abstract 148.
162. Dakeishi, M., Shioya, T., Wada, Y., Shindo, T., Otaka, K., Manabe, M., Nozaki, J.-I., Inoue, S., and Koizumi, A. (2002). Research article. Genetic epidemiology of hereditary hemorrhagic telangiectasia in a local community in the northern part of Japan. *Hum. Mutat.* 19, 140–148.
163. Takahama, H., Noto, S., Ito, M., Nishimoto, H., and Tadokoro M. A case of hereditary hemorrhagic telangiectasia (Rendu-Osler-Weber's disease) with dystrophic calcinosis cutis and retinal lesions. *J. Dermatol.* 29, 512–515.
164. Gemke, G. R., Kaupasa, M. M., Rafal'skii, A. A., and Tabachuk, N. N. [Association of Rendu-Osler disease, polyarthritis and ovarian cancer.] [Russian]. *Klin. Med. (Mosk.)* 72, 65–66.

165. Nichols, K. E., Malkin, D., Garber, J. E., Fraumeni, J. F., Jr., and Li, F. P. (2001). Hypothesis. Germ-line p53 mutations predispose to a wide spectrum of early-onset cancers. *Cancer Epidemiol. Biomarkers Prev.* 10, 83–87.
166. Chompret, A. (2002). The Li-Fraumeni syndrome. *Biochimie* 84, 75–82.
167. Kruse, R., Rutten, A., Hosseiny-Malayeri, H. R., Bisceglia, M., Friedl, W., Propping, P., Ruzicka, T., and Mangold, E. (2001). "Second hit" in sebaceous tumors from Muir-Torre patients with germline mutations in MSH2: Allele loss is not the preferred mode of inactivation. *J. Invest. Dermatol.* 116, 463–465.
168. Rigel, D. S., and Jacobs, M. I. (1980). Malignant acanthosis nigricans: A review. *J. Dermatol. Surg. Oncol.* 6, 923–927.
169. Evans, T. R., Mansi, J. L., and Bevan, D. H. (1996). Trousseau's syndrome in association with ovarian carcinoma. *Cancer* 77, 2544–2549.
170. Maede, Y., Fujiwaki, R., Watanabe, Y., Hata, K., and Miyazaki, K. (1999). Bilateral granulose cell tumor in a patient with blepharophimosis syndrome. *Gynecol. Oncol.* 73, 335–336.
171. Prinssen, H. M., Hoekman, K., and Burger, C. W. (1999). Clostridium septicum myonecrosis and ovarian cancer: A case report and review of the literature. *Gynecol. Oncol.* 72, 116–119.
172. Kukhtevich, A. V., Russkikh, A. V., Kuznetsova, A. I., and Gorbacheva, E. N. [Paraneoplastic syndrome (fever, anemia, migrating thrombophlebitis) in ovarian cancer.] [Russian]. *Ter. Arkh.* 71, 46–48.
173. Smucker, J. D., Roth, L. M., Sutton, G. P., and Hurteau, J. A. (1999). Trisomy 21 associated with ovarian dysgerminoma. *Gynecol. Oncol.* 74, 512–514.
174. Hasle, H., Clemmensen, I. H., and Mikkelsen, M. (2000). [Incidence of cancer in individuals with Down syndrome.] [Dutch]. *Tidsskr. Nor. Laegeforen.* 120, 2878–2881.
175. Neary, B., Young, S. B., Reuter, K. L., Cheeseman, S., and Savarese, D. (1996). Ovarian Burkitt lymphoma: Pelvic pain in a woman with AIDS. *Obstet. Gynecol.* 88, 706–608 (4 Pt 2).
176. Nadal, D., Caduff, R., Frey, E., Hassam, S., Zimmerman, D. R., Seigneurin, J. M., and Pluss, H. J. (1994). Non-Hodgkin's lymphoma in four children infected with the human immunodeficiency virus. Association with Epstein-Barr virus and treatment. *Cancer* 73, 224–230.
177. McCluggage, W. G., Bryson, C., Lamki, H., and Boyle, D. D. (2000). Benign, borderline, and malignant endometrioid neoplasia arising in endometriosis in association with tamoxifen therapy. *Int. J. Gynecol. Pathol.* 19, 276–279.
178. Seoud, M., Salem, Z., Shamseddine, A., Khabbaz, A., Zaatari, G., and Khalil, A. (1999). Papillary serous carcinoma of the ovary following prolonged tamoxifen treatment. *Eur. J. Gynaecol. Oncol.* 20, 237–239.
179. Lacy, J. V., Mink, P. J., Lubin, J. H., Sherman, M. E., Troisi, R., Hartge, P., Schatzin, A., and Schairer, C. (2002). Menopausal hormone replacement therapy and risk of ovarian cancer. *JAMA* 288, 334–341.
180. Noller, K. L. (2002). Estrogen replacement therapy and risk of ovarian cancer. *JAMA* 288, 369.
181. Liu, S., Tunkel, R., Lachmann, E., and Nagler, W. (2000). Paraneoplastic cerebellar degneration as the first evidence of cancer: A case report. *Arch. Phys. Med. Rehab.* 81, 834–836.
182. Greenlee, J. E., Dalman, J., Lyons, T., Clawson, S., Smith, R. H., and Pirch, H. R. (1999). Association of anti-Yo (type I) antibody with paraneoplastic cerebellar degeneration in the setting of transitional cell carcinoma of the bladder: Detection of Yo antigen in tumor tissue and fall in antibody titers following tumor removal. *Ann. Neurol.* 45, 805–809.
183. Lin, J. T., Lachmann, E., and Nagler, W. (2001). Paraneoplastic cerebellar degeneration as the first manifestation of cancer. *J. Womens. Health Gend. Based Med.* 10, 495–502.
184. Geomini, P. M., Dellemijin, P. L., and Bremer, G. L. (2001). Paraneoplastic cerebellar degeneration: Neurological symptoms pointing to occult ovarian cancer. *Gynecol. Obstet. Invest.* 52, 145–146.
185. Forgy, A. P., Ewing, T. L., and Flaningam, J. (2001). Two paraneoplastic syndromes in a patient with ovarian cancer: Nephrotic syndrome and paraneoplastic cerebellar degeneration. *Gynecol. Oncol.* 80, 96–98.
186. Aydiner, A., Gurvit, H., and Baral, I. (1998). Paraneoplastic limbic encephalitis with immature ovarian teratoma—a case report. *J. Neurooncol* 37, 63–66.
187. Trivedi, R., Mundanthanam, G., Amyes, E., Lang, B., and Vincent, A. (2000). Autoantibody screening in subacute cerebellar ataxia. *Lancet* 356, 565–566.
188. Okano, H. J., Park, W. Y., Corradi, J. P., and Darnell, R. B. (1999). The cystoplasmic Purkinje onconeuronal antigen cdr2 down-regulates c-Myc function: Implications for neuronal and tumor cell survival. *Genes. Dev.* 13, 2087–2097.
189. Drlicek, M., Bianchi, G., Bogliun, G., Casati, B., Griswold, W., Kolig, C., Liszka-Setinek, U., Marzorati, L., Wondrusch, E., and Cavaletti, G. (1997). Antibodies of the anti-Yo and anti-Ri type in the absence of paraneoplastic neurological syndromes: A long-term survey of ovarian cancer patients. *J. Neurol.* 244, 85–89.
190. Atoine, J. C., Absi, L., Honnorat, J., Boulesteix, J. M., de Brouker, T., Vial, C., Butler, M., DeCamilli, P., and Michel, D. (1999). Antiamphiphysin antibodies are associated with various paraneoplastic neurological syndromes and tumors. *Arch. Neurol.* 56, 172–177.
191. Albert, M. L., Darnell, J. C., Bender, A., Francisco, L. M., Bhardwaj, N., and Darnell, R. B. (1998). Tumor-specific killer cells in paraneoplastic cerebellar degeneration. *Nat. Med.* 11, 1321–1324.
192. Kaiser, R. (1999). [Paraneoplastic neurologic syndromes. Diagnostic and pathogenic significance of autoantibodies] [German]. *Nervenartz* 70, 688–701.
193. Chabriat, H., Chen, Q. M., Poisson, M., and Delattre, J. Y. (1994). [Paraneoplastic cerebellar degeneration.] [French]. *Rev. Neurol. (Paris)* 150, 105–114.
194. Rosenbaum, T., Gartner, J., Korholz, D., Janssen, G., Schneider, D., Engelbrecht, V., Gobel, U., and Lenard, H. G. (1998). Paraneoplastic limbric encephalitis in two teenage girls. *Neuropediatrics* 29, 159–162.
195. Khwaja, S., Sripathi, N., Ahmad, B. K., and Lennon, V. A. (1998). Paraneoplastic motor neuron disease with type 1 Purkinje cell antibodies. *Muscle Nerve* 21, 943–945.
196. Jongren, J. L., Moll, N. J., Sillevis Smitt, P. A., Vecht, C. J., and Tijssen, C. C. (1998). Anti-Ri positive opsoclonus-myoclonus-ataxia in ovarian duct cancer. *J. Neurol.* 245, 691–692.
197. Taylor, R. B., Mason, W., Kong, V., and Wennberg, R. (1999). Reversible paraneoplastic encephalomyelitis associated with a benign ovarian teratoma. *Can. J. Neurol. Sci.* 26, 317–320.
198. Nokura, K., Yamamoto, H., Okawara, Y., Koga, H., Osawa, H., and Sakai, K. (1997). Reversible limbic encephalitis caused by ovarian teratoma. *Acta Neurol. Scand.* 95, 367–73.
199. Belanescu, I., Colita, D., Moicean, A., Dutu, R., Stanculescu, M., and Voinea, S. (1998). [A case of disseminated intravascular coagulation—a paraneoplastic manifestation of a borderline ovarian tumor.] [Romanian]. *Chirurgia (Bucur)* 93, 331–341.
199a. Jahn, K., Pfefferkorn, T., Gropp, M., Hamann, G., and Pfister, H. W. (1999). [Cerebral ischemia as initial manifestation of neoplastic low-malignancy changes. 2 case reports and review of the literature] [German]. *Nervenarzt* 70, 342–348.
200. Marlier, S., Civatte, M., de Jaureguiberry, J. P., Yao, N., Gisserot, O., Kologo, K., and Jaubert, D. (1999). [Subacute paraneoplastic cerebellar degeneration preceding cerebellar metastasis of ovarian origin. Two rare complications of ovarian cancer.] [French]. *Pressee Med.* 28, 1018.
201. Abrey, L. E., and Dalmau, J. O. (1999). Neurologic complications of ovarian carcinoma. *Cancer* 85, 127–133.
202. Cano, J. R., Catalan, B., and Jara, C. (1998). [Neuropathy due to cisplatin.] [Spanish]. *Rev. Neurol.* 27, 606–610.

203. Pothuri, B., Chi, D. S., Reid, T., Aghajanian, C., Venkatraman, E., Alektiar, K., Bilsky, M., and Barakat, R. R. (2002). Craniotomy for central nervous system metastases in epithelial ovarian cancer. *Gynecol. Oncol.* 87, 133–137.
204. Callen, J. P. (2000). Dermatomyositis. *Lancet* 355, 53–57.
205. Callen, J. P., Jorizzo, J., Greer, K. E., Penneys, N., Piette, W., and Zone, J. J. (1988). "Dermatological Signs of Internal Disease." W. B. Saunders Co., Philadelphia, PA.
206. Kubo, M., Sato, S., Kitahara, H., Tsuchida, T., and Tamaki, K. (1996). Vesicle formation in dermatomyositis associated with gynecologic malignancies. *J. Am. Acad. Dermatol.* 34, 391–394.
207. Whitmore, S. E., Anhalt, G. J., Provost, T. T., Zacur, H. A., Hamper, U. M., Helzlsouer, K. J., and Rosenshein, N. B. (1997). Serum CA-125 screening for ovarian cancer in patients with dermatomyositis. *Gynecol. Oncol.* 65, 241–244.
208. Whitmore, S. E., Rosenshein, N. B., and Provost, T. T. (1994). Ovarian cancer in patients with dermatomyositis. *Medicine (Baltimore)* 73, 153–160.
209. Hill, C. L., Zhang, Y., Sigurgeirsson, B., Pukkala, E., Mellemkjaer, L., Airio, A., Evans, S. R., and Felson, D. T. (2001). Frequency of specific cancer types in dermatomyositis and polymyositis: A population-based study. *Lancet* 357, 96–100.
210. Verducci, M. A., Malkasian, G. D., Friedman, S. J., and Winkelmann, R. K. (1984). Gynecologic carcinoma associated with dermatomyositis-polymyositis. *Obstet. Gynecol.* 64, 695–698.
211. Scaling, S. T., Kaufman, R. H., and Patten, B. M. (1979). Dermatomyositis and female malignancy. *Obstet. Gynecol.* 54, 474–477.
212. Maoz, C. R., Langevitz, P., Livneh, A., Blumstein, Z., Sadeh, M., Bank, I., Gur, H., and Ehrenfeld, M. (1998). High incidence of malignancies in patients with dermatomyositis and polymyositis: An 11-year analysis. *Semin. Arthritis. Rheum.* 27, 319–324.
213. Davis, M. D., and Ahmed, I. (1997). Ovarian malignancy in patients with dermatomyositis and polymyositis: A retrospective analysis of fourteen cases. *J. Am. Acad. Dermatol.* 37, 730–733.
214. Piura, B., Meirovitz, M., Cohen, Y., and Horowitz, J. (1999). Dermatomyositis and peritoneal papillary serous carcinoma. *Eur. J. Obstet. Gynecol. Reprod. Biol.* 82, 93–96.
215. Voravud, N., Dimopoulos, M., Hortobagyi, G., Ross, M., and Theriault, R. (1991). Breast cancer and second primary ovarian cancer in dermatomyositis. *Gynecol. Oncol.* 43, 286–290.
216. Solomon, S. D., and Maurer, K. H. (1983). Letter: Association of dermatomyositis and dysgerminoma in a 16-year-old patient. *Arthr. Rheumatol.* 26, 572–573.
217. Legrain, S., Raguin, G., and Piette, J. C. (1999). Digital necrosis revealing ovarian cancer. *Dermatology* 199, 183–184.
218. Chtourou, M., Aubin, F., Savariault, I., Chabot, P., Manchet, G., Montcuquet, P., and Humbert, P. (1998). Digital necrosis and lupus-like syndrome preceding ovarian carcinoma. *Dermatology* 196, 348–349.
219. Spadaro, A., Riccieri, V., Sili-Scavalli, A., Innocenzi, D., Pranteda, G., and Taccari, E. (1994). [Value of cytological analysis of the synovial fluid in multicentric reticulohistiocytosis. A case.] [French]. *Rev. Rhum. Ed. Fr.* 61(7–8), 554–557.
220. Ruffatti, A., Aversa, S., Del Ross, T., Tonetto, S., Fiorentino, M., and Todesco, S. (1994). Antiphospholipid antibody syndrome associated with ovarian cancer. A new paraneoplastic syndrome? *J. Rheumatol.* 21, 2162–2163.
221. Braverman, I. (1998). "Skin Signs of Systemic Disease," 3rd Edition. W. B. Saunders, Philadelphia, PA.
222. Requena, L., Aguilar, A., Renedo, G., Martin, L., Pique, E., Farina, M., and Escalonilla, P. (1995). Tripe palms: A cutaneous marker of internal malignancy. *J. Dermatol.* 22, 492–495.
223. Reinhold, U., Bruske, T., and Schupp, G. (1996). Paraneoplastic urticaria in a patient with ovarian carcinoma. *J. Am. Acad. Dermatol.* 35, 988–989.
224. Stashower, M., Rennie, T., Turiansky, G., and Gilliland, W. (1999). Ovarian cancer presenting as leukocytoclastic vasculitis. *J. Am. Acad. Dermatol.* 40, 287–289.
225. Cafagna, D., and Ponte, E. (1997). [Pulmonary embolism of paraneoplastic origin.] [Italian]. *Minerva Med.* 88, 523–530.
226. Crandon, A., and Koutts, J. (1983). Incidence of post-operative deep vein thrombosis in gynaecological oncology. *Aust. NZ. J. Obstet. Gynaecol.* 23, 216–219.
227. Padovani, M., Tillie-Leblond, I., Vennin, P., Demarcq, G., and Wallaert, B. (1996). [Paraneoplastic superior vena cava thrombosis disclosing an ovarian tumor.] [French]. *Rev. Mal. Respir.* 13, 598–600.
228. Beauvolsk, P., and Quenneville, G. (1975). [Potentially curable thromboembolic paraneoplastic syndromes.] [French]. *Union Med. Can.* 104, 72–77.
229. Mitsui, T., Aoki, Y., Nagata, Y., Kojima, Y., and Tanaka, K. (2001). Patent foramen ovale complicated by paradoxical embolism and brain infarct in a patient with advanced ovarian cancer. *Gynecol. Oncol.* 83, 608–609.
230. Donovan, J., Prefontaine, M., and Gragoudas, E. (1999). Blindness as a consequence of a paraneoplastic syndrome in a woman with clear cell carcinoma of the ovary. *Gynecol. Oncol.* 73, 424–429.
231. Leys, A., Dierick, H., and Sciot, R. (1991). Early lesions of bilateral diffuse melanocytic proliferation. *Arch. Ophthalmol.* 109, 1590–1594.
232. Harmon, J., Purvin, V., Guy, J., Aptsiauri, N., and Sutton, G. (1999). Cancer-associated retinopathy in a patient with advanced epithelial ovarian carcinoma. *Gynecol. Oncol.* 73, 430–432.
233. Yoon, Y., Cho, E., Sohn, J., and Thirkill, C. (1999). An unusual type of cancer-associated retinopathy in a patient with ovarian cancer. *Korean J. Ophthalmol.* 13, 43–48.
234. Chahud, F., Young, R., Remulla, J., Khadem, J., and Dryja, T. (2001). Bilateral diffuse uveal melanocytic proliferation associated with extraocular cancers: Review of a process particularly associated with gynecologic cancers. *Am. J. Surg. Pathol.* 25, 212–218.
235. Florell, S. R., Bruggers, C. S., Matlak, M., Young, R. H., and Lowichik, A. (1999). Ovarian small cell carcinoma of the hypercalcemic type in a 14 month old: The youngest reported case. *Med. Pediatr. Oncol.* 32, 304–307.
236. Bakri, Y. N., and Akhtar, M. (1993). Gonadal dysgerminoma-seminoma associated with severe hypercalcemia. *Acta Obstet. Gynecol. Scand.* 72, 57–59.
237. Allan, S. G., Lockhart, S. P., Leonard, R. C., and Smyth, J. F. (1984). Paraneoplastic hypercalcemia in ovarian carcinoma. *Br. Med. J.* 288, 1714–1715.
238. Okoye, B. O., Harmston, C., and Buick, R. G. (2001). Dysgerminoma associated with hypercalcemia: A case report. *J. Pediatr. Surg.* 36, E10.
239. Knecht, T. P., Behling, C. A., Burton, D. W., Glass, C. K., and Deftos, L. J. (1996). The humoral hypercalcemia of benignancy. A newly appreciated syndrome. *Am. J. Clin. Pathol.* 105, 487–492.
240. Bruns, D. E., and Bruns, M. E. (1996). Parathyroid hormone-related protein in benign lesions. *Am. J. Clin. Pathol.* 105, 377–379.
241. Stephen, M. R., and Lindop, G. B. (1998). A renin secreting ovarian steroid cell tumor associated with secondary polycythaemia. *J. Clin. Pathol.* 52, 75–77.
242. Girish, T., Lamb, M. P., Rollason, T. P., and Brown, L. J. R. (2001). An endometrioid tumor of the ovary presenting with hyperandrogenism, secondary polycythaemia and hypertension. *Br. J. Obstet. Gynecol.* 108, 330–332.
243. Briggs, N. D., and Katchy, K. C. (1988). Brenner tumour as encountered in a southern Nigerian hospital. *Int. J. Gynaecol. Obstet.* 27, 455–458.
244. Azizlerli, H., Tanakol, R., Terzioglu, T., Alagol, F., and Dizdaroglu, F. (1997). Steroid cell tumor of the ovary as a rare cause of virilization. *Mt. Sinai. J. Med.* 64, 130–135.
245. Montag, T. W., Murphy, R. E., and Belinson, J. L. (1984). Virilizing malignant lipid cell tumour producing erythropoietin. *Gynaecol. Oncol.* 19, 98–103.

246. Roux-Guinot, S., Gorin, I., Vadrot, D., Djid, R., Bethoux, J. P., and Escande, J. P. (2001). [Androgenic alopecia revealing an androgen secreting ovarian tumor.] [French]. *Ann. Dermatol. Venereol.* 128, 1241–1244.
247. Matsuda, K., Maehama, T., and Kanazawa, K. (2002). Strumal carcinoid tumor of the ovary: A case exhibiting severe constipation associated with PYY. *Gynecol. Oncol.* 87, 143–145.
248. Soga, J., Yakuwa, Y., and Osaka, M. (1999). Carcinoid syndrome: A statistical evaluation of 748 reported cases. *J. Exp. Clin. Cancer Res.* 18, 133–141.
249. Franko, D. M., and Berger, M. (2000). Carcinoid heart disease in association with a primary diagnostic role of echocardiography. *Echocardiography* 17, 571–574.
250. Sabatini, T., Rozzini, R., Morandi, G. B., Meriggi, F., and Zorzi, F. (2000). Primary carcinoid tumor of the ovary: Report of an unusual case. *Tumori* 86, 91–94.
251. Kalinsky, E., Cuillerier, E., Lemann, M., Rain, J. D., Menasche, S., Brenot, F., and Jian, R. (1998). [Favorable outcome of a severe carcinoid cardiopathy after complete resection of the primary ovarian tumor.] [French]. *Gastroenterol. Clin. Biol.* 22, 961–963.
252. Khadilkar, U. N., Pai, R. R., Lahiri, R., and Kumar, P. (2000). Ovarian strumal carcinoid—report of a case that metastasized. *Ind. J. Pathol. Microbiol.* 43, 459–461.
253. Soga, J., Osaka, M., and Yakuwa, Y. (2000). Carcinoids of the ovary: An analysis of 329 reported cases. *J. Exp. Clin. Can. Res.* 19, 271–280.
254. Orbetzova, M., Andreeva, M., Zacharieva, S., Ivanoza, R., and Dashev, G. (1997). Ectopic ACTH-syndrome due to ovarian carcinoma. *Exp. Clin. Endocrinol. Diabetes* 105, 363–365.
255. Ball, S. G., Davison, J. M., Burt, A. D., McNicol, A. M., and Baylis, P. H. (1996). Cushing's syndrome secondary to ectopic SCTH secretion from a primary ovarian carcinoma. *Clin. Endocrinol. (Oxf.)* 45, 775–778.
256. Kasperlik-Zauska, A. A., Jeske, W., and Migdalska, B. (1997). [Comment on] Cushing's syndrome secondary to ectopic SCTH secretion from a primary ovarian carcinoma. *Clin. Endocrinol. (Oxf.)* 47, 501–502.
257. Crawford, S. M., Pyrah, R. D., and Ismail, S. M. (1994). Cushing's syndrome associated with recurrent endometrioid adenocarcinoma of the ovary. *J. Clin. Pathol.* 47, 766–768.
258. Maton, P. N., Gardner, J. D., and Jensen, R. T. (1986). Cushing's syndrome in patients with the Zollinger-Ellison syndrome. *N. Engl. J. Med.* 315, 1–5.
259. Hirasawa, K., Yamada, M., Kitagawa, M., Takehira, Y., Tamakoshi, K., Nakamura, T., Kawamura, K., Takagi, M., Murohisa, B., Ozawa, T., Hanai, H., and Kaneko, E. (2000). Ovarian mucinous cystadenocarcinoma as a cause of Zollinger-Ellison syndrome: Report of a case and review of the literature. *Am. J. Gastroenterol.* 95, 1348–1351.
260. Abboud, P., Bart, H., Mansour, G., Pinteaux, A., and Birembaut, P. (2001). Ovarian gastrinoma in multiple endocrine neoplasia type I: A case report. *Am. J. Obstet. Gynecol.* 184, 237–238.
260a. Myhre, A. G., Halonen, M., Eskelin, P., Ekwall, O., Hestrand, H., Rorsman, F., Kämpe, O., and Husebye, E. S. (2001). Autoimmune polyendocrine syndrome type I (APS I) in Norway. *Clin. Enocrinol. (Oxf.)* 54, 211–217.
260b. Elsheikh, M., Dunger, D. B., Conway, G. S., and Wass, J. A. (2002). Turner's syndrome in adulthood. *Endocr. Rev.* 23, 120–140.
260c. Tauchmanova, L., Rossi, R., Pulcrano, M., Tarantino, L., Baldi, C., and Lombardi, G. (2001). Turner's syndrome mosaicism 45X/47XXX: An interesting natural history. *J. Endocrinol. Invest.* 24, 811–815.
260d. Bremer, G. L., Land, J. A., Tiebosch, A., and van der Putten, H. W. (1993). Five different histological subtypes of germ cell malignancies in an XY female. *Gynecol. Oncol.* 50, 247–248.
260e. Mendez, J. P., Ulloa-Aguirre, A., Kofman-Alfaro, S., Mutchinick, O., Fernandez-del-Castillo, C., Reyes, E., and Perez-Palacios, G. (1993). Mixed gonadal dysgenesis: Clinical, cytogenetic, endocrinological, and histopathological findings in 16 patients. *Am. J. Med. Genet.* 15, 263–267.
260f. Telvi, L., Lebbar, A., Del Pino, O., Barbet, J. P., and Chaussain, J. L. (1999). 45,X/46,XY mosaicism: Report of 27 cases. *Pediatrics* 104, 304–308.
261a. Alvarez-Nava, F., Gonzalez, S., Soto, S., Pineda, L., and Morales-Machin, A. (1999). Mixed gonadal dysgenesis: A syndrome of broad clinical, cytogenetic and histopathologic spectrum. *Genet. Couns.* 10, 233–243.
261b. Chu, C. (1999). (Commentary) Y-chromosome mosaicism in girls with Turner's syndrome. *Clin. Endocrinol. (Oxf.)* 50, 17–18.
261c. Vlasak, I., Plochl, E., Kronberger, G., Bergendi, E., Rittinger, O., Hagemann, M., Schmitt, K., Blumel, P., Glatzl, J., Fekete, G., Kadrnka-Lovrencic, M., Borkenstein, M., Hausler, G., and Frisch, H. (1999). Screening of patients with Turner syndrome for "hidden" Y-mosaicism. *Klin. Padiatr.* 211, 30–34.
261d. Lopez, M., Canto, P., Aguinaga, M., Torres, L., Cervantes, A., Alfaro, G., Mendez, J. P., and Kofman-Alfaro, S. (1998). Frequency of Y chromosomal material in Mexican patients with Ullrich-Turner syndrome. *Am. J. Med. Genet.* 5, 120–124.
261e. Mendes, J. R., Strufaldi, M. W., Delcelo, R., Moises, R. C., Vieira, J. G., Kasamatsu, T. S., Galera, M. F., Andrade, J. A., and Verreschi, I. T. (1999). Y-chromosome identification by PCR and gonadal histopathology in Turner's syndrome without overt Y-mosaicism. *Clin. Endocrinol. (Oxf.)* 50, 19–26.
261f. Gravholt, C. H., Fedder, J., Naeraa, R. W., and Muller, J. (2000). Occurrence of gonadoblastoma in females with Turner syndrome and Y chromosome material: A population study. *J. Clin. Endocrinol. Metab.* 85, 3199–3202.
261g. Coutin, A. S., Hamy, A., Fondevilla, M., Savigny, B., Paineau, J., and Visset, J. (1996). [Pure 46XY gonadal dysgenesis] [French] *J. Gynecol. Obstet. Biol. Reprod. (Paris)* 25, 792-796.
261h. Tanaka, Y., Fujiwara, K., Yamauchi, H., Mikami, Y., and Kohno, I. (2000). Pregnancy in a woman with a Y chromosome after removal of an ovarian dysgerminoma. *Gynecol. Oncol.* 79, 519–521.
261i. Wysocka, B., Serkies, K., Debniak, J., Jassem, J., and Limon, J. (1999). Sertoli cell tumor in androgen insensitivity syndrome—a case report. *Gynecol. Oncol.* 75, 480–483.
261j. Watanobe, H., and Kawabe, H. (1997). Pituitary apoplexy developed in a patient with androgen insensitivity syndrome. *J. Endocrinol. Invest.* 20, 497–500.
261k. Giltay, J. C., Ausems, M. G., van Seumeren, I., Zewald, R. A., Sinke, R. J., Faas, B., and de Vroede, M. (2001). Short stature as the only presenting feature in a patient with an isodicentric (Y)(q11.23) and gonadoblastoma. A clinical and molecular cytogenetic study. *Eur. J. Pediatr.* 160, 154–158.
261l. Pierga, J. Y., Giacchetti, S., Vilain, E., Extra, J. M., Brice, P., Espie, M., Maragi, J. A., Fellous, M., and Marty, M. (1994). Dysgerminoma in a pure 45,X Turner syndrome: Report of a case and review of the literature. *Gynecol. Oncol.* 55, 459–464.
261m. Schanne, F. J., Cooper, C. S., and Canning, D. A. (1999). False-positive pregnancy test associated with gonadoblastoma. *Urology* 54, 162.
261n. Zanetta, G., Bonazzi, C., Cantu, M., Binidagger, S., Locatelli, A., Bratina, G., and Mangioni, C. (2001). Survival and reproductive function after treatment of malignant germ cell ovarian tumors. *J. Clin. Oncol.* 19, 1015–1020.
261o. Khi, C., Low, J. J., Tay, E. H., Chew, S. H., and Ho, T. H. (2002). Malignant ovarian germ cell tumors: The KK Hospital experience. *Eur. J. Gynaecol. Oncol.* 23, 251–256.
262. Shulman, L. P., Muram, D., Marina, N., Jones, C., Portera, J. C., Wachtel, S. S., Simpson, J. L., and Elias, S. (1994). Lack of heritability in ovarian germ cell malignancies. *Am. J. Obstet. Gynecol.* 170, 1803–1805.
262a. Blake, K. I., and Gerrard, M. P. (1993). Malignant germ cell tumours in two siblings. *Med. Pediatr. Oncol.* 21, 299–300.

262b. Weinblatt, M., and Kochen, J. (1991). An unusual family cancer syndrome manifested in young siblings. *Cancer* 68, 1068–1070.

262c. Mandel, M., Toren, A., Kende, G., Neuman, Y., Kenet, G., and Rechavi, G. (1994). Familial clustering of malignant germ cell tumors and Langerhans' histiocytosis. *Cancer* 73, 1980–1983.

262d. Yule, S. M., Dawes, P. J., Malcolm, A. J., and Pearson, A. D. (1994). Occurrence of seminoma and dysgerminoma in father and daughter. *Pediatr. Hematol. Oncol.* 11, 211–213.

262e. Mascarello, J. T., Cajulis, T. R., Billman, G. F., and Spruce, W. E. (1993). Ovarian germ cell tumor evolving to myelodysplasia. *Genes Chromosomes Cancer* 7227–7230.

262f. Winther, J. F., Sankila, R., Boice, J. D., Tuinius, H., Bautz, A., Barlow, L., Glattre, E., Langmark, F., Moller, T., Mulvihill, J. J., Olafsdottir, G. H., Ritvane, A., and Olsen, J. H. (2002). [Cancer in siblings of children with cancer.] [Danish]. *Ugeskr. Laeger.* 164, 3073–3079.

262g. Barakat, R. R., and Rubin, S. C. (2002). Perspective: Should we remove a woman's ovaries to prevent ovarian cancer? *Contemp. OB/GYN* 47, 69–78.

263. Boyd, J. (1999). Hereditary gynecological cancers. *In* "Molecular Biology in Reproductive Medicine." (B. C. J. M. Fauser, ed.), p. 111. Parthenon, New York.

264. Fricker, J. P., Muller, D., Cutuli, B., Rodier, J. F., Janser, J. C., Jung, G. M., Mors, R., Petit, T., Haegele, P., and Abecassis, J. (2000). [Germ-line mutations of the BRCA1 gene in northereastern France.] [French]. *Bull. Cancer* 87, 739–744.

265. Borg, A., Dorum, A., Heimdal, K., Maehle, L., Hovig, E., and Moller, P. (1999). BRCA1 1675delA and 1135insA account for one third of Norwegian familial breast-ovarian cancer and are associated with later disease onset than less frequent mutations. *Dis. Markers* 15, 79–84.

266. Claes, K., Machackova, E., De Vos, M., Poppe, B., De Paepe, A., and Messiaen, L. (1999). Mutation analysis of the BRCA1 and BRCA2 genes in the Belgian patient population and identification of a Belgian founder mutation BRCA1 IVS5+3A>G. *Dis. Markers* 15, 69–73.

266a. Schoumacher, F., Glaus, A., Meuller, H., Eppenberger, U., Bolliger, B., and Senn, H. J. (2001). BRCA1/2 mutations in Swiss patients with familial or early-onset breast and ovarian cancer. *Swiss Med. Wkly.* 21, 223–226.

267. Einbeigi, Z., Bergman, A., Kindblom, L. G., Matinsson, T., Meis-Kindblom, J. M., Nordling, M., Suurkula, M., Wahlstrom, J., Wallgren, A., and Karlsson, P. (2001). A founder mutation of the BRCA1 gene in Western Sweden associated with a high incidence of breast and ovarian cancer. *Eur. J. Cancer* 37, 1904–1909.

268. Verhoog, L. C., van den Ouweland, A. M., Berns, E., van Geghel-Landsoen, M. M., van Staveren, I. L., Wagner, A., Bartels, C. C., and Tilanus-Linthorst, M. M. (2001). Large regional differences in the frequency of distincit BRCA1/BRCA2 mutations in 517 Dutch breast and/or ovarian cancer families. *Eur. J. Cancer* 37, 2082–2090.

269. Meindl, A., German Cosortium for Hereditary Breast and Ovarian Cancer (2002). Comprehensive analysis of 989 patients with breast or ovarian cancer provides BRCA1 and BRCA2 mutation profiles and frequencies for the German population. *Int. J. Cancer* 97, 472–480.

270. Montagna, M., Santacatterina, M., Torri, A., Menin, C., Zullato, D., Chieco-Bianchi, L., and D'Andrea, E. (1999). Identification of a 3 kb Alu-mediated BRCA1 gene rearrangement in two breast/ovarian cancer families. *Oncogene*, 18, 4160–4165.

271. Zweemer, R. P., Shaw, P. A., Verheijen, R. M., Ryan, A., Berchuck, A., Ponder, B. A., Risch, H., McLaughlin, J. R., Narod, S. A., Menko, F. H., Kenemans, P., and Jacobs, I. J. (1999). Accumulation of p53 protein is frequent in ovarian cancer associated with BRCA1 and BRCA2 germline mutations. *J. Clin. Pathol.* 52, 372–375.

272. Srivastava, A., McKinnon, W., and Wood, M. E. (2001). Risk of breast and ovarian cancer in women with strong family histories. *Oncology (Huntingt).* 15, 889–902.

273. De Jong, M. M., Nolte, I. M., te Meerman, G. J., Van Der Graaf, W. T. A., Oosterwijk, J. C., Kleibeuker, J. H., Schaapveld, M., and de Vries, E. G. E. (2002). Genes other than BRCA1 and BRCA2 involved in breast cancer susceptibility. *J. Med. Genet.* 39, 225–242.

274. Lu, K. H., and Broaddus, R. R. (2001). Gynecological tumors in hereditary nonpolyposis colorectal cancer: We know they are common—now what? *Gynecol. Oncol.* 82, 221–222.

275. Watson, P., Butzow, R., Lynch, H. T., *et. al.* (2001). Clinical features of ovarian cancer in hereditary nonpolyposis colorectal cancer. *Gyneco.l Oncol.* 82, 223–228.

276. Cohn, D. E., Babb, S., Whelan, A. J., Mutch, D. G., Herzog, T. J., Rader, J. S., Elbendary, A., and Goodfellow, P. J. (2000). Atypical clustering of gynecologic malignancies: A family study including molecular analysis of candidate genes. *Gynecol. Oncol.* 77, 18–25.

277. Peel, D. J., Ziogas, A., Fox, E. A., Gildea, M., Laham, B., Clements, E., and Kolodner, R. D. (2000). Characterization of hereditary nonpolyposis colorectal cancer families from a population-based series of cases. *J. Natl. Cancer Inst.* 92, 1517–1522.

278. Lynch, H. T., and Lynch, J. (2000). Lynch syndrome: Genetics natural history, genetic counseling, and prevention. *J. Clin. Oncol.* 18, 19S–31S.

279. Thorstenson, Y. R., Roxas, A., Kroiss, R., Wagner, T., and Oefner, P. J. (2001). Germline carriers of ATM mutations are prevalent among Austrian hereditary breast and ovarian cancer (HBOC) patients. *Am. J. Hum. Genet.* 69, 205.

CHAPTER

20

A Geneticist Looks at Ovarian Cancer

FRED GILBERT

Department of Pediatrics, Division of Human Genetics
Weill College of Medicine of Cornell University
and
Human Cancer Genetics
Strang Cancer Prevention Center
New York, New York 10021

I. INTRODUCTION

A geneticist looks at ovarian cancer with a perspective that is different from a gynecologist or gynacologic oncologist. The primary focus of the geneticist is on process—how the cancer develops, then on how to identify persons at highest risk to develop the cancer, and then on how to prevent development of the cancer. The primary focus of the oncologist is diagnosis and treatment.

Ovarian cancer is not unlike most solid tumors of adults in its genetic basis. All cancers are genetic disorders, caused by the accumulation of genetic mutations that alter the growth pattern of a primary cell. In ovarian cancer, as in other solid tumors, a mutation can be inherited or develop spontaneously in the somatic target cell, an ovarian epithelial cell. The inherited change or the initial mutation (the "first hit") is, by itself, insufficient to produce malignant transformation of the target cell. Additional gene changes must occur, though the number and nature of the changes are largely unknown, before the ovarian epithelial cell becomes transformed and continues to divide to produce the cancer.

Though the first hit is the same within a family and can be transmitted to successive generations, the subsequent gene changes that contribute to malignant transformation are likely to be different in different family members. The differences in the patterns of mutations that accumulate in the ovarian epithelial cell may contribute to the variation that is seen in the ages at which cancers develop within (and between) families, as well as in the patterns of cancers in other organs that can be seen within (and between) families.

In studies of families, there are three common scenarios in which ovarian cancer is found: site-specific ovarian cancer, where multiple women in successive generations of a family have only ovarian cancer; the breast-ovarian cancer syndrome, in which both ovarian and breast cancers occur in successive generations of a family; and the hereditary nonpolyposis colon cancer (or HNPCC) syndrome, in which gynecologic cancers, including ovarian cancers, can be found in female family members.

In the case of both site-specific ovarian cancer families and the breast-ovarian cancer syndrome, changes in two genes, BRCA1 and BRCA2, have been implicated as the inherited first hits. In the series reported to date, about 90% of the families with BRCA1/BRCA2 mutations as constitutional findings (inherited and present, therefore, in all cells of the body, including germ cells) carry mutations in BRCA1; about 10% involve inherited mutations in BRCA2. In the case of HNPCC families, inherited mutations have been reported in multiple genes of a particular category, called DNA mismatch repair genes, of which there may be six members. Of these, 80% of the mutations are believed to involve two members of this category, designated *hMSH2* and *hMLH1*.

It is important to stress that in the heritable cancer syndromes, a gene change is transmitted from parent to child or occurs as a new mutation in a sperm or egg that gives rise to the child. The gene change then confers a predisposition or susceptibility to development of cancer. Since all of the cells in the body of the individual that is formed from the fertilized embryo inheriting the mutation contain the mutation in single copy, there is a finite possibility for malignant transformation of any cell should the required number and pattern of subsequent gene changes responsible for that transformation occur.

Why do cancers of only a limited number of tissue types actually occur in these families? Why do members of some families in which a BRCA1 mutation is inherited develop only ovarian cancer, while members of other families in which the same BRCA1 mutation is inherited develop both breast and ovarian cancer? Why do female members of some HNPCC families inheriting the same *hMSH2* and *hMLH1* mutations develop ovarian cancers, while other families inheriting the same mutations in the same genes, do not? These are currently unanswered questions. However, for the question concerning the range of cancers in HNPCC families, we can postulate that the particular cancers that appear in any one individual most likely reflect the statistical likelihood of the secondary gene mutations that are necessary for malignant transformation occurring in any one cell of a particular target oran, like the ovary.

It is clear that many members of heritable cancer families will develop more than one cancer in their lifetimes. In the case of women with breast cancer in BRCA1/BRCA2-associated heritable breast and breast-ovarian cancer families, there is a 60% chance of developing cancer in the contralateral breast over a lifetime. This can be compared with the about 20% lifetime risk of developing cancer in the contralateral breast for women with primary breast cancer as a sporadic event (without any family history of breast or ovarian cancers). In BRCA1/BRCA2-mutation positive women, the risk of developing ovarian cancer over a lifetime has varied between 15 and 55% in different series.

In the case of families in which BRCA2 mutations are inherited, there is a risk of many tumor types in addition to breast and ovarian cancer, including cancers of the pancreas, thyroid, colon, and prostrate. In the case of HNPCC families, there are, in addition to colon, gynecologic (ovarian, endometrial), and kidney cancers, an association with brain cancers (primarily glioblastomas) (the association of colon and brain cancer is also called Turcot's syndrome), and with sebaceous neoplasms (called Muir-Torre syndrome).

II. THE ROLE OF THE GENETICIST

For the geneticist seeing a patient with cancer, the first questions concern the age at which the cancer was discovered in the proband (the first person identified in a family with a genetic condition) and whether the cancer is unilateral or bilateral (Table 20.1). The heritable cancer syndromes are notable for a generally earlier age of development of the cancer in affected within the family, and a tendency to bilateral involvement. However, in the case of ovarian cancer, the age at development in heritable cases is not appreciably different from that in nonheritable or sporadic cases—the late 50s. Also, many ovarian cancers in heritable families are discovered after the cancer has spread throughout the abdomen, so whether it is unilateral or bilateral is often difficult to assess.

TABLE 20.1 Algorithm for Genetic Counseling About Cancer Risk Assessment

Step 1:	Patient cancer history (what organ, age at discovery)
Step 2:	Patient family pedigree—particularly cancers by organ and age at development
Step 3:	Determine whether the patient is likely to be part of a heritable cancer family, based on the presence of certain cancers in first and second degree relatives: e.g., recurrent ovarian cancers—site-specific ovarian cancer family; recurrent ovarian and ovarian cancers—breast-ovarian cancer family; and ovarian, colon (<age 55), endometrial cancers—hereditary nonpolyposis colon cancer (HNPCC) family
Step 4:	If does not fit into a cancer family syndrome–no further testing, cancer risks the same as in general population If does fit into a cancer family syndrome—testing using appropriate modality—ovarian and breast-ovarian: BRCA1, BRCA2; HNPCC: *hMSH2*, *hMLH1* (whether limited mutation panel or complete gene sequencing determined by patient's ethnic background)
Step 5:	If mutation testing is NEGATIVE—either not a cancer family or testing has missed the gene or mutation Counsel about significance of result and surveillance options If mutation testing is POSITIVE—then Counsel patient about risks of cancer recurrence/additional primary cancers (breast, ovarian, colon, etc.) Counsel about surveillance options, approaches to prevention and surgical prophylaxis Counsel about risks to other relatives and testing option for them
Step 6:	For identified heritable cancer families (mutation-positive), extended family counseling and testing possible—siblings, adult children, parents, uncles, aunts, cousins

For the geneticist, the next question concerns the diagnosis of cancer in relatives of the proband. The geneticist constructs a family pedigree identifying who in the family has/had cancer and of which cancer types. In the heritable cancer syndromes in adults, the predisposition to cancer development is transmitted from parent to child in a dominant fashion. One expects, therefore, to find examples of cancers in successive generations, with mothers and daughters presenting with ovarian (or breast or colon) cancers. However, what is inherited is a "predisposition" to cancer development—unless the secondary mutations occur in the target cell—that cell will not become transformed. There is a finite possibility that any one individual inheriting a first hit in BRCA1 or *hMSH2*, for example, will not develop cancer in their lifetime. Also, they could die prematurely from another cause, or the mutation transmission could be through a male relative.

The case of males in site-specific ovarian and breast-ovarian cancer families is interesting. There is an incidence of breast cancer in males, but it is less than 1% that in women. It is estimated that about 180,000 cases of breast cancer are identified in women each year in the U.S., while in males, the comparable number is about 1000 cases. At least 10% of male breast cancer appears to involve an inherited susceptibility (a similar percentage to that seen in women). However, virtually all of the heritable male breast cancer risk is associated with mutations in BRCA2; less than 10% is associated with inherited BRCA1 mutations (the major player in breast-ovarian families).

In any event, since a person has two parents, it is important to recognize that any cancer susceptibility gene can be inherited from the paternal, as well as the maternal sides of the family. One, therefore, is concerned with cancers in a proband's siblings, mother, father, aunts, uncles, and grandparents. While studies of heritable ovarian cancers often present pedigrees with affected mother and daughters, it is not uncommon to find a woman with ovarian cancer who has a paternal aunt (father's sister) and paternal grandmother (father's mother) with breast and/or ovarian cancer.

Once one has a family with more than one person with cancer and a pattern of cancers consistent with a heritable cancer syndrome, it is time to decide which test is appropriate. If one is dealing with ovarian alone, or ovarian and breast, then testing for mutations in BRCA1 and BRCA2 is appropriate. If one has a family with ovarian, colon, and other cancers, then it could be BRCA1 or BRCA2, but may more likely be an HNPCC family. The colon cancers in BRCA2-mutation positive families, tend to occur at the same ages as seen in sporadic cases: that is, after age 60. In HNPCC families, the age at which colon cancers are discovered is usually younger—often under age 55. So if one is dealing with a family with ovarian cancers and colon cancers under age 60, then it might be appropriate to start with screening for mutations in *hMSH2* and *hMLH1*.

Once the geneticist decides that he/she is dealing with a likely BRCA1/2 family or an HNPCC family, what kind of testing should be ordered? At the present time, there are two levels of testing available. In the case of BRCA1/2, one can order limited mutation screens or complete gene sequencing. This is because in different ethnic populations, distinct patterns of mutations have been identified. For example, in Jews of Eastern European origin (Ashkenazi Jews), three mutations—BRCA1: 185delAG, 5382insC; BRCA2:6174delT—account for virtually all of the BRCA1/2-associated risk. No other mutations in either BRCA1 or BRCA2 have been reported in more than Ashkenazi Jewish individual or family, and it is very likely that in those rare instances, one is dealing with a mutation introduced into the family by a non-Ashkenazi. Also, in the Scandanavian countries—Finland, Iceland, Norway, etc.—a limited number of founder mutations in BRCA1 and BRCA2 have been reported in the vast majority of heritable family cases. In the case of HNPCC families in Scandanavia, limited numbers of mutations in *hMSH2* and *hMLH1* have been reported as responsible for the disease as well.

The phenomenon of founder mutations giving rise to a disease in a particular racial or ethnic group is well known in genetics. It is presumed to reflect both the fact that for many diseases, the responsible mutations are "ancient," having arisen generations ago and are maintained in a population for different reasons. The reasons include a lack of out-breeding (members of a society choose or are unable to have children with persons outside of the society for social, religious, or geographic reasons); no effect on reproductive fitness (being a carrier of a mutation does not interfere with one's ability to reproduce, because the consequences of that mutation—e.g., cancer—generally develop after a woman finishes having their family); and a selective advantage to carriers (the best example is in sickle cell disease, where carriers for the recessive sickle cell disease are better able to survive infection by the malaria parasite; it has been postulated that a single copy of a BRCA1 or BRCA2 mutation might result in greater proliferation of milk ducts in the breast enhancing the survival potential of children of carrier women).

In any event, if one is concerned about BRCA1 or BRCA2 mutations in an Ashkenazi Jewish family, then one only has to perform testing for the three founder mutations. However, if one is dealing with an Italian, Irish, or Polish non-Jewish woman who is suspected of being part of a heritable ovarian cancer family, one would have to order a complete sequencing of BRCA1 and BRCA2, in order to maximize the potential for identifying a mutation.

Before the gene testing is performed the woman, and often other family members, has to be counseled about the testing, why it is being ordered, what will be done, and what might be the results, and the consequences for that woman and for the family. The geneticist and genetic counselor will discuss the heritable cancer syndromes and why this woman's case seems to fit a heritable cancer pattern. Then which test(s) are being considered will be discussed. The woman will also be told that there are three possible results of the testing: she is found to carry a known pathological mutation (one that introduces a "stop" codon into the gene sequence, called a "nonsense" mutation, resulting in premature truncation of the protein specified by the gene); that she carries a mutation of "unknown significance," that is a gene change that results in an amino acid substitution in the protein specified by the gene called a "missense" mutation; or she is mutation-negative. In the case of "nonsense" mutations, the premature truncation of the protein results in a total loss of activity of that protein; most of the mutations that have been implicated in heritable breast, breast-ovarian, and HNPCC families are nonsense mutations.

In the case of "missense" mutations, the change in a single amino acid in the protein may or may not affect the ability of the protein to function normally. The testing laboratory may be able to exclude a 'missense' mutation as likely to be non-pathologic, if it is found in a percentage of the general population. Many single base pair changes are permitted in genes if they do not affect the gene's function; these can occur in the general population and if they are found in at least 1% of a population, they are called "polymorphisms." Because these data on any one missense mutation are usually limited, it is often difficult to interpret the significance of the finding for a family. One can extend the study to other members of that family with and without cancer: if the mutation is always associated with family members with cancer and only rarely associated with older adult women (over age 75) who have not had ovarian or breast cancer, then the mutation is more likely to be related to the cancer risk. If the mutation is inherited from the side of the family without the cancer risk, then its association with cancer susceptibility is less likely.

What about women who are mutation-negative? There are two possibilities; they are truly mutation-negative, which means that their chances of having inherited a cancer susceptibility gene is decreased, or the mutation actually conferring cancer susceptibility has not been identified. The latter possibility is what is often the most concerning for families. In the families we have studied in which at least 2 first- or second-degree female relatives (mother, sister, aunts) of a woman with ovarian or breast cancer, have breast or ovarian cancer themselves (a minimum of 3 cases), about half (50%) are negative for a BRCA1 or BRCA2 mutation by complete gene sequencing.

To explain a negative result by gene sequencing (which is "complete" in that all exons and surrounding splice site regions are sequenced), one can postulate that the mutation is present in a region of the gene that has not sequenced—either within the introns or outside of the gene sequence entirely (e.g., in a promoter element controlling transcription of the gene)—or involves deletion of an entire exon (which can be missed by sequencing of the exons), or involves another gene entirely. Investigators are still searching for a BRCA3 to account for the families that are negative by the current screening methods.

What do you do with a woman who does not have cancer herself, but is concerned about her risks because her mother or sister or aunt has ovarian cancer? When there are multiple cases of specific cancers in first- (parent, child, sibling) or second-degree (aunt, uncle, grandparent, grandchild) relatives, and the patterns are suggestive of heritable ovarian, breast-ovarian, or HNPCC, one can test a relative with the cancer. If that relative is mutation-positive, then one can test other family members, and if they are mutation-negative, then their cancer risk is essentially that of the general population; if they are mutation-positive, then they face the increased risk of ovarian (up to 55%), breast (up to 85%), or colon (up to 85%) cancer that is specific to the identified gene and mutation.

What if there is no living family member with cancer available for testing? One can test the woman asking the question: if she is mutation-positive, then she faces the individual cancer risks noted previously for specific genes and mutations. If she is mutation-negative, then her cancer risk is decreased, but not to the general population level: there still are the 50% of heritable cancer families in which the responsible 'first hit' gene mutation cannot be identified.

III. THE GENETICIST AND PATIENT FOLLOW-UP

For patients who are in a cancer family and have or have not yet developed cancer and who know their mutation-status, what comes next? The geneticist will discuss future options. One obvious course is surveillance. The patient will learn that there is a risk of recurrence of breast cancer (60% in heritable families versus 20% in sporadic, nonheritable cases); that if she has had breast cancer, she can develop ovarian cancer later in life (up to 55%, depending on the gene and mutation); and she may be at the risk for other cancers—e.g., colon, endometrial, pancreas, thyroid, etc.—depending on the gene mutation.

Surveillance options, therefore, will include breast examinations and mammograms, colonoscopy, and vaginal ultrasound/CA125 (for ovarian cancer). The reality is that mammograms and breast exams are very effective for early detection of breast cancer, and colonoscopy is very effective for early detection of colon cancer, but there is no effective method for early detection of ovarian cancer. Most ovarian cancer cases when discovered have already spread beyond the ovary and the prognosis for survival beyond two years is poor. This may change with better therapy in the future, but the generally poor prognosis with ovarian cancer has led many clinicians to recommend prophylactic oophorectomy for those women at increased risk for ovarian cancer. Since the age at which ovarian cancer develops in the heritable cases is generally greater than 45, the usual recommendation is that the high-risk patient consider prophylactic oophorectomy around age 45 or when she has completed her reproduction.

However, prophylactic oophorectomy does not reduce the risk of ovarian cancer in high-risk women to zero. A small percentage (under 5%, perhaps close to 1%) of mutation-positive women in breast-ovarian cancer families (the only ones for which data are available), will be found to have ovarian cancer following prophylactic oophorectomy. Two hypotheses have been advanced to explain this: they already had a small nidus of ovarian cancer that had spread outside of the ovary before oophorectomy, or the cancer developed in embryonic rest cells (now called "stem cells") that are present in the peritoneum.

IV. THE RELEVANCE OF GENETICS TO THE DOCTOR CARING FOR THE PATIENT WITH OVARIAN CANCER

For physicians primarily responsible for the care of the patient with ovarian cancer, a potentially life-threatening situation, concern for genetics can seem to be a tangential or irrelevant consideration. Would treatment choices be affected by knowing whether the disease was sporadic or associated with the inheritance of a BRCA1-mutation? Would the post-surgery/chemotherapy course be different if the patient had a sporadic cancer or was part of a heritable cancer family? Would the concerns of the patient's family be different if the cancer was sporadic or heritable? The answer to all three questions is a qualified YES.

Treatment choices in ovarian cancer, at the present time, are not different in sporadic versus heritable cases. However, in the case of breast cancer, one might argue that given the high rate of recurrence in heritable versus sporadic disease, mastectomy (even bilateral mastectomy) might be a better choice for the long term than lumpectomy. There are no data to indicate that there is a greater rate of local recurrence in breast cancers that are heritable versus sporadic. But we do know that over time the rate of cancers in the contralateral breast are greater in the heritable category, so it is possible that the rate of development of second primary tumors in the ipsilateral breast may also be higher in the heritable cases—additional studies will answer this question. Bilateral mastectomy at the time of discovery of an initial cancer is now being chosen by women in heritable breast and breast-ovarian cancer families concerned about the higher rate of second breast cancer development.

In women concerned about an increased risk for ovarian cancer, there are data (controversial) that indicate that oral contraceptive use for up to three years will reduce (or delay) the development of breast cancer by a significant degree. In the case of breast cancer risk, we know that estrogen receptor blocking medications, like tamoxifen, will reduce (or delay) the development of breast cancer in BRCA2-mutation positive individuals. Exercise, presumably by lowering plasma estrogen levels, has also been shown to reduce the risk for breast cancer in women in the general population. So, women in site-specific ovarian cancer or breast cancer families, or in breast-ovarian cancer families, could be placed on oral contraceptives to reduce the risk of ovarian cancer, or an oral anti-estrogens to reduce the risk of breast cancer, or be recommended to increase their exercise regimens as a way to reduce their breast cancer risk.

Prophylactic surgery is also an option to reduce the risk of developing cancer. Women who are BRCA1/2-mutation positive have elected to have bilateral mastectomies before they develop breast cancer and at the time they develop cancer in one breast, as prophylaxis. Women who are BRCA1/2-mutation positive or *hMSH2/hMLH1*-mutation positive have elected to have bilateral oophorectomies and hysterectomy at around age 45, before any cancer in the organs have been identified, as prophylaxis.

And for the extended families of an identified mutation carrier, there is information relevant to their care and follow-up and, perhaps, to their reproductive choices. A woman who is part of a site-specific ovarian cancer family, or a man or woman who is part of a breast-ovarian cancer family or an HNPCC family has several options: appropriate gene testing to determine if they are mutation-positive; preventive initiatives including anti-estrogens, contraceptives, exercise (as discussed previously); intensive surveillance (with earlier mammograms beginning 10 years earlier than the earliest age of breast cancer in the family; vaginal ultrasounds and CA125 to monitor for ovarian cancer; colonoscopy to detect early colon cancers); and early pregnancy and prophylactic surgery.

For many women who have ovarian or breast cancer, it becomes important to know their gene mutation status to provide information for their sisters, brothers, and children. Even if the information does not help the proband directly, it can prove extremely valuable to other family members and to the physicians caring for them.

In the future, our knowledge of the genetic basis of diseases, including cancers, will lead to new approaches to treatment. For the present, genetics provides us with a tool to identify persons and families at highest risk to develop certain diseases, including several cancers. Genetics also provides us with the opportunity to institute surveillance, preventive treatments, and prophylactic surgeries that can reduce the clinical consequences for high-risk individuals and families. Knowledge of one's genetic deficiencies can be perceived as a curse, but that same knowledge also provides us with the opportunity to delay or reverse what might seem to be pre-ordained, as with the development of cancer. It, therefore, makes sense for physicians to champion the acquisition of genetic knowledge by their patients who are likely to be at high risk to develop cancers, like ovarian cancer, based on their family histories.

C H A P T E R

21

Gene Therapy of Ovarian Cancer—State-of-the-Art and Future Perspectives

DIRK G. KIEBACK
Department of Obstetrics and Gynecology
Maastricht University Medical Center
NL 6202 AZ Maastricht, Netherlands

ANNETTE HASENBURG
Department of Obstetrics and Gynecology
Freiburg University Medical Center
D-79106 Freiburg, Germany

INGO B. RUNNEBAUM
Department of Obstetrics and Gynecology
Freiburg University Medical Center
D-79106 Freiburg, Germany

XIAO W. TONG
Department of Obstetrics and Gynecology
Tongi University Shanghai
Shanghai, 200065 PR China

DAGMAR-C. FISCHER
Department of Obstetrics and Gynecology
Maastricht University Medical Center
NL 6202 AZ Maastricht, Netherlands

I. INTRODUCTION

Ovarian cancer represents the second most frequent cancer of the female genitale tract. Yearly, about 191,000 cases are diagnosed worldwide (for review see [1] and references therein). Due to the absence of clinical symptoms most cases are detected in advanced stages, e.g., FIGO III and IV. Late onset of primary therapy transduced into a poor 5-year survival rate of less than 40%. In addition to a continous improvement of surgical procedures and the establishment of platinum-based chemotherapy in the first-line situation, large efforts of additional therapeutic approaches either additive to the primary therapy or applied after recurrence of disease have been made. Even though the growing knowledge about the molecular basis of familial and sporadic cancers and the signal transduction pathways altered in cancer cells have resulted in a variety of new molecularly based treatment approaches, gene therapy also remains one of the most attractive tools. Gene therapy relies on the application of either DNA, RNA, or even a synthetic oligonucleotide as a precursor molecule which will be transformed to the therapeutic agent by the recipient cells. Irrespective of the molecule encoded by either form of nucleic acids, one of the major obstacles to overcome is the internalization and further processing of these therapeutic precursor molecules. Furthermore, the target cell to be addressed by gene therapy has to be defined. The ultimate goal of definitive elimination of the cancer cells can be reached in different ways. Besides the replacement of a nonfunctional tumor-suppressor gene by a functional one, inhibition of a constitutively active oncogene, for example, by blocking signal transduction or by inducing an anti-tumor response of the immune system, and gene-directed enzyme prodrug therapy (GDEPT), are concepts to be evaluated for gene therapy of cancer.

First of all, different vector systems and the problems associated with targeting and transgene expression will be discussed. Thereafter, different gene therapy approaches will be presented and finally, concepts are reported, which have already been introduced into clinical trials as well as those which are likely to be introduced into clinical trials in the near future.

II. OVARIAN CANCER

A. Characterstics of the Disease, Etiology, and Gold Standard of Therapy

Ovarian cancer is still among the leading causes of death in Western countries, even though prognosis has been improved during the past 15 years.[2, 3] Due to the absence of effective screening methods and due to the absence of relevant symptoms in early-stage ovarian cancer, the majority of patients present at advanced stages (FIGO III and IV) with ascites and peritoneal carcinomatosis.[4, 5] Despite great progress in first-line therapy, patients with advanced disease are at high risk for recurrence and therefore overall 5-year survival rate is less than 40%.[4, 6–8] The vast majority of ovarian carcinomas are of epithelilian origin (approximately 85%) whereas germ cell tumors and sex cord-stromal tumors arising from germ cells and stroma cells are less frequent (approximately 15% of all ovarian cancers). Biology and treatment response differ between these tumor entities and epithelial ovarian cancer has the worst prognosis. Due to the striking similarity between the histomorphology of epithelial ovarian cancer and Müllerian-duct-derived epithelium, the origin of epithelial ovarian cancer from either remnants of the Müllerian duct or the ovarian surface mesothelial layer has been an issue of controversial discussion.[9, 10] However, the origination of ovarian cancer from ovarian surface epithelial cells is now widely accepted (for review see [11]). The same type of malignancy can also arise from the peritoneal surfaces of the abdomen. The fact that epithelial ovarian cancer appears more differentiated than the "tissue of origin" strongly indicates the complex nature of this malignancy.[12] This observation is a strong hint toward the unique etiology and nature of epithelial ovarian cancer compared to other epithelium-derived cancers, which are in general less differentiated than their tissue of origin. Due to the lack of suitable animal models for human ovarian epithelial cancer little is known about the etiology and early events during cancerogenesis. All information about genetic aberrations and molecular characteristics of epithelial ovarian cancer is mostly generated from established human ovarian tumors and/or human cell lines, thus excluding the possibilty to rank these observations with respect to the time scale of transition from the normal to the malignant state. In addition, up to now only some murine ovarian cancer cell lines, which enable therapeutic studies with syngenic models have been described.[13, 14] Very recently, microarray based high-throughput analysis was used to compare gene expression in normal ovarian surface epithelium cells and in established ovarian cancers.[15–17] Even though, with this technology a better comparison of genetic aberrations between normal epithelial cells and established tumors is possible, the sequence of events during cancerogenesis remains difficult to elucidate.

The incidence of ovarian cancer is high in North America and Western Europe (10/100,000) compared with developing countries or Japan (3/100,000).[1, 6, 18] Besides environmental and dietary influences, ethnic as well as molecular, genetic, and endocrine factors, (e.g., onset of menarche, total number of ovulations, use of oral contraceptives), were shown to be influencing cancer risk (for reference see [1, 6]). The importance of the hormonal environment is stressed by our observation that a polymorphism of the progesterone receptor gene, which affects receptor stability rather than ligand binding, alone or in combination with other factors is also a risk modulator.[19, 20] In addition to the effect of environmental and genetic factors, the risk for ovarian cancer increases with age. The majority of patients is diagnosed between age 50 and 60 (median age 58 years). Above the age of 75 years the incidence is declining. The majority of epithelial ovarian cancers occur sporadically, only 5–10% of cancers are the result of an inherited predisposition, e.g., mutations of BRCA1/BRCA2 or of DNA mismatch repair genes.[21] As mentioned above, there are numerous papers evaluating genetic alterations in either ovarian tumors or ovarian cancer cell lines, but the impact of each of these genetic aberrations on tumorigenesis as well as the ovarian cancer specificity of such events remains unclear. Mutation-induced loss of function of the tumor suppressor gene p53 is the most frequently seen genetic alteration in nearly all cancers and is also described in about 50% of epithelial ovarian cancers.[21–24] This is more likely to reflect the importance of p53 in the prevention of malignant growth than an indicator of a specific role in ovarian cancerogenesis. In addition, directly or indirectly induced overexpression of oncogenes *c-myc*, *k-ras*, as well as members of the epithelial growth factor receptor family, e.g., *erb-B2 (Her2/neu)* and EGF-R occur rather frequently in ovarian cancers.[11, 12, 21, 25–27] However, the contribution of each genetic aberration to oncogenesis still remains to be clarified. Genetic profiling of either established or primary ovarian cancer cell lines [15, 17, 28] and the comparison with normal ovarian surface epithelium is likely to contribute to our understanding of ovarian cancer and will help to define further tools for screening modalities and therapeutic interventions.

Today, primary therapy of epithelial ovarian cancer is based on optimal tumor reductive surgery (surgical debulking; residual tumor should be as little as possible) followed by chemotherapy including paclitaxel and platinum.[29] However, due to the unsatisfactory long-term response of most ovarian cancers to primary chemo- and/or radiotherapy, alternative concepts including gene therapy have to be extensively evaluated.

III. GENE THERAPEUTIC APPROACHES FOR TREATMENT OF CANCER

One prominent feature of cancer cells is their virtually unlimited ability to proliferate. This could be linked to severe disturbances of gene expression as the result of complex genetic aberrations. Numerous studies have shown, that either the overexpression of oncogenes, and the therefore disturbed or constitutively activated signal transduction cascades alone or in combination with the mutation-induced silencing of tumor-suppressor genes are associated with malignant transformation.[23, 24, 30–36] Although the key events which are responsible for these complex changes in cellular behavior are widely unknown, both the overexpression of oncogenes as well as the diminished expression of tumor suppressors are attractive molecular targets for a more causal anti-cancer therapy than the widely used chemotherapeutic agents. The concept of either selective inhibition of oncogene activation or re-establishing of functional tumor suppressors needs proteins as therapeutic agents. Also, there are still severe technical problems with large-scale production and purification of proteins for pharmaceutical use. Therefore, gene therapy becomes especially attractive. Gene therapy is based on the introduction of either DNA or RNA in the recipient cells, thereby enabling the transduced cell to synthesize the desired protein.[37] Even though the concept of genetic therapy as prototype of a tailored and causal treatment is brilliant, a variety of problems are encountered. The transfer of genetic material *in vivo* is not a simple task as nature has developed powerful mechanisms to protect cells from the incorporation of foreign DNA into their genomes. On the other hand, viruses are naturally occurring organisms whose replication solely relies on the transfer of the viral genome into host cells. Thus, it is not surprising, that viruses are at least to a certain extent able to overcome some of those defense mechansims.[38, 39] Viruses appear as suitable shuttle systems for gene therapy. A variety of problems related to the process of genetic modification and/or the intrisic pathogenicity of the parental virus exists. Non-viral delivery systems for cancer gene therapy have been developed recently and even the injection of uncomplexed (naked) DNA was evaluated.[37, 40]

The currently relevant methods to eliminate tumor cells by gene therapy can be summarized as follows.[41–44]

1. *Gene-replacement therapy*: Re-introduction of a functional tumor-suppressor gene (p53, p16, BRCA1) which in turn should help to sensitize cells to chemotherapy and/or radiation therapy
2. *Gene therapy*: Utilized to induce and/or to enhance the anti-tumor response of the immune system (vaccination, introduction of immunostimulatory cytokines together with antigen presentating cells)
3. *GDEPT*: The introduction of a foreign gene enabling the transduced cell to metabolize and thus toxify a prodrug. Examples are the herpes simplex virus-1 derived thymidine kinase (hsv1-tk) or the *E. coli* derived cytosine deaminase (CD)

For any approach the efficient transfer of therapeutic gene(s) to the desired target cells is required. The therapeutic efficacy is likely to depend on the properties of the therapeutic gene as well as on those of the shuttle system. Whereas transduction efficiency and duration of transgene expression are mainly determined by the vector system, the level of transgene expression is a function of the promoter strength. To achieve selective targeting, additional features can be added to either the vector and/or the promoter, controlling the expression of the therapeutic gene. To make the story even more complicated, the response of the immune system toward the therapeutic vector and transgene is important for the clinial outcome. Therefore, the introduction of gene therapy into cancer treatment is a multidisciplinary effort, based on the combined knowledge of virology, cancer biology, and immunology.

A. Methods for Transgene Delivery

Efficient delivery of the transgene is a most important prerequisite for the therapeutic outcome. An overview about the vector systems currently used for gene therapy of cancer is given in Table 21.1.

1. Non-Viral Systems for Transgene Delivery

The introduction of naked foreign DNA is mostly based on a physical transfer into the target cell ("gene gun") and thus restricted to easily accessible or superficial sites. Even though the successful intratumoral application of plasmid DNA has been described,[45–47] to date the intramuscular injection is mainly used for DNA-based vaccination.[48] With systemic administration (iv injection) of noncomplexed naked DNA rapid degradation occurs and the DNA is cleared from the plasma within minutes.

Non-viral gene transfer systems, which are widely used for *in vitro* transformation of eukaryotic cells, rely on the complexation and/or encapsulation of the DNA in artificial liposomes.[37, 40, 49, 50] Liposomes have been successfully used for the delivery of chemotherapeutic agents into tumor cells and are now part of the therapeutic armament in ovarian cancer treatment.[51] In addition, these systems were seen to be rather effective for gene transfer *in vitro*.

TABLE 21.1 Systems for *in vivo* Transgene Delivery

Vector	Ref.
Non-viral vectors	[37, 40]
Retroviral vectors	[39, 56, 59, 61, 85]
Lentiviral vectors	[39]
Adenoviral vectors	[39, 94, 136, 357]
Adeno-associated vectors	[117, 166]
Herpesvirus vectors	[39, 59]
Poxvirus vectors	[39, 59, 169]
Epstein-Barr virus vectors	[39, 59]

However, a variety of problems occurred upon *in vivo* application. These are related to the toxicity of the carrier systems, the targeting of tumor cells, a low transduction efficiency, and thus low levels of transgene expression. Low transgene expression is likely to be a consequence of problems with downstream processing of foreign DNA after endosomal release from the carrier complex. Targeting can be improved, if the carrier system is linked to a ligand or ligand domain binding specifically to a cell-surface receptor of the target cell.

Such non-viral gene delivery systems are continuously improved and very recently several cationic liposome formulations were evaluated *in vitro* and *in vivo* for the utilization in disseminated ovarian cancer gene therapy.[52–54] Based on these preclinical studies, a phase I trial in patients with Her-2/neu expressing breast or ovarian cancer is currently being performed.[55] In this study, a plasmid encoding for the adenoviral E1A gene is delivered via a cationic lipid carrier directly to the peritoneal cavity or the pleural space of patients with advanced metastatic breast and/or epithelial ovarian carcinomas or peritoneal carcinomatosis refractory to standard chemo- and hormone therapy.

Besides this novel approach, retrovirus- or adenovirus-based vectors have been used in clinical trials for gene therapy of ovarian cancer. These vectors are delivered either directly into the peritoneal cavity or indirectly via *ex vivo* transduced cells.

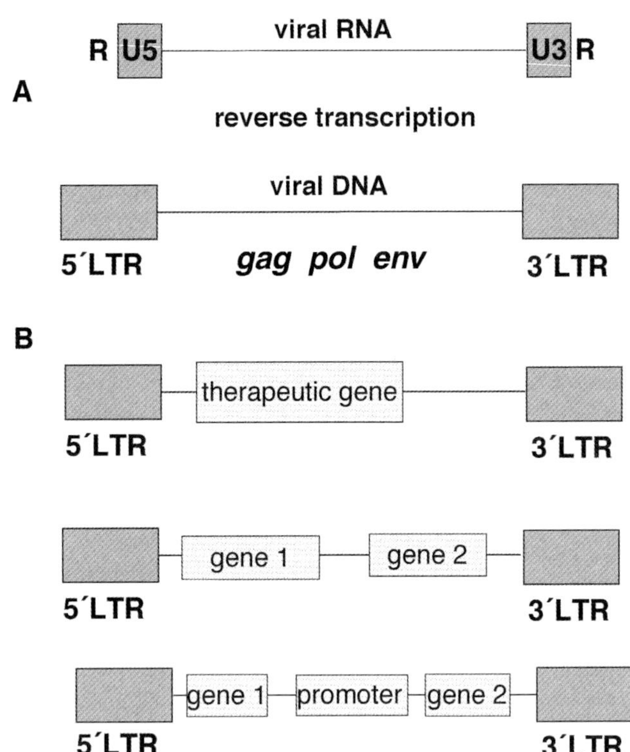

FIGURE 21.1 Schematic representation of the retroviral genome (A) and vectors derived thereof (B). The viral genes *gag*, *pol*, and *env* can be replaced by one or two therapeutic gene(s), expressed under the control of the LTR-viral promoter of an exogeneous promoter, introduced with the transgene. (From Walther, W., and Stein, U. (2000). *Drugs* 60, 249–271; and Galanis, E., Vile, R., and Russell, S. J. (2001). *Crit. Rev. Oncol. Hematol.* 38, 177–192.)

2. Viral Vectors for Transgene Delivery

a. Retrovirus-Based Vectors

Whereas the vast majority (ca. 40%) of current clinical gene therapy trials are based on retroviral transfer of foreign genes into target cells, adenoviral vectors are preferred in the treatment of ovarian cancer.[39] Besides the ability to infect dividing cells exclusively and the risk to introduce insertional mutations with these vectors, their longer research history and the accumulated knowledge about behavior and manipulation of their genome made retrovirus-based vectors especially attractive as a shuttle system. Mainly, replication-deficient vectors are derived from the Moloney murine leukemia virus (MoMLV). According to the host cells susceptible to retroviral infection, ecotropic vectors, which are infectious only for murine cells and amphotropic vectors, being able to infect murine and human cells, are distinguished. The retroviral genome (Fig. 21.1) encodes for three structural genes, *gag* (group specific antigens), *pol* (encoding the reverse transciptase and integrase), and *env* (viral envelope glycoproteins, SU and TM). Whereas the integrase is an enzyme critical for insertion of the viral genome into the genome of the host cell, SU and, TM are necessary for inseration into the host cell membrane. The genome is flanked by the viral long terminal repeats (LTR) which regulate the expression of the viral genome.[56]

All information necessary for viral replication is included in the viral genome, nevertheless the virus strictly depends on a cellular environment for replication. Deletion of *gag*, *pol* and/or *env* and replacing them with foreign gene(s) completely abolishes the ability of the modified virus to replicate and generate retroviral particles. However, if such a crippled virus infects cells which provide the missing genes, replication and packaging of the mutated virus occurs. Thus, the construction of recombinant virus critically depends on the availability of packaging cell lines and/or helper plasmids.[57] In addition, the separation of the parental viral genome into several plasmids reduces the risk that replication competent viral particles occur. Due to a balanced ratio of envelope and genome size, the size of the recombinant genome is limited to that of the wild-type genome. Therefore, the size of the expression cassette replacing *gag*, *pol,* and *env* should not exceed 8 kb. Usually, retroviral vectors are produced with titers of up to 10^6 and 10^7 pfu/ml (plaque forming units per milliliter), but the yield is influenced by the properties of the retroviral particle. The mature replication-deficient retroviral vector is characterized by the inserted gene cassette and by the viral envelope. As both compartments are important not only for production and purification of the vectors but also for determining their therapeutic efficacy, both are targets for improvement of retroviral-based cancer gene therapy. A variety of retroviral vectors besides those carrying only the therapeutic gene under the control of the viral LTR have been constructed (Fig. 21.1; for summary see [39]). Vectors carrying two transgenes, for example, a selectable marker gene and the therapeutic gene, are used rather frequently. In this type of vector, the expression of one or both transgenes can be driven either by the viral LTR or by internal promoters introduced with these transgenes. The selectable marker, e.g., *neo* (neomycin phosphotransferase) or *hgr* (hygromycin phosphotransferase) allows for *ex vivo/in vitro* selection and cloning of transduced cells. In addition, the introduction of a non-viral promoter allows the cell-type specific and/or regulatable gene expression.

The MoMLV-derived amphotropic vectors are internalized by binding of the viral envelope protein to the phosphate transporter Ran-1 (GLVR-2) on the surface of the target cell.[39, 58, 59] However, as this infection is restricted to rapidly dividing cells, nondividing cells are refractory to retroviral infection.[60, 61] Therefore, even in rapidly growing tumors only a fraction of the cell population is susceptible to retroviral infection and resting cells, which are the heart of the problem of recurrence, are not reached. After internalization, the viral genome or, in case of retroviral vectors, the transgene, is reversely transcribed into a double-stranded viral DNA followed by stable integration into the host cell genome and transgene expression. Even though this stable integration is advantageous for long-term expression of the therapeutic gene, it could also result in insertional mutagenesis. To prevent insertional activation of genes in the host genome, retroviral vectors with mutation-induced loss of the promoter/enhancer sequences in the U3 region of the viral 3′-LTR (SIN-vectors) were constructed.[62] With this construct, a dramatic loss of viral titers (ca. 10^4 pfu/ml of virus stocks) during the production is observed and therefore the application of these vectors is limited.[39]

Besides the limited size of the transgene (maximum 8 kb) and problems related to purification and concentration of viral stocks for clinical application, targeting of retroviral vectors and/or therapeutic gene expression need further improvement.[39] Whereas a broad range of cell types is susceptible to an infection with MuMLV-derived vectors, this is restricted to dividing cells thereby lowering transduction efficiencies even in aggressive tumors.[59] However, due to the bystander effect, tumor eradication with GDEPT appears to be possible even with transduction of only 10% of cells.[63]

The goal of the gene therapeutic approach (e.g., gene replacement therapy in combination with chemo- and or radiation therapy, induction of an anti-tumoral immune response, or suicide gene therapy), the target cells, and the desired route of application determine the required stringency of retroviral transduction. For stimulation of the immune system, cells are mainly manipulated *ex vivo/in vitro* and stably transduced cells are selected prior to re-infusion into the patient. For this approach, vectors carrying a selectable marker in addition to the therapeutic gene are preferred. Given that the cell population desired for transduction can be isolated with sufficient purity, selective targeting of the retroviral particle is a minor problem. However, if the *in vivo* application of retroviral vectors is considered, targeting is likely to become a critical issue. Several methods to modify the viral envelope thereby increasing the specificity and also transduction efficiency have been developed (for review see [56, 59]). The replacement of the original viral *env* protein by an *env* sequence from another retrovirus (pseudotyping), the genetic modification of the retroviral envelope protein, either by incorporation of a target-cell-specific ligand or receptor as well as the utilization of bi-specific antibodies as bridging agents have been described.[64–79] However, these manipulations often result in significant reduction of viral titers, and modifications of the viral envelope protein do not necessarily narrow the spectrum of susceptible cell types, especially in view of the potentially systemic application in cancer gene therapy.

Due to the fact that the serum complement system is able to inactivate retroviruses and also retroviral vectors, transduction efficiency of systemically delivered retroviral vectors is generally reduced. In the case of ovarian cancer, gene therapy is applied intraperitoneally, as this is the site of cancer spread and the peritoneal cavity reduces the systemic distribution of the viral vector. Moreover, due to the presence of complement inhibitors in peritoneal fluid, inactivation of retroviral vectors is less likely to occur than in the presence of serum.[80–82] Another approach evaluated for GDEPT in ovarian cancer is the local delivery of vector-producing cells which were stably transfected *ex vivo* with a replication-incompetent virus, thus locally increasing the concentration of the therapeutic protein. Furthermore, an immune response aiding in the elimination of tumor cells is expected.[83, 84]

In addition to problems related to low transduction efficiency and therefore low levels of transgene expression, silencing of gene expression occurs quite often, further reducing the therapeutic effect.[39]

Very recently, the construction of a stable replication-competent murine leukemia derived virus carrying the green fluorescent protein (GFP) as a reporter was described.[85] This construct was seen to be stable and to replicate efficiently *in vitro* and *in vivo*. This is the first example of a stable replication-competent retroviral vector. However, it is too early to speculate on the translation into a therapeutic concept before a therapeutic vector is available for preclinical studies.

To overcome some of the inherent problems of retroviral vectors, lentivirus-based vectors have been developed.[86–88] The lentivirus (HIV-1) is able to infect and integrate into nondividing cells and is naturally targeted to $CD4^+$ cells. Given the complexity of the HIV genome and the pathogenicity of the wild-type virus, extensive studies for biosafety are necessary before application in human gene therapy can be envisoned. At this point, the utilization of lentiviral vectors for treatment of ovarian cancer appears speculative.

b. Adenovirus-Based Vectors

Adenoviruses (Ad) are common nonenveloped DNA viruses and carry a linear double-stranded DNA of about 36 kDa. Based on the hemagglutination properties, 6 serogroups (A to F) are distinguished and at least 49 different serotypes have been described so far.[89, 90] Adenoviruses usually cause rather mild infections affecting either the respiratory tract (subgroups B, C, and E), the gastrointestinal tract (subgroups A and F), or ocular epithelial cells (subgroup D).[91] Even though adenoviruses preferentially infect epithelial cells, a wide variety of different cell types are susceptible to infection. Besides a rather stringent host specificity, the subgroup A members Ad12, Ad18, and Ad31 were seen to be mildly oncogenic in rodents.[92] In humans no association between adenoviral infection and oncogenic transformation has been described.

In contrast to retroviruses, adenoviruses are able to infect quiescent cells and viral replication occurs episomally, thereby nearly totally excluding the risk of insertional mutations. Furthermore, the episomal incorporation of the viral genes limits their transduction to a time span of 4–6 weeks after which they are expelled from the host cell nucleus. Given the extremely low pathogenic potential of the serogroup C members Ad2 and Ad5 together with the broad knowledge about their genome and gene function, both subtypes are attractive candidates as shuttle vectors in human gene therapy. In fact, about 25% of gene therapy clinical trials utilize Ad2- and Ad5-derived vectors.

Adenoviruses are icosahedral particles (diameter 80–110 nm; 20 facets, 12 vertices) with an outer capsid composed of 252 capsomers building 240 hexons (12 per facet) and 12 penton bases (1 per vertix) carrying a noncovalently attached antenna-like fiber.[93, 94] With the exception of serogroup B viruses, each fiber has a distal C-terminal knob domain responsible for binding to the Coxsackie-Adenovirus-receptor (CAR).[90, 93, 95] HLA class I molecules are likely to participate in binding the adenovirus fiber to human epithelial and B lymphoblastoid cells.[96] The penton base consists of five identical subunits, each containing an Arg-Gly-Asp (RGD) sequence known to interact with αv integrins, e.g., integrins αvβ3 (CD51/CD61) and αvβ5.[97–101] Secondary to binding of the adenovirus fiber knob domain to CAR, the fibers dissociate from the penton base, thereby enabling the interaction between integrins αvβ3/αvβ5 and the penton base. This is followed by virus internalization via receptor-mediated endocytosis. Intact virions are released to the cytosol and binding to the nuclear pore complex is required to transfer the viral genome into the nucleus.[98, 99, 102–107] Whereas the expression of CAR as an important prerequisite for adenoviral transduction is widely accepted, the role of integrins is not so clear.[98, 108–116]

The adenovirus genome is encoded by a linear, double-stranded DNA molecule of about 36 kb, which is packed in a densed chromatin-like structure resulting from the interaction between the viral DNA and viral proteins. Both sides of the viral genome are flanked by inverted terminal repeats (ITR, 103 bp each) which function as replication origins.[117, 118] The packaging sequence (Ψ) is located closely upstream to the left ITR (Fig. 21.2). According to the time of expression, three groups of genes, early, intermediate, and late are distinguished and distinct functions have been assigned to most of them (for review see [94, 118] and the references cited therein). The early coding region consists of five transcription units (E1A, E1B, E2, E3, and E4), the intermediate (early delayed) transcription units are the pIX and IVa$_2$ genes, and the late transcription unit (LTU) encodes mostly structural proteins of the capsid and the internal core.[119] It is far beyond the scope of this chapter to present the complex network of adenoviral gene expression. The most prominent features of the early genes are summarized briefly, as at least some of them are used in cancer gene therapy. Gene expression relies on the host cell RNA polymerase II. Viral replication can only start after expression of the early genes, beginning with E1A which is translated immediately after the viral genome has entered the nucleus. Even though, a nonfunctional or missing E1A excludes viral replication, it does not prevent expression of the viral genome.

E1A encodes for two rather similar multifunctional regulatory proteins (243R and 289R, generated by alternative splicing), which either directly or indirectly activate cellular transcription factors and are important for a productive infection of quiescent cells, e.g., inducing cell cycle progression from G1 into S phase.[94, 120] Proteins known to interact with E1A are p300 and p105-Rb, both involved in preventing the G1 to S phase progression of the cell cycle.[34, 36] Within the two conserved regions (CR-1 and CR-2) of E1A for p300 and p105-Rb non-overlapping binding sites have been identified.[120, 121] As E1A can be provided by a separate DNA

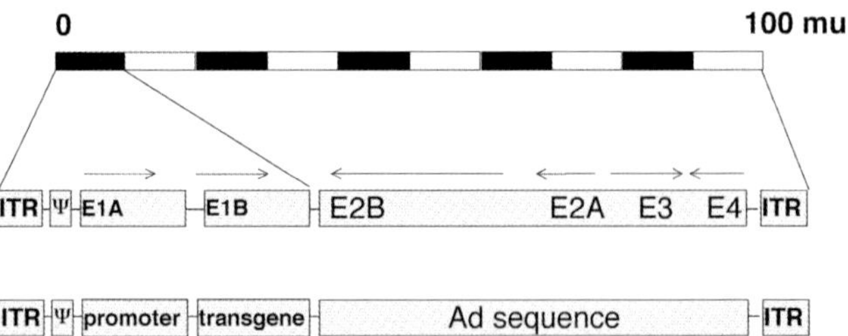

FIGURE 21.2 Schematic representation of the adenoviral genome. The viral genome (about 36 kb) is divided into 100 map units. To generate replication-incompetent adenoviral vectors, the E1A and E1B region are substituted with the transgene and an appropriate promoter. (From Walther, W., and Stein, U. (2000). *Drugs* 60, 249–271; Perricaudet, M., and Stratford-Perricaudet, L. D. (1995). *In* "Viruses in Human Gene Therapy" (J. M.-H. Vos, ed.), pp, 1–32. Academic Press, Durham, NC; and Yeh, P., and Perricaudet, M. (1997). *FASEBJ,* II, 615–623.)

(a helper phage or a transformed cell line), the production of replication-incompetent adenoviral vectors is possible.[122] In case of an infection with wild-type Ad, E1A proteins suppress the anti-viral actions of interferons α and β. In addition, the E1A induced susceptibility of infected cells to cytolysis mediated by tumor necrosis factor-α (TNF-α), natural killer cells (NK cells), and macrophages is, at least in part, counteracted by E1B and E3 encoded proteins.

It is of special interest, that in contrast to the effect in rodent cells, E1A acts as a tumor suppressor in human tumor cells independently of *HER2/neu* oncogene overexpression.[33, 123] Although the molecular mechanisms are not yet fully understood, clinical trials based on either adenoviral or non-viral delivery of E1A expressing plasmids in head and neck and breast and ovarian cancer are under way.[55, 124–126]

The E1B region encodes for two unrelated proteins (55 and 19 kDa) essential for a productive viral infection, as both proteins inhibit apoptosis. The 55-kDa protein is known to inactivate the tumor suppressor p53 and to repress p53 mediated transcription.[127] The 19-kDa protein acts as a negative regulator of E1A gene expression and prevents DNA degradation and TNF-α-mediated lysis of infected cells. Recently, this protein was shown to be a functional homolog of BCL-2, preventing apoptosis by binding to the pro-apoptotic members of the BCL-2 family.[128, 129]

Proteins encoded by the E2 region (E2A and E2B subregions) are mainly involved in the replication of the viral genome. The 72-kDa protein encoded by E2A is also involved in transcriptional control and virus assembly.[119] E2B encodes for a DNA polymerase and an 80-kDa protein, both participating in DNA replication at multiple sites.[130, 131]

E3 encoded proteins are important for adenovirus infected cells in order to escape from the host immune system, even though the E3 locus is not essential for viral growth in tissue culture.[129] Transcription of the E3 region is likely to be independent from E1A as the E3 promoter contains a binding site for the NF-κB transcription factor,[132, 133] which in turn is inducible by cytokines like TNF-α. The E3 encoded gp19 kDa prevents the cytotoxic T-lymphocyte-mediated cell killing as it blocks the translocation of MHC-class I molecules to the cell surface.[134] The 14.7-kDa protein and the 10.4 kDa/14.5 kDa complex (also named E3 RID because of its role in receptor internalization and degradation; RIDα is the 10.4-kDa and RIDβ is the 14.5-kDa protein) inhibit apoptosis mediated by Fas ligand (FasL) or TNF-α.[121, 129, 135] Finally, the E3 11.6-kDa adenovirus death protein (adp) promoting virus release is encoded within this region.[133]

The E4 region encodes seven different polypeptides and regulates gene expression at the transcriptional and post-transcriptional level. This region appears to be essential for viral growth in cell culture, e.g., the propagation of an E4-deleted adenovirus requires a cell line compensating for the E4 defect.[94]

For cancer gene therapy, adenovirus is either used as a vehicle for the desired therapeutic gene(s), or specially designed adenoviral vectors themselves are used as therapeutic agents.

The E1 region and most of E3 genes were deleted in first generation Ad5- and/or Ad2-based vectors, making room for inserts of about 7–8 kb.[136] The human embryonic kidney derived 293 cell line is used for the propagation of E1-deleted adenoviral vectors, as this cell line is stably transformed with a large fragment of Ad5 encoding for the left ITR, the packaging signal sequences, and the complete E1A and E1B regions.[122] With this cell line sufficient amounts of adenoviral vectors (titers >10^{11} pfu/ml) can be produced. However, due to the extensive overlap between the sequences integrated in the 293 cells and the E1-deleted adenoviral backbone, homologous recombinations resulting in replication-competent virus occur, thus increasing the costs for production of virus for clinical application.[137] The unwanted generation of replication-competent adenoviral vectors can be avoided by using the human lung cell line A549, which is transformed with an E1-expression vector.[138] Another possibility is to generate vectors with additional large inserts in the E3 region, giving rise to the creation of vectors with a genome of more than 105% that of the wild-type virus upon homologous recombination. Such large genomes cannot be packaged efficiently and are therefore rather unstable.[139]

Evaluation of first generation replication-deficient vectors in clinical trials have shown that, especially with E3 deleted vectors, systemic application is accompanied by a strong immune reaction, rendering repeated application difficult.[38, 140] In second generation Ad2 and Ad5 vectors additional deletions/mutations are introduced to reduce both the risk for contamination with replication-competent virus and the immune response toward the transduced cells.[39, 137, 141, 142] Even though the recognition and subsequent elimination of transduced cells by the immune system might not be a disadvantage for elimination of the tumor cells, the immune response itself may prevent long-term expression of transgenes in gene replacement therapy and might eventually prevent repeated application of the virus. To overcome these limitations, the construction of an adenoviral vector devoid of all viral coding regions except the ITR and Ψ packaging sequence, often referred to as "gutless vector," was described recently,[143, 144] (for review see [117] and references cited therein). For propagation and amplification of these vectors, cell lines and helper phages providing the function of the adenoviral genome are required making large-scale production and purification rather difficult. Therefore, it will take some time until this type of vector is available for clinical trials.[117]

Despite the ability of adenovirus to infect nondividing cells and the rather high (rather 100%) *in vitro* transduction efficiencies, transduction efficiency *in vivo* rarely exceeds 20%, even when the vector is applied locally, e.g., either via intratumoral injection or, in case of peritoneal carcinomatosis and ovarian cancer, intraperitoneally. However, due to the bystander effect (see Section III.C.3) present in GDEPT this markly reduced transduction efficiency was not seen to reduce or even abolish the therapeutic response.[145–147] In contrast, in gene replacement therapy the bystander effect is much less pronounced, indicating that with this approach low transduction efficiencies are likely to limit the therapeutic effect.[148]

In order to increase the local concentration of the therapeutic vector, thereby increasing the probability for internalization and transgene expression, replication-attenuated adenoviral vectors have been (re-)introduced into clinical trials.[59] There is a rather long history of viral and bacterial agents in cancer treatment (for review see [149, 150]).

The efficient replication of wild-type adenovirus depends on specific interactions between viral proteins and between viral and cellular proteins in order to avoid recognition and premature elimination of infected cells by the immune system as well as premature cytolytic effects. Some of the viral gene products like the E3 encoded adenoviral death protein (adp or E3 11.6 kDa) and the E4 encoded protein E4ORF4 are cytotoxic themselves.[118, 133] On the other hand, deletion of those E3 proteins preventing recognition of infected cells by the immune system induces strong immune response and elimination of the infected cells before viral replication is completed (for review see [149, 150]). Based on the knowledge about the interactions between adenoviral and host cell proteins during the time course of a productive (=cytolytic) infection, replication-competent Ad2, Ad5, and even chimeric Ad2/Ad5 viruses are engineered for utilization as tumor-selective oncolytic agents. With this type of viral oncolytic therapy the transfer of an additional therapeutic gene to the cells is not absolutely required.[39, 59, 142, 149–152] Up to date, two replication-attenuated adenoviruses are evaluated in clincal trials.

First, in case of the Ad5-derived vector, CN 706, replication is restricted to the tumor cells by introduction of a tumor-specific promoter driving the E1A expression. This concept is evaluated for the treatment of prostate-specific antigen (PSA) producing prostate cancer, as E1A expression is driven by minimal enhancer/promoter constructs from the human PSA gene.[153] Similar approaches for the introduction of other tumor- and/or tissue-specific promoters as well as additional modifications of the viral backbone with the goal of enhanced oncolytic activity have recently been reported.[154, 155]

Secondly, another approach is realized with the E1B gene-attenuated adenovirus, also referred to as ONYX-015, Ad *dl1520* or as CI-1042. ONYX-015 is an Ad2/Ad5 chimeric vector with a double mutated E1B region, e.g., a deletionof about 825 bp (bp2496 to bp3323) and a single mutation (C to T) at position 2022 generating a stop codon at the third amino acid of the E1B protein. Thus, the resulting vector is unable to express the E1B encoded 55-kDa protein, which is required for replication of Ad in the presence of functional p53.[156] As in about 50% of all human cancers, loss-of-function mutations are found in p53, this vector is preferentially used to lyse tumor cells lacking functional p53. This approach has been extensively evaluated for the treatment of patients with recurrent head and neck cancer, [157–159] and recently a phase I trial with patients suffering from recurrent ovarian cancer was reported.[160]

Although these replication-attenuated viruses are oncolytic by themselves, the additional inclusion of a therapeutic gene (armed therapeutic virus) is advantagous. The viral replication amplifies the transgene production and, due to the spread of the virus, the number of transduced cells is increasing.[152, 161] The construction and application of a replication-attenuated adenovirus containing a hsv-tk expression cassette (Ad.TK^{RC}) or even a double suicide gene cassette (CD/hsv1-tk) to further improve the therapeutic efficacy was reported.[162–164] The therapeutic efficacy of Ad.TK^{RC} was evaluated in preclinical studies using a mouse model for human cervical cancer, subcutaneous melanoma, and colon carcinoma.[164, 165] In these trials mice receiving Ad.TK^{RC} and ganciclovir (gcv) showed significantly increased long-term survival compared to those treated with Ad.TK^{RC} alone. Moreover, the onset of treatment with gcv relative to start of gene therapy is critical for the therapeutic outcome indicating that sufficient spread of the virus is necessary to efficiently eradicate the tumor.

c. Adenovirus-Associated Virus Vectors (AAV) and other DNA Viruses

Besides the utilization of retroviral and adenoviral vectors for gene therapy, a variety of other DNA viruses are being evaluated (see Table 21.1).

The AAV belongs to the family of parvoviruses and seems not to be associated with any human disease. It requires either an adenovirus or herpesvirus for replication (for a recent review see [166] and references cited therein). Even though AAVs have a rather limited capacity (between 4.1 and 4.5 kb) for the insertion of foreign genes, there are several advantages like a broad range of target cells, low immunogenicity, long-lasting expression of transgenes, and virtually no pathogenic potential making this virus especially attractive for gene replacement therapy of inherited diseases.

Due to the exclusive tropism of herpes simplex virus-1 (HSV-1) for neuronal tissue, this virus has gained special interest in the treatment of malignant brain tumors (for review see [167]). HSV-1 is a large (152 kb) enveloped double-stranded DNA virus capable of accepting about 30 kb of foreign genes. Similar to Ad, HSV-1 does not integrate into the host genome and the cytotoxicity of HSV-1 wild-type can be reduced significantly by deletion of the respective genes. Replication-deficient as well as conditionally replicating HSV-1 vectors have been described.[39, 167]

In GDEPT for ovarian cancer, the thymidine kinase gene encoded by HSV-1 is frequently used as a suicide gene transferred to the tumor cells via either retroviral- or adenoviral-based vectors. There is one recent report on the preclinical evaluation of a replication-competent HSV-1 mutant for the treatment of epithelial ovarian cancer.[168] In this study, irradiated vector producer cells derived from human teratocarcinoma were delivered intraperitoneally to ensure high local concentrations of the viral particles. One major problem associated with the introduction of this approach into a phase I clinical trial is the intraperitoneal application of tumor cells, even lethally irradiated, as carriers for the therapeutic vector. This may not only pose safety concerns but may also make it psychologically difficult to accept for the patients.

Although other viruses like Epstein-Barr virus (EBV), Newcastle disease virus (NDV), reovirus, or poxvirus have gained interest as therapeutic vectors, these viruses are not being utilized for application in ovarian cancer gene therapy.[39, 59, 169]

B. Targeting of Tumor Cells

Effective transgene delivery is ultimately required for the success of any gene therapeutic approach. The main routes of adenoviral and retroviral internalization are known. The receptors for those viruses are often expressed at insufficient densities by the target cell and, equally important, the expression of viral receptors is not restricted to tumor cells. Even though *in vitro* these problems are often overcome by increasing the ratio of viral particles per cell, inadequate targeting and unwanted vector spread can significantly lower the therapeutic efficacy *in vivo*. Systemic vector spread can be reduced by local application of the vector, e.g., using intraperitoneal application in case of ovarian cancer. To further increase transduction efficiency, vectors have also been engineered for improved targeting. This goal can be achieved by either direct or indirect modification of the viral envelope (retroviral vectors) or capsid (adenoviral vectors).[39, 50, 56, 59, 79, 136] Another possibility to restrict transgene expression to target cells is the utilization of target-cell-specific promoters driving the therapeutic gene.[39, 170]

1. Modification of the Viral Envelope in Retroviral Vectors

Several ways to enhance the specificity of retroviral vectors have been realized. Among those are the replacementof the viral env protein with one from another retrovirus (pseudotyping) and the genetic modification of the retroviral envelope protein, either by incorporation of a target-cell-specific ligand or receptor or by utilization of bi-specific antibodies as bridging agents.[64–79] In gene therapy of ovarian cancer, none of these approaches have been realized. This is likely due to the fact that ovarian cancer grows inside the peritoneal cavity for a long time, which in turn provides a suitable compartment for local application of gene therapy. Thus, problems associated with the "nondirected" delivery, e.g., inhibition of virus through complement factors, dilution effects, unwanted transduction, etc., are less pronounced.[81, 171] In two of the clinical phase I trials utilizing retroviral vectors with the *hsv1-tk* gene, *ex vivo* transduced cells were delivered intraperitoneally. The rationale behind these trials was either to eradicate the tumor by combination of the bystander effect and an induced immune response (tumor vaccination) or to achieve high local vector concentrations, thus resulting in sufficient transduction efficiencies to sensitize cells directly to gcv. In the latter case, the bystander effect and the induced immune response improve the therapeutic effect.[83, 84]

2. Modification of the Viral Capsid in Adenoviral Vectors

Similar to retroviral vectors, modifications of the adenoviral capsid have been performed either to reduce unwanted transduction or to increase transduction efficiency for target cells. Techniques include the utilization of bi-specific antibodies, binding to the target cell and to the adenoviral capsid, modification of the viral fiber or penton base by site-directed mutagenesis, or construction of adenoviral vectors utilizing fibers from other adenoviral subtypes.[59, 172–178] Internalization of Ad2 and Ad5 strongly requires the binding of the fiber knob domain to CAR. Subsequently, interaction between integrins $\alpha v\beta 3/\alpha v\beta 5$ and the RGD sequence of the penton base is followed by virus internalization. As expected of adenoviral tropism, CAR is widely expressed on epithelial cells. By contrast, endothelial cells, smooth muscle cells, and fibroblasts virtually do not express CAR and are therefore almost resistent to Ad infection and transduction.[90, 100] For efficient adenoviral transduction of a specific target cell in an enviroment of equally permissive nontarget cells, vector load has to be increased with a concomitant increase of unwanted side effects. In this situation, the utilization of a receptor or ligand that is preferentially expressed on the target cell can be used to enhance the tropism of the vector. A variety of molecules have been described that are suitable for this purpose (for review see [11, 179]). Recently, the expression of the folate receptor and of fibroblast growth factor receptor (FGF-R) by ovarian cancer cells was utilized for targeted adenoviral transduction.[172, 175, 180] The Fab-fragment of a knob domain specific monoclonal antibody was conjugated with folate [172] or a 115 amino acid fragment of the basic fibroblast growth factor (FGF2).[175] Due to binding of the conjugated Fab fragment to the knob domain, direct interaction with CAR was prevented. Instead, the tagged vector bound to the target cell surface via the ligand which was conjugated to the antibody. Subsequent interactions with the viral penton base and cell surface integrins could take place. This approach has been evaluated *in vitro* [172] and in a murine model of ovarian cancer *in vivo*.[175, 180] The goal of re-targeting adenoviral vectors requires prevention of the interaction between the fiber knob domain and CAR of nontargeted cells and at the same time the introduction of a novel ligand with high specificity for the desired target cells. Besides utilizing antibodies for this purpose, a nonbiodegradable polymeric covalent coating of the adenoviral surface resulting in a re-targeting procedure was described recently.[181] The coating procedure completely blocked adenovirus internalization and the binding of anti-adenoviral antibodies which are likely to reduce adenoviral transduction efficiency *in vivo*. Re-targeting to tumor cells was achieved by the covalent binding of FGF2 to the coated adenoviral suface. With this virus, effective internalization and transgene expression was achieved in cells with functional FGF-R. The covalent incorporation of vascular endothelial growth factor (VEGF) in the polymer coat could, for example, allow for the selective targeting of VEGF-R positive cells, e.g., endothelial cells.

Whereas internalization of uncoated adenovirus depends on the interaction with CAR and αvβ3/αvβ5 integrins, these interactions are no longer required for the internalization of FGF2-re-targeted virus. This indicates, that FGF2-mediated internalization involves the cellular pathway of FGF-R.[182]

Another novel strategy increasing transduction efficiency and long-term transgene expression is based on the combination of retroviral and adenoviral properties. An adenoviral vector is used as a carrier for the retroviral genome, combining the high transduction efficiency of Ad and the long-term expression of the transgene introduced by the retrovirus.[183] After successful construction of such chimeric viral vectors a variety of problems remain to be addressed before introduction into clinical trials can be envisioned.

3. Tissue-Specific Promoters for the Selective Expression of Transgenes Transcriptional Targeting

The controlled expression of the transgene is another powerful tool for targeted gene therapy since the viral tropism and the expression of the therapeutic gene together determine the therapeutic outcome. In first generation adenoviral vectors the expression of the transgenes was mainly under the control of strong viral promoters such as the cytomegalovirus-immediate early gene promoter (CMV-IE-promoter) or the Rous-sarcoma virus (rsv) long terminal repeat promoter.[101, 184–187] In the case of first generation retroviral vectors, the respective retroviral promoters were utilized.[56] With this approach, each successfully transduced cell should, in principle, express the transgene at a sufficient level seen in *in vitro* and preclinical *in vivo* studies. However, the risk of *in vivo* silencing of the viral promoters may limit transgene expression.[170] Besides this reduction in transgene expression, the unrestricted expression resulting from poor targeting of the gene delivery system could be disadvantageous, as especially with GDEPT also non-malignant cells are likely to be eliminated. This problems can at least partially be overcome by transcriptional targeting, e.g., the introduction of tissue- and/or tumor-specific promoters driving the transgene expression (for recent reviews see also [170, 188] and references cited therein). Moreover, these promoters can also be used to engineer oncolytic viruses with inherent replication-selectivity.[44, 149, 150, 152, 167, 189]

The regulatory elements (promoter/enhancer) of tumor marker proteins in combination with GDEPT have been seen to be especially suitable for achieving tumor-specific gene expression and for enhancing the therapeutic efficacy in *in vitro* and preclinical animal studies. Important examples are the utilization of CEA-specific regulatory elements in the treatment of colon and lung carcinoma,[190–193] AFP-specific regulatory elements in the treatment of hepatocellular carcinoma,[194–197] tyrosinase promoter for the treatment in melanomas,[198–202] the DF3 enhancer in DF3-positive breast carcinomas,[203] the secretory leukoprotease inhibitor (SLPI) regulatory sequence in epithelial carcinomas,[41, 204] and PSA-specific regulatable elements for the treatment of prostate carcinoma.[205, 206] In addition, the PSA promoter and the surfactant protein B (SPB) promoter have also been utilized to drive adenoviral replication in PSA expressing prostate cancer cells and SPB producing lung cancer cells, respectively.[153, 155] A replication-deficient adenoviral vector expressing hsv-tk under control of the osteocalcin-promoter has been constructed, since osteocalcin was seen to be expressed almost exclusively in osteotropic tumors and differentiated osteoblasts. Based on preclinical studies indicating that eradication of prostate tumor xenografts at subcutaneous and bone sites is possible, a clinical phase I trial in patients with metastatic prostate cancer is currently under way.[207]

Another approach to selective enhancement of transgene expression in CEA-producing cancer cells is the incorporation of the Cre recombinase/*loxP* system. For this purpose, two replication-deficient E1/E3 deleted adenoviral vectors were constructed expressing either Cre recombinase under the control of the CEA promoter or the *hsv1-tk* gene separated from a modified CMV promoter by insertion of the neomycine (*neo*) resistance gene flanked by a pair of loxP sites. These sites are necessary for recognition by Cre recombinase. Expression of Cre recombinase is required for excisional deletion of the *neo* gene resulting in *hsv1-tk* expression.[208] This system prevents suicide gene expression in CEA-negative cells thus minimizing unwanted side effects. One major disadvantage of this system is that the therapeutic effect relies mainly on the expression of two transgenes introduced into the same cell. Given the overall suboptimal transduction efficiency of viral vectors, the simultaneous transduction of one cell with two different vectors seems even more unlikely. Further studies are necessary to show clearly, whether the therapeutic benefit of this system is improved compared to the direct expression of the therapeutic gene under control of the CEA promoter.

The utilization of such tissue-specific promoters for ovarian cancer gene therapy is hampered by the fact that no such ovarian cancer specific gene is available. However, very recently an ovarian-specific promoter (OSP) was derived from a retrovirus-like element specifically expressed in the rat ovary.[209, 210] Most interestingly, this promoter also functions in a variety of transiently transfected human ovarian cancer cell lines indicating that it might be a suitable promoter for driving transgene expression in ovarian cancer gene therapy.

The application of promoter/enhancer elements mentioned above is restricted to tumors expressing the respective marker proteins. In contrast, L-plastin, belonging to a family of genes encoding actin-binding proteins, was seen to be broadly expressed in epithelian neoplasms; while being solely expressed in mature leukocytes of healthy persons.[211–213] Due to the expression of L-plastin by epithelial tumors, the L-plastin promoter appears especially suitable for conferring tumor-specific gene expression to ovarian cancer cells. Consequently, a replication-deficient adenoviral vector expressing the *E. coli* derived, CD under control of the L-plastin promoter was constructed and evaluated *in vitro* and *in vivo* as an approach for treating bladder and ovarian cancer.[214] Whereas in normal peritoneum this vector shows significantly reduced cytotoxicity compared to the commonly used vector expressing the transgene under control of the CMV promoter, these differences were hardly seen in cancer cell lines. Despite the promising results presented in this study, the efficacy for eradication of ovarian cancer cells may be improved by changing the therapeutic gene. The *E. coli* derived, CD converts 5-fluorocytosine to the cytotoxic 5-fluorouracil (5-FU), which is used as an anti-metabolite in chemotherapy for bladder cancer. Unfortunately, the sensitivity of ovarian cancer cells to 5-FU is rather low thus limiting the bystander effect, which is of major importance for efficient elimination of the tumor cells *in vivo*. Therefore, it would be worthwhile to repeat this study using an adenoviral vector harboring *hsv1-tk* instead.

Another possibility would be the utilization of cell-cycle-regulated promoters driving transgene expression in proliferating tumor cells (for review see [170]).

The promoter of the early growth response 1 (*egr*-1) gene or the tissue plasminogen activator (t-PA) which are activated by therapeutic doses of ionizing radiation or the promoter of the P-glycoprotein/multidrug resistance-1 gene (*mdr*-1) which in turn is activated by chemotherapeutic agents are attractive for the timely expression of therapeutic genes which are likely to sensitize or even to enhance the therapeutic effects of the two traditional treatment modalities. Viral vectors expressing tumor necrosis factor-α (TNF-α) or *hsv1-tk* under control of either radiation inducible promoters or the *mdr*-1 promoter have been constructed and evaluated in animal models for malignant gliomas and hepatocellular carcinomas.[215–222]

A common feature of the promoters currently utilized for cancer gene therapy is that they are either active ("on") or inactive ("off"). As a consequence, the amount and activity of the transgene solely depends on the status of the promoter and is inaccessible to exogeneous stimulation and/or repression. Therefore, in addition to tissue-specific promoters, those which can be regulated through exogeneous factors are also under investigation. Regulated gene expression can be achieved either by incorporating endogeneous response elements like steroid-response elements [223] or hypoxia-responsive elements.[224, 225] Steroid receptors are involved in progression and prognosis of breast cancer, and are likely to also be involved in ovarian cancer. They may be utilized to achieve tumor-selective and controlled transgene expression in ovarian cancer.[226–229] A tumor-associated promoter which is not necessarily restricted to a single tumor entity is the transcriptional activator hypoxia-inducible factor-1 (HIF-1). In most solid tumors hypoxia is rather common and hypoxia-responsive elements were utilized to engineer viral vectors for tumor-specific transgene expression.[224, 225, 230] None of those systems has so far been introduced in a clinical phase I trial even though the *in vitro* data look promissing.

In addition to endogeneous systems, chimeric controlled (regulatable) systems are being developed. These systems are based on prokaryotic and eukaryotic elements in combination with transactivators designed for specific interaction with the desired response elements. These are incorporated into the vector together with the therapeutic gene (for review see [231]). Such systems ("gene switches") are widely used for controlled gene expression *in vitro* and in transgenic mice, and gain special interest for application in gene therapy of those disorders, where transgene expression is required at a level close to the overall physiological situation. Examples for the inducible expression of transgenes are the *E. coli* derived tetracycline-repressed system,[232] the progesterone regulatable system,[233] and the *Drosophila* derived ecdysone inducible system.[234] Briefly, one vector or plasmid expresses the transactivator which binds to its exogeneously provided ligand with high affinity followed by the interaction of the ligand-occupied transactivator with the responsive element which is upstream of a minimal promoter driving target gene expression (for review see [235–238]). Whereas the inclusion of endogeneous enhancers of transcription into clinical trials is likely in the near future, the application of exogeneous regulatable systems in human gene therapy is still in its infancy and several problems related to these systems need to be addressed. First, the successful induction of gene expression requires the co-transduction of target cells. Given the low overall transduction efficiencies in cancer gene therapy, it is hard to imagine that stimulatable transgene expression can overcome the disadvantage of an overall reduced number of cells co-transduced with both vectors. Therefore, the concept of this application has been restricted mainly to the *ex vivo* manipulation of cells and to the induction of gene expression in transgenic mice. Secondly, a strong immune response resulting in the elimination of transduced cells is to be expected, because these gene switches are based on the expression of non-mammalian proteins.

Very recently, a high capacity adenoviral vector carrying all elements necessary for exogeneous inducible gene expression was described.[239] All coding sequences of the parental Ad5 were eliminated and replaced by an internal cassette coding for the regulator and the target gene. For forming the regulator, a chimeric protein consisting of a mutated progesterone ligand binding domain was fused to the yeast GAL4DNA binding domain and the p65 activation domain, which is part of the NFκB complex.[233, 240–242] The target gene for expression was the human growth hormone (hGH) coupled to a 17mer GAL4 binding site which in turn was linked to the liver-specific transthyretin promoter to ensure liver-specific expression. Reproducible hGH secretion was observed upon induction with mifepristone (RU486) in mice intravenously injected with this construct. Interestingly, the mifepristone concentrations needed for induction were below those necessary for its antiprogestin effects. Also problems associated with the immune response toward non-mammalian receptor proteins were reduced with this construct, thus increasing the potential therapeutic benefit. Even though the elimination of transduced tumor cells is the major goal of cancer gene therapy, it is a major obstacle in the gene therapy of other diseases.

C. Concepts for Cancer Gene Therapy

A variety of important signal transduction pathways with related inducers and inhibitors as well as aberrations in cancer cells have been described, however, up to now the "key molecule of cancerogenesis" has not been identified.[34] In normal tissues homeostasis is guaranteed by the balanced rates of proliferation and apoptosis. Unrestricted proliferation, most likely as a consequence of oncogene activation in combination with a reduced sensitivity toward apoptotic stimuli is a common feature of cancer cells. The malignant precursor cell of the macroscopic tumor must also have evaded immune recognition (for review see [24, 36, 243–246]). The goal of any gene therapy for cancer is to completely eradicate malignant transformed cells. This can be achieved, at least in theory, by re-introducing tumor suppressor genes or inhibiting oncogenes, by stimulation of an anti-tumor immune response or by introduction of a new feature sensitizing the transduced cell to cytotoxic drugs and/or radiation therapy. Given the complex genetic changes present in tumor cells, it sounds naive to expect that restorage of a single gene would be sufficient to revert the malignant phenotype *in vivo*. However, gene therapeutic approaches may enhnace the efficacy of conventional anti-cancer therapy.

1. Gene Replacement Therapy

a. Restorage of Tumor-Suppressor Gene Function

Until now, at least 24 tumor suppressor genes and their corresponding pathways have been identified (for review see [247] and references cited therein). The most prominent among them is the p53 protein. Inherited mutations of the p53 gene are associated with the Li-Fraumeni syndrom, a familial predispositon to sarcomas, breast, and brain tumors.[248] In about 50% of all human cancers loss of function of the tumor suppressor protein p53 is observed secondary to mutations, even though frequencies vary from below 10% in cervical cancer to 50% in ovarian cancer and to even more than 50% in lung cancer.[22, 23] Inactivation and degradation of p53 protein may also be induced by viral proteins like the E6 oncoprotein from human papilloma virus (HPV). In fact, this is frequently observed in cervical cancer, which is strongly associated with HPV infection.[249–252] Taken together, these findings stress the important role of functional p53 as a "guardian of the genome."[253]

In resting cells, the concentration of p53 is kept rather low (half-life ≈20 min) and the protein is barely detectable using routine immunohistochemistry techniques. In resting cells MDM2, which is the negative regulator of p53, binds to and blocks the transactivation domain of p53. Furthermore, MDM2 has an intrinsic ubiquitin ligase activity which is likely to be involved in p53 degradation. Whereas activated p53 is restrained to the nucleus, relocalization of p53 into the cytoplasm depends on the binding to MDM2 in resting cells.[254, 255] Activation of p53, which exerts its multiple functions as a homotetramer, is accompanied by a sharp increase of protein concentration in the nucleus. This accumulation of p53 is mostly due to reduced degradation. As a consequence of the MDM2-p53 dissociation, export of p53 from the nucleus is blocked. The need of homotetramerization (dimerization of dimers) is likely to explain that mutation-induced loss of one p53 allele may be sufficient to abrogate p53 protein function. The formation of mixed tetramers, containing the wild-type and the mutated protein, a disturbed conformation of the mutated protein and/or the deletion of sites for posttranslational modifications affect p53 function. The mature protein consists of 393 amino acid (aa) and can be divided into four domains with distinct functions. The acidic N-terminal transactivation domain (aa 1–42) is followed by the central sequence-specific DNA-binding domain (aa 102–292), the tetramerization domain (aa 324–355), and the basic C-terminal regulatory domain (aa 363–393). It functions as a sequence-specific transcription factor (see Table 21.2 for transcriptional targets) via its central DNA-binding domain. This requires structural changes of the C-terminal part. In addition, p53 also interacts directly with components of the basal transcriptional machinery via the N- and C-terminal domains. Like MDM2, the Ad E1B 55-kDa protein binds to the N-terminal domain of p53, thereby inhibiting the transcriptional activity of p53.[24, 245, 256] The vast majority of loss-of-function-inducing mutations are found in the central DNA-binding domain, preventing the activation of p53 target genes.[257, 258] In addition, posttranslational protein modifications can be impaired as a consequence of amino acid

TABLE 21.2 Transcriptional Targets for p53

Target gene	Effect
$p21^{WAF1/CIP1}$	
GADD45	Growth arrest
14-3-3σ	
Reprimo	
MDM2	Negative regulator of p53, targets p53 for degradation
KILLER/DR5, p53AIP1, IGF-BP3, *Fas*, *Bax*, PIDD (reactive oxygen species)	Induction of apoptosis, the effectors vary between different cell types

Modified from Somasundaram, K., and El-Deiry, W. S. (2000). *Front. Biosci.* 5, d424–437; Levine, A. J. (1997). *Cell*, 88, 303–331; and Vogelstein, B., Lane, D., and Levine, A. J. (2000). *Nature* 408, 307–310.

TABLE 21.3 Clinical Trials Utilizing Gene Therapy for Treatment of Ovarian Cancer

Therapeutic gene	Vector system	Trial phase	Ref.
HLA-A2, B13, or H-2K	Lipofection	I	[358]
E1A	Lipofection	I	[55]
BRCA1	Retrovirus	I/II	[81, 171]
hsv1-tk	Retrovirus	I	[83]
hsv1-tk	Retrovirus	I	[84]
anti-erbB-2 single chain antibody	Adenovirus	I	[359]
p53	Adenovirus	I/II	[273]
hsv1-tk + Topotecan	Adenovirus	I	[329, 360–362]
hsv1-tk	Adenovirus	I	[308, 330]

For overview on gene therapy trials see also: http://www.wiley.co.uk/wileychi/genmed/clinical/charts3.html.

changes and even deletion-mutants and truncated forms of p53 can be detected. Activation of p53 occurs as a consequence of several stressing events like exposure to DNA-damaging agents (radiation, alkylating agents, etc.), altered ribonucleotide pools, hypoxia, and redox-stress, heat-shock, oncogenic stimuli and other factors.[24, 245, 256, 259] The activation of p53 by this variety of different agents points to p53 as a key molecule integrating different signal transduction pathways. So far, three different upstream effectors have been identified inducing posttranslational modifications of p53 that prevent degradation.[256] Elevated levels of p53 in conjunction with several modifications of the protein enhance the transcriptional activation of downstream effectors. Finally, the transcriptional activation of p53 target genes results in the activation of genes promoting cell cycle arrest or other genes promoting apoptosis. Growth arrest is related to the induction of $p21^{WAF1/CIP1}$ and 14-3-3σ which inhibit the cyclin-dependent kinases (cdk) and sequester cyclin B1-cdk1 complexes outside the nucleus.[245] DNA repair is mediated by induction of GADD-45 and the pro-apoptotic pathways are triggered by induction of *bax*, *fas*, *KILLER/DR5*, *PUMA*, *NOXA*, and *p53AIP1*.[24, 35, 245, 260, 261]

Given the important role of p53 in controlling cell-cycle progression and induction of apoptosis, loss of p53 function is thought to be one of the most important reasons not only for malignant transformation but also for the observed resistance to chemo- and/or radiation therapy.[23, 24, 256] Given the rather high frequency of mutation-induced loss of p53 function in sporadic ovarian cancer, gene replacement of p53 with the rationale of re-enabling the cell to undergo apoptosis is an attractive approach.[43, 262, 263] Based on the preclinical *in vitro* and *in vivo* evaluation of p53 gene replacement therapy for ovarian cancer [264–272] and the results of a phase I clinical trial, p53 gene replacement therapy was recently introduced in a multicenter phase II/phase III trial for primary ovarian cancer (FIGO III) or primary peritoneal carcinomatosis (Table 21.3).[273] However, despite functional p53, numerous tumors are rather resistant to chemo- and or radiation therapy, thus pointing to other mechanisms enabling these cells to escape from growth arrest.[23, 30, 274–277] Indeed, other key regulator molecules like MDM2 and ARF may be mutated in tumors expressing wild-type p53.[255, 278, 279] The *INK4/ARF* locus on chromosome 9p21 is one of the sites mutated most frequently in human cancer. Two genes have been identified that play an important role in cell-cycle progression. Most interestingly, these two gene products are generated through the utilization of alternative reading frames (ARF). The $p16^{INK4a}$ is able to inhibit cyclin-dependent kinase 4 (cdk-4) and links the Rb and p53 pathways. The alternative transcript—$p19^{ARF}$ in mice and $p14^{ARF}$ in humans—is likely to bind to MDM2 thereby preventing p53 degradation.[254, 280] Mutation-induced loss of function of $p16^{INK4a}$ is observed in a variety of human tumors and it was shown recently that overexpression of $p16^{INK4a}$ is associated with replicative senescense.[281, 282] These findings make $p16^{INK4a}$ an attractive candidate for gene replacement therapy.[283] Even though rather little is known about the frequency of mutations affecting $p16^{INK4a}$ in ovarian cancer, there is some evidence that $p16^{INK4a}$ overexpression may be associated with an unfavorable prognosis. Very recently, the efficacy of $p16^{INK4a}$ gene replacement therapy, either alone or in combination with p53 replacement therapy, for ovarian cancer was evaluated *in vitro* and *in vivo* in a mouse model.[284, 285] In this study, adenoviral vectors harboring either p53 or $p16^{INK4a}$ under control of the CMV promoter were utilized alone or in combination. The cell lines tested were p53/$p16^{INK4a}$ wild-type, mutated in both or in only one of the the rapeutic genes evaluated. Whereas the *in vitro* data indicated that the therapeutic efficacy was enhanced by the application of both therapeutic genes, this effect was not seen *in vivo*. By contrast, only survival of mice treated with $p16^{INK4a}$ alone was improved. The comparison of the therapeutic efficacies, especially with respect to the double-transduction, might be hampered by differences in transduction efficiency. Therefore, the construction of a double-gene vector might be advantageous.

Another target for gene replacement therapy is BRCA1, since hereditary loss of function mutations of BRCA1 are present in about 5% of familial breast and ovarian cancer.[286, 287] Although the molecular function of BRCA1 is still not fully understood, overexpression of BRCA1 was shown to inhibit tumor growth *in vitro* and *in vivo*, most likely due to the activation of p53 and subsequent induction of p21. BRCA1 may also induce apoptosis directly.[286, 288–291] Retrovirally mediated overexpression of BRCA1 was shown to inhibit growth of ovarian and breast cancer cells *in vitro*. This was not observed with cell lines from lung or colon carcinoma, indicating that the BRCA1 mediated effects are affected by the cellular microenviroment. Furthermore overexpression of BRCA1 significantly inhibits growth of pre-established tumors in a mouse model of peritoneal carcinoma.[292] These data have been translated into clinical phase I and phase II trials.[81, 171] Patients with therapy-resistant (phase I) and minimal residual disease after first-line chemotherapy (phase II) received intraperitoneal delivery of a retroviral vector with wild-type BRCA1. Patients enrolled in the phase I trial had received already numerous chemotherapies. No significant immune response leading to complement-mediated degradation of the retroviral vehicle was detected, and repeated application of the vector was well tolerated. Since these findings indicated that intraperitoneal delivery of a retroviral vector might be a suitable approach for treatment of ovarian cancer, a phase II trial enrolling patients with minimal residual disease after first-line chemotherapy was initiated. In sharp contrast to the phase I trial, the vector was rapidly degraded upon intraperitoneal delivery and neutralizing antibodies toward the retroviral envelope were induced, thus preventing the therapeutic response. These tremendeous differences affecting the therapeutic outcome were most likely due to the severe suppression of the immune system in the phase I patients induced by several chemotherapeutic regimens.[171] Moreover, these observations stressed the importance of the transgene vehicle and the transgene for the therapeutic outcome. Meanwhile, a second generation of retroviral vectors with improved stability in the presence of human complement has been developed and is being evaluated in preclinical trials.[293]

b. Overexpression of Pro-Apoptotic Genes

Mutations can also impair apoptotic pathways, thereby rendering cells resistant to apoptosis.[294, 295] Apoptosis can be induced via the death-receptor pathway which is triggered by CD95/Fas receptor, tumor necrosis factor receptor-1 (TNF-R1) and other members of the death-receptor superfamily triggering the caspase cascade. In case of DNA damage, apoptosis is initiated mainly by p53 transactivation of Bax, the most prominent pro-apoptotic member of the Bcl-2 family of proteins. Other members of this family include the antiapoptotic proteins Bcl-2 and Bcl-x_L and the pro-apoptotic protein Bak (for review see [35, 260, 296] and references cited therein). Activation of apoptosis via the Bax-pathway releases mitochondrial cytochrome *c* which in turn activates the caspase cascade and results in the orderly dismantling and removal of the cell. Besides activating Bax, p53 can also promote cell surface expression of Fas receptor, and was even shown to directly stimulate mitochondria to produce high levels of toxic reactive oxygen species.[256, 297] In addition, other tumor-suppressor genes like PTEN, APC, and PML also exert their functions via induction of apoptosis.[30, 298, 299]

In ovarian cancer cells expression of Bax was found to be important for paclitaxel induced cell death. Moreover, in about 40% of ovarian cancer specimens low expression of Bax correlates with an impaired response to paclitaxel therapy resulting in a shortend disease-free interval.[300–302] On the basis of these observations, the efficacy of adenovirus-mediated Bax overexpression in human ovarian cancer cells was evaluated *in vitro* and in a preclinical mouse model of peritoneal carcinomatosis.[303] The DF3 promoter was used to drive transgene expression, since high levels of DF3 (MUC1) are detectable in about 75% of epithelial ovarian cancers, while normal mesothelial cells are virtually negative for DF3. Taken together, transgene-induced cytotoxicity correlated well with the DF3 levels and Ad.DF3.Bax significantly improved the survival of mice inoculated with DF3-positive human ovarian cancer cells. Since no information regarding the p53 and Bax status of the cell lines used was given, the interpretation of the data is difficult in view of the complex signaling pathways involving p53 and Bax. It would also be interesting to know whether these gene therapeutic approaches sensitized cells to treatment with paclitaxel. These data are ultimately necessary prior to the evaluation of this approach in a phase I clincal trial.

c. Inhibition of Oncogene Activation

Inhibition of oncogene activation is another possibility to prevent tumor cell proliferation. Due to the contrary molecular mechanisms—mutation-induced loss of function versus mutation-induced activation—oncogene activation cannot be reverted using gene replacement therapy. Instead, oligodesoxynucleotides (ODN), antisense gene encoding vectors, and ribozymes, e.g., RNA molecules with the ability to enzymatically degrade their target mRNA, have been evaluated (for review see [42] and references therein). Even though the initial results obtained *in vitro* were encouraging, severe problems related to the stability and targeting of the therapeutic molecules occurred *in vivo* and, similar to gene replacement therapy, the therapeutic efficacy relies on 100% transduction efficiency.

Another possibility to abolish oncogene-mediated signaling is to mask the oncogene with an antibody, thus preventing signal transduction. This approach was evaluated with the epidermal growth factor receptor (EGF-R) related molecule HER-2 (human EGF-receptor 2; also termed cErbB-2 or *HER-2/neu*) as a target molecule. HER-2 is a 185-kDa transmembraneous glycoprotein with an intracytoplasmatic tyrosine kinase activity pointing to a role in signal transduction from the extracellular enviroment to the cell nucleus.[33, 34, 36] In addition to EGF-R, which is also referred to as HER-1 or erbB-1, and HER-2, HER-3 (erbB-3), and HER-4 (erbB4) have been identified as members of the EGF-R family. In contrast to a rather high homology of the intracytoplasmatic domain, a great diversity of the extracellular ligand-binding domains and the domains flanking the intrinsic tyrosine kinase catalytic core sequence is seen. With the exception of HER-2, which has to be classified as an orphan receptor, ligands binding to the other HER-family members are known. Since signal transduction relies on the tyrosine kinase activity, which in turn occurs only after dimerization or even oligomerization, overexpression of HER-2 is likely to trigger downstream events like cell proliferation regardless of binding of a specific ligand. Moreover, the capability to be independent of an exogeneous supply of growth factors is likely to be a consequence of growth factor receptor overexpression.[304–306] These observations were translated into the concept of blocking HER-2-mediated signaling with a humanized monoclonal antibody (Trastuzumab, rhu4D5, Herceptin®). This treatment approach has been widely evaluated in clinical trials during the last couple of years.[305, 307]

Besides the exogeneous application of a humanized monoclonal antibody it should be possible to transfer the gene encoding an antibody of the desired specificity. For this purpose, the gene encoding a single-chain antibody (sFv) specifically binding to HER-2 was introduced into a replication-deficient adenovirus and expressed under the control of the CMV promoter. A signal sequence sequestering the antibody with its bound target to the endoplasmatic reticulum (ER) was incorporated to prevent the expression of functional HER-2 at the cell surface. Preclinical *in vitro* and *in vivo* experiments with nude mice intraperitoneally inoculated with HER-2 expressing human ovarian cancer cells showed that inhibition of HER-2 expression induced apoptosis and tumor eradication. To further evaluate this concept, a phase I trial was recently announced,[308] but up to now the results have not been published.

2. Induction of An Anti-Tumor Immune Response

One of the requirements for the development of cancer is the ability of the transformed progenitor cell to evade immune recognition as "non-self." This becomes possible most likely due to the low expression of MHC antigens, adhesion molecules, and co-stimulatory signals necessary for complete T-cell activation. Tumor cells may also produce immunosuppressive cytokines and/or molecules of the TNF family of receptors and ligands like the CD95 ligand (CD95L).[296, 309] Consequently, the major goal of cancer immunotherapy is to induce a long-lasting and strong anti-tumor response by the immune system, e.g., tumor cells should be recognized and eliminated as "foreign cells." More importantly, T-cell-mediated (cellular) immune response is required for the rejection of tumors. The application of tumor-specific antibodies is not sufficient to label cells for elimination but has been successful in inhibiting growth-factor-mediated signal transduction (see Section III.C.1.a).[310]

The induction of tumor-specific T cells requires the expression of antigens together with human leukocyte antigen (HLA) molecules on antigen-presenting cells (APC). Whereas intracellular cytoplasmatic proteins are presented on class I HLA and are recognized by $CD8^+$ T cells (cytotoxic T cells), extracellular molecules are presented on class II HLA and are recognized by $CD4^+$ T helper cells. The induction of tumor-specific $CD4^+$ T cells is critical in initiating the elimination of tumor cells via the immune system. Since tumor cells are able to fight this reaction of the immune system, the counterattack of the tumor cells and the enhancement of the natural immune response have to be considered in cancer immuntherapy.[309, 311]

The knowledge about the induction of a cellular immune response has been translated into therapeutic protocols with the intention to induce and/or enhance the naturally occurring weak immune response. The local administration of cytokines, e.g., interferon-γ (IFN-γ) or interleukins (IL) stimulating the invasion and propagation of NK cells, lymphokine-activated cells, monocytes, and macrophages have been used to enhance T-cell response *in vivo*. The transduction of tumor cells with viral vectors harboring either one (mostly IL-2, but other cytokines have been used as well) or even combinations of two T-cell-stimulating cytokines has been evaluated as a gene therapeutic approach (for review see [151, 312] and references therein).

Numerous protocols have been described including gene therapeutic modifications of APC for tumor-specific vaccination and/or *ex vivo* expansion of tumor specific T cells.[311] Even though it is an attractive idea to fight cancer with the weapons of the immune system and the results of animal studies have been encouraging, clincial success is limited to a subset of patients suffering from melanoma or renal cell cancer.[151, 310–315] Since the viral transduction of tumor cells per se is likely to enhance the immunogenicity of the cell, this could add to the therapeutic effects of the transgene.

The fusion of primary ovarian cancer cells with peripheral blood derived autologous or allogeneic human dentric cells was seen to stimulate autologous T cells and induce cytotoxic T lymphocytes *in vitro*.[316] This might be the basis for the development of a vaccine for ovarian cancer patients.

So far only one clinical phase I trial evaluating a gene-modified vaccine for ovarian cancer has opened.[83] Briefly, the human ovarian cancer cell line PA-1 stably transduced with a retroviral vector encoding *hsv1-tk* was irradiated prior to intraperitoneal delivery to patients with recurrent ovarian cancer. Within 24 h after delivery of the vaccine, treatment with gcv was initiated. With this approach elimination of tumor cells as a consequence of bystander killing and the induction of an immune response against the killed tumor cells were expected. Unfortunately, up to now the results of this phase I trial have not been reported. Moreover, the acceptance of tumor cell inoculation by the patients appear to be problematic, even though the cells were genetically modified with a suicide gene and lethally irradiated.

In a recently reported preclincial trial *ex vivo* transduced human fibroblasts derived from ovarian cancer biopsies were utilized for the local administration of IL-12 in a mouse model of ovarian cancer.[315] With this approach, a significant reduction in tumor burden was seen even in a syngenic mouse model and the tumor-derived human fibroblasts were nontumorigenic in nude mice. Taken together, the data indicated, that local administration of IL-12 secreting fibroblasts might be suitable as an additional treatment modality for microscopic disease.

3. GDEPT

The therapeutic effect of gene replacement therapy mainly relies on the (re-)introduction and correct expression of a gene which has lost its function during oncogenesis. A common feature of cancer cells are multiple changes in the gene expression pattern which contribute to the malignant phenotype. The therapeutic efficacy of gene replacement therapy is based on the expectation that a correct expression and function of the transduced protein occurs even in such a disordered cellular environment. It seems rather unlikely that the re-expression of a single protein would be sufficient enough to revert the cellular phenotype. However, gene replacement therapy may at least help to eliminate tumor cells by "classical" cytotoxic drugs and/or radiation therapy.

Recurrent tumors are often almost completely resistant to any combination of chemotherapeutic drugs. Gene therapy offers the possibility to break this resistance and to change the drug sensitivity profile of a cell by introduction of a "new" and preferentially non-mammalian gene. For this purpose, genes are selected that enable the metabolization and thereby toxification of otherwise inert or significantly less harmful compounds. This concept is referred to as "suicide gene therapy" or gene-directed enzyme prodrug therapy (GDEPT).[317] Both, the enzymes as well as the corresponding pro-drug and drug should ideally fulfill a variety of criteria, even though so far none of the proposed combinations for GDEPT meet all of the requirements (for recent reviews see also [161, 318, 319]). Under physiological conditions, the enzyme should have a high catalytic activity (high K_{cat} and low K_m) even at low substrate concentrations. To prevent unwanted activation of the prodrug, the reaction activating the drug should be restricted to the transferred enzyme. In addition, the prodrug should be stable under physiological conditions, and must be able to freely diffuse through the tumor and to cross the tumor cell membrane. The cytotoxicity should differ at least by two orders of magnitude between prodrug and drug.[161, 318] The activated drug should also be highly diffusible or actively taken up by neighboring cells to achieve a bystander effect. On the other hand, the half-life should be short enough to prevent unwanted side effects after escape into the circulation, and, ideally therapeutic efficacy should be independent from proliferation.

Up to now, most of the prodrugs used in GDEPT have been introduced into clinical practice either as anti-cancer or as anti-viral agents and the pharmacological properties of these prodrug/drug pairs are reasonably well known.[319] In addition to the hsv1-tk-gcv/acv and CD-5-FC system, which are already introduced in clinical trials, numerous pairs of enzymes and suitable prodrugs have been evaluated *in vitro* and in preclinical *in vivo* studies. Examples are the *E. coli* derived nitroreductase (NR) together with 5-Aziridinyl-2,4-dinitrobenzamide (CB 1954) the *E. coli* derived purine nucleoside phosphorylase (EC 2.4.2.1) together with 6-thioxanthine or 6-thioguanine or the *Pseudomonas* sp. derived carboxypeptidase G2 (EC 3.4.22.12) together with (2-chloroethyl)(2-mesyloxyethyl)-aminobenzoyl-L-glutamic acid [320–322] (for review see also [161, 318, 319]). As the bystander effect is likely to be a function of the enzyme-prodrug combination, further studies are necessary to provide sufficient evidence that these systems are superior to viral thymidine kinase and cytosine deaminase *in vivo*.

Given the overall unsatisfactory transduction efficiency of gene therapy, one major advantage of GDEPT in comparison to gene replacement therapy is that the therapeutic effect is not restricted to transduced cells. Instead, the bystander effect is most important to achieve significant eradication of tumor cells even in the presence of only 10% (or even lesser amounts) transduced cells. It is now widely accepted that the bystander effect is the sum of (1) the direct cytotoxicity of the activated drug, (2) induction of an hemorrhagic tumor necrosis, and (3) the conversion of the immunoinhibitory environment of the tumor into an immunostimulatory one.[317] Whereas *in vitro* the bystander effect is mainly due to the transfer of the activated prodrug into neighboring nontransduced cells and also the transfer of apoptotic bodies from dead or dying cells ("kiss of death"), the activation of a systemic immune response is critically important for the bystander effect *in vivo*. This is concluded from experiments showing that the bystander effect is significantly reduced in athymic mice.[145, 200] The relative contribution of the immune reaction and of the cytotoxic compound transfer to the bystander effect varies between prodrug/drug combinations, viral vectors, and the localization of the tumor.[145, 146, 200, 323–327]

In published clinical trials utilizing GDEPT for treatment of ovarian cancer, *hsv1-tk* (EC 2.7.1.21) in combination with either acyclovir (acv), gcv or the acyclovir-derived valacyclovir are used exclusively.[83, 84, 308, 328–330] These compounds are guanosine derivatives and their structures and therapeutic profiles are almost identical. The affinity of the *hsv1-tk* for both, gcv (K_m=45 μM) and acv (K_m>400 μM) is much higher than for thymidine (K_m=0.5 μM). The pharmacologically relevant differences are related only to the side effect profiles and the drugs can substitute for each other. However, *hsv1-tk* mutants with significantly enhanced affinity for these synthetic prodrugs have been described. The utilization of an enzyme with improved features is accompanied by an improved ratio of cytotoxicity between pro-drug and drug, and should allow for the reduction of the loading dose of the pro-drug without loss of therapeutic efficacy.[331] The gcv-triphosphate competes with GTP for incorporation into elongating DNA, thereby inhibiting the DNA polymerase and inducing single strand breaks. Therefore, the therapeutic effect is restricted to proliferating cells. Moreover, the triphosphorylated gcv is insoluble in lipid membranes indicating the need for gap junctions for direct transfer of the activated drug to neighboring cells. The important role of gap junctions for the bystander effect has been clearly demonstrated *in vitro* and *in vivo*.[146, 327] Despite the wide utilization of *hsv1-tk*/gcv for cancer gene therapy, the gcv-mediated mechanism of cell killing is still a matter of discussion.[332–336] Onset of hemorrhagic tumor necrosis within 24 h after exposure to activated gcv is characterized by the secretion of pro-inflammatory cytokines (IL-1, IL-6, and TNF-α). These pro-inflammatory cytokines switch the immunoinhibitory microenvironment of the tumor to an immunostimulatory one, thus initiating the considerably longer (weeks) lasting T-cell-mediated immune response.[326, 337] The enhancement of an anti-tumor immune response by incorporation of T-cell-stimulating cytokines like IL-2 or IL-12 into GDEPT is likely to enhance the therapeutic efficacy, however, this is still an issue of controversial discussion.[14, 338, 339] Most interestingly, in one of the first clinical trials addressing ovarian cancer, the therapeutic effect was expected to rely almost exclusively on the bystander effect. Lethally irradiated *ex vivo* transduced tumor cells were intraperitoneally delivered to metabolize systemically applicated gcv.[83] Unfortunately, the results of this trial have not been published.

The eradication of intraperitoneally delivered ovarian cancer cells by application of hsv1-tk suicide gene therapy and gcv is possible even in nude mice, again indicating the complex nature of the bystander effect. These experiments show that cytotoxicity of the activated prodrug may be sufficient for the cure of animals from tumor xenografts.[13, 14, 270, 340–342] However, tumors induced by inoculation of proliferating tumor cells are likely to contain a higher portion of proliferating cells rendering them more sensitive to activated gcv, even in the presence of low transduction efficiencies.

Adenoviral- and retroviral-based hsv1-tk suicide gene therapies have been extensively evaluated *in vitro* and preclinically *in vivo* as well as in clinical phase I trials for several tumor entities including prostate and ovarian cancer [84, 308, 329, 330, 343] for review see also [262, 344].

IV. OVERVIEW OF CLINICAL TRIALS

The concepts outlined above have been translated mostly into phase I clinical trials for the treatment of recurrent ovarian cancer. In Table 21.3 an overview of previous and ongoing studies is presented. Unfortunately, in some cases only the clinical protocol has been announced, but no results are available, thus preventing the evaluation of the approach. Moreover, the primary goal of any phase I clinicial trial is to determine the treatment-induced toxicity rather than a prospective evaluation of therapeutic efficacy. Thus, in phase I clinical trials patients predominantly are enrolled after multiple courses of chemotherapy and a long history of recurrent disease. Since the tumor cells giving rise for the recurrence have been extensively selected against multiple rounds of cytotoxic treatment, their growth patterns and molecular characteristics are hard to compare with those from primary tumors. Moreover, the capacity of the immune system to elicit an anti-tumor response is greatly reduced after multiple courses of chemotherapy. On the other hand, this may enhance transduction efficiency due to the reduced capacity for clearing the viral vehicle.[345]

The immune system was seen to be the most important reason for tremendous differences in the therapeutic response of patients enrolled in phase I and phase II clinical trials for retroviral-mediated gene replacement therapy of BRCA1.[81, 171] An additional layer of complexity is added when gene therapy is combined with conventional chemotherapy, since the therapeutic and even the side effects of the chemotherapeutic agent are likely to interfere not only with the expression and the therapeutic effects of the transgene product but also with the viral vector.[165, 346, 347] To quantify the relative contribution of each therapeutic approach to the net effect is problematic.[348, 349] Even though the *in vitro* and preclinical *in vivo* data suggest that both modalities add to the eradication of the tumor cells, this is still a controversial issue.

The current gold standard of chemotherapy for ovarian cancer consists of paclitaxel and carboplatin or cisplatin.[29] Paclitaxel stabilizes tubulin polymerization, thereby inducing G2/M arrest and apoptosis. Interestingly, the paclitaxel induced apoptosis seems to be enhanced after loss of functional p53, whereas cells harboring functional p53 were able to bypass the paclitaxel induced G2/M block.[350] In contrast, a synergistic effect of adenoviral-mediated p53 gene replacement therapy and paclitaxel has recently been reported.[266] Even though the molecular mechanism is still not clear, subtherapeutic concentrations of paclitaxel may enhance adenoviral internalization, thereby increasing the number of p53 positive cells. However, especially in view of the p53 independent cytotoxicity of paclitaxel the involvement of other mechanisms is likely. The combination of p53 gene replacement therapy with either apoptosis-inducing chemotherapeutics (cisplatin, carboplatin, 5-FU) or radiotherapy was seen to be accompanied by an improved therapeutic response.[271, 346, 351–355] In light of these data it will be interesting to evaluate results of the ongoing clinical phase II/phase III trial combining adenoviral-mediated p53 gene replacement therapy with paclitaxel and carboplatin. This treatment is offered to patients with proven loss of p53 function in the first-line treatment situation.[273]

In addition, adenoviral infection was seen to induce topoisomerase I expression, which in turn renders the cells sensitive to the toposiomerase inhibitor topotecan. This is probably the reason for the observed synergistic effects of both treatment modalities.[165, 356]

Taken together, gene therapy may be developed into a powerful tool in the treatment of ovarian cancer, but much effort is needed to understand the multiple interactions between cancer cells, cancer cells modified by gene therapy, chemotherapeutic agents, and the immune system.

References

1. Runnebaum, I. B., and Stickeler, E. (2001). Epidemiological and molecular aspects of ovarian cancer risk. *J. Cancer Res. Clin. Oncol.* 127, 73–79.
2. Bjørge, T., Engeland, A., Sundfor, K., and Tropé, C. G. (1998). Prognosis of 2,800 patients with epithelial ovarian cancer diagnosed during 1975-94 and treated at the Norwegian Radium Hospital. *Acta Obstet. Gynecol. Scand.* 77, 777–781.
3. Bjørge, T., Engeland, A., Hansen, S., and Tropé, C. G. (1998). Prognosis of patients with ovarian cancer and borderline tumours diagnosed in Norway between 1954 and 1993. *Int. J. Cancer* 75, 663–670.
4. Dauplat, J., Le Bouedec, G., Pomel, C., and Scherer, C. (2000). Cytoreductive surgery for advanced stages of ovarian cancer. *Semin. Surg. Oncol.* 19, 42–48.
5. Lawton, F. G. (1995). Secondary debulking in ovarian cancer: Is it all in the timing? *Curr. Opin. Obstet. Gynecol.* 7, 1–3.
6. Riman, T., Persson, I., and Nilsson, S. (1998). Hormonal aspects of epithelial ovarian cancer: Review of epidemiological evidence. *Clin. Endocrinol.* 49, 695–707.
7. Michel, G., De Iaco, P., Castaigne, D., El-Hassan, M. J., Lobreglio, R., Lhomme, C., Rey, A., and Duvillard, P. (1997). Extensive cytoreductive surgery in advanced ovarian carcinoma. *Eur. J. Gynaecol. Oncol.* 18, 9–15.
8. Eisenkop, S. M., Friedman, R. L., and Wang, H. J. (1998). Complete cytoreductive surgery is feasible and maximizes, survival in patients with advanced epithelial ovarian cancer: A prospective study. *Gynecol. Oncol.* 69, 103–108.
9. McCluskey, L. L., and Dubeau, L. (1997). Biology of ovarian cancer. *Curr. Opin. Oncol.* 9, 465–470.
10. Dubeau, L. (1999). The cell of origin of ovarian epithelial tumors and the ovarian surface epithelium dogma: Does the emperor have no clothes? *Gynecol. Oncol.* 72, 437–442.
11. Auersperg, N., Wong, A. S., Choi, K. C., Kang, S. K., and Leung, P. C. (2001). Ovarian surface epithelium: Biology, endocrinology, and pathology. *Endocr. Rev.* 22, 255–288.
12. Van Niekerk, C. C., Ramaekers, F. C., Hanselaar, A. G., Aldeweireldt. J., and Poels, L. G. (1993). Changes in expression of differentiation markers between normal ovarian cells and derived tumors. *Am. J. Pathol.* 142, 157–177.
13. Al-Hendy, A., Magliocco, A. M., Al-Tweigeri, T., Braileanu, G., Crellin, N., Li, H., Strong, T., Curiel, D., and Chedrese, P. J. (2000). Ovarian cancer gene therapy: Repeated treatment with thymidine kinase in an adenovirus vector and ganciclovir improves survival in a novel immunocompetent murine model. *Am. J. Obstet. Gynecol.* 182, 553–559.
14. Yamaguchi, Y., Takashima, I., Hihara, J., Ohta, K., Shimizu, K., Minami, K., Yoshida, K., and Toge, T. (2000). Co-transduction of herpes simplex virus thymidine kinase gene and human interleukin-2 gene into mouse ovarian cancer cell line, OVHM. *Int. J. Mol. Med.* 6, 185–190.
15. Hough, C. D., Sherman-Baust, C. A., Pizer, E. S., Montz, F. J., Im, D. D., Rosenshein, N. B., Cho, K. R., Riggins, G. J., and Morin, P. J. (2000). Large-scale serial analysis of gene expression reveals genes differentially expressed in ovarian cancer. *Cancer Res.* 60, 6281–6287.
16. Hough, C. D., Cho, K. R., Zonderman, A. B., Schwartz, D. R., and Morin, P. J. (2001). Coordinately upregulated genes in ovarian Cancer. *Cancer Res.* 61, 3869–3876.
17. Welsh, J. B., Zarrinkar, P. P., Sapinoso, L. M., Kern, S. G., Behling, C. A., Monk, B. J., Lockhart, D. J., Burger, R. A., and Hampton, G. M. (2001). Analysis of gene expression profiles in normal and neoplastic ovarian tissue samples identifies candidate molecular markers of epithelial ovarian cancer. *Proc. Natl. Acad. Sci. USA.* 98, 1176–1181.
18. Parkin, D. M., Pisani, O., and Ferlay, J. (1993). Estimates of the worldwide incidence of eighteen major cancers in 1985. *Int. J. Cancer.* 54, 594–606.
19. Rowe, S. M., Coughlan, S. J., McKenna, N. J., Garrett, E., Kieback, D. G., Carney, D. N., and Headon, D. R. (1995). Ovarian carcinoma associated TaqI restriction fragment length polymorphism in Intron G of the progesterone receptor gene is due to an alu sequence insertion. *Cancer Res.* 55, 2743–2745.
20. Runnebaum, I. B., Wang-Gohrke, S., Vesprini, D., Kreienberg, R., Lynch, H., Moslehi, R., Ghadirian, P., Weber, B., Godwin, A. K., Risch, H., Garber, J., Lerman, C., Olipade, O. L., Foulkes, W. D., Karlan, B., Warner, E., Rossen, B., Rebbeck, T., Tonin, P., Dubé, M. -P., Kieback, D. G., and Narod, S. A. (2001). Progesterone receptor varinat increases ovarian cancer risk in BRCA1 and BRCA2 mutation carriers who were never exposed to oral contraceptives. *Pharmacogenetics* 11, 1–4.
21. Aunoble, B., Sanches, R., Didier, E., and Bignon, Y. J. (2000). Major oncogenes and tumor suppressor genes involved in epithelial ovarian cancer (review). *Int. J. Oncol.* 16, 567–576.
22. Hollstein, M., Rice, K., Greenblatt, M. S., Soussi, T., Fuchs, R., Sorlie, T., Hovig, E., Smith-Sorensen, B., Montesano, R., and Harris, C. C. (1994). Database of p53 gene somatic mutations in human tumors and cell lines. *Nucleic Acids Res.* 22, 3551–3555.
23. Weller, M. (1998). Predicting response to cancer chemotherapy: The role of p53. *Cell Tissue Res.* 292, 435–445.
24. Somasundaram, K., and El-Deiry, W. S. (2000). Tumor suppressor p53: Regulation and function. *Front. Biosci.* 5, d424–437.
25. Rodriguez, G. C., Berchuck, A., Whitaker, R. S., Schlossman, D., Clarke-Pearson, D. L., and Bast, R. C. Jr. (1991). Epidermal growth factor receptor expression in normal ovarian epithelium and ovarian cancer. II. Relationship between receptor expression and response to epidermal growth factor. *Am. J. Obstet. Gynecol.* 164, 745–750.

26. Ilekis, J. V., Connor, J. P., Prins, G. S., Ferrer, K., Niederberger, C., and Scoccia, B. (1997). Expression of epidermal growth factor and androgen receptors in ovarian cancer. *Gynecol. Oncol.* 66, 250–254.
27. Tong, X. W., Kieback, D. G., Ramesh, R., and Freeman, S. M. (1999). Molecular aspects of ovarian cancer. *Hematol. Oncol. Clin. N. Am.* 13, 109–133.
28. Ross, D. T., Scherf, U., Eisen, M. B., Perou, C. M., Rees, C., Spellman, P., Iyer, V., Jeffrey, S. S., Van de Rijn, M., Waltham, M., Pergamenschikov, A., Lee, J. C., Lashkari, D., Shalon, D., Myers, T. G., Weinstein, J. N., Botstein, D., and Brown, P. O. (2000). Systematic variation in gene expression patterns in human cancer cell lines. *Nat. Genet.* 24, 227–235.
29. McGuire, W. P., Hoskins, W. J., Brady, M. F., Kucera, P. R., Partridge, E. E., Look, K. Y., Clarke-Pearson, D. L., and Davidson, M. (1996). Cyclophosphamide and cisplatin compared with paclitaxel and cisplatin in patients with stage III and stage IV ovarian cancer. *N. Engl. J. Med.* 334, 1–6.
30. Di Cristofano, A., and Pandolfi, P. P. (2000). The multiple roles of PTEN in tumor suppression. *Cell* 100, 387–390.
31. Tsatsanis, C., and Spandidos, D. A. (2000). The role of oncogenic kinases in human cancer. *Int. J. Mol. Med.* 5, 583–590.
32. Weiner, H. L., and Zagzag, D. (2000). Growth factor receptor tyrosine kinases: Cell adhesion kinase family suggests a novel signaling mechanism in cancer. *Cancer Invest.* 18, 544–554.
33. Klapper, L. N., Kirschbaum, M. H., Sela, M., and Yarden, Y. (2000). Biochemical and clinical implications of the ErbB/HER signaling network of growth factor receptors. *Adv. Cancer Res.* 77, 25–79.
34. Hanahan, D., and Weinberg, R. A. (2000). The hallmarks of cancer. *Cell* 100, 57–70.
35. Hengartner, M. O. (2000). The biochemistry of apoptosis. *Nature* 407, 770–776.
36. Hunter, T. (2000). Signaling - 2000 and beyond. *Cell* 100, 113–127.
37. Mahato, R. I., Smith, L. C., and Rolland, A. (1999). Pharmaceutical perspectives of nonviral gene therapy. *Adv. Genet.* 41, 95–156.
38. Anderson, W. F. (1998). Human gene therapy. *Nature* 392, 25–30.
39. Walther, W., and Stein, U. (2000). Viral vectors for gene transfer: A review of their use in the treatment of human diseases. *Drugs* 60, 249–271.
40. Schatzlein, A. G. (2001). Non-viral vectors in cancer gene therapy: Principles and progress. *Anticancer Drugs* 12, 275–304.
41. Garver, R. I., Jr., Goldsmith, K. T., Rodu, B., Hu, P. C., Sorscher, E. J., and Curiel, D. T. (1994). Strategy for achieving selective killing of carcinomas. *Gene Ther.* 1, 46–50.
42. Walther, W., and Stein, U. (1999). Therapeutic genes for cancer gene therapy. *Mol. Biotechnol.* 13, 21–28.
43. Anklesaria, P. (2000). Gene therapy: A molecular approach to cancer treatment. *Curr. Opin. Mol. Ther.* 2, 426–432.
44. Vile, R. G., Russell, S. J., and Lemoine, N. R. (2000). Cancer gene therapy: Hard lessons and new courses. *Gene Ther.* 7, 2–8.
45. Oshima, Y., Sakamoto, T., Yamanaka, I., Nishi, T., Ishibashi, T., and Inomata, H. (1998). Targeted gene transfer to corneal endothelium in vivo by electric pulse. *Gene Ther.* 5, 1347–1354.
46. Sawamura, D., Ina, S., Itai, K., Meng, X., Kon, A., Tamai, K., Hanada, K., and Hashimoto, I. (1999). In vivo gene introduction into keratinocytes using jet injection. *Gene Ther.* 6, 1785–1787.
47. Hui, K. M., and Chia, T. F. (1997). Eradication of tumor growth via biolistic transformation with allogeneic MHC genes. *Gene Ther.* 4, 762–767.
48. Barry, M. E., Pinto-Gonzalez, D., Orson, F. M., McKenzie, G. J., Petry, G. R., and Barry, M. A. (1999). Role of endogenous endonucleases and tissue site in transfection and CpG-mediated immune activation after naked DNA injection. *Hum Gene Ther.* 10, 2461–2480.
49. Luo, D., and Saltzman, W. M. (2000). Synthetic DNA delivery systems. *Nat. Biotechnol.* 18, 33–37.
50. Maron, D. J., Choi, E. A., and Spitz, F. R. (2001). Gene therapy of metastatic disease: Progress and prospects. *Surg. Oncol. Clin. N. Am.* 10, 449–460.
51. Muggia, F. M. (2001). Liposomal encapsulated anthracyclines: New therapeutic horizons. *Curr. Oncol. Rep.* 3, 156–162.
52. Kikuchi, A., Aoki, Y., Sugaya, S., Serikawa, T., Takakuwa, K., Tanaka, K., Suzuki, N., and Kikuchi, H. (1999). Development of novel cationic liposomes for efficient gene transfer into peritoneal disseminated tumor. *Hum Gene Ther.* 10, 947–955.
53. Xing, X., Zhang, S., Chang, J. Y., Tucker, S. D., Chen, H., Huang, L., and Hung, M. C. (1998). Safety study and characterization of E1A-liposome complex gene-delivery protocol in an ovarian cancer model. *Gene Ther.* 5, 1538–1544.
54. Ueno, N. T., Xia, W., Tucker, S. D., Zhang, S., Lopez-Berestein, G., Huang, L., and Hung, M. C. (1999). Issues in the development of gene therapy: Preclinical experiments in E1A gene delivery. *Oncol. Rep.* 6, 257–262.
55. Hortobagyi, G. N., Hung, M. C., and Lopez-Berestein, G. A. (1998). Phase I multicenter study of E1A gene therapy for patients with metastatic breast cancer and epithelial ovarian cancer that overexpresses HER-2/neu or epithelial ovarian cancer. *Hum Gene Ther.* 9, 1775–1798.
56. Günzburg, W. H., and Salmons, B. (1996). Development of retroviral vectors as safe, targeted gene delivery systems. *J. Mol. Med.* 74, 171–182.
57. Markowitz, D., Goff, S., and Bank, A. (1988). A safe packaging line for gene transfer: Separating viral genes on two different plasmids. *J. Virol.* 62, 1120–1124.
58. Miller, D. G., and Miller, A. D. (1994). A family of retroviruses that utilize related phosphate transporters for cell entry. *J. Virol.* 68, 8270–8276.
59. Galanis, E., Vile, R., and Russell, S. J. (2001). Delivery systems intended for in vivo gene therapy of cancer: Targeting and replication competent viral vectors. *Crit. Rev. Oncol. Hematol.* 38, 177–192.
60. Miller, D. G., Adam, M. A., and Miller, A. D. (1990). Gene transfer by retrovirus vectors occurs only in cells that are actively replicating at the time of infection. *Mol. Cell. Biol.* 10, 4239–4242.
61. McLachlin, J. R., Cornetta, K., Eglitis, M. A., and Anderson, W. F. (1990). Retroviral-mediated gene transfer. *Prog. Nucleic Acid Res. Mol. Biol.* 38, 91–135.
62. Yu, S. F., von Ruden, T., Kantoff, P. W., Garber, C., Seiberg, M., Ruther, U., Anderson,. W. F., Wagner, E. F., and Gilboa, E. (1986). Self-inactivating retroviral vectors designed for transfer of whole genes into mammalian cells. *Proc. Natl. Acad. Sci. USA.* 83, 3194–3198.
63. Ishii-Morita, H., Agbaria, R., Mullen, C. A., Hirano, H., Koeplin, D. A., Ram, Z., Oldfield, E. H., Johns, D. G., and Blaese, R. M. (1997). Mechanism of 'bystander effect' killing in the herpes simplex thymidine kinase gene therapy model of cancer treatment. *Gene Ther.* 4, 244–251.
64. Burns, J. C., Friedmann, T., Driever, W., Burrascano, M., and Yee, J. K. (1993). Vesicular stomatitis virus G glycoprotein pseudotyped retroviral vectors: Concentration to very high titer and efficient gene transfer into mammalian and nonmammalian cells. *Proc. Natl. Acad. Sci. USA.* 90, 8033–8037.
65. Friedmann, T., and Yee, J. K. (1995). Pseudotyped retroviral vectors for studies of human gene therapy. *Nat. Med.* 1, 275–277.
66. Reiser, J., Harmison, G., Kluepfel-Stahl, S., Brady, R. O., Karlsson, S., and Schubert, M. (1996). Transduction of nondividing cells using pseudotyped defective high-titer HIV type 1 particles. *Proc. Natl. Acad. Sci. USA* 93, 15266–15271.
67. Kasahara, N., Dozy, A. M., and Kan, Y. W. (1994). Tissue-specific targeting of retroviral vectors through ligand-receptor interactions. *Science* 266, 1373–1376.
68. Marin, M., Noel, D., Valsesia-Wittman, S., Brockly, F., Etienne-Julan, M., Russell, S., Cosset, F. L., and Piechaczyk, M. (1996). Targeted infection of human cells via major histocompatibility complex class I molecules by Moloney murine leukemia virus-derived viruses displaying single-chain antibody fragment-envelope fusion proteins. *J. Virol.* 70, 2957–2962.

69. Somia, N. V., Zoppe, M., and Verma, I. M. (1995). Generation of targeted retroviral vectors by using single-chain variable fragment: An approach to in vivo gene delivery. *Proc. Natl. Acad. Sci. USA* 92, 7570–7574.
70. Schnierle, B. S., and Groner, B. (1996). Retroviral targeted delivery. *Gene. Ther.* 3, 1069–1073.
71. Schnierle, B. S., Moritz, D., Jeschke, M., and Groner, B. (1996). Expression of chimeric envelope proteins in helper cell lines and integration into Moloney murine leukemia virus particles. *Gene Ther.* 3, 334–342.
72. Jiang, A., Chu, T. H., Nocken, F., Cichutek, K., and Dornburg, R. (1998). Cell-type-specific gene transfer into human cells with retroviral vectors that display single-chain antibodies. *J. Virol.* 72, 10148–10156.
73. Snitkovsky, S., and Young, J. A. (1998). Cell-specific viral targeting mediated by a soluble retroviral receptor-ligand fusion protein. *Proc. Natl. Acad. Sci. USA* 95, 7063–7068.
74. Cosset, F. L., and Russell, S. J. (1996). Targeting retrovirus entry. *Gene Ther.* 3, 946–956.
75. Ott, D., and Rein, A. (1992). Basis for receptor specificity of nonecotropic murine leukemia virus surface glycoprotein gp70SU. *J. Virol.* 66, 4632–4638.
76. Morgan, R. A., Nussbaum, O., Muenchau, D. D., Shu, L., Couture, L., and Anderson, W. F. (1993). Analysis of the functional and host range-determining regions of the murine ectropic and amphotropic retrovirus envelope proteins. *J. Virol.* 67, 4712–4721.
77. Battini, J. L., Heard, J. M., and Danos, O. (1992). Receptor choice determinants in the envelope glycoproteins of amphotropic, xenotropic, and polytropic murine leukemia viruses. *J. Virol.* 66, 1468–1475.
78. Russell, S. J., Hawkins, R. E., and Winter, G. (1993). Retroviral vectors displaying functional antibody fragments. *Nucleic Acids Res.* 21, 1081–1085.
79. Salmons, B., and Gunzburg, W. H. (1993). Targeting of retroviral vectors for gene therapy. *Hum. Gene Ther. 4,* 129–141.
80. Rother, R. P., Squinto, S. P., Mason, J. M., and Rollins, S. A. (1995). Protection of retroviral vector particles in human blood through complement inhibition. *Hum. Gene Ther.* 6, 429–435.
81. Tait. D. L., Obermiller, P. S., Redlin-Frazier, S., Jensen, R. A., Welcsh, P., Dann, J., King, M. C., Johnson, D. H., and Holt, J. T. (1997). A phase I trial of retroviral BRCA1sv gene therapy in ovarian cancer. *Clin. Cancer Res.* 3, 1959–1968.
82. Ayesh, S. K., Azar, Y., Barghouti, I. I., Ruedi, J. M., Babior, B. M., and Matzner, Y. (1995). Purification and characterization of a C5a-inactivating enzyme from human peritoneal fluid. *Blood* 85, 3503–3509.
83. Freeman, S. M., McCune, C., Robinson, W., Abboud, C. N., Abraham, G. N., Angel, C., and Marrogi, A. (1995). The treatment of ovarian cancer with a gene modified cancer vaccine: A phase I study. *Hum. Gene Ther.* 6, 927–939.
84. Link, C. J., Jr., Moorman, D., Seregina, T., Levy, J. P., and Schabold, K. J. (1996). A phase I trial of in vivo gene therapy with the herpes simplex thymidine kinase/ganciclovir system for the treatment of refractory or recurrent ovarian cancer. *Hum. Gene Ther.* 7, 1161–1179.
85. Logg, C. R., Tai, C. K., Logg, A., Anderson, W. F., and Kasahara, N. (2001). A uniquely stable replication-competent retrovirus vector achieves efficient gene delivery in vitro and in solid tumors. *Hum. Gene Ther.* 12, 921–932.
86. Kim, V. N., Mitrophanous, K., Kingsman, S. M., and Kingsman, A. J. (1998). Minimal requirement for a lentivirus vector based on human immunodeficiency virus type 1. *J. Virol.* 72, 811–816.
87. Naldini, L., Blomer, U., Gallay, P., Ory, D., Mulligan, R., Gage, F. H., Verma, I. M., and Trono, D. (1996). In vivo gene delivery and stable transduction of nondividing cells by a lentiviral vector. *Science* 272, 263–267.
88. Zufferey, R., Nagy, D., Mandel, R. J., Naldini, L., and Trono, D. (1997). Multiply attenuated lentiviral vector achieves efficient gene delivery in vivo. *Nat. Biotechnol.* 15, 871–875.
89. Schnurr, D., and Dondero, M. E. (1993). Two new candidate adenovirus serotypes. *Intervirology* 36, 79–83.
90. Roelvink, P. W., Lizonova, A., Lee, J. G., Li, Y., Bergelson, J. M., Finberg, R. W., Brough, D. E., Kovesdi, I., and Wickham, T. J. (1998). The coxsackievirus-adenovirus receptor protein can function as a cellular attachment protein for adenovirus serotypes from subgroups A, C, D, E, and F. *J. Virol.* 72, 7909–7915.
91. Bailey, A., and Mautner, V. (1994). Phylogenetic relationships among adenovirus serotypes. *Virology* 205, 438–452.
92. Wadell, G. (2000). Adenoviruses. *In* "Principles and Practice of Clinical Virology," 4th edition, (A. J. Zuckerman, J. E. Banatvala, and J. R. Pattison, eds.), Chapter 8, pp. 307–327. John Wiley & Sons, New York.
93. Chroboczek, J., Ruigrok, R. W. H., and Cusack, S. (1995). Adenovirus fiber. *Curr. Top. Microbiol. Immunol.* 199, 163–200.
94. Perricaudet, M., and Stratford-Perricaudet, L. D. (1995). Adenovirus-mediated in-vivo gene therapy. *In* "Viruses in Human Gene Therapy," (J.-M. H. Vos, ed.), pp. 1–32. Academic Press, Durham, NC.
95. Bergelson, J. M., Cunnigham, J. A., Droguett, G., Kurt-Jones, E. A., Krithivas, A., Hong, J. S., Horwitz, M. S., Crowell, R. L., and Finberg, R. W. (1997). Isolation of a common receptor for coxsackie B viruses and adenoviruses 2 and 5. *Science* 275, 1320–1323.
96. Hong, S. S., Karayan, L., Tournier, J., Curiel, D. T., and Boulanger, P. A. (1997). Adenovirus type 5 fiber knob binds to MHC class I alpha2 domain at the surface of human epithelial and B lymphoblastoid cells. *EMBO J.* 16, 2294–2306.
97. Nemerow, G. R., Cheresh, D. A., and Wickham, T. J. (1994). Adenovirus entry into host cells. A role for αv integrins. *Trends Cell Biol.* 4, 52–56.
98. Wickham, T. J., Mathias, P., Cheresh, D. A., and Nemerow, G. R. (1993). Integrins alpha v beta 3 and alpha v beta 5 promote adenovirus internalization but not virus attachment. *Cell* 73, 309–319.
99. Wickham, T. J., Filardo, E. J., Cheresh, D. A., and Nemerow, G. R. (1994). Integrin $\alpha v\beta 5$ selectively promotes adenovirus mediated cell membrane permeabilization. *J. Cell Biol.* 127, 257–264.
100. Hidaka, C., Milano, E., Leopold, P. L., Bergelson, J. M., Hackett, N. R., Finberg, R. W., Wickham, T. J., Kovesdi, I., Roelvink, P., and Crystal, R. G. (1999). CAR-dependent and CAR-independent pathways of adenovirus vector-mediated gene transfer and expression in human fibroblasts. *J. Clin. Invest.* 103, 579–587.
101. Wills, K. N., Maneval, D. C., Menzel, P., Harris, M. P., Sutjipto, S., Vaillancourt, M. T., Huang, W. M., Johnson, D. E., Anderson, S. C., Wen, S. F. *et. al.* (1994). Development and characterization of recombinant adenoviruses encoding human p53 for gene therapy of cancer. *Hum. Gene Ther.* 5, 1079–1088.
102. Greber, U. F., Willetts, M., Webster, P., and Helenius, A. (1993). Stepwise dismantling of adenovirus 2 during entry into cells. *Cell* 75, 477–486.
103. Greber, U. F., Singh, I., and Helenius, A. (1994). Mechanisms of virus uncoating. *Trends Microbiol.* 2, 52–56.
104. Greber, U. F., Webster, P., Weber, J., and Helenius, A. (1996). The role of the adenovirus protease in virus entry into the cells. *EMBO J.* 15, 1766–1777.
105. Greber, U. F., Suomalainen, M., Stidwill, R. P., Boucke, K., Ebersold, M. W., and Helenius, A. (1997). The role of the nuclear pore complex in adenovirus DNA entry. *EMBO J.* 16, 5998–6007.
106. Cotton, M., and Weber, J. M. (1995). The adenovirus protease is required for viurs entry into host cells. *Virology* 213, 494–502.
107. Whittaker, G. R., and Helenius, A. (1998). Nuclear import and export of viruses and virus genomes. *Virology* 246, 1–23.
108. Huang, S., Endo, R. I., and Nemerow, G. R. (1995). Upregulation of integrins alpha v beta 3 and alpha v beta 5 on human monocytes and T lymphocytes facilitates adenovirus-mediated gene delivery. *J. Virol.* 69, 2257–2263.
109. Hemmi, S., Geertsen, R., Mezzacasa, A., Peter, I., and Dummer, R. (1998). The presence of human coxsackievirus and adenovirus

receptor is associated with efficient adenovirus-mediated transgene expression in human melanoma cell cultures. *Hum. Gene Ther.* 9, 2363–2373.

110. Teoh, G., Chen, L., Urashima, M., Tai, Y. T., Celi, L. A., Chen, D., Chauhan, D., Ogata, A., Finberg, R. W., Webb, I. J., Kufe, D. W., and Anderson, K. C. (1998). Adenovirus vector-based purging of multiple myeloma cells. *Blood* 92, 4591–4601.
111. Hautala, T., Grunst, T., Fabrega, A., Freimuth, P., and Welsh, M. J. (1998). An interaction between penton base and alpha v integrins plays a minimal role in adenovirus-mediated gene transfer to hepatocytes in vitro and in vivo. *Gene Ther.* 5, 1259–1264.
112. Li, Y., Pong, R. C., Bergelson, J. M., Hall, M. C., Sagalowsky, A. I., Tseng, C. P., Wang, Z., and Hsieh, J. T. (1999). Loss of adenoviral receptor expression in human bladder cancer cells: A potential impact on the efficacy of gene therapy. *Cancer Res.* 59, 325–330.
113. Pickles, R. J., McCarty, D., Matsui, H., Hart, P. J., Randell, S. H., and Boucher, R. C. (1998). Limited entry of adenovirus vectors into well–differentiated airway epithelium is responsible for inefficient gene transfer. *J. Virol.* 72, 6014–6023.
114. Nalbantoglu, J., Pari, G., Karpati, G., and Holland, P. C. (1999). Expression of the primary coxsackie and adenovirus receptor is downregulated during skeletal muscle maturation and limits the efficacy of adenovirus-mediated gene delivery to muscle cells. *Hum. Gene Ther.* 10, 1009–1019.
115. Brüning, A., Kohler, T., Quist, S., Wang-Gohrke, S., Moebus, V. J., Kreienberg, R., and Runnebaum, I. B. (2001). Adenoviral transduction efficiency of ovarian cancer cells can be limited by loss of integrin beta3 subunit expression and increased by reconstitution of integrin alphavbeta3. *Hum. Gene Ther.* 12, 391–399.
116. You, Z., Fischer, D, C., Tong, X., Hasenburg, A., Aguilar-Cordova, E., and Kieback, D. G. (2001). Coxsackievirus-adenovirus receptor expression in ovarian cancer cell lines is associated with increased adenovirus transduction efficiency and transgene expression. *Cancer Gene Ther.* 8, 168–175.
117. Morsy, M. A., and Caskey, C. T. (1999). Expanded-capacity adenoviral vectors—the helper-dependent vectors. *Mol. Med. Today* 5, 18–24.
118. Yeh, P., and Perricaudet, M. (1997). Advances in adenoviral vectors: From genetic engineering to their biology. *FASEB J.* 11, 615–623.
119. Shenk, T. (1996). Adenoviridiae: The viruses and their replication. *In* "Virology," 3rd edition, (Fields, K. D., Knipe, D. M., Howley, P. M., *et al.* eds.), Vol. 2, Chapter 67, pp. 2111–2148, Raven Publishers, Philadelphia.
120. Bayley, S. T., and Mamryk, J. S. (1994). Adenovirus E1A proteins and transformation. *Int. J. Oncol.* 5, 425–444.
121. Shisler, J., Duerksen-Hughes, P., Hermiston, T. M., Wold, W. S., and Gooding, L. R. (1996). Induction of susceptibility to tumor necrosis factor by E1A is dependent on binding to either p300 or p105-Rb and induction of DNA synthesis. *J. Virol.* 70, 68–77.
122. Graham, F. L., Smiley, J., Russell, W. C., and Nairn, R. (1977). Characteristics of a human cell line transformed by DNA from human adenovirus type 5. *J. Gen. Virol.* 36, 59–74.
123. Frisch, S. M. (2001). Tumor suppression activity of adenovirus E1a protein: Anoikis and the epithelial phenotype. *Adv. Cancer Res.* 39–49.
124. Reynolds, T., Alberts, D., Gershenson, D., Gleich, L., Glisson, B., Hanna, E., Huang, L., Hung, M. C., Kenady, D., Ueno, N., Villaret, D., and Yoo, G. (2000). Activity of E1a in human clinical trials. *Proc. Am. Soc. Clin. Oncol.* pp. abstr. 1809.
125. Yoo, G. H., Hung, M. C., Lopez-Berestein, G., LaFollette, S., Ensley, J. F., Carey, M., Batson, E., Reynolds, T. C., and Murray, J. L. (2001). Phase I trial of intratumoral liposome E1a gene therapy in patients with recurrent breast and head and neck cancer. *Clin. Cancer Res.* 7, 1237–1245.
126. Zang, R. Y., Shi, D. R., Lu, H. J., Cai, S. M., Lu, D. R., Zhang, Y. J., and Qin, H. L. (2001). Adenovirus 5 E1a-mediated gene therapy for human ovarian cancer cells in vitro and in vivo. *Int. J. Gynecol. Cancer* 11, 18–23.
127. Martin, M. E., and Berk, A. J. (1998). Adenovirus E1B 55K represses p53 activation in vitro. *J. Virol.* 72, 3146–3154.
128. Adams, J. M., and Cory, S. (1998). The Bcl-2 protein family: Arbiters of cell survival. *Science* 281, 1322–1326.
129. Wold, W. S. M., Doronin, K., Toth, K., Kuppuswamy, M., Lichtenstein, D. L., and Tollefson, A. E. (1999). Immune responses to adenoviruses: Viral evasion mechanisms and their implications for the clinic. *Curr. Opin. Immunol.* 11, 380–386.
130. Fredman, J. N., and Engler, J. A. (1993). Adenovirus precursor to terminal protein interacts with the nuclear matrix in vivo and in vitro. *J. Virol.* 67, 3384–3395.
131. Schaack, J., Ho, W. Y., Freimuth, P., and Shenk, T. (1990). Adenovirus terminal protein mediates both nuclear matrix association and efficient transcription of adenovirus DNA. *Genes Dev.* 4, 1197–1208.
132. Williams, J. L., Garcia, J., Harrich, D., Pearson, L., Wu, F., and Gaynor, R. (1990). Lymphoid specific gene expression of the adenovirus early region 3 promoter is mediated by NF-kappa B binding motifs. *EMBO J.* 9, 4435–4442.
133. Tollefson, A. E., Scaria, A., Hermiston, T. W., Ryerse, J. S., Wold, L. J., and Wold, W. S. (1996). The adenovirus death protein (E3-11.6K) is required at very late stages of infection for efficient cell lysis and release of adenovirus from infected cells. *J. Virol.* 70, 2296–2306.
134. Hermiston, T. W., Tripp, R. A., Sparer, T., Gooding, L. R., and Wold, W. S. (1993). Deletion mutation analysis of the adenovirus type 2 E3-gp19K protein: Identification of sequences within the endoplasmic reticulum lumenal domain that are required for class I antigen binding and protection from adenovirus-specific cytotoxic T lymphocytes. *J. Virol.* 67, 5289–5298.
135. Dimitrov, T., Krajcsi, P., Hermiston, T. W., Tollefson, A. E., Hannink, M., and Wold, W. S. (1997). Adenovirus E3-10.4K/14.5K protein complex inhibits tumor necrosis factor-induced translocation of cytosolic phospholipase A2 to membranes. *J. Virol.* 71, 2830–2837.
136. Descamps, V., Duffour, M. T., Mathieu, M. C., Fernandez, N., Cordier, L., Abina, M. A., Kremer, E., Perricaudet, M., and Haddada, H. (1996). Strategies for cancer gene therapy using adenoviral vectors. *J. Mole. Med.* 74, 183–189.
137. Hehir, K. M., Armentano, D., Cardoza, L. M., Choquette, T. L., Berthelette, P. B., White, G. A., Couture, L. A., Everton, M. B., Keegan, J., Martin, J. M., Pratt, D. A., Smith, M. P., Smith, A. E., and Wadsworth, S. C. (1996). Molecular characterization of replication-competent variants of adenovirus vectors and genome modifications to prevent their occurrence. *J. Virol.* 70, 8459–8467.
138. Imler, J. L., Chartier, C., Dreyer, D., Dieterle, A., Sainte-Marie, M., Faure, T., Pavirani, A., and Mehtali, M. (1996). Novel complementation cell lines derived from human lung carcinoma A549 cells support the growth of E1-deleted adenovirus vectors. *Gene Ther.* 3, 75–84.
139. Bett, A. J., Prevec, L., and Graham, F. L. (1993). Packaging capacity and stability of human adenovirus type 5 vectors. *J. Virol.* 67, 5911–5921.
140. Ali, M., Lemoine, N. R., and Ring, C. J. (1994). The use of DNA viruses as vectors for gene therapy. *Gene Ther.* 1, 367–384.
141. Lusky, M., Christ, M., Rittner, K., Dieterle, A., Dreyer, D., Mourot, B., Schultz, H., Stoeckel, F., Pavirani, A., and Mehtali, M. (1998). In vitro and in vivo biology of recombinant adenovirus vectors with E1, E1/E2A, or E1/E4 deleted. *J. Virol.* 72, 2022–2032.
142. Kovesdi, I., Brough, D. E., Bruder, J. T., and Wickham, T. J. (1997). Adenoviral vectors for gene transfer. *Curr. Opin. Biotechnol.* 8, 583–589.
143. Fisher, K. J., Choi, H., Burda, J., Chen, S. J., and Wilson, J. M. (1996). Recombinant adenovirus deleted of all viral genes for gene therapy of cystic fibrosis. *Virology.* 217, 11–22.
144. Kochanek, S., Clemens, P. R., Mitani, K., Chen, H.-H., Chan, S., and Caskey, C. T. (1996). A new adenoviral vector: Replacement of all

viral coding sequences with 28 kb of DNA independently expressing both full-length dystrophin and β-galactosidase. *Proc. Natl. Acad. Sci. USA* 93, 5731–5736.

145. Freeman, S. M., Abboud, C. N., Whartenby, K. A., Packman, C. H., Koeplin, D. S., Moolten, F. L., and Abraham, G. N. (1993). The "bystander effect": Tumor regression when a fraction of the tumor mass is genetically modified. *Cancer Res.* 53, 5274–5283.
146. Elshami, A. A., Saavedra, A., Zhang, H., Kucharczuk, J. C., Spray, D. C., Fishman, G. I., Amin, K. M., Kaiser, L. R., and Albelda, S. M. (1996). Gap junctions play a role in the "bystander effect" of the herpes simplex virus thymidine kinase/ganciclovir system in vitro. *Gene Ther.* 3, 85–92.
147. Tong, X. W., Block, A., Chen, S. H., Woo, S. L., and Kieback, D. G. (1996). Adenovirus-mediated thymidine kinase gene transduction in human epithelial ovarian cancer cell lines followed by exposure to ganciclovir. *Anticancer Res.* 16, 1611–1617.
148. Rizk, N. P., Chang, M. Y., Kouri, C. E., Seth, P., Kaiser, L. R., Albelda, S. M., and Amin, K. A. (1999). The evaluation of adenoviral p53-mediated bystander effect in gene therapy of cancer. *Cancer Gene Ther.* 6, 291–301.
149. Kirn, D. H. (2000). Replication-selective microbiological agents: Fighting cancer with targeted germ warfare. *J. Clin. Invest.* 105, 837–839.
150. Heise, C., and Kirn, D. H. (2000). Replication-selective adenoviruses as oncolytic agents. *J. Clin. Invest.* 105, 847–851.
151. Agha-Mohammadi, S., and Lotze, M. T. (2000). Immunomodulation of cancer: Potential use of selectively replicating agents. *J. Clin. Invest.* 105, 1173–1176.
152. Hermiston, T. (2000). Gene delivery from replication-selective viruses: Arming guided missiles in the war against cancer. *J. Clin. Invest.* 105, 1169–1172.
153. Rodriguez, R., Schuur, E. R., Lim, H. Y., Henderson, G. A., Simons, J. W., and Henderson, D. R. (1997). Prostate attenuated replication competent adenovirus (ARCA) CN706: A selective cytotoxic for prostate-specific antigen-positive prostate cancer cells. *Cancer Res.* 57, 2559–2563.
154. Hallenbeck, P. L., Chang, Y. N., Hay, C., Golightly, D., Stewart, D., Lin, J., Phipps, S., and Chiang, Y. L. (1999). A novel tumor-specific replication-restricted adenoviral vector for gene therapy of hepatocellular carcinoma. *Hum. Gene Ther.* 10, 1721–1733.
155. Doronin, K., Kuppuswamy, M., Toth, K., Tollefson, A. E., Krajcsi, P., Krougliak, V., and Wold, W. S. (2001). Tissue-specific, tumor-selective, replication-competent adenovirus vector for cancer gene therapy. *J. Virol.* 75, 3314–3324.
156. Bischoff, J. R., Kirn, D. H., Williams, A., Heise, C., Horn, S., Muna, M., Ng, L., Nye, J. A., Sampson-Johannes, A., Fattaey, A., and McCormick, F. (1996). An adenovirus mutant that replicates selectively in p53-deficient human tumor cells. *Science* 274, 373–376.
157. Heise, C., Sampson-Johannes, A., Williams, A., McCormick, F., von Hoff, D. D., and Kirn, D. H. (1997). ONYX-015, an E1B gene-attenuated adenovirus, causes tumor-specific cytolysis and antitumoral efficacy that can be augmented by standard chemotherapeutic agents. *Nat. Med.* 3, 639–645.
158. Ganly, I., Eckhardt, S. G., Rodriguez, G. I., Soutar, D. S., Otto, R., Robertson, A. G., Park, O., Gulley, M. L., Heise, C., Von Hoff, D. D., and Kaye, S. B. (2000). A phase I study of Onyx-015, an E1B attenuated adenovirus, administered intratumorally to patients with recurrent head and neck cancer. *Clin. Cancer Res.* 6, 798–806.
159. Khuri, F. R., Neumunaitis, J., Ganly, I., Arseneau, J., Tannock, I. F., Romel, L, Gore, M., Ironside, J., MacDougall, R. H., Heise, C., Randlev, B., Gillenwater, A. M., Bruso, P., Kaye, S. B., Hong, W. K., and Kirn, D. H. (2000). A controlled trial of intratumoral ONYX-015, a selectively-replicating adenovirus, in combination with cis-platin and 5-fluorouracil in patients with recurrent head and neck cancer. *Nat. Med.* 6, 879–885.
160. Vasey, P. A., Seiden, M., O'Neill, V., Campo, S., Johnston, S., Davis, J., Kirn, D., Kaye, S. B., and Shulman, L. N. (2000). Phase I trial of intraperitoneal ONYX-015 adenovirus in patients with recurrent ovarian cancer. Proc. ASCO 2000, pp. Abstract #1512.
161. Springer, C. J., and Niculescu-Duvaz, I. (2000). Prodrug-activating systems in suicide gene therapy. *J. Clin. Invest.* 105, 1161–1167.
162. Freytag, S. O., Rogulski, R., Paielli, D. L., Gilbert, J. D., and Kim, J. H. (1998). A novel three-pronged approach to kill cancer cells selectively: Concomitant viral, double suicide gene, and radiotherapy. *Hum. Gene Ther.* 9, 1323–1333.
163. Wildner, O., Morris, J. C., Vahanian, N. N., Ford, H. Jr., Ramsey, W. J., and Blaese, R. M. (1999). Adenoviral vectors capable of replication improve the efficacy of HSVtk/GCV suicide gene therapy of cancer. *Gene Ther.* 6, 57–62.
164. Wildner, O., Blaese, R. M., and Morris, J. C. (1999). Therapy of colon cancer with oncolytic adenovirus is enhanced by the addition of herpes simplex virus-thymidine kinase. *Cancer Res.* 59, 410–413.
165. Wildner, O., Blaese, R. M., and Morris, J. C. (1999). Synergy between the herpes simplex virus tk/ganciclovir prodrug suicide system and the topoisomerase I inhibitor topotecan. *Hum. Gene Ther.* 10, 2679–2687.
166. Tal, J. (2000). Adeno-associated virus-based vectors in gene therapy. *J. Biomed. Sci.* 7, 279–291.
167. Martuza, R. L. (2000). Conditionally replicating herpes vectors for cancer therapy. *J. Clin. Invest.* 105, 841–846.
168. Coukos, G., Makrigiannakis, A., Kang, E. H., Caparelli, D., Benjamin, I., Kaiser, L. R., Rubin, S. C., Albelda, S. M., and Molnar-Kimber, K. L. (1999). Use of carrier cells to deliver a replication-selective herpes simplex virus-1 mutant for intraperitoneal therapy of epithelial ovarian cancer. *Clin. Cancer Res.* 5, 1523–1537.
169. Carroll, M. W., and Moss, B. (1997). Poxviruses as expression vectors. *Curr. Opin. Biotechnol.* 8, 573–577.
170. Nettelbeck, D. M., Jérome, V., and Müller, R. (2000). Gene therapy: Designer promoters for tumour targeting. *Trends Genet.* 16, 174–181.
171. Tait, D. L., Obermiller, P. S., Hatmaker, A. R., Redlin-Frazier, S., and Holt, J. T. (1999). Ovarian cancer BRCA1 gene therapy: Phase I and II trial differences in immune response and vector stability. *Clin. Cancer Res.* 5, 1708–1714.
172. Douglas, J. T., Rogers, B. E., Rosenfeld, M. E., Michael, S. I., Feng, M., and Curiel, D. T. (1996). Targeted gene delivery by tropism-modified adenoviral vectors. *Nat. Biotechnol.* 14, 1574–1578.
173. Dmitriev, I., Krasnykh, V., Miller, C. R., Wang, M., Kashentseva, E., Mikheeva, G., Belousova, N., and Curiel, D. T. (1998). An adenovirus vector with genetically modified fibers demonstrates expanded tropism via utilization of a coxsackievirus and adenovirus receptor-independent cell entry mechanism. *J. Virol.* 72, 9706–9713.
174. Krasnykh, V., Dmitriev, I., Mikheeva, G., Miller, C. R., Belousova, N., and Curiel, D. T. (1998). Characterization of an adenovirus vector containing a heterologous peptide epitope in the HI loop of the fiber knob. *J. Virol.* 72, 1844–1852.
175. Rancourt, C., Rogers, B. E., Sosnowski, B. A., Wang, M., Piche, A., Pierce, G. F., Alvarez, R. D., Siegal, G. P., Douglas, J. T., and Curiel, D. T. (1998). Basic fibroblast growth factor enhancement of adenovirus-mediated delivery of the herpes simplex virus thymidine kinase gene results in augmented therapeutic benefit in a murine model of ovarian cancer. *J. Clin. Caner Res.* 4, 2455–2461.
176. Wickham, T. J., Tzeng, E., Shears, L. L. 2nd, Roelvink, P. W., Li, Y., Lee, G. M., Brough, D. E., Lizonova, A., and Kovesdi, I. (1997). Increased in vitro and in vivo gene transfer by adenovirus vectors containing chimeric fiber proteins. *J. Virol.* 71, 8221–8229.
177. Wickham, T. J., Segal, D. M., Roelvink, P. W., Carrion, M. E., Lizonova, A., Lee, G. M., and Kovesdi, I. (1996). Targeted adenovirus gene transfer to endothelial and smooth muscle cells by using bispecific antibodies. *J. Virol.* 70, 6831–6838.
178. Vanderkwaak, T. J., Wang, M., Gomez-Navarro, J., Rancourt, C., Dmitriev, I., Krasnykh, V., Barnes, M., Siegal, G. P., Alvarez, R., and

Curiel, D. T. (1999). An advanced generation of adenoviral vectors selectively enhances gene transfer for ovarian cancer gene therapy approaches. *Gynecol. Oncol.* 74, 227–234.

179. Sudimack, J., and Lee, R. J. (2000). Targeted drug delivery via the folate receptor. *Adv. Drug Deliv. Rev.* 41, 147–162.
180. Printz, M. A., Gonzalez, A. M., Cunningham, M., Gu, D. L., Ong, M., Pierce, G. F., and Aukerman, S. L. (2000). Fibroblast growth factor 2-retargeted adenoviral vectors exhibit a modified biolocalization pattern and display reduced toxicity relative to native adenoviral vectors. *Hum. Gene Ther.* 11, 191–204.
181. Fisher, K. D., Stallwood, Y., Green, N. K., Ulbrich, K., Mautner, V., and Seymour, L. W. (2001). Polymer-coated adenovirus permits efficient retargeting and evades neutralising antibodies. *Gene Ther.* 8, 341–348.
182. Doukas, J., Hoganson, D. K., Ong, M., Ying, W., Lacey, D. L., Baird, A., Pierce, G. F., and Sosnowski, B. A. (1999). Retargeted delivery of adenoviral vectors through fibroblast growth factor receptors involves unique cellular pathways. *FASEB J.* 13, 1459–1466.
183. Reynolds, P. N., Feng, M., and Curiel, D. T. (1999). Chimeric viral vectors—the best of both worlds? *Mol. Med. Today* 5, 25–31.
184. Gorman, C. M., Merlino, G. T., Willingham, M. C., Pastan, I., and Howard, B. H. (1982). The Rous sarcoma virus long terminal repeat is a strong promoter when introduced into a variety of eukaryotic cells by DNA-mediated transfection. *Proc. Natl. Acad. Sci. USA* 79, 6777–6781.
185. Boshart, M., Weber, F., Jahn, G., Dorsch-Hasler, K. F. B., and Schaffner, W. (1985). A very strong enhancer is located upstream of an immediate early gene of human cytomegalovirus. *Cell* 41, 521–530.
186. Foecking, M. K., and Hofstetter, H. (1986). Powerful and versatile enhancer-promoter unit for mammalian expression vectors. *Gene* 45, 101–105.
187. Rosenfeld, M. E., Feng, M., Michael, S. I., Siegal, G. P., Alvarez, R. D., and Curiel, D. T. (1995). Adenoviral-mediated delivery of the herpes simplex virus thymidine kinase gene selectively sensitizes human ovarian carcinoma cells to ganciclovir. *Clin. Cancer Res.* 1, 1571–1580.
188. Walther, W., and Stein, U. (1996). Cell type specific and inducible promoters for vectors in gene therapy as an approach for cell targeting. *J. Mol. Med.* 74, 379–392.
189. Vile, R. G., Sunassee, K., and Diaz, R. M. (1998). Strategies for achieving multiple layers of selectivity in gene therapy. *Mol. Med. Today* 4, 84–92.
190. Osaki, T., Tanio, Y., Tachibana, I., Hosoe, S., Kumagai, T., Kawase, I., Oikawa, S., and Kishimoto, T. (1994). Gene therapy for carcinoembryonic antigen-producing human lung cancer cells by cell type-specific expression of herpes simplex virus thymidine kinase gene. *Cancer Res.* 54, 5258–5261.
191. Richards, C. A., Austin, E. A., and Huber, B. E. (1995). Transcriptional regulatory sequences of carcinoembryonic antigen: Identification and use with cytosine deaminase for tumor-specific gene therapy. *Hum. Gene Ther.* 6, 881–893.
192. Lan, K. H., Kanai, F., Shiratori, Y., Okabe, S., Yoshida, Y., Wakimoto, H., Hamada, H., Tanaka, T., Ohashi, M., and Omata, M. (1996). Tumor-specific gene expression in carcinoembryonic antigen–producing gastric cancer cells using adenovirus vectors. *Gastroenterology* 111, 1241–1251.
193. Lan, K. H., Kanai, F., Shiratori, Y., Ohashi, M., Tanaka, T., Okudaira, T., Yoshida, Y., Hamada, H., and Omata, M. (1997). In vivo selective gene expression and therapy mediated by adenoviral vectors for human carcinoembryonic antigen-producing gastric carcinoma. *Cancer Res.* 57, 4279–4284.
194. Huber, B. E., Richards, C. A., and Krenitsky, T. A. (1991). Retroviral-mediated gene therapy for the treatment of hepatocellular carcinoma: An innovative approach for cancer therapy. *Proc. Natl. Acad. Sci. USA* 88, 8039–8043.
195. Kaneko, S., Hallenbeck, P., Kotani, T., Nakabayashi, H., McGarrity, G., Tamaoki, T., Anderson, W. F., and Chiang, Y. L. (1995). Adenovirus-mediated gene therapy of hepatocellular carcinoma using cancer-specific gene expression. *Cancer Res.* 55, 5283–5287.
196. Ido, A., Nakata, K., Kato, Y., Nakao, K., Murata, K., Fujita, M., Ishii, N., Tamaoki, T., Shiku, H., and Nagataki, S. (1995). Gene therapy for hepatoma cells using a retrovirus vector carrying herpes simplex virus thymidine kinase gene under the control of human alpha-fetoprotein gene promoter. *Cancer Res.* 55, 3105–3109.
197. Kanai, F., Lan, K. H., Shiratori, Y., Tanaka, T., Ohashi, M., Okudaira, T., Yoshida, Y., Wakimoto, H., Hamada, H., Nakabayashi, H., Tamaoki, T., and Omata, M. (1997). In vivo gene therapy for alpha-fetoprotein-producing hepatocellular carcinoma by adenovirus-mediated transfer of cytosine deaminase gene. *Cancer Res.* 57, 461–465.
198. Vile, R. G., and Hart, I. R. (1993). Use of tissue-specific expression of the herpes simplex virus thymidine kinase gene to inhibit growth of established murine melanomas following direct intratumoral injection of DNA. *Cancer Res.* 53, 3860–3864.
199. Vile, R. G., and Hart, I. R. (1993). In vitro and in vivo targeting of gene expression to melanoma cells. *Cancer Res.* 53, 962–967.
200. Vile, R. G., Nelson, J. A., Castleden, S., Chong, H., and Hart, I. R. (1994). Systemic gene therapy of murine melanoma using tissue specific expression of the HSVtk gene involves an immune component. *Cancer Res.* 54, 6228–6234.
201. Diaz, R. M., Eisen, T., Hart, I. R., and Vile, R. G. (1998). Exchange of viral promoter/enhancer elements with heterologous regulatory sequences generates targeted hybrid long terminal repeat vectors for gene therapy of melanoma. *J. Virol.* 72, 789–795.
202. Siders, W. M., Halloran, P. J., and Fenton, R. G. (1998). Melanoma-specific cytotoxicity induced by a tyrosinase promoter-enhancer/herpes simplex virus thymidine kinase adenovirus. *Cancer Gene Ther.* 5, 281–291.
203. Manome, Y., Abe, M., Hagen, M. F., Fine, H. A., and Kufe, D. W. (1994). Enhancer sequences of the DF3 gene regulate expression of the herpes simplex virus thymidine kinase gene and confer sensitivity of human breast cancer cells to ganciclovir. *Cancer Res.* 54, 5408–5413.
204. Robertson, M. W., 3rd, Wang, M., Siegal, G. P., Rosenfeld, M., Ashford, R. S., 2nd, Alvarez, R. D., Garver, R. I., and Curiel, D. T. (1998). Use of a tissue-specific promoter for targeted expression of the herpes simplex virus thymidine kinase gene in cervical carcinoma cells. *Cancer Gene Ther.* 5, 331–336.
205. Cleutjens, K. B., van Eekelen, C. C., van der Korput, H. A., Brinkmann, A. O., and Trapman, J. (1996). Two androgen response regions cooperate in steroid hormone regulated activity of the prostate-specific antigen promoter. *J. Biol. Chem.* 271, 6379–6388.
206. Dannull, J., and Belldegrun, A. S. (1997). Development of gene therapy for prostate cancer using a novel promoter of prostate-specific antigen. *Br. J. Urol.* 79, Suppl. 1, 97–103.
207. Koeneman, K. S., Kao, C., Ko, S. C., Yang, L., Wada, Y., Kallmes, D. F., Gillenwater, J. Y., Zhau, H. E., Chung, L. W., and Gardner, T. A. (2000). Osteocalcin-directed gene therapy for prostate-cancer bone metastasis. *World J. Urol.* 18, 102–110.
208. Kijima, T., Osaki, T., Nishino, K., Kumagai, T., Funakoshi, T., Goto, H., Tachibana, I., Tanio, Y., and Kishimoto, T. (1999). Application of the Cre recombinase/loxP system further enhances antitumor effects in cell type-specific gene therapy against carcinoembryonic antigen-producing cancer. *Cancer Res.* 59, 4906–4911.
209. Godwin, A. K., Miller, P. D., Getts, L. A., Jackson, K., Sonoda, G., Schray, K. J., Testa, J. R., and Hamilton, T. C. (1995). Retroviral-like sequences specifically expressed in the rat ovary detect genetic differences between normal and transformed rat ovarian surface epithelial cells. *Endocrinology* 136, 4640–4649.
210. Selvakumaran, M., Bao, R., Crijns, A. P., Connolly, D. C., Weinstein, J. K., and Hamilton, T. C. (2001). Ovarian epithelial cell

lineage-specific gene expression using the promoter of a retrovirus-like element. *Cancer Res.* 61, 1291–1295.
211. Leavitt, J. (1994). Discovery and characterization of two novel human cancer-related proteins using two-dimensional gel electrophoresis. *Electrophoresis* 15, 345–357.
212. Lin, C. S., Chang, C. H., and Huynh, T. (1997). The murine L-plastin gene promoter: Identification and comparison with the human L-plastin gene promoter. *DNA Cell Biol.* 16, 9–16.
213. Park, T., Chen, Z. P., and Leavitt, J. (1994). Activation of the leukocyte plastin gene occurs in most human cancer cells. *Cancer Res.* 54, 1775–1781.
214. Peng, X. Y., Won, J. H., Rutherford, T., Fujii, T., Zelterman, D., Pizzorno, G., Sapi, E., Leavitt, J., Kacinski, B., Crystal, R., Schwartz, P., and Deisseroth, A. (2001). The use of the L-plastin promoter for adenoviral-mediated, tumor-specific gene expression in ovarian and bladder cancer cell lines. *Cancer Res.* 61, 4405–4413.
215. Hallahan, D. E., Mauceri, H. J., Seung, L. P., Dunphy, E. J., Wayne, J. D., Hanna, N. N., Toledano, A., Hellman, S., Kufe, D. W., and Weichselbaum, R. R. (1995). Spatial and temporal control of gene therapy using ionizing radiation. *Nat. Med.* 1, 786–791.
216. Seung, L. P., Mauceri, H. J., Beckett, M. A., Hallahan, D. E., Hellman, S., and Weichselbaum, R. R. (1995). Genetic radiotherapy overcomes tumor resistance to cytotoxic agents. *Cancer Res.* 55, 5561–5565.
217. Mauceri, H. J., Hanna, N. N., Wayne, J. D., Hallahan, D. E., Hellman, S., and Weichselbaum, R. R. (1996). Tumor necrosis factor alpha (TNF-alpha) gene therapy targeted by ionizing radiation selectively damages tumor vasculature. *Cancer Res.* 56, 4311–4314.
218. Manome, Y., Kunieda, T., Wen, P. Y., Koga, T., Kufe, D. W., and Ohno, T. (1998).Transgene expression in malignant glioma using a replication-defective adenoviral vector containing the Egr-1 promoter: Activation by ionizing radiation or uptake of radioactive iododeoxyuridine. *Hum. Gene Ther.* 9, 1409–1417.
219. Joki, T., Nakamura, M., and Ohno, T. (1995). Activation of the radiosensitive EGR-1 promoter induces expression of the herpes simplex virus thymidine kinase gene and sensitivity of human glioma cells to ganciclovir. *Hum. Gene Ther.* 6, 1507–1513.
220. Kawashita, Y., Ohtsuru, A., Kaneda, Y., Nagayama, Y., Kawazoe, Y., Eguchi, S., Kuroda, H., Fujioka, H., Ito, M., Kanematsu, T., and Yamashita, S. (1999). Regression of hepatocellular carcinoma in vitro and in vivo by radiosensitizing suicide gene therapy under the inducible and spatial control of radiation. *Hum. Gene Ther* 10, 1509–1519.
221. Walther, W., Wendt, J., and Stein, U. (1997). Employment of the mdr1 promoter for the chemotherapy-inducible expression of therapeutic genes in cancer gene therapy. *Gene Ther* 4, 544–552.
222. Weichselbaum, R. R., Hallahan, D. E., Beckett, M. A., Mauceri, H. J., Lee, H., Sukhatme, V. P., and Kufe, D. W. (1994). Gene therapy targeted by radiation preferentially radiosensitizes tumor cells. *Cancer Res.* 54, 4266–4269.
223. Jeng, M. H., Kao, C., Sivaraman, L., Krnacik, S., Chung, L. W. K., Medina, D., Conneely, O. M., and O´Malley, B. W. (1998). Reconstitution of estrogen-dependent transcriptional activation of an adenoviral target gene in selected regions of the rat mammary gland. *Endocrinology* 139, 2916–2925.
224. Shibata, T., Giaccia, A. J., and Brown, J. M. (2000). Development of a hypoxia-responsive vector for tumor-specific gene therapy. *Gene Ther* 7, 493–498.
225. Semenza, G. L. (2001). HIF-1 and mechanisms of hypoxia sensing. *Curr. Opin. Cell Biol.* 13, 167–171.
226. Nandi, S., Guzman, R. C., and Yang, J. (1995). Hormones and mammary carcinogenesis in mice, rats, and humans: A unifying hypothesis. *Proc. Natl. Acad. Sci. USA* 92, 3650–3657.
227. Freedman, R. S., Saul, P. B., Edwards, C. L., Jolles, C. J., Gershenson, D. M., Jones, L. A., Atkinson, E. N., and Dana, W. J. (1986). Ethinyl estradiol and medroxyprogesterone acetate in patients with epithelial ovarian carcinoma: a phase II study. *Cancer Treat. Rep.* 70, 369–373.
228. Kieback, D. G., McCamant, S. K., Press, M. F., Atkinson, E. N., Gallager, H. S., Edwards, C. L., Hajek, R. A., and Jones, L. A. (1993). Improved prediction of survival in advanced adenocarcinoma of the ovary by immunocytochemical analysis and the composition adjusted receptor level of the estrogen receptor. *Cancer Res.* 53, 5188–5192.
229. Nash, J. D., Ozols, R. F., Smyth, J. F., and Hamilton, T. C. (1989). Estrogen and anti-estrogen effects on the groth of human epithelial ovarian cancer in vitro. *Obstet. Gynecol.* 73, 1009–1016.
230. Dachs, G. U., Patterson, A. V., Firth, J. D., Ratcliffe, P. J., Townsend, K. M., Stratford, I. J., and Harris, A. L. (1997). Targeting gene expression to hypoxic tumor cells. *Nat. Med.* 3, 515–520.
231. Agha-Mohammadi, S., and Lotze, M. T. (2000). Regulatable systems: Applications in gene therapy and replicating viruses. *J. Clin. Invest.* 105, 1177–1183.
232. Gossen, M., and Bujard, H. (1992). Tight control of gene expression in mammalian cells by tetracycline-responsive promoters. *Proc. Natl. Acad. Sci. USA* 89, 5547–5551.
233. Wang, Y., DeMayo, F. J., Tsai, S. Y., and O'Malley, B. W. (1997). Ligand-inducible and liver-specific target gene expression in transgenic mice. *Nat. Biotechnol.* 15, 239–243.
234. No, D., Yao, T. P., and Evans, R. M. (1996). Ecdysone-inducible gene expression in mammalian cells and transgenic mice. *Proc. Natl. Acad. Sci. USA* 93, 3346–3351.
235. Allgood, V. E., and Eastman, E. M. (1997). Chimeric receptors as gene switches. *Curr. Opin. Biotechnol.* 8, 474–479.
236. Clackson, T. (1997). Controlling mammalian gene expression with small molecules. *Curr. Opin. Chem. Biol.* 1, 210–218.
237. Harvey, D. M., and Caskey, C. T. (1998). Inducible control of gene expression: Prospects for gene therapy. *Curr. Opin. Chem. Biol.* 2, 512–518.
238. Saez, E., No, D., West, A., and Evans, R. M. (1997). Inducible gene expression in mammalian cells and transgenic mice. *Curr. Opin. Chem. Biotechnol.* 8, 608–616.
239. Burcin, M. M., Schiedner, G., Kochanek, S., Tsai, S. Y., and O'Malley, B. W. (1999). Adenovirus-mediated regulable target gene expression in vivo. *Proc. Natl. Acad. Sci. USA* 96, 355–360.
240. Schmitz, M. L., and Baeuerle, P. A. (1991). The p65 subunit is responsible for the strong transcription activating potential of NF-kappa B. *EMBO J.* 10, 3805–3817.
241. Wang, Y., O'Malley, B. W., Jr., Tsai, S. Y., and O'Malley, B. W. (1994). A regulatory system for use in gene transfer. *Proc. Natl. Acad. Sci. USA* 91, 8180–8184.
242. Wang, Y., Xu, J., Pierson, T., O'Malley, B. W., and Tsai, S. Y. (1997). Positive and negative regulation of gene expression in eukaryotic cells with an inducible transcriptional regulator. *Gene Ther.* 4, 432–441.
243. Hunter, T. (1997). Oncoprotein networks. *Cell* 88, 333–346.
244. Lengauer, C., Kinzler, K. W., and Vogelstein, B. (1998). Genetic instabilities in human cancers. *Nature* 396, 643–649.
245. Levine, A. J. (1997). p53, the cellular gatekeeper for growth and division. *Cell* 88, 323–331.
246. DePinho, R. A. (2000). The age of cancer. *Nature* 408, 248–254.
247. Macleod, K. (2000). Tumor suppressor genes. *Curr. Opin. Genet. Dev.* 10, 81–93.
248. Malkin, D., Li, F. P., Strong, L. C., Fraumeni, J. F., Jr., Nelson, C. E., Kim, D. H., Kassel, J., Gryka, M. A., Bischoff, F. Z., and Tainsky, M. A., *et al.* (1990). Germ line p53 mutations in a familial syndrome of breast cancer, sarcomas, and other neoplasms. *Science* 250, 1233–1238.
249. Werness, B. A., Levine, A. J., and Howley, P. M. (1990). Association of human papillomavirus types 16 and 18 E6 proteins with p53. *Science* 248, 76–79.

250. Scheffner, M., Werness, B. A., Huibregtse, J. M., Levine, A. J., and Howley, P. M. (1990). The E6 oncoprotein encoded by human papillomavirus types 16 and 18 promotes the degradation of p53. *Cell* 63, 1129–1236.
251. Scheffner, M., Munger, K., Byrne, J. C., and Howley, P. M. (1991). The state of the p53 and retinoblastoma genes in human cervical carcinoma cell lines. *Proc. Natl. Acad. Sci. USA* 88, 5523–5527.
252. Storey, A., Thomas, M., Kalita, A., Harword, C., Gardiol, D., Mantovani, F., Breuer, J., Leigh, I. M., Matlashewski, G., and Banks, L. (1998). Role of a p53 polymorphism in the development of human papilloma-virus-associated cancer. *Nature* 393, 229–234.
253. Lane, D. P. (1992). Cancer. p53, guardian of the genome. *Nature* 358, 15–16.
254. Sherr, C. J., and Weber, J. D. (2000). The ARF/p53 pathway. *Curr. Opin. Genet. Dev.* 10, 94–99.
255. Vousden, K. H., and Vande Woude, G. F. (2000). The ins and outs of p53. *Nat. Cell Biol.* 2, E178–E180.
256. Vogelstein, B., Lane, D., and Levine, A. J. (2000). Surfing the p53 network. *Nature* 408, 307–310.
257. Hollstein, M., Sidransky, D., Vogelstein, B., and Harris, C. C. (1991). p53 mutations in human cancers. *Science* 253, 49–53.
258. Ko, L. J., and Prives, C. (1996). p53: Puzzle and paradigm. *Genes Dev.* 10, 1054–1072.
259. Giaccia, A. J., and Kastan, M. B. (1998). The complexity of p53 modulation: Emerging patterns from divergent signals. *Genes Dev.* 12, 2973–2983.
260. Rich, T., Allen, R. L., and Wyllie, A. H. (2000). Defying death after DNA damage. *Nature* 407, 777–783.
261. Vousden, K. H. (2000). p53: Death star. *Cell* 103, 691–694.
262. Roth, J. A., and Cristiano, R. J. (1997). Gene therapy for cancer: What have we done and where are we going? *J. Natl. Cancer Inst.* 89, 21–39.
263. Nielsen, L. L., and Maneval, D. C. (1998). P53 tumor suppressor gene therapy for cancer. *Cancer Gene Ther.* 5, 52–63.
264. Santoso, J. T., Tang, D. C., Lane, S. B., Hung, J., Reed, D. J., Muller, C. Y., Carbone, D. P., Lucci, J. A., 3rd, Miller, D. S., and Mathis, J. M. (1995). Adenovirus-based p53 gene therapy in ovarian cancer. *Gynecol. Oncol.* 59, 171–178.
265. Mujoo, K., Maneval, D. C., Anderson, S. C., and Gutterman, J. U. (1996). Adenoviral-mediated p53 tumor suppressor gene therapy of human ovarian carcinoma. *Oncogene* 12, 1617–1623.
266. Nielsen, L. L., Lipari, P., Dell, J., Gurnani, M., and Hajian, G. (1998). Adenovirus-mediated p53 gene therapy and paclitaxel have synergistic efficacy in models of human head and neck, ovarian, prostate, and breast cancer. *Clin. Cancer Res.* 4, 835–846.
267. Von Gruenigen, V. E., Santoso, J. T., Coleman, R. L., Muller, C. Y., Miller, D. S., and Mathis, J. M. (1998). In vivo studies of adenovirus-based p53 gene therapy for ovarian cancer. *Gynecol. Oncol.* 69, 197–204.
268. Kim, J., Hwang, E. S., Kim, J. S., You, E. H., Lee, S. H., and Lee, J. H. (1999). Intraperitoneal gene therapy with adenoviral-mediated p53 tumor suppressor gene for ovarian cancer model in nude mouse. *Cancer Gene Ther.* 6, 172–178.
269. Wolf, J. K., Mills, G. B., Bazzet, L., Bast, R. C., Jr., Roth, J. A., and Gershenson, D. M. (1999). Adenovirus-mediated p53 growth inhibition of ovarian cancer cells is independent of endogenous p53 status. *Gynecol. Oncol.* 75, 261–266.
270. Von Grueningen, V. E., O'Boyle, J. D., Coleman, R. L., Wilson, D., Miller, D. S., and Mathis, J. M. (1999). Efficacy of intraperitoneal adenovirus-mediated p53 gene therapy in ovarian cancer. *Int. J. Gynecol. Cancer* 9, 365–372.
271. Wu, Q., Kreienberg, R., and Runnebaum, I. B. (2000). Growth suppression of human ovarian carcinoma OV-MZ-2a and OV-MZ-32 cells mediated by gene transfer of wild-type p53 enhanced by chemotherapy in vitro. *J. Cancer Res. Clin. Oncol.* 126, 139–144.
272. Mujoo, K., Zhang, L., Klostergaard, J., and Donato, N. J. (2000). Emergence of cisplatin-resistant cells from the OVCAR-3 ovarian carcinoma cell line with p53 mutations, altered tumorigenicity, and increased apoptotic sensitivity to p53 gene replacement. *Int. J. Gynecol. Cancer* 10, 105–114.
273. Barnard, D. L. (2000). Technology evaluation: Sch-58500, Canji. *Curr. Opin. Mol. Ther.* 2, 586–592.
274. Eliopoulos, A. G., Kerr, D. J., Herod, J., Hodgkins, L., Krajewski, S., Reed, J. C., and Young, L. S. (1995). The control of apoptosis and drug resistance in ovarian cancer: Influence of p53 and Bcl-2. *Oncogene* 11, 1217–1218.
275. Vikhanskaya, F., D'Incalci, M., and Broggini, M. (1995). Decreased cytotoxic effects of doxorubicin in a human ovarian cancer-cell line expressing wild-type p53 and WAF1/CIP1 genes. *Int. J. Cancer* 61, 397–401.
276. Vasey, P. A., Jones, N. A., Jenkins, S., Dive, C., and Brown, R. (1996). Cisplatin, camptothecin, and taxol sensitivities of cells with p53-associated multidrug resistance. *Mol. Pharmacol.* 50, 1536–1540.
277. Gallagher, W. M., Cairney, M., Schott, B., Roninson, I. B., and Brown, R. (1997). Identification of p53 genetic suppressor elements which confer resistance to cisplatin. *Oncogene* 14, 185–193.
278. Ashcroft, M., and Vousden, K. H. (1999). Regulation of p53 stability. *Oncogene* 18, 7637–7643.
279. Adams, P. D., and Kaelin, W. G., Jr. (1998). Negative control elements of the cell cycle in human tumors. *Curr. Opin. Cell Biol.* 10, 791–797.
280. Sharpless, N. E., and DePinho, R. A. (1999). The INK4A/ARF locus and its two gene products. *Curr. Opin. Genet. Dev.* 9, 22–30.
281. Alcorta, D. A., Xiong, Y., Phelps, D., Hannon, G., Beach, D., and Barrett, J. C. (1996). Involvement of the cyclin-dependent kinase inhibitor p16 (INK4a) in replicative senescence of normal human fibroblasts. *Proc. Natl. Acad. Sci. USA* 93, 13742–13747.
282. Dai, C. Y., and Enders, G. H. (2000). p16 INK4a can initiate an autonomous senescence program. *Oncogene* 19, 1613–1622.
283. Schreiber, M., Muller, W. J., Singh, G., and Graham, F. L. (1999). Comparison of the effectiveness of adenovirus vectors expressing cyclin kinase inhibitors p16INK4A, p18INK4C, p19INK4D, p21(WAF1/CIP1) and p27KIP1 in inducing cell cycle arrest, apoptosis and inhibition of tumorigenicity. *Oncogene* 18, 1663–1676.
284. Modesitt, S. C., Ramirez, P., Zu, Z., Bodurka-Bevers, D., Gershenson, D., and Wolf, J. K. (2001). In vitro and in vivo adenovirus-mediated p53 and p16 tumor suppressor therapy in ovarian cancer. *Clin. Cancer Res.* 7, 1765–1772.
285. Murphy, M. E. (2001). The battle between tumor suppressors: Is gene therapy using p16(INK4a) more efficacious than p53 for treatment of ovarian carcinoma? *Clin. Cancer Res.* 7, 1487–1489.
286. Welcsh, P. L., Owens, K. N., and King, M. C. (2000). Insights into the functions of BRCA1 and BRCA2. *TIG* 16, 69–74.
287. Miki, Y., Swensen, J., Shattuck-Eidens, D., Futreal, P. A., Harshman, K., Tavtigian, S., Liu, Q., Cochran, C., Bennett, L. M., Ding, W. *et al.* A strong candidate for the breast and ovarian cancer susceptibility gene BRCA1. *Science* 266, 66–71.
288. Scully, R., and Livingston, D. M. (2000). In search of the tumour-suppressor functions of BRCA1 and BRCA2. *Nature* 408, 429–432.
289. Somasundaram, K., Zhang, H., Zeng, Y. X., Houvras, Y., Peng, Y., Wu, G. S., Licht, J. D., Weber, B. L., and El-Deiry, W. S. (1997). Arrest of the cell cycle by the tumour-suppressor BRCA1 requires the CDK-inhibitor p21WAF1/CiP1. *Nature* 389, 187–190.
290. Zhang, H., Somasundaram, K., Peng, Y., Tian, H., Bi, D., Weber, B. L., and El-Deiry, W. S. (1998). BRCA1 physically associates with p53 and stimulates its transcriptional activity. *Oncogene* 16, 1713–1721.
291. Shao, N., Chai, Y. L., Shyam, E., Reddy, P., and Rao, V. N. (1996). Induction of apoptosis by the tumor suppressor protein BRCA1. *Oncogene* 13, 1–7.

292. Holt, J. T., Thompson, M. E., Szabo, C., Robinson-Benion, C., Arteaga, C. L., King, M. C., and Jensen, R. A. (1996). Growth retardation and tumour inhibition by BRCA1. *Nat. Genet.* 12, 298–302.
293. Tait, D. L., Obermiller, P. S., and Holt, J. T. (2000). Preclinical studies of a new generation retroviral vector for ovarian cancer BRCA1 gene therapy. *Gynecol. Oncol.* 79, 471–476.
294. Reed, J. C. (1999). Mechanisms of apoptosis avoidance in cancer. *Curr. Opin. Oncol.* 11, 68–75.
295. Bunz, F. (2001). Cell death and cancer therapy. *Curr. Opin. Pharmacol.* 1, 337–341.
296. Krammer, P. H. (2000). CD95´s deadly mission in the immune system. *Nature* 407, 789–795.
297. Bennett, M., Macdonald, K., Chan, S. W., Luzio, J. P., Simari, R., and Weissberg, P. (1998). Cell surface trafficking of Fas: A rapid mechanism of p53-mediated apoptosis. *Science* 282, 290–293.
298. Morin, P. J., Vogelstein, B., and Kinzler, K. W. (1996). Apoptosis and APC in colorectal tumorigenesis. *Proc. Natl. Acad. Sci. USA* 93, 7950–7954.
299. Wang, Z. G., Ruggero, D., Ronchetti, S., Zhong, S., Gaboli, M., Rivi, R., and Pandolfi, P. P. (1998). PML is essential for multiple apoptotic pathways. *Nat. Genet.* 20, 266–272.
300. Tai, Y. T., Lee, S., Niloff, E., Weisman, C., Strobel, T., and Cannistra, S. A. (1998). BAX protein expression and clinical outcome in epithelial ovarian cancer. *J. Clin. Oncol.* 16, 2583–2590.
301. Strobel, T., Swanson, L., Korsmeyer, S., and Cannistra, S. A. (1996). BAX enhances paclitaxel-induced apoptosis through a p53-independent pathway. *Proc. Natl. Acad. Sci. USA* 93, 14094–14099.
302. Strobel, T., Swanson, L., Korsmeyer, S., and Cannistra, S. A. (1997). Radiation-induced apoptosis is not enhanced by expression of either p53 or BAX in SW626 ovarian cancer cells. *Oncogene* 14, 2753–2758.
303. Tai, Y. T., Strobel, T., Kufe, D., and Cannistra, S. A. (1999). In vivo cytotoxicity of ovarian cancer cells through tumor-selective expression of the BAX Gene. *Cancer Res.* 59, 2121–2126.
304. Di Fiore, P. P., Pierce, J. H., Kraus, M. H., Segatto, O., King, C. R., and Aaronson, S. A. (2001). erbB-2 is a potent oncogene when overexpressed in NIH/3T3 cells. *Science* 237, 178–182.
305. Prenzel, N., Fischer, O. M., Streit, S., Hart, S., and Ullrich, A. (2001). The epidermal growth factor receptor family as a central element for cellular signal transduction and diversification. *Endocr. Relat. Cancer* 8, 11–31.
306. Yarden, Y., and Sliwkowski, M. X. (2001). Untangling the ErbB signalling network. *Nat. Rev. Mol. Cell Biol.* 2, 127–137.
307. Fendly, B. M., Winget, M., Hudziak, R. M., Lipari, M. T., Napier, M. A., and Ullrich, A. (1990). Characterization of murine monoclonal antibodies reactive to either the human epidermal growth factor receptor or HER2/neu gene product. *Cancer Res.* 50, 1550–1558.
308. Alvarez, R. D., and Curiel, D. T. (1997). A phase I study of recombinant adenovirus vector-mediated intraperitoneal delivery of herpes simplex virus thymidine kinase (hsv-tk) gene and intraveneous ganciclovir for previously treated ovarian and extraovarian cancer patients. *Hum. Gene Ther.* 8, 597–613.
309. Igney, F. H., Behrens, C. K., and Krammer, P. H. (2000). Tumor counterattack—concept and reality. *Eur. J. Immunol.* 30, 725–731.
310. Rosenberg, S. A. (2001). Progress in human tumour immunology and immunotherapy. *Nature* 411, 380–384.
311. Dallal, R. M., and Lotze, M. T. (2000). The dendritic cell and human cancer vaccines. *Curr. Opin. Immunol.* 12, 583–588.
312. Melero, I., Mazzolini, G., Narvaiza, I., Qian, C., Chen, L., and Prieto, J. (2001). IL-12 gene therapy for cancer: In synergy with other immunotherapies. *Trends Immunol.* 22, 113–115.
313. Houghton, A. N., Gold, J. S., and Blachere, N. E. (2001). Immunity against cancer: Lessons learned from melanoma. *Curr. Opin. Immunol.* 13, 134–140.
314. Boon, T., and Old, L. J. (1997). Cancer tumor antigens. *Curr. Opin. Immunol.* 9, 681–683.
315. Sanches, R., Kuiper, M., Penault-Llorca, F., Aunoble, B., D'Incan, C., and Bignon, Y. J. (2000). Antitumoral effect of interleukin-12-secreting fibroblasts in a mouse model of ovarian cancer: Implications for the use of ovarian cancer biopsy-derived fibroblasts as a vehicle for regional gene therapy. *Cancer Gene Ther.* 7, 707–720.
316. Gong, J., Nikrui, N., Chen, D., Koido, S., Wu, Z., Tanaka, Y., Cannistra, S., Avigan, D., and Kufe, D. (2000). Fusions of human ovarian carcinoma cells with autologous or allogeneic dendritic cells induce antitumor immunity. *J. Immunol.* 165, 1705–1711.
317. Freeman, S. M. (2000). Suicide gene therapy. *Adv. Exp. Med. Biol.* 465, 411–422.
318. Greco, O., and Dachs, G. U. (2001). Gene directed enzyme/prodrug therapy of cancer: Historical appraisal and future prospectives. *J. Cell Physiol.* 187, 22–36.
319. Niculescu-Duvaz, I., Spooner, R., Marais, R., and Springer, C. J. (1998). Gene-directed enzyme prodrug therapy. *Bioconjug Chem.* 9, 4–22.
320. Bridgewater, J. A., Springer, C. J., Knox, R. J., Minton, N. P., Michael, N. P., and Collins, M. K. (1995). Expression of the bacterial nitroreductase enzyme in mammalian cells renders them selectively sensitive to killing by the prodrug CB1954. *Eur. J. Cancer* 31A, 2362–2370.
321. Tamiya, T., Ono, Y., Wei, M. X., Mroz, P. J., Moolten, F. L., and Chiocca, E. A. (1996). Escherichia coli gpt gene sensitizes rat glioma cells to killing by 6-thioxanthine or 6-thioguanine. *Cancer Gene Ther.* 3, 155–162.
322. Marais, R., Spooner, R. A., Light, Y., Martin, J., and Springer, C. J. (1996). Gene-directed enzyme prodrug therapy with a mustard prodrug/carboxypeptidase G2 combination. *Cancer Res.* 56, 4735–4742.
323. Dilber, M. S., Abedi, M. R., Christensson, B., Bjorkstrand, B., Kidder, G. M., Naus, C. C., Gahrton,, G., and Smith, C. I. (1997). Gap junctions promote the bystander effect of herpes simplex virus thymidine kinase in vivo. *Cancer Res.* 57, 1523–1528.
324. Gagandeep, S., Brew, R., Green, B., Christmas, S. E., Klatzmann, D., Poston, G. J., and Kinsella, A. R. (1996). Prodrug-activated gene therapy: Involvement of an immunological component in the "bystander effect." *Cancer Gene Ther.* 3, 83–88.
325. Pavlovic, J., Nawrath, M., Tu, R., Heinicke, T., and Moelling, K. (1996). Anti-tumor immunity is involved in the thymidine kinase-mediated killing of tumors induced by activated Ki-ras(G12V). *Gene Ther.* 3, 635–643.
326. Ramesh, R., Marrogi, A. J., Munshi, A., Abboud, C. N., and Freeman, S. M. (1996). In vivo analysis of the "bystander effect": A cytokine cascade. *Exp. Hematol.* 24, 829–838.
327. Touraine, R. L., Vahanian, N., Ramsey, W. J., and Blaese, R. M. (1998). Enhancement of the herpes simplex virus thymidine kinase/ganciclovir bystander effect and its antitumor efficacy in vivo by pharmacologic manipulation of gap junctions. *Hum. Gene Ther.* 9, 2385–2391.
328. Hasenburg, A., Tong, X. W., Rojas-Martinez, A., Nyberg-Hoffman, C., Kieback, C. C., Kaplan, A. L., Kaufman, R. H., Ramzy, I., Aguilar-Cordova, E., and Kieback, D. G. (1999). Thymidine kinase (TK) gene therapy of solid tumors: Valacyclovir facilitates outpatient treatment. *Anticancer Res.* 19, 2163–2165.
329. Hasenburg, A., Tong, X. W., Rojas-Martinez, A., Nyberg-Hoffman, C., Kieback, C. C., Kaplan, A., Kaufman, R. H., Ramzy, I., Aguilar-Cordova, E., and Kieback, D. G. (2000). Thymidine kinase gene therapy with concomitant topotecan chemotherapy for recurrent ovarian cancer. *Cancer Gene Ther.* 7, 839–852.
330. Alvarez, R. D., Gomez-Navarro, J., Wang, M., Barnes, M. N., Strong, T. V., Arani, R. B., Arafat, W., Hughes, J. V., Siegal, G. P., and Curiel, D. T. (2000). Adenoviral-mediated suicide gene therapy for ovarian cancer. *Mol. Ther.* 2, 524–530.
331. Black, M. E., Newcomb, T. G., Wilson, H. M., and Loeb, L. A. (1996). Creation of drug-specific herpes simplex virus type 1

thymidine kinase mutants for gene therapy. *Proc. Natl. Acad. Sci. USA* 93, 3525–3529.
332. Beltinger, C., Fulda, S., Kammertoens, T., Meyer, E., Uckert, W., and Debatin, K. M. (1999). Herpes simplex virus thymidine kinase/ganciclovir-induced apoptosis involves ligand-independent death receptor aggregation and activation of caspases. *Proc. Natl. Acad. Sci. USA* 96, 8699–8704.
333. Melcher, A., Todryk, S., Hardwick, N., Ford, M., Jacobson, M., and Vile, R. G. (1998). Tumor immunogenicity is determined by the mechanism of cell death via induction of heat shock protein expression. *Nat. Med.* 4, 581–587.
334. Thust, R., Tomicic, M., Klocking, R., Voutilainen, N., Wutzler, P., and Kaina, B. (2000). Comparison of the genotoxic and apoptosis-inducing properties of ganciclovir and penciclovir in Chinese hamster ovary cells transfected with the thymidine kinase gene of herpes simplex virus-1: Implications for gene therapeutic approaches. *Cancer Gene Ther.* 7, 107–117.
335. Vile, R. G., Castleden, S., Marshall, J., Camplejohn, R., Upton, C., and Chong, H. (1997). Generation of an anti-tumour immune response in a non-immunogenic tumour: HSVtk killing in vivo stimulates a mononuclear cell infiltrate and a Th1-like profile of intratumoural cytokine expression. *Int. J. Cancer* 71, 267–274.
336. Wei, S. J., Chao, Y., Hung, Y. M., Lin, W. C., Yang, D. M., Shih, Y. L., Chang, L. Y., Whang-Peng, J., and Yang, W. K. (1998). S- and G2-phase cell cycle arrests and apoptosis induced by ganciclovir in murine melanoma cells transduced with herpes simplex virus thymidine kinase. *Exp. Cell Res.* 241, 66–75.
337. Freeman, S. M., Ramesh, R., and Marrogi, A. J. (1997). Immune system in suicide-gene therapy. *Lancet* 394, 2–3.
338. Chen, S. H., Chen, X. H. L., Wang, Y., Kosai, K. I., Finegold, M. J., Rich, S. S., and Woo, S. L. C. (1995). Combination gene therapy for liver metastasis of colon carcinoma in vivo. *Proc. Natl. Acad. Sci.* 92, 2577–2581.
339. Freund, C. T., Sutton, M. A., Dang, T., Contant, C. F., Rowley, D., and Lerner, S. P. (2000). Adenovirus-mediated combination suicide and cytokine gene therapy for bladder cancer. *Anticancer Res.* 20, 1359–1365.
340. Behbakht, K., Benjamin, I., Chiu, H.-C., Eck, S. L., Van Deerlin, P. G., Rubin, S. C., and Boyd, J. (1996). Adenovirus-mediated gene therapy of ovarian cancer in a mouse model. *Am. J. Obstet. Gynecol.* 175, 1260–1265.
341. Tong, X. W., Engehausen, D. G., Freund, C. T. F., Agoulnik, I., Oehler, M. K., Kim, T. E., Hasenburg, A., Guo, Z., Contant, C. F., Woo, S. L. C., and Kieback, D. G. (1999). Comparison of long-term survival of cytomegalovirus promoter versus rous sarcoma virus promoter-driven thymidine kinase gene therapy in nude mice bearing human ovarian cancer. *Hybridoma* 18, 93–97.
342. Tong, X. W., Block, A., Chen, S. H., Contant, C. F., Agoulnik, I., Blankenburg, K., Kaufman, R. H., Woo, S. L. C., and Kieback, D. G. (1996). In vivo gene therapy of ovarian cancer by adenovirus-mediated thymidine kinase gene transduction and ganciclovir administration. *Gynecol. Oncol.* 61, 175–179.
343. Hassan, W., Sanford, M. A., Woo, S. L., Chen, S. H., and Hall, S. J. (2000). Prospects for herpes-simplex-virus thymidine-kinase and cytokine gene transduction as immunomodulatory gene therapy for prostate cancer. *World J. Urol.* 18, 130–135.
344. Rosenberg, S. A., Blaese, R. M., Brenner, M. K., Deisseroth, A. B., Ledley, F. D., Lotze, M. T., Wilson, J. M., Nabel, G. J., Cornetta, K., Economou, J. S., Freeman, S. M., Riddell, S. R., Brenner, M., Oldfield, E., Gansbacher, B., Dunbar, C., Walker, R. E., Schuening, F. G., Roth, J. A., Crystal, R. G., Welsh, M. J., Culver, K., Heslop, H. E., Simons, J., Wilmott, R. W., Boucher, R. C., Siegler, H. F., Barranger, J. A., Karlsson, S., Kohn, D., Galpin, J. E., Raffel, C., Hesdorffer, C., Ilan, J., Cassileth, P., O'Shaughnessy, J., Kun, L. E., Das, T. K., Wong-Staal, F., Sobol, R. E., Haubrich, R., Sznol, M., Rubin, J., Sorcher, E. J., Rosenblatt, J., Walker, R., Brigham, K., Vogelzang, N., Hersh, E., Curiel, D., Evans, C. H., Freedman, R., Liu, J., Simons, J., Flotte, T. R., Holt, J., Lyerly, H. K., Whitley, C. B., Isner, J. M., and Eck, S. L. (2000). Human gene marker/therapy clinical protocols. *Hum. Gene Ther.* 11, 919–979.
345. Bouvet, M., Fang, B., Ekmekcioglu, S., Ji, L., Bucana, C. D., Hamada, K., Grimm, E. A., and Roth, J. A. (1998). Suppression of the immune response to an adenovirus vector and enhancement of intratumoral transgene expression by low-dose etoposide. *Gene Ther.* 5, 188–195.
346. Nguyen, D. M., Spitz, F. R., Yen, N., Cristiano, R. J., and Roth, J. A. (1996). Gene therapy for lung cancer: Enhancement of tumor suppression by a combination of sequential systemic cisplatin and adenovirus-mediated p53 gene transfer. *J. Thorac. Cardiovasc. Surg.* 112, 1372–1377.
347. Tong, X. W., Shine, D. H., Agoulnik, I., Freund, C. T. F., Hasenburg, A., Aguilar-Cordova, E., Woo, S. L. C., and Kieback, D. G. (1998). Adenovirus mediated thymidine kinase gene therapy may enhance sensitivity of ovarian cancer cells to chemotherapeutic agents. *Anticancer Res.* 18, 3421–3426.
348. Chou, T.-C. (1991). The median-effect principle and the combination index for quantitation of synergism and antagonism. *In* "Synergism and Antagonism in Chemotherapy," (T. C. Chou and D. C. Rideout, eds.), pp. 61–102. Academic Press, San Diego CA.
349. Chou, T. C., and Talalay, P. (1984). Quantitative analysis of dose-effect relationships: The combined effects of multiple drugs or enzyme inhibitors. *Adv. Enzyme Regulat.* 22, 27–55.
350. Wahl, A. F., Donaldson, K. L., Fairchild, C., Lee, F. Y., Foster, S. A., Demers, G. W., and Galloway, D. A. (1996). Loss of normal p53 function confers sensitization to Taxol by increasing G2/M arrest and apoptosis. *Nat. Med.* 2, 72–79.
351. Gjerset, R. A., Turla, S. T., Sobol, R. E., Scalise, J. J., Mercola, D., Collins, H., and Hopkins, P. J. (1995). Use of wild-type p53 to achieve complete treatment sensitization of tumor cells expressing endogenous mutant p53. *Mol. Carcinog.* 14, 275–285.
352. Yang, B., Eshleman, J. R., Berger, N. A., and Markowitz, S. D. (1996). Wild-type p53 protein potentiates cytotoxicity of therapeutic agents in human colon cancer cells. *Clin. Cancer Res.* 2, 1649–1657.
353. Blagosklonny, M. V., and El-Deiry, W. S. (1996). In vitro evaluation of a p53-expressing adenovirus as an anti-cancer drug. *Int. J. Cancer* 67, 386–392.
354. Spitz, F. R., Nguyen, D., Skibber, J. M., Meyn, R. E., Cristiano, R. J., and Roth, J. A. (1996). Adenoviral-mediated wild-type p53 gene expression sensitizes colorectal cancer cells to ionizing radiation. *Clin. Cancer Res.* 2, 1665–1671.
355. Gallardo, D., Drazan, K. E., and McBride, W. H. (1996). Adenovirus-based transfer of wild-type p53 gene increases ovarian tumor radiosensitivity. *Cancer Res.* 56, 4891–4893.
356. Romig, H., and Richter, A. (1990). Expression of the type I DNA topoisomerase gene in adenovirus-5 infected human cells. *Nucleic Acids Res.* 18, 801–808.
357. Wilson, J. M. (1997). Adenoviruses as gene-delivery vehicles. *N. Engl. J. Med.* 334, 1185–1187.
358. Hui, K. M., Ang, P. T., Huang, L., and Tay, S. K. (1997). Phase I study of immunotherapy of cutaneous metastases of human carcinoma using allogeneic and xenogeneic MHC DNA-liposome complexes. *Gene Ther.* 4, 783–790.
359. Alvarez, R. D., and Curiel, D. T. (1997). A phase I study of recombinant adenovirus vector-mediated delivery of an anti-erbB-2 single-chain (sFv) antibody gene for previously treated ovarian and extraovarian cancer patients. *Hum. Gene Ther.* 8, 229–242.
360. Hasenburg, A., Tong, X. W., Fischer, D. C., Rojas-Martinez, A., Nyberg-Hoffman, C., Kaplan, A. L., Kaufman, R. H., Ramzy, I.,

Aguilar-Cordova, E., and Kieback, D. G. (2001). Adenovirus-mediated thymidine kinase gene therapy in combination with topotecan for patients with recurrent ovarian cancer: 2.5-year follow-up. *Gynecol. Oncol.* 83, 549–554.

361. Hasenburg, A., Fischer, D. C., Tong, X. W., Rojas-Martinez, A., Kaufman, R. H., Ramzy, I., Kohlberger, P., Orlowska-Volk, M., Aguilar-Cordova, E., and Kieback, D. G. (2002). Adenovirus-mediated thymidine kinase gene therapy for recurrent ovarian cancer: Expression of coxsackie-adenovirus receptor and integrins alphav-beta3 and alphavbeta5. *J. Soc. Gynecol. Investig.* 9, 174–180.

362. Hasenburg, A., Fischer, D. C., Tong, X. W., Rojas-Martinez, A., Nyberg-Hoffman, C., Orlowska-Volk, M., Kohlberger, P., Kaufman, R. H., Ramzy, I., Aguilar-Cordova, E., and Kieback, D. G. (2002). Histologic and immunohistochemical analysis of tissue response to adenovirus-medited herpes simplex thymidine kinase gene therapy of ovarian cancer. *Int. J. Gynecol. Cancer* 12, 66–73.

CHAPTER

22

Speculation and Deductive Reasoning About Ovarian Epithelial Carcinogenesis and New Horizons

ALBERT ALTCHEK
Department of Obstetrics, Gynecology and Reproductive Science
The Mount Sinai School of Medicine and Hospital
New York, New York 10029

LIANE DELIGDISCH
Departments of Pathology, and Obstetrics, Gynecology and Reproductive Science
The Mount Sinai School of Medicine and Hospital
New York, New York 10029

FRÉDÉRIQUE PENAULT-LLORCA
Service d'Anatomia et Cytologie Pathologiques
Clermont-Ferrand Cedex 01, France

ABSTRACT

Deductive reasoning may give insight into why cancer forms in inclusion cysts, the unappreciated role of the stroma, the 10- to 40-year time for cancer to develop, why the psammoma body might be the remnants of wayward cells, the myth of the "evil genius" cancer, why most intraperitoneal metastases are superficial, the mechanisms of multifocal peritoneal carcinomatosis, and a reason for recurrence after a negative "second look."

Recommendations are suggested for improved researcher communication, verifying the diagnosis of dysplasia, coordinating the bits and pieces of genetic findings, improving ultrasound resolution and serum tumor markers, chemoprevention, and prophylactic salpingo-oophorectomy rather than oophorectomy.

I. INTRODUCTION

A. Genes and Chromosomes

Most ovarian carcinomas develop from surface type epithelium. About 90% are "sporadic" and develop from acquired somatic mutations. About 10% result from an inherited tendency with an increased incidence and earlier onset, usually associated with inherited germplasm BRCA1 and BRCA2 mutations.

Theoretically, in human sporadic epithelial carcinogenesis there may be from four to eight genetic changes based on age-specific incidence rates.[1] Nevertheless sporadic ovarian epithelial cancer shows extensive genetic damage involving molecules, genes, and chromosomes. There may be large losses on chromosome 17p and 16q, and gains on 8q 23–24, 3q 26, and 11q, and many translocations. There are usually more gains than losses identified. In addition there is extensive loss of heterozygosity of genetic loci on many chromosomes. With microarray technique there was upgrading of 55 genes and down-regulation of 48 genes.[2] Estimates indicate that more than 100 oncogenes and at least 12 tumor-suppressor (TS) genes have been identified "...and the list keeps growing."[3] Recent comparative genomic hybridization has disclosed that the putative chromosome 17q 21–23 may harbor another tumor-associated gene.[4] Focal adhesion kinase (FAK) is a cytoplasmic tyrosine kinase involved with cell adhesion, motility, and invasion. It was discovered to be overexpressed by oncoprotein activation in ovarian carcinoma.[5] There are differences of opinion. "...although human tumor cells were hypothesized to carry a number of distinct, mutated growth-controlling genes, most tumors appear to carry only a single activated oncogene."[6]

The most common mutation is that of the p53 TS gene which regulates proliferation causing apoptosis in damaged cells which cannot be corrected. Even if only one allele is mutant the p53 suppression can be lost. In stage I cancer there may be 10–20%, rising to a 70% defect in advanced cancer.[2] Thus even the most frequent single genetic abnormality may not be present in about one-third of cases.

Inactivation of p53 gene may not be necessary if there is another G1 growth regulatory gene such as p16 which has been inactivated, or if there is an overexpression of proto-oncogene products such as cyclins and cyclin-dependent kinases.[7]

TS genes have an unfortunate susceptibility to mutate the second gene. Initially there might be a small 10^{-6} per cell generation of a spontaneous mutation. The probability of the second copy mutating is 10^{-12} per cell generation which is too remote. The mutant allele replaces the opposite chromosomal region with a copy of its own mutation. This results in the tumor-suppressing gene going from a heterozygous to homozygous condition together with the adjacent chromosomal region. It is referred to as loss of heterozygosity (LOH) and it implies that there are many undiscovered TS genes.[6]

Historically it was assumed that abnormal chromosomes cause cancer. At present the consensus is that it is gene mutation. A contrary philosophy returns to the original concept that it is chromosomal aneuploidy with alterations of thousands of genes, even though a mutant gene may have started the process. Since the chances are small that an abnormal karyotype will have a growth advantage over normal cells, the "...evolution of a neoplastic cell species is slow and thus clonal, which is comparable to conventional evolution of a new species." "Cancers are clonal for aneuploidy (and certain gene mutations) but not for a particular karyotype."[8] Non-neoplastic aneuploidy has few and small chromosomal changes (as in Down syndrome). There is a threshold of cancer aneuploidy with many or all chromosomes resulting in many complex abnormal cancer phenotypes.[8]

It was suggested that tumor gene changes are not uniform, and do not immediately cause tumors. In addition mutation oncogenes activation causing abnormal enzymes and functions may be balanced by upstream and downstream buffering actions. This hypothesis "...predicts that the normal human cells became aneuploid before tumorgenicity...."[8]

Cultured overtly normal ovarian epithelial cells from women with BRCA1 mutation already show early change of phosphatidylinositol 3-kinase which is often activated in ovarian carcinoma.[9] It is of interest that dysplastic cells in inclusion cysts and deep clefts of ovarian surface epithelium have chromatic abnormalities with enlarged size, irregular surface, and heterogeneous chromatin.[10] This indicates aneuploidy before complete malignancy and raises the question of which came first, aneuploidy or dysplasia.

Many feel it is all a "tempest in a teapot" since there are changes in both genes and chromosomes. Since gene investigation can be pinpointed while chromosomal study is too variable, the latter was not studied as much.

The essential problem of gene and chromosomal changes is that the information comes in a jigsaw puzzle of small pieces at one unknown point in time without understanding the sequence of events, timing, host physiologic changes to counteract the mutations (up- and downstream), relations to other simultaneous occurrences, etc.

Since our common basic knowledge is histopathology, the landmark reference should be dysplasia and the molecular changes should be related to it. Weinstein divided cancer-associated genes into two functional groups. The first controls intracellular circuitry and includes response to external growth stimuli, DNA replication and repair, cell cycle control, and cell fate (differentiation, senescence, and apoptosis). The second group involves the cell surface and extracellular functions, including reaction to extracellular matrix, adjacent cells, cell adhesion, angiogenesis, invasion, and metastasis.[3] Carcinogenesis is not simply the multistage activation of oncogenes and inactivation of TS genes. With mutations the potential carcinoma cell must continue to coordinate intracellular complex functions to survive and multiply. Thus a new bizarre circuitry develops to maintain homeostasis. "This concept could help to explain the long latent period of carcinogenesis and the complex and heterogeneous phenotypes of cancer cells."[3] Cancer is considered a "...global disturbance of the network of regulatory circuitry within cells..." Therefore our analyzing a few genes, transcripts, or proteins or even proteomics still does not give a dynamic view of intracellular cancer circuitry.[3]

B. The Diagnosis of Cancer

There is no genetic diagnosis of cancer since there are no specific precise defects present in all cases.

Individual cell cytology might suggest carcinoma because of an enlarged, irregular nucleus. The only method of increasing the probable diagnosis is by computerized image analysis measuring the nucleus and its texture which will yield an average index number for carcinoma.[10]

The impossibility of genetic diagnosis becomes understandable when we realize that no two first monoclonal cancer cells in two separate individuals are exactly alike. They have been compared to snowflakes [11] where no two are identical but, nevertheless, still identifiable.

In carcinogenesis it is probable that the abnormal mechanism is in place even before the cell acts malignant. Therefore it might be expected that a small percentage of dysplastic cells in an inclusion cyst about to exhibit final transition to carcinoma would have statistical morphometric indication of already being malignant. Presumably in such cells the intracellular aspect has completed the transition. It awaits completion of surface changes for release of cell-to-cell, basement membrane, and matrix restraints to change its relation to surrounding cells.

C. Theoretical Mathematics

If five to seven gene changes are required to produce cancer there might be a mathematical model. This assumes that one gene has many functions because there are many abilities that the transitional cell must randomly acquire to complete the malignant status. This includes resistance to host defense, ability to recruit blood supply, growth advantage, and progressive escape from control by various mechanisms including oncogenes, TS genes, extracellular spread by infiltration, etc. Aside from this each gene may have a dozen variations, and probably each gene mutation might have several defense mechanisms, such as upstream and downstream modifications. There would also be factors of age, ovulation, etc.[11] However, even "in the simplest model, if each gene activation were to occur randomly and independently of the others, the number of cells mathematically required to produce an adult form of cancer would exceed reason."[12] Thus no one would live long enough to develop cancer. It would be like winning a lotto where the chance is impossibly small.

This conclusion is based on a "one-shot" inanimate chance of the fortuitous hitting a specific combination of numbers. It does not take into consideration the biologic aspect of (1) many cells rather than one start the transition journey to malignancy, (2) there is more than one "winning" number of genes and chromosomes, (3) the progressive reduction of odds, and (4) the time factor. Thus the odds are reduced and unfortunately cancer occurs.

D. General Aspects of Carcinogenesis

1. Conceptual Protective Inherent Metabolic Organization Networks

Metabolic organizations are identical in all living organisms in robust and error-tolerant scale-free networks inherently designed to resist random genetic errors. Although these networks are very heterogeneous, their topology is dominated by a few highly connected nodes (or hubs) that link the rest of the less connected nodes to the system. New nodes become attached to already established nodes which characterizes the evolution of biological systems. A few hubs dominate the overall connectivity of the network and thus there is a robustness against random errors of the less connected nodes. In 43 different organisms studied for organization of topography of core cellular metabolic enzyme networks, 4% of all substrates found in all species which were the most highly connected. There was a generic utilization of the same substrate by each species.[13]

2. Biologic Dynamic Factors Acquired Cumulative Mutational Genetic Clones with Growth Advantage

Since mathematical estimates of a cell becoming malignant are so remote why does cancer occur? These estimates are like a lotto based on hitting one number by chance out of millions of possibilities at one time. It assumes that one cell forms the cancer, has a specific definition, that events proceed at the same rate, and that the chance possibilities remain the same. It is true that one cell finally becomes malignant.

Since carcinoma occurs there must be a biologic speed-up involving many cells, time, and progressive reduction of odds. There is a general agreement that sporadic carcinogenesis is a progression of acquired, cumulative mutational genetic clone changes. It has been compared to Darwinian evolution with survival of the fittest extending over thousands or millions of years with only slight periodic random mutations at about the same rate, and sometimes the body becomes more competitive with the change. Thus there is natural selection within each species and eventually a change of species. Rapid great change would be fatal.

With carcinogenesis there is rapid change within one lifetime. The loss of cell control may be fatal to the host. The potential cancer cell has no concern (philosophically speaking) for the host. The only control and selection is the growth advantage compared to normal cells and other clones of transforming cells.

3. The Microenvironment

Recently there has been an appreciation of the competitive microenvironment of even a microscopic tumor with reduced oxygen, low pH, increased lactic acid, reduced nutrition, and increased aerobic glycolysis by transforming cells. This environment stimulates cell mutations, and increases genetic instability, genetic heterogenicity, angiogenesis, and metastasis.[14]

Certain bacteria and viruses have an even faster inherent rate of spontaneous mutation or interchange of genetic material. They apparently always survive the mutations because of their simple life survival requirements. The host may expire but the species survives.

4. The Time Factor

Aside from progressive change by growth selection of new clones, there is an import time factor. Carcinogenesis begins slowly and later with more genetic changes there is an increased rate of change inherently and also with the age factor, which is associated with an increased rate of mutations (or epigenetic changes) and decreased ability to correct it or cause apoptosis.

The time factor for the development of sporadic ovarian cancer might range from 10 to 40 years. This has been shown indirectly by the reduction of cancer in women who took oral contraceptives (OCs) many years previously. Initially it was assumed that incessant ovulation by requiring incessant mitogenic growth stimulus to the ovarian epithelium for repair of the ovulation site was the cause of cancer. When analyzed the effect of ovulation reduction alone did not account for the reduction of cancer. The reduction was traced to the progestin of the OC.[15] It is believed that the progestin might cause apoptosis of abnormal cells. This would reduce the number of cells going toward neoplasia, thereby statistically reducing cancer in later life. Since OCs are taken in the child-bearing age group, perhaps about 18–40, and since carcinoma rates increase during menopause (50–60), the abnormal cells might have formed 10–40 years earlier. The cell abnormality is unknown but has to be acquired, persistent, and accumulative. Presumable additional changes are slow in coming but later increase in pace. The initial change is unknown and might be single nucleotide polymorphisms (SNPs), epigenetic factors, methylation of DNA cystosine, LOH, and gradually global accumulation of genetic defects.[11, 12]

5. Self-Selection Reduction of Odds

Whereas mathematical calculations are compared to winning a lotto, carcinogenesis has a continuous automatic evolution with innumerable random variations constantly developing, however, only those with a growth advantage will survive. With each step toward carcinogenesis there is a reduction of the mathematical odds. In addition each subsequent genetic change is automatically focused toward faster transition by limiting types of mutations. Thus spontaneously by growth selection itself, there is direction towards cancer.[12] This is all by a fortuitous, random biologic phenomenon. As different clones in different inclusion cysts close in on completion they are probably not too apart in time so that with early carcinoma there is often nearby and opposite side ovarian dysplasia.

With germplasm BRCA mutation the process begins at birth and should appear sooner than sporadic cancer, however, even then there is only a few years difference. Presumably despite being present at birth, the ovulatory mitogenic repair stimulus must play an important role especially since OCs reduce the cancer risk "…independent of inherent cancer risk."[15, 16]

E. Monoclonal (Unifocal) and Multiclonal (Multifocal) Similarities

Sporadic ovarian epithelial cancer is monoclonal. Familial, usually BRCA mutational cancer, is multifocal and may be found after prophylactic oophorectomy with the development of primary peritoneal ovarian histology carcinoma.

We believe that even BRCA mutational peritoneal multifocal carcinoma begins like sporadic carcinoma from a single cell, except for the starting point of BRCA mutation, with multiple random changes which persist with growth advantage selection. It must also be unifocal for each malignant site. It presents as multifocal because the peritoneum is huge compared to the ovarian serous surface and therefore there are more opportunities, despite the lack of ovarian stromal stimulation. This would also account for the approximate same time presentation since other random clones were simultaneously going toward malignancy. These concepts could be verified by new different clonal carcinoma cells developing after removal of one ovary with sporadic early ovarian cancer in a young woman or after successful removal of multifocal primary peritoneal carcinomas after prophylactic oophorectomy.

If this concept is correct then dysplasia cells from separate individual inclusion cysts will be different from each other or from a unifocal sporadic cancer.

F. Ovarian Cancer Is Different

1. Peritoneal Spread

Ovarian epithelial surface cancer is different from other "solid neoplasms." Whereas the latter spreads by local infiltration and migration into blood and lymph vessels, the ovarian cancer has an additional and probably earlier route of peritoneal dissemination. Although ovarian cancer develops in inclusion cysts (ICs) it is still close to the surface especially with any enlargement. As soon as intercellular controls are lost (cell-to-cell, basement membrane, matrix), tumor cells can be transported by peritoneal fluid circulation and cause peritoneal death. Probably only a few of the multitude of drifting cells actually implant and grow. Most metastatic colonies remain relatively superficial while the more aggressive ones invade deeply.

We suspect that the absence of metastatic deep penetration is that the malignant cells, although freed from attachment, did not complete their random mutation to develop the full ability to infiltrate tissue, migrate, and enter vessels. They were washed away too soon.

2. Recurrence of Cancer after a Negative "Second-Look"

It is probably not the result of a new cancer since it would take longer than the recurrence which often occurs within two years. We believe it results from the original cancer. Obviously the first cell was not resistant to chemotherapy otherwise it and its initial clone would have been destroyed. It must have been that after the first cell there continued to be further random mutations and one cell formed before the chemotherapy, which was fortuitously resistant. It probably had formed only a small clone because it had a reduced growth advantage compared to the other predominant cells. The latter were destroyed by chemotherapy leaving the field for the small coincidental resistant remaining clone, which had a growth advantage over normal cells. Apparently it takes up to two years to become clinically manifest, perhaps because inherently it was slower growing than the parent cell. Nevertheless, it would continue to mutate thereby selecting faster growing clones. This time estimate would be close to the slightly longer theoretical time from the first cancer cell to clinical disease. Thus our hypothesis is that chemotherapy resistance developed from random mutations after the original cancer cell formed but before chemotherapy.

3. Telomere Length Independence

Telomerase activity is increased in gynecologic cancer (ovary, endometrium, cervix), and stabilizes the length of the telomere; however, unexpectedly there is no relationship between telomere length, stage of disease, or telomerase activity.[17]

Cell cultures of normal ovarian surface epithelium from women with familial breast/ovarian cancer show increased telomeric instability, decreased mean telomeric length, and reduced growth potential which are associated with cellular aging. "Consequently, an accumulation of genetic aberrations due to accelerated cellular aging may contribute to the enhanced susceptibility for malignant transformation and earlier onset in heritable ovarian cancer."[18]

This finding indicates that germ line mutations (presumably BRCA1 and BRCA2) familial cancer has adult molecular instability despite normal histology. However, it is paradoxical since cancers, in general, characteristically re-express telomerase to elongate telomeres thereby causing immortalization. Presumably after an initial shortening of the telomore, it stabilizes and reactivates (and perhaps lengthens) after it becomes dsyplastic histologically or overtly malignant.

II. INCLUSION CYSTS (ICs)

A. Formation of ICs, Preselection toward Malignancy

We believe that most serous ovarian surface epithelial carcinoma arises from dysplastic "surface" epithelial ICs just below the surface rather than from topographic surface epithelium. Eighty-five percent of ovarian cancers originate in the ovarian surface epithelium, and most are serous carcinomas (40%). Later and more detailed descriptions included ICs. The consensus should be reversed. Our hypothesis is based on the presumption that the postmenopausal inclusion cyst epithelium is more active than its origin surface epithelium.

The consensus concept of the first stage of carcinogenesis generally is proliferation. Our view is that the first histologic step in ovarian epithelial carcinogenesis is also proliferation. This simple, logical approach has largely been ignored, however, it explains the mechanism of the formation of significant perimenopausal ICs and the preselection of abnormal cells toward transition to malignancy. Despite the lack of histologic findings indicating increased proliferation, either there should be increased cell division and/or decrease in senescence or apoptosis to result in an increased number of surface epithelium cells and in total area. Usually even normal rates of apoptosis are not observed in routine histology because it is a very rapid process. Therefore a reduced rate would not be detected.

Our ongoing study of ovaries of high risk women discovered that the inclusion cyst lining nuclear-cytoplasmic ratio indicated a young crop of cells. This is in accord with active proliferation with the most active cells invaginating. Apparently this has never been described before and is histologic evidence of increased proliferation of selected areas of surface epithelium even before histologic dysplasia is seen (see Chapter 37, "Prevention of Ovarian Serous Epithelial Carcinoma," Section XVI.B).

Surface epithelium is not uniform. Several types of cells are present in different areas of the same ovary varying from flat to cuboidal to columnar as a simple or focally pseudostratified layer.[19] This implies minor mutations and therefore some cells might have a greater tendency to proliferate.

For the surface to increase there should be an unrecognized molecular change to drive itself or a growth stimulus from the underlying stroma or both. Favoring the first possibility is the protective effect of OCs taken during menstrual life which persists for many decades to reduce the cancer rate in the menopausal years. This indicates an undetected persistent structural epithelial change. The effective agent of OC is progestin,[20, 21] which causes apoptosis of abnormal cells thereby reducing their numbers and reducing the overall chances of transition to malignancy. Thus at the time that the OC was taken there were already undetected molecular abnormal cells.

The original interpretation of the benefit of OCs was that by reducing the repeated growth stimulus for the repair of "incessant ovulation" there was a reduced chance of carcinogenesis.[22] This concept was reinforced by cell cultures becoming malignant after repeated rapid subculturing, possibly because mitosis requires a certain time otherwise there is an increase in mutations.[23] "Incessant ovulation" may be valid, however, deductive reasoning suggested that the reduction of later cancer was greater than could be accounted for by ovulation induction alone. Thus the benefit of high-dose progestin was discovered.

How is the proliferating and enlarging surface area epithelium accommodated? Outward expansion of surface epithelium is not efficient. It would require new capillary growth, and continued outgrowth would require unsupported larger vessels. In addition surface epithelium would be further from the possibility of stromal stimulation. Thus the theoretical benefit of limitless space by outward expansion is canceled.

The logical accommodation of increased surface area is by invaginations and forming a corrugated surface similar to the embryonic brain which fulfills a selective surface increase by gyrations and sulci (tethered to a central site to remain within the skull confine). When the ovary uses this mechanism pathologists have described it as "brain-like" (cerebriform). Crevice and cleft formation of the expanding surface would be ideal since there would not be a need to grow new capillaries (only increased local flow) and there would be a maintenance and possibly increase of stromal growth stimulating substances by diffusion. Since the stroma is relatively firm the invaginating epithelium might secrete a local acting substance to soften the extracellular matrix and permit space for the invaginating epithelium. If this is correct it further indicates that the invaginating clefts already have infiltration-like ability. Continued expansion of the surface epithelium would deepen the crevices and clefts and finally they would be covered over thus completing the formation of the IC.

Since the IC epithelium came from the active proliferating part of the surface (assuming that the surface had varying degrees of proliferation ability), it would be the most likely to continue the possible transition to malignancy. In addition the IC epithelium by being surrounded by stroma would have more contact with stromal stimulation growth factors such as keratocyte and hepatocyte growth factors, TGF-α, TGF-β,[22] than the remaining topographic surface epithelium.

Although most authors use the term "inclusion cysts," Scully refers to them as "inclusion glands." When larger and recognizable macroscopically he names them "inclusion cysts." If it is larger than 1 cm it is referred to as cystadenoma.[19]

Others have suggested that ICs form in the process of surface repair immediately after ovulation "entrapping" cells.[24] This mechanism is improbable since ICs have a dramatic increase at menopause when ovulation has already ceased.

With increasing age the frequency of epithelial inclusion glands (EIGs) increases and they are common in the late reproductive and postmenopausal age groups. EIGs are usually multiple and are spread singly or in small clusters in the superficial cortex. The lining is a single layer of columnar cells and sometimes ciliated suggesting tubal epithelium. Occasionally psammoma bodies (PBs) are in the lumen or adjacent stroma. The cut surface may occasionally have ICs up to several millimeters.[19] The gyriform surface represents invaginations of the surface epithelium forming clefts.

Theoretically there might be two types of ICs with the same histology. Inclusion cysts can be found at all ages beginning with the fetus. They increase with age and particularly at menopause. The earlier forming ICs are presumably from benign intent reasons, while the menopausal crop might have an ominous suggestion.

B. The Overlooked and Unappreciated Stroma

Since carcinoma derives from the epithelium, the stroma has been overlooked, nevertheless, "...the stroma may play a more active role in ovarian tumorigenesis than previously assumed...." [25]

The traditional view is that the postmenopausal ovary is small, smooth, atrophic, and inactive and often not visualized by ultrasound. In fact, although the postmenopausal ovary typically is reduced in size by one-half, there is considerable variation depending in part on the amount of stroma. "Most postmenopausal ovaries have a shrunken gyriform external surface but some have a smooth surface." There may be ICs several millimeters in size.[26]

Stromal secretory activity must play a significant role in carcinogenesis by growth stimulation canceling the controls of normal epithelial cells. Stromal stimulation may be the mechanism of increase in epithelial cell proliferation and formation of crevices and ICs in surface cells with a mutation predisposition toward transition by an unknown subtle change and cannot override the growth stimulus. Even in normal ovaries there is a parallel increase in the development of ICs and stromal activity in menopause.

There is a gradual increase in the amount of ovarian stroma from the fourth to the seventh decades of life. The amount is variable in each individual but usually there are intermediate degrees of modular or diffuse proliferation of the cortical and medullary stroma. There may be atrophy with a thin cortex and stroma ranging to marked stromal proliferation of cortical and medullary stroma.[19]

The reason for the surge in the postmenopausal ovarian stroma is unknown. We suggest that it may be the result of maintained elevated gonadotropic stimulation which is the hallmark of menopause. This concept has been overlooked because follicle stimulating hormone (FSH) added to postmenopausal human surface epithelial cells in culture (*in vitro* and without stroma) inhibited proliferation and luteinizing hormone (LH) had no effect.[27] This is an inherent problem in all focused cell culture studies.

In addition to increased size of the stroma there is unrecognized activity in the postmenopausal ovary. About one-third of women over 55 have an increase in lipid-containing luteinized stromal cells. This is "...probably secondary to elevated levels of circulating gonadotropins...." Enzymatically active stromal cells (EASCs) increase with age and are present in more than 80% of postmenopausal women. Although some are luteinized stromal cells, "...most cannot be distinguished from nonreactive cells with standard histology."[28] "Numerous studies have demonstrated the steroidogenic potential and the gonadal responsiveness of the ovarian stroma in both premenopausal and postmenopausal women."[19] Human stroma cell cultures secrete androstenedione, testosterone, and dehydroepiandrosterone which are stimulated by pituitary gonadotropins and insulin via stromal receptors.[29] Normal postmenopausal women often develop hairs on the chin.

We suggest that investigation of stromal growth factors will also be found to be stimulated by gonadotropins.

Functional abnormalities of receptor tyrosine kinases (RTKs) are considered important in carcinogenesis generally. H-RYK, a newly discovered member of the RTK family, is expressed in the epithelium, stroma, and blood vessels in normal ovaries. It is overexpressed in all three structures in cancer. It induces anchorage-independent growth and tumorgenicity in nude mice, implying that overexpression can be transforming and significant in the pathogenesis of ovarian cancer.[30]

In 63% of epithelial cancer, the stroma secretes a protein which is acidic and rich in cysteine (SPARC). Only 29% of normal ovaries produce SPARC and only premenopausal. SPARC modulates cell adhesion and growth and has a decisive role in tissue remodeling and angiogenesis. It also modulates the mitogenic activity of vascular endothelial growth factor (VEGF) in normal epithelium and possibly malignant transformation. SPARC may contribute to tumor proliferation and invasion. Both SPARC and VEGF increase in cancer, the latter in cancer cells.[31]

Matrix metalloproteinase–2 (MMP-2) is involved with degradation of extracellular matrix, including type IV collagen of basement membrane, tumor invasion, and metastasis. It enables cancer cells to detach and migrate into the peritoneal cavity and also invade into the stroma. It is found in both cancer cells and stromal fibroblasts.[32] TGF–β is a multifunctional peptide which increases MMP thereby enhancing ovarian cancer invasiveness.[33]

The stroma of ovarian cancer overexpresses tenascin, an extracellular matrix (ECM) glycoprotein, especially at the interface with the epithelium suggesting invasion induction. Cell culture shows an effect in adhesion and migration of epithelial cancer.[34] Tenascin is absent in normal menopausal ovaries although it is transiently expressed in developing tissues. "Focal increased expression of tenascin adjacent to tumor cells and vessels may suggest a paracrine role for tenascin in ovarian tumorigenesis."[25]

Grade I serous carcinoma has stromal p53 mutations that were absent in the epithelium. "...stromal oncogene mutations in serous ovarian neoplasms suggest that stromal epithelial interactions rather than epithelial transformation alone may mediate tumor progression."[35]

On a clinical level, with routine transvaginal ultrasound of normal, asymptomatic postmenopausal women about 15% have small simple ovarian cysts, usually smaller than 3 cm. They may disappear, persist, or recur. There was no relation to hormone replacement therapy or time since menopause in a small series. Although there was no pathology examination the cysts may have been unusually large ICs. It further emphasizes that dynamic changes occur in the postmenopausal ovary.[36]

In preoperative postmenopausal women with ultrasound findings of ovarian tumors 3 cm or larger or less than 3 cm with solid parts, simple unilocular ovarian cysts with smooth walls were found in one-third.[37] These may have been exaggerated ICs.

In postmenopausal women, unilocular cystic tumors less than 5 cm were followed and half resolved spontaneously within 60 days.[38]

C. IC Transition toward Malignancy

Separate from the increase with age and especially menopause, there is a difference in reports on whether there is an additional increase of IC in women with a family history of ovarian cancer and/or BRCA mutations. This may be related to the number of sections made (often only one to three slides), possible bias selection in selecting areas for section, small series, extent of family history, BRCA status, age, experience, or bias of investigators, and the theoretical probability that only one aggressive cell of an IC is needed to be the origin of the cancer. Most studies did not find an increase in IC. However, the contralateral ovary of unilateral carcinoma [39] and of prophylactic oophorectomy [40, 41] was reported to have an increase in ICs.

A "cancer-prone phenotype" was described with ICs, deep invaginations of surface epithelium, stromal hyperplasia, epithelial hyperplasia, and surface papillomatosis in an unblinded study of prophylactic oophorectomy.[41]

Normal-appearing epithelial cells in ICs may exhibit subtle abnormalities suggesting the potential for later malignant change. Although CA125 is present in peritoneal mesothelium and other coelomic Mullerian duct derivatives, it is not present in the surface ovarian epithelium in the fetus and adult. CA125 was found in the epithelium of ICs, areas of metaplasia, and papillary excrescences.[42] Normal IC cells stain for tumor markers.[43] There may be tubal metaplasia and expression of HER-2 neu/gene in IC epithelium but absent or slight in surface epithelium.[44] In prophylactic oophorectomy specimens from BRCA heterozygotes, IC nuclear overexpression of p53 was found in 31% showing TP53 mutation and LOH at BRCA. Other normal-appearing IC cells had LOH at BRCA but not TP53 mutations. In sporadic early-stage cancer there were normal-appearing IC cells with TP53 mutation.[45] This suggests that these changes may have started in the IC or possibly even in the proliferating antecedent surface epithelium. p53 protein expression may precede overt cytologic abnormalities in IC in cases with dysplasia.[46]

D. IC and Dysplasia

In cases of prophylactic oophorectomy for familial cancer benign ovary IC epithelium shows increased nuclear size, irregularity, and irregular chromatin texture by computerized image analysis cytometry.[40]

Dysplasia is the missing link in the *de novo* concept of ovarian carcinogenesis. The current concept of ovarian carcinogenesis is that presented by Scully as being *de novo*.[47] This requires an explanation. It is not necessarily *de novo* from nothing preceding, but rather *de novo* to contradict another concept that cancer develops from a preexisting benign neoplasm that was overgrown by the secondary cancer. Thus *de novo* does not contradict a preceding dysplasia concept.

The *de novo* concept is important since it indicates that screening ultrasound cannot discover carcinoma until the ovary is enlarged. This issue was clarified by Scully in 2000 with "...most ovarian epithelial cancers probably arise *de novo* and not from benign, generally large, epithelial lesions that are easily detectable on ultrasonography."[48]

Prophylactic oophorectomy led to the recognition of microscopic ovarian epithelial dysplasia as the putative origin of epithelial carcinoma. Dysplasia was first described histologically and named by Gusberg and Deligdisch.[49] Dysplasia is easily overlooked because of its subtle histologic pattern which was only recently described. Pathologists have been trained to report only cancer or no cancer.

Dysplasia has been considered in the cervix and other epithelia as the precursor to cancer. It has been found in the ovaries of high-risk women [10, 50] and adjacent to carcinoma.[51] A contradictory report [52] concerning the incidence of dysplasia in high-risk cases can be explained by similar factors in the reported incidence of IC due to insufficient tissue studies and age of patient.

The diagnosis of dysplasia may be somewhat subjective especially since there may be small or large areas of different severity. Whereas it is true that individual cellular morphology is most distorted in cancer, invasion is required for the diagnosis of carcinoma. The diagnosis became more precise, objective, and reproducible using histologic interactive morphometry,[53] neural networks,[54] chromatin texture assessment,[55] and a new autocorrelation-based method that emphasized nuclear area and nuclear texture.[10] With this new technology ovarian dysplasia was identified in 77.6% of prophylactic oophorectomy specimens in 31 Ashkenazi Jewish women with BRCA mutations and family history of ovarian or breast cancer.[10] The high incidence of dysplasia may be due to complete examination of the ovary, the new diagnostic technologies, and experience in cellular structural analysis and family history selection. The location of the dysplastic cells in ICs was reported,[54] but morphometric studies of the stroma were not performed.

Dysplasia usually develops in ICs or deep clefts as opposed to surface epithelium. Although not emphasized, illustrations and descriptions of dysplasia from various studies demonstrate this.[19, 45, 49, 54]

In addition to histologic morphologic change, there must be factors which cannot be visualized such as genes, and functional elements such as growth factors, cell functional "upstream" and "downstream" efforts to counteract mutations of oncogenes and/or TS genes, and external factors such as intercellular matrix, stromal paracrine stimulation, autocrine stimulation, etc. Epithelial IC dysplasia exhibits mutational changes in nuclear p53,[46] and for LOH at BRCA. p53 mutation is a very early event in hereditary and sporadic ovarian carcinogenesis.[45, 56] We suspect it may even occur locally in surface epithelium just before or with proliferation or with formation of the IC.

Overtly normal epithelial cell cultures from cancer-prone humans produce CA125.[57, 58] The synucleins (α, β, and γ) are small cytoplasmic proteins that are expressed predominantly in neurons. It is interesting that PBs are present in meningiomas and ovarian neoplasms. No synucleins were found in normal epithelium or stroma. For the first time it was found that at least one type of synuclein was expressed in 87% of ovarian carcinomas, and 42% expressed all 3 synucleins. About 20% of "preneoplastic lesions" (presumably dysplasia) of epithelium ICs, deep invaginations, and psuedostratification stain for γ synuclein. Synuclein expression may occur at a very early stage in ovarian growth abnormalities and carcinogenesis. "...γ synuclein expression dramatically increases the mobility of ovarian tumor cells and may be involved in modulating the cytoskeleton." Three ovaries with hyperplastic stroma had diffuse γ, β, and α synuclein throughout the stroma and epithelial cells. Since there were no suggestions of mutations it was thought "...that the mechanism driving γ synuclein overexpression in ovarian tumors may act at the transcriptional level." Normal breast tissue does not have synucleins. Eighty-two percentage of stage III/IV breast ductal carcinomas expressed β and/or γ synuclein but no α synuclein.[59]

E. Dysplasia in ICs Is the Precursor of Ovarian Surface Epithelial Carcinoma

It is illogical that carcinoma could arise from perfectly normal cells since the change would be too abrupt, carcinogenesis is multistep mutations over time and normal defense mechanisms can counteract a single gene change. There is a progressive continuity of surface proliferation, formation of clefts and ICs, then dysplasia and finally cancer.

Prophylactic oophorectomy specimens (n = 39) and stage I carcinoma (n = 8) from BRCA heterozygotes were examined and subsequently extended to include early-stage sporadic ovarian carcinoma. Benign epithelial IC cells showed TP53 mutation and LOH at BRCA. In stage I cancer all cases had a "...single inclusion cyst containing a morphologic continuum of normal epithelium, dysplastic epithelium (nuclear atypia with multiple cell layers but no stromal invasion), and invasive carcinoma were observed, with BRCA LOH and the same TP53 mutation present in all three morphologic elements of the cyst." "These data suggest that most epithelial ovarian carcinomas arise within inclusion cysts, that a very limited (and probably short-lived) field of dysplasia precedes the transformation of normal epithelium to carcinoma, and that TP53 mutation is a very early event in hereditary and sporadic ovarian carcinomas."[45] This is the most eloquent description of the malignant transformation by using molecular genetic combined with morphologic techniques. It also suggests that dysplasia is common in prophylactically removed ovaries. In addition it confirms the recognition of "dysplasia" since their objective included the recognition of a premalignant lesion which has not been "firmly elucidated." Furthermore it confirms that dysplasia leads to carcinoma.

ICs are the preferred sites of neoplastic progression in ovarian carcinogenesis. Early malignant changes occur more frequently in surface epithelial lined clefts and ICs than on the ovarian surface facing the peritoneal cavity.[58] Incidental microscopic ovarian carcinoma was discovered originating in an inclusion cyst with "metastatic" epithelium in the remainder of ICs of the same ovary in a case report.[60]

Occasionally in early epithelial ovarian cancer there may be found "...continuity between the malignant lesion and normal-appearing surface epithelial cells." There is a general feeling that there are clues that carcinoma forms from preexisting unusual cells in "normal" ovaries in high-risk cases and in the contralateral ovary with unilateral cancer. These cases seem to have increased numbers of ICs, deep invaginations of the surface, and papillomatosis of the surface. In addition there is a hyperactive stroma with hyperthecosis and/or luteal hyperplasia often close to surface proliferative activity.[24]

"Since more ovarian epithelial stromal tumors are located within the ovarian stroma rather than on its surface, at least in their early stages, it is logical to conclude that such tumors arise principally from epithelial inclusion glands rather than directly from the surface epithelium."[44]

III. THE MYTHS OF THE "EVIL GENIUS CANCER CELL" AND THE "SUCCESSFUL CANCER CELL"

As humans we became subjectively involved and frustrated with cancer. We feel it is an "evil genius." The cancer cell is an uncontrolled, genetically unstable cell which rapidly, constantly, and randomly mutates. Growth advantage is the selection factor in developing new clones. It has been considered a reversion or de-differentiation to an unregulated embryonic stem cell.[61] However, even the stem cell has genetic stability. This is different from Darwinian evolution where there are slow, small changes with a requirement to preserve the immortality of the germ cell and the life of the somatic host carrier.

Our humanity and fear cause us to think of the developing cancer cell as speeding directly and relentlessly toward completion of its transition. Our perspective requires correction. Carcinogenesis probably evolves over decades. The inherent basic problem is the small chance of spontaneous random mutation whenever normal cells divide, perhaps once in every replication of one million pairs of DNA synthesis. If uncorrected or if the affected cell is not destroyed then the error persists. If more errors accumulate with time eventually the accumulation rate speeds up. Although the accumulative errors are fortuitous, there is a competitive natural selection process based on growth advantage. Thus certain clones will survive and will evolve toward uncontrolled growth and spread. We notice only the "successful cancer cell." We imagine that it simply went along its journey in a direct logical progression. We forget that for the single "successful" cancer cell perhaps millions or billions of cells might have started the transition toward cancer and "success" is like winning a very "long shot" lottery.

Although not possible to prove, it might be that most normal humans who never had clinical cancer do have varieties of subtle abnormal cells which never went beyond the earliest stage of transition toward malignancy. Some have speculated that if we all lived forever most of us would eventually develop clinical cancer.

IV. PSAMMOMA BODIES (PBs)

A. What Are PBs?

PBs are well-defined microscopic, extracellular calcium phosphate spherules with concentric laminations usually associated with ovarian papillary serous carcinomas and less often in borderline and benign ovarian serous neoplasms, dysplasia, low-grade serous tumors of peritoneum, non-neoplastic serous epithelial proliferations, peritoneal serous endosalpingiosis, and in retroperitoneal nodes related to sloughed cells. They are occasionally present in salpingitis and even in apparently normal ovaries. They stain cyanophilic or basophilic.[62, 63] PBs are seen in "second-look" peritoneal bodies after cancer chemotherapy.

When associated with malignancy PBs may have a coat of neoplastic cells, while in apparently benign situations the coat is of bland cuboidal cells. PBs are occasionally found adjacent to endometrial serous papillary and clear cell carcinoma.[64] PBs are also found in papillary thyroid carcinoma and meningiomas. Presumably there is some unknown factor unique to these neoplasms. Although prominent and frequent, PBs have been ignored because their origin and significance is unknown.

B. Our Hypothesis—Remnants of Potential Neoplasms which Perished at the Time when Vascularization Should have Developed. If Valid it Might Provide a Therapeutic Clue

Since many cells begin the route to neoplasia and since only one is successful perhaps out of potentially millions, there must be many potential tumor cells that perished en route and at different stages of development. Our hypothesis is that potential carcinomas which are stopped in a microscopic cluster at the time when angiogenesis should be occurring may become PBs. They are in greatest number with malignant epithelial serous ovarian cancers compared to low malignant potential or benign neoplasms. The reason might be the greater molecular difference of the wayward cell going toward malignancy, which presents a better target for the body defense mechanism. If the hypothesis is valid then discovery of the mechanism might suggest a therapeutic approach before the development of clinical disease and metastasis.

C. PBs: Possible Mechanisms of Development

Speculation includes genetic-chromosomal combinations incompatible with survival and replication, failure in competitive growth microenvironment, failure to develop a blood supply at the time and size when diffusion was inadequate, and the normal body host defense.

There is a consensus that once a tumor reaches 0.5 mm in diameter (or 0.125 mm in volume), nutrient diffusion is inadequate.[65, 66] Mathematical models suggest that hypoxia is the feedback adaptational signal processing for proliferation of a spherical tumor,[67] and that avascular three-dimensional multicell spheroids result in central necrosis from nutrient deficiency.[68] Present theory is that in response to the local, hostile microenvironment of hypoxia, acidosis, and competition for nutrients the small tumor actively produces specific locally acting angiogenesis growth factor unique to the tumor, which induces proliferation of normal capillaries toward the tumor. We suggest that the locally acting angiogenesis growth factors of the small tumor are nonspecific, universal, and essentially would be similar to the angiogenesis factors which normal tissues would produce when confronted with hypoxia and/or wound healing. If the tumor had to produce an original unique neoplastic angiogenesis factor(s) it would require extensive random mutational changes necessitating many cell generations to accidentally evolve it. In addition, different clones would develop greatly different angiogenesis factors with self-competition problems. With the delay to evolve angiogenesis abilities the tumors would spontaneously die and/or be more susceptible to body defense mechanisms. Therefore logic suggests a simple, immediate solution for the tumor. It has retained the basic life-stressing chemical signals for hypoxia of all normal cells. This does not require the delay to invent a new angiogenesis system. In addition, there is no problem in deceiving the normal body response for angiogenesis. Thus our hypothesis is simple logic. The malignant and normal cells send the same distress signals.

Angiogenesis is a rapid phenomenon. We have observed clinically that in the McIndoe surgical construction of a vagina for Rokitansky syndrome that the split-thickness skin graft covering a deep raw dissected area induces functional capillary growth into the graft within 2–3 days. (Tumors would have an even faster time frame since they are surrounded by capillaries.)

This extraordinary prompt angiogenetic ability may be explained by a new report showing rapid initial recruitment of bone-marrow-derived endothelial and hematopoietic precursor cells to form blood vessels. This was in response to tumor secretion of serum endothelial growth factor (VEGF) affecting two tyrosine kinase receptors VEGFR1 and VEGFR2. Later, by day 14, there was also recruitment from adjacent preexisting capillaries.[69]

Ovarian epithelial tumors have a unique, rapid angiogenesis. Some ovarian cells are programmed to produce VEGF as part of physiologic ovulation angiogenesis and therefore in early malignancy the tumor cells readily produce paracrine and autocrine VEGF.[70] Thus we are not alone in implying that normal cells as well as neoplasms with the stress of hypoxia and/or trauma secrete similar nonspecific VEGF.

PB development might be related to slow microscopic tumor growth or demise perhaps by senescence, apoptosis, and some factor provoking calcium deposit in layers as a primary or secondary event or an unusual component of abnormal epithelial cells. Inhibition by apoptosis (programmed cell death) is an important factor in controlling tumorigenesis. It occurs rapidly. In physiologic situations there is shrinking and blebbing and then the cell is phagocytosed "...either by their nearest neighbor or by professional macrophages." However, during apoptosis in tumors with substantial cell mortality and overload, "...unphagocytosed apoptotic cells undergo secondary necrosis, characteristically swelling and losing membrane integrity." p53 TS gene is inactivated in about 70% of all neoplasms. p53 induces cell growth arrest or apoptosis. During apoptosis there is an increase in intracellular Ca^{2+} which may be the apoptosis trigger.[71] The necrotic unphagocytosed apoptotic cells would be a good target for calcification.

In human ovarian epithelial cancer as the incidence of PBs increases with the progression of carcinogenesis and its grade, there is a parallel increase in apoptotic activity and p53 protein expression.[72]

The similarity between neoplasms of the ovary, thyroid, and meningiomas, all of which promote PBs, consists in the fact that they have papillary tumor components. PBs result from degenerative changes of papillary growths.

Circulating immunoglobulins which react to cancer cell surfaces, especially antimucin antibodies, inhibit the growth of neoplasms. Antibodies to tumor intracellular proteins do not have therapeutic value,[63] suggesting the importance of the cell surface.

There is a suggestive relationship between the thyroid and ovary. Many cases of thyroid papillary carcinoma stain for CA125. Occasionally ovarian papillary carcinoma may stain for thyroglobulin.[73]

Analysis of PBs show bone morphogenic matrix protein-2 (extracellular polypeptide signaling molecule of the TGF-β superfamily) and type IV collagen. These might cause slow growing tumor cells to form PBs.[74]

Osteoponin (OPN), a noncollagenous bone-related protein related to bone mineralization, is found in the calcified areas of PBs. OPN messenger ribonucleic acid is found in CD68-positive macrophages. This suggests that OPN is produced and promptly secreted by macrophages and translocated to PBs to cause calcium phosphate deposition in ovarian serous papillary adenocarcinoma.[75]

D. PBs Value in Identifying Ovarian Source of Metastases

Ovarian serous papillary carcinoma is rarely metastatic to the breast but shows PBs with fine-needle aspiration cytology.[76, 77] Metastatic carcinoma to supraclavicular nodes may also have PBs.[73] Although more numerous in ovarian serous carcinoma, PBs may be found in malignant mesotheliomas especially in papillary areas with laminated hyalinized cores. Despite the rarity of mitotic figures suggesting slow growth it is often fatal.[78] Psammoma bodies are occasionally found in well-differentiated papillary mesothelioma which is usually benign or indolent and occurs in women in the third and fourth decade.[79] PBs are very rare in background cervix cytology but when present are "highly suggestive" of genital tract malignancy, especially of papillary serous ovarian carcinoma in postmenopausal women.[80]

Despite the fact that PBs have been found in dilatation and curettage of the uterus in benign and malignant conditions, the first report of 11 cases of PBs found incidentally by endometrial biopsy showed only benign findings. Nevertheless the advice was to search for a gynecologic neoplasm.[81] Perhaps the fact that positive cervical cytology sometimes indicated a malignant condition is because the cytology could pick up ovarian and peritoneal PBs.

E. Psammocarcinoma

Whereas PBs are found in 11–38% of serous ovarian carcinomas, some rare cases have over 75% of PBs and are called psammocarcinoma. They are usually clinically indolent suggesting that somehow it is associated with the heavy deposit of PBs.[82] One could speculate that an extraordinary efficient defense stopped huge numbers of potential small tumors (especially targeting more virulent types) leaving PBs which could not be absorbed as remnants.

The usual case of psammocarcinoma is discovered in stage III, has no more than moderate cytologic atypia, without destructive invasion of ovarian stroma or intraperitoneal viscera and "...at least 75% of the papillae and nests were associated with, or completely replaced by psammoma body formation." PBs are usually surrounded by a single layer of neoplastic cells and often clustered into larger lobulated calcified masses.[82] Psammocarcinoma is classified as a rare type of micropapillary serous carcinoma.[83] Occasionally a case has an aggressive course.[84]

V. NEW HORIZONS

A. Referral Diagnostic Consultation Service for Ovarian Dysplasia and Registry of Ovarian Dysplasia

There should be a slide referral diagnostic consultation service for ovarian dysplasia. This diagnosis has not been taught to pathologists. We sense the need for a consultation service since slides from reputable institutions considered normal have been found on review to have dysplasia.

There should be a registry of ovarian dysplasia, the putative origin of *de novo* epithelial carcinoma. This should include verification of diagnosis and clinical history.

B. Registry of Prophylactic Oophorectomy

There should be a registry of prophylactic oophorectomy (and now prophylactic salpingo–oophorectomy) to acquire data on possible dysplasia and unexpected microscopic or overt carcinoma, as well as risk of prophylactic surgery, and follow-up for risk of later peritoneal carcinomatosis, breast cancer, or endometrial cancer, etc. This would affect informed consent and clinical management. At prophylactic surgery the ovary should have many sections made at close intervals rather than the unfortunate customary few sections. Aside from careful evaluation of the surface epithelium and ICs the stroma should be studied for activity.

Such registries with clinical records might give clues to when dysplasia develops, what percent might progress to carcinoma and over how long a time, and whether it remains stable and does it ever regress. At present the evidence that dysplasia is the transition from normal to cancer is presumptive based on histology, comparison with other epithelial neoplasms being present in high-risk women, and being adjacent to early carcinoma or in the opposite ovary. There has not been uniformity on the presence of dysplasia in prophylactic oophorectomy. This might be related to few sections, to inexperience in diagnosis, too soon for dysplasia to have developed, age of patient, parity, use of other medications, or year of menopause, statistical factors, patient population, extent of family history, etc.

C. Need for Careful Examination of Prophylactically Removed Ovaries

Ideally with prophylactic oophorectomy the ovaries should be gently handled, the surface should be surveyed by scanning microscopy, and most important there should be almost serial sectioning. This would give reliable estimates of surface crevices, ICs, whether the cysts are in fact round or linear, occurrence of dysplasia, discovery of microscopic cancer, etc. This would give indications as to whether the entire surface or only a patch had proliferated. It would also be a source for investigating subtle changes despite normal histology.

Others have also suggested standardization and that "…without optimized specimen preparation and pathologic examination, use of molecular markers, and collection of epidemiologic information, advances in understanding the pathogenesis of this lethal tumor may be slow."[85]

D. Coordination of Research with Reference to Histology, Dysplasia, and Sequence of Events; Preoperative Progestin before Oophorectomy as a Suggested Sample Cooperative Investigation

Cellular pathology is the framework of our knowledge and the only method of diagnosing cancer. There is no specific biochemical, gene, or chromosomal change that diagnoses cancer. Dysplasia is the putative transition from normal to cancer and is a definable landmark. Research in genetic, biochemical, and molecular disturbances should be identified with the histologic diagnosis in order to determine the timing, sequence, and organization of specific and group molecular functional disturbances. By association with the standard histology framework the changes might be assigned to apparently normal histology, severity of dysplasia, early microscopic carcinoma, invasion, angiogenesis, metastasis, loss of cell control with releasing of surface cells, etc. At present many excellent laboratories do specific studies on one special gene, protein, or growth factor without regard to how it fits into the basic time-histology frame. There is even less attempt to place it in context with immediate adjacent "upstream" and "downstream" effects, defense counter measures, and a possible new molecular functional reorganization. In a sense every change might be expected to induce a corrective counter change. Ideally using a histologic frame with emphasis on dysplasia researchers should coordinate and match investigations using different techniques unique to each laboratory to analyze a change (gene, chromosome, LOH, growth factors, molecular structure, function, etc.) and to relate it to other simultaneous events (direct and secondary). Thus there might be a central information bank organized on a time-histology-clinical map sequence with various multidescriptive investigations being fitted into the map.

Some clinical investigations might be developed with various research collaborators using different techniques to maximize new knowledge with minimum human exposure. With appropriate safeguards it would be of interest to give progestin prior to prophylactic oophorectomy to investigate the theory that progestin causes apoptosis of abnormal epithelial cells by decreasing the expression of TGF–β1 and increasing TGF–β2/3.[21]

There is great benefit in the concept of large registries in general for new and infrequent problems. It gives structure to a prospective study with a central clinical and pathological review with concurrent molecular research.[86]

E. Ovarian Surface Visualization and Topography: Laparoscopic Ultrasound

Occasionally laparoscopy happens to be done in high-risk women before the time of elective oophorectomy. It would be the ideal time to study ovarian surface topography *in vivo* perhaps by magnification, chromatic or enzyme staining, side lighting, and light of different wavelengths. Photodynamic-induced fluorescent laparoscopy has been used in rats to detect small metastatic ovarian epithelial cancers less than 1 mm and is more sensitive than standard white light.[87] Fluorescent stereomicroscopy was similarly successful in detecting green fluorescent protein positive human cancer in nude mice.[88]

In addition sonographic probes could be attached to laparoscopes or rods (as is done for stones in bile ducts) to investigate ICs (as is done on skin by dermatologists) for signs of stromal activity, and for the location of small deep dermoid cysts for cystectomy.

F. Transvaginal Ultrasound Technology

Transvaginal ultrasound is the standard method of detecting and evaluating ovarian enlargement. Although ultrasound is the best method of detecting enlargement it is less reliable in specificity. Morphology is the mainstay of diagnosis. Although with malignancy circulation generally is high volume, and low pressure with irregular vessels, there is often significant overlap in vascular impedance between benign and malignant enlargements.

Unfortunately ultrasound does not detect malignancy until it enlarges the ovary. Therefore the best it can do is relatively early detection if done frequently. Since there is a controversial "cost-benefit" situation and since cancer in infrequent, ultrasound will probably not become a screening test for the general population. Typically it is done for high-risk screening. Those who theorize that discovery and removal of benign ovarian neoplasms will reduce cancer mortality base their concept that cancers form from pre-existing large neoplasms. Most pathologists believe that cancer develops *de novo* (and at present from dysplasia), which is microscopic, and therefore a screening ultrasound will not cause a dramatic reduction in cancer mortality.

To further confuse the picture ultrasound has revealed that about 15% of normal postmenopausal women have unsuspected, benign, small, simple thin-walled ovarian cysts which had not been noted in pathology books. Some cysts disappear with time and may or may not recur, while some remain stationary or infrequently enlarge.

There is general agreement that observer experience and adequate time are critical for ultrasound examination. Investigations are proceeding with transvaginal three-dimensional power Doppler ultrasound that might improve specificity by morphology and vascular characteristics of enlarged ovaries.[89, 90] Ultrasound is more precise than MRI or CT for ovarian and other intra-abdominal masses. It is also less expensive, faster, has no radiation, and is less frightening. Standard transvaginal ultrasound has a higher resolution than three-dimensional sonography or of pelvic MRI. New high-frequency transvaginal sonogram machines will probably be available in late 2002 with an improved measurement resolution to as little as 0.5 mm.

Sonographers have been oriented to measuring the size and internal structure of the ovary. There has been limited interest in the outer surface, in part because of reduced resolution due to surrounding bowel. We are interested in the 'brain-like' surface appearance of some menopausal ovaries (rather than the traditional description of the small, smooth ovary), which may be due to surface area enlargement and associated with papillations, formation of crevices, ICs, and dysplasia. Since the 'brain-like' surface is visible to the naked eye it should be visualized by ultrasound.

G. A New Possible Simple Logical Method to Improve Transvaginal Ultrasound Resolution of the Ovary

We suggest a new, simple, logical, inexpensive modification of the present sonohysterography technique that is used to outline the uterine cavity and outline an endometrial polyp. With usual transvaginal sonography techniques the endometrial polyp often escapes detection or is only vaguely identified as questionable endometrial thickening. With simple sonohysterography the clinical resolution has been vastly improved by the uniform plain background. Therefore we suggest a saline (or lactated Ringer's) solution be instilled into the uterus in larger volume (requiring greater pressure to pass through the tubes) so that the fluid goes into the cul-de-sac to bathe and surround the ovaries with a uniform background thereby greatly improving the clinical resolution. This will give details of surface topography, clefts, and ICs. The sonographer would have to be reoriented to this new examination technique. In addition other solutions with different ultrasound qualities might be developed.

H. New Imaging

Positron emission tomography (PET) scans were more sensitive than conventional CT scans in documenting and predicting early ovarian cancer recurrence.[91]. Whole-body 18 F-fluorodeoxyglucose positron emission tomography (FDG-PET) imaging had a high sensitivity for detecting intraperitoneal and retroperitoneal metastases, with elevated CA125, especially solitary 1.5–2 cm tumors which were difficult to detect using CT or ultrasound.[92]

I. Serum Tumor Markers, CA125, a New Concept of Stimulation Testing

CA125 serum tumor-associated antigen is not reliable for the early detection of ovarian cancer since only about half of stage I cases are positive. Furthermore there may be false-positives from benign conditions such as endometriosis, menstruation, pelvic inflammatory disease, trauma, peritoneal inflammation, ascites, pleural fluid, etc. It is even less reliable during premenopause. Many no longer use it as a screening test because a false-positive may result in unnecessary surgery. It is of value in monitoring ovarian cancer treatment if it is elevated to begin with. It is used in screening high-risk postmenopausal women. Malignancies other than ovarian (endometrium, pancreatic) may also increase serum CA125.

Whereas true ovarian epithelial surface cells have no or little histologic CA125, epithelial surface cells and dysplasia cells in ICs may stain for CA125. Peritoneal, pleural, and pericardial mesothelial lining cells normally stain for CA125. CA125 has a physiologic unknown function and is related to tissues associated with the coelomic cavity. It is interesting that human peritoneal mesothelial cell cultures from ovarian cancer cases shed CA125 at a five times greater rate than ovarian cancer cell cultures.[93]

The first real advance in understanding the CA125 antigen since it was first identified by Bast in 1981 [94] was the molecular cloning of the CA125 ovarian cancer antigen by Yin and Lloyd in 2001.[95] It was found to be a new mucin molecule designated CA125/MUC 16 (gene MUC 16). There is a high serine, threonine, and proline content in an N-terminal region of 9 partially conserved tandem repeats of 156 amino acids each, and a C-terminal region nontandem repeat sequence containing a possible transmembrane region and a potential tyrosine phosphorylation site. It is the peptide core of the CA125 antigen of the new mucin species that has a high carbohydrate content. This type of mucin is secreted to presumably lubricate epithelial and peritoneal tissue. The secretion mechanism from ovarian tumors is unknown but it is stimulated by epidermal growth factor by its receptor, which is a tyrosine kinase.[95]

Despite various approaches serum CA125 has not had significant improvement as a practical marker for early ovarian cancer. Research retrospective serial gradual increases in serum CA125 may anticipate malignancy but is neither practical nor precise for individual or public health use.

Combination serum tumor markers added to CA125 have improved detection but are not popular. Combining three serum tumor markers (OVXI, CA125-II, macrophage-colony stimulating factor (M-CSF)) gave increased sensitivity, however, only CA125-II could separate stage I cancer from normal controls.[96]

In 1996 Balkin and Altchek suggested a novel concept of an active stimulation test for CA125 and other serum tumor markers rather than the customary single static test.[97] In 1998 Gebauer *et al.* reported that in one case of four of ovarian cancer with a normal serum level of CA125, an injection of interferon-α caused a dramatic increase of serum CA125 three days later. Those with preoperative CA125 elevations did not have further elevation. It was thought that the CA125 was newly produced and not simply released.[98]

J. New Serum Tests

A new approach by Petricoin *et al.* is the mass spectroscopy, computer-generated "artificial intelligence" algorithm analysis of ovarian carcinoma serum proteomic patterns with 100% sensitivity, 95% specificity, and a 94% positive predictive value, including stage I. The discriminating proteins or peptides were low-molecular weight of unknown origin.[99] This is understandable since gross chromosomal changes of carcinoma should result in different serum proteins or peptides as a carcinogenic or secondary effect.

A pilot study described the unique increase of serum tumor-derived plasma membrane fragments in both ovarian and endometrial cancer which can differentiate benign from malignant ovarian disease. The shedding occurs continuously and is associated with gelatinolytic activity, mmp-2 and -9, and FasL which suppresses cellular immunity.[100]

There are ongoing investigations of surface-enhanced laser desorption/ionization-mass spectroscopy and liquid chromatography to identify haptoglobin α chain and other proteins as serum tumor biomarkers.[101]

Ovarian carcinoma cells were found in the bone marrow in 21% and in the peripheral blood in 12%. It did not affect survival time. "Even those tumors which are confined to the true pelvis have the same extent of access to the peripheral circulation as more advanced tumors." In addition serum CA125 "...did not correlate with circulating tumor cells."[102]

There is a new concept of metastasis-suppressor proteins or genes which regulate the growth of disseminated cancer cells at the secondary site (metastatic cascade).[103] This has two implications. The first is that there is a difference between reaching the circulation and forming a metastatic lesion. The circulating cancer cell may not have by random selection achieved required additional abilities. The second implication is that with more precise technology this might be developed into a supplementary method of detection.

K. Chemoprevention

The realization that OCs dramatically reduce the subsequent chance of later sporadic and BRCA familial ovarian cancer was an after-the-fact discovery. It has the disadvantage that there is a possibility that it may increase the chance of later familial BRCA breast cancer. Because the decrease of cancer was more than was accounted for by the cessation of ovulation, it was discovered that progestin had an apoptosis effect. This now brings to question how significant is the reduction of ovulation since its effect appears to be dwarfed by the epidemiologic progestin effect.[20]

This suggests numerous experiments such as acute ovarian molecular responses to progestin just prior to prophylactic oophorectomy by mouth or by progestin IUD. It would also be of interest to communicate with women who have had a progestin IUD, or who have had I.M. Provera Depot long-acting progestin for contraception for a retrospective survey of later chance of ovarian cancer. If these were to have beneficial effects and had no disadvantages, they might be a substitute for oophorectomy or be used while waiting for oophorectomy. It also suggests searching for other medications to induce apoptosis.

High levels of progesterone exerted marked inhibitory effects on cell cultures of human ovarian surface epithelium and ovarian cancer.[104] Narod and Boyd wrote "We believe that five years of oral contraceptive pills will significantly reduce the risk of ovarian cancer, without appreciably increasing the risk of breast cancer."[15] However, they feel that if hormone replacement therapy is considered for the menopausal BRCA mutation carrier that "...progesterone should be avoided if possible." "Several studies now indicate that the progesterone component significantly increases the breast cancer risk."[15]

There have been suggestions that vitamin A and its relatives retinoid and fenretinide may reduce epithelial cancer of the ovaries as well as upper aerodigestive tract, skin, lungs, bladder, and breasts.[105]

Retinoic acid analogs (retinoids) bind to retinoic acid receptors which regulate cell growth. All retinoids tested at clinically achievable concentrations when added to ovarian cancer cultures decreased growth fractions, induced differentiation and apoptosis and increased expression of the mucin MUC 1. The latter is involved with cell-adhesion and immune-effector cells.[106] It has been suggested that women about to have prophylactic oophorectomy and those for incidental oophorectomy as part of hysterectomy for other purposes be given retinoids to investigate short-term ovarian changes.[107]

There are conflicting reports of the efficacy of nonsteroidal anti-inflammatory drugs (acetylsalicylic acid, acetaminophen, and a cyclooxygenase-2 inhibitor) in reducing the frequency of ovarian cancer. Cell-culture effect required large doses, unlike bowel cancer cells which are very sensitive to the effect of NSAIDS due to overexpression of COX-2. Since ovarian cancer cells express low levels of COX-1 and COX-2, there may be a different mechanism of reduction of proliferation. Acetaminophen may decrease ovulation.[108]

A contrary study showed that cyclooxygenase-2 (COX-2) is overexpressed in human ovarian cancer cell live culture and in tumor specimens as well as other epithelial cancers. Treatment of culture with COX-2 inhibitors caused growth inhibition and apoptosis, suggesting a possible role in prevention or treatment.[109]

L. Prophylactic Surgery: Prophylactic Salpingo-Oophorectomy Rather than Oophorectomy

For high-risk cases, generally with BRCA mutation carriers and/or a strong family history of hereditary breast-ovarian cancer syndrome, there is a 40–60% lifetime chance (age 70) with BRCA1 mutation of ovarian cancer and a 10–27% chance with BRCA2 mutation.[110] Therefore prophylactic oophorectomy is considered, usually by laparoscopy, after childbearing is completed, and after genetic counseling.

Since cases of occult fallopian tube carcinoma have been reported with prophylactic oophorectomy for BRCA1 mutations [111, 112] and since there is molecular evidence linking primary tubal cancer to BRCA1 mutations,[113] prophylactic bilateral salpingo-oophorectomy is now the procedure of choice.[114] Patients with founder BRCA gene mutations, usually Ashkenazi Jewish, are almost 10 years younger at the time of diagnosis of primary peritoneal and fallopian tube adenocarcinomas than those without mutations.[115] The relative risk for primary fallopian tube carcinoma is increased in BRCA1/2 mutation carriers, however, the absolute risk is low, about 3%, compared to the average risk of 0.0246%.[116] We suspect that primary fallopian tube cancer might be a reflection of primary peritoneal multifocal cancer.

Because unexpected microscopic ovarian carcinoma is sometimes discovered on later serial sections, some have suggested additional simultaneous random omental biopsy and inspection. Although additional prophylactic hysterectomy to remove the intramural tube has been advised,[111] most have not recommended it because of the increased inherent surgical risk. Prophylactic oophorectomy especially when done under age 40 for BRCA1 mutations gave significant risk reduction for later breast cancer despite hormone replacement therapy.[117–119] Ovarian ablation may be an effective form of adjuvant systemic therapy for premenopausal women with early-stage receptor positive breast cancer.[120]

We tend to overlook women with hereditary nonpolyposis, colorectal cancers (HNCC) with mutations of MLH1 and MSH2 DNA mismatch repair genes who have a 10–12% chance of ovarian cancer, and a 43–60% chance of endometrial cancer by age 70.[86, 121] Such ovarian cancers occur at a "markedly earlier age" (mean age 43, general population mean age 59), are usually epithelial, are likely to be well or moderately differentiated, and are more likely to have a synchronous endometrial cancer.[122]

HNPCC-associated endometrial cancer constitutes 5–10% of all endometrial cancers, and like its ovarian counterpart occurs 15 years earlier than sporadic endometrial cancer. Among women with HNPCC syndrome who had more than one lifetime cancer, more than 50% had endometrial or ovarian cancer as the first cancers and therefore require colon surveillance.[86]

Unilateral salpingo-oophorectomy for early stage I cancer to preserve fertility may be followed by carcinoma later presenting in the opposite ovary. Of 44 cases, 4 developed tumor recurrence 8–78 months later. Two were in the contralateral ovary, one was in the contralateral ovary, and one the fallopian tube. Twelve patients achieved 16 term deliveries. The disease-free survival rate was 95.2% at 5 years and 86.3% at 10 years. "Fertility-sparing surgery should be considered a treatment option in women with stage I epithelial ovarian cancer who desire further childbearing."[123]

It would be interesting to know whether the "recurrences" were really recurrences or new primaries and whether they were BRCA mutation carriers who might have an improved survival rate.[124]

References

1. Boyd, J. A., Hamilton, T. C., and Berchuck, A. (2000). Oncogenes and tumor-suppressor genes. *In* "Principles and Practice of Gynecologic Oncology," (W. J. Hoskins, C. A. Perez, and R. H. Young, eds.), pp. 103–128. Lippincott Williams & Wilkins, New York.
2. Lancaster, J. M., Havrilesky, L. J., and Berchuck, A. (2002). Genetic etiology of sporadic ovarian cancer. *In* "Diagnosis and Management of Ovarian Disorders," 2nd Ed. (A. Altchek, L. Deligdisch, and N. Kase, eds.). Academic Press, San Diego, CA.
3. Weinstein, I. B. (2000). Disorders in cell circuitry during multistage carcinogenesis: The role of homeostasis. *Carcinogenesis* 21, 857–864.
4. Watanabe, T., Imoto, I., Kosugi, Y., Ishiwata, I., Inoue, S., Takayama, M., Sato, A., and Inazawa, J. (2001). A novel amplification at 17q21-23 in ovarian cancer cell lines detected by comparative genomic hybridization. *Gynecol. Oncol.* 81, 172–177.
5. Judson, P. L., He, X., Cance, W. G., and Van Le, L. (1999). Overexpression of focal adhesion kinase, a protein tyrosine kinase, in ovarian carcinoma. *Cancer* 86, 1551–1556.
6. Weinberg, R. A. (2001). Cancer: A genetic disorder. *In* "The Molecular Basis of Cancer," (J. Mendelsohn, P. M. Howley, M. A. Israel, and L. A. Liotta, eds.), pp. 3–9. W. B. Saunders, New York.
7. Havrilesky, L. J., Alvarez, A. A., Whitaker, R. S., Marks, J. R., and Berchuck, A. (2001). Loss of expression of the p16 tumor suppressor gene is more frequent in advanced ovarian cancers lacking p53 mutations. *Gynecol. Oncol.* 83, 491–500.
8. Li, R., Sonik, A., Stindl, R., Rasnick, D., and Duesberg, P. (2000). Aneuploidy vs. gene mutation hypothesis of cancer: Recent study claims mutation but is found to support aneuploidy. *Proc. Natl. Acad. Sci. USA* 97, 3236–3241.
9. Wong, A. S., Kim, S. O., Leung, P. C., Auersperg, N., and Pelech, S. L. (2001). Profiling of protein kinases in the neoplastic transformation of human ovarian surface epithelium. *Gynecol. Oncol.* 82, 305–311.
10. Deligdisch, L., Gil, J., Kerner, H., Wu, H. S., Beck, D., and Gershoni-Baruch, R. (1999). Ovarian dysplasia in prophylactic oophorectomy specimens: Cytogenetic and morphometric correlations. *Cancer* 86, 1544–1550.
11. Stephens, J. C., Schneider, J. A., Tanguay, D. A., Choi, J., Acharya, T., Stanley, S. E., Jiang, R., Messer, C. J., Chew, A., Han, J. H., Duan, J., Carr, J. L., Lee, M. S., Koshy, B., Kumar, A. M., Zhang, G., Newell, W. R., Windemuth, A., Xu, C., Kalbfleisch, T. S., Shaner, S. L., Arnold, K., Schulz, V., Drysdale, C. M., Nandabalan, K., Judson, R. S., Ruano, G., and Vovis, G. F. (2001). Haplotype variation and linkage disequilibrium in 313 human genes. *Science* 293, 489–493.
12. Kern, S. E. (2001). Progressive genetic abnormalities in human neoplasia. *In* "The Molecular Basis of Cancer," (J. Mendelsohn, P. M. Howley, M. A. Israel, and L. A. Liotta, eds.), pp. 41–69. W. B. Saunders, New York.
13. Jeong, H., Tombor, B., Albert, R., Oltvai, Z. N., and Barabasi, A. L. (2000). The large-scale organization of metabolic networks. *Nature* 407, 651–654.
14. Bhujwalla, Z. M., Artemov, D., Aboagye, E., Ackerstaff, E., and Giles, R. V. (2001). Physiological environment in cancer vascularization, invasion, and metastases. *In* "The Tumour Microenvironment: Causes and Consequences of Hypoxia and Acidity." (J. Goode, and D. Chadwick, eds.), pp. 23–45. Wiley, New York.
15. Narod, S. A., and Boyd, J. (2002). Current understanding of the epidemiology and clinical implications of BRCA1 and BRCA2 mutations for ovarian cancer. *Curr. Opin. Obstet. Gynecol.* 14, 19–20.
16. Narod, S. A., Risch, H., Moslehi, R., Dorum, A., Neuhausen, S., Olsson, H., Provencher, D., Radice, P., Evans, G., Bishop, S., Brunet, J. S., and Ponder, B. A. (1998). Oral contraceptives and the risk of hereditary ovarian cancer. Hereditary Ovarian Cancer Clinical Study Group. *N. Engl. J. Med.* 339, 424–428.
17. Wang, S. J., Sakamoto, T., Yasuda, S. S., Fukasawa, I., Ota, Y., Hayashi, M., Okura, T., Zheng, J. H., and Inaba, N. (2002). The relationship between telomere length and telomerase activity in gynecologic cancers. *Gynecol. Oncol.* 84, 81–84.
18. Kruk, P. A., Godwin, A. K., Hamilton, T. C., and Auersperg, N. (1999). Telomeric instability and reduced proliferative potential in ovarian surface epithelial cells from women with a family history of ovarian cancer. *Gynecol. Oncol.* 73, 229–236.
19. Scully, R. E., Young, R. H., and Clement, P. B. (1998). Tumors of the ovary, maldeveloped gonads, fallopian tubes, and blood ligament. *In* "Atlas of Tumor Pathology." (J. Rosai, and L. H. Sobin, eds.), p. 9. Armed Forces Institute of Pathology, Washington, D.C.
20. Schildkraut, J. M., Calingaert, B., Marchbanks, P. A., Moorman, P. G., and Rodriguez, G. C. (2002). Impact of progestin and estrogen potency in oral contraceptives on ovarian cancer risk. *J. Natl. Cancer Inst.* 94, 32–38.
21. Rodriguez, G. C., Nagarsheth, N. P., Lee, K. L., Bentley, R. C., Walmer, D. K., Cline, M., Whitaker, R. S., Isner, P., Berchuck, A., Dodge, R. K., and Hughes, C. L. (2002). Progestin-induced apoptosis in the Macaque ovarian epithelium: Differential regulation of transforming growth factor-beta. *J. Natl. Cancer Inst.* 94, 50–60.
22. Bast, R. C., Jr., and Gordon, B. M. (2001). Molecular pathogenesis of ovarian cancer. *In* "The Molecular Basis of Cancer," (J. Mendelsohn, P. M. Howley, M. A. Israel, and L. A. Liotta, eds.), pp. 361–383. W. B. Saunders, New York.
23. Godwin, A. K., Testa, J. R., Handel, L. M., Liu, Z., Vanderveer, L. A., Tracey, P. A., and Hamilton, T. C. (1992). Spontaneous transformation of rat ovarian surface epithelial cells: Association with cytogenetic changes and implications of repeated ovulation in the etiology of ovarian cancer. *J. Natl. Cancer Inst.* 84, 592–601.
24. Godwin, A. K., Schultz, D. C., Hamilton, T. C., and Knudson, A. G., Jr. (2000). Oncogenes and tumor-suppressor genes. *In* "Principles and Practice of Gynecologic Oncology," (W. J. Hoskins, and C. A. Y. R. C. Perez, eds.), pp. 107–148. Lippincott Williams & Wilkins, New York.
25. Ortiz, B. H., Berkowitz, R. S., and Mok, S. C. (2002). Increased expression of the extracellular membrane protein tenascin in ovarian tumors suggests that ovarian stroma may play a role in tumorigenesis. *Gynecol. Oncol.* 84, 507–508.
26. Scully, R. E., Young, R. H., and Clement, P. B. (1998). Tumors of the ovary, maldeveloped gonads, fallopian tubes, and blood ligament. *In* "Atlas of Tumor Pathology," (J. Rosai, and L. H. Sobin, eds.), p. 5. Armed Forces Institute of Pathology, Washington, D.C.
27. Ivarsson, K., Sundfeldt, K., Brannstrom, M., Hellberg, P., and Janson, P. O. (2001). Diverse effects of FSH and LH on proliferation of human ovarian surface epithelial cells. *Hum. Reprod.* 16, 18–23.
28. Scully, R. E., Young, R. H., and Clement, P. B. (1998). Tumors of the ovary, maldeveloped gonads, fallopian tubes, and blood ligament. *In* "Atlas of Tumor Pathology," (J. Rosai, and L. H. Sobin, eds.), p. 8. Armed Forces Institute of Pathology, Washington, D.C.
29. Scully, R. E., Young, R. H., and Clement, P. B. (1998). Tumors of the ovary, maldeveloped gonads, fallopian tubes, and blood ligament. *In* "Atlas of Tumor Pathology," (J. Rosai, and L. H. Sobin, eds.), p. 20. Armed Forces Institute of Pathology, Washington, D.C.
30. Katso, R. M., Manek, S., Biddolph, S., Whittaker, R., Charnock, M. F., Wells, M., and Ganesan, T. S. (1999). Overexpression of H-Ryk in mouse fibroblasts confers transforming ability in vitro and in vivo: Correlation with up-regulation in epithelial ovarian cancer. *Cancer Res.* 59, 2265–2270.
31. Paley, P. J., Goff, B. A., Gown, A. M., Greer, B. E., and Sage, E. H. (2000). Alterations in SPARC and VEGF immunoreactivity in epithelial ovarian cancer. *Gynecol. Oncol.* 78, 336–341.
32. Wu, X., Li, H., Kang, L., Li, L., Wang, W., and Shan, B. (2002). Activated matrix metalloproteinase-2—A potential marker of prognosis for epithelial ovarian cancer. *Gynecol. Oncol.* 84, 126–134.

33. Rodriguez, G. C., Haisley, C., Hurteau, J., Moser, T. L., Whitaker, R., Bast, R. C., Jr., and Stack, M. S. (2001). Regulation of invasion of epithelial ovarian cancer by transforming growth factor-beta. *Gynecol. Oncol.* 80, 245–253.
34. Wilson, K. E., Bartlett, J. M., Miller, E. P., Smyth, J. F., Mullen, P., Miller, W. R., and Langdon, S. P. (1999). Regulation and function of the extracellular matrix protein tenascin-C in ovarian cancer cell lines. *Br. J. Cancer* 80, 685–692.
35. Ortiz, B. H., Tsung, D., Muto, M. G., and Berkowitz, R. S. (2001). Mutations of p53 and Kras are frequent in the stroma of serous ovarian tumors. *Gynecol. Oncol.* 80, 321.
36. Wolf, S. I., Gosink, B. B., Feldesman, M. R., Lin, M. C., Stuenkel, C. A., Braly, P. S., and Pretorius, D. H. (1991). Prevalence of simple adnexal cysts in postmenopausal women. *Radiology* 180, 65–71.
37. Osmers, R. G., Osmers, M., von Maydell, B., Wagner, B., and Kuhn, W. (1998). Evaluation of ovarian tumors in postmenopausal women by transvaginal sonography. *Eur. J. Obstet. Gynecol. Reprod. Biol.* 77, 81–88.
38. van Nagell, J. R. Jr. (2001). Reply. *Gynecol. Oncol.* 80, 422.
39. Mittal, K. R., Zeleniuch-Jacquotte, A., Cooper, J. L., and Demopoulos, R. I. (1993). Contralateral ovary in unilateral ovarian carcinoma: A search for preneoplastic lesions. *Int. J.Gynecol. Pathol.* 12, 59–63.
40. Werness, B. A., Afify, A. M., Bielat, K. L., Eltabbakh, G. H., Piver, M. S., and Paterson, J. M. (1999). Altered surface and cyst epithelium of ovaries removed prophylactically from women with a family history of ovarian cancer. *Hum. Pathol.* 30, 151–157.
41. Salazar, H., Godwin, A. K., Daly, M. B., Laub, P. B., Hogan, W. M., Rosenblum, N., Boente, M. P., Lynch, H. T., and Hamilton, T. C. (1996). Microscopic benign and invasive malignant neoplasms and a cancer-prone phenotype in prophylactic oophorectomies. *J. Natl. Cancer Inst.* 88, 1810–1820.
42. Kabawat, S. E., Bast, R. C., Jr., Bhan, A. K., Welch, W. R., Knapp, R. C., and Colvin, R. B. (1983). Tissue distribution of a coelomic-epithelium-related antigen recognized by the monoclonal antibody OC125. *Int. J. Gynecol. Pathol.* 2, 275–285.
43. Blaustein, A., Kaganowicz, A., and Wells, J. (1982). Tumor markers in inclusion cysts of the ovary. *Cancer* 49, 722–726.
44. Scully, R. E., Young, R. H., and Clement, P. B. (1998). Tumors of the ovary, maldeveloped gonads, fallopian tubes, and blood ligament. *In* "Atlas of Tumor Pathology," (J. Rosai, and L. H. Sobin, eds.), p. 43. Armed Forces Institute of Pathology, Washington, D.C.
45. Pothuri, B., Leitano, M., Barakat, R. R., Akram, M., Bogomolniv, F., *et al.* (2001). Genetic analysis of ovarian carcinoma histogenesis. *Gynecol. Oncol.* 80, 277.
46. Hutson, R., Ramsdale, J., and Wells, M. (1995). p53 protein expression in putative precursor lesions of epithelial ovarian cancer. *Histopathology* 27, 367–371.
47. Bell, D. A., and Scully, R. E. (1994). Early *de novo* ovarian carcinoma. A study of fourteen cases. *Cancer* 73, 1859–1864.
48. Scully, R. E. (2000). Influence of origin of ovarian cancer on efficacy of screening. *Lancet* 355, 1028–1029.
49. Gusberg, S. B., and Deligdisch, L. (1984). Ovarian dysplasia. A study of identical twins. *Cancer* 54, 1–4.
50. Colgan, T. J., Murphy, J., Cole, D. E., Narod, S., and Rosen, B. (2001). Occult carcinoma in prophylactic oophorectomy specimens: Prevalence and association with BRCA germline mutation status. *Am. J. Surg. Pathol.* 25, 1283–1289.
51. Plaxe, S. C., Deligdisch, L., Dottino, P. R., and Cohen, C. J. (1990). Ovarian intraepithelial neoplasia demonstrated in patients with stage I ovarian carcinoma. *Gynecol. Oncol.* 38, 367–372.
52. Casey, M. J., Bewtra, C., Hoehne, L. L., Tatpati, A. D., Lynch, H. T., and Watson, P. (2000). Histology of prophylactically removed ovaries from BRCA1 and BRCA2 mutation carriers compared with noncarriers in hereditary breast ovarian cancer syndrome kindreds. *Gynecol. Oncol.* 78, 278–287.
53. Deligdisch, L., and Gil, J. (1989). Characterization of ovarian dysplasia by interactive morphometry. *Cancer* 63, 748–755.
54. Deligdisch, L., Einstein, A. J., Guera, D., and Gil, J. (1995). Ovarian dysplasia in epithelial inclusion cysts. A morphometric approach using neural networks. *Cancer* 76, 1027–1034.
55. Deligdisch, L., Miranda, C., Barba, J., and Gil, J. (1993). Ovarian dysplasia: Nuclear texture analysis. *Cancer* 72, 3253–3257.
56. Werness, B. A., Parvatiyar, P., Ramus, S. J., Whittemore, A. S., Garlinghouse-Jones, K., Oakley-Girvan, I., DiCioccio, R. A., Wiest, J., Tsukada, Y., Ponder, B. A., and Piver, M. S. (2000). Ovarian carcinoma *in situ* with germline BRCA1 mutation and loss of heterozygosity at BRCA1 and TP53. *J. Natl. Cancer Inst.* 92, 1088–1091.
57. Auersperg, N., Maines-Bandiera, S., Booth, J. H., Lynch, H. T., Godwin, A. K., and Hamilton, T. C. (1995). Expression of two mucin antigens in cultured human ovarian surface epithelium: Influence of a family history of ovarian cancer. *Am. J. Obstet. Gynecol.* 173, 558–565.
58. Auersperg, N., Wong, A. S., Choi, K. C., Kang, S. K., and Leung, P. C. (2001). Ovarian surface epithelium: Biology, endocrinology, and pathology. *Endocr. Rev.* 22, 255–288.
59. Bruening, W., Giasson, B. I., Klein-Szanto, A. J., Lee, V. M., Trojanowski, J. Q., and Godwin, A. K. (2000). Synucleins are expressed in the majority of breast and ovarian carcinomas and in preneoplastic lesions of the ovary. *Cancer* 88, 2154–2163.
60. Aoki, Y., Kawada, N., and Tanaka, K. (2000). Early form of ovarian cancer originating in inclusion cysts. A case report. *J. Reprod. Med.* 45, 159–161.
61. da Costa, L. F. (2001). Return of de-differentiation: Why cancer is a developmental disease. *Curr. Opin. Oncol.* 13, 58–62.
62. Clement, P. B. (1994). Anatomy and histology of the ovary. *In* "Pathology of the Female Genital Tract," (R. J. Kurman, ed.), pp. 563–596. Springer-Verlag, New York.
63. Gercel-Taylor, C., Bazzett, L. B., and Taylor, D. D. (2001). Presence of aberrant tumor-reactive immunoglobulins in the circulation of patients with ovarian cancer. *Gynecol. Oncol.* 81, 71–76.
64. Kurman, R. J., Zaino, R. J., and Norris, H. J. (1994). Endometrial carcinoma. *In* "Pathology of the Female Genital Tract," (R. J. Kurman, ed.), pp. 439–486. Springer-Verlag, New York.
65. Folkman, J. (1995). Angiogenesis in cancer, vascular, rheumatoid and other disease. *Nat. Med.* 1, 27–31.
66. Ellis, L. M., and Fidler, I. J. (2001). Tumor angiogenesis. *In* "The Molecular Basis of Cancer," (J. Mendelsohn, P. M. Howley, M. A. Israel, and L. A. Liotta, eds.), pp. 173–188. W. B. Saunders, New York.
67. Michelson, S., and Leith, J. T. (1994). Dormancy, regression, and recurrence: Towards a unifying theory of tumor growth control. *J. Theor. Biol.* 169, 327–338.
68. Chaplain, M. A., Ganesh, M., and Graham, I. G. (2001). Spatio-temporal pattern formation on spherical surfaces: Numerical simulation and application to solid tumour growth. *J. Math. Biol.* 42, 387–423.
69. Lyden, D., Hattori, K., Dias, S., Costa, C., Blaikie, P., Butros, L., Chadburn, A., Heissig, B., Marks, W., Witte, L., Wu, Y., Hicklin, D., Zhu, Z., Hackett, N. R., Crystal, R. G., Moore, M. A., Hajjar, K. A., Manova, K., Benezra, R., and Rafii, S. (2001). Impaired recruitment of bone-marrow-derived endothelial and hematopoietic precursor cells blocks tumor angiogenesis and growth. *Nat. Med.* 7, 1194–1201.
70. Hazelton, D. A., and Hamilton, T. C. (1999). Vascular endothelial growth factor in ovarian cancer. *Curr. Oncol. Rep.* 1, 59–63.
71. Zornig, M., Baum, W., Heuber, A. D., and Evans, G. (2001). Programmed cell death and senescence. *In* "The Molecular Basis of Cancer," (J. Mendelsohn, P. M. Howley, M. A. Israel, and L. A. Liotta, eds.), pp. 19–40. W. B. Saunders, New York.
72. Chan, W. Y., Cheung, K. K., Schorge, J. O., Huang, L. W., Welch, W. R., Bell, D. A., Berkowitz, R. S., and Mok, S. C. (2000). Bcl-2 and p53 protein expression, apoptosis, and p53 mutation in human epithelial ovarian cancers. *Am. J. Pathol.* 156, 409–417.

73. Keen, C. E., Szakacs, S., Okon, E., Rubin, J. S., and Bryant, B. M. (1999). CA125 and thyroglobulin staining in papillary carcinomas of thyroid and ovarian origin is not completely specific for site of origin. *Histopathology* 34, 113–117.
74. Kiyozuka, Y., Nakagawa, H., Senzaki, H., Uemura, Y., Adachi, S., Teramoto, Y., Matsuyama, T., Bessho, K., and Tsubura, A. (2001). Bone morphogenetic protein-2 and type IV collagen expression in psammoma body forming ovarian cancer. *Anticancer Res.* 21, 1723–1730.
75. Maki, M., Hirota, S., Kaneko, Y., and Morohoshi, T. (2000). Expression of osteopontin messenger RNA by macrophages in ovarian serous papillary cystadenocarcinoma: A possible association with calcification of psammoma bodies. *Pathol. Int.* 50, 531–535.
76. Raptis, S., Kanbour, A. I., Dusenbery, D., and Kanbour-Shakir, A. (1996). Fine-needle aspiration cytology of metastatic ovarian carcinoma to the breast. *Diagn. Cytopathol.* 15, 1–6.
77. Hansen, P. B., Rasmussen, J. V., and Bak, M. (1998). A lump in the breast. A rare first symptom of ovarian cancer. *Ugeskr. Laeger* 160, 2401–2402.
78. Clement, P. B., Young, R. H., and Scully, R. E. (1996). Malignant mesotheliomas presenting as ovarian masses. A report of nine cases, including two primary ovarian mesotheliomas. *Am. J. Surg. Pathol.* 20, 1067–1080.
79. Butnor, K. J., Sporn, T. A., Hammar, S. P., and Roggli, V. L. (2001). Well-differentiated papillary mesothelioma. *Am. J. Surg. Pathol.* 25, 1304–1309.
80. Nicklin, J. L., Perrin, L., Obermair, A., McConachie, I., and Cominos, D. (2001). The significance of psammoma bodies on cervical cytology smears. *Gynecol. Oncol.* 83, 6–9.
81. Fausett, M. B., Zahn, C. M., Kendall, B. S., and Barth, W. H., Jr. (2002). The significance of psammoma bodies that are found incidentally during endometrial biopsy. *Am. J. Obstet. Gynecol.* 186, 180–183.
82. Gilks, C. B., Bell, D. A., and Scully, R. E. (1990). Serous psammocarcinoma of the ovary and peritoneum. *Int. J. Gynecol. Pathol.* 9, 110–121.
83. Burks, R. T., Sherman, M. E., and Kurman, R. J. (1996). Micropapillary serous carcinoma of the ovary. A distinctive low-grade carcinoma related to serous borderline tumors. *Am. J. Surg. Pathol.* 20, 1319–1330.
84. Poggi, S. H., Bristow, R. E., Nieberg, R. K., and Berek, J. S. (1998). Psammocarcinoma with an aggressive course. *Obstet. Gynecol.* 92, 659–661.
85. Sherman, M. E., Lee, J. S., Burks, R. T., Struewing, J. P., Kurman, R. J., and Hartge, P. (1999). Histopathologic features of ovaries at increased risk for carcinoma. A case-control analysis. *Int. J. Gynecol. Pathol.* 18, 151–157.
86. Lu, K. H., and Broaddus, R. R. (2001). Gynecological tumors in hereditary nonpolyposis colorectal cancer: We know they are common—now what? *Gynecol. Oncol.* 82, 221–222.
87. Chan, J. K., Pham, H., Cuccia, D., Kimel, S., and Gu, M. (2001). Early detection of metastatic ovarian cancer using 5-aminolevulinic acid induced pheoresence laparoscopy in a rat model. *Gynecol. Oncol.* 80, 329.
88. Chaudhuri, T. R., and Mountz, J. M. (2001). Early detection of ovarian cancer by light-based imaging. *Gynecol. Oncol.* 80, 330.
89. Cohen, L. S., Escobar, P. F., Scharm, C., Glimco, B., and Fishman, D. A. (2001). Three-dimensional power Doppler ultrasound improves the diagnostic accuracy for ovarian cancer prediction. *Gynecol. Oncol.* 82, 40–48.
90. Guerriero, S., Alcazar, J. L., Ajossa, S., Lai, M. P., Errasti, T., Mallarini, G., and Melis, G. B. (2001). Comparison of conventional color Doppler imaging and power doppler imaging for the diagnosis of ovarian cancer: Results of a European study. *Gynecol. Oncol.* 83, 299–304.
91. Lin, W.-C. M., and Eisenkop, S. M. (2002). Positron emission tomography predicts early recurrence of ovarian cancer. Correlation with secondary cytoreductive surgery. *Gynecol. Oncol.* 84, 506.
92. Murakami, M., Arai, T., Shida, M., Mitamoto, T., Shinozuka, T., *et al.* (2002). Evaluation of whole-body 18 F-fluorodeoxyglucose positron emission tomography imaging for the detection of metastatic tumors in patients with suspected recurrence of malignant ovarian tumors. *Gynecol. Oncol.* 84, 492.
93. Zeimet, A. G., Marth, C., Offner, F. A., Obrist, P., Uhl-Steidl, M., Feichtinger, H., Stadlmann, S., Daxenbichler, G., and Dapunt, O. (1996). Human peritoneal mesothelial cells are more potent than ovarian cancer cells in producing tumor marker CA-125. *Gynecol. Oncol.* 62, 384–389.
94. Bast, R. C., Jr., Feeney, M., Lazarus, H., Nadler, L. M., Colvin, R. B., and Knapp, R. C. (1981). Reactivity of a monoclonal antibody with human ovarian carcinoma. *J. Clin. Invest.* 68, 1331–1337.
95. Yin, B. W., and Lloyd, K. O. (2001). Molecular cloning of the CA125 ovarian cancer antigen: Identification as a new mucin, MUC16. *J. Biol. Chem.* 276, 27371–27375.
96. Haaften-Day, C., Shen, Y., Xu, F., Yu, Y., Berchuck, A., Havrilesky, L. J., de Bruijn, H. W., van der Zee, A. G., Bast, R. C., Jr., and Hacker, N. F. (2001). OVX1, macrophage-colony stimulating factor, and CA-125-II as tumor markers for epithelial ovarian carcinoma: A critical appraisal. *Cancer* 92, 2837–2844.
97. Altchek, A., and Balkin, M. (1996). Detection of neoplasms by hormonal tumor stimulation test. 201270(5,583,110). 12-10-1996; 2-24-1994. U.S. Patent Office.
98. Gebauer, G., Jaeger, W., Thiel, G., and Lang, N. (1998). Increase of serum tumor marker concentrations by interferon-alpha. *Eur. J. Gynaecol. Oncol.* 19, 363–367.
99. Petricoin, E. F., Ardekani, A. M., Hitt, B. A., Levine, P. J., Fusaro, V. A., Steinberg, S. M., Mills, G. B., Simone, C., Fishman, D. A., Kohn, E. C., and Liotta, L. A. (2002). Use of proteomic patterns in serum to identify ovarian cancer. *Lancet* 359, 572–577.
100. Taylor, D. D., Lyons, K. S., and Gercel-Taylor, C. (2002). Shed membrane fragment-associated markers for endometrial and ovarian cancers. *Gynecol. Oncol.* 84, 443–448.
101. Ye, B., Cramer, D. W., Pratomo, V., Skates, S., Leung, S.-M. *et al.* (2002). Identification of the haptoglobin α chain as a diagnostic ovarian cancer biomarker by enhanced laser desorption/ionization mass spectometry. *Gynecol. Oncol.* 84, 512.
102. Marth, C., Kisic, J., Kaern, J., Trope, C., and Fodstad, O. (2002). Circulating tumor cells in the peripheral blood and bone marrow of patients with ovarian carcinoma do not predict prognosis. *Cancer* 94, 707–712.
103. Yoshida, B. A., Sokoloff, M. M., Welch, D. R., and Rinker-Schaeffer, C. W. (2000). Metastasis-suppressor genes: A review and perspective on an emerging field. *J. Natl. Cancer Inst.* 92, 1717–1730.
104. Syed, V., Ulinski, G., Mok, S. C., Yiu, G. K., and Ho, S. M. (2001). Expression of gonadotropin receptor and growth responses to key reproductive hormones in normal and malignant human ovarian surface epithelial cells. *Cancer Res.* 61, 6768–6776.
105. Lotan, R., and Hong, W. K. (2001). Molecular mechanisms of chemoprevention and differentiation therapy. *In* "The Molecular Basis of Cancer," (J. Mendelsohn, P. M. Howley, M. A. Israel, and L. A. Liotta, eds.), pp. 621–643. W. B. Saunders, New York.
106. Guruswamy, S., Lightfoot, S., Gold, M. A., Hassan, R., Berlin, K. D., Ivey, R. T., and Benbrook, D. M. (2001). Effects of retinoids on cancerous phenotype and apoptosis in organotypic cultures of ovarian carcinoma. *J. Natl. Cancer Inst.* 93, 516–525.
107. Veronesi, U., and Decensi, A. (2001). Retinoids for ovarian cancer prevention: Laboratory data set the stage for thoughtful clinical trials. *J. Natl. Cancer Inst.* 93, 486–488.
108. Mills, G. B. (2002). Mechanisms underlying chemoprevention of ovarian cancer. *Clin. Cancer Res.* 8, 7–10.
109. Krivak, T. C., Gardner, G. J., Seidman, J. D., Hamel, J., Linnoila, I. *et al.* (2002). The role of cyclooxygenase-2 in epithelial cancer. *Gynecol. Oncol.* 84, 505.

110. Lynch, H. T., and Casey, M. J. (2001). Current status of prophylactic surgery for hereditary breast and gynecologic cancers. *Curr. Opin. Obstet. Gynecol.* 13, 25–30.
111. Paley, P. J., Swisher, E. M., Garcia, R. L., Agoff, S. N., Greer, B. E., Peters, K. L., and Goff, B. A. (2001). Occult cancer of the fallopian tube in BRCA-1 germline mutation carriers at prophylactic oophorectomy: A case for recommending hysterectomy at surgical prophylaxis. *Gynecol. Oncol.* 80, 176–180.
112. Aziz, S., Kuperstein, G., Rosen, B., Cole, D., Nedelcu, R., McLaughlin, J., and Narod, S. A. (2001). A genetic epidemiological study of carcinoma of the fallopian tube. *Gynecol. Oncol.* 80, 341–345.
113. Zweemer, R. P., van Diest, P. J., Verheijen, R. H., Ryan, A., Gille, J. J., Sijmons, R. H., Jacobs, I. J., Menko, F. H., and Kenemans, P. (2000). Molecular evidence linking primary cancer of the fallopian tube to BRCA1 germline mutations. *Gynecol. Oncol.* 76, 45–50.
114. Boyd, J. (2001). BRCA: The breast, ovarian, and other cancer genes. *Gynecol. Oncol.* 80, 337–340.
115. Levine, D. A., Yee, C., Marshall, D. S., Olivera, N., Bogomolniv, F. *et al.* (2002). Frequency of BRCA founder mutations among Ashkenazi Jewish patients with primary peritoneal and fallopian tube adenocarcinoma. *Gynecol. Oncol.* 84, 493.
116. Quillin, J. M., Boardman, C. H., Bodurtha, J., and Smith, T. (2001). Preventive gynecologic surgery for BRCA1/2 carriers—information for decision-making. *Gynecol. Oncol.* 83, 168–170.
117. Rebbeck, T. R., Levin, A. M., Eisen, A., Snyder, C., Watson, P., Cannon-Albright, L., Isaacs, C., Olopade, O., Garber, J. E., Godwin, A. K., Daly, M. B., Narod, S. A., Neuhausen, S. L., Lynch, H. T., and Weber, B. L. (1999). Breast cancer risk after bilateral prophylactic oophorectomy in BRCA1 mutation carriers. *J. Natl. Cancer Inst.* 91, 1475–1479.
118. Eisen, A., Rebbeck, T. R., Lynch, H. T., Lerman, C., Ghadirian, P. *et al.* (2000). Reduction in breast cancer risk following bilateral prophylactic oophorectomy in BRCA1 and BRCA2 mutation carriers. *Am. J. Hum. Gene.* 67(Suppl. 2), 58.
119. Weber, B. L., Punzalan, C., Eisen, A., Lynch, H. T., Narod, S. A. *et al.* (2002). Ovarian cancer risk reduction after bilateral prophylactic oophorectomy (BPO) in BRCA1 and BRCA2 mutation carriers. *Am. J. Hum. Gene.* 67(Suppl. 2), 59.
120. Davidson, N. E. (2001). Ovarian ablation as adjuvant therapy for breast cancer. *J. Natl. Cancer Inst. Monogr.* 67–71.
121. Aarnio, M., Sankila, R., Pukkala, E., Salovaara, R., Aaltonen, L. A., de la Chapelle, A., Peltomaki, P., Mecklin, J. P., and Jarvinen, H. J. (1999). Cancer risk in mutation carriers of DNA-mismatch-repair genes. *Int. J. Cancer* 81, 214–218.
122. Watson, P., Butzow, R., Lynch, H. T., Mecklin, J. P., Jarvinen, H. J., Vasen, H. F., Madlensky, L., Fidalgo, P., and Bernstein, I. (2001). The clinical features of ovarian cancer in hereditary nonpolyposis colorectal cancer. *Gynecol. Oncol.* 82, 223–228.
123. Schilder, J. M., Thompson, A. M., Depriest, P. D., Ueland, F. R., Cibull, M. L. *et al.* (2002). Outcome of reproductive-age women with stage IA or IC invasive epithelial ovarian cancer treated with fertility-sparing surgery. *Gynecol. Oncol.* 84, 491.
124. Boyd, J., Sonoda, Y., Federici, M. G., Bogomolniy, F., Rhei, E., Maresco, D. L., Saigo, P. E., Almadrones, L. A., Barakat, R. R., Brown, C. L., Chi, D. S., Curtin, J. P., Poynor, E. A., and Hoskins, W. J. (2000). Clinicopathologic features of BRCA-linked and sporadic ovarian cancer. *JAMA* 283, 2260–2265.

C H A P T E R

23

In Vitro Fertilization, Stem Cells, Cloning, and the Future of Assisted Reproductive Technologies

LISA SPIRYDA
Department of Obstetrics and Gynecology
Brigham & Women's Hospital
Boston, Massachusetts 02115

AMY ANTMAN
Harvard Medical School
Boston, Massachusetts 02115

ELIZABETH S. GINSBURG
Assisted Reproductive Technologies Program
Brigham & Women's Hospital
Boston, Massachusetts 02115

I. CURRENT *IN VITRO* FERTILIZATION PROCEDURES

Over twenty years ago Steptoe and Edwards [1, 2] reported the first pregnancy and birth of an *in vitro* fertilized human egg. Since then, tens of thousands of births have been achieved successfully through assisted reproductive technologies. *In vitro* fertilization (IVF) was a technique initially used in women with tubal damage and now has been expanded to help women with other causes of infertility including endometriosis, failed tuboplasty, poor prognosis pelvic disease, male infertility, or unexplained infertility. *In vitro* fertilization involves several steps: superovulation, follicle aspiration, fertilization, and embryo transfer.

A. Superovulation

In a natural menstrual cycle, follicle stimulating hormone (FSH) is synthesized by the anterior pituitary and stimulates oocyte (egg) differentiation and maturation. FSH binds to specific ovarian cell membrane receptors and subsequently increases conversion of androgens to estrogens, directing morphological and cellular events. This leads to acquisition of the antral cavity, induction of luteinizing hormone (LH) receptors on granulosa cells as well as the activation of various enzymes leading to induction of intracellular signaling pathways.[3–5] The anterior pituitary also produces LH. The main function of LH is to support the follicular growth initiated by FSH. The preovulatory LH surge ultimately results in the oocyte meiosis, maturation, follicular rupture, and subsequent oocyte expulsion (i.e., ovulation). Additionally, LH contributes to the formation and maintenance of the corpus luteum.[6, 7]

Superovulation involves exploitation of the natural hypothalamic-pituitary-ovarian pathway through the administration of exogenous gonadotropins (i.e., LH and FSH). In IVF, exogenous gonadotropins are used to induce ovulation with stimulation of multiple ovarian follicles or superovulation.

Gonadotropins were initially extracted in the 1950s from human pituitaries. This preparation fell out of favor because of the limited supply of human pituitaries and potential transmission of viruses to the recipient.[8, 9] In the early 1960s, human menopausal gonadotropins (hMG) were extracted from urine of postmenopausal women.[10] The bioactivity of LH and FSH in this preparation was 1:1 and each ampule contains 75 IU of each compound. These preparations contain many residual urinary proteins creating the need for intramuscular injection in most cases.[11, 14]

Refinement of purification techniques of the above crude urinary products led to the development of purified and highly purified FSH extracts containing less than 0.0001 IU of LH. These preparations contained significantly less of the contaminating urinary proteins and can be given by subcutaneous injection. Since these extracts are purified through elution through immunoaffinity columns, gonadotropin levels between batches are inconsistent and theoretically would not result in reproducible ovulation induction responses.[12]

The advent of DNA recombinant technology techniques led to the production of recombinant FSH and LH.[11] Chinese hamster ovary (CHO) cells have been engineered to express human recombinant genes of both gonadotropins. The FSH derived from the CHO cells has been shown to be identical to human pituitary FSH, with correct amino acid sequence, post-translational modifications, and glycosylation sites. Advantages of recombinant FSH are numerous. First, the FSH isoform profile is controlled leading to excellent batch-to-batch consistency. Secondly, since this preparation is highly purified it is free of any contaminating proteins and has high specific activity.[13–15] Therefore, somewhat lower amounts of this preparation are required for ovulation induction, and it can be administered subcutaneously. In several studies recombinant FSH has been shown to yield higher pregnancy rates than urinary gonadotropins.[16, 17]

One potential disadvantage is that the recombinant preparations are devoid of LH. Women who are infertile secondary to hypogonadotropic amenorrhea generally also produce very low levels of LH. These women require exogenous LH to maintain adequate estradiol biosynthesis as well as follicular development for superovulation. HMG preparations containing LH and FSH are used for ovulation induction in these patients. Soon, recombinant LH will be available for use in combination with recombinant FSH.[18]

The role of gonadotropin releasing hormone agonists (GnRH) in superovulation has been less well defined. This hormone is normally produced by the hypothalamus in a pulsatile manner, causing release of LH and FSH from the pituitary gland. GnRH agonists inhibit endogenous gonadotropin synthesis in the pituitary after an initial flare or increase in LH and FSH synthesis. This enables maximum ability to manipulate and control the cycle.[19, 20] Administration of GnRH prevents premature ovulation and luteinization of follicles. This in turn has been shown to increase clinical pregnancy rates per IVF cycle as well as lowering cancellation rates.[21]

GnRH antagonists were recently approved for controlled ovarian hyperstimulation in IVF. In addition to competitively inhibiting the GnRH receptor, this antagonist also binds to the LH receptor, preventing the LH surge. This in turn leads to lower amounts of FSH required for each ovulation cycle. Additionally, it has been reported that there is a lower incidence of ovarian hyperstimulation syndrome (as described in Section I.B) than when GnRH agonists are used. There is still much debate and a learning curve in utilizing GnRH antagonists as a standard protocol because of questions related to the possibility of lower embryo implantation rates and possibly ongoing pregnancy rates.[22–24]

B. Follicle Monitoring

The ovarian response to the exogenous gonadotropins is monitored biochemically with the measurement of estradiol levels. This is an indirect assessment of granulosa cell development. Additionally, transvaginal ultrasound is used to assess follicular diameter. Once an adequate cohort of follicles is deemed mature, human chorionic gonadotropin (hCG) is administered in lieu of LH to stimulate final oocyte maturation and ovulation. Recombinant LH for the final follicular maturation has currently completed phase III trials.[25–27]

One potentially life-threatening condition that may occur as a sequelae of superovulation following hCG administration is ovarian hyperstimulation syndrome (OHSS). In this condition the severe ovarian enlargement secondary to multiple large follicular cysts and extravasation of fluid from the intravascular spaces leads to hypovolemia, ascites, and in severe cases hemoconcentration with attendant risks of thromboemboli formation, disseminated intravascular coagulation, and acute respiratory distress syndrome.[28] Treatment is mainly conservative with intravenous hydration and administration of colloids to maintain intravascular volume. Paracentesis with removal of the exudative ascitic fluid is done for patient comfort only and is not therapeutic. Severe cases may require intensive care unit monitoring. It appears that OHSS may be avoided through the use of recombinant LH for induction of ovulation. LH has a shorter half-life than hCG and may have comparable oocyte retrieval rates and subsequent pregnancy rates.[27] Therefore, hCG may not be used for final follicular maturation and ovulatory triggering in the future.

C. Follicle Retrieval

Thirty-six hours following induction of ovulation, oocytes are retrieved most commonly through needle aspiration with transvaginal ultrasound guidance. Generally, prior to the procedure, the patient receives intravenously general anesthesia or sedation, or a regional anesthetic. A needle attached to the transvaginal ultrasound probe is then introduced and passed transvaginally into each follicle. The contents are aspirated during visualization with the ultrasound probe (Fig. 23.1).

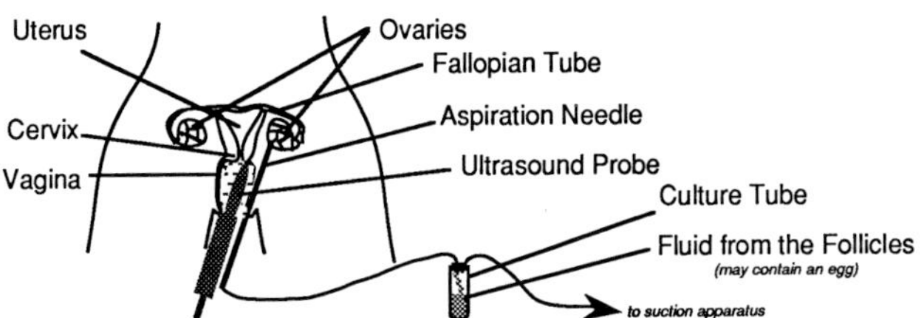

FIGURE 23.1 Schematic diagram of follicular aspiration in transvaginal, ultrasound-guided IVF oocyte retrieval.

D. Fertilization

Fertilization occurs in the laboratory by inseminating oocytes with spermatozoa in a small volume of culture media approximately four to six hours following embryo retrieval. Embryos are then cultured for two or three days to generate a cleavage stage embryo or five days (some programs allow them to divide for up to six days) to generate a blastocyst, the embryonic stage at which implantation occurs (Fig. 23.2). One major advantage of blastocyst transfer is that potentially fewer embryos may need to be transferred for each successful pregnancy. Several studies have shown that implantation rates are higher for the more advanced embryos with excellent pregnancy rates.[29–32] Therefore generally only 2 blastocysts are transferred, compared to up to 4 day 2 or 3 embryos. The blastocyst transfer, therefore, decreases the risk of triplet or quadruplet pregnancy (high-order multiple gestations). Twinning rates are high with both day 5 and cleavage stage transfers, with programs across the country reporting that 20–50% of IVF pregnancies result in twinning. The major drawback in transferring day 5 embryos as demonstrated in the previously mentioned studies, is that only 40–60% of embryos may survive in culture for 5 days. Therefore, a couple may have apparently good quality embryos on day 2 or 3 which fail to continue dividing (for unknown reasons) after day 3, possibly leaving no viable embryos for transfer back into the uterus. Currently rigorous protocols are employed to determine which embryos will be allowed to attempt to develop in culture to the blastocyst stage. Other reported risks in small trials of blastocyst transfers have been increased risk of monozygote twinning of 5%. In addition, more males may result. With day 5 transfer fewer embryos are available for cryopreservation due to the fact that some embryos do not continue to divide to day 5.[33, 34]

E. Male Infertility and Intracytoplasmic Sperm Injection

Since the advent of assisted reproductive technology, male infertility that can be attributed by moderate to severe oligospermia, asthenospermia (low sperm motility), and teratospermia (abnormal sperm morphology) can be circumvented by fertilization of retrieved oocytes through intracytoplasmic sperm injection (ICSI) from sperm collected from an ejaculated sample, epididymis, or testis.[35–37] The ICSI technique involves direct injection of sperm into the cytoplasm of the mature haploid human oocyte through the zona pellucida, delivering the male genome directly into the oocyte. Fertilization rates of approximately 60% or more are achieved through this technique.[38–40]

Concerns about safety have been raised because the sperm that fertilized the oocyte is selected by the operator and not by the natural selection process in the reproductive tract. No differences in congenital abnormalities have been found and performance testing by two years of age shows no differences between conventional IVF groups, ICSI, and natural cycles.[41, 42] However, it has been consistently shown that ICSI conceived children do have slightly higher rates of chromosomal abnormalities, fairly equally distributed between autosomal and sex chromosomes at an approximate rate of 2.5–3.5%.[43–46] In part this is due to the fact that men with severe oligospermia and azospermia have a higher frequency of chromosomal abnormalities in both somatic cells and spermatozoa. It has been recommended that the severely oligospermic male should undergo karyotyping and Y chromosome microdeletion analysis prior to ICSI and that couples should be appropriately counseled of the risks of transmission.[47]

F. Embryo Transfer

The final step in IVF is to place the embryos back into the uterus through the cervical os. The number of embryos that are transferred are based on a clinic-specific paradigm based on age, stage of embryo (cleavage stage versues blastocyst), and quality of embryos.[48] Factors known to adversely effect on transfer are traumatic transfer causing uterine contractions, blood or mucus on catheter tip, and bacterial contamination. To optimize the endometrial cavity for implantation, progesterone is given at the time of embryo transfer and continued through at least part of the first trimester. Implantation rates are lower in women as age increases due to increasing rates of aneuploidy in their oocytes.[49, 50]

A technique that may increase implantation rates is called assisted hatching. Failure of the cells of the embryo to hatch through the zona pellucida may be secondary to intrinsic abnormalities in the blastocyst, the zona pellucida, or the endometrium. Assisted hatching is generally performed on cleavage stage embryos on day 3 after retrieval, by creating a small gap in the zona either through chemical or mechanical means. Randomized, controlled trials indicate that clinical pregnancy rates are improved in women over 38 who have failed several IVF cycles.[51, 52] Monozygote twinning has been reported to occur at increased rates in assisted hatching.[53]

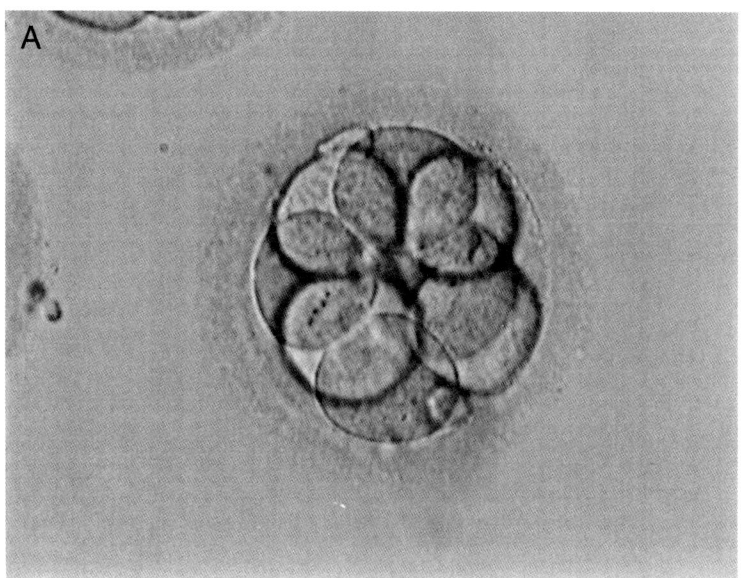

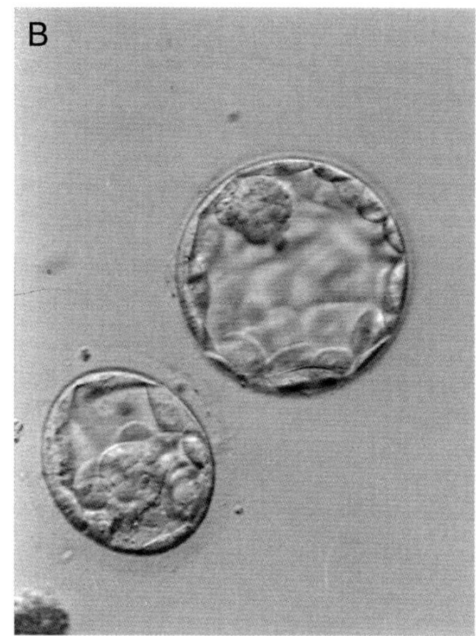

FIGURE 23.2 (A) Human 8-cell embryo on day 3 after oocyte retrieval. The zona pellucida is the halo surrounding the outer membrane of the embryo. (B) Human blastocysts day 5 after oocyte retrieval. The larger expanded blastocyst on the right has an easily identified inner cell mass at 11 o'clock. The smaller blastocyst on the left is in an earlier stage of development.

G. Chemotherapy and Future Fertility

It is well known that chemotherapy has a deleterious effect on ovarian function. Currently, there are several paradigms to preserve future fertility. It has been shown that women who have undergone chemotherapy treatment do not respond as well to ovulation induction agents.[54] In preliminary studies GnRH analogs administered during chemotherapy in adolescent patients has shown promise in preserving oocyte function and fertility.[55] The most proven protocols involve ovulation induction, retrieval, and fertilization of oocytes prior to chemotherapy treatment and radiation for cancer. These embryos are then cryopreserved for future use when cancer treatment is complete.[54] Although pregnancies have been achieved with cryopreserved oocytes, techniques are not reproducible, and very few pregnancies have occurred since the early 1980s.[56, 57] Currently the techniques to cryopreserve oocytes are being perfected and the hope for the future is ovarian tissue or oocyte banking in an anologous manner to sperm banking.[58]

II. STEM CELLS AND IVF

Since the advent of assisted reproductive technology, the standard use of IVF to assist infertile couples to conceive has enabled us to create human embryos *in vitro* fairly easily. The role of these embryos in creating stem cells has received much attention in both the popular and scientific press.

The potential utility of these pluripotent cells to treat and potentially cure a wide array of diseases through cell transplantation therapies is not a new theory. As early as 1928, unsuccessful attempts were made to cure type I diabetes mellitus through transplantation of fetal pancreatic tissue.[59] More recently, the development of stem cells from a variety of sources has led to the rapid progression in stem cell research for therapeutic applications. This research has also lead to many political, legal, and ethical debates regarding potential sources and ultimate applications of these cells and their role in assisted reproductive technologies.

A. Definition of Stem Cells

Stem cells are cells with the capacity for prolonged or unlimited capacity for self-renewal in an undifferentiated state, which have the capacity to develop into at least one type of highly differentiated descendent. Stem cells can be isolated from many adult tissue types.[60] Stem cell isolation has been most successful in cells from tissues undergoing rapid cell turnover, senescence, and replacement such as epithelia, the hematopoietic system, and germ cells as well as in some tissues that have a more limited cellular regeneration, e.g., hepatocytes.[60]

Adult stem cells are usually considered multipotent, meaning that they may develop into many different, but not all cell types. Usually adult stem cells are able to develop into cells of tissues embryologically related (i.e., transdetermination or transdifferentiation).[60]

Embryonically derived stem cells are pluripotent. These cells can self-renew indefinitely while in an undifferentiated state and have the developmental potential to differentiate into any cell type given the correct growth conditions. It is important to note that these cells are not totipotent, i.e., they have not been shown to differentiate into extra-embryonic tissues such as placenta nor can they develop into a complete embryo by themselves. The three main sources of human pluripotent stem cells are preimplantation human embryos (ES cells), embryonal (primordial) germ cells (EG), and human germ cell tumors or teratocarcinomas (EC cells).[60, 61]

Primordial EG have been developed from gonadal ridges of 5–9 week embryos obtained as a result of a therapeutic abortion, as first established in mice in the 1980s.[62, 63] Embryonic stem cells, on the other hand, are derived from blastocyst-stage embryos. In unmanipulated embryos, the inner cell mass develops into the ectoderm which in term ultimately differentiates into the three germ cell layers during gastrulation. When these inner cell mass cells are removed from their native environment they can survive in culture and proliferate indefinitely while maintaining a stable karyotype. As discussed previously, blastocyst-stage embryos are obtained through maturation of cleavage-stage embryos produced by IVF five to six days following oocyte retrieval.[61, 64, 65]

The potential for EG and ES cells to be pluripotent has been confirmed in both *in vitro* and *in vivo* systems. Cell lines have been shown to retain the ability to differentiate into all three germ cell layers. Studies in mice have found that if mouse blastocysts are injected with either EG or ES cells, and then transferred back to the mouse uterus, the resulting offspring are chimeras with descendents of the injected stem cells represented in all cell types including the germ cell lines.[60]

EC cell lines are derived from teratocarcinomas.[66, 67] Although these cells have been successfully used in animal transplantation models of stroke and are currently undergoing phase I trials, there are underlying concerns about the use of these cells because of the possibility of transmitting defective genetic material.[68] These cells do not have the pluripotent potential or plasticity demonstrated by the EG and ES cell lines. For example, when these cells are injected into blastocysts, the germ line cells do not have EC cells, in contrast to what occurs with the injection of EG and ES cells.[60]

B. Potential Applications

It has become increasingly clear that embryonic stem cells have distinct advantages over adult-derived stem cells. ES and EG cells are isolated more easily in single cell type populations, multiply more readily in the laboratory, and are more proficient in producing very specialized cell types including neurons and pancreatic islet cells. ES and EG cells play a vital role in understanding how cells differentiate, and can provide much information on secondary pathways and regulators of cell differentiation.[59, 61, 69]

The most publicized use of stem cells is to replace cells damaged, degenerating, or destroyed by diseases, such as pancreatic islet cells in type 1 diabetes mellitus or glial cells in multiple sclerosis or hematopoietic cells from the bone marrow destroyed by chemotherapy or radiation. *In vitro* studies have repeatedly shown that cells grown under the control of specific growth factors can differentiate into cardiomyocytes, epithelial cells, and neurons. Hematopoietic precursors have been derived through co-culture of ES cells with irradiated bone marrow stromal cells with no additional growth media. These precursors have the potential to develop into many different lineages including erythroid, macrophage, and granulocyte cell populations. The ultimate use of specialized cells derived from stem cell lines will be determined by the technical ability to transplant these differentiated cells into humans with specific diseases. Work in animal models has shown that transplantation of pluripotent stem cells can successfully treat a variety of disorders including Duchenne muscular dystrophy, spinal cord injuries, and heart failure and are currently being applied to clinical models.[61, 70, 71]

Progeny cells appear to behave as specific cell types expressing specific proteins and displaying specific phenotypes. Unfortunately, endodermal cells have been more difficult to develop *in vitro*. There has been a long quest to successfully develop pancreatic islet cells. It has been difficult to define the signaling that induces pancreatic cell differentiation and activation of gene transcription. Most recently, Mckay *et al.* have described a method of inducing mouse ES cells into pancreas-like cells that have the ability to produce insulin in response to glucose, although in lower concentrations than natural pancreatic tissue.[72–74]

One example of the current clinical state-of-the-art is typified by a study in which transplantation of glial cell precursors derived from mouse ES cells was performed. These cells were transplanted into dorsal columns of the spinal cord of myelin-deficient mice. Two weeks posttransplantation, numerous myelin sheaths were found in several of the mice. The myelin precursors were not restricted to the implantation site and were found elsewhere. These cells differentiated into oligodendrocytes and astrocytes. The oligodendrocytes found within the myelin sheaths were normal in ultrastructural appearance, which is in contrast to the abnormal host oligodendrocytes.[75–78] However, long-term survival and functional studies have yet to be done.

C. Stem Cells and Organ Development

Development of specific organs through the use of stem cells has been an active area of research. This could potentially obliterate the need for organ donation. Currently many models used in developing organs utilize polymer scaffolds. Functional bladders have been formed by co-culturing uroepithelial cells and smooth muscle cells on a polymer shaped as a bladder. This synthetic structure was initially implanted into dogs and was functional for almost a year,[79] and is currently in use for bladder reconstruction in humans as well. It can be hypothesized that through the correct combination of extracellular matrix and stem cells induced to form specific different cell types, one could develop specific tissues and organs. This has been attempted for many tissues, including blood vessels, heart muscle, pancreas, cartilage, and liver to name a few, and has been most successful in clinical trials in bone, skin, and cornea.[80] The future of stem cells in tissue engineering will likely also not only include reconstruction of specific organs, but also gene targeting and replacement of aberrant cells in a specific organ. One example would be in islets cells of the pancreas leading to the reversal of diabetes.[81] This era of *de novo* organogenesis and gene transfer through the use of stem cells will likely play an important role in organ replacement in the next decade.

D. Stem Cells and Study of Gene Function and Therapy

An important use for ES cells is in the study of gene function. Currently the best method to study specific gene functions involves experimentation with transgenic mice who are bred with and without specific genes. Although transgenic mice models provide useful information about genes through specific overexpression or deletion, experiments are laborious and require long time commitments and high costs because of the need to follow the life span of animals. In addition, results are often inconclusive even after long studies. ES cells may ultimately provide an easier model reducing unnecessary animal testing.[61, 70, 82]

Gene therapy is another potential area where stem cells could be useful. For example, in patients with a single known gene defect such as those with the thalassemias. Currently, gene replacement therapy has been limited by both difficulties delivering the genes to the targeted tissue as well as the integration of the gene into the appropriate location in the patient's genome, which must occur in order for controlled expression of the gene. Through examining which ES cells most efficiently express a specific gene, optimal integration sites could be found. These optimized cells would then be induced to differentiate and then introduced into the host tissue. The new gene product would then be appropriately expressed, correcting the genetic disease permanently.[61, 69, 81]

E. Complications of Stem Cell Technology

No new technology is without complications. Most problems arise because pure cell populations are not obtained prior to transplantation, and once these cells are successfully transplanted, they do not behave as a native cell. This has been a stumbling block in human stem cell research.

Human pluripotent cell lines retain a broad pattern of multilineage gene expression even in the presence of a specific growth factor or hormone. Several different cell populations arise including undifferentiated cells, partially differentiated cells, and as several different populations of well-differentiated cells. It has been repeatedly shown in mouse models that when undifferentiated or partially differentiated cells are transplanted back into mice, tumors called teratomas can form in the recipient.[61, 82] Future research will have to focus on developing effective protocols for purification of lineage-specific ES cells.

Another potential concern related to transplanting ES cells is the risk of rejection. The immunogenicity of ES cells appears to correlate with the expression of specific major histocompatibility complexes that develop as cells differentiate. In order to circumvent this and achieve a homogenous population of cells, gene-targeting experiments have begun. These involve the introduction of a tissue-specific promoter creating a genetically manipulated cell expressing a foreign, but specific protein. Since ES cells are grown and manipulated in culture, they could be genetically manipulated to suppress the expression of a particular MHC antigen, rendering it immunologically inert. Alternatively, ES cells could be engineered to express MHC antigens identical to host cells.[61]

F. Legal and Ethical Issues Concerning Stem Cells

There has been much legal and political debate over stem cell research because EG cells are obtained from aborted tissue and ES cells can be harvested from embryos left over from IVF or even specifically engineered for these purposes. President Bush put in place a moratorium on creating new stem cell lines and has limited research to existing stem cell lines.

Opponents of this policy argue that there are very few stem cell lines available in the U.S. for public research. Most stem cell lines are owned and distributed by large biotech firms that charge individual scientists exorbitant fees for the use of these lines for research. On a more basic level, stem cells cannot undergo indefinite proliferation. After many passages cells loose their pluripotency. This raises the concern that in a few years there will be no pluripotent stem cell lines for research.

Ethical questions also arise regarding stem cell research. The most widely debated is what should be done with the discarded IVF-created embryos. Can stem cells be generated from these embryos? Who should decide their fate—individual couples or the government through legislation? Once a couple consents to allow their discarded embryos be used for research, could they then direct or select what types of research in which the embryos were used?

III. CLONING AND IVF

Since the cloning of Dolly the sheep in 1997, the popular press has focused the cloning debate on the ethical concerns surrounding cloning a deceased individual.[83] This is clearly not the only or most important application of cloning. In the U.S., as well as most European countries, cloning of embryos to create a human life has been banned.

A. What Is Cloning?

Cloning is the derivation of genetically identical individuals or entities from a single individual. In mammals this can theoretically be achieved in several ways. One is by transferring genetic material from a somatic cell into an enucleated oocyte. Alternatively, this can be achieved through embryo splitting. This latter technique involves splitting an eight-cell embryo into four two-cell daughter cells with identical genetic information. Once these embryos are generated, they can either be transferred to a receptive uterus or maintained *in vitro* to generate stem cells.

B. Complications Observed in Cloned Mammals

The success of cloning is highly species dependent. Cloning has been successfully done for generations in plants by simply clipping a branch of a plant and growing it in water. Cloning in mammals has been more difficult and problematic. First of all, cloning is a very inefficient process resulting in spontaneous abortions secondary to poor implantation or possibly chromosomal abnormalities. Only about 1–2% of cloned embryos have led to delivery in sheep, cows, and mice. In particular, many of the cattle had severe placental malformations. Additionally, it has been reported that many of the offspring that do survive have a higher rate of developmental or congenital abnormalities. It has been surmised that cloned mammals lack telomerases to correct DNA material and have shorter telomeres because genetic material is obtained from older somatic cells.[84] The animal would therefore have a shorter life span, one similar to that of animal from which the nucleus was derived. This has been confirmed in cloned sheep, like Dolly. This has not been found to occur in several cloned cows as well as in offspring of Dolly, so this issue is still up for debate.[85–87]

Only the nuclear DNA of the somatic cell and not the mitochondrial DNA is transferred. However, certain required genes are only expressed by maternally derived mitochondrial DNA. This raises the question about imprinted genes.[88, 89] Although two copies of the imprinted genes are obtained from maternal and paternal genetic material, only one is specifically required. If the incorrect gene is expressed, abnormalities may arise (i.e., Prader-Willi syndrome). It remains to be seen how imprinted genes are affected by cloning since both copies are obtained from the same individual.[82]

C. Potential Applications of Cloning

There are many potential uses for cloning that do not involve reproductive cloning. One is embryonic cloning that involves creation of an embryo by conventional IVF techniques followed by enucleation of the blastomeres. These nuclei are then transferred into several enucleated oocytes, generating identical embryos for transfer into a receptive uterus leading to pregnancy and identical offspring. This would be most useful in generating genetically identical animals for research protocols. This could also be used for women with poor responses to superovulation in IVF creating more embryos and increasing the likelihood of pregnancy.

Another potential use of cloning is to create stem cells. Therapeutic cloning involves somatic cell-nuclear transfer as discussed above, but the created embryo is never transferred to a uterus, creating stem cells that are maintained in culture. Stem cells can then be generated which are antigenically identical to the donor of the somatic cell. Such cells could be manipulated and ultimately used for organ transplantation. This theoretically raises the possibility that a stem cell line could be created for every individual. Although different from cloning an embryo for the purpose of creating human life, it still raises many ethical issues regarding the use and creation of human embryos and their subsequent destruction.[90]

Lastly, another application of this technique is in couples with known genetic abnormalities, or in older women whose oocytes have a plethora of abnormal chromosomes due to aging. It has been proposed that stem cells could be harvested from blastocyst-staged embryos of the couple derived from IVF. These stem cells could then be theoretically genetically manipulated through homologous recombination as mentioned above, creating a population of stem cells with corrected genes. The nuclei of these stem cells could then be transferred into an enucleated oocyte from that mother, or another source, resulting in a chromosomally normal child.[82] Additionally, this technique can be used in preimplantation genetic diagnosis where couples are known to be carriers of specific diseases.[91, 92] Currently, preimplantation diagnosis involves removal of single cells from day 3 embryos, analysis of the cells, and transfer of only unaffected embryos, but cannot correct abnormal genes identified. However, stem cell technology again raises many ethical and legal barriers because it involves initially creating an embryo, albeit one potentially incompatible with life or with high morbidity and mortality, to create another human life with corrected genetic information.

D. Conclusions

This is an exciting time in assisted reproductive technology. Undoubtedly, in the next 25 years there will be many advances we only dream of now. It is likely that IVF pregnancy rates will approach 90% with single embryo transfer due to better embryo screening, genetic manipulation of embryos, and possibly the routine use of cloning to increase embryo numbers. Over the next century it can be anticipated that ovarian tissue and oocyte cryopreservation will become standard techniques. Additionally it can be anticipated that genetic manipulation and generation of stem cells, perhaps using cloning as well, may make it possible to create tissue and organ differentiation *in vitro*, creating an unlimited source for transplantation. Manipulation of genes and stem cell technologies may some day render many of the diseases common today of historical interest only.

References

1. Stepoe, P. C., and Edwards, R. G. (1976). Reimplantation of a human embryo with subsequent tubal pregnancy. *Lancet* 1, 880–882.
2. Stepoe, P. C., and Edwards, R. G. (1978). Birth after the reimplantation of a human embryo. *Lancet* 2, 366.
3. Hsueh, A. J., Adashi, E. Y., Jones, P. B., and Welsh, T. H., Jr. (1984). Hormonal regulation of the differentiation of cultured ovarian granulosa cells. *Endocr. Rev.* 5(1), 76–127.
4. Dorrington, J. H., and Armstrong, D. T. (1979). Effects of FSH on gonadal functions. *Recent Prog. Horm. Res.* 35, 301–342.
5. Zeleznik, A. J., and Hillier, S. G. (1984). The role of gonadotropins in the selection of the preovulatory follicle. *Clin. Obstet. Gynecol.* 27, 927–940.
6. Richards, J. S. (1994). Hormonal control of gene expression in the ovary. *Endocr. Rev.* 15(6), 725–751.
7. Fink, G. (1989). Gonadotropin secretion and its control. *In*: "The Physiology of Reproduction," Vol. 1. (E. Knobil, and J. D. Neill, eds.), pp. 1349–1377. Raven Press, New York.
8. Gemzell, C. A., Dicfaluzy, E., and Tillinger, K. G. (1960). Human pituitary follicle-stimulating hormone I: Clinical effect of a partly purified preparation. *Ciba Found. Colloq. Endocrinol.* 13, 191–200.
9. Goujard, J., Entat, M., Maillard, F., Mugnier, E., Rappaport, R., and Job, J. C. (1988). Evaluation of risks related to human growth hormone (hGH) treatment. Results of an epidemiologic survey conducted in France of patients treated from 1959 to 1985. *Arch. Fr. Pediatr.* 46, 411–416.
10. WHO (1973). Agents stimulating gonadal function in the human. Report of a WHO scientific group. *WHO Tech Rep Ser* 514–929.
11. Shoham, Z., and Insler, V. (1996). Recombinant Technique and gonadotropins production: New era in reproductive medicine. *Fertil. Steril.* 66(2), 187–201.
12. Bergh, C., Howles, C. M., Borg, K., Hamberger, L., Josefsson, B., Nilsson, L., and Wikland, M. (1997). Recombinant human follicle stimulating hormone (r-hFSH; Gonal-F) versus highly purified urinary FSH (Metrodin HP): Results of a randomized comparative study in women undergoing assisted reproductive techniques. *Hum. Reprod.* 12(10), 2133–2139.
13. Porchet, H. C., Le Cotonnec, J. Y., Canali, S., and Zanolo, G. (1993). Pharmaco-kinetics of recombinant human follicle stimulating hormone after intravenous, intramuscular, and subcutaneous administration in monkeys, and comparison with intravenous administration of urinary follicle stimulating hormone. *Drug Metab. Dispos.* 21, 144–150.
14. Keene, J. L., Matzuk, M. M., Otani, T., Fauser, B. C., Galway, A. B., Hsueh, A. J. *et al.* (1989). Expression of biologically active human follitropin in Chinese hamster ovary cells. *J. Biol. Chem.* 264, 4769–4775.
15. Galway, A. B., Hseuh, A. J., Keene, J. L., Yamoto, M., Fauser, B. C., and Boime, I. (1990). In vitro and in vivo bioactivity of recombinant human follicle-stimulating hormone and partially deglycosy-lated variants secreted by transfected eukaryotic cell lines. *Endocrinology* 127, 93–100.
16. Daya, S., Gunby, J., Hughes, E. G., Collins, J. A., and Sagle, M. A. (1995). Follicle-stimulating hormone versus human gonadotropin for in vitro fertilization cycles: A meta-analysis. *Fertil. Steril.* 64, 747–752.
17. Out, H. J., Driessen, S. G., Mannaerts, B. M., and Coelingh-Bennink, H. J. (1997). Recombinant follicle-stimulating hormone yields higher pregnancy rates in in vitro fertilization than urinary gonadotropins. *Fertil. Steril.* 68, 138–142.
18. Hull, M., Corrigan, E., Piazzi, A., and Loumaye, E. (1994). Recombinant human luteinizing hormone: An effective new gonadotropin preparation. *Lancet* 344, 334–335.
19. Dodson, W. C. (1990). Gonadotropin releasing analogues as adjuctive therapy in ovulation induction. *Semin. Reprod. Endocrinol.* 8, 198.
20. Dodson, W. C., Hughs, C. L., Whitesides, D. B., and Haney, A. F. (1987). The effect of leuprolide acetate on ovulation induction with human menopausal gonadotropins in polycystic ovarian syndrome. *J. Clin. Endocrinol. Metab.* 65, 95.
21. Hughs, E. G., Fedorkow, D. M., Daya, S., Sagle, M. A., Van de Koppel, P., and Collins, J. A. (1994). The routine use of gonadotropin-releasing hormone agonists prior to in vitro fertilization and gamete intrafallopian trnsfer: A meta-analysis of randomized controlled trials. *Fertil. Steril.* 61, 1068–1076.
22. Blumenfeld, Z. (2001). Gonadotropin-releasing hormone antagonists instead of agonists: A change for the better? *Fertil. Steril.* 78, 443–444.
23. Hernandez, E. (2000). Embryo Implantation: The Rubicon for GnRH antagonists. *Hum. Reprod.* 15, 1211–1216.
24. Kol, S. GnRH antagonists in ART: Lower embryo implantation? (2000). *Hum. Reprod.* 15, 1881–1882.
25. Driscoll, G. L., Tyler, J. P., Hangan, J. T., Fisher, P. R., Birdsall, M. A., and Knight, D. C. (2000). A prospective, randomized, controlled, double-blind, double-dummy comparison of recombinant and urinary HCG for inducing oocyte maturation and follicular luteinization in ovarian stimulation. *Hum. Reprod.* 15(6), 1305–1310.
26. Andersen, C. Y., Ziebe, S., Guoliang, X., and Byskov, A. G. (1999). Requirements for human chorionic gonadotropin and recombinant human luteinizing hormone for follicular development and maturation. *J. Assist. Reprod. Genet.* 16(8), 425–430.
27. The European Recombinant LH Study Group, Human recombinant luteinizing hormone is as effective as, but safer than, urinary human chorionic gonadotropin in inducing final follicular maturation and ovulation in in vitro fertilization procedures: Results of a multicenter double-blind study. (2001). *J. Clin. Endocrinol. Metab.* 86(6), 2607–2618.
28. Whelan, J. G., and Vlabos, N. F. (2000). The ovarian hyperstimulation syndrome. *Fertil. Steril.* 73(5), 883–896.
29. Gardner, D. K., Vella, P., Lane, M., Wagley, L., Schlenker, T., and Schoolcraft, W. B. (1998). Culture and transfer of human blastocysts increase implantation rates and reduces the need for multiple embryo transfers. *Fertil. Steril.* 69, 84–88.
30. Gardner, D. K., Schoolcraftm, W. B., Wagley, L., Schlenker, T., Stevens, J., and Hesla, J. (1998). A prospective randomized trial of blastocyst culture and transfer in in vitro fertilization. *Hum. Reprod.* 13, 3434–3440.

31. Da Motta, E. L. A., Alegretti, J. R., Baracat, E. C., Olive, D., and Serafini, P. C. (1998). High implantation and pregnancy rates with transfer of human blastocysts developed in preimplantation stage one and blastocyst media. *Fertil. Steril.* 70, 659–663.
32. Milki, A. A., Hinckley, M. D., Fisch, J. D., Dasig, D., and Behr, B. (2000). Comparison of blastocyst transfer with day 3 embryo transfer in similar patient populations. *Fertil. Steril.* 73(1), 126–129.
33. Tsirigotis, M. (1998). Blastocyst stage transfer: Pitfalls and benefits. *Hum. Reprod.* 13, 3285–3289.
34. Behr, B., Fisch, J. D., Racowsky, C., Miller, K., Pool, T. B., and Milki, A. A. (2000). Blastocyst-ET and monozygotic twinning. *J. Assist. Reprod. Genet.* 17(6), 349–351.
35. Girardi, S. K., and Schlegel, P. N. (1996). Microsurgical epididymal sperm aspiration: Review of techniques, preoperative considerations, and results. *J. Androl.* 17(1), 5–9.
36. Schlegel, P. N., Palermo, G. D., Goldstein, M., Menendez, S., Zaninovic, N., Veeck, L. L., and Rosenwaks, Z. (1997). Testicular sperm extraction with intracytoplasmic sperm injection for nonobstructive azoospermia. *Urology* 49(3), 435–440.
37. Janzen, N., Goldstein, M., Schlegel, P. N., Palermo, G. D., and Rosenwaks, Z. (2000). Use of electively cryopreserved microsurgically aspirated epididymal sperm with IVF and intracytoplasmic sperm injection for obstructive azoospermia. *Fertil. Steril.* 74(4), 696–701.
38. Schlegel, P. N., and Girardi, S. K. (1997). In vitro fertilization for male factor infertility. *J. Clin. Endocrinol. Metab.* 82(3), 709–716.
39. Palermo, G. D., Cohen, J., Alikani, M., Adler, A., and Rosenwaks, Z. Intracytoplasmic sperm injection: A novel treatment for all forms of male factor infertility. *Fertil. Steril.* 63(6), 1231–1240.
40. Tarlatzis, B. C., and Bili, H. (2000). Intracytoplasmic sperm injection. Survey of world results. *Ann. N. Y. Acad. Sci.* 900, 336–344.
41. Bonduelle, M., Joris, H., Hofmans, K., Liebaers, I., and Van Steirteghem, A. (1998). Mental development of 201 ICSI children at 2 years of age. *Lancet* 351(9115), 1553.
42. Bonduelle, M., Camus, M., De Vos, A., Staessen, C., Tournaye, H., Van Assche, E., Verheyen, G., Devroey, P., Liebaers, I., Van Steirteghem, A. (1999). Seven years of intracytoplasmic sperm injection and follow-up of 1987 subsequent children. *Hum. Reprod.* 14 Suppl. 1, 243–264.
43. Aboulghar, H., Aboulghar, M., Mansour, R., Serour, G., Amin, Y., and Al-Inany, H. (2001). A prospective controlled study of karyotyping for 430 consecutive babies conceived through intracytoplasmic sperm injection. *Fertil. Steril.* 76(2), 249–253.
44. Meschede, D., Lemcke, B., Exeler, J. R., De Geyter, C., Behre, H. M., Nieschlag, E., and Horst, J. (1998). Chromosome abnormalities in 447 couples undergoing intracytoplasmic sperm injection—prevalence, types, sex distribution and reproductive relevance. *Hum. Reprod.* 13(3), 576–582.
45. Peschka, B., Leygraaf, J., Van der Ven, K., Montag, M., Schartmann, B., Schubert, R., van der Ven, H., and Schwanitz, G. (1999). Type and frequency of chromosome aberrations in 781 couples undergoing intracytoplasmic sperm injection. *Hum. Reprod.* 14(9), 2257–2263.
46. Rubio, C., Gil-Salom, M., Simon, C., Vidal, F., Rodrigo, L., Minguez, Y., Remohi, J., and Pellicer A. (2001). Incidence of sperm chromosomal abnormalities in a risk population: Relationship with sperm quality and ICSI outcome. *Hum. Reprod.* 16(10), 2084–2092.
47. Johnson, M. D., (1998). Genetic risks of intracytoplasmic sperm injection in the treatment of male infertility: Recommendations for genetic counseling and screening. *Fertil. Steril.* 70(3), 397–411.
48. Racowsky, C., Jackson, K. V., Cekeniak, N. A., Fox, J. H., Hornstein, M. D., and Ginsburg, E. S. (2000). The number of eight cell embryos is a key determinant for selecting day 3 or day 5 transfer. *Fertil. Steril.* 73, 558–564.
49. Balen, A. H., MacDougall, J., and Tan, S. L. (1993). The influence of the number of embryos transferred in 1060 in-vitro fertilization pregnancies on miscarriage rates and pregnancy outcome. *Hum. Reprod.* 8(8), 1324–1328.
50. Schoolcraft, W. B., Surrey, E. S., and Gardner, D. K. (2001). Embryo transfer: Techniques and variables affecting success. *Fertil. Steril.* 76(5), 863–870.
51. Cohen, J., Alikani, M., Trowbridge, J., and Rosenwaks, Z. (1992). Implantation enhancement by selective assisted hatching using zona drilling of human embryos with poor prognosis. *Hum. Reprod.* 7(5), 685–691.
52. Magli, M. C., Gianaroli, L., Ferraretti, A. P., Fortini, D., Aicardi, G., and Montanaro, N. (1998). Rescue of implantation potential in embryos with poor prognosis by assisted zona hatching. *Hum. Reprod.* 13(5), 1331–1335.
53. Hershlag, A., Paine, T., Cooper, G. W., Scholl, G. M., Rawlinson, K., and Kvapil, G. (1999). Monozygotic twinning associated with mechanical assisted hatching. *Fertil. Steril.* 71(1), 144–146.
54. Ginsburg, E. S., Yanushpolsky, E. H., and Jackson, K. V. (2001). In vitro fertilization for cancer patients and survivors. *Fertil. Steril.* 75(4), 705–710.
55. Pereyra Pacheco, B., Mendez Ribas, J. M., Milone, G., Fernandez, I., Kvicala, R., Mila, T., Di Noto, A., Contreras Ortiz, O., and Pavlovsky, S. (2001). Use of GnRH analogs for functional protection of the ovary and preservation of fertility during cancer treatment in adolescents: A preliminary report. *Gynecol. Oncol.* 81(3), 391–397.
56. Porcu, E., Fabbri, R., Seracchioli, R., Ciotti, P. M., Magrini, O., and Flamigni, C. (1997). Birth of a healthy female after intracytoplasmic sperm injection of cryopreserved human oocytes. *Fertil. Steril.* 68(4), 724–726.
57. Yoon, T. K., Chung, H. M., Lim, J. M., Han, S. Y., Ko, J. J., and Cha, K. Y. (2000). Pregnancy and delivery of healthy infants developed from vitrified oocytes in a stimulated in vitro fertilization-embryo transfer program. *Fertil. Steril.* 74(1), 180–181.
58. Kim, S. S., Battaglia, D. E., and Soules, M. R. (2001). The future of human ovarian cryopreservation and transplantation: Fertility and beyond. *Fertil. Steril.* 75(6), 1049–1056.
59. Edwards, B. E., Gearhart, J. D., and Wallach, E. E. (2000). The human pluripotent stem cell: Impact on medicine and society. *Fertil. Steril.* 74(1), 1–7.
60. Vogel, G. (2001). Stem Cell Policy: Can Adult Stem Cells Suffice? *Science* 292(5523), 1820–1822.
61. Odorico, J. S., Kaufman, D. S., and Thomson, J. A. (2001). Multilineage differentiation from human embryonic stem cell lines. *Stem Cells* 19(3), 193–204.
62. Shamblott, M. J., Axelman, J., Wang, S., Bugg, E. M., Littlefield, J. W., Donovan, P. J., Blumenthal, P. D., Huggins, G. R., and Gearhart, J. D. (1998). Derivation of pluripotent stem cells from cultured human primordial germ cells. *Proc. Natl. Acad. Sci. USA* 95(23), 13726–13731.
63. Matsui, Y., Zsebo, K., and Hogan, B. L. (1992). Derivation of pluripotential embryonic stem cells from murine primordial germ cells in culture. *Cell* 70(5), 841–847.
64. Thomson, J. A., Itskovitz-Eldor, J., Shapiro, S. S., Waknitz, M. A., Swiergiel, J. J., Marshall, V. S., and Jones, J. M. (1998). Embryonic stem cell lines derived from human blastocysts. *Science* 282(5391), 1145–1147.
65. Thomson, J. A., Kalishman, J., Golos, T. G., Durning, M., Harris, C. P., Becker, R. A., and Hearn, J. P. (1995). Isolation of a primate embryonic stem cell line. *Proc. Natl. Acad. Sci. USA* 92(17), 7844–7848.
66. Illmensee, K., and Mintz, B. (1976). Totipotency and normal differentiation of single teratocarcinoma cells cloned by injection into blastocysts. *Proc. Natl. Acad. Sci. USA* 73(2), 549–553.
67. Mintz, B., and Illmensee, K. (1975). Normal genetically mosaic mice produced from malignant teratocarcinoma cells. *Proc. Natl. Acad. Sci. USA* 72(9), 3585–3589.
68. Borlongan, C. V., Tajima, Y., Trojanowski, J. Q., Lee, V. M., and Sanberg, P. R. (1998). Transplantation of cryopreserved human embryonal carcinoma-derived neurons (NT2N cells) promotes functional recovery in ischemic rats. *Exp. Neurol.* 149(2), 310–321.

69. Amit, M., Carpenter, M. K,, Inokuma, M. S., Chiu, C. P., Harris, C. P., Waknitz, M. A., Itskovitz-Eldor, J., and Thomson, J. A. (2000). Clonally derived human embryonic stem cell lines maintain pluripotency and proliferative potential for prolonged periods of culture. *Dev. Biol.* 227(2), 271–278.
70. Van der Kooy, D., and Weiss, S. (2000). Why stem cells? *Science* 287(5457), 1439–1442.
71. Watt, F. M., and Hogan, B. L. M. (2000). Out of Eden: Stem cells and their niches. *Science* 287(5457), 1427–1439.
72. Assady, S., Maor, G., Amit, M., Itskovitz-Eldor, J., Skorecki, K. L., and Tzukerman, M. (2001). Insulin production by human embryonic stem cells. *Diabetes* 50(8), 1691–1697.
73. Eshavaria, M., and Pang, K. (2000). Manipulation of pancreatic stem cells for cell replacement therapy. *Diabetes Technol. Ther.* 2(3), 453–460.
74. Lumelsky, N., Blondel, O., Laeng, P., Velasco, I., Ravin, R., and McKay, R. (2001). Differentiation of embryonic stem cells to insulin-secreting structures similar to pancreatic islets. *Science* 292(5520), 1389–1394.
75. Herrera, J., Yang, H., Zhang, S. C., Proschel, C., Tresco, P., Duncan, I. D., Luskin, M., and Mayer-Proschel, M. (2001). Embryonic-derived glial-restricted precursor cells (GRP cells) can differentiate into astrocytes and oligodendrocytes in vivo. *Exp. Neurol.* 171(1), 11–21.
76. Franceschini, I. A., Feigenbaum-Lacombe, V., Casanova, P., Lopez-Lastra, M., Darlix, J. L., and Dalcq, M. D. (2001). Efficient gene transfer in mouse neural precursors with a bicistronic retroviral vector. *J. Neurosci. Res.* 65(3), 208–219.
77. Liu, S., Qu, Y., Stewart, T. J., Howard, M. J., Chakrabortty, S., Holekamp, T. F., and McDonald, J. W. (2000). Embryonic stem cells differentiate into oligodendrocytes and myelinate in culture and after spinal cord transplantation. *Proc. Natl. Acad. Sci. USA* 97(11), 6126–6131.
78. Brustle, O., Jones, K. N., Learish, R. D., Karram, K., Choudhary, K., Wiestler, O. D., Duncan, I. D., and McKay, R. D. (1999). Embryonic stem cell-derived glial precursors: A source of myelinating transplants. *Science* 285(5428), 754–756.
79. Oberpenning, F., Meng, J., Yoo, J. J., and Atala, A. (1999). De novo reconstitution of a functional mammalian urinary bladder by tissue engineering. *Nat. Biotechnol.* 17(2), 149–155.
80. Bianco, P., and Robey, P. G. (2001). Stem cells in tissue engineering. *Nature* 414(6859), 118–121.
81. Ramiya, V. K., Maraist, M., Arfors, K. E., Schatz, D. A., Peck, A. B., and Cornelius, J. G. (2000). Reversal of insulin-dependent diabetes using islets generated in vitro from pancreatic stem cells. *Nat. Med.* 6(3), 278–282.
82. Solter, D. (1999). Cloning and embryonic stem cells: A new era in human biology and medicine. *Croat. Med. J.* 40(3), 309–318.
83. Wilmut, I., Schnieke, A. E., McWhir, J., Kind, A. J., and Campbell, K. H. (1997). Viable offspring derived from fetal and adult mammalian cells. *Nature* 385(6619), 810–813.
84. Signer, E. N., Dubrova, Y. E., Jeffreys, A. J., Wilde, C., Finch, L. M., Wells, M., and Peaker, M. (1998). DNA fingerprinting Dolly. *Nature* 394(6691), 329–330.
85. Shiels, P. G., Kind, A. J., Campbell, K. H., Waddington, D., Wilmut, I., Colman, A., and Schnieke, A. E. (1999). Analysis of telomere lengths in cloned sheep. *Nature* 399(6734), 316–317.
86. Tian, X. C., Xu, J., and Yang, X. (2000). Normal telomere lengths found in cloned cattle. *Nat. Genet.* 26(3), 272–273.
87. Vogel, G. (2000). In contrast to Dolly, cloning resets telomere clock in cattle. *Science* 288(5466), 586–587.
88. Steinborn, R., Schinogl, P., Zakhartchenko, V., Achmann, R., Schernthaner, W., Stojkovic, M., Wolf, E., Muller, M., and Brem, G. (2000). Mitochondrial DNA heteroplasmy in cloned cattle produced by fetal and adult cell cloning. *Nat. Genet.* 25(3), 255–257.
89. Evans, M. J., Gurer, C., Loike, J. D., Wilmut, I., Schnieke, A. E., and Schon, E. A. (1999). Mitochondrial DNA genotypes in nuclear transfer-derived cloned sheep. *Nat. Genet.* 23(1), 90–93.
90. Munsie, M. J., Michalska, A. E., O'Brien, C. M., Trounson, A. O., Pera, M. F., and Mountford, P. S. (2000). Isolation of pluripotent embryonic stem cells from reprogrammed adult mouse somatic cell nuclei. *Curr. Biol.* 10(16), 989–992.
91. Geraedts, J. P., Harper, J., Braude, P., Sermon, K., Veiga, A., Gianaroli, L., Agan, N., Munne, S., Gitlin, S., Blenow, E., de Boer, K., Hussey, N., Kanavakis, E., Lee, S. H., Viville, S., Krey, L., Ray, P., Emiliani, S., Hsien Liu, Y., and Vermeulen, S. (2001). Preimplantation genetic diagnosis (PGD), a collaborative activity of clinical genetic departments and IVF centres. *Prenat. Diagn.* 21(12), 1086–1092.
92. Munne, S. (2001). Preimplantation genetic diagnosis of structural abnormalities. *Mol. Cell. Endocrinol.* 183 Suppl. 1, S55–S58.

P A R T III

CONTEMPORARY MANAGEMENT

C H A P T E R

24

Polycystic Ovarian Syndrome

ALAN B. COPPERMAN
Division of Reproductive Endocrinology
Department of Obstetrics, Gynecology and Reproductive Science
The Mount Sinai School of Medicine and Hospital
New York, New York 10029

TANMOY MUKHERJEE
Department of Obstetrics, Gynecology and Reproductive Science
The Mount Sinai School of Medicine and Hospital
New York, New York 10029

NATHAN G. KASE
Department of Obstetrics, Gynecology and Reproductive Science
The Mount Sinai School of Medicine and Hospital
New York, New York 10029

I. INTRODUCTION AND HISTORICAL OVERVIEW

Polycystic ovarian syndrome (PCOS) was first described in 1935 by Stein and Leventhal as a syndrome of amenorrhea, virilization, and bilaterally enlarged multicystic ovaries. Today PCOS is recognized as a heterogeneous syndrome involving chronic anovulation accompanied by hyperandrogenism, with clinical manifestations including hirsutism, acne, androgen-dependent alopecia, and frequently, but not always, obesity (Table 24.1).[1] In addition to increased testosterone and androstenedione, elevated mean serum concentrations of luteinizing hormone (LH) are common in all reported series of women with the PCOS,[2, 3] although the prevalence of frankly elevated concentrations of any of these hormones depends on both the criteria for diagnosis and the method of measurement.

PCOS is one of the most common endocrine disorders, affecting approximately 6% of women of reproductive age,[3] and is the leading cause of anovulatory infertility, accounting in some studies for as many as 75% of cases.[4] In one study of anovulatory women, ultrasound examination revealed that 26% of amenorrheic and 86% of oligomenorrheic women had polycystic ovaries.

After initial onset in the peripubertal years, affected women eventually develop signs and symptoms of elevated androgen levels, as well as menstrual irregularity and amenorrhea,

TABLE 24.1 1990 National Institutes of Health Consensus Diagnosis for Polycystic Ovarian Syndrome

Irregular menstrual cycles/anovulation
Hyperandrogenism (acne, mild hirsutism) or hyperandrogenemia (elevated serum DHAS or T)
Exclusion of other medical conditions (abnormalities of thyroid, adrenal, or pituitary)

without a well-defined cause of androgen excess.[5] Although the underlying etiology of PCOS is unknown, there is growing consensus that it is part of a general metabolic/endocrine disorder, the key features of which include insulin resistance, androgen excess, and abnormal gonadotropin secretion.

With the use of high-resolution ultrasound, morphology has re-emerged as a syndrome-amplifying characteristic.[6, 7] However, this appearance has neither the sensitivity nor the specificity to confirm a diagnosis of PCOS. In fact, in patients with polycystic ovaries on ultrasound, the spectrum of findings ranges from hirsutism and normal menses to hyperandrogenism without hirsutism or irregular menses to the full syndrome.[3, 8] More than 90% of anovulatory women with idiopathic hirsutism have polycystic ovaries.[9, 10] Even among normal women not referred for menstrual or infertility complaints, polycystic-appearing ovaries are found on transvaginal ultrasound in 22%, including 86% of those with irregular cycles but also 7% of those with regular cycles.[11] The annual incidence of infertility caused by PCOS is 41 per million population for overt PCOS, and 139 per million for occult (nonhirsute) PCOS.[4]

In the last decade, it has become clear that the metabolic derangements in PCOS are not limited to the sex steroids, and there has been a new focus on the insulin resistance and compensatory hyperinsulinemia found in many of these patients.[12, 13] Recently, point mutations in the insulin receptor gene that cause insulin resistance appear to be associated with the PCOS phenotype.[14] Obesity-induced insulin resistance contributes synergistically to the degree of hyperinsulinemia, but even nonobese patients with PCOS have decreased insulin sensitivity.[12] Ovulatory women with hyperandrogenism, hirsutism, and polycystic ovaries accompanied by normal menstrual cycles display normal insulin sensitivity in response to glucose administration,[15] suggesting that insulin resistance may be the primary process leading to anovulation. The implications of these findings on the management of PCOS and the question of whether PCOS is part of a larger syndrome with dyslysidemia, atherogenesis, and increased risk of cardiovascular disease [16] is under intense study.

Current management of PCOS is reactive and focuses on correction and containment of symptoms such as infertility, amenorrhea, oligomenorrhea, and hirsutism. As many as five major systems may be involved in the development of PCOS [14, 17]: the hypothalamic-pituitary axis, the ovary, peripheral tissues, the adrenal gland, and the metabolic clearance system. However, by the time the patient is seen clinically, the initiating etiology is obscured or undeterminable. Therefore, even with correction of the presenting problem, e.g., infertility, chronic therapy must be sustained in order to prevent potential long-term consequences of the chronic anovulation and metabolic disturbances that are often associated with the syndrome.

II. PATHOGENESIS OF ANOVULATION

In order for a woman to ovulate normally, there must be coordination of several interactive systems: the central hypothalamic-pituitary axis, which directs the ovary, the local responses within the ovary, and the feedback signals that synchronize ovarian and pituitary functions. Several hypotheses have been proposed to explain the defect of PCOS, including a primary hypothalamic defect, inherent pituitary gonadotrope dysfunction, abnormal sex steroid feedback, abnormal sensitivity to feedback, and local follicle steroidogenic and maturation defects.

A. Central Defects

In regard to the hypothalamic-pituitary axis, an intrinsic defect in gonadotropin secretion (LH and FSH), has been demonstrated, characterized by an increase in both immunoreactive and bioactive LH, a decreased pulse amplitude and slightly increased pulse frequency of LH, as well as an elevated LH/FSH ratio.

The prevalence of gonadotropin abnormalities is high in women with PCOS. The positive relationship between LH pulse frequency and both pool LH and LH to FSH ratio supports the hypothesis that a rapid frequency of GnRH secretion may play a key etiologic role in the gonadotropin defect in PCOS patients.[19] The increased LH pulse frequency in PCOS women, independent of body mass index (BMI) has been well-established.[20–22]

In many women with PCOS, GnRH pulse frequency is significantly increased. Waldstreicher *et al.* [20] measured LH pulse frequency in 12 women with PCOS and in 21 ovulating women during the follicular phase. In women with normal ovulatory cycles, the mean LH interpulse interval was 90 min in the early follicular phase. In women with PCOS, the mean LH interpulse interval was 60 min. The LH pulse frequency correlated positively with circulating estradiol.

Normal pituitary ovulatory responses to the follicle's steroid signals require sustained availability of pulsatile secretion of the gonadotropin releasing hormone (GnRH) within a critical range. Thus, for example, the teenager between menarche and the onset of ovulation cannot generate a normal cycle without full frequency and amplitude of GnRH secretion, which may be inhibited by such factors as stress, anxiety, borderline anorexia nervosa, or acute weight loss after a crash diet. It is possible that there is excessive suppression of GnRH due to the increased activity of corticotropin-releasing hormone (CRH) seen in response to stress.[23] If GnRH is only partially suppressed, homeostatic pituitary-ovarian function is maintained, and the patients will be anovulatory. Second, it has been suggested that a primary central nervous system alteration that induces PCOS. Indeed, adolescent girls with PCOS have disordered diurnal secretory patterns of LH, suggesting that a neuroendocrine abnormality may be involved.[24] A number of potential neuroendocrine changes have been suggested in PCOS, including decreases in central dopaminergic tone, but these may be secondary to tonic estrogen feedback rather than primary lesions.

A study by Faure *et al.* sought to evaluate the acute effect of daily subcutaneous injections of the GnRH agonist Buserelin on serum concentration of LH (evaluated by radioimmunoassay (iLH), and by bioassay (bioLH), FSH, estradiol, and testosterone in 20 women with a diagnosis of PCOS. They observed a pituitary hyperresponsiveness in PCOS subjects, and concluded that such acute pituitary responses are not seen when a similar treatment is administered to endocrinologically normal women. The authors suggested that their observations favored the role of an intrinsic central defect in the pathogenesis of PCOS.[25]

Although the presence of the abnormality in gonadotropin secretion has been known for decades,[2, 18] whether the role played by hypothalamic pituitary dysfunction in the etiology of PCOS is causative or reactive remains unclear.

B. Local Processes

Historically, the thesis that the underlying disorder of folliculogenesis in women with PCOS is intrinsic to the ovary has had wide support. Microscopic examination of the ovary reveals islands of luteinized theca cells indicative of LH hyperstimulation, as well as stimulation of other trophic factors such as insulin and IGF-I. In fact, steroidogenic hyperactivity of the theca cells and hypofunction of the granulosa cells are classic findings in this syndrome.[13, 26] Previous studies had shown that androgen production was increased in primary ovarian thecal cells from PCOS patients.[27] The overproduction of steroid hormones in thecal cells from women with PCOS includes increased levels of testosterone, 17α-hydroxyprogesterone, and progesterone. Because increased androgen production in PCOS thecal cells is present even after 20–40 population doublings, it supports the notion that increased androgen production is an intrinsic defect of PCOS ovarian thecal cells.

Chronic LH stimulation undoubtedly induces thecal cell hyperscretion of androgens. The thecal cell hyperactivity can be demonstrated *in vivo* by hyperresponsiveness of 17-hydroxyprogesterone to GnRH agonist challenge.[13] The abnormal regulation of 17-hydroxylase and 17,20-lyase activity in the ovary and thus the hyperandrogenism found in PCOS patients may therefore represent an intrinsic abnormality of ovarian theca-interstitial cell function.[28] Despite repeated efforts, however, the sustained impact of LH excess as the primary cause of the excess response of thecal cells derived from PCOS patients cannot be ruled out. Granulosa cells of PCOS patients *in vitro* also show steroid biosynthetic dysfunction. Granulosa cells derived from arrested follicles are few in number but are also nearly devoid of P450 aromatase activity. The cells themselves may be normal, as they are highly responsive to FSH *in vitro* and *in vivo*,[29] and the low aromatase activity may be secondary to inadequate FSH action.

Under both basal and cAMP-stimulated conditions, CYP17, cholesterol scc, 3β- and 17β-HSD mRNA, and enzymatic expression were increased in PCOS thecal cells compared with normal thecal cells. However, StAR mRNA levels were unaffected in the PCOS thecal cells. These studies suggest that selective alterations in steroidogenic enzyme expression occur in PCOS and are not a result of overall increase in cAMP activity (since StAR is also cAMP regulated).

A number of putative paracrine factors are also thought to interact with FSH in the control of ovarian steroidogenesis.[5] The relative importance of these factors remains to be determined, but the presence of the insulin-like growth factors and their binding proteins, as well as the mechanism of control of the latter through the local production of proteases, suggests a role for this system in folliculogenesis.

Taken together, these data suggest that proliferation of granulosa cells from anovulatory polycystic ovaries is diminished or inhibited, and their steroidogenetic function (aromatase) is inherently impaired due to chronically low FSH, elevated LH, and possibly excess insulin or IGF availability (Fig. 24.3).[27]

C. Abnormal Feedback

As noted above, neuroendocrine abnormalities may play a role in the pathophysiology of polycystic ovaries. Hypersecretion of LH, for example, may be related to the increase in infertility and miscarriage rates found in women with PCOS.[30] These patients have a gonadotropin profile characterized by an elevated amplitude of LH pulsations in association with normal to low levels of FSH and a fast frequency of pulsatile LH secretion.[31] Many theories have been suggested for the etiology of pituitary oversecretion of LH. These include increased pulsatility of GnRH, hypothalamic dysfunction, altered pituitary sensitivity to GnRH, hyperinsulinemic stimulation of the pituitary gland, and perturbed ovarian-pituitary feedback of steroid hormones.

None of these hypotheses fully explains the phenomenon of LH hypersecretion, and there has been much debate in the literature on this subject.[32] There has been, however, some *in vivo* and *in vitro* evidence that suggests that disordered ovarian-pituitary feedback is central to the problem, possibly through a perturbed secretion of nonsteroidal ovarian hormones.[33]

A major question still remaining is whether the neuroendocrine abnormality is primary or secondary to abnormal ovarian feedback by androgens, or more likely, estrogens. Some evidence suggests that the pattern of secretion of LH and FSH from the pituitary may reflect solely an increased frequency of GnRH stimulation, but there is little evidence of a specific primary abnormality of neurotransmitters. Subsequent studies in which the various subgroups of PCOS are carefully delineated will be required to clarify these relationships and in so doing provide patients with optimal therapeutic choices.[31]

From a clinician's point of view, misdirecting and disruptive steroid feedback does play a significant role in the pathogenesis (see Section II.D) and pathophysiology of the chronic anovulation of PCOS. The nonoscillating gonadotropin secretion levels, the static moderately elevated concentrations of estradiol, the arrested maturation of antral follicles and their accumulation *can all be transiently but effectively reversed* in most instances by either the anti-estrogen redirecting instructions of Clomid or the superimposition of increased FSH sufficient for adequate cyclic recruitment and generation of ovulatory follicles. These observations, recorded in many thousands of successful inductions of ovulation cycles in PCOS patients provide unequivocal evidence that inherent, resistant disease in any component of the hypothalamic-pituitary-ovarian system is relatively uncommon in PCOS. More likely, the unusual feedback characteristics of PCOS (inhibins, estradiol, insulin, testosterone) combine to at once induce relatively high LH (modest positive feedback), relatively low FSH (modest negative feedback), which when combined with nonoscillatory interactions, lead to functional chronic anovulation and morphologic PCOS.

D. Adrenal Defects

Over 50% of patients with the PCOS demonstrate excess levels of adrenal androgens, particularly dehydroepiandrosterone sulfate (DHAS).[34] Nonetheless, the mechanism for the adrenal androgens excess remains unclear. It has been noted that in PCOS the pituitary and ovarian responses to their respective trophic factors (i.e., GnRH and LH, respectively) are exaggerated, and it is therefore possible that the excess adrenal androgens also arise from dysfunction of the hypothalamic-pituitary-adrenal axis.

The adrenal glands can contribute to hyperandrogenism in PCOS as indicated by selective venous catheterization studies, elevations of serum DHAS levels, and studies in which ovarian or adrenal steroid production has been suppressed. Indeed, patients with the nonclassical, late-onset form of adrenal 21-hydroxylase deficiency display clinical, biochemical, and ovarian morphological features indistinguishable from PCOS.[35] But even in the absence of a definable adrenal enzyme defect, women with PCOS often show increased responses to exogenous ACTH in DHA, 17-OH progesterone, 17-hydroxypregnenolone, and androstenedione.[13, 36] That these responses do not conform to a pattern for a single adrenal enzyme defect suggests, instead, generalized hyperresponsiveness of the zona reticularis of the adrenal cortex. Interestingly, insulin has been shown to increase adrenal responsiveness to ACTH.[37, 38]

Investigators have suggested that PCOS patients be classified by their response to ACTH.[34] One group would identify those who possess exaggerated pituitary secretion of ACTH in response to hypothalamic CRH, with a second group showing excess sensitivity/responsivity of adrenal androgens to ACTH stimulation and a third group which combines both elements. Clearly, there are patients with PCOS in which plasma ACTH and cortisol levels are significantly higher and the plasma ACTH reaction to administration of hCRH is higher than in controls. Based on the response to hCRH, patients with PCOS could be classified into these three categories.[39] However, it is not clear whether increased responsivity to ACTH is secondary to increased zona reticularis mass or to cellular differences in P450c17 alpha activity, particularly of the delta 4 pathway.[34]

Finally, since adrenal androgen excess affects approximately 25% of PCOS patients, it is possible that adrenal androgen excess may be a genetic trait. The adrenal androgen response to ACTH is highly individualized, and the relative response seems to be constant over time. In addition, there is a strong familial component to adrenal androgen levels in PCOS patients compared to normal individuals. It is possible that the tendency to overproduce adrenal androgens is an inherited risk factor for the development of PCOS. Overall, few hyperandrogenic patients actually have isolated deficiencies of 3β-hydroxysteroid dehydrogenase, 21-hydroxylase, and 11-hydroxylase. The ovarian hormonal secretion in PCOS can affect adrenal androgen secretion and metabolism, although this factor accounts for only part of this abnormality. More likely, the adrenal androgen excess results from a generalized hyperresponsiveness of the adrenal cortex to ACTH, but without an increase in CRH or ACTH sensitivity.

These considerations aside, clinically glucocorticoid administration may improve the ovulatory function in some patients, but the results are modest and cannot be predicted by the circulating androgen levels.[40]

E. Chronic Anovulation and PCOS

From the foregoing, the initiating etiology that leads to chronic anovulation may be at any site in the cascade of HPO endocrine signal interactions, but also includes intrusion into the system by disease or dysfunction of the adrenal cortex (hyperandrogenism, hypercotrisolism), tumor- or drug-induced prolactin excess, and abnormalities of metabolic clearance (liver, kidney disease). All may be associated with PCOS. But in this sea of possibilities, is there a specific isolatable ovarian cause of PCOS?

The two most common causes of secondary amenorrhea are ovarian failure (10% of patients) and PCOS (30% of patients). Ovarian failure differs from PCOS. In the former there is a depletion of all ovarian follicles resulting in the cessation of normal ovarian cyclicity (ovarian failure). Ovarian failure before age 40 is termed premature ovarian failure. Loss of all ovarian follicles results in a marked increase in the serum FSH level secondary to a loss of both estrogen and inhibin-feedback inhibition of FSH. Therefore, ovarian failure is most accurately diagnosed by measuring the patient's serum FSH level. In women with complete ovarian failure, the FSH level will usually be greater than 25 mIU/ml. In women with incipient ovarian failure, the FSH levels can fluctuate markedly between 15 and 25 mIU/ml. Measurements of FSH and estradiol levels during menses for 3 months will often assist the physician in gauging the permanency of the ovarian failure.

Anovulation in women with PCOS is also characterized by arrested growth, but not permanent loss of antral follicles. A relative lack of FSH may contribute to the persistence of anovulation but is unlikely, by itself, to be a major cause of it. Granulosa cells from anovulatory women with polycystic ovaries hypersecrete estradiol, compared with size-matched follicles from normal ovaries or polycystic ovaries from ovulatory women. This phenomenon appears to reflect a condition of advanced maturation of medium-sized antral follicles. The underlying basis for the abnormalities in anovulatory PCOS remains uncertain, but it is possible that there are intrinsic differences in folliculogenesis between polycystic and normal ovaries which affect preantral as well as antral follicles.

Nevertheless, a primary intrinsic ovarian etiology of PCOS is uncommon, and the syndrome once identified, can be treated and controlled. Even once a "definitive" diagnosis is made, it is challenging to find the entry point to the "vicious cycle" of PCOS, in which anovulation begets hyperandrogenism which increases LH secretion and suppresses FSH.

The diagnostic criteria for PCOS proposed by the National Institutes of Health include hyperandrogenism and chronic anovulation but exclude other causes such as congenital adrenal hyperplasia, prolactinoma, androgen-secreting tumors, and Cushing's syndrome. It is therefore important to exclude other obvious pathologies before giving the patient such a diagnosis (see Table 24.1).

III. OVARIAN MORPHOLOGY

A. Gross Morphology and Histology

The classic picture of the polycystic ovary, as described by Stein and Leventhal, is one containing numerous follicles in varying early stages of development and atresia, surrounding dense stromal tissue (Figs. 24.1–24.2). Grossly, polycystic ovaries are enlarged bilaterally, and the capsule is smooth and pearly white but thickened (Fig 24.1A). On cut section, the ovary exhibits 8–10 discrete subcapsular follicles, 4–8 mm in diameter and peripherally arrayed to resemble a necklace (Fig 24.1B). Sometimes there is a corpus luteum or corpus albicans. The cysts, typically lined with a few layers of granulosa cells, are not atretic but a robust luteinized theca cell mantle may be prominent (Fig 24.1C).

For years, it was believed that the thick sclerotic capsule actually functioned as a mechanical barrier to ovulation. It is now known that the polycystic ovary is a consequence of the loss of ovulation and the persistence of a state of anovulation. The surface area can be doubled, with a volume increasing 2.8 times normal. While the same numbers of primordial follicles are present, the number of growing and atretic follicles is doubled, with each ovary containing up to 100 immature follicles. The thickness of the tunica is increased

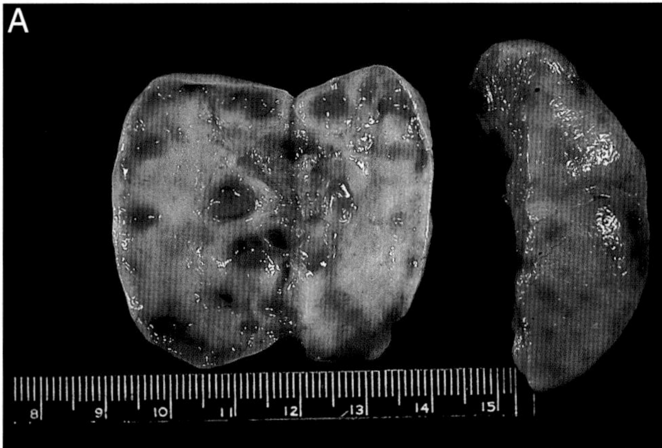

FIGURE 24.1A Polycystic ovary, enlarged in size, with smooth, thickened capsule and multiple peripherally arrayed cysts.

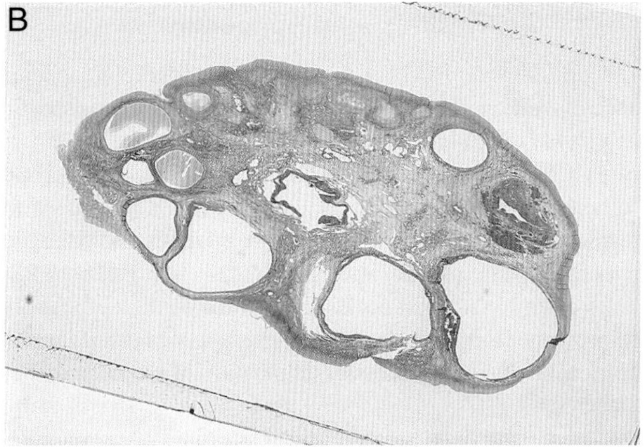

FIGURE 24.1B Polycystic ovary, whole mount. Note the dilated follicle cysts. Hematoxylin-Eosin×10.

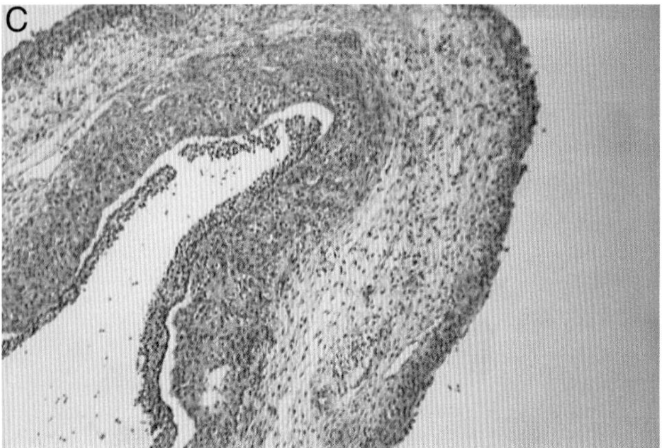

FIGURE 24.1C Cyst wall lined by few granulosa cell layers and, underneath, a luteinized theca interna. Hematoxylin-Eosin × 100

by 50%, and a one-third increase in cortical stromal thickness and a fivefold increase in subcortical stroma are seen.[41]

B. Histochemistry

Connective tissue of human ovarian capsule associated with polycystic ovarian syndrome (PCOS) has been analyzed and has been found to mainly consist of type I collagen and acid glycosaminoglycans, such as dermatan sulfate, heparan sulfate, and chondroitin 4- and 6-sulfate (Fig. 24.2).[42] Although their concentration and constituent ratio in the PCO capsule are found to be similar to those that are normal, their total amounts in whole capsule with PCO are higher than in normal ones, because of the enlarged ovary and the thickened capsule. Furthermore, collagen solubility for pepsin in the PCO capsule is greater than normal. The results suggest that the same or similar factors involved in activation of connective tissue growth in the ovarian capsule such as androgen, IGF, EGF underlie anovulation as well.

C. Ultrasound Appearance

Consideration has been given to the sonographic appearance of ovarian morphology as a distinguishing characteristic of PCOS (Fig. 24.2).[43] With this approach, the diagnosis of PCOS is based on the finding of more than 8 discrete follicles in the ovary, with the follicles less than 10 mm in diameter and usually peripherally arrayed around an enlarged hyperechogenic ovarian stroma. Typically, the multiple follicles resemble a "pearl necklace" on ultrasound examination. Improvements in ultrasound assessment using a transvaginal approach have allowed better delineation of multiple follicular cysts.

Attempts have been made to evaluate ovarian morphology as assessed sonographically with clinical presentation of PCOS patients. In patients with PCOS, the number of small subcapsular follicles correlates with uterine and ovarian blood flow and with specific hormonal parameters. One study performed ultrasonographic evaluation on 30 patients with PCOS and showed 5–10 (group I; n = 14) or >10 (group II; n = 16) small follicles. These patients underwent ultrasonographic (ovarian volume and stroma echodensity; number, diameter, and distribution of follicles) and color Doppler (uterine and intraovarian vessels) analyses, and hormonal assay. In group II, significantly lower pulsatility index values than in group I were observed in the ovarian stromal arteries. The Ferriman-Gallwey score for hirsutism, plasma androstenedione level, and LH/FSH ratio results were significantly higher in group II than in group I. Androstenedione plasma levels correlated with the number of small follicles. Furthermore, the LH/FSH ratio correlated with both the number of small follicles and the stromal artery pulsatility index. The combined assessment of ovarian morphology by transvaginal ultrasound and color Doppler may provide insight into the pathological state of polycystic ovary syndrome.[44]

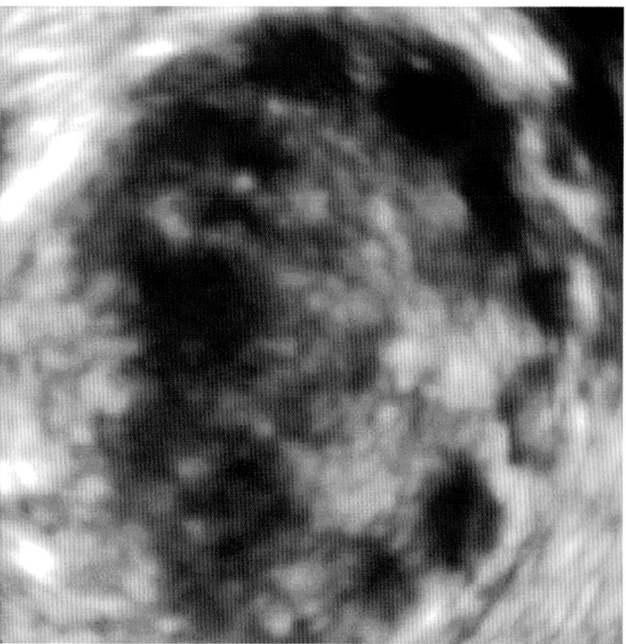

FIGURE 24.2 Sonographic appearance of PCOS. A Three-Dimensional transvaginal sonogram of a "Polycystic ovary" (Kretz, Medison USA, 7.5 Mhz). Note the "string of pearls" configuration of the circumferential pre-antral follicles.

Other investigators have produced similar findings. Compared to controls, women with PCOS had larger ovaries and thicker stroma, increased impedance in the uterine arteries, increased stromal vascularity with decreased impedance that persisted throughout the menstrual cycle, and a lack of luteal conversion.[45]

In summary, the human ovary is a dynamic organ that continually changes in size and activity through life, as an integral part of the changes that the female is going through before, during, and after her reproductive life. Following the rapid increase in the use of transvaginal scan in recent years, the measurement of ovarian volume has become quick, accurate, and cost-effective. Ovarian volume is an important tool in screening, diagnosis, and monitoring the treatment of conditions such as PCOS, ovarian cancer, and adolescent abnormalities. In reproductive medicine, measurement of ovarian volume plays an important but not definitive role in the assessment of ovarian reserve and prediction of response to superovulation.[46]

D. Stromal Hyperthecosis

Alterations in the microendocrine environment of the ovary are associated with specific morphological changes. While predictable morphologic expressions of hormonal changes accompany commencement of menopause, several disease states are associated with ovarian dysfunction. These diseases include PCOS and hyperthecosis (islands of luteinized theca cells within the ovarian stroma), both associated with androgenization. Ovarian tumors may also be associated with morphological and clinical alterations. Even some apparently endocrinologically inactive ovarian tumors may be associated with morphologic evidence of stromal activation. Endocrinologically active ovarian tumors with considerable stromal compartments may induce clinical manifestations of either masculinization or feminization as a consequence of differential productions of androgens and estrogens.[47] It has also been found that a significant degree of insulin resistance exists in women with hyperthecosis and that insulin stimulates ovarian stromal androgen synthesis and thus may play a role in the pathogenesis of ovarian hyperthecosis and its clinical consequences.[48]

E. Hyperplasia of Thecal/Stromal Cells

The most striking feature of the PCOS ovary is the hyperplasia of the thecal stromal cells and an increased stromal area. There is also an increased number of small antral follicles, as well as primary and secondary follicles. The hyperplastic theca interna seen in polycystic ovaries may be responsible for the 17-hydroxyprogesterone secretion.[49] Thus, there is a high degree of correlation between ultrasonographic evidence of PCOS and the presence of the endocrine disturbances and clinical findings that mark the syndrome.[50–52] Nonetheless, any attempt to understand the body of literature examining management of PCOS is hindered by the variation, over time and across institutions, in the definition of the syndrome.

IV. THE HORMONAL PROFILE OF PCOS

Functional hyperandrogenism occurs in approximately 50% of women with PCOS. The exact cause of hyperandrogenism is unclear but accumulating evidence suggests a role for dysregulation of adrenal and ovarian 17,20-lyase. Studies examining ACTH responses in PCOS females have been conflicting.[34, 53–55] However, in those studies utilizing dexamethasone to produce a basal state, ACTH stimulation increased 17-OH progestesterone in PCOS women in comparison to control subjects.[56] Hyperinsulinemia in hyperandrogenic anovulatory women potentiates ovarian hyperandrogenism by enhancing LH secretion, augmenting 17-hydroxylase and, 17,20-lyase activity, as well as suppressing sex hormone binding globulin (SHBG) concentration and capacity. Dysfunctional steriod synthesis is a key component of hyperandrogenic anovulation which is caused by a type of insulin resistance that is independent and additive to that of obesity alone. Although the mechanisms governing insulin action on ovarian steroidogenesis are uncertain, abnormalities of intracellular insulin signaling or cytochrome P450c17 (alpha) activity may render the 17-hydroxylase/17, 20-lyase enzyme complex more sensitive to LH (Fig. 24.3). Hyperinsulinemia in hyperandrogenic anovulatory women is accompanied by truncal obesity characterized by an increased amount of abdominal fat (i.e., greater waist to hip ratio). Upper body obesity is an important independent risk factor for cardiovascular disease and diabetes.

Although genetic and environmental factors affect fat distribution, sex steroids, particularly androgens, regulate lipid metabolism, suggesting yet another link between the hormonal and metabolic abnormalities of hyperandrogenic anovulation. The insulin resistance in at least 50% of PCOS women appears

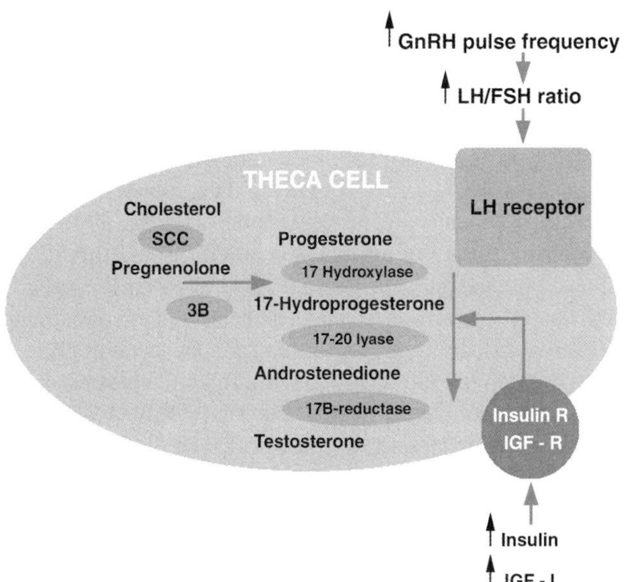

FIGURE 24.3 Cytochrome P450. Diagrammatic depiction linking the accelerated GnRH/LH pulsatile activities and extraovarian factors (insulin/IGF-1) in the development of hyperandrogenism by ovarian theca cells.

to be related to excessive serine phosphorylation of the insulin receptor. A factor extrinsic to the insulin receptor, presumably a serine/threonine kinase,[57] causes this abnormality and is an example of an important new mechanism for human insulin resistance related to factors controlling insulin receptor signaling. Serine phosphorylation appears to modulate the activity of the key regulatory enzyme of androgen biosynthesis, P450c17. It is thus possible that a single defect produces both the insulin resistance and the hyperandrogenism in some PCOS women. It appears that insulin is acting through its own receptor (rather than the IGF-I receptor) in PCOS to augment not only ovarian and adrenal steroidogenesis but also pituitary LH release.

PCOS may originate as an adrenal cortex disorder manifested early in sexual maturation in the form of an exaggerated adrenarche. Many studies have shown that children with premature or exaggerated adrenarche are at high risk of developing PCOS-like functional ovarian hyperandrogenism at puberty. These findings, plus the observation that hyperandrogenemia in adolescent girls is accompanied by neuroendocrine-metabolic features very much like those found in adult PCOS strongly support the exaggerated adrenarche hypothesis.

The key event of adrenarche is the initiation of adrenal androgen secretion of DHA, DHAS, and androstenedione through the activation of 17,20-lyase activity of the P450c17. Premature hypersecretion of adrenal androgen precursors provides substrate for transformation to potent androgens and estrogens in the target cells of the reproductive axis, where they act locally through androgen and estrogen receptors.

Free IGF-I levels have recently been shown to increase during childhood and peak during the transition from adrenarche to early puberty. When combined with concurrent elevations of GH, insulin, and gonadotropin secretion, it is understandable how girls who develop insulin resistance might incur the burdens of incremental androgen biosynthesis by the adrenal and ovary.[36] To assess the potential contribution of leptin (another puberty related hormone) to the pathogenesis of PCO, Mantzoros *et al.* [64] measured leptin levels in obese women with PCO and in controls to determine if alterations in hyperinsulinemia produced by administration of the insulin-sensitizing agent troglitazone had an effect on serum leptin levels. Baseline leptin levels were not different between PCO and control subjects and remained unchanged after treatment with troglitazone. They concluded that leptin levels in patients with PCO do not differ from controls and that increased circulating insulin due to insulin resistance does not appear to alter circulating leptin levels in women with PCO.

V. INSULIN RESISTANCE, HYPERINSULINEMIA, AND HYPERANDROGENISM

Insulin synthesis and secretion occurs in pancreatic islet cells. Insulin has many sites of action, including the liver,

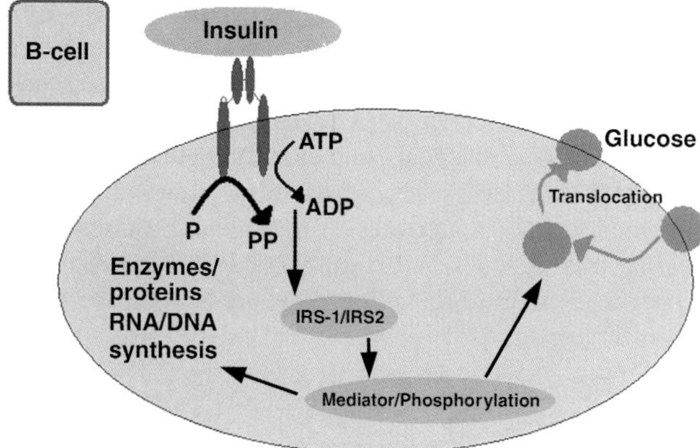

FIGURE 24.4 Pathways of Insulin action. The extramembrane domain of the insulin receptor is the binding for insulin. The transmembrane and intracellular domains of the receptor express tyrosine kinase (TYR) activity and undergo autophosphorylation when activated by signals from the extramembrane domain of the receptor. Subsequent intracellular action involves insulin substrate receptor (IRS)-1, initiating signal cascades that lead to stimulation of enzymatic systems, protein synthesis, and gene expression.

where it inhibits gluconeogenesis, skeletal muscle, where it increases glucose uptake, and adipose tissue, where it increases glucose uptake and inhibits lipolysis (visceral fat is more resistant to anti-lipolytic effects than subcutaneous fat). Also notable are the systemic anabolic effects whereby insulin increases amino acid uptake, RNA, DNA, protein synthesis, and cell growth. Insulin's primary effect in the ovary is to stimulate ovarian steroidogenesis which may be explained by the remarkable similarity between the insulin receptor and the receptor for insulin-like growth factor I (Fig. 24.4).[70]

There is a strong correlation between the degree of hyperinsulinemia and hyperandrogenism.[71, 72] Insulin binding to the IGF-I receptor then augments thecal androgen synthesis in response to LH. Accordingly, the insulin resistance characteristic of obesity and the resultant relative hyperinsulinemia induces excess androgen in these women. However, obesity and hyperinsulinemia are both prominent features of the metabolic picture in PCOS, and the degree of hyperinsulinemia is positively correlated with the degree of obesity.[73]

As a result, correction of hyperinsulinemia to decrease androgenicity and improve the efficacy of ovulation inducing treatment has received increasing utilization. Diazoxide, metformin, and troglitazone have all been shown to decrease androgen production and serum free testosterone in women with PCOS [74–78] even in those who are lean.[76] Ovulatory menses are restored in many women on these agents, [77, 78] and with metformin therapy, spontaneous pregnancies have been reported in previously anovulatory women.[78]

Some women with PCOS are profoundly insulin resistant and have deficient insulin-mediated glucose uptake that is comparable to that observed in type 2 diabetes. Current studies suggest that insulin binding to the insulin receptor (IR) remains normal in PCOS, suggesting a post-binding defect in IR-mediated signal transduction in affected tissues.

But a circulating factor may also induce insulin resistance. There has been recent interest in the relationship between a small (114 amino acids) newly discovered protein called resistin that is secreted by abdominal fat cells. The primary function of resistin appears to be as a signaling molecule in inducing tissues to be less sensitive to the action of insulin. Resistin secretion is enhanced in the extra-large fat cells of obese animals, and this may account for the strong association between human obesity and type 2 diabetes (over 80% of the people with type 2 diabetes are obese). Resistin levels are increased in diet-induced obesity as well as in genetic models of obesity and insulin resistance. In adipocytes, neutralization with resistin antiserum enhanced insulin-stimulated glucose uptake, and recombinant resistin blunted insulin action. The administration of resistin to mice impaired glucose tolerance (IGT) without reducing insulin levels, and decreased sensitivity to the effects of insulin.

Allthough first identified and its action studied in mice, resistin has now been found in humans. This protein may eventually be part of the explanation of how obesity predisposes people to diabetes, and in particular women, to PCOS.[79]

However, even nonobese patients with PCOS have decreased insulin sensitivity.[12] Furthermore, women with hyperandrogenism, hirsutism, and polycystic ovaries accompanied by normal menstrual cycles have been shown to have normal insulin sensitivity and responses to glucose administration,[15] suggesting that insulin resistance may be the primary process leading to anovulation.

VI. GENETIC ASPECTS

Estimates of the prevalence of PCO in the general population have ranged from 2–20%. The vast majority of these reports have studied white populations in Europe, used limited definitions of the disorder, and/or used biased populations, such as those seeking medical care. To estimate the prevalence of this disorder in the U.S. and address these limitations, Knochenhauer *et al.* [60] prospectively determined the prevalence of PCO in a reproductive-aged population of 369 consecutive women (174 white and 195 black; aged 18–45 years) examined at the time of their preemployment physicals. In these unselected women the prevalence of hirsutism varied from 2–8% depending on the chosen cut-off Ferriman-Gallwey (F-G) score, with no significant difference between white and black women. Using an F-G score of 6 or more as indicative of hirsutism, 3.4% of blacks and 4.7% of whites had PCO, suggesting that PCO may be one of the most common reproductive endocrine disorders of women.

Heritability of PCOS has been inferred from studies of the syndrome in various populations (ethnic groups, twins, and PCOS families). These data suggest that the condition is passed down through either sex, according to an autosomal dominant model of genetic transmission. While specific gene mutations affecting androgen synthesis, insulin secretion, and insulin activity, which could explain most of the endocrine and metabolic symptoms have been sought, their unequivocal identification has remained elusive. Clearly acquired risk factors (either during prenatal or postnatal life), seem to convert an occult PCOS proclivity or susceptibility into a clinically manifest syndrome.[58]

The inheritance of some cases of PCOS is consistent with an autosomal dominant inheritance pattern in PCOS families, perhaps caused by the same gene. Although the diagnosis of PCOS often represents a heterogeneous collection of women, several of the adrenal cortical enzyme abnormalities can resemble a PCOS-like clinical picture. Adult-onset 21-hydroxylase deficiency, partial 17α-hydroxylase, and 3β-ol-dehydrogenase may each be accompanied by PCO symptomatology. There was no such genetic influence in families of women without PCOS. Sisters of PCOS probands with polycystic ovarian morphology were more likely to have menstrual irregularity and had larger ovaries and higher serum androstenedione and dehydroepiandrosterone-sulfate levels than sisters without PCOS. This suggests a spectrum of clinical phenotype in PCOS families. These data are consistent with a role for genetic differences in androgen synthesis, metabolism, or action in the pathogenesis of PCOS.[59] Complicating matters is that both autosomal and X-linked patterns of inheritance have been described in PCOS and available pedigree analyses do not discrimate between these two modes of inheritance. The major difficulty lies in the methods of diagnosing PCOS and using ultrasound criteria alone may be misleading.

Carey *et al.* described an autosomal dominant syndrome of polycystic ovaries and premature male-patterned baldness (PMPB),[61] and later suggested an association with a change in the 5′ promoter region of the CYP17 gene (202110), which modified the expression of the syndrome in some families but did not appear to be the primary genetic defect.[62]

Govind *et al.* [59] screened first-degree relatives of women affected by PCO to obtain evidence for the genetic basis of polycystic ovaries and PMPB. Of the relatives of 29 PCO probands, 15 of 29 (52%) mothers, 6 of 28 (21%) fathers, 35 of 53 (66%) sisters, and 4 of 18 (22%) brothers were assigned affected status. First-degree female and male relatives of affected individuals had a 61 and 22% chance of being affected, respectively. Of all sibs of PCO probands, 39 of 71 were affected, giving a segregation ratio of 39/32 (55%), which is consistent with autosomal dominant inheritance for PCO/PMPB. Thus the inheritance of PCO and PMPB is consistent with an autosomal dominant mode in PCO families. Sisters of PCO probands with polycystic ovarian morphology were more likely to have menstrual irregularity and had larger ovaries and higher serum androstenedione and dehydroepiandrosterone sulfate levels than sisters without PCO, suggesting a spectrum of clinical phenotypes in PCO families. Men with PMPB had higher serum testosterone than those without. The authors concluded that these data are consistent with a role for genetic differences in androgen synthesis, metabolism, or action in the pathogenesis of PCO.

Gharani *et al.* [63] presented linkage and association data indicating a strong relationship between CYP11A (118485) locus and PCOS with hyperandrogenism.

In preliminary family studies, Legro *et al.* [66, 67] found that some female first-degree relatives of women with PCOS have hyperandrogenemia. They hypothesized that this may be a genetic trait suitable for linkage analysis and examined 115 sisters of 80 probands with PCOS from unrelated families. PCOS was diagnosed by the combination of elevated serum androgen levels and six or fewer menses per year with the exclusion of secondary causes. The diagnostic criteria for PCOS were fulfilled in 22% of the sisters. In addition, 24% of the sisters had hyperandrogenemia and regular menstrual cycles. Probands, sisters with PCOS, and hyperandrogenemic sisters had elevated serum LH levels compared with control women. The familial aggregation of hyperandrogenemia in PCOS kindreds suggested that it is a genetic trait which can be used to assign affected status in linkage studies designed to identify PCOS genes.

Urbanek *et al.* [68] tested a carefully chosen collection of 37 candidate genes for linkage and association with PCOS or hyperandrogenemia in 150 families. The strongest evidence for linkage was with the follistatin gene for which affected sisters showed increased identity by descent (72%). After correction for multiple testing, the follistatin findings were still highly significant. Although the linkage results for CYP11A were also nominally significant ($p = 0.02$), they were not significant after correction. In 11 candidate gene regions, at least 1 allele showed nominally significant evidence for population association with PCOS in the transmission/disequilibrium test. The strongest effect in this test was observed in the insulin receptor (INSR) region but was not significant after correction. Odunsi and Kidd [69] have also supported these conclusions.

While the exact mode of inheritance of PCOS remains unclear at the moment, further elucidation of the disease process may provide valuable linkage data and clarify modes of transmission. Better diagnostic criteria and stringent adherence to these criteria are essential to eventual understanding of PCOS inheritance. The need for such clarification is obvious: the full blown syndrome of hyperandrogenism, chronic anovulation, and polycystic ovaries affects 5–10% of all premenopausal women. These women are likely to be obese, hirsute, and hyperinsulinemic and are at increased risk of type II diabetes, dyslipidemia, athersclerosis, coronary artery disease, hypertension, and endometrial cancer.

VII. CLINICAL CONSEQUENCES OF PCOS

Untreated PCOS may be regarded as a disorder that progresses until the time of menopause. An approach to treating a patient who presents with PCOS begins with a thorough history and identification of both medical issues and the patient's principal concerns. A thorough history should include menstrual history, recent weight changes, hirsutism (including type and frequency of depillation techniques, acne, galactorrhea, polyuria/polydipsia, fertility, cold intolerance and constipation, and a dietary assessment). Physical examination should include blood pressure, weight:height ratio, BMI, Ferriman-Gallwey scale, presence of abdominal striae, scalp hair pattern, thyromegaly, galactorrhea, and skin evaluation. Because of the high prevalence of IGT or type II diabetes in obese young women with PCOS, it is logical to perform a standard 75g oral glucose tolerance test routinely in such patients (Table 24.2).

Table 24.2 Two hour Glucose Tolerance Testing

2 hour glucose tolerance testing (75 mg glucose)[a]
Clinical symptoms of diabetes, plus random plasma glucose ≥200 mg/dl
Fasting plasma glucose ≥126 mg/dl
Plasma glucose ≥200 mg/dl

[a]From the American Diabetes Association, 1997.

A pelvic sonogram is often performed during the first visit, and includes preantral follicle count and ovarian volume measurements. If there are risk factors including prolonged amenorrhea or dysfunctional uterine bleeding, endometrial biopsy must even be part of the initial assessment.

Ongoing studies lend support to the hypothesis that women with the syndrome are at increased risk for the development of cardiovascular disease.[80] More importantly, the long-term effects of unopposed estrogen place women with the syndrome at considerable risk for endometrial cancer, endometrial hyperplasia and, perhaps, breast cancer.[81] The risk of endometrial cancer is three times higher in women with PCOS than in normal women. In addition, small observational studies have suggested that chronic anovulation during the reproductive years is associated with a three to four times increased risk of breast cancer in the postmenopausal years. Still other studies have failed to find an association with increased rates of breast cancer. Although no evidence shows that outcomes are improved, mammography and endometrial sampling to search for underlying estrogen-stimulated cancer should be considered in high-risk women with dysfunctional uterine bleeding.[82] Because the syndrome is also associated with lipid abnormalities, PCO women would benefit from identification of dyslipidemia, and if present steps to prevent cardiovascular disease and the other sequelae of long-standing hypertension and diabetes mellitus should be undertaken.

A. Hyperandrogenism

Masculinization is defined as clinical evidence of excess androgen action in women. It includes acne and alopecia in addition to hirsutism. True virilization is defined as temporal balding, deepening of the voice, increased muscle bulk, and clitoromegaly, and is the clinical consequence of severe hyperandrogenism. Masculinization results from the effects of either increased androgen production or increased sensitivity to androgen at target tissues. The spectrum of hyperandrogenic conditions ranges from a subtle increase in terminal facial hair to true virilization. Because of genetic differences in target tissue number and sensitivity to androgens, hyperandrogenism may exist without clinical evidence of its presence.

Androgens are steroid hormones synthesized and secreted directly by the adrenal glands and gonads.[86–88] Potent androgens are also converted from precursors in peripheral tissues, including skin and fat cells. Androgens are defined specifically in bioassay systems by their ability to induce growth and secretion by the prostate and seminal vesicles and to bind tightly to prostatic cytosolic androgen receptors. Like insulin and growth hormone, androgens are anabolic because they cause nitrogen retention.

In humans, testosterone is the biologically important extracellular androgen. It is metabolized into biologically active but vastly disparate products. These biologically active metabolites include the even more potent androgen, dihydrotestosterone (DHT), formed intracellularly through the 5α-reduction of testosterone, and is locally active, and estradiol (E_2), formed through the aromatization of testosterone, which may have local as well as distant, endocrine effects.

B. Hirsutism

The most commonly appreciated expression of hyperandrogenism is excess terminal hair in women. Hirsutism is defined as the transformation of vellus (fine, soft, unpigmented) to terminal (coarse, pigmented, longer) hair in androgen-dependent hair areas (e.g., upper lip, chin, chest, upper back, pubis, inner thighs). Although the hormonal environment influences the conversion of vellus hairs to terminal hairs, the total number of hair follicles is genetically determined and is not changed by hormones. Racial and ethnic (but not sex) differences exist in total follicle number; for example, white persons have more follicles than Asians, and persons of Mediterranean descent have more follicles than those of Northern European descent. The total hair follicle number influences the severity of the expression of hirsutism in hyperandrogenic women. For example, one-fourth to one-third of women of non-Scandinavian European origin may normally have terminal hair on the upper lip, periareolar area, or linea alba, whereas such hair must be considered abnormal in Asian and Scandinavian women.[89–91] Unlike those areas, the upper abdomen, sternum, back, and shoulders are distinctly unusual sites for terminal hair in women and should be cause for further evaluation, regardless of genetic background. Finally, hirsutism must be differentiated from hypertrichosis, which is a generalized increase in vellus (lanugo in the neonate) but not terminal hair. Hypertrichosis may be associated with certain drugs, metabolic disorders, or malignancy.

C. Alopecia

Androgen stimulation of the pilosebaceous unit in most parts of the body produces increased hair diameter, pigmentation, rate of growth, and sebaceous gland secretion. Conversely, androgen stimulation of androgen-sensitive hair follicles on the scalp decreases the diameter and rate of hair growth, especially in the temporal area (male pattern baldness). Diffuse hair thinning can also be a sign of mild hyperandrogenism in women.[92]

D. Acne

Increased production of sebum leads to acne in susceptible persons; if it is chronic, it can produce scarring. Occasionally, acne is the only sign of severe hyperandrogenism.[95, 96]

E. Menstrual Irregularity and Infertility

Hyperandrogenism is often associated with chronic anovulation that results in menstrual irregularity.[4] The anovulatory state can be associated with chronic, unopposed estrogen stimulation of the endometrium, resulting in endometrial hyperplasia, erratic heavy menstrual bleeding, and even endometrial carcinoma.[97] In addition, the reduced frequency of ovulation is associated with decreased opportunities for conception. Hyperandrogenism probably has an impact on fertility in addition to anovulation. Many studies suggest a decreased conception rate in spite of induced ovulation, and some suggest an increased risk for spontaneous miscarriage in hyperandrogenic women.[3, 98] The mechanisms for this androgen action remain to be determined.

Since anovulatory cycles are the source of infertility in PCOS, the objective in managing these patients is the induction of ovulation. After establishing that a patient is anovulatory and screening for easily treated sources of anovulation (i.e., measuring TSH and prolactin), the approach to the patient with PCOS should involve the use of progressively more aggressive treatment strategies until ovulation is established and pregnancy can be achieved. It is important to mention here the distinction between ovulation induction and controlled ovarian hyperstimulation (COH). While the ultimate goal for ovulation induction may appear to be a truism, the induction of ovulation, it is only the single or double follicle that is desired. Conversely, COH is used in patients to induce a multiple follicular response (i.e., in patients with unexplained infertility, or in preparation for an ovum retrieval and subsequent *in vitro* fertilization).

Use of gonadotropins (FSH and LH or FSH alone) provides a more targeted, if not more aggressive, approach to ovulation induction. Urinary human menopausal gonadotropin (hMG), which contains both FSH and LH, has been used for many years. Because the LH in women with PCOS is often already elevated, it has been theorized that purified FSH would be more effective than hMG. In fact, no randomized controlled trials have shown a significant difference between hMG and urinary FSH in pregnancy rate in patients with PCOS.[99]

To reduce the risk of over-stimulating a patient, some sacrifice in fecundity rate is necessary. It may, at times, even be necessary to cancel cycles. However, with intensive monitoring and the proper choice of dosage regimen, ovarian hyperstimulation syndrome can be mild, and rates of both hyperstimulation and cycle cancellation can be kept to a minimum. (Amaru and Copperman, personal communication.)

F. Endometrial Hyperplasia

Patients with PCOS often have multiple risk factors for the development of endometrial hyperplasia and even endometrial cancer. The risk factors include obesity, nulliparity, hypertension, and diabetes mellitus. There is an increased risk of endometrial cancer in hyperandrogenic women (RR = 3.1), and the endometrial effects of hyperinsulinemia may also be significant.[83, 84]

A host of evidence is now available to suggest that chronic unopposed estrogen exposure, as occurs in PCOS, will lead to the development of endometrial hyperplasia and even frank carcinoma. Epidemiologic studies have shown an increased risk for endometrial cancer in women with chronic anovulation. Because abundant adipose tissue represents a large compartment for peripheral aromatization of androgen to estrogen, the high incidence of obesity in PCOS patients may represent the key factor in the genesis of endometrial neoplasia.[85] Early detection is very advantageous. The tumors that are found are usually of low grade and well-differentiated and are successfully treated surgically.

G. Obesity

Obesity has consistently been demonstrated to have a detrimental effect upon the female reproductive system. Obesity has been divided into two types, central or upper body obesity (this involves hypertrophy of fat cells with insulin resistance and hyperandrogenism, and is associated with a waist to hip ratio of >0.85), and lower body (not associated with insulin resistance or high androgen levels). The presence and degree of obesity affects a host of clinical and endocrinological parameters, and predicts the degree of insulin resistance and the phenotypic expression of PCOS. Weight loss has been shown to result in an improvement in menstrual function, a decrease in the clinical androgenic profile, and significant increase in spontaneous pregnancy rates. Conversely, obesity is associated with poor pregnancy outcome and miscarriage in both women with PCOS, and in those with normal ovarian morphology. Effective nutritional counseling should be offered at all stages of the female reproductive life cycle.[100]

Though obesity is not a prerequisite for the diagnosis of PCOS, it is a common feature of these patients. In obese women, weight loss alone may lead to spontaneous ovulation and pregnancy.[101] Both the presence of obesity and body weight positively correlate with the dose of clomiphene required to induce ovulation,[102–104] perhaps because obese patients are more likely to be hyperinsulinemic.[73] Obese patients may also have worse outcomes in terms of rates of ovulation and pregnancy loss when treated with low-dose gonadotropins.[105] Like stimulation with clomiphene, gonadotropin treatment of obese women with PCOS may require a higher dose and longer cycles.[106] For all the above reasons, calorie restriction and weight reduction are good first steps in the management of PCOS. The occurrence of a continuous spectrum of gonadotropin abnormalities varying with body fat suggests that nonobese and obese patients with PCOS do not represent distinct pathophysiologic subsets of this disorder.[19]

H. Dyslipidemia

Obtaining a lipid profile is advisable in women with PCOS, as is surveillance of the blood pressure. Several lines of evidence suggest that a subset of women may be at increased risk of cardiovascular disease because of unfavorable alterations in insulin action and/or production, accompanying altered apolipoprotein metabolism and altered androgenicity and/or estrogenicity.[93] A number of cardiovascular disease risk factors, including central obesity, insulin resistance (with associated hyperinsulinemia), dyslipidemia, and/or diabetes mellitus, tend to cluster in these women. Studies indicate that androgen excess may be a signal of increased risk for coronary artery disease, even in younger women. If androgenicity and insulin resistance are early warning signs of increasing risk of morbidity and mortality, these patients are prime candidates for preventive medicine. In women having coronary angiography, those with more extensive coronary artery disease were more likely to have polycystic ovaries on ultrasonography than were those with less extensive disease. Visualization of polycystic ovaries by sonography was associated with distinct metabolic and endocrine abnormalities. Further study is required to evaluate whether surgery or hormone replacement therapy can modify the risk.[94]

VIII. THERAPEUTIC OPTIONS

A. Goals of Therapy

Except in the rare occurrence of an androgen-secreting tumor, therapy for hyperandrogenic women is directed at the patient's primary symptoms and personal goals. An elevated serum androgen level is not required to initiate treatment because hyperandrogenic symptoms demonstrate that there is increased androgen use by the target tissue.

In all obese women, weight reduction can substantially improve hyperandrogenism and anovulation.[101] Medical therapy may consist of suppressing LH or ACTH release to reduce glandular secretion interfering with androgen synthesis, increasing SHBG to decrease androgen bioavailability, or decreasing local androgen availability by inhibiting 5α-reductase activity or blocking androgen action with wider spectrum androgen receptor antagonists. In addition, many cosmetic therapies are available for the symptoms of hirsutism, acne, and alopecia. Nonpharmacologic techniques are particularly useful in conjunction with pharmacologic therapy.

It is essential to ensure that the patient has realistic expectations about the time course and the results of therapy. Once a hair follicle has been transformed by androgen exposure to produce a terminal hair, biochemical control of hyperandrogenism will not result in restoration of vellus hair growth. However, biochemical control will result in a slowing of the rate of hair growth and a decrease in hair diameter and color. Clinical effects on hair growth are not evident until 3–6 months of therapy, and maximal effects are not seen for up to 1 year. In most women it takes approximately 1 year for the effects of therapy for alopecia to result in clinically evident changes because of the cyclic nature of scalp hair growth. Conversely, improvements in acne and seborrhea can be seen within 1–2 months on therapy. Eradication of terminal hairs requires electrolysis or repeated laser treatments. Because these modalities are expensive, we recommend that the patient wait until biochemical control has been achieved (3–6months) before adding these therapies.

B. Nonpharmacologic Approaches

Techniques used to manage hirsutism include depilation with shaving, tweezers, waxes, or creams; electrocoagulation with diathermy; electrolysis with direct current; repeated bleaching; and laser therapy. Male pattern baldness may be managed surgically with full-thickness, hair-bearing punch autografts obtained from resistant occipital follicles.

In addition, because obesity can unmask or aggravate hyperandrogenic syndromes and insulin resistance associated with PCOS is often observed and has significant health consequences, weight loss should be strongly encouraged from the outset in all overweight patients. Weight loss results in decreased androgen production and insulin levels and increased SHBG levels, occasionally leading to the complete resolution of symptoms and the resumption of ovulatory menses. As little as a 7% reduction in body weight can lead to a significant decrease in androgen levels and to the resumption of ovulatory menses in obese women with PCOS.[101]

C. Endometrial Protection

Women with chronic anovulation and continued estrogen production, such as women with PCOS, are at risk for endometrial neoplasia because of the unopposed estrogen effect.[107, 108] Thus, regular endometrial shedding must be induced in amenorrheic, hyperandrogenic women with intermittent oral progestin administration (e.g., 5 mg medroxyprogesterone acetate orally for 14 days every 1–2 months). The exact frequency of withdrawal bleeding to prevent endometrial hyperplasia has not been established in patients with PCOS. However, duration of each intervention (14 days) is critical to endometrial control. Progesterone withdrawal must be provided, in addition to agents for controlling hyperandrogenism, if the latter do not restore regular menses.

D. Oral Contraceptives

Estrogen and progestin are more effective in combination than either agent is alone in suppressing LH-dependent hyperandrogenemia. Although at least 50 μg ethinyl estradiol (EE) or the equivalent is required to suppress LH, lower estrogen levels (approximately 35 μg EE) can increase serum SHBG and decrease ACTH-dependent adrenal DHAS production.[109] Thus, low-dose oral contraceptive pills (30–35 μg EE) are usually effective in controlling hirsutism and acne and are FDA approved for this purpose. Contraceptive pills also induce cyclic uterine withdrawal bleeding, suppress hyperplasia, and provide contraception. In women in whom estrogens are contraindicated, high-dose medroxyprogesterone has been used alone with some efficacy. Progesterone inhibits 5α-reductase activity, which decreases target-tissue androgen use.

In nonsmoking patients with clinically mild to moderate hyperandrogenism who are 35 years of age or younger and who do not have contraindications, oral contraceptive pills with 35 μg EE may be used as first-line therapy. Antiandrogen therapy is usually needed if hirsutism is moderate to severe or if alopecia has developed. The major risks inherent in the use of oral contraceptive pills are related primarily to their estrogen content. Risks include thromboembolic phenomena early in use, gallbladder disease, and exacerbation of hypertension and migraine headaches. Phlebitis, hypertension, and cholelithiasis are relative contraindications to oral contraceptive use. Cigarette smoking significantly increases the risk for thromboembolic phenomena during oral contraceptive use and must be discouraged. Oral contraceptive agents may worsen insulin resistance in hyperandrogenic women.[110, 111]

E. Glucocorticoids

Glucocorticoids are used to suppress ACTH-dependent adrenal androgen secretion. They are most commonly indicated for the treatment of congenital adrenal hyperplasia (CAH), though they are not used as commonly with nonclassical forms of congenital adrenal hyperplasia.[112] Fertility rates may also be improved by glucocorticoid therapy in conjunction with ovulation induction in hyperandrogenic women who do not have CAH, possibly related to decreasing negative androgen effects on the uterus, follicle, or hypothalamic-pituitary axis.

Glucocorticoid replacement, usually with 0.25–0.5 mg oral dexamethasone at bedtime, is the specific therapy for women with nonclassical congenital adrenal hyperplasia. Clinical improvement may be expected to occur any time between 3 and 12 months after the institution of therapy. Dexamethasone is the glucocorticoid of choice because it is virtually devoid of mineralocorticoid activity and can be given in a single bedtime dose.

F. Antiandrogens

Antiandrogens act primarily by interfering with target tissue binding of androgens to their intracellular receptor. They may be used alone or in combination with oral contraceptive pills for masculinizing signs that are not responsive to a single agent. Antiandrogens can improve insulin sensitivity slightly in women with PCOS.[37]

1. Spironolactone

The diuretic spironolactone is not approved by the FDA for use in hirsutism. Nevertheless, it has potent antiandrogen action in high dosages (75–200 mg a day) by interfering with androgen synthesis by inhibiting 17α-hydroxylase/17, 20-lyase activity (P450c17) and by competitively inhibiting intracellular testosterone and DHT receptor binding. Moreover, spironolactone may inhibit 5α-reductase activity. Comparative studies have shown spironolactone to have similar efficacy to cyproterone acetate,[113] flutamide,[114] and finasteride.[115]

A starting dosage of 50–100 mg twice a day is recommended.[116] If side effects do not develop, a maximal dosage of 100 mg twice daily can be used to control hyperandrogenism. A clinical response may be expected to occur approximately 3–6 months after therapy is started. Spironolactone has been used for many years and has an excellent safety profile. Side effects include dysfunctional bleeding (56%) but not electrolyte disturbances. Spironolactone should not be given during pregnancy because of the potential to interfere with the normal masculinization of a male fetus. Its teratogenic potential is particularly important because spironolactone can lead to a resumption of ovulation in women with PCOS.[117]

2. Cyproterone Acetate

The antiandrogen cyproterone acetate is highly effective in the treatment of acne and hirsutism. It also competitively inhibits intracellular androgen receptor function, but it has only 18.6% of the activity of spironolactone. The decrease in LH-dependent androgen synthesis is attributed to the progestational activity of cyproterone and the EE that is administered with it to provide contraception and further suppress LH. This drug is not available in the U.S., despite its apparent safe use in Europe. Because it is a progestin, large doses can suppress the hypothalamic-pituitary-adrenal axis. In approximately 10% of patients, the drug is discontinued because it causes fatigue, weight gain, and loss of libido. A clinical response in hirsutism may be expected to occur in 50–90% of patients roughly 2–3 months after cyproterone acetate is started. The relapse rate 6 months after withdrawal of the drug ranges from 40–80%. Acne and seborrhea improve in approximately 60% of patients. It is also teratogenic because of its antiandrogenic actions, and it is always administered in combination with EE in premenopausal women.

3. Flutamide

Flutamide is a pure antiandrogen that is used primarily in the medical management of prostate cancer. Preliminary clinical trials in hirsutism using 100 mg a day have been promising. Dosages of 250 mg a day have resulted in decreased hirsutism and the resumption of ovulatory menses in adolescents with PCOS. Side effects include liver toxicity, and case reports of hepatic failure leading to transplantion or death have been reported in men and in at least one woman administered flutamide for hirsutism.[118] Flutamide is not FDA approved for the treatment of hirsutism. Given this safety profile, flutamide should be considered only for women in whom all other therapies have failed.

G. Other Agents

1. 5α-Reductase Inhibitors

Without binding to the androgen receptor, 5α-reductase inhibitors block the conversion of testosterone to DHT. However, there are at least two different isoforms of the 5α-reductase enzyme that are differentially distributed in androgen-sensitive tissues. For example, finasteride was developed for the treatment of prostate hypertrophy, and it was not thought to affect skin 5α-reductase significantly. Recent studies demonstrate that finasteride has an efficacy similar to that of 100 mg/day spironolactone for the treatment of hirsutism.[115] These agents are also teratogenic because they cross the placenta and inhibit fetal 5α-reductase activity, potentially resulting in ambiguous genitalia in a male fetus. These agents are not FDA approved for the treatment of hirsutism.

2. Ketoconazole

Technically, the antifungal agent ketoconazole is not an antiandrogen because it blocks the synthesis of androgens through the suppression of P450-dependent adrenal and gonadal enzymes such as P450c17. This results in a reduction in serum testosterone levels, whereas 17-hydroxyprogesterone levels increase. Ketoconazole is not FDA approved for the treatment of hirsutism. However, in a study of 9 hirsute women treated with 400–1200 mg/day, clinical improvement was apparent at 6 months.[119] Low-dose therapy (400 mg a day) is recommended after a 1-month induction period on 1200 mg a day. Untoward effects include nausea, pruritus, and hepatocellular dysfunction.

3. GnRH Agonists (GnRHa)

Long-acting GnRH agonists decrease LH secretion (and, therefore, LH-dependent androgen secretion) by producing gonadotropin desensitization. GnRHa may be used in women in whom primary therapy with oral contraceptive pills or antiandrogens fails. When nafarelin acetate was administered to 6 hirsute women as a nasal spray at a dosage of 500 μg twice daily, biochemical control occurred in 4 of the women within 1–3 months.[120] This drug also may be useful for women with idiopathic hirsutism because it decreases androgen delivery to target tissue. Indeed, it was as effective as high-dose cyproterone acetate in one study.[51] An important side effect of these agents is osteoporosis because both estrogen and androgen levels are decreased. The major limitation is that GnRHa treatment is expensive, costing up to $400–500 per month. The FDA has not approved GnRHa for the treatment of hyperandrogenism. Osteoporosis may be minimized by supplementation with a low-dose estrogen preparation and periodic progesterone withdrawal.[121, 122]

4. Cimetidine

Cimetidine is a weak androgen receptor antagonist. A controlled clinical study has not found cimetidine to be effective in the treatment of hyperandrogenism.[123, 124]

5. Insulin-Lowering and Insulin-Sensitizing Agents

Troglitazone and metformin lower biologically available testosterone levels by approximately 25% in women with PCOS.[77, 78, 125] Testosterone reduction correlates with and apparently depends upon the reduction in insulin levels.[57] While it is reasonable to expect that this improvement in hyperandrogenemia will also be associated with an improvement in hirsutism, this remains to be documented in prolonged trials. Resumption of ovulation has been reported in women receiving these agents alone or in combination with clomiphene citrate.[125] Metformin is not consistently effective at lowering insulin levels in PCOS.[126] Few studies have been conducted on troglitazone in PCOS,[127–130] but preliminary data suggest that troglitazone may improve the ovulatory dysfunction, hirsutism, hyperandrogenemia, and insulin resistance of PCOS in a dose-related fashion, with a minimum of adverse effects. Metformin can cause lactic acidosis in persons with compromised renal function, and it commonly causes gastrointestinal side effects such as nausea and diarrhea, but these usually do not lead to discontinuation of the drug among patients with PCOS. Troglitazone is well tolerated, but it has been associated with several cases of fatal hepatic necrosis. It is unknown whether this hepatic failure can be predicted by surveillance of liver function tests. Neither of these agents is FDA approved for use in hyperandrogenism.

Finally, evidence suggests that some actions of insulin are mediated by putative inositolphosphoglycan (IPG) mediators, also known as second messengers. Insulin may stimulate ovarian androgen production via the IPG signaling system, thereby increasing thecal androgen biosynthesis. In support of this concept, administration of D-chiro-inositol has been suggested in an attempt to improve glucose tolerance, decrease serum androgens, and improve ovulation in PCOS.[131]

6. Ovarian Surgery

In 1939, after removing wedges of ovarian tissue for pathologic analysis, Stein and Cohen observed that ovulatory function and regular menses were restored in all seven patients, and two even became pregnant.[132] For years, ovarian wedge resection via laparotomy was standard therapy for infertile women with PCOS, until it was observed that though ovulation was restored, postoperative adhesions replaced hormonal with mechanical infertility.[133, 134] Ovarian wedge resection results in transient decreases in androgen levels.[135] Thus, this procedure is used only as a last resort in infertile women and not for control of hyperandrogenism. Oophorectomy may be considered to manage women with tumors or for those in whom pharmacologic therapy has failed or is contraindicated.

The success of ovulation-inducing agents has virtually eliminated the use of ovarian wedge resection surgery. Newer surgical techniques such as ovarian drilling (Figure 24.5) often provide temporary results but do not address the underlying metabolic disturbances in patients with polycystic ovary syndrome. A significant percentage of women who undergo ovarian cautery or laser vaporization via laparoscopic techniques have spontaneous restoration of ovulation with subsequent pregnancy, but postoperative complications, including adhesion formation, continue to overshadow the potential benefits of these surgical interventions.[82, 101] Most authors, therefore, now agree that a surgical approach should not be the first line of treatment for PCOS. However, in a woman who has failed to become pregnant with both clomiphene and gonadotropins, operative management may be a viable option alone or as an adjunct to medical therapy.

7. Dopamine Agonists

Although a unique approach to lowering LH might be feasible through dopamine enhancement, placebo-controlled trials have shown that bromocriptine is no more effective than placebo in controlling hyperandrogenism.[136]

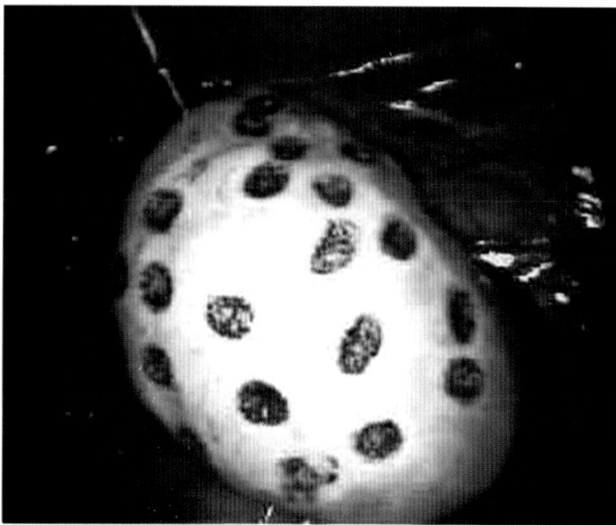

FIGURE 24.5 Ovarian Drilling. A Laparoscopic view following ovarian cautery using a monopolar needle for the surgical management of clomiphene citrate resistant anovulation in a patient with Polycystic ovarian syndrome.

IX. SUMMARY

Understanding the pathophysiology of PCOS and consequently its management has evolved significantly over the last sixty years. Treatment options have become more sophisticated and not only have pregnancy rates risen, but great strides have been made to counter the long-term deletrious effects on the health of women with PCOS. As we gain further insight into the pathophysiology of this complicated syndrome, including elucidating the roles of insulin resistance, insulin-like growth factors, and inhibins, our management techniques should be broadened as well as fine tuned. Newer drugs will be studied and developed, and existing drugs will be purified and produced at lower cost. As much as possible, our goal should be to replace anecdotal practices with evidence-based medicine derived from well-designed, randomized controlled studies. The commitment to minimize harm must stand side by side with the commitment to advance research and technological expertise as we strive to achieve optimal long-term outcome in patients with PCOS.

In conclusion, PCOS is a complex disorder with several potential mechanisms of action. It is a disease that may involve multiple organ systems. PCOS appears to be influenced by genetic and environmental factors, and its evaluation and management therefore requires a detail-oriented approach.

References

1. Franks, S., Adams, J., Mason, H., and Polson, D. (1985). Ovulatory disorders in women with polycystic ovary syndrome. *Clin. Obstet. Gynaecol.* 12(3), 605–632.
2. Yen, S. S., Vela, P., and Rankin, J. (1970). Inappropriate secretion of follicle-stimulating hormone and luteinizing hormone in polycystic ovarian disease. *J. Clin. Endocrinol. Metab.* 30(4), 435–442.
3. Franks, S. (1995). Polycystic ovary syndrome. *N. Engl. J. Med.* 333(13), 853–861.
4. Hull, M. G. (1987). Epidemiology of infertility and polycystic ovarian disease: Endocrinological and demographic studies. *Gynecol. Endocrinol.* 1(3), 235–245.
5. Bachmann, G. A. (1998). Polycystic ovary syndrome: Metabolic challenges and new treatment options. *Am. J. Obstet. Gynecol.* 179(6 Pt 2), S87–S88.
6. Parisi, L., Tramonti, M., Derchi, L. E., Casciano, S., Zurli, A., and Rocchi, P. (1984). Polycystic ovarian disease: Ultrasonic evaluation and correlations with clinical and hormonal data. *J. Clin. Ultrasound* 12(1), 21–26.
7. Swanson, M., Sauerbrei, E. E., and Cooperberg, P. L. (1981). Medical implications of ultrasonically detected polycystic ovaries. *J. Clin. Ultrasound* 9(5), 219–222.
8. Polson, D. W., Mason, H. D., Saldahna, M. B., and Franks, S. (1987). Ovulation of a single dominant follicle during treatment with low-dose pulsatile follicle stimulating hormone in women with polycystic ovary syndrome. *Clin. Endocrinol.(Oxf)* 26(2), 205–212.
9. Adams, J., Polson, D. W., and Franks, S. (1986). Prevalence of polycystic ovaries in women with anovulation and idiopathic hirsutism. *Br. Med. J. (Clin. Res. Ed.)* 293(6543), 355–359.
10. Polson, D. W., Sagle, M., Mason, H. D., Adams, J., Jacobs, H. S., and Franks, S. (1986). Ovulation and normal luteal function during LHRH treatment of women with hyperprolactinaemic amenorrhoea. *Clin. Endocrinol. (Oxf)* 24(5), 531–537.
11. Polson, D. W., Adams, J., Wadsworth, J., and Franks, S. (1988). Polycystic ovaries—a common finding in normal women. *Lancet* 1(8590), 870–872.
12. Dunaif, A., Segal, K. R., Futterweit, W., and Dobrjansky, A. (1989). Profound peripheral insulin resistance, independent of obesity, in polycystic ovary syndrome. *Diabetes* 38(9), 1165–1174.
13. Ehrmann, D. A., Barnes, R. B., and Rosenfield, R. L. (1995). Polycystic ovary syndrome as a form of functional ovarian hyperandrogenism due to dysregulation of androgen secretion. *Endocr. Rev.* 16(3), 322–353.
14. Barbieri, R. L. (1991). Polycystic ovarian disease. *Annu. Rev. Med.* 42, 199–204.
15. Robinson, S., Kiddy, D., Gelding, S. V., Willis, D., Niththyananthan, R., Bush, A. *et al.* (1993). The relationship of insulin insensitivity to menstrual pattern in women with hyperandrogenism and polycystic ovaries. *Clin. Endocrinol. (Oxf)* 39(3), 351–355.
16. Dahlgren, E., Janson, P. O., Johansson, S., Lapidus, L., and Oden, A. (1992). Polycystic ovary syndrome and risk for myocardial infarction. Evaluated from a risk factor model based on a prospective population study of women. *Acta Obstet. Gynecol. Scand.* 71(8), 599–604.
17. Barbieri, R. L. (1990). Hyperandrogenic disorders. *Clin. Obstet. Gynecol.* 33(3), 640–654.
18. Yen, S. S., Vela, P., Rankin, J., and Littell, A. S. (1970). Hormonal relationships during the menstrual cycle. *JAMA* 211(9), 1513–1517.
19. Taylor, A. E., McCourt, B., Martin, K. A., Anderson, E. J., Adams, J. M., Schoenfeld, D. *et al.* (1997). Determinants of abnormal gonadotropin secretion in clinically defined women with polycystic ovary syndrome. *J. Clin. Endocrinol. Metab.* 82(7), 2248–2256.
20. Waldstreicher, J., Santoro, N. F., Hall, J. E., Filicori, M., and Crowley, W. F., Jr. (1988). Hyperfunction of the hypothalamic-pituitary axis in women with polycystic ovarian disease: Indirect evidence for partial gonadotroph desensitization. *J. Clin. Endocrinol. Metab.* 66(1), 165–172.
21. Laughlin, G. A., and Yen, S. S. (1996). Nutritional and endocrine-metabolic aberrations in amenorrheic athletes. *J. Clin. Endocrinol. Metab.* 81(12), 4301–4309.
22. Morales, A. J., Laughlin, G. A., Butzow, T., Maheshwari, H., Baumann, G., and Yen, S. S. (1996). Insulin, somatotropic, and luteinizing hormone axes in lean and obese women with polycystic ovary syndrome: Common and distinct features. *J. Clin. Endocrinol. Metab.* 81(8), 2854–2864.

23. Voutilainen, R., Franks, S., Mason, H. D., and Martikainen, H. (1996). Expression of insulin-like growth factor (IGF), IGF-binding protein, and IGF receptor messenger ribonucleic acids in normal and polycystic ovaries. *J. Clin. Endocrinol. Metab.* 81(3), 1003-1008.
24. Zumoff, B., Freeman, R., Coupey, S., Saenger, P., Markowitz, M., and Kream, J. (1983). A chronobiologic abnormality in luteinizing hormone secretion in teenage girls with the polycystic-ovary syndrome. *N. Engl. J. Med.* 309(20), 1206–1209.
25. Faure, N., and Lemay, A. (1988). Acute pituitary-ovarian response during chronic luteinizing hormone-releasing hormone agonist administration in polycystic ovarian syndrome. *Clin. Endocrinol. (Oxf)* 29(4), 403–410.
26. Erickson, G. F., Hsueh, A. J., Quigley, M. E., Rebar, R. W., and Yen, S. S. (1979). Functional studies of aromatase activity in human granulosa cells from normal and polycystic ovaries. *J. Clin. Endocrinol. Metab.* 49(4), 514–519.
27. Mason, H., and Franks, S. (1997). Local control of ovarian steroidogenesis. *Baill. Clin. Obstet. Gynaecol.* 11(2), 261–279.
28. White, D., Leigh, A., Wilson, C., Donaldson, A., and Franks, S. (1995). Gonadotrophin and gonadal steroid response to a single dose of a long-acting agonist of gonadotrophin-releasing hormone in ovulatory and anovulatory women with polycystic ovary syndrome. *Clin. Endocrinol. (Oxf)* 42(5), 475–481.
29. Fauser, B. C., and Van Heusden, A. M. (1997). Manipulation of human ovarian function: Physiological concepts and clinical consequences. *Endocr. Rev.* 18(1), 71–106.
30. Conway, G. S., Honour, J. W., and Jacobs, H. S. (1989). Heterogeneity of the polycystic ovary syndrome: Clinical, endocrine and ultrasound features in 556 patients. *Clin. Endocrinol. (Oxf)* 30(4), 459–470.
31. Hall, J. E. (1993). Polycystic ovarian disease as a neuroendocrine disorder of the female reproductive axis. *Endocrinol. Metab. Clin. N. Am.* 22(1), 75–92.
32. Balen, A. H. (1993). Hypersecretion of luteinizing hormone and the polycystic ovary syndrome. *Hum. Reprod.* 8 Suppl. 2, 123–128.
33. Balen, A. H., and Jacobs, H. S. (1994). A prospective study comparing unilateral and bilateral laparoscopic ovarian diathermy in women with the polycystic ovary syndrome. *Fertil. Steril.* 62(5), 921–925.
34. Azziz, R., Black, V., Hines, G. A., Fox, L. M., and Boots, L. R. (1998). Adrenal androgen excess in the polycystic ovary syndrome: Sensitivity and responsivity of the hypothalamic-pituitary-adrenal axis. *J. Clin. Endocrinol. Metab.* 83(7), 2317–2323.
35. Lobo, R. A., and Goebelsmann, U. (1980). Adult manifestation of congenital adrenal hyperplasia due to incomplete 21-hydroxylase deficiency mimicking polycystic ovarian disease. *Am. J. Obstet. Gynecol.* 138(6), 720–726.
36. Lucky, A. W., Rosenfield, R. L., McGuire, J., Rudy, S., and Helke, J. (1986). Adrenal androgen hyperresponsiveness to adrenocorticotropin in women with acne and/or hirsutism: Adrenal enzyme defects and exaggerated adrenarche. *J. Clin. Endocrinol. Metab.* 62(5), 840–848.
37. Moghetti, P., Tosi, F., Castello, R., Magnani, C. M., Negri, C., Brun, E. *et al.* (1996). The insulin resistance in women with hyperandrogenism is partially reversed by antiandrogen treatment: Evidence that androgens impair insulin action in women. *J. Clin. Endocrinol. Metab.* 81(3), 952–960.
38. Moghetti, P., Castello, R., Negri, C., Tosi, F., Spiazzi, G. G., Brun, E. *et al.* (1996). Insulin infusion amplifies 17 alpha-hydroxycorticosteroid intermediates response to adrenocorticotropin in hyperandrogenic women: Apparent relative impairment of 17,20-lyase activity. *J. Clin. Endocrinol. Metab.* 81(3), 881–886.
39. Kondoh, Y., Uemura, T., Ishikawa, M., Yokoi, N., and Hirahara, F. (1999). Classification of polycystic ovary syndrome into three types according to response to human corticotropin-releasing hormone. *Fertil. Steril.* 72(1), 15–20.
40. Moran, C., and Azziz, R. (2001). The role of the adrenal cortex in polycystic ovary syndrome. *Obstet. Gynecol. Clin. N. Am.* 28(1), 63–75.
41. Hughesdon, P. E. (1982). Morphology and morphogenesis of the Stein-Leventhal ovary and of so- called "hyperthecosis." *Obstet. Gynecol. Surv.* 37(2), 59–77.
42. Mori, Y., Hasumi, F., Ito, A., Shiina, K., and Hirakawa, S. (1984). Collagen and glycosaminoglycans in the human ovarian capsule with polycystic ovarian disease. *Gynecol. Obstet. Invest.* 18(5), 244–251.
43. Adams, J., Franks, S., Polson, D. W., Mason, H. D., Abdulwahid, N., Tucker, M. *et al.* (1985). Multifollicular ovaries: Clinical and endocrine features and response to pulsatile gonadotropin releasing hormone. *Lancet* 2(8469–70), 1375–1379.
44. Battaglia, C., Genazzani, A. D., Salvatori, M., Giulini, S., Artini, P. G., Genazzani, A. R. *et al.* (1999). Doppler, ultrasonographic and endocrinological environment with regard to the number of small subcapsular follicles in polycystic ovary syndrome. *Gynecol. Endocrinol.* 13(2), 123–129.
45. Dolz, M., Osborne, N. G., Blanes, J., Raga, F., Abad-Velasco, L., Villalobos, A. *et al.* (1999). Polycystic ovarian syndrome: Assessment with color Doppler angiography and three-dimensional ultrasonography. *J. Ultrasound Med.* 18(4), 303–313.
46. Lass, A., and Brinsden, P. (1999). The role of ovarian volume in reproductive medicine. *Hum. Reprod. Update* 5(3), 256–266.
47. Haney, A. F. (1987). Endocrine and anatomical correlations in human ovarian pathology. *Environ. Health Perspect.* 73, 5–14.
48. Nagamani, M., Van Dinh, T., and Kelver, M. E. (1986). Hyperinsulinemia in hyperthecosis of the ovaries. *Am. J. Obstet. Gynecol.* 154(2), 384–389.
49. Laatikainen, T., Apter, D., Andersson, B., and Wahlstrom, T. (1983). Follicular fluid steroid levels and ovarian steroid secretion in polycystic ovarian disease. *Eur. J. Obstet. Gynecol. Reprod. Biol.* 16(4), 283–291.
50. O'Driscoll, J. B., Mamtora, H., Higginson, J., Pollock, A., Kane, J., and Anderson, D. C. (1994). A prospective study of the prevalence of clear-cut endocrine disorders and polycystic ovaries in 350 patients presenting with hirsutism or androgenic alopecia. *Clin. Endocrinol. (Oxf)* 41(2), 231–236.
51. Carmina, E., Wong, L., Chang, L., Paulson, R. J., Sauer, M. V., Stanczyk, F. Z. *et al.* (1997). Endocrine abnormalities in ovulatory women with polycystic ovaries on ultrasound. *Hum. Reprod.* 12(5), 905–909.
52. Scarpitta, A. M., and Sinagra, D. (2000). Polycystic ovary syndrome: An endocrine and metabolic disease. *Gynecol. Endocrinol.* 14(5), 392–395.
53. Ditkoff, E. C., Fruzzetti, F., Chang, L., Stancyzk, F. Z., and Lobo, R. A. (1995). The impact of estrogen on adrenal androgen sensitivity and secretion in polycystic ovary syndrome. *J. Clin. Endocrinol. Metab.* 80(2), 603–607.
54. Sahin, Y., and Kelestimur, F. (1997). 17-Hydroxyprogesterone responses to gonadotrophin-releasing hormone agonist buserelin and adrenocorticotrophin in polycystic ovary syndrome: Investigation of adrenal and ovarian cytochrome P450c17alpha dysregulation. *Hum. Reprod.* 12(5), 910–913.
55. Sahin, Y., Ayata, D., and Kelestimur, F. (1997). Lack of relationship between 17-hydroxyprogesterone response to buserelin testing and hyperinsulinemia in polycystic ovary syndrome. *Eur. J. Endocrinol.* 136(4), 410–415.
56. Ehrmann, D. A., Rosenfield, R. L., Barnes, R. B., Brigell, D. F., and Sheikh, Z. (1992). Detection of functional ovarian hyperandrogenism in women with androgen excess. *N. Engl. J. Med.* 327(3), 157–162.
57. Dunaif, A. (1997). Insulin resistance and the polycystic ovary syndrome: Mechanism and implications for pathogenesis. *Endocr. Rev.* 18(6), 774–800.
58. Crosignani, P. G., and Nicolosi, A. E. (2001). Polycystic ovarian disease: Heritability and heterogeneity. *Hum. Reprod. Update* 7(1), 3–7.
59. Govind, A., Obhrai, M. S., and Clayton, R. N. (1999). Polycystic ovaries are inherited as an autosomal dominant trait: Analysis of 29 polycystic ovary syndrome and 10 control families. *J. Clin. Endocrinol. Metab.* 84(1), 38–43.
60. Knochenhauer, E. S., Key, T. J., Kahsar-Miller, M., Waggoner, W., Boots, L. R., and Azziz, R. (1998). Prevalence of the polycystic ovary

syndrome in unselected black and white women of the southeastern United States: A prospective study. *J. Clin. Endocrinol. Metab.* 83(9), 3078–3082.

61. Carey, A. H., Chan, K. L., Short, F., White, D., Williamson, R., and Franks, S. (1993). Evidence for a single gene effect causing polycystic ovaries and male pattern baldness. *Clin. Endocrinol. (Oxf)* 38(6), 653–658.
62. Carey, A. H., Waterworth, D., Patel, K., White, D., Little, J., Novelli, P. *et al.* (1994). Polycystic ovaries and premature male pattern baldness are associated with one allele of the steroid metabolism gene CYP17. *Hum. Mol. Genet.* 3(10), 1873–1876.
63. Gharani, N., Waterworth, D. M., Batty, S., White, D., Gilling-Smith, C., Conway, G. S. *et al.* (1997). Association of the steroid synthesis gene CYP11a with polycystic ovary syndrome and hyperandrogenism. *Hum. Mol. Genet.* 6(3), 397–402.
64. Mantzoros, C. S., Dunaif, A., and Flier, J. S. (1997). Leptin concentrations in the polycystic ovary syndrome. *J. Clin. Endocrinol. Metab.* 82(6), 1687–1691.
65. Franks, S., Gharani, N., Waterworth, D., Batty, S., White, D., Williamson, R. *et al.* (1997). The genetic basis of polycystic ovary syndrome. *Hum. Reprod.* 12(12), 2641–2648.
66. Legro, R. S., Driscoll, D., Strauss, J. F., 3rd, Fox, J., and Dunaif, A. (1998). Evidence for a genetic basis for hyperandrogenemia in polycystic ovary syndrome. *Proc. Natl. Acad. Sci. USA* 95(25), 14956–14960.
67. Legro, R. S., Spielman, R., Urbanek, M., Driscoll, D., Strauss, J. F., 3rd, and Dunaif, A. (1998). Phenotype and genotype in polycystic ovary syndrome. *Recent Prog. Horm. Res.* 53, 217–256.
68. Urbanek, M., Legro, R. S., Driscoll, D. A., Azziz, R., Ehrmann, D. A., Norman, R. J. *et al.* (1999). Thirty-seven candidate genes for polycystic ovary syndrome: Strongest evidence for linkage is with follistatin. *Proc. Natl. Acad. Sci. USA* 96(15), 8573–8578.
69. Odunsi, K., and Kidd, K. K. (1999). A paradigm for finding genes for a complex human trait: Polycystic ovary syndrome and follistatin. *Proc. Natl. Acad. Sci. USA* 96(15), 8315–8317.
70. Myers, L. E., Silva, S. V., Procunier, J. D., and Little, P. B. (1993). Genomic fingerprinting of "*Haemophilus somnus*" isolates by using a random-amplified polymorphic DNA assay. *J. Clin. Microbiol.* 31(3), 512–517.
71. Buyalos, R. P., Geffner, M. E., Bersch, N., Judd, H. L., Watanabe, R. M., Bergman, R. N. *et al.* (1992). Insulin and insulin-like growth factor-I responsiveness in polycystic ovarian syndrome. *Fertil. Steril.* 57(4), 796–803.
72. Chang, R. J., Nakamura, R. M., Judd, H. L., and Kaplan, S. A. (1983). Insulin resistance in nonobese patients with polycystic ovarian disease. *J. Clin. Endocrinol. Metab.* 57(2), 356–359.
73. DeFronzo, R. A., and Ferrannini, E. (1991). Insulin resistance. A multifaceted syndrome responsible for NIDDM, obesity, hypertension, dyslipidemia, and atherosclerotic cardiovascular disease. *Diabetes Care* 4(3), 173–194.
74. Nestler, J. E., Barlascini, C. O., Matt, D. W., Steingold, K. A., Plymate, S. R., Clore, J. N. *et al.* (1989). Suppression of serum insulin by diazoxide reduces serum testosterone levels in obese women with polycystic ovary syndrome. *J. Clin. Endocrinol. Metab.* 68(6), 1027–1032.
75. Nestler, J. E., and Jakubowicz, D. J. (1996). Decreases in ovarian cytochrome P450c17 alpha activity and serum free testosterone after reduction of insulin secretion in polycystic ovary syndrome. *N. Engl. J. Med.* 335(9), 617–623.
76. Nestler, J. E., and Jakubowicz, D. J. (1997). Lean women with polycystic ovary syndrome respond to insulin reduction with decreases in ovarian P450c17 alpha activity and serum androgens. *J. Clin. Endocrinol. Metab.* 82(12), 4075–4079.
77. Dunaif, A., Scott, D., Finegood, D., Quintana, B., and Whitcomb, R. (1996). The insulin-sensitizing agent troglitazone improves metabolic and reproductive abnormalities in the polycystic ovary syndrome. *J. Clin. Endocrinol. Metab.* 81(9), 3299–3306.
78. Velazquez, E. M., Mendoza, S., Hamer, T., Sosa, F., and Glueck, C. J. (1994). Metformin therapy in polycystic ovary syndrome reduces hyperinsulinemia, insulin resistance, hyperandrogenemia, and systolic blood pressure, while facilitating normal menses and pregnancy. *Metabolism* 43(5), 647–654.
79. Steppan, C. M., Bailey, S. T., Bhat, S., Brown, E. J., Banerjee, R. R., Wright, C. M., Patel, H. R., Ahima, R. S., and Lazar, M. A. (2001). The hormone resistin links obesity to diabetes. *Nature* 409, 307–312.
80. Talbott, E., Guzick, D., Clerici, A., Berga, S., Detre, K., Weimer, K. *et al.* (1995). Coronary heart disease risk factors in women with polycystic ovary syndrome. *Arterioscler. Thromb. Vasc. Biol.* 15(7), 821–826.
81. Ron, E., Lunenfeld, B., Menczer, J., Blumstein, T., Katz, L., Oelsner, G. *et al.* (1987). Cancer incidence in a cohort of infertile women. *Am. J. Epidemiol.* 125(5), 780–790.
82. Goudas, V. T., and Dumesic, D. A. (1997). Polycystic ovary syndrome. *Endocrinol. Metab. Clin. N. Am.* 26(4), 893–912.
83. Gibson, M. (1995). Reproductive health and polycystic ovary syndrome. *Am. J. Med.* 98(1A), 67S–75S.
84. Burkman, R. T., Jr. (1995). The role of oral contraceptives in the treatment of hyperandrogenic disorders. *Am. J. Med.* 98(1A), 130S–136S.
85. Rose, P. G. (1996). Endometrial carcinoma. *N. Engl. J. Med.* 335(9), 640–649.
86. Konishi, I., Koshiyama, M., Mandai, M., Kuroda, H., Yamamoto, S., Nanbu, K. *et al.* (1997). Increased expression of LH/hCG receptors in endometrial hyperplasia and carcinoma in anovulatory women. *Gynecol. Oncol.* 65(2), 273–280.
87. Longcope, C. (1986). Adrenal and gonadal androgen secretion in normal females. *Clin. Endocrinol. Metab.* 15(2), 213–228.
88. Longcope, C., Baker, R., and Johnston, C. C., Jr. (1986). Androgen and estrogen metabolism: Relationship to obesity. *Metabolism* 35(3), 235–237.
89. Ragonesi, F. P., Lo Mastro, F., Arena, V., and Ermini, M. (1995). Treatment of female hyperandrogenism: Estroprogestinic therapy at low dose in an inversal sequential scheme. *Acta Eur. Fertil.* 26(4), 141–143.
90. Ichikawa, Y., Asai, M., Masahashi, T., Wu, M. C., Ohsawa, M., Narita, O. *et al.* (1988). [Clinical assessment of body hair growth in Japanese women. The relationship between a grade of hirsutism and the menstrual status]. *Nippon Sanka Fujinka Gakkai Zasshi* 40(11), 1719–1724.
91. Carmina, E., Koyama, T., Chang, L., Stanczyk, F. Z., and Lobo, R. A. (1992). Does ethnicity influence the prevalence of adrenal hyperandrogenism and insulin resistance in polycystic ovary syndrome? *Am. J. Obstet. Gynecol.* 167(6), 1807–1812.
92. Futterweit, W. (1998). Endocrine therapy of transsexualism and potential complications of long-term treatment. *Arch. Sex. Behav.* 27(2), 209–226.
93. Wild, R. A. (1995). Obesity, lipids, cardiovascular risk, and androgen excess. *Am. J. Med.* 98(1A), 27S–32S.
94. Birdsall, M. A., Farquhar, C. M., and White, H. D. (1997). Association between polycystic ovaries and extent of coronary artery disease in women having cardiac catheterization. *Ann. Intern. Med.* 126(1), 32–35.
95. Lucky, A. W., McGuire, J., Rosenfield, R. L., Lucky, P. A., and Rich, B. H. (1983). Plasma androgens in women with acne vulgaris. *J. Invest. Dermatol.* 81(1), 70–74.
96. Lucky, A. W. (1983). Endocrine aspects of acne. *Pediatr. Clin. N. Am.* 30(3), 495–499.
97. Aiman, J., Forney, J. P., and Parker, C. R. (1986). Androgen and estrogen secretion by normal and neoplastic ovaries in premenopausal women. *Obstet. Gynecol.* 68(3), 327–332.
98. Balen, A. H., Tan, S. L., MacDougall, J., and Jacobs, H. S. (1993). Miscarriage rates following in vitro fertilization are increased in women with polycystic ovaries and reduced by pituitary desensitization with buserelin. *Hum. Reprod.* 8(6), 959–964.
99. Hughes, E. G., Fedorkow, D. M., Daya, S., Sagle, M. A., Van de Koppel, P., and Collins, J. A. (1992). The routine use of gonadotropin-releasing hormone agonists prior to in vitro fertilization and gamete intrafallopian transfer: A meta-analysis of randomized controlled trials. *Fertil. Steril.* 58(5), 888–896.

100. Pettigrew, R., and Hamilton-Fairley, D. (1997). Obesity and female reproductive function. *Br. Med. Bull.* 53(2), 341–358.
101. Kiddy, D. S., Hamilton-Fairley, D., Bush, A., Short, F., Anyaoku, V., Reed, M. J. *et al.* (1992). Improvement in endocrine and ovarian function during dietary treatment of obese women with polycystic ovary syndrome. *Clin. Endocrinol.(Oxf)* 36(1), 105–111.
102. Lobo, R. A., Paul, W., March, C. M., Granger, L., and Kletzky, O. A. (1982). Clomiphene and dexamethasone in women unresponsive to clomiphene alone. *Obstet. Gynecol.* 60(4), 497–501.
103. Lobo, R. A., Granger, L. R., Davajan, V., and Mishell, D. R., Jr. (1982). An extended regimen of clomiphene citrate in women unresponsive to standard therapy. *Fertil. Steril.* 37(6), 762–766.
104. Lobo, R. A., Gysler, M., March, C. M., Goebelsmann, U., and Mishell, D. R., Jr. (1982). Clinical and laboratory predictors of clomiphene response. *Fertil. Steril.* 37(2), 168–174.
105. Hamilton-Fairley, D., Kiddy, D., Watson, H., Sagle, M., and Franks, S. (1991). Low-dose gonadotrophin therapy for induction of ovulation in 100 women with polycystic ovary syndrome. *Hum. Reprod.* 6(8), 1095–1099.
106. Dale, O., Tanbo, T., Lunde, O., and Abyholm, T. (1993). Ovulation induction with low-dose follicle-stimulating hormone in women with the polycystic ovary syndrome. *Acta Obstet. Gynecol. Scand.* 72(1), 43–46.
107. Wood, G. P., and Boronow, R. C. (1976). Endometrial adenocarcinoma and the polycystic ovary syndrome. *Am. J. Obstet. Gynecol.* 124(2), 140–142.
108. Chuang, J. T., and Woeppel, C. J. (1971). Endometrial carcinoma associated with Stein-Leventhal syndrome. *N. Y. State J. Med.* 71(11), 1231–1234.
109. Wild, R. A., Umstot, E. S., Andersen, R. N., Ranney, G. B., and Givens, J. R. (1983). Androgen parameters and their correlation with body weight in one hundred thirty-eight women thought to have hyperandrogenism. *Am. J. Obstet. Gynecol.* 146(6), 602–606.
110. Korytkowski, M. T., Mokan, M., Horwitz, M. J., and Berga, S. L. (1995). Metabolic effects of oral contraceptives in women with polycystic ovary syndrome. *J. Clin. Endocrinol. Metab.* 80(11), 3327–3334.
111. Korytkowski, M. T., Berga, S. L., and Horwitz, M. J. (1995). Comparison of the minimal model and the hyperglycemic clamp for measuring insulin sensitivity and acute insulin response to glucose. *Metabolism* 44(9), 1121–1125.
112. Spritzer, P., Billaud, L., Thalabard, J. C., Birman, P., Mowszowicz, I., Raux-Demay, M. C. *et al.* (1990). Cyproterone acetate versus hydrocortisone treatment in late-onset adrenal hyperplasia. *J. Clin. Endocrinol. Metab.* 70(3), 642–646.
113. Erenus, M., Yucelten, D., Gurbuz, O., Durmusoglu, F., and Pekin, S. (1996). Comparison of spironolactone-oral contraceptive versus cyproterone acetate-estrogen regimens in the treatment of hirsutism. *Fertil. Steril.* 66(2), 216–219.
114. Erenus, M., Gurbuz, O., Durmusoglu, F., Demircay, Z., and Pekin, S. (1994). Comparison of the efficacy of spironolactone versus flutamide in the treatment of hirsutism. *Fertil. Steril.* 61(4), 613–616.
115. Erenus, M., Yucelten, D., Durmusoglu, F., and Gurbuz, O. (1997). Comparison of finasteride versus spironolactone in the treatment of idiopathic hirsutism. *Fertil. Steril.* 68(6), 1000–1003.
116. Rittmaster, R. S. (1999). Antiandrogen treatment of polycystic ovary syndrome. *Endocrinol. Metab. Clin. N. Am.* 28(2), 409–421.
117. Evron, S., Shapiro, G., and Diamant, Y. Z. (1981). Induction of ovulation with spironolactone (Aldactone) in anovulatory oligomenorrheic and hyperandrogenic women. *Fertil. Steril.* 36(4), 468–471.
118. Wysowski, D. K., Freiman, J. P., Tourtelot, J. B., Horton, M. L., 3rd. (1993). Fatal and nonfatal hepatotoxicity associated with flutamide. *Ann. Intern. Med.* 118(11), 860–864.
119. Martikainen, H., Heikkinen, J., Ruokonen, A., and Kauppila, A. (1988). Hormonal and clinical effects of ketoconazole in hirsute women. *J. Clin. Endocrinol. Metab.* 66(5), 987–991.
120. Andreyko, J. L., Bhavnani, B. R., Nisker, J. A., Walker, W. H., and Woolever, C. A. (1986). Role of serum androgens and sex hormone binding globulin capacity in the evaluation of hirsutism in women. *Clin. Biochem.* 19(1), 58–61.
121. Rittmaster, R. S. (1995). Clinical review 73: Medical treatment of androgen-dependent hirsutism. *J. Clin. Endocrinol. Metab.* 80(9), 2559–2563.
122. Rittmaster, R. S. (1995). Gonadotropin-releasing hormone (GnRH) agonists and estrogen/progestin replacement for the treatment of hirsutism: Evaluating the results. *J. Clin. Endocrinol. Metab.* 80(12), 3403–3405.
123. Bednarek-Tupikowska, G., Milewicz, A., Bohdanowicz-Pawlak, A., Bidzinska, B., and Szymczak, J. (1993). [Treatment of hyperandrogenic manifestations in polycystic ovary syndrome]. *Pol. Tyg. Lek.* 48(27–28), 620–623.
124. Loy, R., and Seibel, M. M. (1988). Evaluation and therapy of polycystic ovarian syndrome. *Endocrinol. Metab. Clin. N. Am.* 17(4), 785–813.
125. Nestler, J. E., Jakubowicz, D. J., Evans, W. S., and Pasquali, R. (1998). Effects of metformin on spontaneous and clomiphene-induced ovulation in the polycystic ovary syndrome. *N. Engl. J. Med.* 338(26), 1876–1880.
126. Crave, J. C., Fimbel, S., Lejeune, H., Cugnardey, N., Dechaud, H., and Pugeat, M. (1995). Effects of diet and metformin administration on sex hormone-binding globulin, androgens, and insulin in hirsute and obese women. *J. Clin. Endocrinol. Metab.* 80(7), 2057–2062.
127. Azziz, R., Ehrmann, D., Legro, R. S., Whitcomb, R. W., Hanley, R., Fereshetian, A. G. *et al.* (2001). Troglitazone improves ovulation and hirsutism in the polycystic ovary syndrome: A multicenter, double blind, placebo-controlled trial. *J. Clin. Endocrinol. Metab.* 86(4), 1626–1632.
128. Ehrmann, D. A. (1998). Attenuation of hyperinsulinemia in polycystic ovary syndrome: What are the options? *J. Endocrinol. Invest.* 21(9), 632–635.
129. Cavaghan, M. K., Ehrmann, D. A., Byrne, M. M., and Polonsky, K. S. (1997). Treatment with the oral antidiabetic agent troglitazone improves beta cell responses to glucose in subjects with impaired glucose tolerance. *J. Clin. Invest.* 100(3), 530–537.
130. Ehrmann, D. A., Schneider, D. J., Sobel, B. E., Cavaghan, M. K., Imperial, J., Rosenfield, R. L. *et al.* (1997). Troglitazone improves defects in insulin action, insulin secretion, ovarian steroidogenesis, and fibrinolysis in women with polycystic ovary syndrome. *J. Clin. Endocrinol. Metab.* 82(7), 2108–2116.
131. Nestler, J. E., Jakubowicz, D. J., and Iuorno, M. J. (2000). Role of inositolphosphoglycan mediators of insulin action in the polycystic ovary syndrome. *J. Pediatr. Endocrinol. Metab.* 13(Suppl. 5), 1295–1298.
132. Stein, I., and Cohen, M. (1939). Surgical treatment of bilateral polycystic ovaries—amenorrhea and sterility. *Am. J. Obstet. Gynecol.* 38, 465–480.
133. Toaff, R., Toaff, M. E., and Peyser, M. R. (1976). Infertility following wedge resection of the ovaries. *Am. J. Obstet. Gynecol.* 124(1), 92–96.
134. Weinstein, D., and Polishuk, W. Z. (1975). The role of wedge resection of the ovary as a cause for mechanical sterility. *Surg. Gynecol. Obstet.* 141(3), 417–418.
135. Katz, M., Carr, P. J., Cohen, B. M., and Millar, R. P. (1978). Hormonal effects of wedge resection of polycystic ovaries. *Obstet. Gynecol.* 51(4), 437–444.
136. Buvat, J., Buvat-Herbaut, M., Marcolin, G., Racadot, A., Fourlinnie, J. C., Beuscart, R. *et al.* (1986). A double blind controlled study of the hormonal and clinical effects of bromocriptine in the polycystic ovary syndrome. *J. Clin. Endocrinol. Metab.* 63(1), 119–124.

CHAPTER

25

General Concepts of Endocrine Manipulation of Assisted Reproduction

SOZOS J. FASOULIOTIS
Department of Obstetrics and Gynecology
Hebrew University–Hadassah Medical Center
Jerusalem, 91120, Israel

NERI LAUFER
Department of Obstetrics and Gynecology
Hebrew University–Hadassah Medical Center
Jerusalem, 91120, Israel

I. OVULATION INDUCTION: AN OVERVIEW

The goal of "controlled ovarian hyperstimulation" (COH) for ovulation induction for the assisted reproductive technologies (ART) is to develop several mature eggs in the hopes that at least one will result in pregnancy.[1] This aim can be accomplished in a number of ways using medications, either singly or in combination (Table 25.1).

Clomiphene citrate (CC) binds to the estrogen receptor and exhibits both agonist and antagonist properties.[2] Patients using CC require little monitoring. It is given orally for 5 days in the early follicular phase, and generally causes ovulation 7 days after the last dose via a spontaneous LH surge in a "closed loop" feedback.

Human menopausal gonadotropins (hMG) are drugs, which contain equal concentrations of LH and FSH (Pergonal®, Serono, Randolph, MA; Humegon®, Organon, West Orange, NJ) or contain purified FSH (Metrodin®, Serono, Randolph, MA) alone, or highly purified urinary FSH (u-hFSH HP, Metrodin HP, Serono Laboratories, Aubonne, Switzerland). Until recently, all available human FSH pharmaceutical preparations were extracted from postmenopausal urine. However, biotechnology has made available a recombinant preparation of FSH (rFSH) for medical use. Intramuscular injection of hMG begins in the early follicular phase and is continued daily until follicular development is judged to be adequate. Human chorionic gonadotropin (hCG) is then administered to mimic the native LH surge and cause ovulation. HMG causes direct stimulation of follicular development on the ovary itself. HMG can be administered in excess. This is an example of an "open loop" feedback system where the body cannot control or limit further ovarian stimulation since it is being administered exogenously. To avoid excessive ovarian stimulation the growth and development of ovarian follicles are carefully monitored by serial transvaginal ultrasonography, and frequent serum E_2 sampling.

Gonadotropin releasing hormone (GnRH) also referred to as luteinizing releasing hormone (LHRH) can be used to induce follicular development given intravenously or subcutaneously in a pulsatile fashion. It stimulates the synthesis and release of LH and FSH [3] from the anterior pituitary gland. This is used when patients lack native pulsatile GnRH activity or lack a functional hypothalamic-pituitary portal system, which prevents delivery of endogenous GnRH to the pituitary (Table 25.2).

Native GnRH is a decapeptide with a half-life of 2 min; however, it can be altered chemically to produce long-acting agonists. When GnRH agonists are first administered, the pituitary responds by releasing both LH and FSH (flare-up effect). However, continued administration over time causes GnRH receptor downregulation, pituitary desensitization, and a fall in gonadotropin levels, and the ovary

TABLE 25.1 Medications Used for Controlled Ovarian Hyperstimulation

1. Clomiphene citrate
2. Human menopausal gonadotropins, hMG (menotropins)
    a. Pergonal®; Humegon®; Menogon®- FSH/LH
    b. Metrodin®- FSH
    c. Metrodin HP®- highly purified FSH
3. Recombinant FSH
    a. Gonal-F®
    b. Puregon®
4. Human chorionic gonadotropin, hCG
5. Gonadotropin releasing hormone (GnRH)
6. Gonadotropin releasing hormone agonist (GnRHa)
7. Gonadotropin releasing hormone antagonist
    a. Ganirelix®
    b. Cetrorelix®
8. Growth hormone (GH)

TABLE 25.2 Candidates for Pulsatile GnRH Therapy

1. Absence of native GnRH pulsation
    Kallman's syndrome
    Hypothalamic lesion
2. Hypothalamic amenorrhea
    Weight loss
    Exercise
    Stress induced
    Anorexia nervosa
3. Pituitary stalk transection

becomes dormant.[4–6] Thus, a pharmacologic yet reversible hypophysectomy can be achieved.[7] GnRH agonists are commonly used with hMG for COH for ART. The agonists can be administered by intramuscular or subcutaneous injection or by intranasal spray.[8]

Growth hormone (GH) increases ovarian levels of insulin-like growth factor I (IGF-I), which enhances the action of gonadotropins on the developing follicle.[9]

Finally, GnRH antagonists are compounds that directly inhibit the release of pituitary gonadotropins and do not cause release of hormone stores prior to suppression. With the first generation of GnRH antagonists, allergic side effects due to induced histamine release hampered the clinical development of these compounds. However, modern GnRH antagonists such as Cetrorelix (Cetrotide®, Asta-Medica, Dresden, Germany) and Ganirelix (Orgalutran®, NV Organon, Oss, The Netherlands) appeared to have resolved these problems and, thus, have become available for medical use in ovulation induction protocols.

TABLE 25.3 Indications for Medical Induction of Ovulation

1. Oligo/anovulation
2. Empiric therapy
    Endometriosis
    Male Factor
    Unexplained Infertility
3. Assisted reproductive technology(ART)
    In Vitro Fertilization (IVF)
    Gamete Intrafallopian Transfer (GIFT)
    Zygote Intrafallopian Transfer (ZIFT)

Each medication regimen also imparts a different set of risks and benefits that can be tailored to the situation at hand.

Medical induction of ovulation can be performed for any of several indications (Table 25.3). When the ovaries of women with oligo/anovulation, or those of women undergoing empiric therapy are stimulated for ovulation induction, the physician cannot control the actual number of oocytes that are released for potential fertilization.

The approach to COH for ART, like *in vitro* fertilization (IVF) and gamete intrafallopian transfer (GIFT), differs markedly from ordinary ovulation induction, based on the degree of ovarian stimulation. Patients undergoing IVF or GIFT can have large numbers of oocytes recruited without undue fear of high-order pregnancies because the number of oocytes or embryos returned to her can be controlled. The physician can choose to return 3 or 4 of these embryos to the patient and cryopreserve the remaining embryos for transfer at a later date. Whereas ordinary medical induction of ovulation is therefore directed toward developing a few mature oocytes, COH for ART begins with the goal of developing the maximum number of mature oocytes.

II. CLOMIPHENE CITRATE

Clomiphene citrate (CC), an orally active, nonsteroidal triphenylethylene derivative [10–11] was approved for clinical use in 1967 (Fig. 25.1). CC alone was commonly prescribed for ovulation induction in the early and mid-1980s.[12–14] CC acts by binding to the estrogen receptor; in some tissues this results in pro-estrogenic effect and in others it exhibits a distinctly anti-estrogenic effect [Table 25.4]. However, serum LH elevation may occur during the early follicular phase,[15] which may impair fertilization,[16–18] and cause subclinical pregnancy loss.[19] Approximately 80% of those receiving the drug can be expected to ovulate.[20]

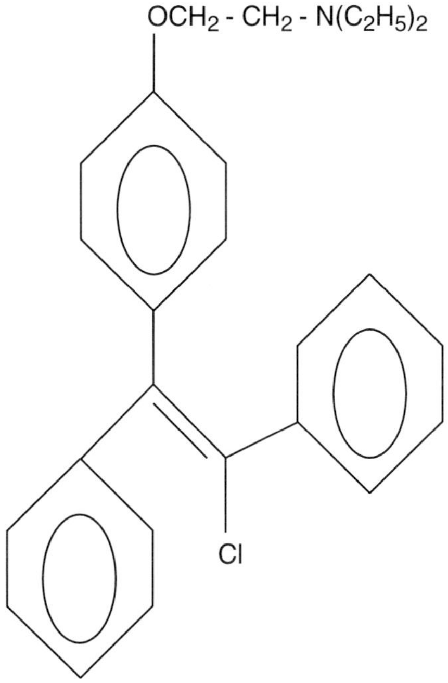

FIGURE 25.1 The molecular structure of clomiphene.

Adding human menopausal gonadotropin to CC resulted in an increase of follicles and oocytes retrieved,[21–24] however, the antiestrogenic effects persisted on mucus production.[25] The combined use of CC and hMG accounted for 21.2% of all stimulation protocols for assisted reproduction in 1988.[26] Furthermore, this combination is often used as a second-line treatment, with encouraging results, for low responders in assisted reproduction.[27]

One other persistent problem was the occurrence of an LH surge prior to the achievement of adequate follicular development resulting in resumption of meiosis [28] and granulosa and theca cell luteinization [29–30] with production of progesterone [31] and endometrial transformation. Inadequate oocyte development prevents the gamete from being fertilized and therefore a "premature" LH surge cancels the cycle. The 13% clinical pregnancy rate for IVF-ET and the 31% rate for GIFT achieved with CC/hMG must be viewed, therefore, in light of the 32% cycle cancellation rate. CC/hMG was used in only 8.5% of all stimulation protocols for ART in 1990.[32]

On the basis of the theory that hyperinsulinemia impedes ovulation and may be an important contributor to the pathophysiology of polycystic ovarian syndrome (PCOS), a new therapeutic option for PCOS women and infertility has been proposed, and includes the use of insulin sensitizers (metformin, and possibly rosiglitazone and pioglitazone) with or without CC. It is postulated that insulin sensitizers might improve the endocrine imbalances associated with PCOS, resulting in an increase in ovulatory menstrual cycles and pregnancy. Recent research suggests that metformin may increase the number of ovulatory cycles in women with PCOS especially in conjunction with clomiphene, however, additional randomized studies are needed to confirm the beneficial effect of insulin sensitizers on ovulation and pregnancy rates among women with PCOS.[33]

TABLE 25.4 Sites of Action and Effects of Clomiphene Citrate

Site	Estrogenic	Antiestrogenic
Hypothalamus		Vaitukaitis [102]
Pituitary	Czygan [103]	Vaitukaitis [102]
	Hashimoto [104]	
	Ravid [105]	
Ovary		Laufer [106, 107]
		Marut [108]
		Nakano [109]
		Westfahl [110]
Endometrium	Clark [111]	Kokko [112]
		Wall [113]
		Kistner [114]
		Van Campenhout [115]
		Lamb [116]
		Yen [117]
		Garcia [118]
		Belasch [119]
Cervix		Riley [120]
		Lamb [121]
		Maxson [122]
		Van Campenhout [115]
Vagina	Natrajan [123]	Pildes [125]
	Markus [124]	Van Campenhout [115]
Bone	Beall [126]	
	Goulding [127]	
	Stewart [128]	

III. HUMAN MENOPAUSAL GONADOTROPINS

HMG, sometimes called menotropins, are available in ampules containing 75 IU of LH and 75 IU of FSH or as 150 IU of purified FSH. HMG acts to stimulate follicular development directly. Intramuscular injection of hMG begins on menstrual cycle day 3 and is continued daily until follicular development is judged to be adequate by serial serum E_2 levels (≥500–1500 pg/ml) and repeated measurement of mean follicular diameter by transvaginal ultrasonography (at least one follicle 14–18 mm).[34–38] A dose of 10,000 IU of hCG should be administered to mimic the native LH surge and cause ovulation once the patient's serum E_2 nears 1000 pg/ml with one or more follicles ≥14–18 mm.

Use of hMG routinely drives the serum E_2 serum concentration well above the natural cycle peak of 300 pg/ml. Those with a low serum E_2 response (≤50 pg/ml) after 5 days of hMG therapy, which routinely corresponds to cycle day 8, had a lower fertilization rate than patients with an initial E_2 of 51–150 pg/ml.[39] A decline in serum E_2 following hCG administration is predictive of a poor cycle outcome.[40–42] The predictive value does not apply when GnRH agonist is added to regimens containing hMG.[43]

An inopportune LH surge which occurs with CC/hMG [44] treatment also arises with hMG alone with late luteal biopsy abnormalities in 27%,[45] and premature luteinization.[46] Since endometrial biopsy is an invasive technique, many investigators have sought noninvasive alternatives for endometrial evaluation.

Transvaginal ultrasonography images the endometrium during monitoring of follicular development. Endometrial thickness on the day after hCG administration of patients who conceived via IVF found no change,[47] or slight thickness to 8.6 mm,[48] or a significant thickness ≥13 mm. Serum E_2 and progesterone (P) levels were not predictive of endometrial thickness.[49]

Endometrial thickness per se did not discriminate between normal and out-of-phase biopsies; however, increased echogenicity may represent stromal edema (Fig. 25.2), which was used to predict histologically normal endometrial development.[50] The most serious complication associated with the use of hMG is the ovarian hyperstimulation syndrome (OHSS). OHSS encompasses a spectrum from mild ovarian enlargement and supraphysiologic serum E_2 and P to a potentially lethal disease marked by massive extravascular exudate accumulation combined with severe intravascular volume depletion, hemoconcentration,[51] increased blood viscocity, coagulation abnormalities, and diminished renal function. Fortunately, the severe form is a rare occurrence, largely due to well-established risk factors (Table 25.5). Of foremost concern are the presence of multiple small (2–8 mm) and intermediate sized (9–15 mm) follicles and elevated serum E_2 concentration above 1500 pg/ml.

Development of the full-blown syndrome is contingent upon either exogenously administered hCG or endogenous, pregnancy-derived hCG stimulation. Exogenous hCG

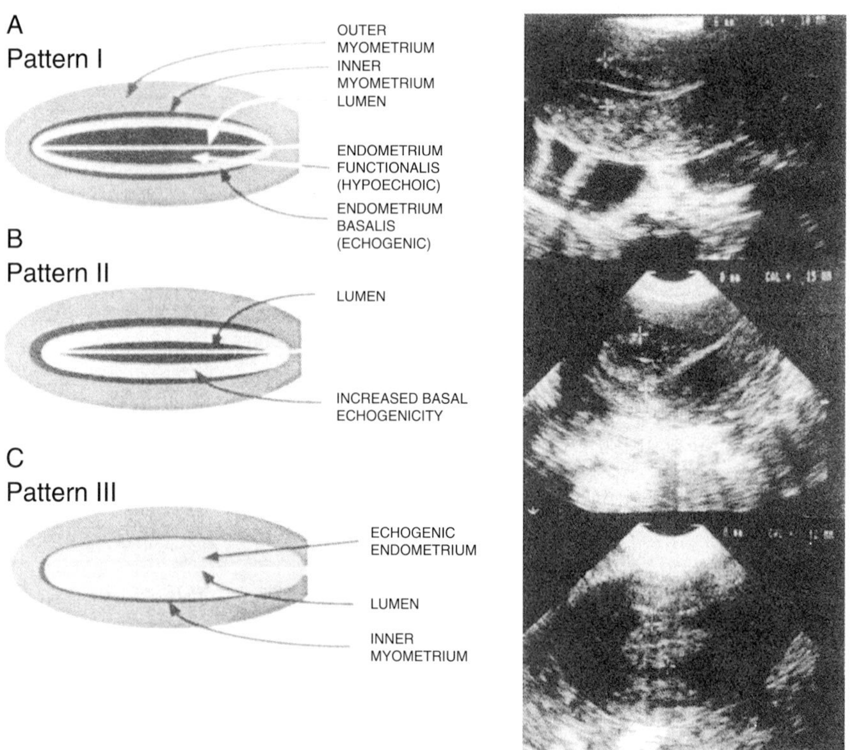

FIGURE 25.2 (A) Pattern I is characteristic of the late follicular phase. The midline echo represents the endometrial lumen. This is surrounded by a hypoechoic area and an echogenic basalis. (B) Pattern II is a transitional phase. There is increased echogenicity of the basalis, but still a hypoechoic functionalis. (C) Pattern III demonstrates echogenicity of the entire functionalis. (From Grunfeld *et al.* (1991). *Obstet. Gynecol.* 78, 200–204.)

TABLE 25.5 Risk Factors for OHSS

Young age (<35 years)
Asthenic habitus
Polycystic Ovary Syndrome
High Serum E_2 (>4000 pg/ml)
Multiple immature and intermediate follicles
"Necklace" sign on Ultrasonography
Luteal hCG supplementation
GnRHa Protocol
Pregnancy

administration may be avoided. Endogenous, pregnancy-derived hCG can also be avoided by advising the patient to abstain form conception during this cycle. Moderate and mild disease can occur even within acceptable guidelines of E_2 concentration and follicle number. The peak effects are seen 7–10 days after hCG administration and generally abate with menses. If pregnancy is achieved, the syndrome may worsen initially and persist for several weeks.

Although the pathophysiology of this syndrome remains unclear, it seems likely that the release of vasoactive substance secreted by the ovaries under hCG stimulation plays a key role in triggering this syndrome. The underlying mechanism responsible for the clinical manifestations of OHSS appears to be an increase in capillary permeability of the ovarian vessels and other mesothelial surfaces. There is a continuous effort to find the exact factors responsible for the increased vascular permeability. Several factors including histamine, serotonin, prostaglandins, prolactin, and a variety of other substances have been implicated in the past. However, only scant data support an important role for any of these factors. Recent evidence suggests that several other factors including the angiotensin-renin cascade, various cytokines such as interleukin-6 (IL-6), interleukin-8 (IL-8), or interleukin-2 (IL-2), tumor necrosis factor (TNF), vascular endothelial growth factor (VEGF), endothelin-I and Von Willebrand factor may play a modulatory role in ovarian physiology and in the pathogenesis of ovarian hyperstimulation syndrome.[52–54]

Since the pathogenesis of OHSS has not been clearly elucidated, management is generally empiric. Pharmacologic therapies have had little effect on its clinical course. The renin-angiotensin system may have a major role in the pathogenesis of OHSS.[55] Angiotensin-converting enzyme inhibitors (ACE) or angiotensin antagonists may ultimately prove to be effective therapeutically. The drawback to ACE inhibitor therapy is its reported harmful effect on early pregnancy.

Patients with moderate ascites and mild hemoconcentration may be treated with bedrest and copious liquid intake while monitoring their urine output, hematocrit, and serum electrolytes, and may be candidates for paracentesis and/or plasma expanders if respiratory or renal function are compromised.

IV. RECOMBINANT FSH

While hMG nay be used as a source of FSH, it has low specific activity and contains significant amounts of LH (as well as other proteins), which is thought to interfere with poor oocyte quality, reduced fertilization rates, lower embryonic viability, and early pregnancy wastage. The development of other urine-derived FSH preparations (urofollitropin and highly purified urofollitropin), which contain significantly reduced or negligible quantities of LH, has resulted in higher pregnancy rates than with hMG. Nevertheless, all urinary-derived preparations have the drawback of requiring the collection of large quantities of urine from multiple donors, leading to variability in supply and, perhaps most importantly, batch-to-batch inconsistency.[56]

Recently, by using recombinant DNA technology, pure recombinant human FSH preparations were produced by inserting the genes encoding for α- and β-subunits of FSH into expression vectors that are transfected into a Chinese hamster ovary cell line. The use of mammalian cells for this purpose is necessary because glycosylation is required to ensure full biological activity of the protein. This technology has three advantages: FSH production is independent of urine collection, a constant FSH supply is ensured, and batch-to-batch consistency can be guaranteed. The highly effective purification process yields FSH preparations with a specific activity of 10,000 IU FSH/mg protein, thus these recombinant products are the most biochemically pure for clinical use, which confer safety and tolerability advantages.[57]

There are two rFSH preparations currently available for clinical use: follitropin alpha (Gonal-F®, Ares-Serono, Geneva, Switzerland) and follitropin beta (Puregon®, NV Organon, Oss, The Netherlands), which are devoid of any LH activity and extraneous human protein. Although both preparations have been developed using the same technique, the posttranslation glycosylation process and purification procedures are not identical. The purification procedure used for follitropin alpha includes the use of immunochromatographic methods, whereas purification of follitropin beta does not involve immunological methods.

Initial clinical studies in IVF established the efficacy and safety of rFSH in stimulating follicular development, with or without concurrent GnRH agonists, and showed that rFSH was at least as effective as uFSH or hMG. Retrospective and prospective comparisons of rFSH with highly purified FSH now suggest that rFSH may be more effective in stimulating follicular development, without any increase in the risk of OHSS. In a multicenter prospective randomized trial, significantly more oocytes were retrieved following controlled ovarian superovulation using Puregon.[58] Similar findings have been reported with the use of Gonal.-F.[59] However, pregnancy rates were not found to differ significantly between recombinant and urinary FSH. Especially, in the multicenter phase 3 trial using Puregon, significantly higher ongoing pregnancy rates were observed after including the transfer of frozen-thawed embryos. From these data, it can be concluded that no differences are observed in the fresh cycles, since only a limited number of embryos are replaced. However, in the presence of a cryopreservation program, the ongoing pregnancy rate is significantly increased after the replacement of frozen-thawed embryos. The rationale for this observation is the presence of more viable and better quality embryos after administering rFSH.

Furthermore, in a recent meta-analysis evaluating recombinant versus urinary FSH in assisted reproduction, the common odds ratio for clinical pregnancy per started cycle, obtained by pooling the data using a fixed-effects model, was 1.20 [95% confidence interval (CI), 1.02–1.42, $p=0.03$] in favor of rFSH. The risk difference represented a 3.7% (95% CI, 0.5–6.9%) increase in clinical pregnancy rate per cycle started with rFSH, compared with uFSH. The overall conclusion from this study was that the use of rFSH in assisted reproduction is preferred over uFSH.[60]

V. GONADOTROPIN RELEASING HORMONE AGONIST (GnRHa)

GnRHa can achieve a pharmacologic and reversible hypophysectomy.[61–64] The use of GnRH agonists in superovulation protocols was first described in 1984. GnRH agonists prevent the untimely pituitary gonadotropin surge in response to rising serum estradiol levels from the multiple ovarian follicles, thereby reducing the chance of spontaneous ovulation and cycle cancellation and allowing continuation of stimulation in cases of asynchronous follicular growth. Other advantages of using GnRHa in ovarian stimulation protocols include improved timing and convenience with regard to oocyte collection and embryo transfer, and simplification of planning for the patient, laboratory staff, and physician.[65]

Pituitary suppression typically requires a minimum of 10 days of GnRHa administration, which may be given on either day 21 or day 3.[66–69] GnRHa is given until suppression down to serum $E_2 < 40$ pg/ml, and then hMG is started electively.

The term "long protocol" with a GnRHa given on the preceding day 21 implies the existence of a "short protocol" (Fig. 25.3). The 'flare-up' or short protocol differs from its long counterpart in that pituitary desensitization is not achieved prior to initiating hMG. In the flare-up protocol, GnRHa is initiated on cycle day 1, or day 2, and hMG is either co-administered from the onset, or begun within the ensuing 2 or 3 days.[70–72] The initial response of the pituitary to GnRHa administration, is the release of its stored LH and FSH. Co-administration of hMG during this phase causes the ovary to perceive an intense stimulatory signal. Continued GnRHa administration, however, is inhibitory and protects against an inopportune spontaneous LH surge.

The choice of a long protocol versus a flare-up protocol for patients entering an IVF program is controversial.[73–74] Several prospective randomized studies have compared short and long protocols, and have shown significantly better results with the long protocol. Results of these studies have been confirmed in a recent meta-analysis, which also confirmed the superiority of the long protocol over the ultrashort protocol. However, evidence suggests that the short protocol may be superior to the long protocol for women who were low responders to ovarian stimulation in previous treatment cycles.[75]

A third variant of GnRHa administration exists. This is the so-called "ultrashort protocol" (Fig. 25.4). GnRHa is administered in only the first 3–4 days of the menstrual cycle

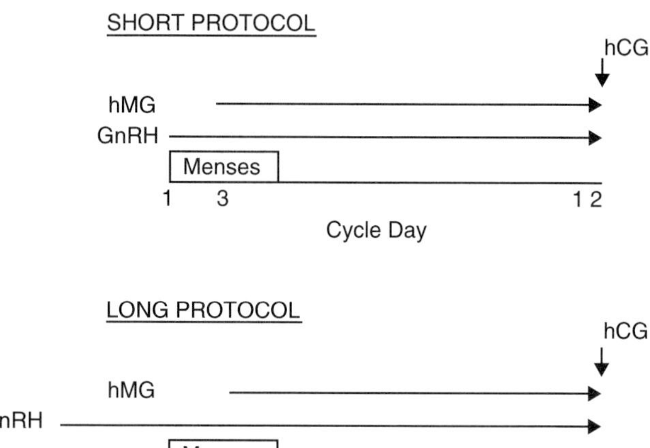

FIGURE 25.3 Schematic representation of two GnRH-agonist protocols. The "short" or "flare-up protocol" introduces GnRH agonist with the onset of menstruation. The "long protocol" calls for administration of GnRH agonist as early as cycle day 21 of the preceding cycle. In this approach, gonadal suppression is achieved prior to addition of hMG.

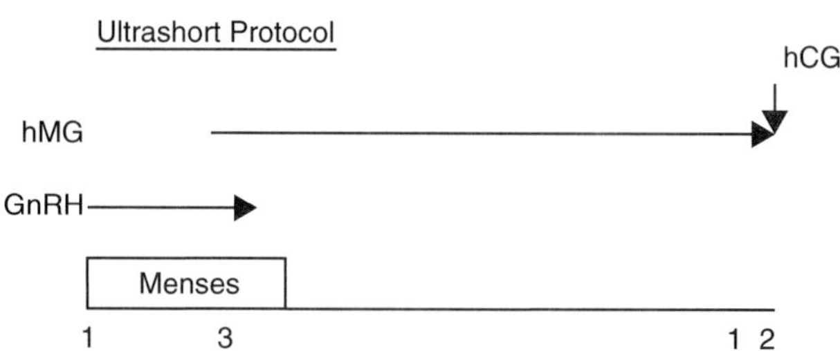

FIGURE 25.4 Schematic representation of the "ultrashort protocol." GnRH agonist is administered during the first 3 or 4 days of the menstrual cycle and then discontinued.

and then discontinued. The effect of this brief exposure to GnRHa may be enough to protect against a premature spontaneous LH surge.[76–77]

Despite reducing premature ovulation with GnRHa and hMG, premature luteinization of the endometrium seen with CC/hMG and hMG alone is not reduced.[78]

IVF cycles stimulated with GnRHa/hMG appear to have an increased incidence of OHSS. Ovarian cysts found at baseline may cause confusion.[80–81]

VI. GONADOTROPIN RELEASING HORMONE ANTAGONISTS

In parallel with the development of GnRH agonists, other analogs were synthesized which also bind to pituitary GnRH receptors but are not functional in inducing the release of gonadotropins. These compounds, the GnRH antagonists, are far more complex than GnRH agonists, with modifications in the molecular structure not only introducing D-amino acids at positions 6 and 10, but also at positions 1, 2, 3, and 8. GnRH antagonists currently in use in ovulation induction include the Cetrorelix (Cetrotide®, Asta-Medica, Dresden, Germany) and the Ganirelix (Orgalutran®, NV Organon, Oss, The Netherlands) (Fig. 25.5).

Significant advantages of GnRH antagonists to GnRH agonists involve their ability of immediately suppressing the pituitary gonadotropins by GnRH receptor competition and permit flexibility in the degree of pituitary-gonadal suppression. Moreover, discontinuation of GnRH antagonist treatment leads to a rapid and predictable recovery of the pituitary-gonadal axis. In women undergoing ovarian stimulation, GnRH antagonist treatment is required for only a few days when a premature LH surge is imminent. Also, in GnRH antagonists' treatment protocols a GnRH agonist may be used to trigger ovulation instead of hCG decreasing thus significantly the cancellation rate and minimizing the risk for developing OHSS.[82]

Initial studies have shown that Cetrorelix has proved to be reliable in preventing the onset of premature LH surges during hMG stimulation, by daily injections (0.25 mg) from 5 or 6 days of stimulation onward or by a single injection (3 mg) on stimulation day 7 (Fig. 25.6). Pregnancy rates of about 30% per transfer seemed to be very promising.[83] Furthermore, in an effort to establish the minimum effective dosage of the GnRH antagonists during ovulation induction multicenter phase 3 studies were performed, which established the safety and efficacy of both Cetrorelix and Ganirelix at its minimum effective dose of 0.2 mg/day according to the multiple-dose protocol.[84] While clinical experience with GnRH antagonists in IVF treatment thus far has been encouraging and demonstrates a high efficacy in preventing the LH surge, several concerns have been raised regarding the safety aspects of GnRH antagonists on extra-pituitary structures such as the ovary, oocyte, granulosa cell, endometrium and embryo, since the discovery of extra-pituitary GnRH receptors in human, may have a possible detrimental effect on implantation rates.[85] Furthermore, comparative trials of GnRH antagonists and agonists have not yet shown a significant advantage of the former. However, it is anticipated that by optimization of the treatment protocol and by specific small dose adjustments to suit individual patient response, GnRH antagonists will be comparable with the agonists in terms of cycle outcome, and will soon be a significant addition to the ART pharmacology arsenal.[86]

VII. GH AND OVULATION INDUCTION

Growth-promoting peptides such as insulin, GH and insulin-like growth factor might have an important role in normal follicular development.

Isolated GH deficiency can delay the onset of puberty.[87] The effect of GH on the ovaries is mediated by somatomedin C, which is similar to insulin (also termed insulin-like

	1	2	3	4	5	6	7	8	9	10
GnRH	pyro-GLU	HIS	TRP	SER	TYR	GLY	LEU	ARG	PRO	Gly-NH2
Cetrorelix	Ac-D-Nal(2)	D-Phe(4Cl)	D/PAL	SER	TYR	D/CIT	LEU	ARG	PRO	D-Ala-NH2
Ganirelix	Ac-D-Nal(2)	D-Phe(4Cl)	D/PAL	SER	TYR	D-hArg(Et2)	LEU	L-hArg(Et2)	PRO	D-Ala-NH2

D-Ala: D-alanine; D/CIT; D-citrulline; D-hArg: D-homoarginine; L-hArg; L-homoarginine; D-Nal; (2-naphthyl)-D-alanine; D/PAL; (3-pyridyl)-D-alanine; D-Phe: D-phenylalanine;

FIGURE 25.5 Structure of GnRH antagonists of the third generation, Cetrorelix and Ganirelix, compared with GnRH itself. Amino acid substitutions have been made at positions 1, 2, 3, 6, 8, and 10.

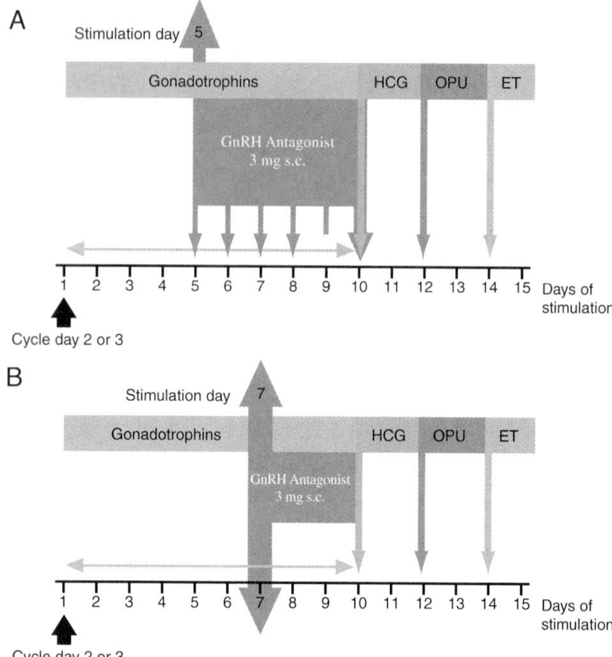

FIGURE 25.6 (A) Multiple dose schedule; (B) Single dose schedule.

growth factor I) and produced by ovarian granulosa cells.[88] Ovarian IGF-I, in addition to FSH and LH, may play an important role in follicular development.[89–94]

GH might act by direct action on GH receptors, by a systemic increase in IGF-I levels or by increasing intraovarian IGF-I (Fig. 25.7).

There is little doubt that IGF-I regardless of origin facilitates or augments the action of gonadotropins on the ovary. The finding that GH may have a direct gonadotropic effect on human granulose cells independent of FSH or IGF-I suggests a physiologic GH seems to be a helpful adjunct in ovulation induction.[95–99]

Most IVF units today use combined long GnRHa/hMG protocols in normal ovulating women [100] to prevent premature ovulation or luteinization and induce better follicular recruitment. The addition of GH did not improve results.[101]

VIII. SUMMARY

We have come to understand that each treatment we prescribe has distinct benefits but also a companion set of liabilities. The combination of medications gives us the ability to modulate our desired effect. We are therefore able to narrowly define the therapeutic goal for a specific patient and select the best available treatment for her. Our knowledge of the events that cause a follicle to develop to maturity continues to evolve. Further understanding of the physiology of oocyte maturation combined with advances in pharmaceuticals will undoubtedly lead to improved treatment options.

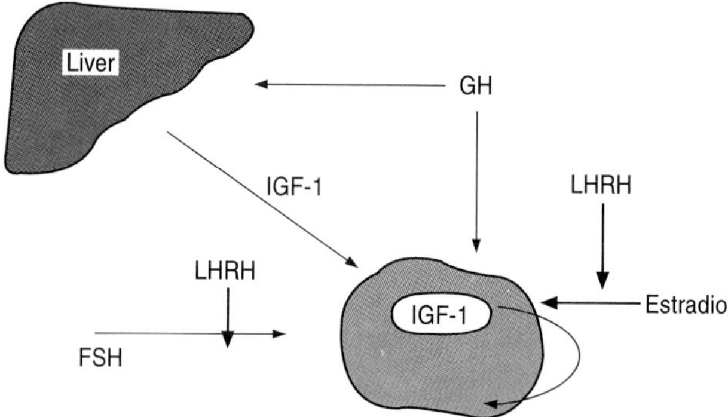

FIGURE 25.7 The effect of growth hormone on IGF-I production.

References

1. Ovulation Drugs: A Guide for Patients. (1990). Birmingham, AL. The American Fertility Society, p. 8.
2. Adashi, E. Y. (1984). Clomiphene citrate: Mechanism(s) and site(s) of action—a hypothesis revisited. *Fertil. Steril.* 42, 331–344.
3. Schriock, E. D., and Jaffe, R. B. (1986). Induction of ovulation with gonadotropin releasing hormone. *Obstet. Gynecol. Surv.* 41, 414–423.
4. Dodson, W. C. (1989). Role of gonadotropin releasing hormone agonists in ovulation induction. *J. Reprod. Med.* 34, 76–80.
5. Moghissi, K. S. (1990). Gonadotropin releasing hormones—clinical applications in gynecology. *J. Reprod. Med.* 35, 1097–1107.
6. Santen, R. J., and Bourguignon, J. P. (1987). Gonadotropin-releasing hormone: Physiological and therapeutic aspects, agonists and antagonists. *Horm. Res.* 28, 88–103.
7. Filicori, M., and Flamigni, C. (1988). GnRH agonists and antagonists current clinical status. *Drugs* 35, 63–82.
8. Penzias, A. S., Shamma, F. N., Gutmann, J. G. *et al.* (1992). Nafarelin versus leuprolide in ovulation induction for in vitro fertilization: A randomized clinical trial. *Obstet. Gynecol.* 79, 739–742.
9. Davoren, J. B., and Hsueh, A. J. W. (1986). Growth hormone increases ovarian levels of immunoreactive somatomedin C/Insulin like growth factor I in vivo. *Endocrinology* 118, 888–890.
10. Allen, R. E., Palopoli, F. P., Schumann, E. L. *et al.* (1959). US Patent 2: 914, 561.
11. Ernst, S., Hite, G., Cantrell, J. S. *et al.* (1976). Stereochemistry of geometric isomers of clomiphene: A correction of the literature and a reexamination of structure–activity relationships. *J. Pharmacol. Sci.* 65, 148–159.
12. Edwards, R. G., Steptoe, P. C., and Purdy, J. M. (1980). Establishing full term human pregnancies using cleaving embryos growth in vitro. *Br. J. Obstet. Gynecol.* 87, 737–743.
13. Fritz, M. A., and Speroff, L. (1982). The endocrinology of the menstrual cycle: The interaction of folliculogenesis and neuroendocrine mechanisms. *Fertil. Steril.* 38, 508–513.
14. Gronow, M. J. (1985). Ovarian hyperstimulation for successful in vitro fertilization and embryo transfer. *Acta Obstet. Gynecol. Scand. Suppl.* 131, 12–14.
15. Shoham, Z., Borenstein, R., Lunenfeld, B. *et al.* (1990). Hormonal profiles following clomiphene citrate therapy in conception and non-conception cycles. *Clin. Endocrinol.* 33, 271–278.

16. Stanger, J. D., and Yovich, J. L. (1985). Reduced in vitro fertilization of human oocytes from patients with raised basal luteinizing hormone levels during the follicular phase. *Br. J. Obstet. Gynecol.* 92, 385–393.
17. Homburg, R., Armar, N. A., Eshel, A. *et al.* (1988). Influence of serum luteinizing hormone concentrations on ovulation, conception and early pregnancy loss in polycystic ovary syndrome. *Br. Med. J.* 297, 1024–1026.
18. Howles, C. M., Macnamee, M. C., Edwards, R. G. *et al.* (1986). Effect of high tonic levels of luteinizing hormone on outcome of in vitro fertilization. *Lancet* ii, 521–522.
19. Bateman, B. G., Kolp, L. A., Nunley, W. C. *et al.* (1992). Subclinical pregnancy loss in clomiphene citrate treated women. *Fertil. Steril.* 57, 25–27.
20. Induction of ovulation. 4th Ed. (1989). *In* "Clinical Gynecologic Endocrinology and Infertility," (L. Speroff, R. H. Glass, and N. G. Kase, eds.), p. 591. Williams & Wilkins, Baltimore, MD.
21. Lopata, A. (1981). Concepts in human in vitro fertilization and embryo transfer. *Fertil. Steril.* 36, 669–673.
22. Marrs, R. P., Vargyas, J. M., Shangold, S. M. *et al.* (1984). The effect of time of initiation of clomiphene citrate on multiple follicle development for human in vitro fertilization and embryo transfer procedures. *Fertil. Steril.* 41, 682–687.
23. Quigley, M. M., Maklad, N. F., and Wolf, D. P. (1983). Comparison of two clomiphene citrate dosage regimens for follicular recruitment in an in vitro fertilization program. *Fertil. Steril.* 40, 178–183.
24. Quigley, M. M., Schmidt, C. L., Beauchamp, P. J. *et al.* (1984). Enhanced follicular recruitment in an in vitro fertilization program: Clomiphene alone versus a clomiphene/human menopausal gonadotropin combination. *Fertil. Steril.* 42, 25–33.
25. Diamond, M. P., Maxson, W. S., Vaughn, W. K. *et al.* (1986). Antiestrogenic effect of clomiphene citrate in a multiple follicular stimulation protocol. *J. In Vitro Fertil. Embryo Transfer* 3, 106–109.
26. Medical Research Internationai and the Society for Assisted Reproductive technology, The American Fertility Society. (1990). In Vitro Fertilization and Embryo Transfer in the United States: 1988 results from the IVF-ET registry. *Fertil. Steril.* 53, 13–19.
27. Fasouliotis, S. J., Simon, A., and Laufer, N. (2000). Evaluation and treatment of low responders in assisted reproductive technology: A challenge to meet. *J. Assist. Reprod. Genet.* 17, 357–373.
28. Catt, K. J., and Dufau, M. L. (1991). Gonadotropic hormones: Biosynthesis, secretion, receptors, and actions. *In* "Reproductive Endocrinology," 3rd Ed. (S. C. C. Yen, and R. B. Jaffe, eds.), pp. 105–155. W. B. Saunders, Philadelphia, PA.
29. WHO Task Force on Methods for the Determination of the Fertile period. (1980). Temporal relationships between ovulation and defined changes in the concentration of plasma estradiol-17β, luteinizing hormone, follicle stimulating hormone and progesterone. *Am. J. Obstet. Gynecol.* 138, 383–390.
30. Collins, W., Jurkovic, D., Bourne, T. *et al.* (1991). Ovarian morphology, endocrine function and intrafollicular blood flow during the peri-ovulatory period. *Hum. Reprod.* 6, 319–324.
31. Yen, S. C. C. (1991). The human menstrual cycle: Neuroendocrine regulation. *In* "Reproductive Endocrinology." 3rd Ed. (S. C. C. Yen, and R. B. Jaffe, eds.), pp. 273–308. W. B. Saunders, Philadelphia, PA.
32. Medical Research International and the Society for Assisted Reproductive technology, The American Fertility Society. (1992). In Vitro Fertilization and Embryo Transfer in the United States: 1990 results from the IVF-ET registry. *Fertil. Steril.* 57, 15–24.
33. Kim, L. H., Taylor, A. E., and Barbieri, R. L. (2000). Insulin sensitizers and polycystic ovary syndrome: Can a diabetes medication treat infertility? *Fertil. Steril.* 73, 1097–1098.
34. Jones, G. E. S. (1984). Update in in-vitro fertilization. *Endocr. Rev.* 1, 62–79.
35. Haining, R. V., Jr., Levin, R. M., Berhman, H. R. *et al.* (1979). Plasma estradiol window and urinary estriol glucuronide determination for monitoring menotropin induction of ovulation. *Obstet. Gynecol.* 54, 442–445.
36. Seibel, M. M., McArdle, C. R., Thompson, I. E. *et al.* (1981). The role of ultrasound in ovulation: A critical appraisal. *Fertil. Steril.* 36, 573–577.
37. Navot, D., Margalioth, E. J., Laufer, N. *et al.* (1987). Periovulatory 17β-estradiol pattern in conception and non-conception cycles during menotropin treatment of anovulatory infertility. *Fertil. Steril.* 47, 234–237.
38. Shapiro, S. S. (1988). Clinical parameters influencing success in IVF. *In* "In Vitro Fertilization and Embryo Transfer, a Manual of Basic Techniques." (D. P. Wolf ed.), pp. 397–398. Plenum Press, New York.
39. Herschlag, A., Asis, M. C., Diamond, M. P. *et al.* (1990). The predictive value and management of cycles with low initial estradiol levels. *Fertil. Steril.* 53, 1064–1067.
40. Laufer, N., DeCherney, A. H., Tarlatzis, B. C. *et al.* (1986). The association between preovulatory serum 17β-estradiol pattern and conception in human menopausal gonadotropin-human chorionic gonadotropin stimulation. *Fertil. Steril.* 46, 73–76.
41. Lopata, A. (1983). Concepts in human in vitro fertilization and embryo transfer. *Fertil. Steril.* 40, 289–301.
42. Jones, H. W., Jr., Acosta, A., Andrews, M. C. *et al.* (1983). The importance of the follicular phase to success and failure in vitro fertilization. *Fertil. Steril.* 40, 317–321.
43. Penzias, A. S., Shamma, F. N., Gutmann, J. N. *et al.* (1992). Luteinizing response to human chorionic gonadotropin does not predict outcome in GnRH agonist/human menopausal gonadotropin stimulated IVF cycles. *J. Assist. Reprod. Genet.* 9, 244–247.
44. Baukloh, V., Fischer, R., Naether, O. *et al.* (1990). Patterns of serum luteinizing hormone surges in stimulated cycles in relation to injections of human chorionic gonadotropin. *Fertil. Steril.* 53, 69–75.
45. Reshef, E., Segars, J. H., Jr., Hill, G. A. *et al.* (1990). Endometrial inadequacy after treatment with human menopausal gonadotropin/human chorionic gonadotropin. *Fertil. Steril.* 54, 1012–1016.
46. Birkenfeld, A., Mor-Joseph, S., Ezra, J. *et al.* (1990). Preovulatory luteinization during induction of follicular maturation with menotrophin and menotrophin-clomiphene combination. *Hum. Reprod.* 5, 561–564.
47. Fleischer, A. C., Herbert, C. M., Sacks, G. A. *et al.* (1986). Sonography of the endometrium during conception and non-conception cycles of in vitro fertilization and embryo transfer. *Fertil. Steril.* 46, 442–447.
48. Gonen, Y., Casper, R. F., Jacobson, W. *et al.* (1989). Endometrial thickness and growth during ovarian stimulation: A possible predictor of implantation in in vitro fertilization. *Fertil. Steril.* 52, 446–450.
49. Rabinowitz, R., Laufer, N., Lewin, A. *et al.* (1986). The value of ultrasonographic endometrial measurement in the prediction of pregnancy following in vitro fertilization. *Fertil. Steril.* 45, 824–828.
50. Grunfeld, L., Walker, B., Bergh, P. A. *et al.* (1991). High-resolution endovaginal ultrasonography of the endometrium: A non-invasive test for endometrial adequacy. *Obstet. Gynecol.* 78, 200–204.
51. Navot, D., Bergh, P. A., and Laufer, N. (1992). Ovarian hyperstimulation syndrome in the new reproductive technologies: Prevention and treatment. *Fertil. Steril.* 58, 249–261.
52. Abramov, Y., Schenker, J. G., Lewin, A., Friedler, S., and Barak, V. (1996). Plasma inflammatory cytokines correlate to the ovarian hyperstimulation syndrome. *Hum. Reprod.* 11, 1381–1386.
53. Abramov, Y., Barak, V., Nisman, B., and Schenker, J. G. (1997). Vascular endothelial growth factor plasma levels correlate to the clinical picture in severe ovarian hyperstimulation syndrome. *Fertil. Steril.* 67, 261–265.
54. Elchalal, U., and Schenker, J. G. (1997). The pathophysiology of ovarian hyperstimulation syndrome-views and ideas. *Hum. Reprod.* 12, 1129–1137.

55. Navot, D., Margalioth, E. J., Laufer, N. *et al.* (1987). Direct correlation between plasma rennin activity and severity of the ovarian hyperstimulation syndrome. *Fertil. Steril.* 48, 57–64.
56. Out, H. J., Bennink, H., and Laat, W. (1999). What are the clinical benefits of recombinant gonadotropins? The development of recombinant FSH (Puregon®): A scientific business. *Hum. Reprod.* 14, 2189–2190.
57. Recombinant Human FSH study Group (1995). Clinical assessment of recombinant human follicle-stimulating hormone in stimulating ovarian follicular development before in vitro fertilization. *Fertil. Steril.* 63, 77–86.
58. Out, H. J., Mannaerts, B. M. J. L., Driessen, S. G. A. J. *et al.* (1995). A prospective, randomized, assessor-blind, multicentre study comparing recombinant and urinary follicle stimulating hormone (Puregon versus Metrodin) in in vitro fertilization. *Hum. Reprod.* 10, 2534–2540.
59. Bergh, C., Howles, C. M., Borg, K. *et al.* (1997). Recombinant human follicle stimulating hormone (r-hFSH; Gonal-F®) versus highly purified urinary FSH (Metrodin HP®): Results of a randomized comparative study in women undergoing assisted reproductive techniques. *Hum. Reprod.* 1997, 2133–2139.
60. Daya, S., and Gunby, J. (1999). Recombinant versus urinary follicle stimulating hormone for ovarian stimulation in assisted reproduction. *Hum. Reprod.* 14, 2207–2215.
61. Dodson, W. C. (1989). Role of gonadotropin releasing hormone agonists in ovulation induction. *J. Reprod. Med.* 34 (Suppl.), 76–80.
62. Moghissi, K. S. (1990). Gonadotropin releasing hormones–clinical applications in gynecology. *J. Reprod. Med.* 35, 1097–1107.
63. Santen, R. J., and Bourguignon, J. P. (1987). Gonadotropin-releasing hormone: Physiological and therapeutic aspects, agonists and antagonists. *Horm. Res.* 28, 88–103.
64. Filiconi, M., and Flamigni, C. (1988). GnRH agonists and antagonists: Current clinical status. *Drugs* 35, 63–82.
65. Laufer, N., Simon, A., Hurwitz, A. *et al.* (1996). In vitro fertilization. *In* "Infertility: A Comprehensive Text," 2nd ed. (M. M. Seibel, ed.), pp. 703–749. Appleton & Lange, Stamford, CT.
66. Porter, R. N., Smith, W., Craft, I. L. *et al.* (1984). Induction of ovulation for IVF using buserelin and gonadotropins. *Lancet* 2, 1284–1288.
67. Pellicer, A., Simon, C., Miro, F. *et al.* (1989). Ovarian response and outcome of IVF in patients treated with GnRH analogues in different phases of the menstrual cycle. *Hum. Reprod.* 4, 285–288.
68. Rosen, G. F., Cassidenti, D. L., Stone, S. C. *et al.* (1992). Comparing mid-luteal and early follicular phase down regulation with leuprolide acetate. Presented at the 40th Annual Meeting of the Pacific Coast Fertility Society, Indian Wells, CA, April 8–12, Abstract P–19.
69. Seifer, D. B., Thornton, K. L., DeCherney, A. H. *et al.* (1991). Early pituitary desensitization and ovarian suppression with leuprolide acetate is associated with in vitro fertilization-embryo transfer success. *Fertil. Steril.* 56, 500–503.
70. Howles, C. M., Macnamee, M. C., Edwards, R. G. *et al.* (1987). Short term use of an LHRH agonist to treat poor responders entering an IVF programme. *Hum. Reprod.* 2, 655–659.
71. Owen, E. J., Davies, M. C., Kingsland, C. R. et al. (1989). The use of a short regimen of buserelin, a GnRH agonist, and hMG in assisted conception cycles. *Hum. Reprod.* 4, 749–755.
72. Matthews, C. D., Warnes, G. M., Norman, R. J. *et al.* (1991). The leuprolide flare regimen for in vitro fertilization/gamete intrafallopian transfer and embryo cryopreservation. *Hum. Reprod.* 6, 817–822.
73. Acharya, U., Small, J., Randall, J. *et al.* (1992). Prospective study of short and long regimens of gonadotropin-releasing agonist in in vitro fertilization program. *Fertil. Steril.* 57, 815–818.
74. Tan, S. L., Kingsland, C., Campbell, S. *et al.* (1992). The long protocol of administration of gonadotropin-releasing hormone agonist is superior to the short protocol for ovarian stimulation for in vitro fertilization. *Fertil. Steril.* 57, 810–814.
75. Buckett, W. M., and Tan, L. S. (1988). Use of GnRH Agonists in Ovulation Induction. *In* " Treatment of Infertility: The New Frontiers" (M. Filicori, and C. Flamigni, eds.), pp. 135–138. Communications Media for Education, New Jersey.
76. Martikainen, H., Ronnberg, L., Tapanainen, J. *et al.* (1990). Endocrine responses to gonadotropins after LHRH agonist administration on cycle days 1–4: Prevention of premature luteinization. *Hum. Reprod.* 5, 246–249.
77. Macnamee, M. C., Howles, C. M., Edwards, R. G. *et al.* (1989). Short term LHRH agonist treatment: Prospective trial of a novel ovarian stimulation regimen for IVF. *Fertil. Steril.* 52, 264–269.
78. Navot, D., Bergh, P. A., Guzman, I. *et al.* (1992). Complete endometrial maturation arrest, a novel abnormality in cycles with hormonal hyperstimulation. Presented at the 39th Annual Meeting of the Society for Gynecological Investigation, San Antonio, TX, March 18–21, Abstract 226.
79. Zeevi, D., Younis, J. S., and Laufer, N. (1991). Ovulation induction—new approaches. *Assist. Reprod. Rev.* 1, 2–8.
80. Penzias, A. S., Jones, E. E., Seifer, D. B. *et al.* (1992). Baseline ovarian cysts do not affect clinical response to controlled ovarian hyperstimulation for in vitro fertilization. *Fertil. Steril.* 57, 1017–1021.
81. Feldberg, D., Ashkenazi, J., Dicker, D. *et al.* (1989). Ovarian cyst formation: A complication of gonadotropin releasing hormone agonist therapy. *Fertil. Steril.* 51, 42–47.
82. Mannaerts, B., and Gordon, K. (2000). Embryo implantation and GnRH antagonists. GnRH antagonists do not activate the GnRH receptor. *Hum. Reprod.* 15, 1882–1883.
83. Felberbaum, R., and Diedrich, K. (1998). Use of GnRH antagonists in ovulation induction. *In* "Treatment of Infertility: The New Frontiers" (M. Filicori, and C. Flamigni, eds.), pp. 135–138. Communications Media for Education, New Jersey.
84. The ganirelix dose-finding group (1998). A double blind, randomized, dose-finding study to assess the efficacy of the gonadotropin-releasing hormone antagonist ganirelix (Org 37462) to prevent premature luteinizing hormone surges in women undergoing ovarian stimulation with recombinant follicle stimulating hormone (Puregon®). *Hum. Reprod.* 13, 3023–3031.
85. Hernandez, R. R. (2000). Embryo implantation: The Rubicon for GnRH antagonists. *Hum. Reprod.* 15, 1211–1216.
86. Kol, S. (2000). Embryo implantation and GnRH antagonists. GnRH antagonists in art: Lower embryo implantation? *Hum. Reprod.* 15, 1881–1882.
87. Steikholislam, B. M., and Stempfel, R. S., Jr. (1972). Hereditary isolated somatotropin deficiency: Effects of human growth hormone administration. *Pediatrics* 49, 362–371.
88. Adashi, E. Y., Resnik, C. E., Hernandez, E. R. *et al.* (1989). Potential relevance of insulin-like growth factor I to ovarian physiology: From basic science to clinical application. *Semin. Reprod. Endocrinol.* 7, 94–101.
89. Adashi, E. Y., Resnik, C. E., D'Ercole, A. J. *et al.* (1985). Insulin-like growth factors as intraovarian regulators of granulose cell growth and function. *Endocr. Rev.* 6, 400–414.
90. Adashi, E. Y., Resnik, C. E., Svoboda, M. E. *et al.* (1986). Follicle-stimulating hormone enhances somatomedin-C binding to cultured rat granulose cell: Evidence of cAMP-dependence. *J. Biol. Chem.* 261, 3923–3928.
91. Hutchinson, L. A., Findlay, J. K., and Herington, A. C. (1988). Growth hormone and insulin-like growth factor I accelerate PMSG induced differentiation of granulose cells. *Mol. Cell. Endocrinol.* 55, 61–71.
92. Adashi, E. Y., Resnik, C. E., Svoboda, M. E. *et al.* (1985). Somatomedin C synergizes with FSH in the acquisition of projection biosynthetic capacity by cultured rat granulose cells. *Endocrinology* 116, 2134–2140.
93. Jia, X. C., Kalmijin, J., and Hseuh, A. J. (1986). Growth hormone enhances follicle stimulating hormone-induced differentiation of cultured rat granulose cells. *Endocrinology* 118, 1401–1419.

94. Erickson, C. F., Gabriel, V. G., and Magoffin, D. A. (1989). Insulin-like growth factor regulates aromatase activity in human granulose and granulose luteal cells. *J. Clin. Endocrinol. Metab.* 69, 716–721.

95. Mason, H. D., Martikainen, H., Beard, R. W. *et al.* (1990). Direct gonadotropic effect of growth hormone on estradiol production by human granulose cells in vitro. *J. Endocrinol.* 126, R1–R4.

96. Homburg, R., Eshel, A., Abdalla, J. I. *et al.* (1988). Growth hormone facilitates ovulation induction by gonadotropins. *Clin. Endocrinol.* 29, 113–119.

97. Owens, E. J., West, C., Torresani, T. *et al.* (1989). Insulin-like growth factors in women receiving growth hormone in addition to clomiphene and human menopausal gonadotropins for IVF-ET. 6th World Congress of In Vitro Fertilization and Alternate Assisted Reproduction. Jerusalem, Israel. April 2–7, p. 28.

98. Volpe, A., Coutkos, G., Barreca, A. *et al.* (1989). Ovarian response to combined growth hormone-gonadotropin treatment in patients resistant to induction of superovulation. *Gynecol. Endocrinol.* 4, 125–131.

99. Menashe, Y., Lunenfeld, B., Pariente, C. *et al.* (1990). Effect of growth hormone on ovarian responsiveness II. Joint Meeting of the European Society of Human Reproduction and Embryology, Milan, Italy, August 29–September 1, Abstract 190.

100. Jacobs, H. S. (1989). Latest development in growth hormone facilitation of ovulation induction. 6th World Congress of In Vitro Fertilization and Alternate Assisted Reproduction. Jerusalem, Israel. April 2–7, p. 11.

101. Younis, J. S., Simon, A., Koren, R. *et al.* (1992). The effect of growth hormone supplementation on in vitro fertilization outcome: A prospective randomized placebo controlled double-blind study. *Fertil. Steril.* 58, 575–580.

102. Vaitukaitis, J. L., Bermudez, J. A., Cargille, C. M. *et al.* (1971). New evidence for an anti-estrogenic action of clomiphene citrate in women. *J. Clin. Endocrinol. Metab.* 32, 503–509.

103. Czygan, P. J., and Schultz, K. D. (1972). Studies on the anti-estrogenic and estrogen like action of clomiphene citrate in women. *Gynecol. Invest.* 3, 126–133.

104. Hashimoto, T., Miyai, K., Izumi, K. *et al.* (1976). Effect of clomiphene citrate on basal and LHRH-induced gonadotropin secretion in post-menopausal women. *J. Clin. Endocrinol. Metab.* 42, 593–601.

105. Ravid, R., Jedwab, G., Persitz, E. *et al.* (1977). Gonadotropin release in ovariectomized patients. Suppression by clomiphene or low doses of ethinylestradiol. *Clin. Endocrinol.* 6, 333–338.

106. Laufer, N., Reich, R., Braw, R. *et al.* (1982). Effect of clomiphene citrate on preovulatory rat follicles in culture. *Biol. Reprod.* 27, 463–471.

107. Laufer, N., Pratt, B. M., DeCherney, A. H. *et al.* (1983). The in vivo and in vitro effects of clomiphene citrate on ovulation, fertilization and development of cultured mouse oocytes. *Am. J. Obstet. Gynecol.* 147, 633–639.

108. Marut, E. L., and Hodgen, G. D. (1982). Antiestrogenic action of high dose clomiphene in primate: Pituitary augmentation but with ovarian attenuation. *Fertil. Steril.* 38, 100–104.

109. Nakano, R., Nakayama, T., Iwao, M. *et al.* (1982). Inhibition of ovarian follicle growth by a chemical antiestrogen. *Horm. Res.* 16, 230–236.

110. Westfahl, P. K. and Resko, J. A. (1983). Effects of clomiphene on luteal function in the nonpregnant cynomologous macaque. *Biol. Reprod.* 29, 963–970.

111. Clark, J. H., McCormack, S. A., Kling, R. *et al.* (1980). Effect of clomiphene and other triphenylethylene derivatives on the reproductive tract in the rat and baboon. *In* "Hormones and Cancer" (S. Jacobelli, R. J. B. King, H. R. Lindner, and M. E. Lippman, eds.), pp. 295–310. Raven Press, New York.

112. Kokko, E., Janne, O., Kauppila, A. *et al.* (1981). Cyclic clomiphene citrate treatment lowers cytosol estrogen and progestin receptor concentrations in the endometrium of postmenopausal women on estrogen replacement therapy. *J. Clin. Endocrinol. Metab.* 52, 345–351.

113. Wall, J. A., Franklin, R. R., and Kaufman, R. H. (1964). Reversal of benign and malignant endometrial changes with clomiphene. *Am. J. Obstet. Gynecol.* 88, 1072–1080.

114. Kistner, R. W., Lewis, J. L., and Steiner, G. J. (1966). Effects of clomiphene citrate on endometrial hyperplasia in the premenopausal female. *Cancer* 19, 115–119.

115. Van Campenhout, J., Simard, R., and Leduc, B. (1968). Antiestrogenic effect of clomiphene in the human being. *Fertil. Steril.* 19, 704.

116. Lamb, B. J., Colliflower, W. W., and Williams, J. W. (1972). Endometrial histology and conception rates after clomiphene citrate. *Obstet. Gynecol.* 39, 389–396.

117. Yen, S. C. C., Vla, P., and Ryan, K. J. (1970). Effect of clomiphene citrate in polycystic ovary syndrome: Relationship between serum gonadotropin and corpus luteum function. *J. Clin. Endocrinol. Metab.* 31, 7–13.

118. Garcia, J., Jones, G. S., and Wentz, A. C. (1977). The use of clomiphene citrate. *Fertil. Steril.* 28, 707–717.

119. Belasch, J., Vanrell, J. A., Duran, M. *et al.* (1983). Luteal phase evaluation after clomiphene–chorionic gonadotropin induced ovulation. *Int. J. Fertil.* 28, 104–109.

120. Riley, G. M., and Evans, T. N. (1964). Effects of clomiphene citrate on anovulatory ovarian function. *Am. J. Obstet. Gynecol.* 89, 97–102.

121. Lamb, B. J., and Guderian, A. M. (1966). Clinical effects of clomiphene on anovulation. *Obstet. Gynecol.* 28, 505–512.

122. Maxson, W. S., Pittaway, D. E., Herbert, C. M. *et al.* (1984). Antiestrogen effect of clomiphene citrate: Correlation with serum estradiol concentrations. *Fertil. Steril.* 42, 356–359.

123. Natrajan, P. K., and Greenblatt, R. B. (1979). Clomiphene citrate: Induction of ovulation. *In* "Induction of Ovulation" (R. B. Greenblatt, ed.), pp. 35–61. Lea & Febiger, Philadelphia, PA.

124. Markus, S. L. (1965). Biologic effects of clomiphene citrate in the castrate Rhesus monkey. *Am. J. Obstet. Gynecol.* 93, 990–995.

125. Pildes, R. B. (1965). Induction of ovulation with clomiphene. *Am. J. Obstet. Gynecol.* 91, 466–471.

126. Beall, P. T., Misra, L. K., Young, R. L. *et al.* (1984). Clomiphene protects against osteoporosis in the mature ovariectomized rat. *Calcif. Tissue Int.* 36, 123–129.

127. Goulding, A., and Fisher, L. (1991). Preventive effects of clomiphene citrate on estrogen deficiency osteopenia elicited by LHRH agonist administration in the rat. *J. Bone Miner. Res.* 6, 1177–1180.

128. Stewart, P. J., and Stern, P. H. (1986). Effects of the antiestrogens tamoxifen and clomiphene on bone resorption in vitro. *Endocrinology* 118, 125–129.

129. Blumenfeld, Z., and Lunenfeld, B. (1989). The potentiating effect of growth hormone on follicle stimulating with human menopausal gonadotropin in a panhypopituitary patient. *Fertil. Steril.* 52, 328–331.

130. Homburg, R., West, C., Torresani, T. *et al.* (1990). Co-treatment with human growth hormone and gonadotropins for induction of ovulation: A controlled trial. *Fertil. Steril.* 53, 254–260.

131. Homburg, R., West, C., Torresani, T. *et al.* (1990). A comparative study of single-dose growth hormone therapy as an adjuvant to gonadotropin treatment for ovulation induction. *Clin. Endocrinol.* 32, 781–785.

132. Volpe, A., Cookos, G., Artini, P. G. *et al.* (1990). Pregnancy following growth hormone-pulsatile GnRH treatment in a patient with hypothalamic amenorrhea. *Hum. Reprod.* 5, 345–347.

133. Burger, H. G., Kovac, G. T., Polson, D. M. *et al.* (1991). Ovarian sensitization to gonadotropin by human growth hormone. *Clin. Endocrinol.* 35, 119–122.

CHAPTER

26

Endometriosis

W. PAUL DMOWSKI

Institute for the Study and Treatment of Endometriosis
Oak Brook, Illinois 60523
and
Rush Medical College
Chicago, Illinois 60612

I. PATHOPHYSIOLOGY, SYMPTOMS, AND DIAGNOSIS

Endometriosis is one of the few disorders with unknown etiology and poorly understood pathogenesis. It primarily affects women in their reproductive years, although it has been described in teenagers shortly after menarche, and in women after menopause. Spontaneous, as well as experimentally induced endometriosis has also been described in several species of menstruating primates. Estrogenic stimulation, but not necessarily menstrual cycles, appears to be the *sine que non* for this disease. Individual reports of lesions histologically similar to endometriosis in men following orchiectomy and treated with estrogens are also on record. The prevalence of endometriosis in the general female population is considered to be in the range of 5–10% and the incidence figure of 0.33% has been quoted.[1] It is considered that approximately 5 million women in the U.S. are affected by this disease.[2] The first reference to symptoms characteristic of endometriosis dates back to 1500 BC, although the term "endometriosis" was introduced relatively recently by Sampson.[3]

A. Pathophysiology

The earliest gross and histologic description of endometriosis dates back to the turn of the 19th century.[4] Advanced endometriotic lesions, typically cystic in character, were at that time common operative findings and were variously described as "adenomyomas," "cystic adenomas," "cystic adenofibromas," "cystomyomas," or "endometriomas"; each term suggesting a neoplastic origin. Indeed, according to the initial concept, endometriosis was considered a form of benign neoplasia and because of its spread pattern, was frequently referred to as "a benign cancer." John Sampson, an American gynecologist who studied endometriosis extensively at the beginning of the 20th century, was the first to indicate that endometriotic lesions cannot be classified as "true tumors" and proposed the term "endometriosis Mullerianosis."[3] Histologic similarity between ectopic and eutopic endometrium was apparent to Sampson. He also demonstrated that endometrial cells and tissue fragments shed during menses are viable and can be identified in the lumen of fallopian tubes. This suggested to Sampson that endometrial cells and tissue fragments are "regurgitated in a retrograde fashion" with the menstrual flow into the peritoneal cavity, where they implant and develop into endometriotic lesions. This concept, subsequently referred to as the Sampson's Theory on Histogenesis of Endometriosis received support from clinical and experimental data and became generally accepted. For more than half a century, it coexisted with the older theory of coelomic metaplasia, which postulated that endometriotic lesions develop through the metaplastic transformation of mesothelial cells, and which also was supported by clinical and experimental evidence. The cause(s) of "retrograde tubal regurgitation" or "metaplastic transformation" and therefore the etiologic factor(s) in the development of endometriosis were, however, less clear. Sampson suggested that the retrograde tubal transport occurs only in some women and invariably leads to the development of endometriosis. To prevent this process it became generally recommended that procedures such as tubal insufflations or hysterosalpingograms should not be performed during menstrual bleeding and for the same reason coitus should also be avoided. Frequent pregnancy-associated periods of amenorrhea were considered to decrease the likelihood of the endometrial shedding and retrograde transport and therefore the risk for development of endometriosis. In the process of metaplasia, a variety of factors, such as infectious stimuli, hormonal secretions, or menstrual toxins were considered to play a role as causative agents.

During the early 1980s, four reports by separate investigators were published demonstrating alterations in both cellular and humoral immunity in women with endometriosis.[5–8] It was proposed that endometriosis may reflect a deficient cell-mediated immunity [7] or alternatively may represent a form of an autoimmune disease.[6, 8] An extensive research on the mechanisms of interaction between eutopic and ectopic endometrial cells and the immune system followed. Available data strongly suggest that eutopic endometrial cells in women with endometriosis may differ from those of healthy controls.[9] At the end of the cycle, in the healthy endometrium just prior to menses, the process of apoptosis or programmed cell death reaches its maximum. Shed endometrial cells, even when misplaced into ectopic locations, are programmed to apoptose, do not survive, and do not implant. In women with endometriosis, endometrial apoptosis at the time of menses is significantly decreased, while proliferation of the endometrial cells, according to *in vitro* studies, is stimulated. Thus in endometriosis, misplaced eutopic endometrial cells can survive and implant when transported to ectopic locations. Furthermore, apoptosis is significantly lower in ectopic than eutopic endometrium, suggesting ectopic preselection of apoptosis-resistant cells.[10]

Apoptosis of the endometrial cells appears to be under the control of endometrial monocytes/macrophages and their secretory products, more specifically TNF-α. It is interesting to note that TNF-α in some cells, and perhaps also in the endometrial cells, may activate apoptosis or alternatively a proliferative/inflammatory response, depending upon specific conditions.[11] It is therefore possible that in women with endometriosis, abnormal signal transduction between monocytes/macrophages and endometrial cells leads to persistent proliferation/inflammation and decreased apoptosis in the eutopic endometrium and that cells with these characteristics survive when misplaced into ectopic locations. In support of this concept, we have demonstrated in the *in vitro* co-culture system that autologous peripheral blood monocytes in women with endometriosis stimulate eutopic endometrial cell proliferation, while a suppressive effect is noted in healthy controls.[12] The same differential effect, depending on the origin of the endometrial cells, was noted when supernatant from the autologous monocyte culture and more interestingly when TNF-α was added to the endometrial cell culture.[13]

Misplaced endometrial cells have been identified, with equal frequency in the peritoneal cavities of women with and without endometriosis and apoptosis could be only one of the factors that prevent their implantation in healthy women. It has also been suggested that misplaced endometrial cells undergo cytotoxic destruction by natural killer (NK) cells, cytotoxic T lymphocytes (CTL) and monocyte/macrophages.[14] In women with endometriosis, ectopic endometrium resists immune cytotoxicity, secretes several immunosuppressive factors, and responds with proliferation to the immune cell products such as TNF-α. Moreover, ectopic endometrial cells in endometriosis produce a variety of growth factors and growth regulatory cytokines contributing to their uncontrolled growth. Growth autonomy of endometriotic cells in some cases, may also be the result of their ability to produce estrogens for their own use and display abnormally estradiol and progesterone receptors.[9]

Activation of the humoral arm of the immune system in women with endometriosis may be a secondary event, a response to the ectopic implantation of the endometrial cells. Abnormal autoantibodies against endometrial cells or cell-derived antigens such as phospholipids, histones, or nucleotides have been demonstrated in about 60% of affected women by several investigators using different assays.[8, 15] These autoantibodies are of IgG, IgA, and IgM isotype and have been identified in the circulation, in follicular and other body fluids, and in tissues. It has been reported that the concentration of these autoantibodies may be higher in stage I and II than stage III and IV endometriosis. The above would suggest that abnormal autoantibodies may play a role in limiting progression of this disease. Abnormal autoantibodies have also been implicated as a cause of infertility and poor reproductive performance associated with endometriosis.

B. Symptoms

Chronic pelvic pain symptoms are characteristic of endometriosis. However, they are not pathognomonic of the disease and may be associated with other pelvic disorders and sometimes without identifiable cause. Chronic pelvic pain is a common gynecological problem accounting for approximately 10% of gynecologic visits, 40% of laparoscopies, and 12% of hysterectomies.[16, 17] A telephone survey of over 5000 women of reproductive age, indicated that 14.7% complained of some form of pelvic pain within the prior 3 months.[18] A variety of gynecologic and nongynecologic disorders may be associated with chronic pelvic pain symptoms. Endometriosis may be diagnosed in 4–65%, depending on the patient's selection criteria and the laparoscopists' experience.[19] In one of such studies, histologically confirmed endometriosis was demonstrated in 32% of women with chronic pelvic pain while other pathologic conditions in an additional 51%.[20] There was no identifiable cause of pelvic symptoms in 17% and in a control group of asymptomatic women undergoing tubal ligation, 15% had endometriosis. In addition to pelvic pains, women with endometriosis may also report symptoms suggesting involvement of other organs, a variety of generalized symptoms without apparent organic cause referred to as "somatizations," and psychological symptoms suggestive of clinical depression. Infertility is also a major problem associated with endometriosis.

1. Chronic Pelvic Pain Symptoms

Chronic pelvic pain symptoms, that is symptoms lasting for more than 6 months, are reported by about 60–96% of women with endometriosis and are frequently described as a triad of dysmenorrhea, pelvic pain unrelated to menstrual bleeding, and dyspareunia. Dysmenorrhea, typically acquired and progressive, is reported by 28–63%, deep dyspareunia by 12–27%, and pelvic pain by 10–30%. The frequency and intensity of pelvic pain symptoms is individually variable and may not be related to the staging of the disease.[21–23] Women with minimal endometriosis may have severe symptoms requiring strong analgesics; while those with severe disease may be asymptomatic. It has been suggested that dysmenorrhea may be related to the number and location of endometriotic implants,[24] while chronic pelvic pains and dyspareunia to deep infiltrating lesions, ovarian endometriomas, and adhesions.[25, 26] In the same patient, pelvic pain symptoms tend to be progressive in character consistent with the progressive nature of the disease. However, as indicated earlier, pelvic pain symptoms may be present in women without endometriosis and asymptomatic women may have endometriotic lesions. According to one study, dysmenorrhea was as prevalent in infertile women with as without endometriosis.[27] Its severity was, however, greater in endometriosis. Pelvic pains was more prevalent only in women with stage III/IV, while deep dyspareunia was prevalent regardless of the disease stage.

2. Symptoms Suggesting Involvement of Other Organs

In addition to the involvement of the reproductive system and pelvic peritoneum, endometriotic lesions may also be present on the serosa of other pelvic organs such as urinary bladder or bowel. Accordingly, in addition to pelvic pain symptoms, other symptoms such as dysuria, pressure on the bladder, intestinal cramps, abdominal pains, or dyschezia may also be present. With extension of the lesions into the urinary or intestinal tract mucosa the patient may experience hematuria or hematochezia usually of a catamenial pattern and at times symptoms of urinary or bowel compression. Endometriotic implants and associated fibrosis may interfere with the bowel function and occasionally nodular endometriosis may partially or completely obstruct the bowel. Accordingly, the patient may present with the symptoms of partial or complete bowel obstruction.[28] Endometriotic lesions in extra pelvic locations may or may not be associated with pelvic endometriosis but usually cause local swelling, bleeding, and a variety of pain symptoms from the affected organs. Typically, the symptoms and findings are exacerbated during the menstrual period. Cyclic dyspnea, pleural effusion, catamenial hemoptysis, or catamenial pneumo- or hemothorax indicate pulmonary endometriosis. Cyclic headaches or seizures may be caused by lesions in the brain. Cyclic pain, tenderness, or swelling are commonly associated with endometriosis in surgical scars of the abdomen, perineum, or vagina, or with umbilical or inguinal endometriosis. Neurologic symptoms and findings of a catamenial pattern, such as low back pain, leg or sciatic pain, sensory loss, leg weakness, and foot drop have been associated with endometriotic lesions in the retroperitoneal space involving or compressing on the nerves, most frequently sciatic.[29–31] The resulting pain symptoms, as well as sensory and motor deficits may be quite diverse. Endometriotic lesions have been described in almost every tissue and organ of the body. We can therefore conclude that regardless of location, any lesion that changes in relation to the menstrual cycle and any symptom of a catamenial pattern should be considered as suggestive of endometriosis.

3. The Mechanism of Pain Symptoms in Endometriosis

The mechanism(s) through which endometriotic lesions cause pain is unclear. It has been suggested that superficial endometriotic lesions release prostaglandins, inflammatory mediators such as kinins, histamine, interleukins, or other noxious agents. Red petechial implants seem to produce higher levels of PgF2α than brown or black lesions [32] and seem to be associated with more pain on palpation.[33] Tender rectovaginal nodules containing endometriotic lesions and fibrotic components often have a close histological relationship to nerve fibers, most likely afferent sympathetic nerves, which transmit painful stimuli to the superior hypogastric plexus, dorsal horn of the spinal cord, and higher levels.[34] A significant number of women with endometriosis complain of debilitating gastrointestinal symptoms such as chronic abdominal pains, nausea, vomiting, bowel hyperactivity, abdominal cramps, bloating and distention, and bouts of diarrhea or constipation which are usually diagnosed as the irritable bowel syndrome (IBS). IBS frequently coincides with endometriosis and it is quite likely that the bowel irritability may be secondary to hemosiderin deposits on the peritoneal surfaces, a typical finding in endometriosis. However, it has also been suggested that women with endometriosis may suffer from a neuromuscular dysfunction of the gastrointestinal tract, which may also involve other hollow viscera including the reproductive system.[35] The authors' postulated that a biochemical imbalance in the eicosanoid system resulting in the abnormal production of PgE2 and PgF2α may be a common factor responsible for both gastrointestinal and reproductive system symptoms. Occasionally, the origin of pelvic pain symptoms is difficult to establish and peripheral neuropathy is suspected. This has been reported when endometriotic lesions or associated fibrosis involving pelvic nerves, or because of the phenomenon of viscerosomatic convergence.[29, 36]

4. Somatizations of Endometriosis

More than 50% of women with endometriosis and chronic pelvic pain report a wide range of general symptoms of a catamenial pattern such as low-grade fever, general malaise, fatigue, dizziness, generalized pains and aches, nausea, vomiting, and diarrhea, which have no apparent organic cause and which typically have been referred to as "somatizations" of endometriosis.[37] However, it is possible that lack of medical explanation for somatizations may only reflect the state of our knowledge. We have demonstrated that peripheral blood monocytes and peritoneal macrophages in women with endometriosis produce at rest and especially when stimulated higher levels of several cytotokines including TNF-α, IL-6, and IL-8, than monocytes of healthy women.[38] Moreover, Karck *et al.* [39] reported in women with endometriosis higher PgE2 and PgF2α release by peritoneal macrophages, suggesting that the same may also apply to the peripheral monocytes. It is therefore possible that at least some of the generalized symptoms associated with endometriosis may be related to abnormal cytokine and prostaglandin production by the peripheral monocytes/macrophages in women this disease. Somatizations are usually associated with an increased risk for major depression and anxiety disorders and many somatizing patients report a history of sexual or physical abuse.[40] Furthermore, one of the characteristic features of chronic pain is psychologic depression. Women with chronic pelvic pain had significantly higher scores using Beck Depression Inventory than asymptomatic women.[41] This is not unusual, considering that patients with chronic pain almost always are clinically depressed and invariably score high when undergoing psychologic testing. Sometimes it is unclear what comes first, the pain or the depression.

5. Infertility

The association between endometriosis and primary or secondary infertility is unclear and frequently questioned. In the general population, the prevalence of infertility is about 15%, but in women with endometriosis it has been estimated at 30–40% although formal studies are lacking. The estimated risk of infertility is 19.5 × greater in women with endometriosis than in those without.[42] However, infertility in women with endometriosis is relative and spontaneous conceptions are known to occur. The probability of conception appears to be inversely related to the severity of the disease. The exact mechanism(s) of infertility in endometriosis are unknown. In severe endometriosis, periovarian and peritubal adhesions and/or ovarian endometriomas interfere mechanically with conception. The effect of mild endometriosis on fertility is, however, controversial. Monthly fecundity rates in women with untreated mild endometriosis undergoing artificial donor insemination were lower by comparison to healthy controls according to some studies [43, 44] but were not different according to others.[45, 46] In minimal or mild endometriosis, several mechanisms of infertility have been suggested and a variety of substances capable of interfering with ovulation, endocrine function, gamete/embryo transport, oocyte fertilization, embryo development, and implantation have been identified.[47] It has been proposed that secretory products of the ectopic endometrial and/or immune cells interfere with the reproductive system and cause infertility. These substances have been variously identified as cytokines, growth factors, prostaglandins, reactive oxygen species, autoantibodies, etc. About 60% of women with endometriosis produce autoantibodies against endometrial cells or cell-derived antigens. These autoantibodies may play a role in the pathogenesis of endometriosis or may alter reproductive performance through the interference with oocyte fertilization and/or embryo implantation. In a retrospective analysis, monthly fecundity in women undergoing donor insemination was 2% when minimal endometriosis was present, as compared to 11% in controls without endometriosis.[43] Another retrospective analysis compared 343 donor insemination cycles in women with stage I/II endometriosis to 212 such cycles in women without endometriosis.[48] It demonstrated similar average monthly fecundity rates in stages I and II endometriosis (5.2 and 6.5%, respectively), significantly below 14% monthly fecundity of controls. Berube *et al.*,[49] in a prospective cohort study evaluated spontaneous conception after diagnostic laparoscopy in minimal or mild endometriosis as compared to unexplained infertility. Spontaneous monthly fecundity rate was 2.52% in endometriosis and 3.48% in unexplained infertility. Collins *et al.* [50] in a cohort of more than 2000 infertile couples followed at 11 clinics for over 1 year, reported on the probability of spontaneous live births according to the diagnostic category. Live birth rate was 0.68% per cycle in stage I/II, 0.1% in stage III/IV, and 0.52% combined live birth rate per cycle in all patients with endometriosis. Altogether, these data indicate that fertility is significantly impaired in women with endometriosis. Average monthly fecundity rates appear to be about 2% in stage I/II and about 1% in stage III/IV endometriosis.

C. Diagnosis

All endometriotic lesions begin with ectopic implantation of misplaced endometrial cells or tissue fragments. This occurs on the peritoneal surfaces, or along the lymphatic or vascular channels. After implantation the cells proliferate into microscopic then macroscopic implants and become visible through the endoscopic instruments or to the naked eye. Endometriotic implants assume the appearance of nonpigmented or pigmented vesicles, plaques, or nodules, surrounded by varying degrees of fibrotic reaction. The color of the lesions, from clear or white to red, bluish, and dark brown, reflects the degree of vascularization, fibrosis, and hemoglobin/hemosiderin deposits. Fibrosis appears to be the result of a local immune reaction aimed to limit the extent of the lesion. Some endometriotic implants present as exophytic, soft fleshy nodules with little if any fibrosis. Others take the appearance of fibrotic nodules extending deep under the peritoneal surfaces. Cyclic changes in the ectopic, although not necessarily in phase with the eutopic endometrium, result in periodic bleeding and development of cystic lesions filled with old blood, which over time acquires the appearance and consistency of liquid chocolate, thus the name "chocolate cysts." Bleeding and inflammatory reaction associated with endometriosis result in the development of at times extensive adhesive disease. On pelvic examination, endometriotic lesions are typically tender to palpation, assuming the consistency of fibrotic nodules varying in size and shape and typically located in the posterior cul-de-sac. In stage I/II endometriosis, the findings may be limited to adnexal and cul-de-sac tenderness, scarring, and nodules. The uterus may be fixed in retroversion and tender to palpation. It has been suggested that pelvic examination, if performed during menses, facilitates diagnosis of deep infiltrating endometriosis.[51] In advanced endometriosis, ovarian enlargement by endometriomas and fixation by adhesions may be palpable. The imaging studies using pelvic ultrasound with transvaginal or abdominal transducers, CTscans, and magnetic resonance can easily identify endometriomas 10 mm or larger as round-shaped, smooth-walled cystic lesions, usually unilocular and without papillary projections, containing homogeneous hypoechoic or low-level echoe contents.[52–55] Transvaginal sonography, especially when correlated with pelvic examination findings, seems to be 88% effective in differentiating endometriomas from other ovarian masses.[53] Infiltrating rectovaginal or bladder endometriosis can also be identified with transvaginal or transrectal sonography, but the nature of the infiltrating lesion will still need to be determined histologically.[54, 55] The usefulness of CA125 antigen and other tumor marker measurements in endometriosis has been studied extensively. The results have not been encouraging. However, tumor marker measurements combined with transvaginal ultrasonography, pelvic examination findings, and careful assessment of the medical/surgical history and symptomatology may provide a valuable tool in the diagnosis and management of endometriosis.The definitive diagnosis of endometriosis requires visual identification of the lesions and histologic confirmation. Microscopic examination should demonstrate endometrial glands and stroma with hemosiderin-laden macrophages. There is a recent tendency to allow laparoscopic diagnosis without histologic confirmation of the disease. Considering that appearance of endometriotic lesions may be atypical, that other intraperitoneal lesions may be similar in appearance, and that interpretation depends on the experience of the laparoscopist and the quality of his/her equipment, this trend is without a question, a matter of concern.

Endometriotic lesions in most women progressively increase in size resulting in the increasing severity of symptoms.[25, 56] However, the rate of progression is individually variable and in some patients, the stage of the disease does not seem to change on repeat laparoscopies. It is unclear why endometriosis in some women is a self-limited, while in others a rapidly progressive disease. Repeat laparoscopies in women and in baboons with stage I/II endometriosis demonstrated that without treatment some endometriotic lesions may disappear while new ones appear in different locations.[57, 58] This suggests that the natural course of endometriosis in each patient reflects the balance between the opposing forces. On one hand, retrograde dissemination of the endometrial cells and factors that increase the retrograde transport, such as an obstruction to the menstrual flow, lead to the development of new lesions and progression of the disease. While on the other hand, local and systemic immune response leads to the resorption of old lesions, healing of the disease, and fibrosis. In some women, these two events are evenly balanced and the disease seems nonprogressive even though new lesions in new locations appear while the old regress. A change in that balance, which may be temporary, may lead to rapid progression or alternatively to the resolution of the disease. It is well recognized clinically that in women with endometriosis secondary to congenital or acquired obstruction to the menstrual flow, surgical release of such obstruction is followed by spontaneous resolution of endometriotic lesions.

II. MANAGEMENT OF ENDOMETRIOSIS

Endometriosis, in most women, is a progressive disease. Its growth and spread are stimulated by the cyclic secretion of ovarian hormones. There is no cause-directed therapy because the etiology of the disease is unknown. Currently available treatment methods are based on resection or ablation of visible endometriotic lesions or suppression of the endometriotic growth through endocrine manipulations. The majority of women require repeated medical and/or surgical interventions and ultimately may undergo a definitive treatment, that is hysterectomy and oophorectomy. The choice of treatment should depend on the intensity of symptoms, stage of the disease, and factors such as age, fertility status, desire for its preservation, and previous treatment history. Prior to the selection of treatment, alternative therapeutic approaches—medical, surgical, and combined—their advantages and disadvantages, specific indications and contraindications, and side effects and risks, need to be discussed with the patient. Treatment of endometriosis is typically focused in four distinct directions:

1. Management of pelvic pain symptoms related to endometriosis
2. Management of infertility in a patient with endometriosis
3. Management of ovarian endometriomas
4. Prevention of endometriosis recurrence

A. Management of Pelvic Pain Symptoms Related to Endometriosis

Women with chronic pelvic pain need a thorough diagnostic evaluation to identify the cause of their symptoms. Identification of endometriotic lesions is not enough and a cause-and-effect relationship between the disease and pelvic symptoms needs to be established. Careful history, physical examination, laboratory tests, imaging studies, and occasionally psychologic evaluation are necessary. If a prolonged pain relief followed prior medical or surgical treatment, the association is obvious. If there was little or no relief, other causes of pelvic pain need to be identified. In diagnostically difficult cases a trial of treatment is usually helpful. For this purpose, we recommend a short 4–6-week course of ovarian suppression with danazol or one of the GnRH agonists (GnRHa), which should bring a significant symptomatic improvement. If there is no improvement, in spite of amenorrhea, hypoestrogenic symptoms, and peripheral estradiol levels below 60 pg/ml, other causes of pelvic pain need to be considered. Pelvic pain mapping during laparoscopy performed under local anesthetic and conscious sedation may be helpful.[33] Occasionally, peripheral neuropathies may cause pelvic pain symptoms and may be difficult to diagnose. Peripheral nerve blocks may be required to establish the cause of pelvic symptoms.

1. Symptomatic Management

Most women with chronic pelvic pain and stage I/II endometriosis can benefit from the symptomatic management, especially if the symptoms are mild or if medical or surgical treatment is contraindicated. Symptomatic management can also be combined with ovarian suppression. This management requires modification of three separate aspects of pain perception; the peripheral signal, its transmission along the nerve pathways, and its interpretation by the central nervous system. The best strategy is to begin with the simplest and least invasive analgesics. To be clinically effective they need to be administered on a time rather than pain-contingent basis. Dysmenorrhea and other pelvic pain symptoms may respond to nonsteroidal anti-inflammatory drugs (NSAIDs) which suppress prostaglandin synthesis and are a good starting point for the analgesic regimen. They can effectively control symptoms but their effect is individually variable and several preparations may have to be tried. To achieve the best response, treatment should begin a day or two before the onset of symptoms (usually related to menses) and should continue for 3–7 days (usually through the duration of the menstrual flow). NSAIDs decrease tissue inflammation and decrease transmission of the peripheral pain signal. They are usually well tolerated and have few and manageable side effects. For moderate to severe pain, narcotics alone or in combination with antiprostaglandins may be used. They decrease pain transmission and pain perception thereby increasing pain thresholds. In general, medications that affect pain signal transmission at different sites of the pain pathway act synergistically. This means that less of each drug will be needed resulting in a better response and fewer side effects. Several long- and short-acting narcotics such as codeine, morphine, oxycodone, meperidine, and methadone are available. They should be carefully titrated to relieve pain and limit side effects. Transdermal Fentanyl patches deliver the drug continuously for 72 h. They are available in several doses and may be beneficial when other methods of pain control have been exhausted. Tricyclic antidepressants such as amitriptyline, block the reuptake of norepinephrine and inhibit pain transmission by activating descending inhibitory pathways in the spinal cord. They may provide pain relief at lower doses than those required to treat depression.[59] Amitriptyline also helps to restore sleep and thereby increase pain tolerance in women with chronic pelvic pain, who are frequently sleep deprived. Clonidine, by stimulating α_2 noradrenergic receptors also activates inhibitory pathways in the spinal cord producing analgesia.[60] Treatment of depression is an important component of chronic pelvic pain management and antidepressants such as selective serotonin reuptake inhibitors appear to decrease the perception of pain even in the absence of depression. They also greatly improve the quality of life by improving personal relationships and changing behavioral and emotional response to painful stimuli.

Other approaches to the management of chronic pelvic pain may include transcutaneous electrical nerve stimulation (TENS), applied to the peripheral nervous system.[61]

According to the gate control theory, pain and other stimuli such as TENS, heat, or cold, compete for transmission through the same pathways at the level of the spinal cord and one impulse may inhibit another. A concept of viscerosomatic convergence proposes that strong noxious, visceral stimuli irritate somatic afferent fibers in the dorsal root ganglia resulting in pain reference to anterior abdominal dermatomes. Similarly, strong noxious somatic stimuli as in peripheral neuropathies may irritate visceral afferent fibers resulting in a false perception of visceral pain. Thus, peripheral nerve blocks may be beneficial in both peripheral neuropathies and in visceral pain. Many women with chronic pelvic pains find marked symptomatic relief through a regular program of physical exercise. It is possible that endogenous endorphins released during exercise block central nervous system perception of pelvic symptoms. It has been suggested that low central nervous system β-endorphin concentrations in endometriosis may be the cause of increased pain perception (decreased pain threshold) in women with this disease.[62] Other approaches to pain management such as acupuncture, biofeedback, reflexolgy, hypnosis, and visualization may also decrease transmission and perception of pain stimuli and some patients may find them acceptable and effective. Symptomatic management of chronic pelvic pain symptoms to be effective requires close collaboration between the patient and her physician. Patients who are well informed and who thoroughly understand their condition usually respond better to the symptomatic management. Support groups, counseling, and education are therefore extremely helpful. Furthermore, a multidisciplinary approach that recognizes the importance of emotional and behavioral responses as the modulators of pain perception usually offers the best results.

2. Oral Contraceptives (Estrogen/Progestogen Preparations)

Combination type oral contraceptives suppress ovarian activity, i.e., ovarian follicular development, ovulation, and corpus luteum function. They suppress endometrial proliferation and decrease the length and amount of the menstrual flow. There is also a decrease in prostaglandin production in the reproductive system, which may contribute to the decrease in dysmenorrhea and pelvic pain symptoms. With or without concomitant symptomatic management, oral contraceptives should be considered as the first line of treatment in women with stage I/II endometriosis and pelvic pain symptoms. They may be administered according to three different regimens: standard 28-day cycle, long 3–4 month cycle, and continuously. Most effective oral contraceptives are those with strongly progestational properties.

Standard 28-day cycle is the usual form of oral contraceptive use: 21 days of active pills followed by 7 days of placebo. The degree of symptomatic improvement and the frequency of side effects depend on the pharmaceutical product. The objective is to decrease the length and amount of the menstrual flow by about 50%. A significant improvement in dysmenorrhea, dyspareunia, and pelvic pain was reported during 6 cycles of treatment with ethinyl estradiol 0.02–0.03 mg and desogestrel 0.15 mg in all patients.[63] Side effects included spotting (25%), headaches (21%), mood changes (18%), and breast tenderness (18%). However, there is no medical justification for the 28-day cycle and most women with dysmenorrhea and pelvic pain symptoms would rather have less frequent menstruations. To establish a 3–4 month cycle with withdrawal bleeding (WTB) 3–4 times a year, we recommend ethinyl estradiol 0.03–0.05 mg with norgestrel 0.3–0.5 mg. We usually begin with the lower dose and a standard 28-day cycle. The number of active-pill days is then increased gradually by 7 until a 3–4 month cycle is achieved. Irregular breakthrough bleeding (BTB) may be a problem and the dose of oral contraceptives may have to be increased. With this regimen, there is a significant decrease in dysmenorrhea and other pelvic pain symptoms, while side effects are usually minor. After discontinuation of cyclic oral contraceptives, pelvic pain symptoms usually return with the same intensity as before. Continuous administration of oral contraceptives in high doses induces a state of hyperhormonal amenorrhea and along with it a multitude of symptoms and findings resembling changes that occur during pregnancy. This method of treatment has been referred to as pseudopregnancy. Various oral contraceptives have been recommended for this purpose. Those found most effective have strong progestational properties, such as norgestrel 0.5 mg with ethinyl estradiol 0.05 mg. The usual treatment consists of 1 tablet daily, continuously for 6–9 months with an increase by 1 tablet for each episode of BTB. Thus, the lowest effective dose is determined for each patient. Oral contraceptives suppress pituitary FSH and LH and ovarian estradiol and progesterone production. However, exogenous estrogens and progestogens administered as the pseudopregnancy regimen bind to estrogen and progesterone receptors in both eutopic and ectopic endometrium, inducing initial hypertrophy, vascular congestion, edema, and decidual transformation. Later during the course of treatment, endometrial atrophy and resorption of endometriotic lesions have been observed. Symptomatic improvement during pseudopregnancy is variable and depends on the completeness of amenorrhea. In some patients, especially at the beginning of treatment, symptoms of endometriosis may be exacerbated when endometriotic lesions enlarge. Clinically, oral-contraceptive-induced pseudopregnancy is considered less effective than regimens inducing immediate endometrial atrophy such as danazol or GnRH agonists. Side effects, risks, and contraindications to pseudopregnancy are the same as for oral contraceptives.

3. Oral or Parenteral Progestogens

Exogenous progestogens act synergistically with endogenous estrogens suppressing ovarian function and inducing hyperhormonal amenorrhea and decidual endometrial changes that are similar to those observed with continuous estrogen/progestogens. However, ovarian suppression is rather inconsistent with variable estradiol levels and BTB is a frequent occurrence. To control BTB, some clinicians recommend supplemental use of low-dose estrogens, thus converting to a typical estrogen/progestogen regimen. Progestogens recommended for the treatment of endometriosis and its symptoms include: medroxyprogesterone acetate (MPA) in its oral or depot form, norethindrone, norethindrone acetate, megestrol acetate, dydrogesterone, and gestrinone. The dose as with estrogen/progestogen preparations is individually determined in a stepwise fashion. Amenorrhea is usually achieved with 40 mg/day of oral MPA, 40 mg/day of megestrol acetate, 30 mg/day of norethindrone, or 15 mg/day of norethindrone acetate. Depot MPA has been effective in a dose of 100–200 mg monthly. Side effects of progestogens alone are fewer and generally better tolerated than those of estrogen/progestogen preparations. Depot MPA has variable and prolonged absorption and delayed clearance. Progestogens alone may be recommended as an alternative to estrogen/progestogens in women with contraindications to GnRHa or danazol.

4. Treatment with Danazol

Danazol is a synthetic steroid derivative, structurally related to 17α-ethinyl testosterone (ethisterone). Biologic properties of this compound, clinical applications, and effectiveness have been reviewed in several publications.[64–66] As a steroid, danazol binds to receptor proteins in various cells bringing about a multitude of biological effects. At the hypothalamopituitary level, danazol inhibits the midcycle FSH and LH surge and lowers basal FSH and LH levels. Suppression of FSH and LH leads to suppression of ovarian steroidogenesis and to lower peripheral estrogen and progesterone concentrations. This seems to be further magnified *in vivo* by the direct, inhibitory effect of danazol on multiple enzymes of ovarian and adrenal steroidogenesis demonstrated *in vitro*. Without estrogenic and progestational stimulation, endometrium undergoes atrophy, which may be further enhanced by the direct binding of danazol to endometrial androgen and/or progesterone receptors. As an attenuated androgen, danazol binds to androgen receptors in a variety of tissues resulting in androgenic/anabolic effects. In the peripheral circulation, danazol displaces testosterone from the sex hormone binding globulin (SHBG) and through its effect on the liver lowers SHBG, increasing free testosterone fraction. In the bioassay system, androgenic/anabolic effects of danazol are 200× lower then those of testosterone, but administered together both steroids have a synergistic effect, which is most likely secondary to the increase in free testosterone levels. Danazol also modulates humoral and cell-mediated immunity both *in vivo* and *in vitro*. *In vitro*, danazol suppresses macrophage-dependent T-cell activation of B cells, as well as B-cell IgG production. *In vivo*, it lowers the concentration of abnormal autoantibodies and decreases immunoglobulin levels. Both *in vitro* and *in vivo* danazol reverses functional endometriosis-associated changes in the peripheral lymphocytes, NK cells, and monocyte/macrophages.

Danazol was introduced to the management of endometriosis in the mid 1970s. It is recommended in the dose of 400 mg twice a day or approximately 12 mg/kg/day for a period of 4–6 months, beginning on the first day of menstruation. In some patients, the dose of danazol may be lowered to 400–600 mg/day after the onset on amenorrhea. However, lower dose regimens may not completely suppress ovarian function and in some patients, may be the cause of poor clinical response. At the full dose, danazol maintains serum estradiol levels between 20 and 50 pg/ml. Higher estradiol levels indicate incomplete ovarian suppression and suggest either poor absorption of the drug from the gastrointestinal system or poor patient compliance. In some patients, ovarian suppression on a twice a day regimen may be incomplete because of rapid danazol clearance. In such cases, administration schedule of 200 mg 4 times a day, may be a better approach. The length on danazol therapy should be adjusted individually on the basis of the initial stage of the disease and the clinical response. In patients with superficial peritoneal implants and no endometriomas, a 3- to 4-month course of amenorrhea should be adequate. The lesions usually regress completely and there is little or no evidence of residual disease. If small (less than 3 cm) endometriomas are present, the patient may require a 6-month course of therapy. In women with large endometriomas, the lesions may regress during the 6–9 months of treatment, but do not disappear completely. Surgical resection may be necessary at the end of medical treatment. Symptomatic improvement usually begins during the first month of danazol treatment along with the onset of amenorrhea. Complete relief of symptoms has been reported by more than 90% of patients and clinical improvement by more than 80%. Laparoscopic resolution of endometriosis has been observed in 70–90% of cases. Several comparative studies between danazol and different GnRHa reviewed recently demonstrated a comparable symptomatic improvement and comparable resolution of the disease with both regimens.[67] Danazol is well tolerated by most patients. Its major side effects are related to its androgenic/anabolic properties. Paradoxically, they appear to be more frequent and more intense at the lower dose of the drug. It is likely that on a low-dose regimen, there is incomplete suppression of ovarian steroidogenesis, continuing production of testosterone, and resulting increase in free testosterone levels. Thus a common practice of lowering the dose of danazol to decrease the intensity of side effects may have the opposite effect and may also lower its clinical effectiveness.

5. GnRHa

GnRHa are synthetic derivatives of the decapeptide GnRH. Multiple compounds, varying in potency have been synthesized by substitution of amino acids in positions 6, 10, or both. Those with half-life longer than the native GnRH, when administered continuously, downregulate pituitary GnRH receptors within 5–10 days and induce a state of pituitary suppression at times referred to as "medical hypophysectomy." Before FSH and LH suppression, there is usually a brief period to gonadotropin release, the so called "flare effect" which may result in ovarian stimulation, development of ovarian follicles, and an increase in estradiol levels. GnRHa are not active orally and need to be administered intranasally (IN), subcutaneously (SC), or intramuscularly (IM). The degree of hypoestrogenism induced with GnRHa varies and depends on the analog, its dose, and the route of administration. With some regimens, estradiol levels can be maintained in the range of 20–50 pg/ml. With others, and especially with the depot preparations, estrogens are suppressed to a castrate range. The initiation of GnRHa therapy is usually recommended in the midluteal phase or with the onset of menses. Midluteal administration reduces the flare effect and facilitates ovarian suppression. There is, however, a risk that the drug could be administered during early pregnancy and contraception should be recommended during the entire cycle. Leuprolide acetate (Lupron) is available in the injectable form only. It can be administered daily SC or every 4 weeks IM as 3.75 or 7.5 mg depot injections of lyophilized leuprolide acetate in microspheres incorporated into a biodegradable copolymer of polylactic and polyglycolic acids (Lupron Depot). Gradual degradation of the copolymer provides for a slow release of GnRHa. Lupron depot is also available as IM injections of 11.25 and 22.5 mg every 3 months. Nafarelin acetate (Synarel) is available as IN 200 μg per spray solution. It is recommended in a twice daily dose of 200 μg sprayed into the nostrils by a metered dose pump. Nafarelin is readily absorbed through the nasal mucosa and has a half-life of 4 h. Goserelin (Zoladex) can be administered monthly as an SC pellet through a 16-gauge needle. The site of the injection in the lower abdominal wall may be prepared with a local anesthetic. The agonist has a sustained release from a biodegradable matrix containing 3.6 mg of goserelin. Buserelin can be administered either IN in a divided dose of 900–1200 μg/day or SC in a daily dose of 200–400 μg of buserelin acetate. The response to GnRHa may not be consistent and some patients may require higher doses. This is especially so with IN preparations, absorption of which may be affected by nasal congestion. The degree of GnRHa-induced ovarian suppression may need to be evaluated periodically with serum estradiol levels and if necessary GnRHa dose may have to be adjusted. It is not clear at what level of endogenous estrogens there is optimal suppression of endometriosis and whether severe hypoestrogenism is more effective. Studies with danazol suggest that serum estradiol levels during treatment should remain below 60 pg/ml to bring about suppression of the disease, yet above 20 pg/ml to avoid undesirable hypoestrogenic side effects. It is possible that different tissues respond to different estrogen thresholds and that the 20–60 pg/ml range is optimal.[68] Currently recommended length of treatment with GnRHa is 6 months. However, a shorter course of treatment in women with minimal or mild endometriosis may be adequate.

Treatment with GnRHa effectively controls symptoms of endometriosis and reduces the size of the lesions. Complete resolution of pelvic pain symptoms is usually observed in more than 50% of patients and a significant decrease in frequency and intensity in over 90%. There is a decrease in the size of endometriotic lesions and a decline in laparoscopic score of endometriosis by about 50%. All GnRHa appear to be equally effective in this respect.[67, 69, 70] Also, comparative studies between GnRHa and danazol or gestrinone indicate similar degrees of clinical effectiveness.[67, 71] Side effects of GnRHa are primarily the result of the hypoestrogenic state. Hot flashes, night sweats, vasomotor instability, decreased breast size, and vaginal dryness are the most common and can be expected in as many as 90% of patients treated. Development of hypoestrogenic symptoms actually indicates the effectiveness of the drug in inducing ovarian suppression. In women with a history of clinical depression or migraine headaches, these symptoms may become more severe. However, side effects are rarely severe enough to cause discontinuation of therapy. Severe hypoestrogenism (estradiol levels consistently below 20 pg/ml) may be associated with increased calcium mobilization from the bones and may lead to osteoporosis. A decrease in bone density of 5–6% may be expected during the course of treatment, but is usually reversible within 6–12 months after discontinuation of the regimen.[72] Treatment with GnRHa may be combined with low-dose estrogen and/or progestogen as an add-back therapy.[73] Such combinations decrease or eliminate hypoestrogenic symptoms and may prevent undesirable side effects of GnRHa, allowing in some patients prolonged management of chronic pelvic pain symptoms and prevention of disease recurrence. We prefer to combine GnRHa with transdermal estradiol delivery systems. Peripheral estradiol levels with such regimens can be measured and adjusted individually by changing the dose of the delivery system.

6. New Therapeutic Agents

Future developments in the medical management of endometriosis should lead to more effective and shorter courses of treatment. Several approaches are currently being investigated. One involves the use of GnRH analogs with antagonistic properties. GnRH antagonists are capable of inducing immediate and more profound pituitary suppression without the initial flare effect characteristic of GnRHa. Although earlier antagonists had unacceptable side effects, newer products appear to be well tolerated and are currently in clinical trials. GnRH antagonists may shorten the course of treatment and may offer other advantages in the management of symptomatic endometriosis.[74] Another strategy involves direct inhibition of estrogenic and/or progestational effects on the endometrium. A significant symptomatic improvement and decrease in the size of endometriotic lesions along with 50% reduction in peripheral estradiol levels was reported in a patient with aggressive postmenopausal endometriosis treated with an aromatase inhibitor.[75] This report is quite interesting considering that some endometriotic lesions are capable of biosynthesis of estrogens for their own autonomous growth. Antiprogesterone (RU486) has also been used effectively in the management of endometriosis and its symptoms and newer antiprogestogens are currently being developed and some have entered clinical trials.[76] Another approach to the management of endometriosis and its symptoms may involve local delivery of therapeutic agents. Vaginal and intrauterine delivery of danazol was found effective in controlling symptoms of endometriosis and suppressing the disease without detectable systemic effects.[77, 78] Another report on the levonorgestrel-releasing IUD was equally encouraging.[79] Women with severe dysmenorrhea, pelvic pain, and deep dyspareunia experienced significant symptomatic improvement along with the decrease in the size of rectovaginal endometriotic lesions. Local drug delivery systems/IUDs may offer many advantages in the management of endometriosis without undesirable side effects and may be especially beneficial in women with a symptomatic disease who wish to delay pregnancy. Another possible future approach in the management of endometriosis may involve an entirely new class of therapeutic agents, the immunomodulators. If endometriosis is a disease of the immune system, drugs with immunomodulatory properties may have therapeutic applications and may offer a completely new strategy for the management of endometriosis and/or associated infertility.

7. Surgical Management of Endometriosis and Chronic Pelvic Pain

Surgical resection or ablation of endometriotic lesions via laparoscopy or laparotomy has been a traditional approach to the management of this disease. Laparoscopy offers major advantages over laparotomy, which include better visualization of peritoneal surfaces, magnification of small lesions, minimal intraoperative trauma resulting in fewer postoperative adhesions, low morbidity, and fast recovery. Experienced laparoscopic surgeons using sophisticated laparoscopic equipment and a variety of power sources, can resect/electrocoagulate/ablate even extensive endometriosis and adhesions. However, there is a long learning curve and limited tactile perception of the lesions. Laparotomy for resection of advanced endometriosis, especially when there is bowel involvement, may therefore still be necessary depending on the expertise of the surgeon and complexity of the case. The surgical objective, regardless of the approach, is complete removal of endometriotic lesions and adhesions, restoration of pelvic anatomy, and in some patients with pelvic pain, uterosacral and/or presacral nerve ablations. Chronic pelvic pain appears to be associated predominantly with deep infiltrating endometriosis when endometriotic lesions penetrate more than 5 mm under the peritoneal surfaces. It has been suggested that resection of such lesions is more complete than electrocoagulation or laser ablation and that it provides a better symptomatic improvement.[80] Certainly, only a superficial destruction of deep lesions regardless by what modality is less than optimal and may lead to persistence of the disease or symptoms or their rapid recurrence. The entire lesion should be resected or destroyed with whatever modality the laparoscopist is accustomed to. Unfortunately, such surgical procedures are limited to those lesions that are visible and accessible to the surgeon. Microscopic or deep subperitoneal implants may be less apparent and are frequently left behind. Similarly, endometriotic lesions involving vital organs are usually left untouched by less experienced laparoscopists. Resection or ablation of ovarian endometriosis requires careful, ovarian tissue-sparing surgical techniques. It needs to be kept in mind that most oocytes, and especially those within primordial follicles, are located just under the ovarian surface and can be easily destroyed by excessive electrocautery or laser or may be resected along with endometriotic lesions. A decreased ovarian reserve, poor response to stimulation, and ultimately premature menopause may be the outcome in such cases.[81, 82] Most patients following resection or ablation of endometriosis and adhesions report improvement in their symptoms. Significant improvement or relief of symptoms was reported by over 80% of patients treated laparoscopically with ablation or electrocautery of endometriotic lesions in numerous uncontrolled clinical trials.[83, 84] In a double-blind prospective study, comparing the effect of diagnostic laparoscopy to laparoscopic laser surgery combined with uterosacral nerve ablation (LUNA), 62.5% of women who underwent laser ablation had significant improvement in pain at 6 months of follow-up as compared to 22.6% of controls.[85] At 1 year, 90% of those who responded continued to have symptomatic improvement.[57]

In women with persistent pelvic pain symptoms, LUNA, or presacral neurectomy (PSN) may be considered. However, the effectiveness of these procedures is questionable and proper patient selection may be essential. Patients selected for this procedure should have intractable central pelvic pain that does not respond to conservative therapy and cannot be treated medically. LUNA involves ablation or resection of approximately 1.5–2 cm of uterosacral ligaments at their attachment to the cervix. Ureters should be identified during this procedure and care should be taken to avoid their injury. PSN involves interruption of the sympathetic innervation to the uterus at the level of the superior hypogastric plexus. For this purpose, the peritoneum over the sacral promontory is incised and the retroperitoneal space is dissected. Whitish fibers forming the superior hypogastric plexus are identified and excised. Care should be taken not to injure the ureters or blood vessels. In a randomized prospective study, 81% of women with intractable dysmenorrhea who underwent LUNA reported relief of pain 3 months after surgery while no relief was reported by those who underwent diagnostic laparoscopy.[86] However, 1 year after LUNA, the pain returned in almost half of the patients who experienced relief at 3 months after surgery. In a retrospective study, after laparoscopic PSN, a complete relief of symptoms was reported in 52% of patients, while some improvement in 92%.[87] However, a randomized prospective trial failed to show any benefit of the procedure.[88]

B. Management of Infertility in a Patient with Endometriosis

Endometriosis in a reproductive age woman is associated with about tenfold decrease in monthly fecundity and about 50% of women with endometriosis seek infertility treatment. Currently available medical treatment of endometriosis inhibits ovarian function and ovulation, preventing pregnancy during the course of therapy, while ovarian surgery decreases the number of ovarian follicles, lowers ovarian reserve, and also decreases fertility. Treatment of infertility with ovarian stimulation raises estradiol levels and if repeated during several consecutive cycles, may accelerate progression of endometriosis and also compromise fertility. The effect of endometriosis and its treatment on fertility and the effect of fertility treatment on endometriosis need to be considered in managing infertility associated with endometriosis. The optimal approach offers the best chances for conception in the shortest time frame with lowest side effects and lowest costs.

1. Effect of Medical Suppression of Endometriosis on Fertility

Numerous retrospective uncontrolled clinical studies dating back to the 1960s reported higher pregnancy rates in women with endometriosis after treatment with estrogen/progestogen induced pseudopregnancy. Similarly, in the 1970s, reports were published indicating increased chances for pregnancy after treatment with danazol. These studies typically referred to crude pregnancy rates during variable observational periods. Kistner, who reported an overall pregnancy rate of 50.8% in 186 patients during a 12-month follow-up, stated that "a pregnancy rate of approximately 50% may be expected following pseudopregnancy in patients whose only abnormality is surface ovarian endometriosis without endometriomas or tubo-ovarian adhesions."[89] A somewhat higher pregnancy rate in the range of 50–83% was reported by several investigators after danazol treatment.[90] Subsequently, during the 1980s, comparative studies between danazol and several GnRHa reported 12-month cumulative pregnancy rates ranging between 24 and 63% and not different between these two regimens.[67] Life table analysis was not used and monthly fecundity rates were not calculated in these studies, but an average monthly pregnancy rate can be estimated as ranging between 2.3 and 6.3%. Even though these numbers are higher than in untreated endometriosis, a meta-analysis by Hughes *et al.*, [91] suggests that ovarian suppression is not an effective treatment of infertility associated with endometriosis.

2. Effect of Surgical Treatment of Endometriosis on Fertility

Advances in laparoscopic techniques during the 1980s and 1990s greatly facilitated surgical management of even advanced endometriosis at the time of diagnosis. Numerous retrospective studies were published comparing pregnancy rates following resection of the disease via laparoscopy or laparotomy, often using expectant or medical management in controls. Crude pregnancy rates ranged between 20 and 75% during the follow-up period of 5–37 months.[83] The results also suggested somewhat better chances for pregnancy following surgical resection than medical suppression or expectant management. Unfortunately, none of these studies were randomized and all appeared to have problems with patient selection bias. In one report, monthly fecundity was 6.3% in stage I/II endometriosis without treatment, 4.8% after laparoscopic ablation, and 5.7% after treatment with danazol.[48] No significant differences between the groups but significantly below 14% average monthly fecundity of controls. Other reports suggested higher pregnancy rates after surgical treatment than after medical suppression [92, 93] and better results following laparoscopic resection than laparotomy.[94, 95] Adamson *et al.*,[96] in a retrospective analysis of 100 consecutive patients with endometriomas, assigned to either laser laparoscopy or laparotomy, reported comparable pregnancy rates in both groups. Average monthly fecundity during the first year was 2.1% in laparotomy and 2.7% in the laparoscopy group and 2.7 and 2%, respectively, during the second year. As one would expect, slightly higher postoperative pregnancy rates were reported in a less advanced disease [97] but according to another report,[98] no significant differences were detected between different stages of the disease. It appears, however, that chances for conception after re-operation for recurrent endometriosis are quite dismal.[99] The first randomized controlled trial to evaluate the effect of surgery on fertility in women with endometriosis was published relatively recently.[100]

It compared monthly fecundity rate after laparoscopic resection or ablation of visible endometriotic lesions to diagnostic laparoscopy alone in 341 infertile women with stage I/II endometriosis. Monthly fecundity rate was 4.7% in the laparoscopic surgery group, significantly higher than 2.4% in those who underwent diagnostic laparoscopy alone.

3. Controlled Ovarian Hyperstimulation/Insemination (COH/AIH) in the Management of Infertility in Women with Endometriosis

Anovulation and different forms of ovulatory dysfunction have been reported repeatedly in as many as 70% of women with endometriosis. There is also evidence suggesting alterations in gamete/embryo transport. Consequently, ovulation induction with clomiphene citrate and/or hMG combined with artificial insemination have been used routinely in the management of infertility in women with endometriosis. A meta-analysis of 962 cycles of COH/AIH in endometriosis demonstrated a monthly fecundity rate of 13%.[101] Tummon *et al.*,[102] in a randomized controlled trial, compared the effect of COH/AIH against no treatment in women with stage I/II endometriosis. Live birth rate was 11% per cycle in COH/AIH cycles as compared to 2% in no treatment cycles. These data indicate that in stage I/II endometriosis, ovulation induction and artificial insemination may improve chances for pregnancy, but may not completely restore fertility, further underscoring the role of multiple mechanisms of infertility in endometriosis. It is unclear to what extent COH/AIH improve fertility in women with stage III/IV endometriosis. Furthermore, the possible accelerating effect of ovarian stimulation on progression of endometriosis needs to be considered.

4. Treatment of Infertility with *in vitro* Fertilization/Embryo Transfer (IVF/ET) in Women with Endometriosis

During the process of IVF/ET ovaries are hyperstimulated, oocytes are aspirated from the follicles then fertilized *in vitro*, and developing embryos are transferred into the uterus. These procedures correct endocrine and ovulatory dysfunctions and abnormal ovum pick-up or gamete transport mechanisms, compensate for abnormal fertilization, eliminate potentially adverse effect of the intraperitoneal environment, and identify problems of early embryonic development, all factors considered instrumental in subfertility associated with endometriosis. The results of IVF/ET should therefore be comparable in women with and without endometriosis. Indeed most of the reports indicate that endometriosis does not lower the IVF/ET outcome.[103] There is no adverse effect of mild endometriosis on ovarian response to stimulation and the number of eggs retrieved, although this may not be necessarily so in advanced endometriosis. Most reports agree that endometriosis has no adverse effects on oocyte fertilization, even though some studies suggest that oocyte quality, fertilization rates, and quality of the embryos are decreased. Lower implantation and pregnancy rates have been reported by some programs and may be the result of the autoimmune phenomena. Use of corticosteroids or heparin/aspirin in such cases has been recommended. The possibility that peritoneal environment in women with endometriosis may adversely affect chances for pregnancy was suggested by Guzick *et al.*[104]. The authors compared the results of 114 GIFT procedures in women with endometriosis to 214 such procedures in unexplained or mild male factor infertility. In endometriosis, pregnancy and delivery rates per retrieval were 32.5 and 23.7%, respectively, versus 47.2 and 35.5% in controls. If peritoneal environment was the detrimental factor in endometriosis, the authors suggested that IVF/ET would be more effective than GIFT. According to the most recent CDC/SART National Summary, live birth rates with assisted reproductive techniques (ART) in endometriosis are 25.8% per cycle, similar to those in other infertility disorders.[105]

5. Management of Infertility in Women with Endometriosis; Recommendations

The review of literature quoted above indicates that spontaneous fecundity in stage I/II endometriosis is about 2% and in stage III/IV less than 1% per cycle. Chances for spontaneous pregnancy are therefore minimal, decreasing rapidly with age and progression of the disease. Therefore, standard recommendation of 12 months of coital exposure before treatment of infertility should be reconsidered for women with endometriosis and the couple should be treated aggressively, especially if wife's age is over 35. Surgical resection of endometriosis should certainly be attempted at the time of diagnostic laparoscopy. It doubles the fecundity and may improve the peritoneal environment. After surgery, COH/AIH can further improve chances for conception but should be attempted for no more than 3–4 cycles. If there is no pregnancy, in spite of good ovulatory response, IVF/ET should be considered. It is unlikely that COH/AIH for more than four cycles will be effective and the risk of reactivation of the disease is of a concern. In women with stage III/IV endometriosis, and especially in those with a significant adhesive disease, consideration should be given to an earlier IVF/ET attempt, especially if the wife is over 35. Medical treatment with danazol or GnRHa should be considered in women with chronic pelvic pain symptoms and especially in those under 35 or as a preoperative suppression prior to the resection of ovarian endometriomas. In women over 35 with longstanding infertility and recurrent endometriosis, and especially in those with extensive adhesive disease, it is unlikely that COH/AIH will be effective and IVF/ET needs to be considered as the initial approach.

C. Management of Ovarian Endometriomas

Preoperative diagnosis of ovarian endometriomas is facilitated by transvaginal ultrasonography and other imaging techniques, which provide characteristic appearance of the lesions. However, endometriomas need to be differentiated from functional ovarian cysts and from ovarian neoplasia. Patient's age, history and physical, prior diagnosis of endometriosis, and tumor marker levels are helpful. However, transvaginal ultrasonography allows the best assessment of the ovaries and lesions. The size and location of endometriomas and of healthy ovarian tissue can be determined and surgical approach can be planned. Repeat sonographic examinations demonstrate changes in the cyst, which may further indicate its nature. Occasionally, preoperative diagnosis may be difficult and diagnostic laparoscopy or exploratory laparotomy are performed. Preoperative procedures should include a thorough bowel prep because of the risk of bowel involvement and intraoperative consultation with gynecologic oncologist or general surgeon may be required. Provisions should also be made to convert laparoscopy into laparotomy if needed. Ovarian endometriomas, especially those larger than 3 cm in diameter, destroy significant portions of the ovaries. Ovarian cortex with healthy ovarian tissue and oocyte-containing follicles are typically stretched, sometimes paper-thin, over the endometriotic cyst. The ovary is usually adherent to the surrounding pelvic structures and often to the bowel. When the cavity of endometrioma is entered, a fragment of the ovary with cortex and subcortical follicles may remain attached to the bowel or to other pelvic structures. This may further compromise patients fertility or lead to ovarian remnant syndrome. Management of ovarian endometriomas therefore requires specific strategy. The goal in all women is complete resection of the disease with preservation of healthy ovarian tissue in some, while in others with complete resection of the ovaries and definitive surgery.

If ovarian endometrioma is diagnosed at the time of laparoscopy, the extent of endometriosis and adhesions needs to be carefully evaluated and possible involvement of other organs determined. A decision needs to be made whether to proceed with laparoscopic resection, convert to laparotomy, or use ovarian suppression and defer surgical treatment. Laparoscopic resection should be as complete as possible. All endometriotic lesions need to be resected or ablated and the ovaries need to be carefully freed from adhesions and mobilized. Endometriomas with a thick fibrotic capsule can sometimes be resected from the ovaries without releasing their contents. Most of the time, however, the cavity of endometrioma is entered during resection, releasing characteristic chocolate-like contents. These should be aspirated, and the capsule of endometrioma should be carefully stripped from the healthy ovarian tissue using bland and sharp dissection, traction, and countertraction. Hemostasis is then secured with bipolar electrocautery. Care should be taken to preserve as much as possible of the ovarian cortex with underlying follicles. After resection of endometriomas, we like to close its cavity and reconstruct the ovary using fine absorbable sutures. Careful, nontraumatic techniques should be used and hemostasis should be complete. A variety of adhesion-preventing membranes are available and may prevent postoperative adhesions. An alternative to resection is fenestration of endometrioma and drainage of its contents. The capsule then can be electrocoagulated or laser ablated and the patient can be placed on ovarian suppression to prevent recurrence of the lesion.[106–108] There is, however, no agreement as to the effectiveness of this approach. Some claim better results with laparoscopic fenestration and coagulation than resection,[109] while others just the opposite.[110] Simple drainage, regardless whether followed by ovarian suppression or not, seems ineffective and recurrence of endometriomas is quite rapid.[111, 112] In a prospective, randomized trial, symptomatic improvement was better and posttreatment pregnancy rates were higher when cystectomy rather than drainage and coagulation of endometriomas were performed.[113] If endometrioma is diagnosed at the time of exploratory laparotomy, it should be resected along with the capsule using careful microsurgical techniques and ovaries should be reconstructed with fine absorbable sutures. Care should be taken to completely resect the disease and to prevent postoperative adhesions. If resection of the disease is incomplete, the patient may be placed on ovarian suppression immediately after surgery. Occasionally after aspiration of large ovarian endometriomas, healthy ovarian tissue cannot be identified. In such cases, unilateral oophorectomy or alternatively, drainage of endometrioma followed by 3–4 months of ovarian suppression and second laparoscopic resection may have to be considered.

If the diagnosis is assured, the best management of ovarian endometriomas is ovarian suppression followed by laparoscopic resection. After 3–4 months of ovarian suppression, blood supply to the pelvic organs is significantly decreased and there is less inflammation and tissue edema, which improves hemostasis and facilitates surgery. The ovaries are inactive and contain no developing follicles or corpora lutea, which makes resection of endometriomas easier with optimal preservation of the ovarian tissue. Ovarian suppression also facilitates stripping of the endometrioma capsule, which becomes more fibrotic and less edematous. Danazol or GnRHa are preferable to oral contraceptives for preoperative ovarian suppression. The latter usually increases blood supply to the pelvic organs resulting in tissue edema and decidualization of the endometriotic lesions, which in turn make surgery more difficult. During a longer, 4–6 months, ovarian suppression endometriomas may decrease in size with proportional increase in the volume of healthy ovarian tissue. This further facilitates resection of endometriosis and preservation of the ovary.[114]

In women who have completed their families or are not interested in pregnancy, who are in their forties and have recurrent bilateral disease, definitive surgery, i.e., hysterectomy and bilateral oophorectomy should be considered. While performing oophorectomy, care should be taken to completely resect the diseased ovaries without leaving fragments of the ovarian cortex. Under the ovarian cortex, especially in young women, there are numerous primordial follicles. Each one of these follicles under increased FSH and LH stimulation can mature and produce estradiol and progesterone levels not different than those observed during the normal menstrual cycle. Estradiol at these levels can stimulate residual endometriotic lesions and recurrence of the disease. Residual ovarian fragments following hysterectomy and bilateral salpingo-oophorectomy may be multiple and attached to the bowel or pelvic organs in various locations. They may reactivate at different times, making such cases extremely difficult to manage clinically.[115, 116] To prevent this complication, a careful retroperitoneal approach should be used to completely resect the ovaries, which are often tightly adherent to the peritoneal surfaces. We recommend that this procedure is performed by a gynecologic oncologist experienced in retroperitoneal dissection for pelvic cancer.

D. Prevention of Endometriosis Recurrence

One of the major concerns in the management of endometriosis is prevention of its recurrence. Current treatment methods, regardless whether medical or surgical, do not change the pathogenesis of the disease and the same mechanisms for its development remain. With the first menstrual cycle after treatment, the process of gradual recurrence begins. After danazol treatment, recurrence rates were higher during the first year (23%), then varied between 2 and 9% annually with a cumulative 37-month recurrence rate of 39%.[117] After GnRHa, a 5-year cumulative recurrence was 53.4%.[118] In a comparative analysis of time to recurrence, pain-free interval was 6.1 months after danazol, and slightly longer than 5.2 months after GnRHa.[119] After laparoscopic resection, a 24-month cumulative recurrence rate was 27%.[120] The highest recurrence rates have been reported in advanced endometriosis, especially in women with endometriomas. Beretta *et al.* [113] reported a 24-month recurrence of symptoms as high as 20 and 75%, depending whether resection or fenestration was performed. Donnez *et al.* [112] demonstrated recurrence of endometriomas to the same size within 12 weeks after drainage, while Vercellini *et al.* [111] reported the same within 6 months after drainage, regardless whether GnRHa were or were not used postoperatively. Considering that recurrence rates are higher during the first year and in women with advanced endometriosis, it is quite likely that they represent incomplete resolution of the disease during medical treatment and persistence of endometriotic lesions after surgery. Recurrence of endometriosis or reactivation of residual lesions is stimulated by the cyclic secretion of ovarian hormones. The cyclic pattern of estradiol secretion with midcycle peak at 200–400 pg/ml is required for the reproductive function but also seems to be a significant factor in endometriosis recurrence. Women undergoing ovarian stimulation after treatment of the disease have even higher serum estradiol levels, which may further accelerate the recurrence. Suppression of estradiol delays the recurrence and lowers its risk. It has been suggested that peripheral estradiol levels above 60 pg/ml are required to stimulate the disease.[68] On the other hand, experience with estrogen replacement therapy indicates that estradiol levels between 40 and 60 pg/ml are adequate for the normal metabolic function and prevention of hypoestrogenic changes.

In women who desire to conceive after treatment of endometriosis, aggressive management of infertility should be initiated. If ovarian stimulation is attempted, the number of stimulation cycles needs to be carefully controlled and chances for pregnancy optimized using ARTs. In women who do not plan to conceive but want to preserve their fertility, two strategies are available. One involves the use of strongly progestational oral contraceptives in a standard 28-day fashion or preferably in a 3- to 4-month cycle. Decreased menstrual flow, symptomatic control, and endometrial thickness between 6 and 8 mm are indicators of the effective management. An alternative approach involves the use of GnRHa with estrogen add-back. For this purpose, we prefer leuprolide depot in a 3-month regimen combined with 0.025–0.075 mg transdermal estradiol patch. Peripheral estradiol levels should be maintained between 40 and 60 pg/ml and endometrial thickness should be monitored about 1–2 times a year with transvaginal ultrasound. The thickness of the eutopic endometrium reflects the degree of estrogenic stimulation and changes in the ectopic endometrium. When less than 6 mm, the patient remains amenorrheic. If it is above 8 mm, we induce WTB 1–2 times a year with oral progestogens. Such GnRHa add-back regimen provides good control of endometriosis symptoms and probably delays or prevents recurrence of the disease. At this time, however, there are no published data to demonstrate the effectiveness of this approach.

References

1. Houston, D. E., Noller, K. L., Melton L. J., III, Selwyn B. J., and Hardy R. J. (1987). Incidence of pelvic endometriosis in Rochester, Minnesota, 1970–1979. *Am. J. Epidemiol.* 125, 959–969.
2. Ballweg, M. L. (1993). Public testimony to the US Senate Committee on Labor and Human Resources. Subcommittee on Aging, May 5, 1993.
3. Sampson, J. A. (1925). Heterotropic or misplaced endometrial tissue. *Am. J. Obstet. Gynecol.* 10, 649–668.
4. Von Recklinghausen, F. (1895). Die Adenomyome und cystadenome der uterus und tubenwandung. *Berli. klin. Wochenschr.* 8, 530.
5. Startseva, N. V. (1980). Clinico-immunological aspects of genital endometriosis. *Akush. Ginekol. (Moscow)* 3, 23–26.

6. Weed, J. C., and Arguembourg, P. C. (1980). Endometriosis: Can it produce an autoimmune response resulting in infertility? *Clin. Obstet. Gynecol.* 23, 885–893.
7. Dmowski, W. P., Steele, R. W., and Baker, G. F. (1981). Deficient cellular immunity in endometriosis. *Am. J. Obstet. Gynecol.* 141, 377–383.
8. Mathur, S., Peress, M. R., Williamson, H. O., Youmans, C. D., Maney, S. A., Garvin, A. J., Rust, P. F., and Fundenburg, H. H. (1982). Autoimmunity to endometrium and ovary in endometriosis. *Clin. Exp. Immunol.* 50, 259–266.
9. Braun, D. P., and Dmowski, W. P. (1998). Endometriosis: Abnormal endometrium and dysfunctional immune response. *Curr. Opin. Obstet. Gynecol.* 10, 365–369.
10. Dmowski, W. P., Gebel, H., and Braun, D. P. (1998). Decreased apoptosis and sensitivity to macrophage mediated cytolysis of endometrial cells in endometriosis. *Hum. Reprod.* 4, 696–701.
11. Pena, L. A., Fuks, Z., and Kolesnick, R. (1997). Stress-induced apoptosis and the sphingomyelin pathway. *Biochem. Pharmacol.* 53, 615–621.
12. Braun, D. P., Muriana, A., Gebel, H., Rotman, C., Rana, N., and Dmowski, W. P. (1994). Monocyte-mediated enhancement of endometrial cell proliferation in women with endometriosis. *Fertil. Steril.* 61, 78–84.
13. Braun, D. P., Gebel, H., Muriana, D., Rotsztejn, D., Rana, N., Rotman, C., and Dmowski, W. P. (1992). Differential Endometrial Cell (EC) Proliferation in Response to Peripheral Blood Monocytes (PBM), Peritoneal Macrophages (PM) and the Macrophage-Derived Cytokines in Patients with Endometriosis (EN). 1992 Abstracts of the Scientific Oral and Poster Sessions; 48th Annual Meeting of The American Fertility Society. S77.
14. Dmowski, W. P. (1995). Immunological aspects of endometriosis. *Int. J. Gynecol. Obstet.* 1, S3–S10.
15. Gleicher, N., El-Roeiy, A., Confino, E., and Friberg, J. (1987). Is endometriosis an autoimmune disease? *Obstet. Gynecol.* 70, 115–122.
16. Reiter, R. C. (1990). A profile of women with chronic pelvic pain. *Clin. Obstet. Gynecol.* 33, 117–118.
17. Howard, F. M. (1993). The role of laparoscopy in the evaluation of chronic pelvic pain: Promise and pitfall. *Obstet. Gynecol. Surv.* 48, 10–46.
18. Mathias, S. D., Kuppermann, M., Liberman, R. F., Lipschutz, R. C., and Steege, J. F. (1996). Chronic pelvic pain: Prevalence, health-related quality of life, and economic correlates. *Obstet. Gynecol.* 87, 321–327.
19. Mahmood, T. A., and Templeton, A. A. (1991). Prevalence and genesis of endometriosis. *Hum. Reprod.* 6, 544–549.
20. Kresch, A. J., Seifer, D. B., and Sachs, L. B. (1984). Laparoscopy in 100 women with chronic pelvic pain. *Obstet. Gynecol.* 64, 672–674.
21. Vercellini, P., Trespidi, L., De Giorgi, O., Cortesi, I., Parazzini, F., and Crosignani, P. G. (1996). Endometriosis and pelvic pain: Relation to disease stage and localization. *Fertil. Steril.* 65, 299–304.
22. Fukaya, T., Hoshiai, H., and Yajima, A. (1993). Is pelvic endometriosis always associated with chronic pain? A retrospective study of 618 cases diagnosed by laparoscopy. *Am. J. Obstet. Gynecol.* 169, 719–722.
23. Rock, J. A. (1993). Endometriosis and pelvic pain. *Fertil. Steril.* 60, 950–951.
24. Perper, M. M., Nezhat, F., Goldstein, H., Nezhat, C. H., and Nezhat, C. (1995). Dysmenorrhea is related to the number of implants in endometriosis patients. *Fertil. Steril.* 63, 500–503.
25. Koninckx, P. R., Meuleman, C., Demeyere, S., Lesaffre, E., and Cornillie, F. (1991). Suggestive evidence that pelvic endometriosis is a progressive disease, whereas deeply infiltrating endometriosis is associated with pelvic pain. *Fertil. Steril.* 55, 759–765.
26. Porpora, M. G., Koninckx, P. R., Piazze, J., Natili, M., Colagrande, S., and Cosmi, E. V. (1999). Correlation between endometriosis and pelvic pain. *J. Am. Assoc. Gynecol. Laparosc.* 6, 429–434.
27. Fedele, L., Bianchi, S., Boccioline, L., Di Nola, G., and Parazzini, F. (1992). Pain symptoms associated with endometriosis. *Obstet. Gynecol.* 79, 767–769.
28. Dmowski, W. P., Rana, N., and Jafari, N. (2001). Postlaparoscopic small bowel obstruction secondary to unrecognized nodular endometriosis of the terminal ileum. *J. Am. Assoc. Gynecol. Laparosc.* 8, 161–166.
29. Fedele, L., Bianchi, S., Raffaelli, R., Zanconato, G., and Zanette, G. (1999). Phantom endometriosis of the sciatic nerve. *Fertil. Steril.* 72, 727–729.
30. Hibbard, J., and Schreiber, J. R. (1984). Footdrop due to sciatic nerve endometriosis. *Am. J. Obstet. Gynecol.* 149, 800–801.
31. Salazar-Grueso, E., and Roos, R. (1986). Sciatic endometriosis: A treatable sensorimotor mononeuropathy. *Neurology* 36, 1360–1363.
32. Vernon, M. W., Beard, J. S., Graves, K., and Wilson, E. A. (1986). Classification of endometriotic implants by morphologic appearance and capacity to synthesize prostaglandin F. *Fertil. Steril.* 46, 801–806.
33. Demco, L. (1998). Mapping the source and character of pain due to endometriosis by patient-assisted laparoscopy. *J. Am. Assoc. Gynecol. Laparosc.* 5, 241–245.
34. Anaf, V., Simon, P., Nakadi, I. E., Fayt, I., Buxant, F., Simonart, T., Peny, M. O., and Noel, J. C. (2000). Relationship between endometriotic foci and nerves in rectovaginal endometriotic nodules. *Hum. Reprod.* 15, 1744–1750.
35. Mathias, J. R., Franklin, R., Quast, D. C., Fraga, N., Loftin, C. A., Yates, L., and Harrison, V. (1998). Relation of endometriosis and neuromuscular disease of the gastrointestinal tract: New insights. *Fertil. Steril.* 70, 81–88.
36. Perry, C. P. (2000). Peripheral neuropathies causing chronic pelvic pain. *J. Am. Assoc. Gynecol. Laparosc.* 7, 281–287.
37. Walker, E. A. (1997). Medically unexplained physical symptoms. *Clin. Obstet. Gynecol.* 40, 589–601.
38. Braun, D. P., Gebel, H., House, R., Rana, N., and Dmowski, W. P. (1996). Spontaneous and induced synthesis of cytokines by peripheral blood monocytes in patients with endometriosis. *Fertil. Steril.* 65, 1125–1129.
39. Karck, U., Reister, F., Schafer, W., Zahradnik, H. P., and Breckwoldt, M. (1996). PGE2 and PGF2α release by human peritoneal macrophages in endometriosis. *Prostaglandins* 51, 49–60.
40. Badura, A. S., Reiter, R. C., Altmaier, E. M., Rhomberg, A., and Elas, D. (1997). Dissociation, somatization, substance abuse, and coping in women with chronic pelvic pain. *Obstet. Gynecol.* 90, 405–410.
41. Waller, K. G., and Shaw, R. W. (1995). Endometriosis, pelvic pain, and psychological functioning. *Fertil. Steril.* 63, 796–800.
42. Strathy, J. H., Molgaard, C. A., Coulam, C. B., and Melton, L. J. (1982). Endometriosis and Infertility: A laparoscopic study of endometriosis among fertile and infertile women. *Fertil. Steril.* 38, 667–672.
43. Jansen, R. P. (1986). Minimal endometriosis and reduced fecundability: Prospective evidence from an artificial insemination by donor program. *Fertil. Steril.* 46, 141–143.
44. Hammond, M. G., Jordan, S., and Sloan, C. S. (1986). Factors affecting pregnancy rates in a donor insemination program using frozen semen. *Am. J. Obstet. Gynecol.* 155, 480–485.
45. Portuondo, J. A., Echanojauregui, A. D., Herran, C., and Alijarte, I. (1983). Early conception in patients with untreated mild endometriosis. *Fertil. Steril.* 39, 22–25.
46. Rodriguez-Escudero, F. J., Neyro, J. L., Corcostegui, B., and Benito, J. A. (1988). Does minimal endometriosis reduce infertility? *Fertil. Steril.* 50, 522–524.
47. Halme, J., and Surrey, E. S. (1990). Endometriosis and infertility: The mechanisms involved. *In* "Current Concepts in Endometriosis" (D. Chadha, and V. Buttram, Jr., eds.), pp. 157–178. Alan R. Liss, New York.
48. Toma, S. K., Stovall, D. W., and Hammond, M. G. (1992). The effect of laparoscopic ablation or danocrine on pregnancy rates in patients with stage I or II endometriosis undergoing donor insemination. *Obstet. Gynecol.* 80, 253–256.

49. Berube, S., Marcoux, S., Langevin, M., Maheux, R., and The Canadian Collaborative Group on Endometriosis. (1998). Fecundity of infertile women with minimal or mild endometriosis and women with unexplained infertility. *Fertil. Steril.* 69, 1034–1041.
50. Collins, J. A., Burrows, E. A., and Wilan, A. R. (1995). The prognosis for live birth among untreated infertile couples. *Fertil. Steril.* 64, 22–28.
51. Koninckx, P. R., Meuleman, C., Oosterlynck, D., and Cornillie, F. J. (1996). Diagnosis of deep endometriosis by clinical examination during menstruation and plasma CA125 concentration. *Fertil. Steril.* 65, 280–287.
52. Guerriero, S., Ajossa, S., Mais, V., Risalvato, A., Lai, M. P., and Melis, G. B. (1998). The diagnosis of endometriosis using colour doppler energy imaging. *Hum. Reprod.* 13, 1691–1695.
53. Mais, V., Guerriero, S., Ajossa, S., Angiolucci, M., Paoletti, A. M., and Melis, G. B. (1993). The efficiency of transvaginal ultrasonography in the diagnosis of endometrioma. *Fertil. Steril.* 60, 776–780.
54. Fedele, L., Bianchi, S., Portuese, A., Borruto, F., and Dorta, M. (1998). Transrectal ultrasonography in the assessment of rectovaginal endometriosis. *Obstet. Gynecol.* 91, 776–780.
55. Fedele, L., Bianchi, S., Raffaelli, R., and Portuese, A. (1997). Preoperative assessment of bladder endometriosis. *Hum. Reprod.* 12, 2519–2522.
56. Dmowski, W. P., Lesniewicz, R., Rana, N., Pepping, P., and Noursalehi, M. (1997). Changing trends in the diagnosis of endometriosis; A comparative study of women with pelvic endometriosis presenting with chronic pelvic pain or infertility. *Fertil. Steril.* 67, 238–243.
57. Sutton, C., Pooley, A. S., Ewen, S. P., and Haines, P. (1997). Follow-up report on a randomized controlled trial laser laparoscopy in the treatment of pelvic pain associated with minimal to moderate endometriosis. *Fertil. Steril.* 68, 1070–1074.
58. D'Hooghe, T. M., Bambra, C. S., Raeymaekers, B. M., and Koninckx, P. R. (1996). Serial laparoscopies over 30 months show that endometriosis in captive baboons (Papio anubis, Papio cynocephalus) is a progressive disease. *Fertil. Steril.* 65, 645–649.
59. Judd, F. K., Burrows, G. D., and Holwill, B. J. (1987). The psychiatrist in the management of chronic pain. *In* "Handbook of Chronic Pain Management" (G. Burrows, D. Elton, and G. V. Staley, eds.), p. 301. Elsevier, Amsterdam.
60. Eisenach, J. C., Lysak, S. Z., and Viscomi, C. M. (1989). Epidural clonidine analgesia following surgery: Phase 1. *Anesthesiology* 71, 640.
61. Dawood, M. Y. (1990). Transcutaneous electrical nerve stimulation (TENS) for the treatment of primary dysmenorrhea: A randomized crossover comparison with placebo TENS and ibuprofen. *Obstet. Gynecol.* 75, 656–660.
62. Vercellini, P., Sacerdote, P., Panerai, A. E., Manfredi, B., Bocciolone, L., and Crosignani, P. G. (1992). Monocellular cell B-endorphin concentration in women with and without endometriosis. *Obstet. Gynecol.* 79, 743–746.
63. Vercellini, P., Trespidi, L., Colombo, A., Vendola, N., Marchini, M., and Crosignani, P. G. (1993). A gonadotropin-releasing hormone agonist versus a low-dose oral contraceptive for pelvic pain associated with endometriosis. *Fertil. Steril.* 60, 75–79.
64. Barbieri, R. L., and Ryans, K. J. (1981). Danazol: Endocrine pharmacology and therapeutic applications. *Am. J. Obstet. Gynecol.* 141, 453–463.
65. Dmowski, W. P. (1988). Danazol-induced pseudomenopause in the management of endometriosis. *Clin. Obstet. Gynecol.* 31, 829–839.
66. Dmowski, W. P. (1990). Danazol a synthetic steroid with diverse biologic effects. *J. Reprod. Med.* 35, 69–75.
67. Lessey, B. A. (2000). Medical management of endometriosis and infertility. *Fertil. Steril.* 73, 1089–1096.
68. Barbieri, R. L. (1992). Hormone treatment of endometriosis: The estrogen threshold hypothesis. *Am. J. Obstet. Gynecol.* 166, 740–745.
69. Hurst, B. S., and Schlaff, W. D. (1992). Treatment options for endometriosis. *In* "Infertility and Reproductive Medical Clinics of North America" (D. L. Olive, ed.), pp. 645–655. W. B. Saunders, Philadelphia, PA.
70. Cheung, T., Lo, K. W., Lam, C. W., Lau, W., and Lam, P. G. (2000). A crossover study of triptorelin and leuprorelin acetate. *Fertil. Steril.* 74, 299–305.
71. The Gestrinone Italian Study Group. (1996). Gestrinone versus a gonadotropin-releasing hormone agonist for the treatment of pelvic pain associated with endometriosis: A multicenter, randomized, double-blind study. *Fertil. Steril.* 66, 911–919.
72. Dawood, M. Y. (1993). Impact of medical treatment of endometriosis on bone mass. *Am. J. Obstet. Gynecol.* 168, 674–684.
73. Surrey, E. S. (1995). Steroidal and nonsteroidal "add-back" therapy: Extending safety and efficacy of gonadotropin-releasing hormone agonists in the gynecologic patient. *Fertil. Steril.* 64, 673–685.
74. Wong, S. L., Dmowski, W. P., DePaoli, A., Gray, M. E., and Martha, P. M. for the FASTER Study Group. (2000). Comparative pharmacodynamic effects of Abarelix Depot-F vs. Lupron Depot in women with endometriosis-associated pain. *Fertil. Steril.* 74, S118.
75. Takayama, K., Zeitoun, K., Gunby, R. T., Sasano, H., Carr, B. R., and Bulun, S. E. (1998). Treatment of severe postmenopausal endometriosis with an aromatase inhibitor. *Fertil. Steril.* 69, 709–713.
76. Kettel, L. M., Murphy, A. A., Morales, A. J., Ulmann, A., Baulieu, E. E., and Yen, S. S. (1996). Treatment of endometriosis with the antiprogesterone mifepristone (RU486). *Fertil. Steril.* 65, 23–28.
77. Igarashi, M., Iizuka, M., Abe, Y., and Ubuki, Y. (1998). Novel vaginal danazol ring therapy for pelvic endometriosis, in particular deeply infiltrating endometriosis. *Hum. Reprod.* 13, 1952–1956.
78. Igarashi, M., Abe, Y., Fukuda, M., Ando, A., Miyasaka, M., and Yoshida, M. (2000). Novel conservative medical therapy for uterine adenomyosis with a danazol-loaded intrauterine device. *Fertil. Steril.* 74, 412–413.
79. Vercellini, P., Aimi, G., Panazza, S., DeGiorgi, O., Pesole, A., and Crosignani, P. G. (1999). A levonorgestrel-releasing intrauterine system for the treatment of dysmenorrhea associated with endometriosis: A pilot study. *Fertil. Steril.* 72, 505–508.
80. Redwine, D. B. (1991). Conservative laparoscopic excision of endometriosis by sharp dissection: Life table analysis of reoperation and persistent or recurrent disease. *Fertil. Steril.* 56, 628–634.
81. Loh, F. H., Tan, A. T., Kumar, J., and Ng, S. C. (1999). Ovarian response after laparoscopic ovarian cystectomy for endometriotic cysts in 132 monitored cycles. *Fertil. Steril.* 72, 316–321.
82. Hock, D. L., Sharafi, K., Dagostino, L., Kemmann, E., and Seifer, D. B. (2001). Contribution of diminished ovarian reserve to hypofertility associated with endometriosis. *J. Reprod. Med.* 46, 710.
83. Cook, A. S., and Rock, J. A. (1991). The role of laparoscopy in the treatment of endometriosis. *Fertil. Steril.* 55, 663–680.
84. Chapron, C., Dubuisson, J. B., Frital, X., Fernandez, B., Poncelet, C., Beguin, S., and Pinelli, L. (1999). Operative management of deep endometriosis infiltrating the uterosacral ligaments. *J. Am. Assoc. Gynecol. Laparosc.* 6, 31–37.
85. Sutton, C. J., Ewen, S. P., Whitelaw, N., and Haines, P. (1994). Prospective, randomized, double-blind, controlled trial of laser laparoscopy in the treatment of pelvic pain associated with minimal, mild, and moderate endometriosis. *Fertil. Steril.* 62, 696–700.
86. Lichten, E. M., and Bombard, J. (1987). Surgical treatment of primary dysmenorrhea with laparoscopic uterine nerve ablation. *J. Reprod. Med.* 32, 37–41.
87. Nezhat, C., and Nezhat, F. (1992). A simplified method of laparoscopic presacral neurectomy for the treatment of central pelvic pain due to endometriosis. *Br. J. Obstet. Gynecol.* 99, 659–663.
88. Candiani, G. B., Fedele, L., and Vercellini, P. (1992). Presacral neurectomy for the treatment of pelvic pain associated with endometriosis: A controlled study. *Am. J. Obstet. Gynecol.* 167, 100–103.

89. Kistner, R. W. (1975). Management of endometriosis in the infertile patient. *Fertil. Steril.* 26, 1151–1166.
90. Dmowski, W. P. (1993). Endometriosis. "Office Gynecology" (R. H. Glass. ed.), pp. 359–380. Williams & Wilkins, Baltimore , MD.
91. Hughes, E. G., Fedorkow, D. M., and Collins, J. A. (1993). A quantitative overview of controlled trials in endometriosis-associated infertility. *Fertil. Steril.* 59, 963–970.
92. Badawy, S. Z., ElBakry, M. M., Samuel, F., and Dizer, M. (1988). Cumulative pregnancy rates in infertile women with endometriosis. *J. Reprod. Med.* 33, 757–760.
93. Adamson, G. D., and Pastas, D. J. (1994). Surgical treatment of endometriosis-associated infertility: Meta-analysis compared with survival analysis. *Am. J. Obstet. Gynecol.* 171, 1488–1505.
94. Fayez, J. A., and Collazos, L. M. (1990). Comparison between laparotomy and operative laparoscopy in the treatment of moderate and severe stages of endometriosis. *Int. J. Fertil.* 35, 272–279.
95. Busacca, M., Fedele, L., Bianchi, S., Candiani, M., Agnoli, B., Raffaelli, R., and Vignali, M. (1998). Surgical treatment of recurrent endometriosis: Laparotomy versus laparoscopy. *Hum. Reprod.* 13, 2271–2274.
96. Adamson, G. D., Subak, L. L., Pasta, D. J., Hurd, S. J., Franque, O., and Rodriguez, B. D. (1992). Comparison of CO_2 laser laparoscopy with laparotomy for treatment of endometriomata. *Fertil. Steril.* 57, 965–973.
97. Donnez, J., Lemaire-Rubbers, M., Karaman, Y., Nisolle-Pochet, M., and Casanas-Roux, F. (1987). Combined (hormonal and microsurgical) therapy in infertile women with endometriosis. *Fertil. Steril.* 48, 239–242.
98. Guzick, D. S., Silliman, N. P., Adamson, G. D., Buttram, V. C., Canis, M., Malinak, L. R., and Schenken, R. S. (1997). Prediction of pregnancy in infertile women based on the American Society for Reproductive Medicine's revised classification of endometriosis. *Fertil. Steril.* 67, 822–829.
99. Candiani, G. B., Fedele, L., Vercellini, P., Bianchi, S., and DiNola, G. (1991). Repetitive conservative surgery for recurrence of endometriosis. *Obstet. Gynecol.* 77, 421–424.
100. Marcoux, S., Maheux, R., Berube, S., and The Canadian Collaborative Group on Endometriosis. (1997). Laparoscopic surgery in infertile women with minimal or mild endometriosis. *N. Engl. J. Med.* 337, 217–222.
101. Peterson, C. M., Hatasaka, H. H., Jones, K. P., Pousin, A. M., Carrell, D. T., and Urry, R. L. (1994). Ovulation induction with gonadotropins and IUI compared with in vitro fertilization and no therapy: A prospective, nonrandomized, cohort study and meta-analysis. *Fertil. Steril.* 62, 535–544.
102. Tummon, I. S., Asher, L. J., Martin, J. S., and Tulandi, T. (1997). Randomized controlled trial of superovulation and insemination for infertility associated with minimal or mild endometriosis. *Fertil. Steril.* 68, 8–12.
103. Dmowski, W. P. (1995). Endometriosis and *in vitro* fertilization. "Assisted Reproduction Reviews," Vol.5, pp. 74–81. Williams & Wilkins, Baltimore, MD.
104. Guzick, D. S., Yao, Y. S., Berga, S. L., Krasnow, J. S., Stovall, D. W., Kubik, C. J., and Zeleznik, A. J. (1994). Endometriosis impairs the efficacy of gamete intrafallopian transfer: Results of a case-control study. *Fertil. Steril.* 62, 1186–1191.
105. U.S. Dept. of Health and Human Services, Center for Disease Control and Prevention. (2000). 1998 assisted reproductive technology success rates, national summary and fertility clinic reports. CDC. SART. 22.
106. Daniell, J. F., Kurtz, B. R., and Gurley, L. D. (1991). Laser laparoscopic management of large endometriomas. *Fertil. Steril.* 55, 692–695.
107. Sutton, C. J., Ewen, S. P., Jacobs, S. A., and Whitelaw, N. L. (1997). Laser laparoscopic surgery in the treatment of ovarian endometriomas. *J. Am. Assoc. Gynecol. Laparosc.* 4, 319–323.
108. Fayez, J. A., and Vogel, M. F. (1991). Comparison of different treatment methods of endometriomas by laparoscopy. *Obstet. Gynecol.* 78, 660–665.
109. Hemmings, R., Bissonnette, F., and Bouzayen, R. (1998). Results of laparoscopic treatments of ovarian endometriomas: Laparoscopic ovarian fenestration and coagulation. *Fertil. Steril.* 70, 527–529.
110. Saleh, A., and Tulandi, T. (1999). Reoperation after laparoscopic treatment of ovarian endometriomas by excision and by fenestration. *Fertil. Steril.* 72, 322–324.
111. Vercellini, P., Vendola, N., Bocciolone, L., Colombo, A., Rognoni, M. T., and Bolis, G. (1992). Laparoscopic aspiration of ovarian endometriomas—effect with postoperative gonadotropin releasing hormone agonist treatment. *J. Reprod. Med.* 37, 577–580.
112. Donnez, J., Nisolle, M., Gillerot, S., Anaf, V., Clerckx-Braun, F., and Casanas-Roux, F. (1994). Ovarian endometrial cysts: The role of gonadotropin-releasing hormone agonist and/or drainage. *Fertil. Steril.* 62, 63–66.
113. Beretta, P., Franchi, M., Ghezzi, F., Busacca, M., Zupi, E., and Bolis, P. (1998). Randomized clinical trial of two laparoscopic treatments of endometriomas: Cystectomy versus drainage and coagulation. *Fertil. Steril.* 70, 1176–1180.
114. Rana, N., Thomas, S., Rotman, C., and Dmowski, W. P. (1996). Decrease in the size of ovarian endometriomas during ovarian suppression in stage IV endometriosis—role of preoperative medical treatment. *J. Reprod. Med.* 41, 384–392.
115. Dmowski, W. P., Radwanska, E., and Rana, N. (1988). Recurrent endometriosis following hysterectomy and oophorectomy: The role of residual ovarian fragments. *Intern. J. Gynecol. Obstet.* 26, 93–103.
116. Rana, N., Rotman, C., Hasson, H. M., Redwine, D. B., and Dmowski, W. P. (1996). Ovarian remnant syndrome after laparoscopic hysterectomy and bilateral salpingo-oophorectomy for severe pelvic endometriosis. *J. Am. Assoc. Gynecol. Laparosc.* 3, 423–426.
117. Dmowski, W. P., and Cohen, M. R. (1978). Antigonadotropin (danazol) in the treatment of endometriosis. *Am. J. Obstet. Gynecol.* 130, 41–48.
118. Waller, K. G., and Shaw, R. W. (1993). Gonadotropin-releasing hormone analogues for the treatment of endometriosis: Long-term follow-up. *Fertil. Steril.* 59, 511–515.
119. Miller, J. D., Shaw, R. W., Casper, R. F., Rock, J. A., Thomas, E. J., Dmowski, W. P., Surrey, E., Malinak, L. R., and Moghissi, K. (1997). Historical prospective cohort study of the recurrence of pain after discontinuation of treatment with danazol or a gonadotropin-releasing hormone agonist. *Fertil. Steril.* 70, 293–296.
120. Busacca, M., Bianchi, S., Agnoli, B., Candiani, M., Calia, C., DeMarinis, S., and Vignali, M. (1999). Follow-up of laparoscopic treatment of stage III-IV endometriosis. *J. Am. Assoc. Gynecol. Laparosc.* 6, 55–58.

C H A P T E R

27

Menopause

NATHAN G. KASE

Department of Obstetrics, Gynecology and Reproductive Science
The Mount Sinai Medical Center
Mount Sinai School of Medicine and Hospital
New York, New York 10029

I. INTRODUCTION

Menopause, derived from the Greek *men* (month) and *pausis* (cessation), is defined as the point in life when women experience permanent cessation of menstruation due to irreversible loss of "ovarian activity." More precisely, the collective follicle capacity of the ovaries to secrete adequate estradiol diminishes to the point at which proliferation of the endometrium adequate to produce menstruation is no longer achievable. But to women menopause is justifiably more than just loss of menses or even reproductive competence. Although some ovarian steroid function continues transiently beyond this critical point and limited extragonadal production of estrogen may persist (which in certain circumstances can be elevated sufficiently to produce dysfunctional even pathological postmenopausal bleeding), at menopause the ability of the ovaries to function as endocrine organs capable of providing sufficient hormone to sustain the estrogen-dependent biologic aspects of a wide variety of tissues has also ceased. Estrogen modulates a broad array of nonreproductive functions including bone and mineral metabolism,[1] cardiac and vascular function [2] as well as cognition and memory,[3] and the risk of progression of age-related neurodegenerative diseases.[4, 5]

The global and long-term consequences of this prolonged hypoestrogen state and the various reactive strategies available to meet these challenges are the subject of this chapter. Accordingly, it will deal with the demographics and epidemiology of menopause, the complex and paradoxical endocrinology of the perimenopausal transition, and the "burdens" of acute and prolonged hypoestrogenism, as well as the benefits/risks of hormonal replenishment. Finally, a consideration of alternative therapies will be offered.

From this review it should be clear that while the postmenopausal years represent a hormone deficiency state, it is not in itself a disease. Rather, menopause should be viewed as an opportunity to apply interventions which not only modify and correct acute short-term symptomatic difficulties but provide ongoing preventive and supportive health care by the identification, prevention, and correction of emerging quality and duration of life health issues. At the very least, in addition to sustained general medical care, institution of corrective lifestyle measures, such as smoking cessation, positive nutritional and exercise programs confer unequivocal benefits to this population.[6, 7]

II. THE AGING OF THE WORLD'S POPULATION

A detailed review of the demographic and epidemiologic impact of the increasing size of the elderly population experienced in the second half of the last century and projected to *continue* into the first half of this century is beyond the scope of this review. However, Speroff *et al.* [8] have summarized the signal issues. We are now a society unlike any other in recorded history—we can expect to reach old age. Whereas in 1900 in the U.S. life expectancy was only 49 years, the estimated life expectancy in 2000 was 79.7 years for women and 72.9 for men. Furthermore, once attaining the age of 65 current life expectancy for men is 80.5 and women 84.3 years. Should these trends continue eventually two-thirds of the population will survive to 85 or more, as many as 90% will live past 65 years, and a majority will be women. Not only are more women growing older, more are living longer.

Given these data, and with the stability of the median and average age of menopause (52 years) across many decades, women and their health providers must plan for as much as 30 years will be lived in the postmenopausal, physiologically hypoestrogenic state. It is currently estimated that women reach age 50 at about 3–4 thousand per day and will continue at this rate into the first third of this century.

III. OVARIAN FOLLICLE ENDOWMENT, ATTRITION, AND EXHAUSTION

Senescence of the ovary is the cause of menopause and is directly related to the fact that the ovary is endowed with a finite, nonrenewable, postmitotic pool of dormant primordial follicles. Defined endocrinologically, menopause is the consequence of the irreversible depletion and final exhaustion of ovarian follicles, which results in permanent loss of gonadal estradiol secretion and the end of "physiologic" (ovarian follicle generated and controlled) menstruation.

A. Factors Controlling Follicle Reserve and Attrition

Menopause is linked to the complete loss of the primordial follicle reserve. Although the fundamental factors controlling first the imposition of follicle arrest and then the variable retention in the resting pool or even the timing and rate of reactivation and exit from that pool are unknown, certain genetic and nongenetic observations inform (as well as confuse) the understanding of these crucial processes.

1. Genetic Factors

Various lines of study have defined a primary genetic basis for the timing of follicle depletion and menopause. Mothers and daughters as well as identical twins experience menopause at the same ages. A study of 275 monozygotic and 353 dizygotic female twin pairs yielded a heritability (h^2) for age at menopause of 63%. The significance of this genetic effect was not altered by adjustment for confounders. Both early and late menopause were found to be significantly influenced by genetic factors.[9]

That accelerated follicle atresia occurs *in utero* in 45x Turner's syndrome implies that in order to avoid atresia both X chromosomes must be active in germ cells. The occurrence of premature ovarian failure in mosaicisms (45x/46xx; 46xx/47xxx) [10, 11] has intensified interest in identifying factors on the X chromosome which govern normal ovarian follicle maintenance and control. For example, a review of 118 cases of balanced X autosome translocations and 31 cases of balanced inversions revealed critical involvement of regions on the X chromosome (Xq13–q22, Xq22–26).[12] At least 8 different genes on Xq21 are involved in premature ovarian failure.[13] Not all gene defects altering the number and attrition rate of the ovarian follicle pool are located on the X chromosome. A genetic mutation of FOXL2, a gene on chromosome 3, has been identified as a cause of premature ovarian failure and a variety of defects in eyelid development.[14] FOXL2 protein is a transcription factor which controls activation and inactivation of other downstream genes involved in both eyelid formation and the size and retention of the ovarian follicle pool. Finally, the finding of altered FSH receptor isoforms in anovulation and premature ovarian failure suggests other genetic factor involvement.

2. Nongenetic Factors

Multiple studies have consistently documented that age of menopause is earlier by an average of 1.5 years as a consequence of smoking.[15] In addition, sufficient evidence exists to believe that Body Mass Index (BMI) is a factor: undernourished women, thin women, and vegetarians experience earlier menopause.[16] On the other hand, consumption of alcohol is associated with later menopause. There is no correlation between age of menopause and age of menarche, race, height, or duration or intensity of physical labor.

The best data on age of menopause are found in the Massachusetts Women's Health Study.[17] Initiated in 1981 this important study observed 2570 women aged 45–55 over a 4-1/2 year interval and showed the median age for menopause was 51.3 years. Only current smoking was identified as a cause of earlier menopause (1.5 years); no impact was seen in the use of oral contraception (OC), socioeconomic factors, or marital status. (As opposed to median age, i.e., half the women reached menopause by 51.3 years in the Massachusetts study, in the longitudinal study of Treloar [18] the average age of menopause was 50.7 years with a 95% range of 44–56 years.)

Other epidemiologic studies suggest that nongenetic biologic factors influence follicle development and menopausal timing. For example, women of reproductive age who have undergone unilateral oophorectomy or chemotherapy do have an earlier onset of menopause, especially if these procedures occur later in reproductive life.[19] In addition, evidence suggests steroidal contraception lends protection to the ovarian follicle pool in these adverse circumstances. On the other hand, OC use does not delay menopause but women with many pregnancies and hence fewer cycles are delayed in menopause timing.[20, 21] Finally, with respect to follicle "usage" neither women who have undergone repeated cycles of gonadotropin induction of ovulation nor women with dizygotic twins experience earlier menopause.[22]

These considerations aside, the physiologic principles involved in the rate and timing of human ovarian follicle exhaustion provide a framework to define and understand the clinical issues involved in the female climacteric, and arrange these biologic changes into perimenopausal and early and late menopausal phenomena.

IV. DEFINITIONS: MENOPAUSE, PERIMENOPAUSE, AND THE MENOPAUSAL TRANSITION

The World Health Organization (WHO) [23] has established the following definitions. *Menopause* is defined as the date "of the final menstrual period" retrospectively designated as one year without flow in appropriately aged women (over 40 years). For *perimenopause* the WHO definition "includes the period of years immediately before the menopause (when the endocrinological, biological, and clinical features of approaching menopause commence) and the first year after the menopause." To reduce confusion generated by the one-year overlap inherent in these definitions, the term *menopausal transition* is used to define the one year of amenorrhea that at once ends the perimenopause and begins menopause. This compromise has reasonable biologic grounds for its application. First, very few women abruptly end their menstrual life and enter menopause in a single month. A blurred transition is also appropriate since prior to complete exhaustion a limited number of active follicles do transiently exist at the time of menopause but collectively cannot secrete sufficient estradiol to induce menses.

On the other hand, it will be seen that perimenopause is a very different biologic and clinical entity than simply (and incorrectly) the decade marked by intermittent but relentless withdrawal of ovarian function which blends imperceptibly into menopause and the years beyond. To the contrary, perimenopause must now be viewed as a state of *accelerated follicle activation and endocrine hyperactivity*, an "endogenous hyperstimulation syndrome" [24] with unique clinical implications and dramatically contrasts with the follicle exhaustion and permanent ovarian inactivity that defines the biology and clinical consequences of menopause.

V. PERIMENOPAUSE

Although the definition of *the end* of perimenopause as established by WHO is clear—twelve months of amenorrhea—the *start* of perimenopause is less certain. Currently perimenopause is defined as the period preceding menopause, which is characterized by menstrual irregularity (both in cycle length and amount of flow) and increasing months of amenorrhea. During this time anovulatory cycles become more prevalent and cycle length increases. Perimenopause begins when previously normal ovulatory cycles become less frequent and cycle lengths change.

The longitudinal studies of menstrual cycles by Treloar [18] and the Massachusetts Women's Health Study [17] support this concept. When women are in their 40s beginning 2–8 years before menopause and prior to the emergence of frank anovulation, menstrual cycle intervals become variable, first shortened and then lengthened. Cycle variability uniformly precedes menopause regardless of the age when menses cease and whether menopause is early or late. The duration of the follicle phase is the major determinant of overall cycle length. Taken together perimenopause is characterized by average age of onset → 46 years, age of onset for

95% of women → 39–51 years, average duration → 5 years, and duration for 95% of women → 2–8 years.

As will be seen, *endocrine changes* are more specific landmarks of the initiation of perimenopause. These precede cycle interruption and may not be manifest clinically.[24]

A. Endocrinology of Perimenopause

Perimenopause is a unique endocrinologic state. During this 2–8 year interval while anovulatory cycles become progressively more prevalent, ovarian follicles undergo an increase rate of reactivation and loss prior to eventual total depletion. This acceleration appears to begin when the total number of remaining follicles reaches approximately 25,000 (at about 37–38 years of age) and correlates with a subtle but real increase in FSH and a decrease in inhibin. As more follicles grow, collectively these follicles secrete higher levels of estradiol per cycle. Contrary to conventional wisdom, longitudinal studies demonstrate that normal even high estradiol levels persist throughout perimenopause and only decline in the transitional year prior to defined menopause,[25] Fig. 27.1.

To identify the changes in feedback that might account for *both* increased FSH and estradiol, the elements responsible for the overall "tone" of feedback, i.e., concentrations of dimeric inhibin A, inhibin B, activin A, and total and free follistatin as well as serum FSH and estradiol have been measured in the follicle phase and midluteal phase in older and younger normal cycling women.[26, 27] Taken together these studies suggest that the *net increase in FSH stimulatory feedback* which exists in perimenopausal women results from a *decrease* in inhibin B and an *increase* in activin A leading to increased serum FSH. Furthermore, the follicle phase decrease in inhibin B is the earliest marker of the beginning of perimenopause and the decline in follicle number and function accompany reproductive aging.

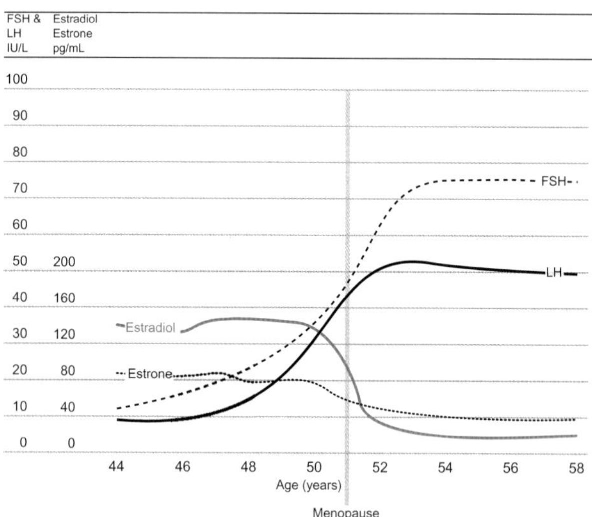

FIGURE 27.1 The perimenopausal transition. In perimenopause, FSH levels rise despite persistent relatively high levels of estrogen. Only in the months prior to formal menopause do estrogen levels decline. After menopause FSH and LH continue to rise whereas estrogen remains low.

1. Summary of Endocrine Changes in Perimenopause [24]

a. Menstrual Characteristics

1. *Menstrual cycles*: At first regular, ovulatory but shorter cycles, shorter follicle phases with gradually evolving ovulatory disturbances, progressive anovulation, cycle lengthening, eventual oligoamenorrhea.
2. *Menstrual flow*: Progressive increase in amount and duration with intermittent menometrorrhagia with spotting alternating with flooding.

b. Hormonal Characteristics

1. *Inhibin*: Inhibin B is the earliest marker of perimenopause and declines before FSH increases. Gradually both inhibin A and B decrease to menopause when both fall below the sensitivity of most assays.
2. *FSH*: Early gradual then accelerated rise through perimenopause.
3. *LH*: Variable levels at first but begin sustained elevation just before menopause.
4. E_2: At first higher concentrations only in the early follicle phase of shortened cycles, evolving to include both the follicle phase and persisting during flow in anovulatory cycles. For over half of perimenopause estradiol levels are either normal or intermittently higher than normal for the entire duration of the cycle, however prolonged. Immediately prior to "defined" menopause estradiol levels decline.
5. *Progesterone*: Normal luteal values at first but swiftly declining as ovulatory dysfunction and anovulatory cycles evolve.

Prior characterization of perimenopause as a state of "endogenous ovarian hyperstimulation" [24] accurately describes the endocrinology of this period, i.e., high FSH, high estradiol, low progesterone, and accelerated but transient appearance of numerous but small active follicles.

B. Clinical Characteristics of Perimenopause

The endocrinologic changes across perimenopause become dramatically real clinically. As Santoro [28] and others have shown, mean estradiol levels both in follicular and premenstrual phases are significantly higher than younger women (and approximately 10% of measurements are extremely high exceeding normal midcycle peak levels) and 50% or more of the cycles are anovulatory, one can understand the resulting perimenopausal "syndrome" of heavy prolonged unpredictable menses, dysfunctional uterine bleeding, menometrorrhagia, breast tenderness and enlargement, fluid retention, new onset of migraine headaches, and new and unpredictable mood swings as the major burdens of many perimenopausal women.

Furthermore, the reduced number and function of the granulosa cells of this remaining cohort of aging follicles (exhibited in the early reduction in inhibin levels as well as IGF) [29] is undoubtedly responsible for the reduced fertility and fecundity of perimenopausal women. Resistance to induced ovulation compounds the already reduced spontaneous ovulatory function. But even with conception, higher rates of early spontaneous abortion and fetuses with major anomalies (note the high rate of meiotic spindle abnormalities and fractured zona pellucida recovered from IVF cycles, diminished fertilization, and decreased implantation rates even in exogenous steroid endometrial supplementation cycles) suggest defects in both oocyte and its nurturing mantle of granulosa cells.

Less clear is the relationship between the endocrinology of perimenopause and changes such as vasomotor symptoms (VMS) and adverse psychosocial and emotional experiences as well as the initiation of bone loss in this period of a woman's life.

1. Menstrual Flow and Cycle Related Symptoms

Menstrual flooding has been estimated to be the major cause of visits to physicians by menopausal women.[30] Furthermore, Ballinger [31] found heavy flow was significantly associated with high estradiol levels late in the cycle. The prevalence of menorrhagia in 45% of women in early and 48% in late perimenopause is not unexpected in women with high estrogen and low progesterone levels. Thickened endometrial stripes on transvaginal ultrasound, the higher frequency of endometrial polyps, and the appearance and/or growth of submucous fibroids predisposes and abets the dysfunctional bleeding in these women. Predictably, the incidence of D&C and hysterectomy peaks in this age group.

2. VMS in Perimenopause

Perimenopausal VMS, both day and night time episodic flushing and sweating, has been extensively reviewed.[32] VMS occur in 11–60% of menstruating perimenopausal women. How can VMS, the hallmark signal of declining estrogen, be such a frequent feature of the high estrogen state of perimenopause? Several points only intensify this apparent contradiction of the received wisdom (i.e., VMS are "classic symptoms of estrogen deficiency").

1. Standard replacement doses of estrogen therapy are only effective in eliminating VMS in late peri- and postmenopause (when estrogen concentrations are declining or low). Standard hormone replenishment therapy does not control perimenopausal VMS. However, the higher steroid content of standard birth control pills (combined E plus P) do control perimenopausal VMS.
2. Intermittent VMS are seen in early perimenopause around midcycle as well as prior to and during menses. While suggesting that VMS may result from acute reduction in previously excessively high estradiol levels, sustained levels of E_2 (in implant therapy) as well as the hyperstimulation associated with hMG/hCG ovulation induction can also lead to VMS.
3. There is a relationship between high estradiol levels, VMS, and the appearance of affective disorders commonly seen in PMS.
4. Unreplaced Turner's syndrome patients do not experience VMS, but once given estrogen and then withdrawn VMS will develop.
5. Postpartum women do not usually experience VMS despite the acute and dramatic withdrawal from exceedingly high steroid levels (both E and P for 9 months), but in this instance accompanied by prolonged *suppression* of FSH.

The prevalence of VMS throughout perimenopause is not understood. Clinical observations suggest that VMS may appear at both high as well as sharply declining estradiol concentrations and when hypothalamic activity (GnRH) is increased. Despite these uncertainties two points are clear. VMS occurs in perimenopause and is highly associated with a decreased quality of life [33] especially when accompanied by sleep deprivation. It is important to note, however, that women in other countries and in different cultures either report fewer and less intense hot flashes than the U.S. Some cultures do not even have a name for the experience.

3. Trabecular Bone Loss begins in Perimenopause [34]

After reaching peak bone mass in the early 20s and plateauing at age 35, bone loss begins in perimenopause and dramatically accelerates after menopause and reflects increased bone turnover without reciprocal increase in bone formation. Many variables including hereditary proclivity and lifestyle factors (exercise, deficient dietary intake of calcium and vitamin D, cigarette smoking, caffeine or alcohol abuse) are probably involved in the initiation of bone loss despite high levels of estradiol. Lack of consistent normal ovulation in perimenopause and the accompanying marked reduction in serum progesterone may aggravate this situation. Finally, the increased rate of bone loss in perimenopause may relate to elevated cortisol production secondary to VMS, sleep disruption, and emotional stress of the approaching end of reproductive life.

C. Therapeutic Considerations for Perimenopause

Perimenopause is characterized by elevated FSH, high oscillating estradiol levels, reduced inhibin, and inconsistent ovulation. These levels of FSH and estrogen coupled with diminished or absent progesterone explain the morbidities associated with this phase of a woman's life: menorrhagia, breast enlargement and pain, increased PMS, migraine headaches, fibroid size, and the reactive risks of operative solutions.

For these reasons appropriate therapy for perimenopause, in addition to the vitally important lifestyle enhancements of exercise and nutritional corrections, should include 10–12 days of cyclic progesterone in the last 2 weeks of the cycle. Medroxyprogesterone acetate and/or 19 norprogestins offer convenient once-a-day dosage as opposed to the multiple dose per day micronized progesterone requires. Increasingly, physicians are returning to low-dose combined OC regimens (with ≤35 µg ethinyl estradiol and a progestin) in nonsmoking, nonhypertensive women in perimenopause.[25] The utility of this at once suppressive and nonoscillating therapy is demonstrated by the substantial list of benefits perimenopausal women accrue from using this strategy. These include noncontraceptive benefits (although perimenstrual women still need some birth control) such as[35]:

- Menstrual cycle control with avoidance of menometrorrhagia
- Less endometrial cancer, ovarian cancer
- Elimination of VMS, reduced dysmenorrhea
- Prevention of bone loss
- No change in fibroids
- Reduced ovarian cysts
- Reduced benign breast disease
- Possibly diminished burdens of rheumatoid arthritis
- Increased, but imperfect resistance to STDs
- Improved lipoprotein profile
- Control of acne and hirsutism in addition to effective contraception.

Some perimenopausal women use monophasic OCs continuously for 3–6 months or even longer to electively eliminate cyclic flow entirely and without observable disadvantages.

After age 50–52, an elevated FSH above 30 m IU/ml at the conclusion of a 7-day OC-pill-free interval indicates the almost certain presence of ovarian exhaustion and the menopausal state. Other strategies, including hormone replenishment, may then be considered.

VI. MENOPAUSE

In this chapter, the WHO definition of menopause has been adopted as a reasonable, clinically applicable descriptor: permanent loss of menstrual function for 12 months in appropriately aged women. A variety of longitudinal studies have defined an age range between 45–56 years but outliers invariably exist. *The Guinness Book of Records* documents a pregnancy in a 57-year-old American woman.

Contrary to perimenopause in which the definition, age of initiation, and endocrinology is complex and at times clinically paradoxical, menopause displays consistent and explicit interdependence of its endocrinology and the resulting clinical manifestations. Although straightforward, the prolonged hypoestrogenic state presents short- and long-term consequences that extend beyond a focused impact on the reproductive system and includes multisystem dysfunctions which weigh heavily on overall life expectancy and quality of life issues.

A. Endocrinology of Menopause [35]

Within a year after the final lapse in menstrual function, ovarian follicle exhaustion is complete (Fig. 27.1). FSH and LH continue to rise, achieving a 10- to 20-fold increase in FSH and a tripling of LH by 3 years postmenopause. Thereafter hypergonadotropism persists at gradually diminishing levels but always remaining in the castrate range.

1. Estrogens [36, 37]

The circulating levels of estradiol in postmenopause are invariably below 30 pg/ml and usually in the 10–20 pg/ml range. This estradiol does not arise from direct gonadal secretion but is produced at extragonadal sites from estrone which in turn is derived from conversion of circulating androgen precursors such as androstenedione. At 30–70 pg/ml the circulating level of estrone is higher than estradiol and in terms of sheer availability is considered the estrogen of the postmenopausal years. As can be seen in Tables 27.1 and 27.2, the estrogen production rate in the postmenopausal woman is entirely derived from nongonadal androgen conversion to estrogen (the production rates of estrogen in both intact and oophorectomized postmenopausal women are the same—0.045 mg/day (45 µg/24 h).

Although estrogen secretion from the ovaries does not continue after menopause, substrate availability for conversion to estrogen can materially increase biologically active estrogen levels. Therefore available estrogen will vary among women and in the same woman over time and reflect the influence of several factors. For example, body weight has a positive correlation with circulating levels of total and free estrone and estradiol.[38] As weight increases, the aromatase capacity increases in filled fat cells and the percent conversion of androstenedione to total estrone increases. In addition, with obesity sex hormone binding globulin (SHBG) levels decrease thereby providing greater substrate availability and higher concentrations of free biologically active estrone

TABLE 27.1 Blood Production Rates of Steroids

	Reproductive age	Postmenopausal	Oophorectomized
Androstenedione	2–3 mg/day	0.5–1.5 mg/day	0.4–1.2 mg/day
Dehydroepiandrosterone	6–8	1.5–4.0	1.5–4.0
Dehydroepiandrosterone sulfate	8–16	4–9	4–9
Testosterone	0.2–0.25	0.05–0.18	0.02–0.12
Estrogen	0.350	0.045	0.045

After menopause the production of androstenedione, testosterone, and estrogens declines significantly. However, note that oophorectomy has no effect on postmenopausal estrogen production indicating the entire availability of estrogen is due to extragonadal conversion from androgen. The decline in dehydroepiandiosterone and its sulfate is dramatic (the "adrenopause") and is exclusively related to diminished adrenocortical secretion.

TABLE 27.2 Changes in Circulating Hormone Levels at Menopause

	Premenopause	Postmenopause
Estradiol	40–400 pg/ml	10–20 pg/ml
Estrone	30–200 pg/ml	30–70 pg/ml
Testosterone	20–80 ng/dl	15–70 ng/dl
Androstenedione	60–300 ng/dl	30–150 ng/dl

Concentrations of all steroids decline after menopause. However, testosterone levels remain relatively stable reflecting both continued gonadal secretion and extra glandular conversion of precursors.

and estradiol. Aromatization of androgen to estrogen is not limited to adipose tissue. Almost every tissue, notably brain, skin, gastrointestinal tract, muscle, and liver possesses aromatase activity.

In addition to aromatization, precursor androgen may vary dramatically as a result of increased input or diminished clearance, i.e., increased ACTH, excess adrenal cortical function, or alterations in androgen clearance and metabolism as in liver disease. As a result of these factors a single acute stress may cause vaginal bleeding and chronic stress in an obese postmenopausal woman may increase and sustain estrogen sufficiently to cause endometrial proliferation and hyperplasia as well as dysfunctional uterine bleeding and cancer.

2. Androgens [36, 37]

The postmenopausal ovary primarily secretes androstenedione and testosterone. Nevertheless, after menopause the serum concentration of androstenedione decreases to one-half the level seen in premenopause and most of that androstenedione is secreted by the adrenal glands. Dehydroepiandroesterone (DHEA) and its sulfate (DHEAS) originate entirely from the adrenal cortex and decline markedly with aging. In the decade after menopause the circulating levels of these androgens decrease by 70–75% compared to concentrations seen in younger menstruating women in adult reproductive life. Whereas in "adrenarche" DHEA-DHEAS increase prior to puberty, there is an age-related decline in these steroids called "adrenopause." Furthermore, as adrenarche appears to have no influence on the timing of puberty, neither does adrenopause govern the initiation of ovarian senescence.

On the other hand, while overall testosterone concentrations decrease in postmenopause by 25%, the early postmenopausal ovary continues to secret important quantities of this steroid. Despite the disappearance of follicles, elevated LH drives the remaining ovarian stromal tissue to sustained testosterone synthesis and secretion. Evidence for this important contribution to overall testosterone production is seen in the significant decrease in its concentration following suppression of gonadotropin with GnRH agonist. However, testosterone production also depends importantly on the peripheral conversion of androstenedione. Although oophorectomized postmenopausal women have lower testosterone than intact women with ovaries, in both groups the total testosterone production rate and concentration is markedly lower due to the 50% reduction in precursor androstenedione production. Nevertheless, testosterone availability in the virtual absence of estrogen may cause cosmetic liabilities in facial hirsutism and scalp alopecia.

Eventually years after menopause even the ovarian stroma is exhausted and despite persistent high levels of gonadotropins, no further ovarian secretion of androgen occurs.

B. Clinical Manifestations of Menopause

With these considerations the clinical manifestations of the endocrinology of the postmenopausal woman can be classified in three categories.

1. Those which are associated with *estrogen excess* such as dysfunctional uterine bleeding, endometrial hyperplasia, and endometrial cancer reflecting increased endogenous

estrogen production in the absence of endogenous progesterone.

2. Those which are associated with *estrogen lack* such as VMS and atrophy of estrogen-dependent tissues such as vagina, urethra, and bladder. As will be seen, some manifestations of estrogen deprivation (hypoestrogenism) cluster in the early postmenopausal years (such as VMS) and still others (atrophy) may predominate in the last postmenopause.
3. Finally, it is fair to say that as much as endogenous endocrine factors carry clinical burdens, so too are the difficulties associated with attempted correction of menopausal issues with *exogenous* hormones. Accordingly, a consideration of the clinical benefits and risks of hormone replenishment is an essential part of any comprehensive dissertation on menopause.

1. Problems of Estrogen Excess

As discussed at length in Section V, among the problems that arise in menopause is the frequency of dysfunctional uterine bleeding. Although the clinician is always appropriately concerned about the possibility of underlying neoplasia, in fact the most common cause is endogenous estrogen stimulation of endometrial growth in the absence of adequate anti-estrogen, anti-mitotic availability of progesterone and the periodic shedding which follows its withdrawal. Whereas the bleeding problems of perimenopause reflect *anovulation*, in postmenopause abnormal bleeding arises from prolonged, sustained, not necessarily markedly elevated concentrations of *extragonadal production* of estrogen in the total absence of endogenous progesterone.

There are four mechanisms by which endogenous estrogen can reach clinically important levels in the postmenopausal woman:

1. Increased precursor androgen (functional and nonfunctional endocrine tumors) or stress (i.e., *increased production*) or failed metabolism and *decreased clearance* of precursors such as in liver disease
2. Increased *utilization* of precursor androgen substrate due to *increased aromatization* such as in obesity, hyperthyroidism, and liver disease
3. Decreased levels of SHBG leading to increased biologic impact by increased availability of *free* unbound estrogen
4. Rarely, increased direct secretion of estrogen by estrogen-secreting tumors such as granulosa cell tumors

2. Management and Therapeutic Considerations of Estrogen Excess

In all postmenopausal women who experience vaginal bleeding whether off or on hormone replenishment therapy, evaluation for specific organic causes, i.e., neoplasia, is mandatory. In addition to a careful history and physical examination to rule out general medical disease (thyroid, liver, and renal) and extrauterine (vulva, vagina, urethra) sources of bleeding, a transvaginal ultrasound measurement of endometrial thickness, presence of polyps, or submucous fibroids is essential. In many instances, however, the clinician may need (or prefer) direct histologic appraisal by office suction biopsy. If the uterus is distorted by intramural fibroids or the office endometrial biopsy result is ambiguous, i.e., tissue insufficient for diagnosis, then an under anesthesia formal D&C with hysteroscopy is required.

The principal symptom of endometrial cancer is abnormal vaginal bleeding. However, carcinoma will be found in only 1–2% of postmenopausal endometrial biopsies.[39, 40] Normal endometrium is retrieved in 50%, polyps in 3%, hyperplasia in 15%, and atrophic endometrium in around 30%. The persistence of abnormal bleeding demands re-evaluation; approximately 10% of patients with benign findings initially will subsequently develop significant pathology in 2 years.[41]

When dysfunctional uterine bleeding is associated with endometrial proliferation or hyperplasia, progestin therapy must be initiated or if currently in use the dosage and duration must be increased. If hyperplasia was present, follow-up biopsy after 3 months of appropriate therapy is required to confirm the initial diagnosis and the effectiveness of therapy. The presence of atypia or dysplasia at any time requires hysterectomy.

On the other hand, if atrophic endometrium is found either continuous combined hormone therapy (E plus P) or simple reassurance and observation for recurrence may be all that is necessary.

In postmenopausal women with dysfunctional uterine bleeding due to estrogen excess, ovarian cancer must be considered and specifically ruled out. For this reason alone most clinicians choose transvaginal ultrasound imaging of the pelvic organs in all such cases. Nonpalpable otherwise asymptomatic ovarian cysts are common in postmenopause and are readily detected by ultrasound. Cysts that are less than 5 cm in diameter, without septations or solid components demonstrating a thin regular wall have a very low potential for malignant disease and can be managed with serial ultrasounds.[42] If growth occurs or solid elements emerge then surgery must be done. With a strong family history of breast or ovarian cancer, independent of BRCA1 or 2 status, surgical intervention is prudent.

C. Problems of Estrogen Deficiency

A full understanding of the biologic and clinical impact of the prolonged hypoestrogenic state of postmenopause must incorporate the influence of three variables:

1. *Aging versus hypoestrogenism*: Since postmenopause evolves and persists over at least 30 years or more of the

terminal portion of a woman's life, the impact of aging must be distinguished from the manifestations of prolonged hypoestrogenism. Furthermore, the degree to which each influence and/or interacts with the other needs to be evaluated.

2. *Early versus late postmenopause in the duration of estrogen lack*: The impact of the speed and slope of deceleration of the early decline in estrogen concentration must be distinguished from the effects of prolonged hypoestrogenism. Each lead to early specific symptoms (VMS, accelerating osteopenia) and late postmenopausal effects (atrophy, emergence of cardiovascular, CNS, and vision impairments).
3. *Reproductive and nonreproductive system involvement*: In addition to the impact of aging and early and late estrogen deficiency, it is clear that the postmenopause is not simply manifested by reproductive system decline (amenorrhea and atrophy) but also is dramatically involved in a variety of nonreproductive organ systems critical to life expectancy and overall quality of life issues.

D. What Portion of Postmenopausal Problems are Due to Aging and/or which Are Due to Hypoestrogenism?

Three sources of data provide a reasonable basis for separating the contributions of aging and the superimposition of hypoestrogenism to the burdens and risks of the postmenopausal woman, as well as providing insights on the significant synergistic effects these jointly impose.

1. Premature Ovarian Failure (POF)

Young women with POF display a significantly higher risk for osteoporosis and cardiovascular disease. Two-thirds of women with normal karyotypes and spontaneous POF show a decreased bone mineral density compared to similar aged menstruating women; this reduction in bone mineral density has been associated with a 2.6-fold increased risk of hip fracture.[43, 44]

A survey of more than 19,000 women aged 25–100 years of age indicates that ovarian failure occurring before 40 years of age is associated with a significantly increased overall mortality (OR = 2.14 95% CI 1.15–3.9). Specific age-adjusted odds ratios were variably increased: coronary heart disease OR = 1.29 (CI 0.61–2.74); stroke OR = 3.07 (CI 1.34–7.03); cancer OR 1.83 (CI 0.73–4.79).[45, 46]

2. Consequences of Human Mutations in Synthesis and Action

Although very small in number and complicated by genetic and compensatory function, studies of mutations of CYP 19, the gene encoding aromatase, and mutations of the estrogen alpha receptor shed light on the biologic impact of low estrogen independent of aging.[47] These include

1. Bone age extremely low for chronologic age
2. Severe osteoporosis
3. Increased bone turnover
4. Insulin resistance, impaired glucose tolerance
5. Early coronary artery calcification despite low LDL cholesterol
6. Heterosexual psychosexual orientation

3. The Effect of ERT/HRT in Postmenopause

Hormone replenishment relieves many consequences of estrogen deprivation in the reproductive system, i.e., the vagina as well as nonreproductive systems (VMS, CNS). However, as will be seen in Section VII, in most systems while the effect of estrogen replenishment may be substantial, a significant portion of recipients show limited or no salutory modification of system dysfunction. Still other studies, largely observational, demonstrate a preponderance of prevention/delaying/modifying effects and not reversal of established disease as a consequence of hormone therapy.[48]

Taken together, low estrogen and aging impose additive impact on most body systems. In general the loss of estrogen appears to lead to either earlier appearance and/or acceleration of dysfunctional states.

E. Specific Symptoms, Signs, and System Changes in Postmenopause

1. VMS

The vasomotor flush or "flash" is experienced to some degree by most postmenopausal women and is the hallmark of early postmenopause (Table 27.3). The experience involves the sudden onset of flushing of head, neck, chest, and back areas of the skin, accompanied by feeling of intense body heat and concluded often by perfuse sweating. The event is variable in duration (seconds to minutes), in frequency, and in timing (day or night or both). It is a common sign, involves perimenopause, and extends into a good portion of the early postmenopause.[49] The physiology of VMS is not understood. Based on observations in hypogonadal and hypophysectomized women, experiences of hormone-treated and nontreated women, and its presence in perimenopause, VMS is thought to be initiated in the hypothalamus (which is involved in temperature regulation as well as gonadotropin control) and is brought about by oscillating declines of estrogen concentrations in current or formerly hormone-replete women. Standard estrogen replacement either totally or at least very substantially relieves postmenopausal VMS and diminishes the "domino" effects associated with them (i.e., sleep deprivation and mood swings).

TABLE 27.3 Consequences of Estrogen Loss

Symptoms (early)	Hot Flushes Insomnia Irritability Mood Disturbances
Physical changes (intermediate)	Atrophy Skin
Dysfunction/disease (intermediate to late)	Osteoporosis CVD Cognitive losses Dementia

The effectiveness of estrogen therapy is so consistent, failure is in itself a clinical bioassay for the existence of other uncommon causes of VMS. In such cases "chasing" the symptom with higher and higher doses of estrogen is usually unrewarding except in the initial phases of higher dosing. The clinician must consider other causes of VMS (i.e., thyroid disease, pheochromocytoma, carcinoid, leukemia, cancer).[50] That VMS may be associated with stressful events and/or a component of a psychosomatic disorder as well as having a high (but transient) response to a placebo must be part of the assessment of refractory VMS.

2. Atrophic Changes

a. Genitourinary Atrophy

This leads to a variety of symptoms that affect the ease and quality of postmenopausal life. The extremely low estrogen production in postmenopause results in atrophy of the vaginal mucosa with the appearance of vaginitis, pruritus, dyspareunia, and eventually even vaginal stenosis. In addition, estrogen insufficiency extends to the lower urinary tract, i.e., urethritis with dysuria, urinary incontinence, and urinary frequency.[51] Recurrent urinary tract infections are common. On the other hand, the consequences of vaginal relaxation such as cystocele, rectocele, and uterine prolapse are not caused by estrogen deprivation. However, cystitis and urethritis, which underlie urge incontinence, compound the problems of anterior wall relaxation and urinary stress incontinence. Otherwise minor or asymptomatic prolapse may become symptomatic because of low estrogen and to the extent this is a factor, the problem can be relieved by estrogen replacement. Vulvar dystrophies, such as lichen sclerosis atrophicus is not estrogen-loss related.

b. Skin

A decline in skin collagen content and skin thickness occurs with aging and can be diminished if not avoided by estrogen replenishment. The result is a clinically significant arrest or avoidance of wrinkling. The effect of estrogen on collagen is evident in both skin and bone.[52] Bone mass and collagen decline in parallel after menopause and estrogen treatment reduces collagen turnover and improves collagen quality.

c. Muscle Mass and Strength

Both aging men and women experience a steady reduction in muscle strength and mass. Many factors other than diminished gonadal steroids contribute to this decline including human growth hormone and the limitation of physical activity imposed by disease, dysfunction, and socioeconomic factors. Clearly this form of atrophy with its consequences of diminished independence, decreased balance, and higher risk of falls has substantial clinical importance. Although estrogen depletion has been reported to increase postmenopausal women's strength, confounding variables affecting the study population limits applicability of this information. This is an aging, not an estrogen related, change.

3. Psychophysiologic Effects [53]

Several lines of evidence indicate that menopause does *not* impose a deleterious effect on mental health. The psychiatric literature and surveys of the general population indicate that menopause is not associated with an increased risk of depression. The diagnostic entity "involutional melancholia" has been abandoned. Furthermore, evidence for a direct causal relationship between declining estrogen and psychologic disorder does not exist. Other factors must lead to the high frequency of complaints such as insomnia, fatigue, nervousness, headaches, depression, irritability, joint and muscle pain, dizziness, and palpitations these women experience. Complicating this situation is the strong impression shared by physicians and their patients that estrogen replenishment has a dramatic effect in relief of this broad spectrum of difficulties.

Part of the answer may lie in the alleviation of the 'domino' burdens of sleep deprivation as estrogen abolishes VMS. Estrogen improves the quality of sleep, decreases the time to onset of sleep, and increases the rapid eye movement (REM) sleep time. Overall quality of life can be improved by retrieval of more satisfying and longer duration of sleep and alleviation of VMS.

4. Sexuality and Postmenopause [54, 55]

Despite the fact that women live longer, are healthier, better educated and have more leisure time, spend more time on grooming and physical appearance, and have had their consciousness raised regarding their sexuality, aging, and in particular menopause has been identified as a life event at which diminished sexual interest, competence, and prospects for satisfaction begins. Although this is not true of many women, several factors underlie this real reduction of sexual experience and pleasure in aging postmenopausal women. A combination of illness, absence or infirmity of a partner, VMS and sleeplessness, vaginal atrophy and diminished lubrication with attending dyspareunia all contribute to the intensity of this problem. Although HRT relieves much of the mechanical barriers to pleasure, libidinous interest is not altered. The loss of ovarian secretion of testosterone has been advanced as a cause of diminished libido. Replacement therapy by testosterone gels and patches are currently being evaluated. In one study [56] only preparations that drove testosterone serum concentrations above normal range and with time could produce androgenic side effects increased libido above control placebo effects. What is not a factor in this complicated problem is any residual prejudice that older women are neither interested nor let alone actually do "it." The wish is there and orgasmic pleasure can be realized; but even with elimination of adverse mechanical factors, the libidinous drive seems to diminish with age. Efforts to reverse this undesirable condition pharmacologically are underway.[57]

5. Cognitive Function [58]

Estrogen protects the CNS and its function and presumably its plasticity by several mechanisms. It increases synapses and neuronal growth, especially in the size and density of dendritic spines. Estrogen protects against neuronal oxidative cytotoxicity and reduces the concentration of amyloid protein in the deposits associated with Alzheimer's disease neurofibrillary tangles. It enhances cerebral blood flow, which increases glucose and oxygen provision and insures efficient clearance of neuronal metabolic waste products. Cognitive decline and dementia prevalence are signs of aging in men but more so in postmenopausal women suggesting some endocrine relationship.[59, 60]

Assessment of the degree to which estrogen deprivation is a factor in these expressions of neuronal aging is complicated by a variety of factors most prominent of which is that estrogen efficacy can only be seen in those burdened by the menopausal syndrome.[61] In these women estrogen does improve verbal memory, vigilance, reasoning, and motor speed. There is suggestive evidence that estrogen replenishment can delay or attenuate Alzheimer's disease, but most studies have structural limitations that leave uncertainty as to the validity of estrogen's impact on dementias, in general, and Alzheimer's disease, specifically.

6. Osteopenia and Osteoporosis [62–64]

Osteoporosis, the most prevalent bone problem in the elderly, involves decreased bone mass but with retention of a normal ratio of mineral to matrix. It is associated with an increased risk of fractures even with little or no trauma. Osteopenia is a term used to indicate the state of evolving bone loss and microarchitectural deterioration of bone tissue, which has not yet declined to the low levels of bone mineral density defined as osteoporotic. The bone loss characteristic of osteoporosis reflects an imbalance in the components of the bone remodeling process within each bone remodeling unit. Whereas localized bone loss (osteoclast activity) precedes and normally is balanced by bone formation (osteoblast activity), in osteoporosis formation does not keep pace with reduction. The multiplicity of genetic environmental, endocrinological, and pathological behavioral factors that promote this imbalance are shown in Fig. 27.2.

Osteoporosis is a major and growing public health problem in the U.S. (Table 27.4). But, as dramatic as the overall statistics are, the individual risks and costs are indeed staggering. Hip fracture, for example, is associated with significant mortality and morbidity.[65] Approximately 16% of patients with a hip fracture die within the first 3 months after injury due to heart failure, pulmonary embolism, or pneumonia. But even with survival the residual loss of personal integrity, dignity, and quality of life, i.e., loss of job, loss of recreational opportunities, loss of mobility, decreased independent living,

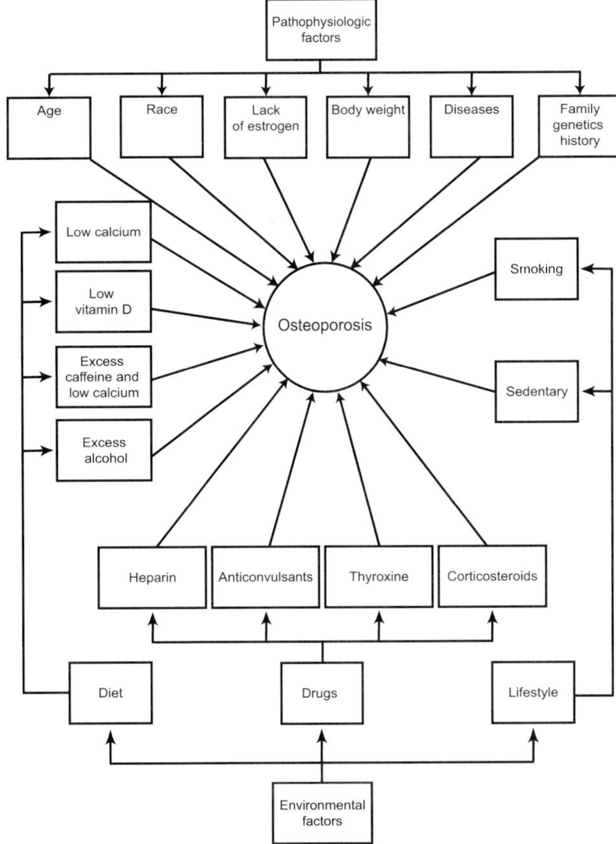

FIGURE 27.2 The multiplicity of factors involved in osteoporosis. These include genetic, environmental, dietary, lifestyle, and hormonal elements, many of which may exist in combination in an individual patient. The impact of smoking, diet, exercise, and hormone (estrogen) is emphasized. Not shown is the crucial development of maximal bone "reserve" during adolescence.

TABLE 27.4 Osteoporosis—A Major U.S. Public Health Challenge in Women

Affects more than 25 million women
Responsible for 1.5 million total fractures/year
250,000 hip fractures annually in women
33% of white postmenopausal women will experience hip fractures
25% of white postmenopausal women will have lumbar compression fractures
25% of African-American women will have hip fractures
Estimated annual costs in women = $11.0 billion affects more than 25 million women

and ability for self-care, pain and suffering inherent in problems with gait, bowel, and pulmonary function and a reduction in sexual possibilities taken together are a daunting and severely discouraging reality.

The risk of fracture for the individual woman depends on two factors: the bone mass she achieved at maturity and the subsequent rate of bone loss she experiences over the remainder of her life. The combination of a low bone mass to begin with, and the acceleration of bone loss with age and a loss of estrogen is additive and together create the greatest risk of osteoporosis and fracture.[66]

It is now recognized that only a narrow window of opportunity exists in which to build bone mass. Almost all bone in the hip and vertebral bodies will be in place in young women by late adolescence. After age 18–20, total skeletal mass continues to increase but at a far slower pace, and ceases by age 30. Thereafter a slow decline in bone mass begins at the rate of approximately 0.7% per year. However, after menopause, as estrogen declines the disproportionate bone remodeling process accelerates. As a result, up to 5% of trabecular bone (spine, hip) and 1–1.5% of total bone mass is lost per year after menopause. This accelerated loss will continue for 10–15 years after which the rate diminishes but continues as age-related loss (parallel to the male slope of decline). Taken together in the 20-year interval following menopause, there will be a 50% loss in trabecular bone and a 30% reduction in cortical bone.[67, 68]

As will be seen, antiresorptive therapy, diet, and physical exercise can stabilize and, to a degree, even reverse some of this loss. Careful review of all potential contributors to bone loss and serial bone mineral densities by dual-energy X-ray absorptiometry (DEXA) monitoring in at-risk individuals are essential management practices. What cannot be undone is the adverse impact of behavioral and dietary practices in adolescence.

7. Cardiovascular Disease (CVD) [69]

Diseases of the heart are the leading cause of death for women in the U.S. (Fig. 27.3), outpacing all malignancies combined, cerebrovascular disease (part of the same arteriosclerotic process), and motor vehicle accidents. Since 1984, the number of CVD deaths in women has exceeded those occurring in men. The impact of myocardial infarction (MI) is not solely a late-age phenomenon: 20,000 women under the age of 65 die of MI each year in the U.S. Sadly for women and even their physicians the perception of their cardiovascular risk is very different from the reality. The death rate from coronary artery disease in women is roughly three times greater than rates seen in breast or lung cancer. Female survivors of a first MI face the prospects of a second infarct in 31%, a stroke in 18%, and sudden death in 16%.[70] Arteriosclerotic cardiovascular disease is a process worth preventing.

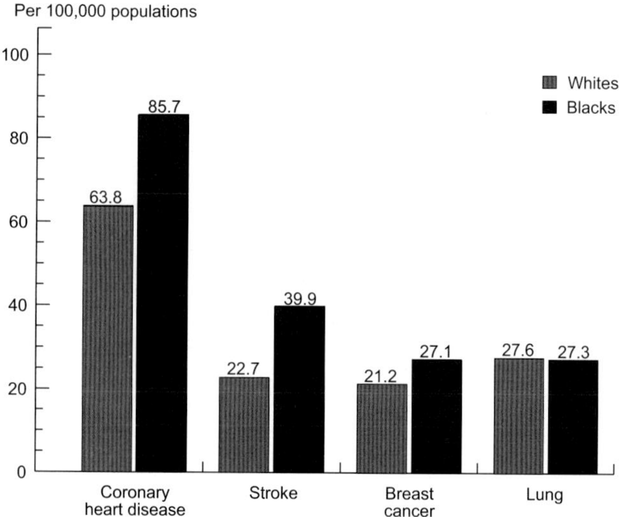

FIGURE 27.3 Age-adjusted mortality rates for U.S. women, 1993. Cardiovascular disease (coronary heart disease and stroke) is significantly higher than breast or lung cancer combined.

Men and women share the same risk factors: smoking, high blood pressure, diabetes mellitus, obesity (particularly central abdominal fat), and dyslipidemia. When controlling for these risk factors, the risk of a male developing coronary heart disease is 3.5 times greater than a female. However, with increasing age, and particularly after menopause, the female "advantage" is gradually lost and CVD becomes the leading cause of death in older women.[71–73]

Why are women protected from CVD during the reproductive years? The reasons for this gender disparity are complex but a significant contribution to this protection is the presence of estrogen. Effects of estrogen include elevation of HDL cholesterol and reduced total cholesterol, as well as LDL cholesterol levels. Total cholesterol and LDL cholesterol rise rapidly after menopause and at about age 60 these levels are higher than in men just at the time when coronary heart disease rates double for women.[74] However, the strongest predictor of coronary heart disease in women is a low HDL cholesterol concentration (<50 mg/dl).

A decrease in HDL cholesterol by as little as 10 mg/dl increases coronary heart disease risk by 40–50%. On the other hand, women with HDL cholesterol concentrations above 55 mg/dl have virtually no increased risk of heart disease even in the presence of total cholesterol elevations.[75, 76]

The protective effects of estrogen are not confined to the salutory balance of circulating lipids.[77] Probably of even greater importance contributing to the gender difference in CVD prevalence and age of onset are direct estrogen effects on the endothelium. Perhaps 65–75% of the cardioprotective effect of estrogen is believed to result from lipid-independent effects on the heart and blood vessels (particularly the endothelium) and on plaque formation. Estrogen increases nitric oxide and prostacyclin PGI2 yielding vasodilation and decreases endothelin-I, a powerful vasoconstrictor.

Respectively, these changes account for beneficial vasodilation and diminished vasoconstriction and platelet aggregation and adhesion.

8. The Relation between Progression of the Atherogenesis and Bone Loss in Postmenopause

The probable link between progressive atherogenesis and bone loss in aging women derives from two lines of clinical investigation and a series of basic scientific observations.

First, Mundy *et al.* [78] demonstrated stimulation of bone formation *in vitro* and in rodents by statins. Thereafter several clinical studies showed hMG-CoA reductase inhibitors (statins) could increase bone mineral density [29] and reduce risk of fractures in postmenopausal women.[80, 81] Second, following Demer *et al.*, observation of disadvantageous skeletal changes in atherosclerosis [82] focus on the linkage of the two processes was given further impetus by the finding of the inverse relationship between bone density and carotid atherosclerosis in postmenopausal women.[83] Most recently progression of atherosclerosis and bone loss was confirmed.[84] The biological plausibility of the association was suggested by the demonstration that lipid oxidation products induce opposite effects on calcification of vascular cells and bone cell differentiation.[85] Finally, the ability of estradiol to inhibit both IL-6 production by osteoblasts [86] and T-cell production of TNF-α [87] (both factors in bone loss and atherogenesis) adds credibility to the thesis that the hypoestrogenicity of postmenopause is materially involved in both atherogenesis and osteoporosis.

9. Miscellaneous Considerations

Finally, a miscellany of disorders has been tentatively designated as largely aging related but the processes and the functional impairment they impose may be compounded by prolonged hypoestrogenism. These include age-related visual changes such as macular degeneration and lens opacity, Parkinson's disease, osteoarthritis, and the insulin resistance of type II diabetes mellitus.

VII. THE BENEFITS AND RISKS OF HORMONE REPLENISHMENT IN THE POSTMENOPAUSAL WOMAN

A. Postmenopausal Hormone Replacement: Opportunities and Challenges

Hormone replacement therapy (HRT) is a major element in the array of clinical management and preventive health-care strategies available to physicians and their postmenopausal patients. As noted the potential impact of the hypoestrogenic state and its pharmacologic repletion ranges well beyond the reproductive organs and involves the functional status of most organ systems. Although much has been learned about this pervasively important clinical topic, the lack of definitive data in crucial areas continues to provoke discussion, controversy, and uncertainty for physicians and patients alike.

This portion of this chapter is devoted exclusively to hormone replacement issues. In general the term "HRT" will apply to combined estrogen and progestin replenishment whereas estrogen replacement therapy only will be designated as "ERT." Except as noted this analysis deals with oral administration of these agents. Where the method of administration, i.e., cyclic, continuous, or sequential, is important, then specific considerations will be dealt with. The critical importance of sustained general medical care, corrective lifestyle measures, nutritional and exercise programs, although not discussed in this section, confer unequivocal well-documented benefits and are essential features of quality care in this population.

B. The Current Status of ERT/HRT

The "received wisdom" expressed in evidence-based reviews,[88, 89] statements of the American Association of Clinical Endocrinologists (AACE),[90] guidelines of the American College of Obstetricians and Gynecologists (ACOG),[91] educational documents of the Association of Professors of Gynecology and Obstetrics (APGO),[92] and leading text in the field [8] stipulate the relative benefits and burdens of HRT. Specific secondary references dealing with each topic can be found in these reviews.

1. Acute Interventions

The effective use of ERT/HRT in the sustained relief of vasomotor instability (hot flushes and sweats) is well supported by controlled randomized trials (Table 27.5). In addition, a variety of epidermal atrophic conditions are ameliorated by this therapy. These include dyspareunia and pruritus secondary to vulval, introtial, and vaginal atrophy; urinary difficulties such as urgency, urethritis, and cystitis; as well as general skin atrophy. Patients often attribute a variety of psychophysiologic burdens to the lack of hormone production in menopause (including but not limited to fatigue, nervousness,

TABLE 27.5 Benefits of ERT/HRT

Acute interventions
Reduction of vasomotor symptoms
Improves duration and quality of sleep
Corrects genitourinary atrophy
Improved cognition

headache, depression, irritability, joint and muscle pain, dizziness, and palpitations). While replenishment of hormone is associated with dramatic relief of many of these subjective complaints, the reduction in hot flush frequency, restoration of duration and quality of sleep, as well as a substantial placebo effect probably account for much of these benefits.

Finally, but not consistently, a variety of cohort and case-controlled trials show both current and past users of HRT score significantly higher in mental state examinations, in short-term visual and verbal memory tests, and in their capacity to learn new associations. Nine randomized controlled trials and eight cohort studies [93] were recently reviewed. Although the study populations and outcome measures differ, and most of the studies have methodologic shortcomings, this compilation offers provisional conclusions about the effects of postmenopausal estrogen therapy on cognition and risk of dementia. While estrogen does not appear to enhance asymptomatic women's performance consistently on formal cognitive testing, in symptomatic women postmenopausal estrogen improved cognitive performance especially in tests of verbal memory, vigilance, reasoning, and motor speed. Inconsistent effects were seen in verbal recall, working memory, complex attention, mental tracking, mental status, and verbal function.

2. Prevention of Disease (Table 27.6)

a. CVD [94]

Some 35 observational studies report an approximately 50% decrease in cardiac disease events in postmenopausal women using ERT/HRT. There is good evidence for the biologic plausibility of a cause and effect relationship supporting these findings. These include estrogen-induced beneficial changes on lipid profile, reduced insulin resistance, improved cardiac contractility and coronary artery blood flow, decreased platelet aggregation, low-density lipoprotein oxidation inhibition, increased coronary vasodilation responses, and decreased plaque formation.

There is strong support for a preventive *cardioprotective* (prevention of initial cardiovascular events) effect of exogenous hormone replenishment in postmenopausal women. However, concerns have arisen with respect to the *adverse* impact of HRT in older women with *established* CVD (secondary prevention). The Heart and Estrogen/Progestin Replacement Study (HERS) [95] was a randomized, double-blind, placebo-controlled secondary prevention clinical trial which sought to determine whether daily treatment with combined continuous HRT (conjugated equine estrogen 0.625 mg and medroxyprogesterone acetate 2.5 mg) could reduce recurrent events in women with preexisting heart disease. In this study 2763 women (average age 66.7 years) were randomized to treatment and placebo groups and studied over just under 5 years. No overall difference was noted between the two groups. However, after a dramatic increase in events in the treatment group in the first 8 months of the study, a significant protective effect (statistically significant for trend) emerged with increased duration of treatment. (Table 27.7). The authors attributed this favorable effect to advantageous changes in the lipid levels in hormone recipients.

The Women's Health Initiative (WHI) informed participants that in the first 2 years of the study slightly more than 1% of the participants have suffered events (heart attacks, stroke, venous thrombosis and pulmonary embolism) regardless of whether taking hormones or placebo, but the frequency of events was slightly higher in users versus controls. Furthermore, as in HERS, the initial increased differential risk seemed to disappear after 2 years of use.

Important clinical lessons emerge from these reports. A small but significant subpopulation of older women are at acute risk for induced cardiovascular events as they initiate HRT. At the moment there is no well-defined method to distinguish these vulnerable individuals. For HRT to be

TABLE 27.6 Benefits of ERT/HRT

Prevention of disease
Cardiovascular disease[a]
Osteoporosis and fracture
Alzheimer's Disease[a]
Colorectal cancer
Tooth loss
Age-related macular degeneration

[a]see text.

TABLE 27.7 The Heart and Estrogen/Progestin Replacement Study (HERS) Coronary Heart Disease Events

Year	Treated	Placebo	Relative risk–Confidence interval
1	57	38	1.52 (1.01–2.29)
2	47	48	1.00 (0.67–1.49)
3	35	41	0.87 (0.55–1.37)
4	33	49	0.67 (0.43–1.04)

From Hulley, S., Grady, D., Bush, T. *et al.* (1998). *JAMA* 280, 605–613.

effective in diminishing cardiovascular risk it appears it must be started early in menopause before adverse changes in vascular status are established. Finally, in individuals with identifiable risk factors, specific therapies (e.g., statins) must be employed in conjunction with HRT to maximize primary prevention. In women with established cardiovascular disease ERT/HRT should not be used for the sole purpose of secondary prevention.

b. Osteoporosis and Fractures

DEXA testing is the best way to diagnose bone loss and identify those at risk for osteoporosis and fracture. Once normal trabecular bone architecture is lost it cannot be restored even if bone mineral content is replenished. For osteopenic bone densities (those with T scores between −1.0 and 2.5), prevention strategies are recommended. For DEXA scans with T scores greater than −2.5 (the WHO definition of osteoporosis) antiabsorptive and anabolic treatment (when available) options are mandatory (Table 27.8). For women with osteopenia, standard measures include appropriate calcium intake up to 1500 mg, and vitamin D, as well as HRT.[96] Bone formation is stimulated by a combination of gravitational and weight-bearing forces such as the low repetitive muscle activity combined with weight load found in walking, jogging, or low-impact aerobics.[97, 98]

HRT can stabilize the osteoporotic process as well as prevent it from occurring. Estrogen inhibits bone resorption, increases intestinal calcium absorption, and increases renal conservation of calcium. HRT with adequate calcium and vitamin D confers a 50–80% reduction in primary arm, hip, and vertebral fractures. However, therapy must be sustained; the protective effect of estrogen is lost after 5 years of discontinuation of therapy. Oral alveolar bone loss (with consequent tooth loss) is strongly correlated with osteoporosis and shares equally in HRT protection.

TABLE 27.8 How to Evaluate Bone Mineral Density Report

	Definition based on bone mineral density
Normal	0 to −1 S.D. from the reference standard (84% of the population)
Osteopenia	−1 to −2.5 S.D.
Osteoporosis	Below −2.5 S.D.

T Score—Standard deviations between patient and average peak young adult bone mass. The more negative, the greater the risk of fracture.

Z Score—Standard deviations between patient and average bone mass for same age and weight. A Z score lower than −2.0 (2.5% of normal population of same age) requires diagnostic evaluation for causes other than postmenopausal bone loss.

c. Alzheimer's Disease (AD) [93]

Preliminary cohort and case-controlled studies have indicated that AD and related dementias occurred as much as 60% less frequently in estrogen users. Furthermore, this positive impact was greater with increasing dose and duration of use. Concomitant estrogen therapy enhances the beneficial response to cholinesterase inhibitor administration in women with AD. Biologic support for these observations derives from the ability of estrogen to stimulate neurotrophic factors in the CNS, protect neurons from β-amyloid toxicity *in vitro*, and stimulate axonal regeneration and synaptogenesis *in vivo* and especially dendritic spine density.

Although these promising early studies on the possibility of prevention or delay of AD await results of larger randomized placebo-controlled clinical trials, such as the WHI Memory Study, and the Women's International Study of Long Duration Oestrogen Use After Menopause (WISDOM Trial), the hopes for HRT's capacity to reduce the rate of deterioration of women with established AD has been questioned.

In a randomized double-blind multicenter clinical trial [99] ERT versus placebo did not slow disease progression nor did it improve global cognitive or functional outcomes in women (average age 75 years) with documented mild to moderate AD. But if ERT does not appear to slow the progression of established AD, the question of whether estrogen can prevent or delay the onset of AD or diminish its severity remains open. Näslund *et al.* [100] have shown that brain tissue levels of β-amyloid peptide were elevated in early dementia and increased as clinical dementia rating scores worsened. Importantly, deposition of β-amyloid could be found in individuals *before* clinical AD was evident or diagnosed. Finally, amyloid plaques appeared first in brain areas where estrogen is known to have its greatest functional morphologic impact; with progression of disease other sites less sensitive to hormone become involved.

A recent analysis of 2 cohort and 10 case-controlled studies suggest that HRT users have a 34% *decreased* risk of AD (95% CI 18–47%) (Fig. 27.4). As noted there are limitations in the studies in which this estimate is based. The validity of surrogate information on HRT use and duration, whether respondents themselves correctly remember HRT use, or if compliance issues interfered with regular usage, and finally the distorting influence of the "healthy user effect" all undermine the strength of these positive conclusions.[93]

d. Colorectal Cancer

Most but not all cohort and case-controlled studies have reported a significantly reduced incidence and mortality of colorectal cancers in current HRT users. There is no known biological basis for this finding but if confirmed the potential benefit is significant. This cancer exceeds ovary or uterine cancer incidence and mortality in women.

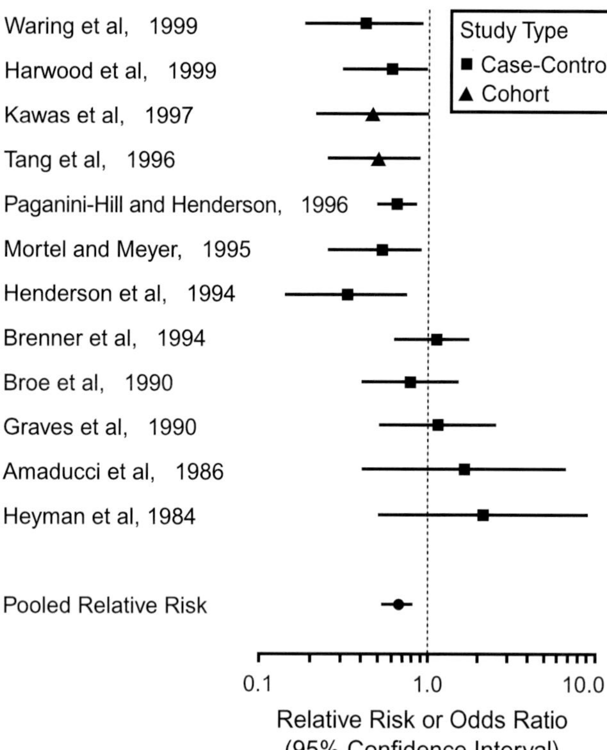

FIGURE 27.4 Results of meta-analysis of dementia studies and the impact of hormone therapy. Particularly in the more recent studies and overall risk of dementia is reduced approximately 30% in HRT users. See Reference 93 for secondary references.

C. Hazards of ERT/HRT (Table 27.9)

1. Breast Cancer [101, 102]

This vitally important woman's issue in the sheer magnitude of its scope (1 in 8 women will develop breast cancer in her lifetime), and in her perception of the magnitude of that risk and its physical, emotional, and behavioral impact on self-image and self-confidence is the single most important consideration determining whether a patient decides to start or continue HRT use. That exogenous estrogen could stimulate a receptor-positive tumor in an estrogen-dependent organ is the entirely reasonable, biologically plausible basis for patient and physician concern. Analysis of the various risk increments associating breast cancer with various indicators of increased estrogen availability or impact (endogenous, exogenous, duration, gender, genetics, and surrogate markers such as bone density) are displayed in Table 27.10.[91] In addition, it has been shown that normal human mammary epithelial cells spontaneously escape senescence and with this potential for continued or resumed growth have the opportunity to acquire gain in function, or loss of inhibition mutations and telomeric sequence erosion creating prolonged possibilities for cancer transformations.[103] In fact, sufficient evidence does exist to indicate that an increased risk of breast cancer is associated with long duration of HRT use.

TABLE 27.9 Hazards of ERT/HRT

Breast cancer[a]
Endometrial cancer
VTE
Gallbladder disease

[a]see text.

However, after over 50 case-controlled and cohort studies and at least 7 meta-analyses worldwide, the explicit epidemiologic data on this relationship are neither sufficiently consistent nor uniform in assisting the individual in assembling a personal benefit/risk ratio which balances issues such as quality of life, CVD risk, and osteopenia against HRT-related breast cancer risk.[8] Until very recently the most useful insights came from a careful collaborative combined re-analysis of 50 studies on the relationship of HRT and breast cancer.[104] The findings were

- Ever users of postmenopausal hormones had an overall increased relative risk of breast cancer of 1.14
- Current users for 5 or more years had a relative risk of 1.35 (CI 1.21–1.49) and the risk increased with increasing duration of use
- Current and recent users had evidence of having only localized disease (no metastases) and ever users had less metastatic disease
- There was no effect of a family history of breast cancer
- There was no increased relative risk in past users
- The increased relative risk in current and recent users was greater in women with lower body weights

These conclusions support the notion not only that estrogen accelerates the growth of a malignant locus already in place but also leads to early detection (improved survival rates, lower frequency of late stage disease, better differentiated tumors, and importantly the increased risk disappears within 4 years of discontinuing therapy).

Greater specificity in these issues has come from two recent reports [105, 106] and a careful clinical review.[102] In the report from the Breast Cancer Detection Demonstration Project,[105] the risk of breast cancer detection associated with postmenopausal hormone regimens of estrogen alone or in combination with progestin was compared to nonusers over a 15-year observation period (Table 27.11). By definition the only relative risk achieving statistical significance existed in current or recent users (within 4 years of diagnosis) of estrogen-progestin. These were recipients of cyclic progestin for less than 15 days (mostly 10 days) and included 26 cases using HRT for less than 4 years and 22 cases receiving HRT for 4 or more years. Insufficient numbers of women used continuous nonsequential progestin to provide comparative data. A substantial portion of cases included

TABLE 27.10 Hormonally Mediated Indicators of the Risk of Breast Cancer

Indicator	Risk group		Relative risk[a]
	Low	High	
Sex	Male	Female	150.0
Age (year)	30–34	70–74	17.0
Age at menarche (year)	>14	<12	1.5
Use of oral contraceptives	Never	Previous or current	1.07–1.2
Age at birth of first child (year)	<20	≥30	1.9–3.5
Breastfeeding (month)	≥16	0	1.37
Parity	≥5	0	1.4
Age at oophorectomy (year)	<35	—[b]	30
Age at natural menopause (year)	<45	≥55	2.0
Estrogen therapy	Never	Current	1.2–1.4
Estrogen-progestin therapy	Never	Current	1.4
Postmenopausal BMI	<22.9	>30.7	1.6
Family history of breast cancer	No	Yes	2.6
Serum estradiol concentration	Lowest quartile	Highest quartile	1.8–5.0
Breast density on mammography	0	≥75	6.0
Bone density	Lowest quartile	Highest quartile	2.7–3.5

[a]The relative risk was calculated with the low-risk group as the reference group.
[b]There is no association between the risk of breast cancer and oophorectomy performed at 35 years of age or older.

TABLE 27.11 ERT and HRT: Relation to Breast Cancer Diagnosis—Breast Cancer Detection Demonstration Project 1980–1995 (n=46,355)

	No. of cases	Relative risk (95% CI)
Ever users of *E* only	805	1.1 (1.0–1.3)
Ever users of estrogen-progestin	101	1.3 (1.0–1.6)
Current and recent users *E* only	375	1.2 (1.0–1.4)
Current and recent users estrogen-progestin	93	1.4 (1.1–1.8)

Schairer, C., Lubin, J., Troisi, R., Sturgeon, S., Brinton, L., and Hoover, R. (2000). *JAMA* 283, 485–491.

TABLE 27.12 ERT and HRT: Relation to Breast Cancer Diagnosis—Los Angeles Case Control Study 1987–1992 (n=1897)

	Odds ratio (OR)	Confidence interval (CI)
ERT	1.05	(0.97–1.5)
HRT (total)	1.24	(1.07–1.45)
HRT (sequential)	1.38	(1.13–1.68)
HRT (continuous combined)	1.09	(0.88–1.35)

Ross, R. K., Paganini-Hill, A., Won, P. C., and Pike, M. C. (2000). *J. Natl. Cancer Inst.* 92, 328–332.

in situ and small (<2 cm) node-negative disease. Of interest, all risk was restricted to recent or current use; no risk was noted if greater than 4 years had elapsed after termination of hormone therapy independent of prior duration or type of HRT employed. As in other studies, increased risk was limited to lean women (BMI <24.4). No effect of race, family history, or history of benign breast disease was noted. The particular provocative influence of high-dose cyclic sequential progestin utilization was confirmed in the Los Angeles County study reported by Ross *et al.* (Table 27.12).[106] In this report women receiving continuous estrogen-progestin regimens as well as those taking only estrogen did not demonstrate a significantly increased risk of breast cancer. On the other hand, the increased incidence of cancer detection found in overall HRT usage was due to the significant increase displayed in women receiving sequential E plus P regimens.

Santen and colleagues have reviewed the biological epidemiological and clinical data regarding the effects of progestins on the breast and breast cancer.[102] Figures 27.5 and 27.6. summarize the results of the Collaborative Group on Hormonal Factors in Breast Cancer calculations of the

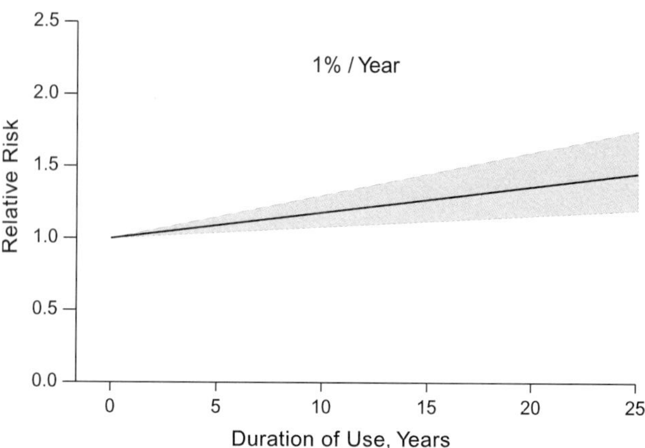

FIGURE 27.5 Estimated increase in RR of breast cancer over 25 years in users of ERT only. (From Santen, R. J., Pinkerton, J., McCartney, C., and Petroni, G. R. (2000). *J. Clin. Endocrinol. Metab.* 86, 16–23.)

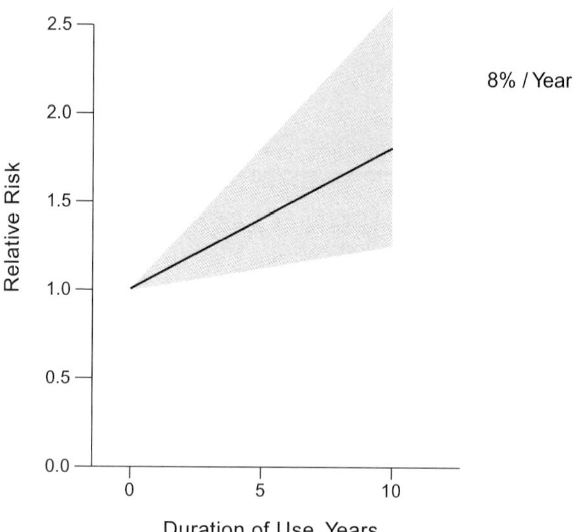

FIGURE 27.6 Estimated increase in RR of breast cancer over a 10-year period in users of sequential cyclic HRT (estrogen and sequential progestin). (From Santen, R. J., Pinkerton, J., McCartney, C., and Petroni, G. R. (2000). *J. Clin. Endocrinol. Metab.* 86, 16–23.)

impact of the cyclic addition of progestin HRT regimens in *lean* women (BMI <25).

How do these studies influence ERT/HRT practice? The limited strength of the association between ERT and breast cancer is reassuring. If there is any real increase in risk it is small, appears only over a long duration of exposure, and results in increased detection of *in situ* or small non-metastatic lesions exclusively in vulnerable (lean) populations of women. However, the disadvantageous effect of progestin regimens on risk requires clinical implementation. These include broader application of combined nonsequential HRT in which progestin dosage is minimized, and wider utilization of intrauterine and vaginal progestin methodologies in which mainly local (endometrial) and not systemic effects are induced. As Santen *et al.* [92] note: "We conclude that no definitive proof exists to establish causal relationship between progestins and breast cancer risk. However, a wide range of biologic and clinical data provides strong supportive evidence for such an effect." The protection to endometrium afforded by current continuous HRT methodologies is sufficient to make endometrial ablation or hysterectomy unwarranted.

2. Endometrial Cancer

Forty case-controlled and cohort studies indicate the risk of endometrial cancer in women using estrogen only therapy (unopposed by progestin as in HRT) increases 2–10 times the expected incidence of 1:1000 postmenopausal women per year. The risk increases with duration and dose of estrogen but that increment is eliminated (but not completely) by the addition of progestin. Any prolonged profuse untimely unusual bleeding in women on HRT must be reviewed by biopsy and/or transvaginal ultrasound.

3. Ovarian Cancer

Largely on the basis of the substantial long-term reduction in ovarian cancer rates in recipients of combined OC, by extension HRT was not thought to be a risk factor in ovarian cancer in postmenopausal women. However, serial reports from the Cancer Prevention Study II of the American Cancer Society recently updated [107] now show a relationship between long-term use of ERT and ovarian cancer mortality. Of a total of 211, 581 postmenopausal women who completed a baseline questionnaire in 1982, 944 ovarian cancer deaths were recorded in 14 years of follow-up. Analysis revealed that women who used postmenopausal ERT for 10 or more years were at increased risk of fatal ovarian cancer (RR = 2.20; 95% CI 1.53–3.17). This risk in ovarian cancer mortality was observed for both baseline users and for long-term users who had discontinued therapy within the previous 15 years. Estrogen use for less than 10 years was not associated with increased risk. Annual age-adjusted ovarian cancer death rates per 100,000 women were 64.4 for baseline users of 10 or more years compared to 26.4 for never users. No data were available on the risk for HRT users. Given the low lifetime risk for ovarian cancer (1.7%) benefit/risk analysis in the individual context is essential.

4. Venous Thrombosis and Pulmonary Embolism (VTE)

Four case-controlled studies and 1 cohort study have shown a 2–3.6-fold increased risk of deep vein thrombosis in current but not past users of HRT. Similar increments were seen in studies employing the selective estrogen receptor modulators (SERMS) raloxifene and tamoxifen. The risk appears confined to individuals starting therapy and the risk increment disappears after one year of use. The actual risk of VTE is very low because of the low frequency of the event: if relative risk is increased by a factor of 3, this would be associated with an increased incidence of VTE of approximately 2 cases per 10,000 women per year of HRT use.

D. The Absolute and Relative Contraindications to ERT/HRT

The absolute contraindications to the use of ERT/HRT are listed in Table 27.13. In addition, several conditions (Table 27.14) are defined as relative contraindications since these disorders can be worsened in some recipients of ERT/HRT. In these circumstances administration of hormone should be done only after details of the accrued benefits and risks are understood by the patient. For example, close surveillance is indicated for patients with seizure disorders and migraine headaches. The latter may actually improve if a daily continuous combined method of treatment is employed. Individuals with a history of liver disease, gallbladder disease, or hypertriglyceridemia can use transdermal ERT administration, thereby avoiding the adverse "first pass" liver impact of oral therapy. Finally, spirometry of asthmatics may worsen with ERT/HRT. In at least one prospective study the use of postmenopausal hormone was associated with a 50% risk of developing adult-onset asthma and that increased risk was related to dose and duration of therapy.

E. Conditions in which ERT/HRT Is not Contraindicated

ERT/HRT can be beneficially administered with appropriate monitoring with little risk of inducing deterioration in a variety of clinical conditions (Table 27.15). For example, the doses of hormone employed in HRT will not activate endometriosis nor will fibroid tumors enlarge with such therapy. A history of successfully treated cervical, ovarian, or stage I, grade I endometrial cancer is not a contraindication to HRT.

TABLE 27.13 Contraindications to ERT/HRT

Known or suspected pregnancy
Known or suspected breast cancer
Estrogen dependent neoplasia
Undiagnosed abnormal genital bleeding
Active thrombophlebitis or thromboembolic disorders

TABLE 27.14 Relative Contraindications for ERT/HRT

Migraine headache
Gallbladder disease
Asthma
Liver disease
Risk of breast cancer

TABLE 27.15 Conditions That Are NOT Contraindications to ERT/HRT

Controlled hypertension
Diabetes mellitus
Arthritis
Uterine fibroids
Endometriosis
Benign breast disease
Treated cervical, ovarian, and stage I, grade I endometrial cancer

Postmenopausal hormone therapy does not appear to aggravate *rheumatoid arthritis* nor does it induce flares in disease activity. On the other hand, the impact of HRT on the symptom burden of *osteoarthritis* is uncertain. While some radiographic studies suggest protective effects and diminished symptoms, others relate increased bone density (an HRT effect) to greater severity of osteoarthritic burdens. Studies using MRI measurements of knee cartilage volume and adjusting for years of menopause, BMI, smoking, and age at menopause showed that ERT increased cartilage significantly compared to controls.[112] In prospective studies, postmenopausal women with *noninsulin-dependent diabetes mellitus*, ERT improved all glucose metabolic parameters including insulin resistance and lipoprotein profile.

Finally, no relationship has been established between the use of ERT/HRT and adverse influences on *hypertension*. In both normotensive and controlled hypertensive women, studies have either shown no effect or small but statistically significant decrease in blood pressure with hormone therapy. In both diabetes and hypertension detection of and periodic assessment for underlying evolving atherogenic CVD is mandatory.

F. Side Effects of ERT/HRT

Among the participants in the Kaiser Surveys [108] older women were 2.5 times (35%) more likely than younger women (14%) to cite osteoporosis prevention or treatment as their main reason for initiating HRT. In comparison younger women reported relief of VMS as their main or additional indication (60%). However, the continuation rate at one year was 52% for younger women and only 38% for older women. In both age groups side effects were the most frequent reasons for stopping HRT; vaginal bleeding was the most frequently cited reason for abandoning therapy (Table 27.16).

TABLE 27.16 Current State of Menopause Management: Reasons for Discontinuing HRT

Main reason for stopping	Age 50–55 years (n=180)	Age ≥65 years (n=174)
Uterine bleeding	29%	52%
Breast tenderness	3%	18%
Concern about health risk other than breast cancer	9%	3%
Headaches	7%	<1%
Weight gain	6%	2%
Depression	4%	1%
Bloating/swelling	4%	1%
Concern about breast cancer	7%	1%
No longer needed	2%	1%

Adapted from Ettinger, B. *et al.* (1999). *Menopause* 6, 282.

1. HRT Related Bleeding

There are two mechanisms by which HRT can cause vaginal bleeding. In cyclic sequential regimens progestin withdrawal bleeding occurs as would be expected physiologically. This flow is usually modest in duration and quantity. Any abnormality requires investigation by biopsy. It invariably follows progestin withdrawal, is well tolerated, and does not lead to discontinuation of therapy. Indeed some women specifically request this regimen ("it makes me feel young to menstruate") but most women prefer any safe alternative that eliminates menses.

This consideration led to the widespread use of continuous combined HRT without a pill-free internal and without hormone withdrawal. The results for most women after one year of use is a very gratifying induced amenorrhea. However, as many as 20% or more of long-term users continue to bleed or spot intermittently on a variety of regimens and despite repeated confirmation of the absence of a provocative cause or disease. In these resistant cases return to sequential therapy, or application of the newly approved long-lasting progestin containing intrauterine device may be necessary. Some patients may choose endometrial ablation or even laparoscopically assisted hysterectomy to solve their problem and retain benefits of ERT.

2. Weight Gain

A variety of longitudinal studies have demonstrated that weight gain experienced by middle aged women bore *no* relation to menopause, or the use of HRTs. Rather, weight increases were strongly related to behavioral factors, particularly diminished exercise and increased ethanol consumption.[109]

G. ERT/HRT Dosage

The presence of side effects reflecting both progestin and estrogen content has led to evaluation of lower dose formulations as replacement therapy. Recent studies of low-dose estrogen-only therapy (0.3 mg) show sustained bone protection benefits and reduced endometrial growth.[110] A number of "minimum dose" formulations will become available in the U.S. to combat the challenge of defection from HRT. The efforts to lower dosage will be accelerated by the findings of the Nurses' Health Study that postmenopausal hormone use not only continues to show a decreased risk for major coronary events in women without previous heart disease, but that 0.3 mg of oral conjugated estrogen daily yields a reduction similar to that seen in the standard 0.625 mg level. Furthermore, estrogen at daily doses of 0.625 or greater and in combination with progestin may increase the risk of stroke.[111] Finally, and in response to the appeal of a lower dose customized formulation, transdermal estradiol delivery systems now provide a wide range of dosage content (ranging as low as 0.025–0.1 mg estradiol. The absence of first pass through the liver permits "customizing" dosage by using accurate blood concentrations of estradiol to guide therapeutic decisions.

VIII. ERT/HRT THERAPY: CONCLUSIONS

In its efficacy in acute interventions and the capacity to modify and prevent a broad spectrum of diseases, the overall *benefit* of ERT/HRT in the postmenopausal woman is sustained. Almost all normal healthy hypoestrogenic women will benefit from these therapies and with appropriate surveillance can be used for decades. With the dimension of breast cancer risk clarified (probably far less than the current perceived estimate) and greater precision regarding differential primary and secondary cardiovascular risk prevention (in the latter instance less than previously determined), ERT/HRT remains a powerful important strategy for healthcare in women. However, it is clear that despite defined benefits there are real and perceived risks and burdens. Accordingly, the decision to undertake HRT, when to start, at what age, with what regimen, and with what agents remains a matter of individualization based not only on current medical knowledge but also personal preferences and medical and family histories of individual patients. Use of complementary strategies, such as the addition of statins, is clearly an important contribution to what had previously been a monochromatic view of preventive therapeutics in aging women.

IX. ALTERNATIVES TO THE USE OF ERT/HRT IN POSTMENOPAUSAL WOMEN [113]

In choosing between estrogen and possible alternatives, the wide range of ERT/HRT benefits achieved in a single comprehensive therapy (VMS, atrophy, heart, bone, CNS, vision, colon cancer, tooth loss) has great appeal. Nevertheless, as has been seen large numbers of women abandon this therapy and still others cannot use HRT due to disease (e.g., previous breast cancer).[114] Furthermore, physicians and their patients are concerned over the potential of incremental problems of progestins such as breast cancer, stroke, VTE, and gallstones.

Fortunately, specific interventions are available although application may require concurrent use of multiple agents.

A. Prevention of CVD

If the likelihood of developing CVD is considered substantial based upon risk factors, modification of those lifestyle risks, exercise, and addition of hMG-CoA reductase inhibitors ('statins') and aspirin may be necessary. Furthermore, SERMS such as raloxifene and tamoxifen should also be considered given their application in breast cancer patients or those viewed as high risk.

1. Lipid Profile Effects

The only head to head comparisons show both estrogen and statins have beneficial impact (Fig. 27.7). Each lower LDL (statin >E), each raise HDL but oral estrogen increases triglycerides whereas statins lower this important contributor to atherogenesis. On the other hand, E lowers lipoprotein (a) but statin is associated with a modest increment. On balance the SERMS show similar but less advantageous changes as estrogen.

2. Primary and Secondary Prevention of Coronary Artery Events

It has already been shown that estrogen alone should not be initiated with the sole intent of preventing secondary events. With respect to primary prevention and improvement of survival head to head comparisons are difficult. While data on estrogen are impressive (30–50% reduction) these conclusions were drawn from entirely observational studies subject to potentially significant bias. Only the statins have been demonstrated by proper randomized trials (some with sufficient numbers of women) to prevent primary and secondary myocardial events and at the roughly comparable rate of 30%. Statins therefore are clearly an appropriate, often preferable, alternative to estrogen for women at cardiovascular risk.

B. Prevention and Treatment of Osteoporosis

Santen and Pinkerton [113] have summarized data on the comparative effects of placebo, alendronate, tamoxifen, raloxifene, nasal calcitonin, and estrogen on percent change from baseline in bone mineral density assessed by DEXA scan. In contrast to loss on placebo all agents showed increases with bisphonates having the greatest effect (Fig. 27.8).

How do these data translate to primary fracture prevention? Head to head comparisons needed to answer this question do not exist and one must resort to comparing efficacy data reported in different trials. Epidemiologic studies suggest a relative reduction of fracture rate of 55% with estrogen even in older women. For alendronate the decrease in spine and hip fracture is 50% but for nasal calcitonin the decrease is seen primarily in lumbar (35%), in spine, but not in the hip. For raloxifene a respectable 38–52% reduction is noted. Based upon these data alendronate, nasal calcitonin, and raloxifene could serve as adequate alternatives to estrogen for prevention and treatment of osteoporosis.

As opposed to the prevailing therapies to counter and possibly correct osteopenia and osteoporosis—all of which are *antiresorptive* rather than bone formation stimulants—parathyroid hormone (PTH) (1–34) has been shown to restore bone mass and strength.

Given in daily subcutaneous injections, PTH (1–34) produces predominantly bone formation with no balancing resorptive impact. In a large (1637 postmenopausal women with prior vertebral fractures) prospective randomized study (ref) subcutaneous PTH (20 μg/day, 40 μg/day versus placebo) was administered daily over a 21-month period.[115] PTH increased bone mineral density of the spine 9% (20 μg)

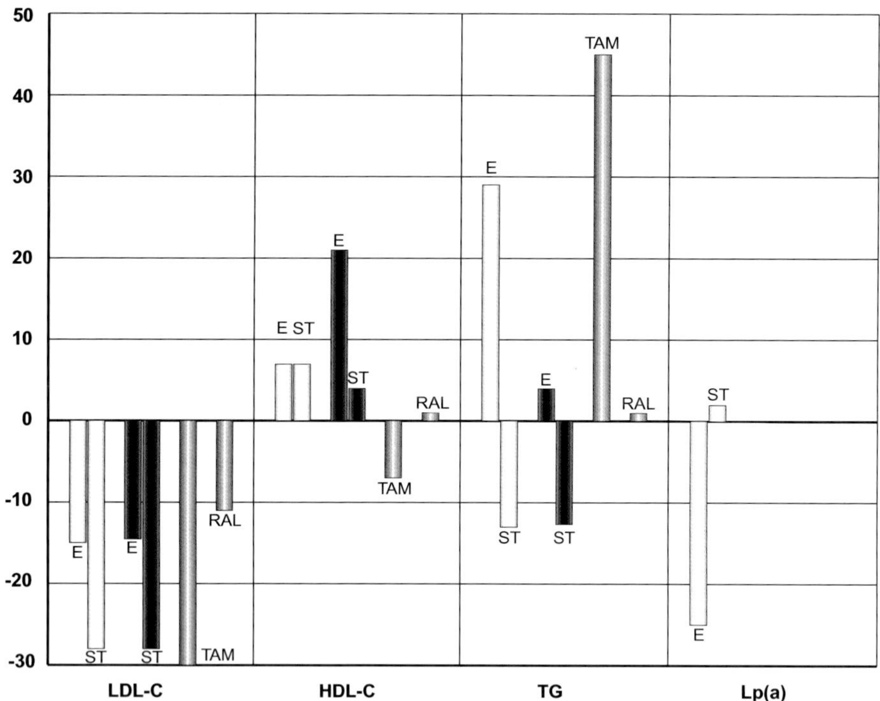

FIGURE 27.7 Comparative effects of estrogens, SERMs, and stations on lipid levels. All preparations lower LDL cholesterol and in comparative studies (back to back bars) statins (ST) and tamoxifen (TAM) are most effective. With regard to HDL cholesterol with the exception of TAM all raise these concentrations to some degree with the greatest effect achieved with estrogen. Statins lower triglycerides (TG) whereas oral estrogens and SERM raise TG concentrations. (From Pinkerton, J. V., and Santen, R. (1999). *Endocr. Rev.* 20, 308–320.)

and 13% (40 μg) more than placebo, and reduced the risk of new fractures by 65 and 69%, respectively, compared to placebo—benefits which exceed all other available treatments in similar patients. Nonvertebral fractures were reduced by 35 and 40%, respectively. Clearly the possibility of swiftly restoring bone density and strength with PTH followed by protective antiresorption therapy is now a reality.

C. Urogenital Atrophy

No agent other than local application of estrogen rings and creams provide prevention or reversal of urogenital atrophy. Dose and frequency must be monitored since transvaginal systemic absorption occurs (much like transdermal) particularly early when the vaginal mucosa is thin.

D. VMS

As noted earlier the use of placebo consistently reduces the number and severity of hot flashes by 25–30%. Against this background vitamin E and transdermal clonidine 0.1 mg show 30 and 40% above baseline improvement, respectively. Megesterolacetate 40 mg daily, however, is almost as effective as estrogen with an 80% improvement over baseline.

Selective serotonin reuptake inhibitors (SSRIs) decrease VMS more than placebo. Phytoestrogens in large quantities of soy milk are helpful particularly in perimenopause and early postmenopause.

E. Phytoestrogens and Herbs as Alternatives to ERT/HRT

Alternative "medicines" used for menopause include phytoestrogens, herbs, and nutritional supplements. Herbs used for VMS and mood swings include black and blue cohosh, evening primrose oil, chasteberry, and licorice. Vitamin E is recommended as a dietary supplement. A recent review article [116] on these materials' safety and efficacy found minimal effects. In the few randomized trials conducted, none proved better than placebo.[117–120]

On the hand, evidence is accumulating that the *phytoestrogens*, a diverse group of nonsteroidal plant compounds which behave as estrogens and occur naturally in most plants, fruits, and vegetables, may provide tangible health benefits to postmenopausal women. This large, complex, often contradictory but expanding literature has been exhaustively reviewed by Glazier and Bowman.[116] For readers desirous of specific secondary references, this review is highly recommended.

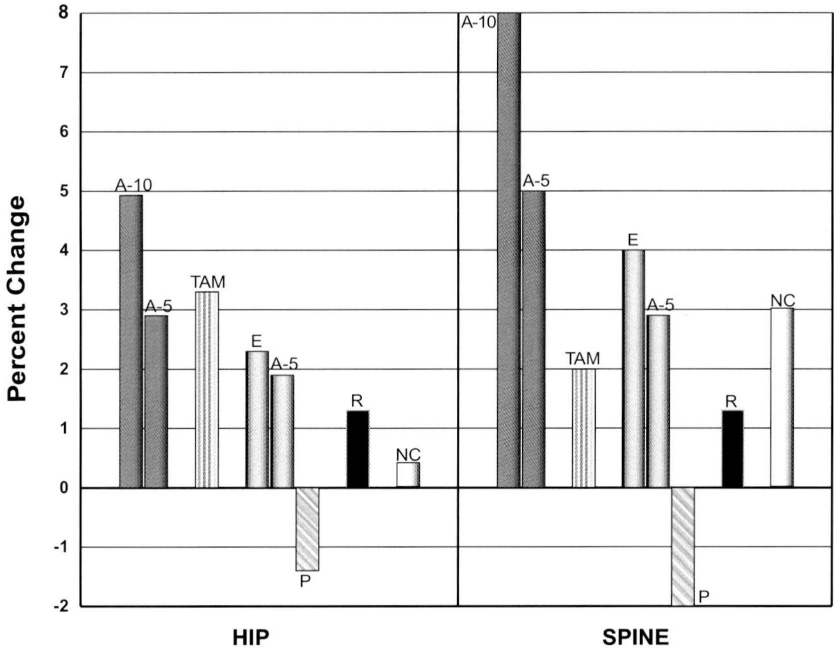

FIGURE 27.8 Comparative effect of alendronate (A), tamoxifen (TAM), estrogen (E), raloxifene (R), nasal calcitonin (NC), and placebo (P) utilization and resulting percent change in bone mineral density (BMD) in hip and spine. With the exception of placebo all agents have positive impact on hip and spine. In general greater effect is seen in the lumbar spine than hip, with alendronate and estrogen yielding greatest benefit. (From Pinkerton, J. V., and Santen, R. (1999). *Endocr. Rev.* 20, 308–320.)

The authors accessed English language MEDLINE, CINAHL, and Cochrane databases from 1966 through 1999, as well as the lay literature via the Internet on this entire subject.

Epidemiologic observational studies form the basis on which to consider supplemental dietary phytoestrogens in the possible risk reduction of certain diseases. For example, rates of colon, breast cancer, and cardiovascular diseases are much lower in Southeast Asia than in the U.S. Although confounding factors such as genetic and psychologic, cultural definitions and beliefs play important roles in these disparities, studies of the impact of migration to the U.S. show Japanese women develop increased incidence of these "western" diseases within one to two generations after coming to the U.S. Because the Asian diet on average results in the ingestion of between 20 and 150 mg of soy per day compared to women in the U.S. whose diet provides at most 1–3 mg/day, interest has focused on soy and in particular its phytoestrogen content as the missing protective factor in western diets.

1. Breast Cancer

Because phytoestrogens share structural similarities with estrogens, theoretically one would expect ingestion might lead to increased risk of breast cancer. However, in countries where phytoestrogen consumption is high, incidence of breast cancer is extremely low.

Although there are no experimental human studies there are some efforts to discern a link between soy intake and breast cancer risk. The uncertainty of the evidence is best demonstrated in citing three studies: urinary excretion of phytoestrogens was less in women with breast cancer compared with matched control women without disease [121]; urinary excretion of five different isoflavones was significantly lower in women with breast cancer in another case-controlled study [122]; but daily supplement of isoflavones (45 mg/day versus placebo) in a randomized placebo-controlled study showed increased breast lobular epithelial growth and increased progesterone receptor expression compared to placebo.[123]

Owing to conflicting evidence, further research is needed to confirm the action, if any, of phytoestrogens on the risk of breast cancer in either pre- or postmenopausal (high and low endogenous estrogen environments) women.

2. CVD

Although the majority of studies do demonstrate reduction of total cholesterol and LDL cholesterol secondary to ingestion of soy protein, there are no studies of the long-term effects of soy on coronary heart disease prevention. The risk of heart disease in Asian countries is significantly lower than in the U.S., but the Asian diet is also lower in saturated fat. One primate study [124] showed a diet high in soy reduced atherosclerotic vascular changes. On balance, although there is no direct evidence soy related avoidance of primary or secondary CVD events in women, low fat, high vegetable, legume, and fruit diets are clearly beneficial to men and women with respect to CVD prevention.

3. Osteoporosis

Again, the extent to which the disparity in osteopenia and osteoporosis incidence in Asian women (50% less common) compared to women consuming a western diet is due to genetics or diet is untested and unknown. Few controlled trials have been performed to study the general relationships of phytoestrogens and osteoporosis. Because of its unique bone and collagen enhancing nonestrogenic properties, ipriflavone, a synthetic nonhormonal preparation produced from the isoflavone daidzein, has been evaluated in several double-blind human studies. Although some have shown beneficial effects, a large recent randomized control trial revealed no benefit from the product. Furthermore, many recipients developed lymphocytopenia.[125]

4. Vasomotor Reactions

Whereas the influence of phytoestrogens in a variety of other systems is equivocal, the few controlled studies examining the effects of phytoestrogens on menopausal symptoms do show a statistically significant reduction of hot flashes achieved by relatively high levels of daily ingestion (45–60 mg/day).

5. Adverse Effects

Aside from the adverse hematologic impact of the synthetic ipriflavone, "there is no definitive evidence that the consumption of phytoestrogens at the levels normally encountered in the diet is likely to be harmful in adults."[116]

F. Conclusions on Alternative Medicines

Although evidence for the health benefits of a low saturated fat, high fruit, vegetable, and legume diet are well established, the specific influence of the phytoestrogen content of these diets on the accrued benefits are suggested but not established. The opinion here, and shared with others is that the "clinically proven benefits of prescribed ERT far outweigh those of phytoestrogens. Therefore there is insufficient evidence to recommend the use of phytoestrogens in place of traditional ERT, or to make recommendations to women about specific phytoestrogen products."[116]

X. WHAT NEXT?

Undoubtedly lower dose combinations of oral HRT, testosterone gels, and patches appropriate for the postmenopausal female and more specific SERMs are on the immediate horizon. Additionally, the customizing possibilities of estrogen patches in wide dose ranges and steady absorption/transfer characteristics will soon permit "test and treat" matches of dose, serum estradiol, and symptomatic objectives.

Finally, a unique new steroid derivative of the 19-nortestosterone family, tibolone, will come on the U.S. market. In a single daily dose of 2.5 mg, tibolone protects bone and controls VMS. Because it is metabolized into three steroid isomers with varying estrogenic, progestogenic, and androgenic properties it can provide specific effects at specific tissues; estrogen effects on bone, vagina, and relief of hot flushes; and progestogenic and androgenic to induce endometrial atrophy with better control of breakthrough bleeding. But nothing is perfect—there is a moderate reduction in HDL-cholesterol on tibolone.

XI. FINAL THOUGHTS

It is hoped that this review of human menopause has conveyed two clinically important messages.

First, women entering the fifth decade of life enjoy the prospect—as no other generation before them—for a longer and potentially fuller, healthier life. Clinicians who interact with these midlife women have the remarkable opportunity, and significant obligation, to offer currently available health-care strategies which can materially extend life and improve the health of their patients. Individualization of these plans is clearly necessary and will lead to compliance with understanding, satisfaction, and confidence for both the patient and her physician.

Second, this happy outlook is not merely one of the usual "pep talk" platitudes which generally conclude clinical reviews of this kind. Rather, it is an entirely feasible and predictable outcome because it is based on firm evidence-based endocrinologic insights that have unequivocally established, clarified, and characterized the three stages of the process of human ovarian "senescence" on the climacterium. These three stages—perimenopause, the early postmenopause, and the late postmenopause—possess uniquely different clinical presentations, uniquely different biology and endocrinology, and uniquely different clinical challenges, each demanding a uniquely different management strategy and each supported by an array of therapeutic options to meet these challenges and realize the full quality of life potential of our patients.

In the July 17, 2002 issue of *JAMA* [126] the Writing Group for the Women's Health Initiative (WHI) provided the clinical data on which the National Heart, Lung, and Blood Institute of the NIH made the decision to halt the combined hormone replacement therapy (HRT-Prempro) arm of the WHI randomized placebo-controlled study evaluating HRT use in postmenopausal women. This arm of the study assessed the effect of HRT (CEE (Premarin 0.625 mg) plus medroxy progesterone acetate (Provera 2.5 mg) daily) use in healthy postmenopausal women with a uterus compared with matched controls receiving a placebo.

While intended to last 8.5 years, the combined HRT arm was halted at 5.2 years primarily because of an increased risk of invasive breast cancer in the women receiving combined HRT. The increased risk was small (an increase of 8 cases per 10,000 women per year taking combined HRT compared to women taking a placebo). The arm of the study of estrogen-only use in women who had previously undergone hysterectomy, is continuing with no reported increased risk of breast cancer.

In addition to the breast cancer risk increment, combined HRT recipients also incurred a small but significant increased risk of cardiovascular events including coronary heart disease, stroke, and pulmonary embolism. Again, the absolute increased risk for individuals was small: estimated to be 7 more coronary heart disease events (37 versus 30) per 10,000 women per year, 8 additional cases of stroke (29 versus 21), and 8 additional cases of pulmonary embolism (16 versus 8) per 10,000 women per year.

On the other hand, combined HRT recipients had fewer hip fractures (10 versus 15), fewer total fractures, and reduced colon cancer (10 versus 16) per 10,000 woman per year. There was no overall mortality differences between the two groups.

To date, this study is the largest, most statistically valid, rigorously designed, and well analyzed randomized controlled trial to examine the impact of HRT in healthy postmenopausal women.[127] In both its positive and negative findings, it confirms but does not add substantially new information to the results of observational studies previously reported.

Accordingly, for a discussion of the impact of this report and previous studies with similar information on HRT use, the reader is referred to the discussion of dosage covered in Section VII. G in this chapter.

References

1. Lindsay, R. (1996). The menopause and osteoporosis. *Obstet. Gynecol.* 87 [Suppl.], 16S–19S.
2. Wild, R. A. (1996). Estrogen: Effects on the cardiovascular tree. *Obstet. Gynecol.* 87 [Suppl.], 27S–35S.
3. Sherwin, B. B. (1996). Hormones, mood, and cognitive functioning in postmenopausal women. *Obstet. Gynecol.* 87[Suppl.], 20S–26S.
4. Sherwin, B. B. (1997). Estrogen effects on cognition in menopausal women. *Neurology* 48 [Suppl.], S21–S26.
5. Tang, M.-X., Jacobs, D., Stern, Y., Marder, K., Schofield, P., Gurland, B., Andrews, H., and Mayeux, R. (1996). Effect of oestrogen during menopause on risk and age at onset of Alzheimer's disease. *Lancet* 348, 429–432.
6. Stampfer, M. J., Hu, F. B., and Manson, J. E. *et al.* (2000). Primary prevention of coronary heart disease in women through diet and lifestyle. *N. Engl. J. Med.* 343, 16–22.
7. National Osteoporosis Foundation. (1998). Physician Guide to Prevention/Treatment of Osteoporosis. National Osteoporosis Foundation. Washington, D.C.
8. Speroff, L., Glass, R., and Kase, N. (1999). "Clinical Gynecologic Endocrinology and Infertility," 6th Edition, pp. 644–767. Williams & Wilkins Co., Baltimore.
9. Sneeden, H., MacGregor, A. J., and Spector, T. D. (1998). Genes Control the Cessation of a Woman's Reproductive Life: A Twin Study of Hysterectomy and Age of Menopause. *J. Clin. Endocrinol. Metab.* 83, 1875–1880.
10. Sarto, G. E. (1974). Cytogenetics of 50 patients with Primary Amenorrhea. *Am. J. Obstet. Gynecol.* 119, 14–23.
11. Rebar, R. W., and Cedars, M. I. (1990). Clinical features of young women with hypergonadotropic amenorrhea. *Fertil. Steril.* 53, 804–810.
12. Therman, E., Laxova, R., and Susman, B. (1990). The critical region on the human Xq. *Hum. Genet.* 85, 455–461.
13. Sala, C., Arrigo, G., and Torri, G. *et al.* (1997). Eleven X-chromosome breakpoints associated with premature ovarian failure (POF) map to 15-Mb YAC contig spanning Xq 21. *Genomics* 40, 123–131.
14. Crisponi, L., Deiana, M., and Loi, A. *et al.* (2001). The putative forkhead transcription factor FOXL2 is mutated in blepharo-phemosis/ptosis/epicanthus inversion syndrome. *Nat. Genet.* 27, 159–166.
15. McKinlay, S. M., Bifano, N. L., and McKinlay, J. B. (1985). Smoking and age at menopause. *Ann. Intern. Med.* 103, 350–356.
16. Tylavsky, F. A., and Anderson, J. J. (1988). Dietary factors in bone health of elderly lactoovovegetarian and omnivorous women. *Am. J. Clin. Nutr.* 48 [3 Suppl.], 842–849.
17. McKinlay, S. M., Brambilla, D. J., and Posner, J. G. (1992). The normal menopause transition. *Maturitas* 14, 103–115.
18. Treloar, A. E. (1981). Menstrual cyclicity and the pre-menopause. *Maturitas* 3, 249–264.
19. Gosden, R. G., and Faddy, M. J. (1994). Ovarian aging follicle depletion and steroidogenesis. *Exp. Gerontol.* 29, 265–274.
20. Fauser, B. C., and Van Heusden, A. M. (1997). Manipulation of human ovarian function: Physiologic concepts and clinical consequences. *Endocr. Rev.* 18, 71–106.
21. Van Noord, P. A., Dubas, J. S., and Dorland, M. *et al.* (1997). Age of natural menopause in a population based screening cohort: The role of menarche, fecundity and lifestyle factors. *Fertil. Steril.* 68, 95–102.
22. McGee, E. A., and Hsueh, A. J. W. (2000). Initial and cyclic recruitment of ovarian follicles. *Endocr. Rev.* 21, 200–214.
23. WHO Scientific Group (1996). Research on the menopause in the 1990s. A report of the WHO Scientific Group. World Health Organization, Geneva, Switzerland. 866, 1–79.
24. Prior, J. (1998). Perimenopause: The complex endocrinology of the menopause transition. *Endocr. Rev.* 19, 397–428.
25. Barbieri, R. L., Berga, S. L., Chang, R. J. and Santoro, N. F. (2001). Managing the perimenopause. APGO educational series on women's health issues. Association of Professors of Gynecology and Obstetrics. Washington, D.C.
26. Reane, N., Wyman, T., Phillips, D., de Kretser, D., and Padmanabhan, V. (1998). Net increase in stimulation input resulting from a decrease in inhibin B and an increase in activin A may contribute in part to the rise in follicular phase FSH of aging cyclic women. *J. Clin. Endocrinol. Metab.* 83, 3302–3307.
27. Santoro, N., Adel, T., and Skurnich., H. (1999). Decreased inhibin tone and increased activin A secretion characterize reproductive aging in women. *Fertil. Steril.* 71, 658–662.
28. Santoro, N., Brown, J. R., Adel, T., and Skurnich, H. (1996). Characterization of reproductive hormone dynamics in the perimenopause. *J. Clin. Endocrinol. Metab.* 81, 1495–1501.

29. Klein, N. A., Battaglia, D. A., and Woodruff, T. K. *et al.* (2000). Ovarian follicular concentrations of activin follistatin inhibin IGF-I, IGF-II, IGF-BP-2, IGF BP-3 and VEGF in spontaneous menstrual cycles of normal women of advanced reproductive age. *J. Clin. Endocrinol. Metab.* 85, 4520–4525.
30. Neugarten, B. L., and Kraines, R. J. (1964). Menopausal symptoms in women of various ages. *Psychosom. Med.* 27, 266–275.
31. Ballinger, C. B., Browining, N. C., and Smith, A. H. W. (1987). Hormonal profiles and psychologic symptoms in perimenopausal woman. *Maturitas* 9, 235–251.
32. Kronenberg, F. (1990). Hot flashes: Epidemiology and physiology. *Ann. N. Y. Acad. Sci.* 592, 52–86.
33. Groeneveld, F. P. M. J., Bareman, F. P., and Barenesen, R. *et al.* (1996). Vasomotor symptoms and well being in the climacteric years. *Maturitas* 23, 293–299.
34. Siemenda, C., Loncope, C., Peacock, M., Johnston, C., and Hui, S. (1996). Sex steroids, bone mass and bone loss. *J. Clin. Invest.* 97, 14–21.
35. Speroff, L., Glass, R., and Kase, N. (1999). Menopause and the perimenopausal transition. *In* "Clinical Gynecologic Endocrinology and Infertility," 6th Edition, pp. 969–970. Lippincott Williams & Wilkins, Philadelphia, PA.
36. Longcope, C., Jaffe, W., and Griffing, G. (1981). Production rates of androgens and estrogens in postmenopausal women. *Maturitas* 3, 215–223.
37. Judd, H. L., Judd, G. E., Lucas, W. E., and Yen, S. S. C. (1974). Endocrine function of the postmenopausal ovary: Concentrations of androgens and estrogens in ovarian and peripheral vein blood. *J. Clin. Endocrinol. Metab.* 39, 1020–1024.
38. Jiroutek, M. R., Chen, M. H., Johnston, C. C., and Longcope, C. (1998). Changes in reproductive hormones and sex hormone-binding globulin in a group of postmenopausal women measured over 10 years. *Menopause* 5, 90–94.
39. Einerth, Y. (1982). Vacuum curettage by the Vabra method. A simple procedure for endometrial assessment. *Acta Obstet. Gynecol. Scand.* 61, 373–376.
40. Gebbie, A. E., Glasier, A., and Sweeting, V. (1995). Incidence of ovulation in perimenopausal women before and during hormone therapy. *Contraception* 52, 221–222.
41. Feldman, S., Shapter, A., Welch, W. R., and Berkowitz, R. S. (1994). Two-year follow-up of 263 patients with post/perimenopausal vaginal bleeding after initial biopsy. *Gynecol. Oncol.* 55, 56–59.
42. Kroon, E., and Andolf, E. (1995). Diagnosis and follow-up of simple ovarian cysts detected by ultrasound in postmenopausal women. *Obstet. Gynecol.* 85, 211–214.
43. Aneste, J. N., Kalantandou, S. N, and Kimzey, L. M. *et al.* (1998). Bone loss in young women with karyotypically normal spontaneous premature ovarian failure. *Obstet. Gynecol.* 91, 12–15.
44. Cummings, S. R., Black, D. M., and Nevitt, M. C. *et al.* (1993). Bone density at various sites for prediction of hip fractures. *Lancet* 341, 72–75.
45. Van Der Schouw, Y. T., Van Der Graaf, Y., and Steyerberg, E. W. *et al.* (1996). Age at menopause as a risk of cardiovascular mortality. *Lancet* 347, 714–718.
46. Snowdon, D. A., Kane, R. L., and Beeson, W. L. *et al.* (1989). Is early natural menopause a biological marker of health and aging? *Am. J. Public Health* 79, 709–714.
47. Grumbach, M. M., and Auchus, R. J. (1999). Estrogen: Consequences and implications of human mutations in synthesis and action. *J. Clin. Endocrinol. Metab.* 84, 4677–4694.
48. Hammond, C. (1998). http://www.menopausalhealth. Duke University School of Medicine.
49. Freedman, R. R. (1998). Biochemical, metabolic, and vascular mechanisms in menopausal hot flashes. *Fertil. Steril.* 70, 332–337.
50. Mohyi, D., Tabassi, K., and Simon, J. (1997). Differential diagnosis of hot flashes. *Maturitas* 27, 203–214. Review.
51. Raz, R., and Stamm, W. E. (1993). A controlled trial of intravaginal estriol in postmenopausal women with recurrent infections. *N. Engl. J. Med.* 329, 753–756.
52. Holland, E. F., Studd, J. W., Mansell, J. P., Leather, A. T., and Bailey, A. J. (1994). Changes in collagen composition and cross-links in bone and skin of osteoporotic postmenopausal women treated with percutaneous estradiol implants. *Obstet. Gynecol.* 83, 180–183.
53. Ballinger, C. B. (1990). Psychiatric aspects of the menopause. *Br. J. Psychiatry* 156, 773–787. Review.
54. Greendale, G. A., Hogan, P., and Shumaker, S. (1996). For the Postmenopausal Estrogen/Progestin Interactions (PEPI) Investigators. Sexual Functioning in Postmenopausal Women. *J. Women's Health* 5, 445.
55. George, L. K., and Weiler S. J. (1981). Sexuality in middle and late life. The effects of age, cohort, and gender. *Arch. Gen. Psychiatry* 38, 919–923.
56. Shifren, J. L., Braunstein, G. D., and Simon, J. A. *et al.* (2000). Transdermal testosterone treatment in women with impaired sexual function after oophorectomy. *N. Engl. J. Med.* 343, 682–688.
57. Meston, C. M., and Frohlich, P. F. (2000). The neurobiology of sexual function. *Arch. Gen. Psychiatry* 57, 1012–1030.
58. McEwen, B. S., Alves, S. E., Bullock, K., and Weiland, N. G. (1997). Ovarian Steroids and the Brain: Implications for cognition and aging. *Neurology* 48 [Suppl.7], 8S–15S.
59. Mayeux, R. (2001). Can estrogen or selective estrogen-receptor modulators preserve cognitive function in elderly women? *N. Engl. J. Med.* 344, 1242–1244.
60. Shaywitz, S. E., Shaywitz, B. A., and Pugh, K. R. *et al.* (1999). Effect of estrogen on brain activation patterns in postmenopausal women during working memory tasks. *JAMA* 281, 1197–1202.
61. LeBlanc, E. S., Janowsky, J., Chan, B. K. S., and Nelson, H. D. (2001). Hormone replacement therapy and cognition. Systemic review and meta-analysis. *JAMA* 285, 1493–1496.
62. Melton, L. J., Thamer, M., and Ray, N. F. (1997). Fractures attributable to osteoporosis: Report from the National Osteoporosis Foundation. *J. Bone Miner. Res.* 12, 16–23.
63. Lindsay, R. (1996). The Menopause and osteoporosis. *Obstet. Gynec.* 87 [Suppl.], 16S–19S.
64. Turner, R. T., Riggs, B. L., and Spelsberg, T. C. (1994). Skeletal effects of estrogen. *Endocr. Rev.* 15, 275–300. Review.
65. Browner, W. S., Pressman, A. R., Nevitt, M. C., and Cummings, S. R. (1996). For the study of osteoporotic fractures group. Mortality following fractures in older women. The study of osteoporotic fractures. *Arch. Intern. Med.* 156, 1521–1525.
66. Riis, B. J., Hansen, M. A., Jensen, A. M., Overgarrd, K., and Christiansen, C. (1996). Low bone mass and fast rate of bone loss at menopause: Equal risk factors for a 15-year follow-up study. *Bone.* 19, 9–12.
67. Ettinger, B. (1988). Prevention of osteoporosis: Treatment of estradiol deficiency. *Obstet. Gynecol.* 72 [5 Suppl.] 12S–17S.
68. Lindsay, R. (1993). Prevention and treatment of osteoporosis. *Lancet* 341, 801–805.
69. Cardiovascular Disease in Women (1998). Pathophysiology diagnosis and treatment. APGO Educational Series on Women's Health Issues. R. L. Barbieri, ed. March.
70. The American Heart Association. http://www.amhrt.org.
71. Rich-Edwards, J. W., Manson, J. E., Hennekens, C. H. and Buring, J. E. (1995). The primary prevention of coronary heart disease in women. *N. Engl. J. Med.* 332, 1758–1765.
72. Hanson, J. J. S. (1994). Modifiable risk factors for coronary heart disease in women. *Am. J. Crit. Care* 3, 177–186.
73. Kannel, W. B., and Wilson, P. W. F. (1995). Risk factors that attenuate the female coronary advantage. *Arch. Intern. Med.* 155, 57–61.
74. Matthews, K. A., Meilahn, E., Kuller, L. H., Kelsey, S. F., Caggiula, A. W., and Wing, R. R. (1989). Menopause and risk factors for coronary heart disease. *N. Engl. J. Med.* 321, 641–646.

75. Brunner, D., Weisbort, J., Meshulam, N., Schwartz, S., Gross, J., Saltz-Rennert, H., Altman, S., and Loebl, K. (1987). Relation of serum total cholesterol and high-density lipoprotein cholesterol per incidence of definite coronary events: Twenty-year follow-up of the Donolo-Tel Aviv Prospective Coronary Artery Disease Study. *Am. J. Cardiol.* 59, 1271–1276.
76. Jacobs, Jr., D. R., Mebane, I. L., Banduvila, S. I., Criqui, M. H., and Tryoler, H. A. (1990). High density lipoprotein cholesterol as a predictor of cardiovascular disease mortality in men and women: The follow-up study of the Lipid Research Clinics Prevalence Study. *Am. J. Epidemiol.* 131, 32–47.
77. Chowienczyk, P. J., Watts, G. F., Cockcroft, J. R., Brett, S. E., and Ritter, J. M. (1994). Sex difference in endothelial function in normal and hypercholesterolemic subjects. *Lancet* 344, 305–306.
78. Mundy, G., Garrett, R., Harris, S., Chan, J., Chen, D., Rossini, G., Boyce, B., Zhao, M., and G. Gutierrez. (1999). Stimulation of Bone formation in Vitro and in Rodents by Statins. *Science* 286, 1946–1949.
79. Edwards, C. J. (2000). Oral statins and increased bone mineral density in postmenopausal women. *Lancet* 355, 2218.
80. Chan, A. K., (2000). Inhibitors of HMG-CoA reductase and risk of fractures among older women. *Lancet* 355, 2185–2188.
81. Wang, P. S., Solomon, D. H., Mogun, H., and Avron, J. (2000). HMG-CoA reductase inhibitors and the risk of hip fractures in elderly patients. *JAMA* 283, 3211–3216.
82. Demer, L. (1995). A skeleton in the artherosclerosis closet. (1995). *Circulation* 92, 2029–2032.
83. Uyama, O., Yoshimoto, Y., Yamamoto, Y., and Kawai, A. (1997). Bone changes and carotid atherosclerosis in postmenopausal women. *Stroke* 28, 1730–1732.
84. Hak, A. E., Huibert, Pols, H. A. P., van Hemert, A. M., Hofman, A., and Witteman, J. C. M., (2000). Progression of aortic calcification is associated with metacarpal bone loss during menopause. *Arterioscler. Thromb. Vasc. Biol.* 20, 1926–1931.
85. Parhami, F., Morrow, A. D., Balucan, J., Leitinger, N., Watson, A. D., Tintut, Y., Berliner, J. A., and Demer, L. L. (1997). Lipid oxidation products have opposite effects on calcifying vascular cell and bone cell differentiation: A possible explanation for the paradox of arterial calcification in osteoporotic patients. *Arterioscler. Thromb. Vasc. Biol.* 17, 680–687.
86. Girasole, G. *et al.* (1992). 17β-estradiol inhibits IL-6 production by bone marrow–derived stromal cells and osteoblasts in vitro. *J. Clin. Invest.* 89, 883–891.
87. Cenci, S., Weitzmann, M. N., Roggia, C., Namba, N., Novack, D. Woodring, J., and Pacifici, R. (2000). Estrogen deficiency induces bone loss by enhancing T-cell production of TNF-α. *J. Clin. Invest.* 106, 1229–1237.
88. Santoro, N., Col, N. F., and Eckman, M. H. *et al.* (1999). Therapeutic controversy: Hormone replacement therapy—where are we going? *J. Clin. Endocrinol. Metab.* 84, 1798–1812.
89. Hammond, C. (2000). http://www.menopausalhealth. Duke University School of Medicine.
90. AACE Medical Guidelines for Clinical Practice for Management of Menopause. (1999). *Endocr. Pract.* 5, 355–366.
91. Hormone replacement therapy (1998). ACOG Educational Bulletin: Number 247.
92. APGO Educational Series on Women's Health Issues. (1998). Maximizing Menopausal Health. Opportunities for Intervention.
93. LeBlanc, E. S., Janowsky, J., Chan, B. K. S., and Nelson, H. D. (2001). Hormone replacement therapy and cognition: Systemic review and meta-analysis. *JAMA* 285, 1496–1499.
94. Hammond, C. H. (2000). Potential and proven benefits of menopausal hormone replacement: Evidence based observations. Transactions AGOS Vol. XVIII, p 93. Mosby Inc., St. Louis.
95. Hulley, S., Grady, D., and Bush, T. *et al.* (1998). Randomized trial of estrogen plus progestin for secondary prevention of coronary heart disease in postmenopausal women. Heart and Estrogen/progestin Replacement Study (HERS) Research Group. *JAMA* 280, 605–613.
96. Dawson-Hughes, B., Harris, S. S., Krall, E. A., and Dallal, G. E. (1997). Effect of calcium and vitamin D supplementation on bone density in men and women 65 years of age and older. *N. Engl. J. Med.* 337, 670–676.
97. Frielander, A. L., Genant, H. K., Sadowsky, S., Byl, N. N., and Gluer, C. C. (1995). A two-year program of aerobics and weight training enhances bone mineral density of young women. *J. Bone Miner. Res.* 10, 574–585.
98. Kerr, D., Morton, A., Dick, I., and Prince, R. (1996). Exercise effects on bone mass in postmenopausal women are site specific and load dependent. *J. Bone Miner. Res.* 11, 218–225.
99. Mulnard, R. A., Cotman, C. W., and Kawas, C. *et al.* (2000). Estrogen replacement therapy for treatment of mild to moderate Alzheimer's disease: A randomized controlled trial. Alzheimer's Disease Cooperative Study. *JAMA* 282, 1007–1015.
100. Näslund, J., Haroutunian, V., and Mohs, R. *et al.* (2000). Correlation between elevated levels of amyloid beta-peptide in the brain and cognitive decline. *JAMA* 283, 1571–1577.
101. Clemens, M., and Goso, P. (2001). Estrogens and the risk of breast cancer. *N. Engl. J. Med.* 344, 276–285.
102. Santen, R. J., Pinkerton, J., McCartney, C., and Petroni, G. R. (2001). Risk of breast cancer with progestins in combination with estrogens as hormone replacement therapy. *J. Clin. Endocrinol. Metab.* 86, 16–23.
103. Romanov, S. R., Korakiewicz, B. K., Holst, C. R., Stampfer, M. R., Haupt, L. M., and Tisty, T. D. (2001). Normal human mammary epithelial cells spontaneously escape senescence and acquire genomic changes. *Nature* 490, 633–637.
104. Collaborative Group on Hormonal Factors in Breast Cancer (1997). Breast Cancer and hormone replacement: Collaborative reanalysis of data from 51 epidemiological studies of 52,705 women with breast cancer and 108,411 women without breast cancer. *Lancet* 350, 1047–1059.
105. Schairer, C., Lubin, J., and Troisi, R. *et al.* (2000). Menopausal estrogen and estrogen-progestin replacement therapy and breast cancer risk. *JAMA* 283, 485–491.
106. Ross, R. K., Paganini-Hill, A., and Won, P. C. *et al.* (2000). Effect of hormone replacement therapy on breast cancer risk: Estrogen versus estrogen plus progestin. *J. Natl. Cancer Inst.* 92, 328–332.
107. Rodriguez, C., Patel, A. V., Calle, E. E., Jacob, E. J., and Thun, M. J. (2001). Estrogen replacement therapy and ovarian cancer mortality in a large prospective study of U.S. women. *JAMA* 285, 1460–1465.
108. Ettinger, B., Pressman, A., and Silver, P. (1999). The effect of age on reasons for initiation and discontinuation of hormone replacement therapy. *Menopause* 6, 282–289.
109. Crawford, S. L., Casey, V. A., and McKinlay, S. H. (2000). A longitudinal study of weight and the menopausal transition: Results from the Massachusetts Women's Health Study. *Menopause* 7, 96–104.
110. Genant, H. K., Weiss, S., Lucas, J., Akin, M., Emkey, R., and McNancy-Flint, H. *et al.* (1997). Low dose esterified estrogen therapy: Effects on bone, plasma estradiol concentration, endometrium and lipids. *Arch. Intern. Med.* 157, 2609–2615.
111. Grodstein, F., Manson, J. E., Colditz, G. A., Willett, W. C., Speizer, F. E., and Stampfer, M. J. (2000). A prospective, observational study of postmenopausal hormone therapy and primary prevention of cardiovascular disease. *Ann. Intern. Med.* 133, 933–941.
112. Wluka, A. E., Davis, S. R., Bailey, M., Stuckey, S. L., and Cicuttini, F. M. (2001). Users of oestrogen replacement therapy have more knee cartilage than non-users. *Ann. Rheum. Dis.* 60, 332–336.
113. Pinkerton, J. V., and Santen, R. (1999). Alternatives to the use of estrogen in postmenopausal women. *Endocr. Rev.* 20, 308–320.
114. Consensus statement: Treatment of estrogen deficiency symptoms in women surviving breast cancer (1998). *J. Clin. Endocrinol. Metab.* 83, 1993–2000.

115. Neer, R. M., Arnaud, C. D., and Zanchetta, J. R. *et al.* (2001). Effect of parathyroid hormone (1–34) on fractures and bone mineral density in postmenopausal women with osteoporosis. *N. Engl. J. Med.* 344, 1434–1441.
116. Glazier, M. G., and Bowman, M. A. (2001). A review of the evidence for the use of phytoestrogens as a replacement for traditional estrogen replacement therapy. *Arch. Int. Med.* 161, 1161–1172.
117. Seidel, M. M., and Stewart, D. E. (1998). Alternative treatments for menopausal symptoms: Systemic review of scientific and lay literature. *Can. Fam. Physician* 44, 1299–1308.
118. Blatt, M. H. G., Weisbader, H., and Kupperman, H. S. (1953). Vitamin E and climacteric syndrome. *Arch. Int. Med.* 91, 792–799.
119. Khoo, S. K., Mundo, C., and Battistutta, D. (1990). Evening primrose oil and treatment of PMS. *Med. J. Aust.* 153, 189–192.
120. Hiruta, J. D., Swierz, L. M., Zell, B., Small, R., and Ettinger, B. (1997). Does Don Quai have estrogen effects in postmenopausal women? A double blind placebo controlled trial. *Fertil. Steril.* 68, 981–986.
121. Ingram, D., Sanders, K., Kolybala, M., and Lopez, D. (1997). Case-control study of phytoestrogens and breast cancer. *Lancet.* 9083, 990–994.
122. Zheng, W., Dai, Q., and Custer, L. J. *et al.* (1999). Urinary excretion of isoflavonoids and the risk of breast cancer. *Cancer Epidemiol. Biomarkers Prev.* 8, 35–40.
123. McMichael-Phillips, D. F., Harding, C., and Morton, M. *et al.* (1998). Effects of soy protein supplementation on epithelial proliferation in the histologically normal breast. *Am. J. Clin. Nutr.* 685, 1431S–1435S.
124. Honore, E. K., Williams, J. K., Anthony, M. S., and Clarkson, T. B. (1997). Soy isoflavones enhance coronary vascular reactivity in atherosclerotic female macaques. *Fertil. Steril.* 67, 148–154.
125. Alexandersen, P., Toussaint, A., and Christiansen, M. D. (2001). Ipriflavone in the treatment of postmenopausal osteoporosis: A randomized controlled trial. *JAMA* 285, 1482–1488.
126. The Writing Group for WHI (2002). Risks and benefits of estrogen plus progestin in healthy postmenopausal women: Principal results from the Women's Health Initiative randomized control trial. *JAMA* 288, 321–333.
127. Response to Women's Health Initiative study results by The American College of Obstetricians and Gynecologists. A Clinical Advisory. August 9, 2002, ACOG.

CHAPTER

28

Laparoscopic Surgery of Benign Ovarian Disorders

M. CANIS
Department of Obstetrics, Gynecology, and Reproductive Medicine Polyclinique CHU 63003 Clermont-Ferrand, France

A. WATTIEZ
Department of Obstetrics, Gynecology, and Reproductive Medicine Polyclinique CHU 63003 Clermont-Ferrand, France

R. BOTCHORISHVILI
Department of Obstetrics, Gynecology, and Reproductive Medicine Polyclinique CHU 63003 Clermont-Ferrand, France

B. RABISCHONG
Department of Obstetrics, Gynecology, and Reproductive Medicine Polyclinique CHU 63003 Clermont-Ferrand, France

C. HOULLE
Department of Obstetrics, Gynecology, and Reproductive Medicine Polyclinique CHU 63003 Clermont-Ferrand, France

H. MANHES
Polyclinique "La Pergola" 03200 Vichy, France

G. MAGE
Department of Obstetrics, Gynecology, and Reproductive Medicine Polyclinique CHU 63003 Clermont-Ferrand, France

J. L. POULY
Department of Obstetrics, Gynecology, and Reproductive Medicine Polyclinique CHU 63003 Clermont-Ferrand, France

M. A. BRUHAT
Department of Obstetrics, Gynecology, and Reproductive Medicine Polyclinique CHU 63003 Clermont-Ferrand, France

I. INTRODUCTION

The laparoscopic treatment of adnexal masses became the gold standard within the last few years. However, the procedures have been rarely extensively described. They are generally summarized as a "stripping" procedure without any detail. Nevertheless, a good laparoscopic technique and adequate surgical management are required to ensure optimal patient care.

The debate is not over between the pioneers who claim that laparoscopic surgery can be proposed to most patients when adequately performed and the conservatives who argue that these procedures should be reserved for expert laparoscopic surgeons.

Obviously any significant and reliable improvement of the preoperative evaluation would be a major step forward in the surgical management of adnexal masses.

II. RISKS OF LAPAROSCOPY IN OVARIAN SURGERY

Most of the 41 cases of abdominal wall metastasis were reported in patients with advanced disease and ascites.[1–4]

Four national surveys of laparoscopic management of adnexal masses [5–9] confirmed that the pre- and intraoperative diagnosis of ovarian cancer may be difficult and that an inadequate laparoscopic procedure may worsen the prognosis. However, the "dissemination" diagnosed at restaging laparotomies may be attributed to several problems.

1. The peritoneal cavity may have not been fully inspected during the initial laparoscopy as the diagnosis of cancer was missed.
2. The laparoscopic approach may have been inadequate: the tumor was morcellated in 55% of the cases reported by Kinderman *et al.*,[8] and endobags were not available in 1991 when Maiman *et al.* published their results.[5]

These data suggested that inadequate laparoscopic procedures may be dangerous. However, inadequate procedures by laparotomy also appeared to worsen the prognosis. Indeed, the 20% incidence of upstaging reported in the French survey [7] was similar to the results found at restaging after inadequate surgical management by laparotomy.[10–13] Previously the complications were attributed to the surgeons [14] whereas today we attribute blame more to the surgical approach.

Some cases of intraperitoneal dissemination after laparoscopic procedures reported as adequate may be more worrying.[2, 15, 16] We reported one case of pelvic dissemination, 3 weeks after a laparoscopic adnexectomy performed with minimal tumor manipulation and using an endobag.[2] The pelvic dissemination found at restaging, 3 weeks after the initial procedure, remained poorly understood as the tumor was a well-differentiated serous cystadenocarcinoma. Definitive conclusions cannot be proposed from these case reports, the prognosis of a cancer being more related to the biology of the tumor than to the surgical approach.[17] Is this complication rare as suggested by the literature or instead, rarely reported?[18]

Reviewing experimental studies, we proposed the following conclusions [19]:

1. Conflicting results have been reported on the incidence of trocar site metastasis when comparing CO_2 laparoscopy and laparotomy depending on the model used
2. Tumor growth after laparotomy is greater than after endoscopy
3. Tumor dissemination is worse after CO_2 laparoscopy than after laparotomy
4. Some of the disadvantages of CO_2 laparoscopy may be treated using local or intravenous treatments or avoided using other endoscopic exposure methods, such as gasless laparoscopy

From experimental data it appeared that the laparoscopic treatment of gynecologic cancer has potential advantages and disadvantages. The risk of dissemination appeared high when a large number of malignant cells are present so that adnexal tumors with external vegetations and bulky lymph nodes may be considered as contraindications to CO_2 laparoscopy. The advantages of gasless laparoscopy should not be overestimated as a recent study showed a significantly lower tumor load and port site metastasis after CO_2 laparoscopy than after gasless laparoscopy.[20]

III. ROLES OF SURGERY IN THE MANAGEMENT OF ADNEXAL MASSES

The goal of surgery is complete and immediate treatment of the mass.[5] Benign tumors should be treated using ovarian preserving procedures, malignant tumors should be staged according to the rules of oncologic surgery as soon as possible. However, if only one adnexa is involved and if the diagnosis of cancer cannot be confirmed by frozen sections, an adnexectomy followed by restaging is an acceptable mode of management used in many gynecologic oncological departments, particularly in young patients.[21]

If an apparently benign mass is later found to be malignant, the delay between the laparoscopic diagnosis and the staging procedure should be as short as possible, ideally less than 8 or 17 days according to Kinderman *et al.* and Lehner *et al.*,[8, 22] respectively.

A delayed staging after unilateral adnexectomy seems acceptable,[21] whereas biopsy or partial resection followed by a delayed adnexectomy and restaging are probably associated with a higher risk of postoperative dissemination.

As recommended, 10 years ago, the ability to immediately and completely treat an ovarian cancer is a prerequisite to the laparoscopic management of adnexal masses.

IV. THE RISKS INDUCED BY A LAPAROSCOPIC PUNCTURE

From the techniques described by laparotomy, we were taught the concept that an adequate cystectomy should be performed without puncture or rupture to avoid spillage of intracystic malignant ovarian tumors. Because of the technical disadvantages of the laparoscopic approach, this rule which was difficult to follow by laparotomy appears as a major disadvantage of laparoscopy. However, some comments can be proposed about this problem.

1. The puncture of a stage Ia ovarian cancer is rare, in our experience of 1600 cases managed in our department we encountered 32 cases of invasive ovarian cancer and only 4 stage Ia were punctured to achieve the diagnosis of cancer. Unfortunately most cases of cancer are obvious before the puncture. (Figs. 28.1–28.6).[23]
2. We know that the puncture of a low malignant potential tumor has no incidence on the prognosis when the tumor is removed immediately by laparotomy.[24–29]
3. Several multivariate analyses suggested that the puncture of an early invasive ovarian cancer has no incidence on the prognosis.[30–34] Recently Vergote *et al*. reviewed a series of 1500 patients and concluded that surgical puncture significantly worsens the prognosis.[35] However, this was a retrospective multicentric study, patients were included during a 25-year period, and the staging procedures were not similar in all centers. So that the debate is not over. A rupture is not the catastrophic event described by Williams in 1973.[36] The surgical puncture should be avoided whenever possible, but if an adequate technique is used, the risks are probably minimal since the number of malignant cells in an ovarian tumor is low as illustrated by the difficulties of the cytologic diagnosis of ovarian cancer.[37] Moreover, these data were reported in patients managed by laparotomy suggesting that the risks are also encountered by laparotomy, so that these results cannot be used to blame the laparoscopic approach.[36]

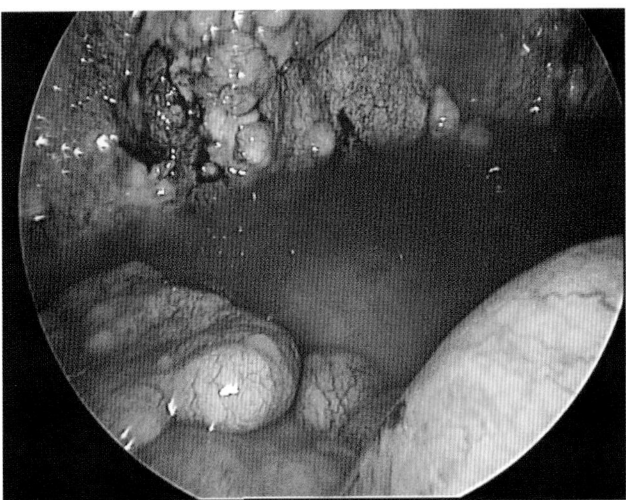

FIGURE 28.1 An obvious peritoneal carcinomatosis.

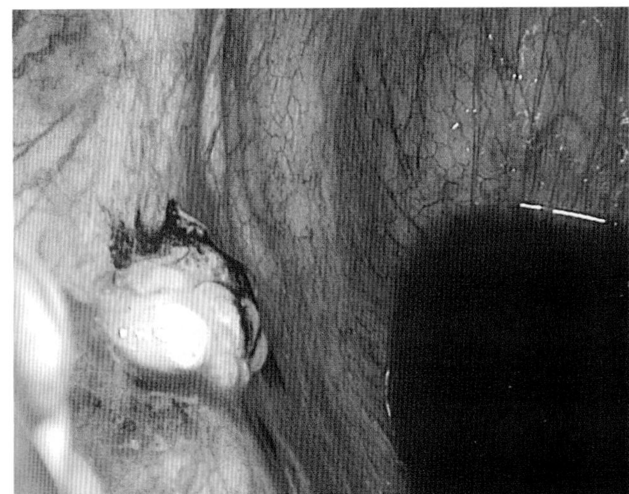

FIGURE 28.3 Peritoneal metastases were obvious.

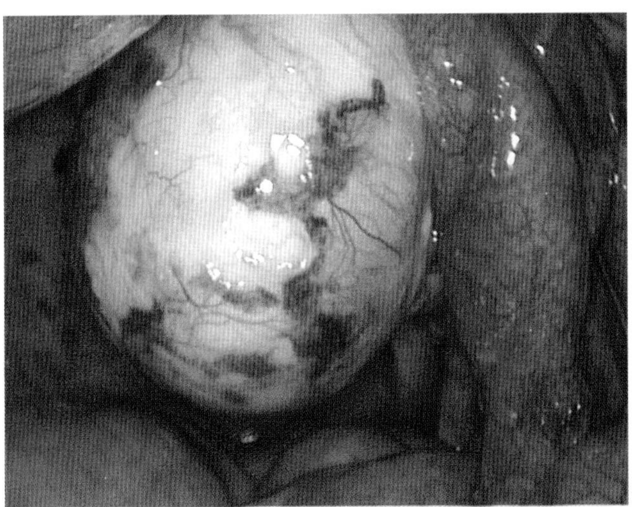

FIGURE 28.2 A puncture was not necessary to diagnose this endometriod carcinoma.

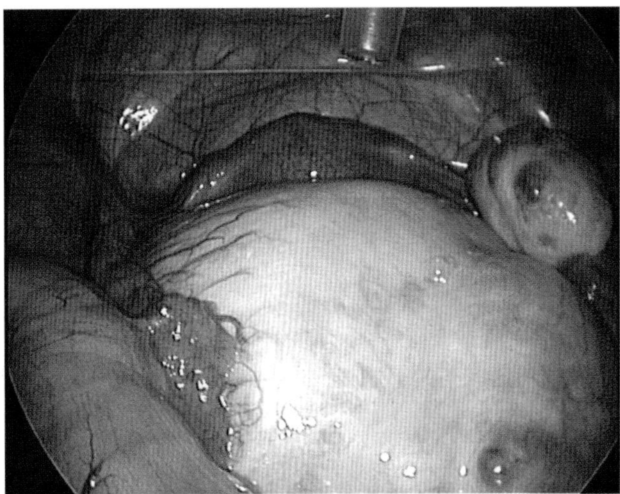

FIGURE 28.4 A puncture was not necessary in this case.

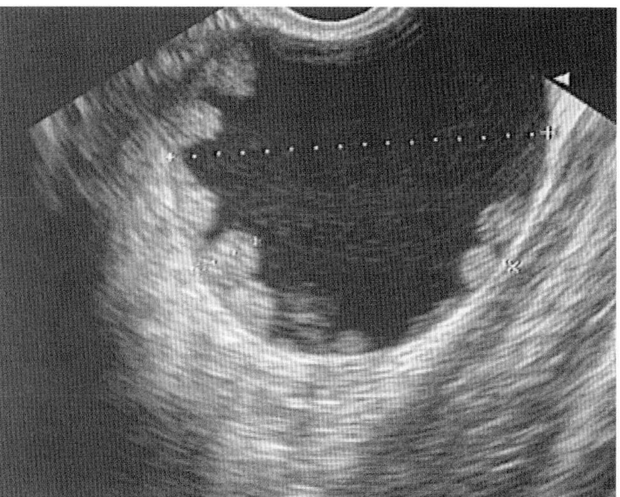

FIGURE 28.5 Intracystic vegetations obvious at ultrasound.

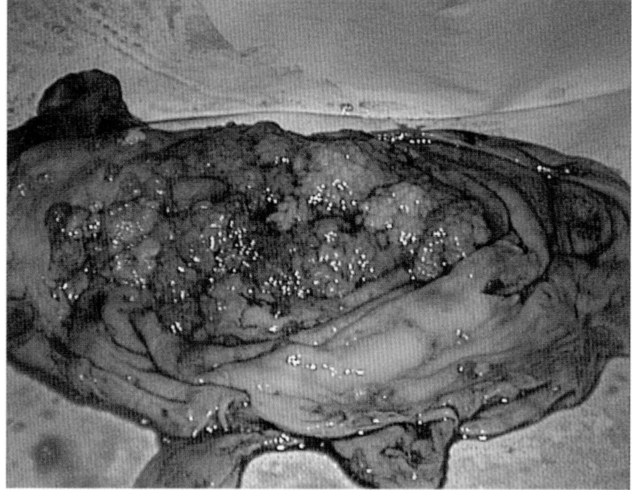

FIGURE 28.6 Intracystic vegetations were confirmed at macroscopy.

4. It is difficult to achieve an ovarian cystectomy without puncture or rupture particularly when the cyst is large (>8 cm); and this may be impossible when treating an early ovarian cancer. Indeed if a tumor is malignant, it invades the cleavage plane and cannot be separated from the surrounding ovarian tissue without rupture. In these cases cystectomy without rupture is a dream, not a reality. The rupture induced by a traditional technique by laparotomy may be worse than a careful laparoscopic puncture.
5. Laparoscopic cystectomy is much easier and faster after a puncture than when trying to remove the cyst intact.

V. THE TECHNIQUE OF LAPAROSCOPY

A. To Enter the Abdomen

The initial steps of the laparoscopy have been described elsewhere.[38] However, a specific technique should be used to manage large adnexal cysts in order to avoid blind punctures with the Veress needle or with the umbilical trocar. To treat a cyst of more than 8 cm, pneumoperitoneum is created in the left hypochondrium with a Veress needle inserted perpendicular to the abdominal wall. In very large masses, up to 20 cm, the first trocar may be inserted above the umbilicus or with an open laparoscopy technique.

A very large mass is not a contraindication to the laparoscopic approach as long as a reliable preoperative endocystic examination has been obtained. As very large masses are often not well examined using ultrasound, we routinely use a second imaging technique, preferably an MRI, in these patients to confirm that the mass is entirely or almost entirely cystic.

If there are large solid contents inside the mass, the laparoscopic approach may be considered to inspect the upper abdomen. In contrast, large solid contents should be considered as an absolute contraindication for laparoscopic treatment, since *ovarian morcellation is always an unacceptable surgical mistake*.

B. The Ancillary Ports

Ancillary trocars should be inserted perpendicular to the abdominal wall. This is particularly important when treating an adnexal mass. Indeed if a cancer is diagnosed or missed during the laparoscopic procedure, a restaging procedure will be required. As trocar site metastases have been reported,[39] an excision of the trocar sites is recommended when performing a restaging. However, the information obtained from an excision, performed perpendicular to the abdominal wall, is reliable only if the trocars were inserted in the same way.

VI. THE TREATMENT OF THE CYST

A complete removal of the cyst wall should be achieved. Pathologic examination of the entire cyst wall is required to make a reliable pathologic diagnosis. An ablation of the cyst wall with laser or bipolar coagulation cannot be considered as a valid treatment, except in selected cases such as endometriomas in young infertile patients. However, a large biopsy should be performed before the ablation. *The key steps in the management of an ovarian mass are the diagnosis and the choice between adnexectomy and ovarian cystectomy.*

VII. THE LAPAROSCOPIC DIAGNOSIS [40]

First, a peritoneal fluid sample and/or peritoneal washings for cytological examination are aspirated from the posterior cul-de-sac, or from the paracolic gutters and the vesicouterine cul-de-sac, when the pouch of Douglas is obliterated by adhesions or filled by a large adnexal mass. Thereafter the cystic ovary, pelvic peritoneum, contralateral ovary, paracolic gutters, diaphragm, omentum, liver, and bowel are carefully inspected. The value of this inspection has been confirmed by Possover *et al.* who reported that metastases easily accessible to laparoscopic inspection were always present in patients with metastasis of the small bowel and of the mesentery.[41] If signs of malignancy such as ascites, peritoneal metastases, or extracystic ovarian vegetations are found, the mass should be treated as suspicious or malignant.

In the remaining cases an intracystic evaluation is required to rule out malignancy. Several techniques may be used to perform this essential step of the surgical diagnosis (Table 28.1). Adnexal masses are punctured only when assumed to be benign from the initial laparoscopic inspection and from the preoperative workup.

This is simple when managing adnexal masses nonsuspicious at ultrasound. In this group the incidence of malignancy is low, and the false negatives are explained by two situations:

1. A solid tumor is found on the surface of the cystic mass or beside the cystic lesion identified by ultrasound
2. Very small vegetations (less than 1mm in diameter) not visible at ultrasound are present inside the cyst and may be identified only at laparoscopy using an endocystic inspection with the magnification provided by the laparoscope.

The situation is more difficult when the adnexal mass was suspicious at ultrasound. Indeed most masses are benign (Table 28.2) and conservative treatment would be possible in most cases whereas a routine adnexectomy is unacceptable. From the results of ultrasound examinations performed preoperatively in our department (Table 28.2), we propose the following management of this sometimes difficult clinical situation.

Young patients (<40 years old) (Fig. 28.7)

The laparoscopic inspection allows a reliable diagnosis of:

1. Functional cysts which are identified using previously reported macroscopic signs (Table 28.3)
2. Endometriomas which are recognized from the ovarian adhesions and the peritoneal implants (Fig. 28.8)
3. Suspicious paraovarian cysts whose solid contents may be seen through the cyst wall.

Moreover teratomas may be diagnosed from the preoperative ultrasonographic examination, CT scan, or MRI.

In the remaining cases, which represent less than 10% of the patients aged less than 40 years, the management should be

TABLE 28.1 Techniques for Intracystic Examination

Preoperative
Abdominal ultrasound
Vaginal ultrasound
CT scan or MRI
Intraoperative
Laparoscopic inspection without puncture
Laparoscopic ultrasound
Ovarioscopy (a second endoscope is required)
Laparoscopic intracystic inspection (an incision is required)
Postoperative
Macroscopic pathologic examination

TABLE 28.2 Pathologic Diagnosis According to Age and the Ultrasonographic Appearance

Age	Nonsuspicious masses[a]				Suspicious or solid masses[b]			
	<40 n (%)	≥40–<50 n (%)	≥50 n (%)	Total n (%)	<40 n (%)	≥40–<50 n (%)	≥50 n (%)	Total n (%)
Functional	94 (22.5)	28 (15.9)	2 (2.0)	124 (17.9)	23 (11.7)	7 (10.8)	3 (4.8)	33 (10.2)
Serous	87 (20.9)	62 (35.2)	70 (70.7)	219 (31.6)	18 (9.2)	6 (9.2)	26 (41.9)	50 (15.5)
Paraovarian	53 (12.7)	17 (9.7)	10 (10.1)	80 (11.6)	3 (1.5)	2 (3.1)	1 (1.6)	6 (1.9)
Mucinous	53 (12.7)	19 (10.8)	9 (9.1)	81 (11.7)	9 (4.6)	5 (7.7)	8 (12.9)	22 (6.8)
Dermoid	20 (4.8)	0 (0.0)	2 (2.0)	22 (3.2)	103 (52.6)	16 (24.6)	9 (14.5)	128 (39.6)
Endométrioma	105 (25.2)	48 (27.3)	5 (5.1)	158 (22.8)	26 (13.3)	25 (38.5)	1 (1.6)	52 (16.1)
LMP	4 (1.0)	2 (1.1)	1 (1.0)	7 (1.0)	6 (3.1)	1 (1.5)	5 (8.1)	12 (3.7)
Cancer	1 (0.2)	0 (0.0)	0 (0.0)	1 (0.1)	8 (4.1)	3 (4.6)	9 (14.5)	20 (6.2)
Total	417	176	99	692	196	65	62	323

[a]Nonsuspicious masses means entirely cystic masses, entirely cystic masses with echogenic fluid, and cyst with one or several thin septae.
[b]Suspicious masses at ultrasound means thick septae, vegetations, and mixed tumors.

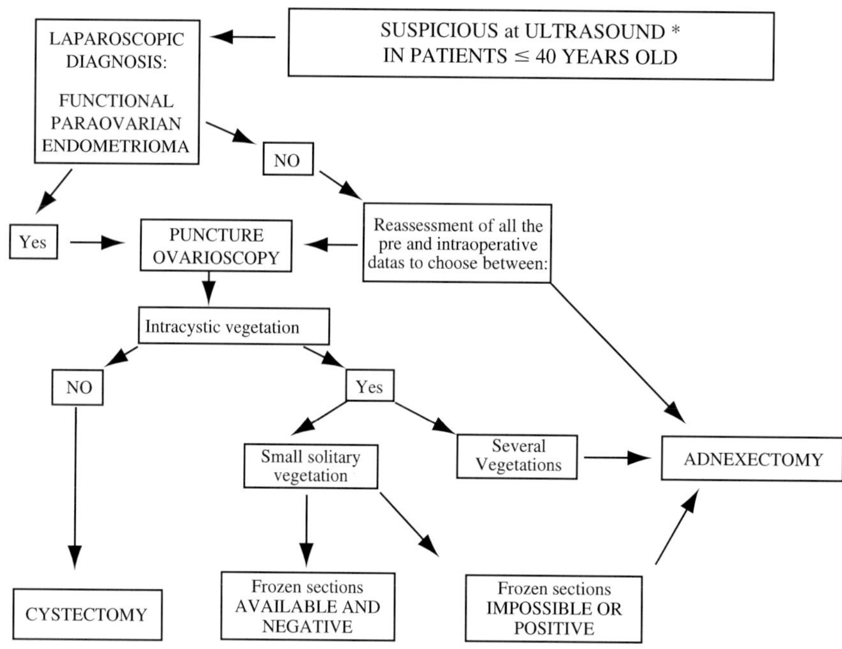

FIGURE 28.7 Management of masses suspicious at ultrasound in young patients.

TABLE 28.3 Laparoscopic Criteria to Distinguish Functional Cyst and of Benign Ovarian Neoplasm

	Benign neoplasm	Functional
Utero-ovarian ligament	Lengthened	Normal
Cyst wall	Thick	Thin
Cyst vessels	Comb-like from the hilum	Scanty, coral-like
Fluid	Clear, chocolate	Saffran yellow
Internal appearance	Smooth	Retinal-like aspect
Cystectomy	Possible	"Impossible"

adapted to each case:

1. If only one small intracystic papillary formation was found at ultrasound, endocystic examination with frozen section may allow a conservative treatment (Fig. 28.7)
2. In contrast, if there were numerous papillary formations, if the tumor was mixed or mainly solid, if numerous vessels with a low resistance index were found or if the tumor is very large, an adnexectomy without puncture is the reasonable treatment.

Puncture is not a routine, it should be discussed cautiously as an essential step of the management with potential but unknown prognosis consequences which cannot justify a routine adnexectomy.

In patients aged 40–50 years, laparoscopy remains an important diagnostic tool given the frequency of functional and paraovarian cysts and of endometriomas (Table 28.2), but difficult situations should be managed by adnexectomy.

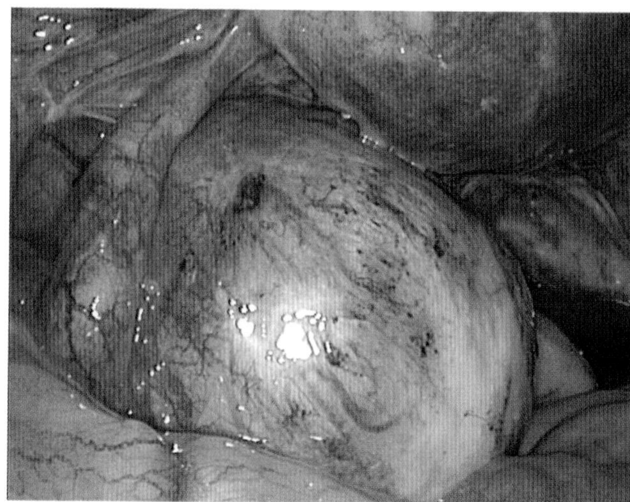

FIGURE 28.8 A typical ovarian endometrioma. Peritoneal lesions are associated. Brown deposits are visible of the surface of the cyst. The ovarian vessels are stretched to the midline as the ovary is fixed to the broad ligament by dense adhesions, which explains this appearance of the vessels.

In postmenopausal patients and patients over 50 years old, where the incidence of malignant tumors is high (22.6%), laparoscopic diagnosis is helpful to inspect the diaphragm and the upper abdomen. All benign masses are treated by bilateral adnexectomy. As the incidence of malignancy is high, frozen sections should be available and an immediate staging laparotomy should be possible when managing this group of patients.

VIII. LAPAROSCOPIC PUNCTURE: THE TECHNIQUE

Care should be taken to minimize spillage when puncturing a cyst. Briefly, the adnexa is grasped and stabilized with an atraumatic forceps placed on the utero-ovarian ligament. The puncture should be performed perpendicular to the ovarian surface and, as discussed in Section IX, it should be located on the antimesenteric border of the ovary. Small cysts are aspirated with a needle connected to a 20- or 50-ml syringe. Cysts of more than 5 cm are punctured with a 5 mm conical trocar and emptied with an aspiration lavage device 5 mm in diameter. A 5-mm conical trocar is used for the following reasons:

1. The penetration of cone-shaped instruments depends on the perforating effect of the instrument and on the elasticity of the cyst wall, so that the puncture is more watertight than when performed with a cutting instrument
2. A 5-mm reusable conical trocar can be inserted through a 5.5-mm disposable trocar, so no trocar changes are necessary after the puncture (Fig. 28.9)
3. A large aspirating device is used for the aspiration of the cyst contents.

As a puncture performed with the currently available instruments cannot be completely watertight; other devices are currently being developed to decrease the risks associated with a puncture. The first possibility is to introduce a large bag in the abdomen, to put the bag in the pelvis, and the adnexa in the bag, so that the cyst fluid will be collected in the bag if any leakage occurs. This technique is not effective when managing very large adnexal masses or in patients with significant pelvic adhesions.

IX. INSPECTION OF THE CYST FLUID AND INTRACYSTIC EXAMINATION

The cyst fluid is examined macroscopically and sent for cytological examination (Fig. 28.10). The cyst and the pelvic cavity are then washed many times with small volumes of fluid to avoid contamination of the upper abdomen. Then the cyst is opened with scissors and the internal cyst wall carefully inspected. If signs of malignancy are found, the mass should be diagnosed and managed as suspicious or malignant.

A. Other Situations Should be Discussed

Very large cysts (>10 cm) are aspirated, inserting the second puncture trocar high enough to allow visual control of the puncture site.

In most cases, *endometriomas* are fixed to the broad ligament by adhesions located close to the ovarian hilum (Fig. 28.8). As these adhesions generally involve the endometrioma itself, the cyst will often be ruptured while freeing the ovary. The puncture should not be performed before ovariolysis. Indeed a puncture performed on the posterior surface of the ovary is an unnecessary trauma as an incision located on the anterior surface is almost always required to treat the cyst. In endometriomas, ovariolysis should be the first step and a puncture is performed only when the cyst has not been ruptured.

In *multilocular mucinous cyst* with less than 3 mm septae, puncture is often difficult, since several punctures are necessary to empty the mass. When there are more than 3 different cystic cavities, conservative treatment is rarely possible (see below) and probably involves a high risk of early recurrence as small mucinous cysts may be missed around the main ones.

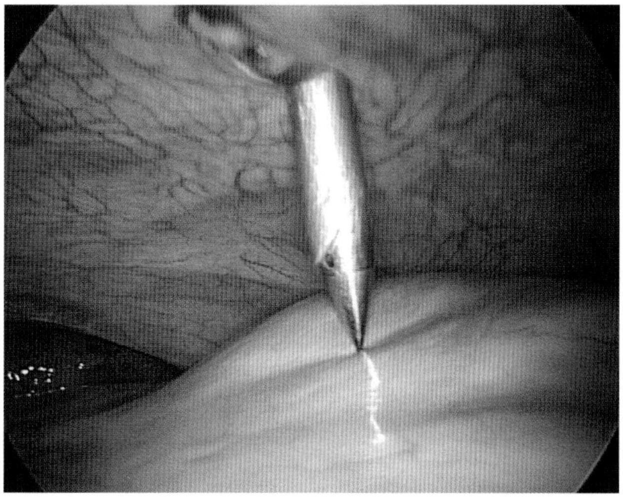

FIGURE 28.9 A puncture using a 5-mm conical trocar inserted perpendicular to the cyst surface.

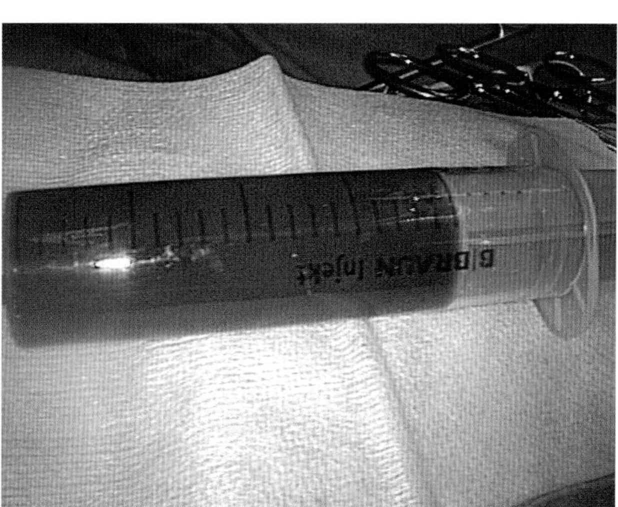

FIGURE 28.10 An example of turbid fluid found in a low malignant potential tumor, the color is close to that found in an endometrioma.

Therefore in large multilocular cystic masses, adnexectomy should be discussed with the patient before surgery.

Concerning *ovarian teratoma*, we unfortunately confirmed that the laparoscopic puncture and or rupture of a teratoma may induce a granulomatous peritonitis. This complication is uncommon (1.1%; 2 cases out of 178 teratomas punctured in our experience).[42] Moreover, from the data collected at incidental and or routine second-look laparoscopy we found that adhesion formation is not uncommon after the laparoscopic treatment of ovarian teratoma. In contrast, adhesion formation appeared uncommon after the laparoscopic treatment of other types of benign ovarian neoplasm (Table 28.4), suggesting that the cyst contents rather than the laparoscopic procedure explained postoperative adhesion *de novo* formation. Therefore the spillage of teratoma content should be avoided whenever possible. An accurate preoperative diagnosis is essential to help the surgical management. Although many ovarian teratomas are diagnosed by ultrasonographic examination, it may be worth confirming the diagnosis with a second imaging technique to identify the fatty tissue inside the cyst. Indeed if fatty tissue is found, the diagnosis of teratoma is probable, malignancy is unlikely, and cystectomy without puncture can be performed. Both CT scan and MRI with fat suppression sequences can be used to identify the fatty tissue.

TABLE 28.4 Adhesions after Laparoscopic Cystectomy: 20 Patients, 22 Treated Adnexa, 17 Contralateral Adnexa

Group	n	Diameter (mm)	Adhesion score[a]
All	22	70.4±37 (30–180)	2.7±5.9 (0–24)
IPC[b]	15	68.7±42 (30–180)	2.4±6.1 (0–24)
EAC[c]	7	74.3±27 (50–120)	3.3±5.9 (0–16)
Teratomas	13	68.4±33 (30–140)	4.6±7.2 (0–24)
Other pathologic Dg[d]	9	73.3±45 (30–180)	0.0±0.0
Contralateral Ad[e]	17	—	0.0±0.0

[a]This adhesion score at second-look laparoscopy was calculated using the AFS classification.
[b]Intraperitoneal cystectomy.
[c]Cystectomy by minilaparotomy.
[d]Other pathologic diagnoses.
[e]Contralateral adnexa.

On the other hand a cystectomy without rupture cannot be achieved in large masses of more than 8 cm, in the 10-cm diameter pelvic cavity. Therefore teratomas of more than 8 cm are emptied with a 10-mm aspiration device. A very large teratoma is not a contraindication for conservative treatment. If a laparotomy seems reasonable to preserve the ovary, then a laparotomy should be performed (Fig. 28.11).

X. TREATMENT TECHNIQUES

A. Benign Ovarian Neoplasms

After puncture, the pressure in the ovary decreases and the cyst wall and the remaining ovarian stroma, which present different degrees of elasticity, retract differently and open the cleavage plane spontaneously (Figs. 28.12–28.16). So careful inspection of the ovarian incision will allow identification

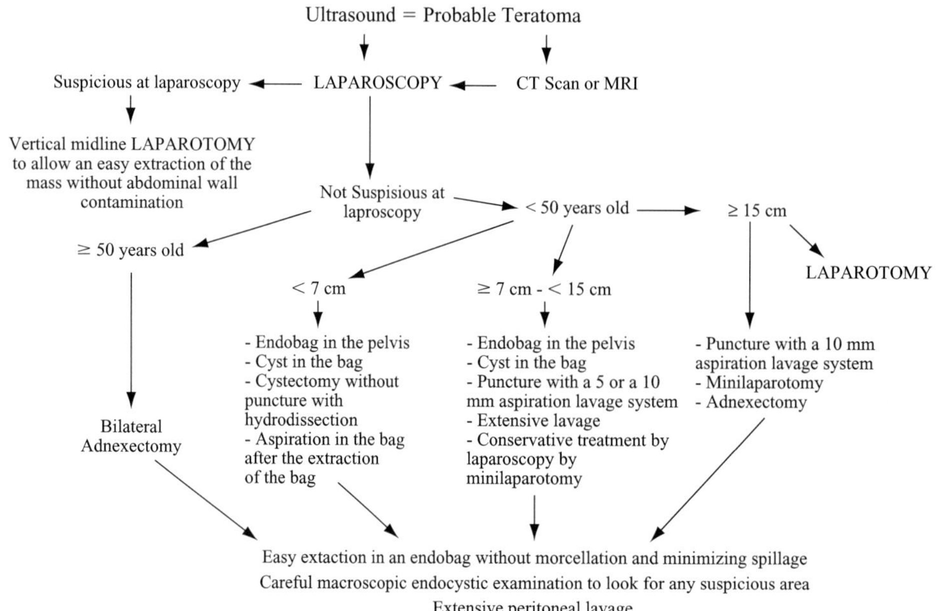

FIGURE 28.11 Management of teratomas.

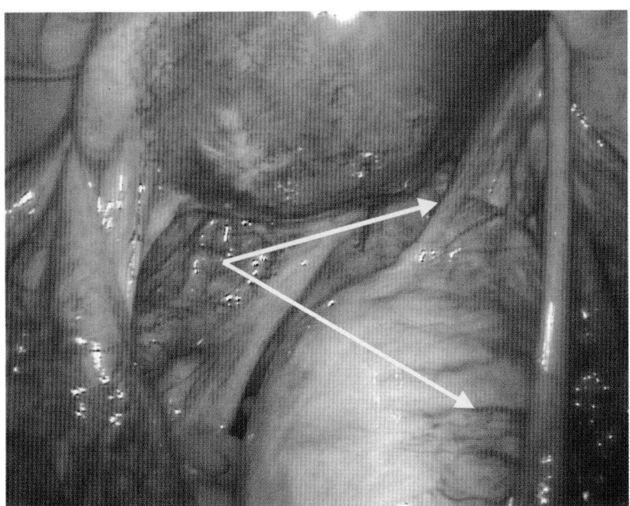

FIGURE 28.12 An example of a benign serous cystadenoma. Note the lengthened utero-ovarian ligament and the vessels of the hilum.

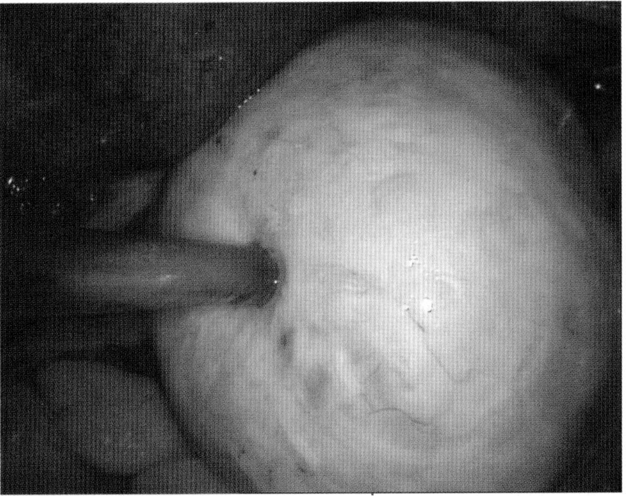

FIGURE 28.13 The cyst is puctured with a 5-mm needle.

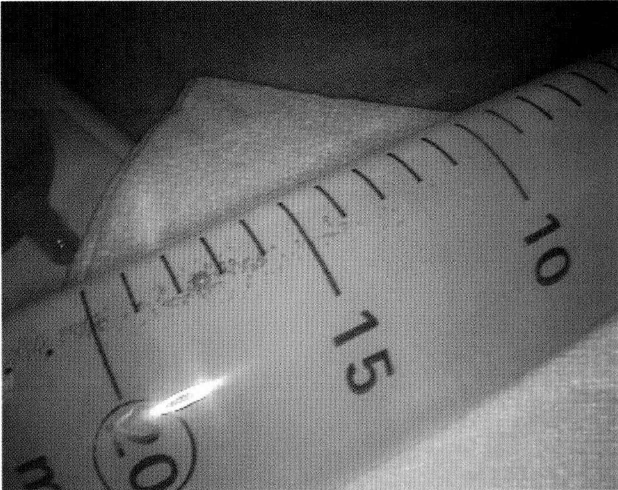

FIGURE 28.14 The fluid is inspected, i.e., a typical serous fluid.

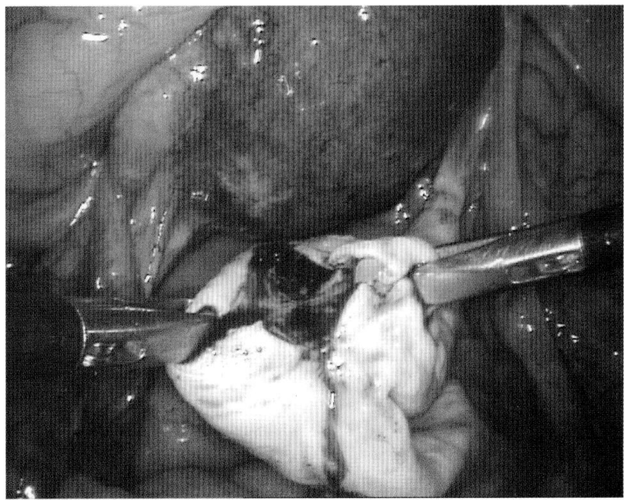

FIGURE 28.15 The cyst is opened on the antimesenteric border of the ovary.

of this plane. To achieve a laparoscopic ovarian cystectomy effective grasping forceps are required. Three effective grasping forceps should be available to treat large cysts. This procedure is simple. However, a strict technique and some rules are required to make it reliable to ensure that the cyst wall is entirely removed without any tearing.

The procedure should be performed under permanent visual control, therefore the cleavage plane should always be exposed implying that:

1. When pulling forceps in opposite directions one should use short and slow movements and move the forceps on the cyst wall and on the remaining ovarian tissue often enough to obtain a perfect exposure.
2. Hemostasis should be perfomed during the dissection, first because bleeding may obscure the cleavage plane and second because the hemostasis is often more difficult at the end of the procedure when the ovarian tissue is retracted.

To avoid ovarian damage, one should follow the "best" cleavage plane. This plane is identified when the outside surface of the cyst wall is white. If there is red tissue on the cyst wall, however, one is probably removing some healthy ovarian tissue (Figs. 28.17 and 28.18).

B. Paraovarian Cysts

As the cyst wall is thin and covered only by the peritoneum, the cyst fluid can be seen through the cyst wall so that the cyst appears blue. If there are abnormal intracystic

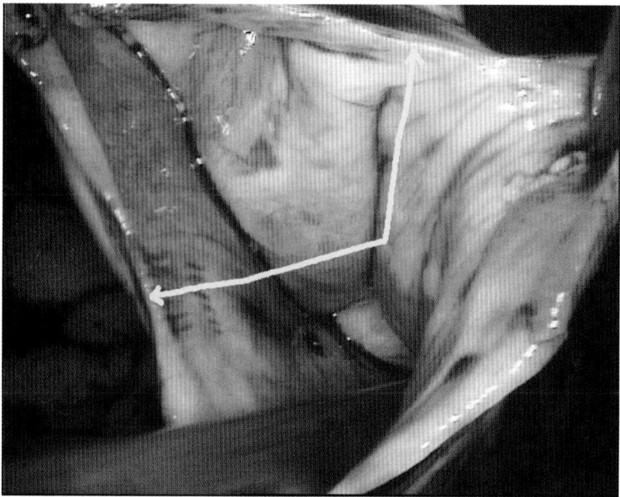

FIGURE 28.16 The endocystic examination is performed. The cleavage plane can be seen on the borders of the incision.

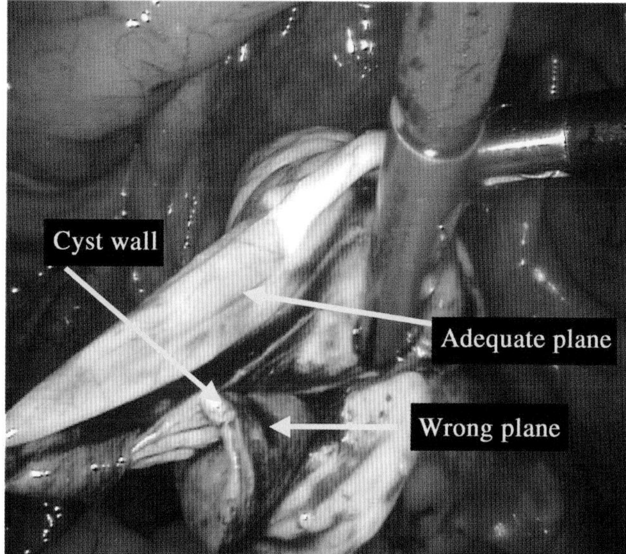

FIGURE 28.17 The dissection is performed with grasping forceps, the plane is correct in the upper part of the dissection, the cyst wall is white, the plane is too far from the cyst in the lower part as the cyst surface is pink.

areas (vegetations), the cyst wall is thicker and appears white, so that intracystic evaluation can often be achieved without puncture.

When treating these cysts, it is important to open the peritoneum and to identify the cleavage plane before the puncture. For small cysts, if the puncture is performed first, it may be difficult to find the cyst in the retroperitoneal space. Paraovarian cysts may often be removed and treated without puncture. However, large ones should be punctured after identification of the plane.

C. Endometriomas

Small ovarian endometriomas of less than 3 cm should be treated with a CO_2 laser or with bipolar coagulation, it is generally not possible to identify a cleavage plane in these small cysts.

The treatment of larger endometriomas is controversial. In our department we perform a cystectomy. In IVF, we obtained satisfactory pregnancy rates and number of ovocytes in most cases, except in patients who underwent several treatments for ovarian endometriomas. So the impaired ovarian function sometimes reported after ovarian cystectomy may be the consequence of the damage induced by the disease rather than the consequence of the surgical procedure. In the ovarian cortex biopsied around an endometrioma, Maneschi *et al.* found a lower number of follicles and of vessels than in the ovarian cortex biopsied around teratoma.[43]

The dissection of an ovarian endometrioma is often difficult and includes several steps. Along the rupture induced by the adhesiolysis, the cleavage plane is difficult to identify just as if the cyst itself was stuck on the broad ligament. To identify the plane it is necessary to enlarge the incision. Thereafter, the initial steps of the dissection are easy. When about one-third

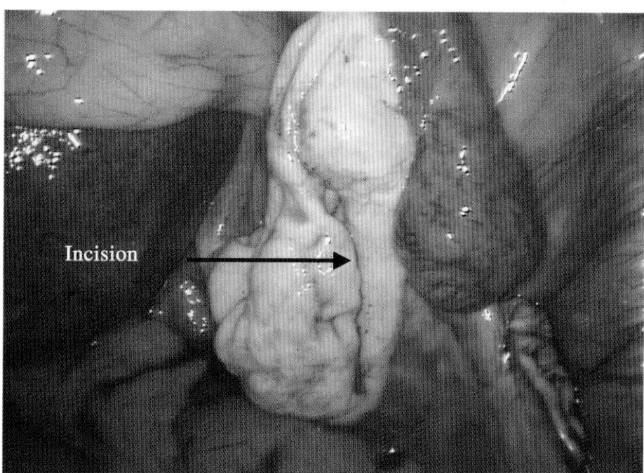

FIGURE 28.18 A final view, the incision was adequate on the antimesenteric border of the ovary, so that the shape of the ovary is spontaneously approximated at the end of the procedure, no suture will be used.

to one-half of the endometrioma has been dissected, other difficulties are encountered. Red fibrotic tissue is seen on the surface of the cyst, meaning that some ovarian tissue is being removed. If the dissection is continued in this plane bleeding and possibly damage to the ovarian vessels will occur. To avoid this, one should stay close to the cyst wall. The procedure is guided by the color of the cyst wall; when it is white, the plane is correct, when it is red, the plane is wrong, and the plane should be identified using scissors and bipolar coagulation (Figs 28.19 and 28.20).

Adhesions are the main problem in the treatment of ovarian endometriomas; we showed previously that postoperative

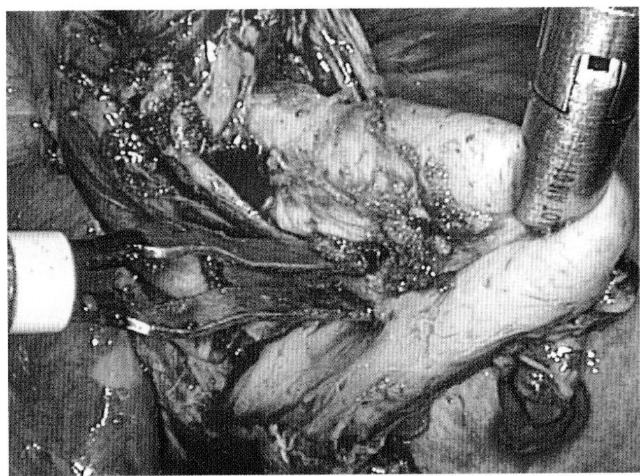

FIGURE 28.19 Red fibers visible on the surface of the endometrioma are coagulated to identify the correct cleavage plane.

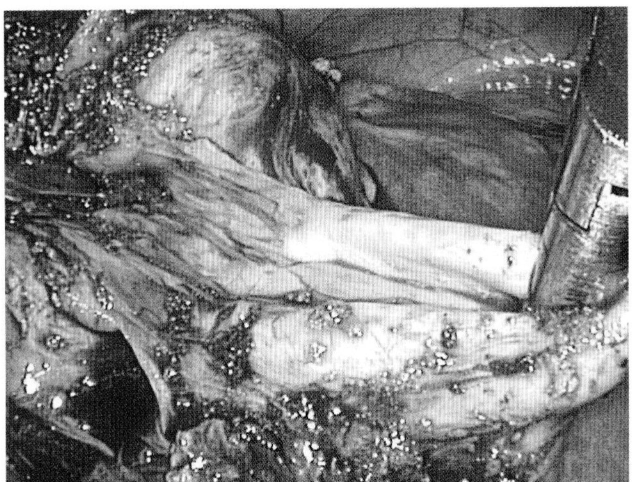

FIGURE 28.20 After the section of these fibers, the correct plane is developed pulling on both forceps.

TABLE 28.5 Adhesions after the Laparoscopic Treatment of Large Endometrioma

		Adnexal adhesion score		
Group	**n**	**Lap. treat**	**Second-look**	**p**
All Cases	53	12.7±10.8	10.4±10	>0.1
Stage III	15	6.1±5.9	5.8±5.6	>0.7
Stage IV	38	15.2±11.3	12.1±10.8	>0.1
Diameter <6 cm	32	14.9±11.3	11.3±10.9	>0.07
Diameter ≥6 cm	21	9.2±9.3	8.9±8.6	>0.8
Unilateral	31	12.6±11.4	9.4±9.7	>0.1
Bilateral	22	12.7±10.2	11.8±10.5	>0.4
Treated adnexa				
Ovarian adhesion score ≤4	19	3±2.4	6.5±7.4	>0.1
Ovarian adhesion score ≥8	34	18.1±9.9	12.5±10.7	<0.01
Contralateral adnexa				
All cases	21	3.9±8.6	2.6±4.2	>0.6
Adnexal adhesion score ≤4	17	0.5±1.3	1.4±2.7	>0.08

TABLE 28.6 Mean Number of Ovocytes Obtained During IVF Cycles

Indication	**n cases**	**n Ovocytes**
Tubal infertility	253	8.43
Endometriosis		
Without previous endometrioma	83	8.22
After the treatment of an endometrioma	67	8.49
After the treatment of an endometrioma by cystectomy	34	7.96
N.S.		

adhesion formation is uncommon but that adhesion reformation occurs in more than 90% of the adnexae (Table 28.5).[44] The number of ovocytes was not lower after the laparoscopic treatment of an ovarian endometrioma (Table 28.6).

D. Teratomas

In this group, other techniques of laparoscopic cystectomy may be used.

"Transparietal cystectomy" is a cystectomy performed by minilaparotomy after a laparoscopic diagnosis. In our group, this technique was used for all the cysts before 1985. Today it is used only for the treatment of large teratomas. After puncture and drainage of the cyst with a 5- and/or 10-mm aspirating device, a 3 cm low transverse incision is performed. The fascia and the muscles are opened using a classical surgical technique. Then the cyst and the ovary are grasped through the peritoneum which is incised while pulling the ovary against the abdominal wall, thus facilitating the extraction of the ovary. Thereafter the drainage of the cyst is finished using the 3-cm incision and the ovary is extracted through the abdominal wall. The cystectomy is performed using a classic surgical technique. The ovary is released in the peritoneal cavity without any suture and the abdominal wall is closed.

As protection of the abdominal wall is difficult or impossible, this technique should not be used in the treatment of suspicious masses.

E. Cystectomy without Puncture (Fig. 28.21)

The ovary is grasped on the antimesenteric surface with an atraumatic forceps. A small superficial incision of the ovarian cortex is performed with scissors. Then aquadissection is used through this small incision. Thereafter the incision is enlarged carefully. The plane is identified with atraumatic grasping forceps or with scissors. Most cases of rupture occur while enlarging the incision even though the cleavage plane has already been identified. To avoid rupture and or to minimize its consequences, our suggestions are

1. To perform the dissection without grasping the cyst and without pushing it
2. To move the instruments away from the cyst
3. To put the cyst in a large bag before dissection
4. To be able to aspirate immediately and effectively the cyst contents

In our department this procedure is successful in about 50% of the cases,[42] it is not used for cysts of more than 7 cm in diameter (Fig. 28.11).

XI. LAPAROSCOPIC ADNEXECTOMY

This procedure is simple when the enlarged ovary has stretched the adnexal ligaments making hemostasis of the adnexal vessels both easy and safe as the distance between the infundibulopelvic ligament and the ureter is increased.

In contrast adnexectomy and or oophorectomy may be very difficult when the ovary is fixed to the broad ligament by dense adhesions. In such cases an excision of the posterior leaf of the broad ligament is required to ensure a complete excision of the ovarian tissue and to avoid both the risks of recurrences and of ovarian remnant syndrome (Figs. 28.22 and 28.23). To achieve that, the ureter should be identified at the pelvic brim and dissected up to the uterine vessels. When the ovary is stuck to the broad ligament, identification of the ureter on the pelvic brim does not imply that the entire ovary may be safely excised without further ureteral dissection. Indeed, complete dissection of the ureter is required. This dissection is particularly important and difficult in patients with endometriosis, as endometriosis frequently invades the retroperitoneal space and the ureter may be involved in the fibrosis induced by the implants.

Hemostasis of the adnexal vessels can be achieved either with bipolar coagulation or with suturing techniques according to the surgeon's preferences. Although much more expensive, the stapling devices present no advantages. In our department, bipolar coagulation is used in more than 95% of

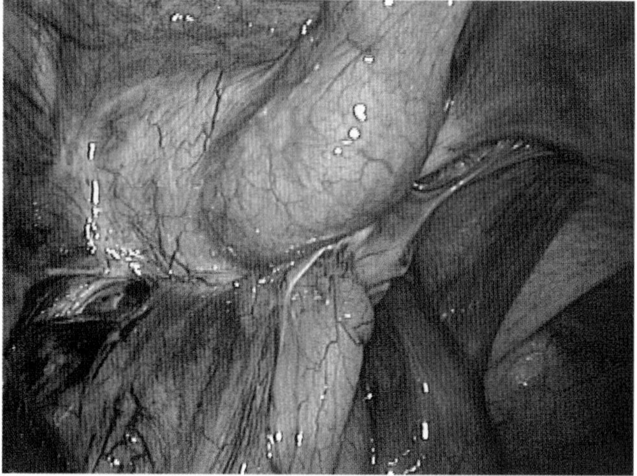

FIGURE 28.22 A suspicious adnexal mass with dense adhesions to the broad ligament. To achieve an adnexectomy, the ureter should be dissected and the peritoneum of the broad ligament excised.

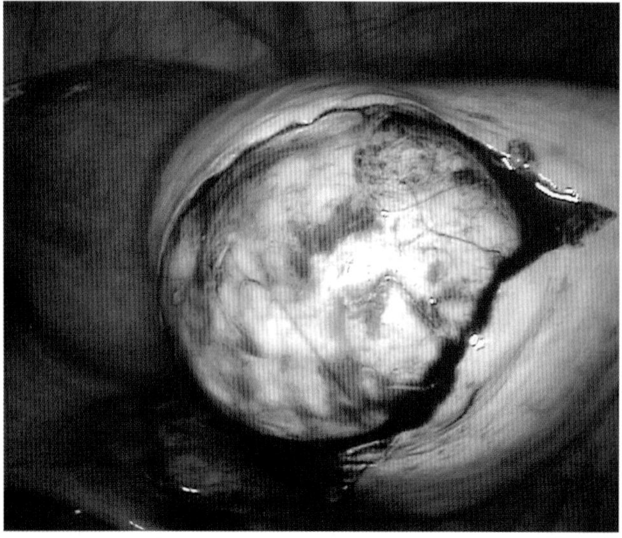

FIGURE 28.21 An example of cystectomy without puncture, a small teratoma can be seen.

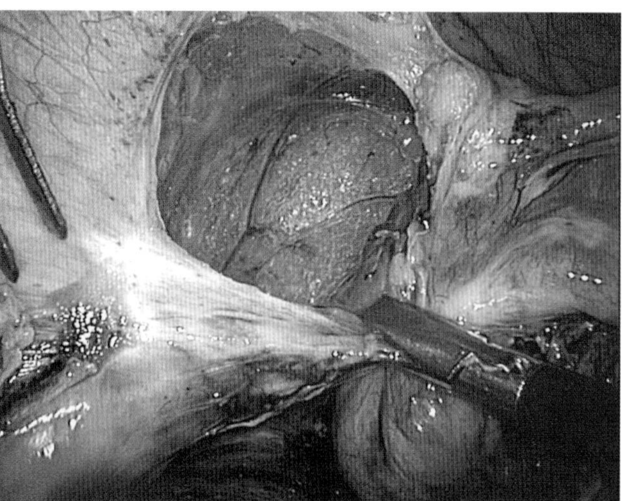

FIGURE 28.23 The retroperitoneal space is opened to allow an easy identification of the ureter and a safe excision of the peritoneum of the broad ligament.

the cases. This technique is safe as no postoperative bleeding has been observed over the last 5 years. To make hemostasis of the infundibulopelvic ligament easier, it is important to open the peritoneum between the ovarian vessels and the round ligament. In this way, the ovarian vessels can be stretched much more effectively than when covered by the peritoneum. Moreover, the coagulation is more effective as it is applied on the ovarian vessels itself and not on the peritoneum which would retract, thus decreasing the effects of the electric current on the vessels.

XII. EXTRACTION OF THE CYST WALL AND/OR OF THE MASS

We reported one case of abdominal wall endometriosis which occurred on a trocar site after the laparoscopic treatment of an active endometrioma.[40] As this complication is uncommon, we assumed that this was induced by a part of the cyst wall left in the abdominal wall while extracting it. This complication which occurred when endobags were not available, showed that the abdominal wall should always be protected when extracting an adnexal mass.

Several techniques can be used. Currently, we use an endobag in most cases. An endobag (Fig. 28.24) should be

1. Large enough to allow the extraction of masses of 8 cm and more, but smaller bags should be available to allow the extraction of small cysts without enlarging the skin incision
2. Easy to open in the abdomen, and it should remain spontaneously open in the peritoneum
3. Long enough to allow an easy extraction of the bag in obese patients
4. Solid enough to prevent rupture when the surgeon is pulling through the abdominal wall
5. Transparent to allow visual control of the punctures performed in the bag. We used endobags designed by Storz.

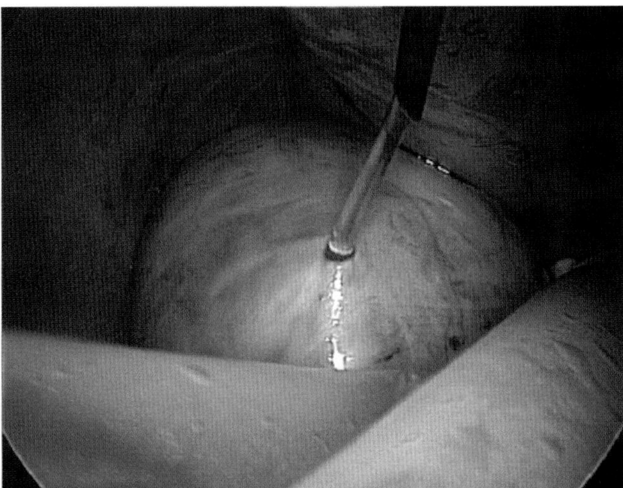

FIGURE 28.24 A mucinous cyst in a large endobag adequate for an easy extraction.

The bag is extracted either through a 10-mm port inserted in an appendectomy scar or through the umbilical incision.

An endobag is required even if the mass is extracted through the vagina. Large masses should be punctured or drained to be extracted. We puncture the mass through the abdominal wall after the extraction of the neck of the bag. A puncture performed in a bag still in the peritoneal cavity increases the risk of spillage. However, when puncturing through the abdominal wall, visual control is required to ensure that the puncture is performed inside the bag and not through it. This is easy in thin patients with a 10-mm incision whereas a larger incision is required in obese patients. It is sometimes necessary to put a 10-mm trocar in the bag to identify the surface of the cyst before the puncture.

One of the port sites or the posterior fornix may be used for extraction of the bag. The colpotomy should be performed by laparoscopy using the instrument designed by the Lausanne group, which allows the posterior fornix to be opened and the bag grasped without losing the pneumoperitoneum.[45]

When an adnexectomy is associated with a hysterectomy, the adnexectomy is performed first. The mass is placed in a bag which is closed and placed in a paracolic gutter. Extraction takes place after the hysterectomy.

XIII. SHOULD WE SUTURE OR NOT?

Our answers to this question are based on the following ideas:

1. Ovarian nonclosure is a valuable technique, as shown by several experimental studies. In rabbit models nonclosure of an ovarian surgical incision is less adhesiogenic than a microsurgical closure.[46, 47]
2. The shape of the ovary needs to be approximated to allow satisfactory healing and to prevent postoperative adhesion. In experimental studies, the ovaries were bivalved so that the shape of the ovary was spontaneously approximated at the end of the procedure.
3. Adhesion formation is increased at the surface of the ovary, when compared to the peritoneum.[48]
4. Ischemia reduces plasminogen activator concentration and increases adhesion formation, so if sutures are used, they should be placed inside the ovary, not on the ovarian surface.

From these results and our experience, some rules may be proposed to improve laparoscopic cystectomy. As in these experimental models, the ovarian puncture and the ovarian incision should be peformed on the antimesenteric surface of the ovary, as far away as possible from the fimbria, so that the edges of the incision will be grossly approximated when the ovary falls back in the posterior cul-de-sac (Fig. 28.18). The puncture site should be included in the ovarian incision. The cystectomy should be performed using only one incision, which should be large enough to avoid any additional tear of the ovarian cortex. Meticulous hemostasis should be achieved. Finally, the shape of the ovary may be approximated using a minimal resection of the remaining ovarian tissue or a superficial coagulation of the ovarian stroma to induce an inversion of the ovary, just as coagulation of the serosa is used to obtain eversion of the distal part of the tube. When the incision is adequate, ovarian sutures are not necessary, but when the shape of the ovary is not spontaneously approximated at the end of the procedure, one or two intraovarian sutures should be used to facilitate the ovarian healing.

XIV. LIMITS OF LAPAROSCOPY

The following ideas should be kept in mind while deciding the surgical management.

1. The treatment of an ovarian tumor should be complete and immediate.
2. At laparoscopy, one cannot distinguish benign vegetations from malignant ones.
3. When treating macroscopically suspicous adnexal masses by laparoscopy one accepts to treat ovarian cancers and low malignant tumors by laparoscopy.[2]
4. Frozen sections should not be used to decide the treatment of the ovary or to choose between laparoscopy and laparotomy. When taking a biopsy for frozen sections, the surgeon is doing the most difficult part of the diagnosis. Most false-negatives of frozen sections are explained by inadequate biopsies.[49, 50] The only exception to this rule is a young patient with a small and solitary vegetation. In this situation, a biopsy is reliable as there is only one suspicious area and the incidence of malignancy is low, below 10%.[51]
5. In contrast, frozen sections are required to decide staging procedures and the treatment of the contralateral adnexa. Whenever possible this treatment should be performed during the same anesthesia, as 20% of the patients may refuse a restaging.[21]
6. Morcellation of an ovarian tumor is always an unacceptable surgical mistake.
7. Most adnexal masses suspicious at ultrasound are benign even in postmenopausal patients (Table 28.2). Despite the progresses of ultrasound, recent external validations of the best models described to distinguish the benign and the malignant adnexal mass clearly showed that the diagnostic performance of these models are never as good as reported in the initial publication.[52, 53] When the sensitivity is around 0.90, the specificity varied between 0.45 and 0.60. So that if the laparoscopic approach is reserved for nonsuspicious masses, many patients would undergo unnecessary vertical midline laparotomies.
8. A reliable surgical diagnosis is required to decide the treatment of adnexal masses suspicious at ultrasound and to avoid transversal laparotomies for ovarian cancer.
9. There are no long-term follow-up data after the laparoscopic treatment of ovarian cancer.

We propose a simple scheme for management.

1. Adnexal masses suspicious at ultrasound should be surgically diagnosed by laparoscopy.
2. Adnexal masses suspicious at surgery should be treated by laparotomy.
3. At laparotomy suspicious masses should be treated by adnexectomy and then managed according to the results of frozen sections. As already discussed above, young patients with a solitary vegetation are the only exception to this rule.
4. High-risk patients such as postmenopausal patients with adnexal masses suspicious at ultrasound should be managed in oncology departments.

The clinical consequences of these simple rules are summarized in Table 28.7. The theoretical incidences of laparotomy and of adnexectomy were calculated using data obtained in our department. The same methods may be used to evaluate the consequences of this management in each department.

TABLE 28.7a Calculated Incidence of Laparotomy: Based on the Data from Patients Treated in our Department between 1992 and 1994

Data used to calculate the theoretical incidence of laparotomy	**Total**
Total number of patients	516
n Cancer and borderline tumors	28
n Benign masses suspicious at surgery	59
Including n masses >6 cm	22
Including n masses >6 cm and/or with external vegetations	36
n Benign masses nonsuspicious at surgery	429
n Laparotomies for technical difficulties	9
Results: n and rate of laparotomy,[a] if it was indicated for all benign masses suspicious at surgery	97 (18.8%)
Benign masses suspicious at surgery >6 cm	60 (11.6%)
Benign masses suspicious at surgery >6 cm and/or with external vegetations	55 (14.3%)

[a]This result includes all the malignant tumors (cancer, borderline) and all the laparotomies for technical reasons.

TABLE 28.7b Calculated Incidence of Adnexectomy among Benign Masses in Patients <40 Years Old: Based on the Data from the Patients Treated in our Department between 1992 and 1994

Data used to calculate the theoretical incidence of adnexectomy	Total
Total number of patients	248
n Benign masses suspicious at surgery	24
Laparotomy in nonsuspicious masses	3
Adnexectomy for technical problem in nonsuspicious masses	10
Results: n and rate of adnexectomy,[a] if it was indicated for all benign masses suspicious at surgery	37 (14.9%)
Incidence in the department between 1992 and 1994 in the same group of patients	24 (9.6%)

[a]This result includes all the malignant tumors (cancer, borderline) and all the laparotomies for technical reasons.

TABLE 28.8a Treatment According to the Pathologic Diagnosis in Patients <40 Years Old, in Nonsuspicious Masses <8 cm

Pathology	n	Laparotomy (n%)	Adnexectomy (n%)	Cystectomy (n%)
Functional	83	1 (1.2)	5 (6.0)	77 (92.8)
Serous	47	0	6 (12.7)	41 (87.3)
Paraovarian	28	0	0	28 (100.0)
Mucinous	24	0	1 (4.2)	23 (95.8)
Teratoma	63	1 (1.6)	2 (3.2)	60 (95.2)
Endometrioma	158	3 (1.9)	5 (3.1)	150 (94.9)
Other	9	0	0	9 (100)
Total	412	5 (1.2)	19 (4.6)	388 (94.2)

TABLE 28.8b Treatment According to the Pathologic Diagnosis in Patients <40 years old, in Nonsuspicious Masses >8 cm

Pathology	n	Laparotomy (n%)	Adnexectomy (n%)	Cystectomy (n%)
Functional	7	0	0	7 (100.0)
Serous	6	1	1	4 (66.6)
Paraovarian	8	0	0	8 (100.0)
Mucinous	18	0	6	12 (66.6)
Teratoma	26	1	3	22 (84.6)
Endometrioma	15	0	1	14 (93.3)
Others	2	0	0	2
Total	82	2 (2.4)	11 (13.4)	69 (84.1)

XV. PLEA AGAINST OOPHORECTOMY

It can be seen from Table 28.8 that whatever the pathologic diagnosis and the diameter, most patients can be treated conservatively. A diameter >10 cm should not be an indication for oophorectomy. Conservative surgery has always been the main objective of the pioneers of laparoscopic ovarian surgery.

References

1. Canis, M., Mage, G., Wattiez, A. *et al.* (1993). Tumor implantation after laparoscopy. *In* "Proceedings of the Twentieth Annual Meeting of the American Association of Gynecologic Laparoscopist, Las Vegas, Nevada, November 13–17 1991,"(R. B. Hunt, ed.), pp. 41–45. The association of Gynecologic Haparoscopists.
2. Canis, M., Pouly, J. L., Wattiez, A., Mage, G., Manhes, H., and Bruhat, M. A. (1997). Laparoscopic management of adnexal masses suspicious at ultrasound. *Obstet. Gynecol.* 89, 679–683.
3. Van Dam, P. A., DeCloedt, J., Tjalma, W. A. A., Buytaert, P., Becquart, D., and Vergote, I. B. (1999). Trocar implantation metastasis after laparoscopy in patients with advanced ovarian cancer. *Am. J. Obstet. Gynecol.* 181, 536–541.
4. Leminen, A., and Lehtovirta, P. (1999). Spread of ovarian cancer after laparoscopic surgery: Report of eight cases. *Gynecol. Oncol.* 75, 387–390.
5. Maiman, M., Seltzer, V., and Boyce, J. (1991). Laparoscopic excision of ovarian neoplasms subsequently found to be malignant. *Obstet. Gynecol.* 77, 563–565.
6. Blanc, B., Boubli, L., D'Ercole, C., and Nicoloso, E. (1994). Laparoscopic management of malignant ovarian cysts: A 78-case national survey part 1: Preoperative and laparoscopic evaluation. *Eur. J. Obstet. Gynecol. Reprod. Biol.* 56, 177–180.
7. Blanc, B., D'Ercole, C., Nicoloso, E., and Boubli, L. (1994). Laparoscopic management of malignant ovarian cysts: A 78-case national survey part 2: Follow up and final treatment. *Eur. J. Obstet. Gynecol. Reprod. Biol.* 61, 147–150.
8. Kinderman, G., Maassen, V., and Kuhn, W. (1995). Laparoscopic management of ovarian malignomas. *Geburtshilfe Frauenheilkd* 55, 687–694.
9. Wenzl, R., Lehner, R., Husslein, P., and Sevelda, P. (1996). Laparoscopic survey in cases of ovarian malignancies: An Austria-wide survey. *Gynecol. Oncol.* 63, 57–61.
10. Young, R. C., Decker, D. G., Wharton, J. T., Piver, M. S., Sindelar, W. F., Edwards, B. K., and Smith, J. P. (1983). Staging laparotomy in early ovarian cancer. *JAMA* 250, 3072–3076.
11. Soper, J. T., Johnson, P., Johnson, V., Berchuk, A., and Clarke-Pearson, D. L. (1992). Comprehensive restaging laparotomy in women with apparent early ovarian carcinoma. *Obstet. Gynecol.* 80, 949–953.
12. Stier, E. A., Barakat, R. B., Curtin, J. P., Brown, C. L., Jones, W. B., and Hoskins, W. J. (1996). Laparotomy to complete staging of presumed early ovarian cancer. *Obstet. Gynecol.* 87, 737–740.
13. Helawa, M. E., Krepart, G. V., and Lotocki, R. (1986). Staging laparotomy in early epithelial ovarian carcinoma. *Am. J. Obstet. Gynecol.* 154, 282–286.
14. McGowan, L., Lesher, L. P., Norris, H. J., and Barnett, M. (1985). Mistaging of ovarian cancer. *Obstet. Gynecol.* 65, 568–572.
15. Wang, P. H., Yuan, C. C., Chao, K. C., Yen, M. S., Ng, H. T., and Chao, H. T. (1997). Squamous cell carcinoma of the cervix after laparoscopic surgery. A case report. *J. Reprod. Med.* 42, 801–804.
16. Cohn, D. E., Tamimi, H. K., and Goff, B. A. (1997). Intraperitoneal spread of cervical cancer after laparoscopic lymphadenectomy. *Obstet. Gynecol.* 89, 864.

17. Berek, J. S. (1995). Ovarian cancer spread: Is laparoscopy to blame? *Lancet* 346, 200.
18. Chew, D. K., Borromeo, J. R., and Kimmelstiel, F. M. (1999). Peritoneal mucinous carcinomatosis after laparoscopic anterior resection for early rectal cancer: Report of a case. *Dis. Colon. Rectum* 42, 424–426.
19. Canis, M., Botchorishvili, R., Wattiez, A., Pouly, J. L., Mage, G., Manhes, H., and Bruhat, M. A. (2000). Cancer and laparoscopy, experimental studies a review. *Eur. J. Obstet. Gynecol. Reprod. Biol.* 91, 1–9.
20. Gutt, C. N., Riemer, V., Kim, Z. G., Jacobi, C. A., Paolucci, V., and Lorenz, M. (1999). Impact of laparoscopic colonic resection on tumor growth and spread in an experimental model. *Br. J. Surg.* 86, 1180–1184.
21. Sevelda, P., Vavra, N., Schemper, M., and Salzer, H. (1990). Prognostic factors for survival in stage I epithelial ovarian carcinoma. *Cancer* 65, 2349–2352.
22. Lehner, R., Wenzl, R., Heinzl, H., Husslein, P., and Sevelda, P. (1998). Influence of delayed staging laparotomy after laparoscopic removal of ovarian masses later found malignant. *Obstet. Gynecol.* 92, 967–971.
23. Canis, M., Botchorishvili, R., Manhes, H., Wattiez, A., Mage, G., Pouly, J. L., and Bruhat, M. A. (2000). Management of adnexal masses: Role and risk of laparoscopy. *Semin. Surg. Oncol.* 19, 28–35.
24. Hart, W. R., and Norris, H. J. (1973). Borderline and malignant tumors of the ovary: Histologic criteria and clinical behaviour. *Cancer* 31, 1031–1045.
25. Katzenstein, A. L. A., Mazur, M. T., Morgan, T. E., and Kao, M. S. (1978). Proliferative serous tumors of the ovary. Histologic features and prognosis. *Am. J. Surg. Pathol.* 2, 339–355.
26. Colgan, T. J., and Norris, H. J. (1983). Ovarian epithelial tumors of low malignant potential: A review. *Int. J. Gynecol. Pathol.* 1, 367–382.
27. Tasker, M., and Langley, F. A. (1985). The outlook for women with borderline epithelial tumors of the ovary. *Br. J. Obstet. Gynecol.* 92, 969–973.
28. Kliman, L., Rome, R. M., and Fortune, D. W. (1986). Low malignant potential tumors of the ovary: A study of 76 cases. *Obstet. Gynecol.* 68, 338–344.
29. Hopkins, M. P., Kumar, N. B., and Morley, G. W. (1987). An assessment of the pathologic features and treatment modalities in ovarian tumors of low malignant potential. *Obstet. Gynecol.* 70, 923–929.
30. Dembo, A. J., Davy, M., Stenwig, A. E., Berle, E. J., Bush, R. S., and Kjorstad, K. (1990). Prognostic factors in patients with stage I epithelial ovarian cancer. *Obstet. Gynecol.* 75, 263–273.
31. Finn, C. B., Luesley, D. M., Buxton, E. J., Blackledge, G. R., Kelly, K., Dunn, J. A., and Wilson, S. (1992). Is stage I epithelial ovarian cancer overtreated both surgically and systemically? Results of a five-year cancer registry review. *Br. J. Obstet. Gynecol.* 99, 54–58.
32. Vergote, I. B., Kaern, J., Abeler, V. M., Pettersen, E. O., De Vos, L. N., and Trpé, C. G. (1993). Analysis of prognostic factors in stage I epithelial ovarian carcinoma: Importance of degree of differentiation and desoxyribonucleic acid ploidy in predicting relapse. *Am. J. Obstet. Gynecol.* 160, 40–52.
33. Sjovall, K., Nilsson, B., and Einhorn, N. (1994). Prognostic incidence of intraoperative rupture of malignant ovarian tumor with immediate surgical treatment. "Proceedings of the 1st European Congress on Gynecologic Endoscopy," (M. A. Bruhat, ed.), pp. 107–108. Blackwell, London.
34. Kodama, S., Tanaka, K., Tokunaga, A., Sudo, N., Takahashi, T., and Matsui, K. (1997). Multivariate analysis of prognostic factors in patients with ovarian cancer stage I and II. *Int. J. Obstet. Gynecol. Obstet.* 56, 147–153.
35. Vergote, I., De Brabanter, J., Fyles, A., Bertelsen, K., Einhorn, N., Sevelda, P., Gore, M. E., Kaern, J., Verrelst, H., Sjovall, K., Timmerman, D., Vandewalle, J., Van Gramberen, M., and Trope, C. G. (2001). Prognostic importance of degree of differentiation and cyst rupture in stage I invasive epithelial ovarian carcinoma. *Lancet* 357, 176–182.
36. Williams, T. J., Symmonds, R. E., and Litwak, O. (1973). Management of unilateral and encapsulated ovarian cancer in young women. *Gynecol. Oncol.* 1, 143–148.
37. Moran, O., Menczer, J., Ben-Baruch, G., Lipitz, S., and Goor, E. (1993). Cytologic examination of ovarian cyst fluid for the distinction between benign and malignant tumors. *Obstet. Gynecol.* 82, 444–446.
38. Bruhat, M. A., Mage, G., Pouly, J. L., Manhes, H., Canis, M., and Wattiez, A. (1992). "Operative Laparoscopy." McGraw-Hill, INC Health Professions Division, New York.
39. Hsiu, J. G., Given, F. T., and Kemp, G. M. (1986). Tumor implantation after diagnostic laparoscopic biopsy of serous ovarian tumors of low malignant potential. *Obstet. Gynecol.* 68S, 90S–93S.
40. Canis, M., Mage, G., Pouly, J. L., Wattiez, A., Manhes, H., and Bruhat, M. A. (1994). Laparoscopic diagnosis of adnexal cystic masses: A 12 year experience with long term follow up. *Obstet. Gynecol.* 83, 707–712.
41. Possover, M., Mader, M., Zielinski, J., Pietrzak, K., and Hettenbach, A. (1995). Is laparotomy for staging early ovarian cancer an absolute necessity. *J. Am. Assoc. Gynecol. Laparosc.* 2, 285–287.
42. Canis, M., Candiani, M., Giambelli, F., Wattiez, A., Pouly, J. L., Mage, G., Manhes, H., and Bruhat, M. A. (1997). Laparoscopic management of ovarian teratoma. *Int. J. Gynecol. Obstet.* 2, 47–53.
43. Maneschi, F., Marasa, L., Incandela, S., Mazzarese, M., and Zupi, E. (1993). Ovarian cortex surrounding benign neoplasm: A histologic study. *Am. J. Obstet. Gynecol.* 169, 388–393.
44. Canis, M., Mage, G., Wattiez, A., Chapron, C., Pouly, J. L., and Bassil, S. (1992). Second-look laparoscopy after laparoscopic cystectomy of large ovarian endometriomas. *Fertil. Steril.* 3, 617–619.
45. Spuhler, S. C., Sauthier, P. G., Chardonnens, E. G., and De Grandi, P. (1994). A new vaginal extractor for laparoscopic surgery. *J. Am. Assoc. Gynecol. Laparosc.* 1, 401–404.
46. Wiskind, A. K., Toledo, A. A., Dudley, A. G., and Zusmanis, K. (1990). Adhesion formation after ovarian wound repair in New Zealand white rabbits: A comparison of microsurgical closure with ovarian non closure. *Am. J. Obstet. Gynecol.* 163, 1674–1678.
47. Brumsted, J. R., Deaton, J., Lavigne, E., and Riddick, D. H. (1990). Postoperative adhesion formation after wedge resection with and without ovarian reconstruction in the rabbit. *Fertil. Steril.* 53, 723–726.
48. Pittaway, D. E., Maxson, W. L., and Daniell, J. F. (1983). A comparison of the CO_2 laser and electrocautery on postoperative intraperitoneal adhesion formation in rabbits. *Fertil. Steril.* 40, 366–368.
49. Obiakor, I., Maiman, M., Mittal, K., Awobuluyi, M., DiMaio, T., and Demopoulos, R. (1991). The accuracy of frozen sections in the diagnosis of ovarian neoplasms. *Gynecol. Oncol.* 43, 61–63.
50. Twaalfhoven, F. C. M., Peters, A. A. W., Trimos, J. B., Hermans, J., and Fleuren, G. J. (1990). The accuracy of frozen section diagnosis of ovarian tumors. *Gynecol. Oncol.* 41, 189–192.
51. Granberg, S., Wikland, M., and Jansson, I. (1989). Macroscopic characterization of ovarian tumors and the relation to the histological diagnosis: Criteria to be used for ultrasound evaluation. *Gynecol. Oncol.* 35, 139–144.
52. Aslam, N., Banerjee, S., Carr, J. V., Savvas, M., Hooper, R., and Jurkovic, D. (2000). Prospective evaluation of logistic regression models for the diagnosis of ovarian cancer. *Obstet. Gynecol.* 96, 75–80.
53. Mol, B. W., Boll, D., De Kanter, M., Heintz, A. P., Sijmons, E. A., Oei, S. G., Bal, H., and Brolmann, H. A. (2001). Distinguishing the benign and malignant adnexal mass: An external validation of prognostic models. *Gynecol. Oncol.* 80, 162–167.

CHAPTER

29

The Management of Malignant Ovarian Neoplasms in the Young Patient

LYNDA ROMAN

Department of Obstetrics and Gynecology
University of Southern California School of Medicine
and
USC Women's and Children's Hospital
Los Angeles, California 90033

I. INTRODUCTION

The nature of ovarian neoplasms in the young patient (25 years of age or less) varies substantially from that seen in the general population. Overall, approximately 90% of ovarian cancers are epithelial, and the median age at diagnosis is 63. In patients under age 21, approximately 66% of ovarian neoplasms are germ cell tumors, 17% are surface epithelial tumors, and 12% are sex cord-stromal tumors. In children under age 10, germ cell and stromal tumors predominate. The risk of malignancy in a pelvic mass is approximately 5% in women under age 30,[1, 2] and 20% in patients under age 20.[3]

In general, ovarian malignancies occurring in young patients are sporadic. Among malignant tumors in children, only 2–5% are gynecologic, most are ovarian, and most occur at puberty.[4] Children with malignant ovarian neoplasms have an increased incidence of congenital anomalies. Familial clustering has been reported but it is rare.[3]

In caring for the young patient with an ovarian malignancy, there are several key clinical issues to consider, including the desire to preserve fertility, the preservation of hormonal function, and, given the long life expectancy, the possibility of future morbidity as a result of antineoplastic treatment.

II. PATHOLOGY

Approximately two-thirds of ovarian malignancies in young patients will be germ cell in nature. In data reported from the University of Texas M.D. Anderson Cancer Center series,[5] the median age of patients with germ cell tumors varied from 16–20 years (depending on the histology). The most common malignant germ cell tumor is the dysgerminoma.[6] Seventy-five percent of dysgerminomas occur in women under age 25 and 10% occur in the prepubertal population. The risk of dysgerminoma is increased in patients with intersex disorders. In the presence of a dysgenetic gonad (containing a Y chromosome), there is a 20–25% chance of developing a gonadoblastoma and a malignant germ cell tumor (usually dysgerminoma) by age 20.[3]

Immature teratomas and endodermal sinus tumors (also known as yolk sac tumors) each account for approximately 20% of malignant germ cell tumors. Approximately 10% of malignant germ cell tumors will be of mixed histology, with dysgerminoma and endodermal sinus tumor being the most common combination observed. Far less common are embryonal carcinomas and choriocarcinomas.

Malignant stromal-cell tumors account for 17–20% of ovarian cancers seen in young women.[4] The most common malignant stromal tumor occurring in the young female is the granulosa cell tumor, of which 90% are of the juvenile type. Juvenile granulosa cell tumors are associated with a high likelihood of isosexual precocious puberty when they occur in the prepubertal period due to their production of estrogen.

Rarely, a juvenile granulosa cell tumor will produce androgens and thus lead to virilization. Juvenile granulosa cell tumors are associated with Potter's disease, Ollier's disease (multiple enchondromatosis), and Maffucci's syndrome (enchondromatosis with hemangiomas).[7–9]

Sertoli-Leydig cell tumors are uncommon stromal tumors, but when they occur they are most likely to occur in young women. The average age is 25. Common presenting complaints are menstrual irregularities and abdominopelvic symptoms attributable to the presence of a large pelvic mass. Some degree of virilization occurs in up to 50% of patients.[10–11] The diagnosis of Sertoli Leydig cell tumor should be the first consideration whenever virilization occurs in a young female with a pelvic mass.

Epithelial cancers, the most common cancer in the general population, account for only 4.5–12.5% of cancers in the young patient.[4] Tumors of low malignant potential (LMP), which account for only 15% of epithelial cancers overall, are the most common epithelial malignancy seen in young women. Frankly invasive epithelial cancers are extremely rare in women under age 25.

III. CLINICAL CONSIDERATIONS

Whenever a young patient presents with a pelvic mass, ovarian cancer is always a part of the differential diagnosis. Features that raise the suspicion of malignancy are the presence of a large (>10 cm), cystic/solid mass on pelvic sonogram, the presence of precocious puberty, or an abnormal tumor marker profile (see further in this section).

Diagnostic considerations in the young patient with a pelvic mass include functional cysts (which tend to be less than 10 cm in size); an ovarian benign or malignant tumor; pelvic inflammatory disease; an ectopic pregnancy; a mesenteric cyst; a pelvic kidney; tumors arising from other organs such as a neuroblastoma or a Wilm's tumor; a urachal cyst; bowel reduplication; or congenital anomalies such as hydrocolpos, hematocolpos, hematometra, syndrome of absent kidney, double uterus, and double vagina with unilateral obstruction.

Diagnostic modalities include physical examination, pelvic sonography, and tumor marker analysis.

In general, ovarian tumors tend to be abdominal in location in preburtal children. In adolescents and young women, ovarian tumors will often be located in the pelvis. Features such as a nodular surface or lack of mobility on examination are concerning for the presence of malignancy. In terms of laterality, it is uncommon for ovarian malignancies to be bilateral in the young patient (see Section IV). The patient should also be evaluated for the stigmata of hormone overproduction, which would raise the suspicion for a malignant stromal tumor, as discussed in the Section II. Should there by any suspicion of a malfunctioning gonad or an intersex disorder, karyotyping should be performed to rule out a dysgenetic gonad.

Pelvic sonography is an invaluable tool in evaluating the patient with a abdominopelvic mass. Ovarian malignancies are associated with the presence of solid components within the mass. Germ cell tumors tend to appear as large (usually greater than 10 cm), primarily solid masses with cystic components. Stromal cell tumors tend to appear as solid masses on sonogram, though they can also occasionally have a cystic component. Epithelial malignancies tend to appear as cystic tumors containing solid papillations, which extrude from the tumor wall or from septae within the tumor.[12] Sonographic characteristics such as a unilocular tumor, the presence of echodense (characteristic of fat which is highly suggestive of a benign cystic teratoma), or a hemorrhagic tumor (suggesting a corpus luteum or an endometrioma) all are associated with benign diagnoses.

Tumor marker determination can also be a valuable diagnostic tool. Germ cell tumors are commonly associated with elevation of either LDH (dysgerminomas), AFP (endodermal sinus tumors), or hCG (choriocarcinomas) (Table 29.1).

TABLE 29.1 Tumor Markers in Ovarian Malignancies

	hCG	AFP	LDH	CA125	Inhibin	Estradiol	Testosterone
Dysgerminoma	±	–	+	±	–	–	–
EST	–	+	±	±	–	–	–
Embryonal	+	±	±	±	–	–	–
IT	±	–	–	±	–	–	–
Mixed	±	±	±	±	–	–	–
LMP	–	–	–	±	–	–	–
Epithelial	–	–	–	±	–	–	–
GCT	–	–	–	±	–	±	±
SLCT	–	±	–	±	±	±	±

CA125 is most likely to be elevated in the serous and endometrioid subtypes. EST = endodermal sinus tumor; IT = immature teratoma; LMP = low malignant potential; GCT = granulosa cell tumor; and SLCT = Sertoli-Leydig cell tumor.

Granulosa cell tumors are associated with elevation of serum inhibin and Sertoli-Leydig cell tumors are associated with elevation in serum testosterone and/or serum DHEAS. Serum LDH, AFP, and hCG should be performed in any young patient with a solid/cystic tumor, especially if it is larger than 5 cm. The hormonal markers should be performed if the history or examination is suggestive of hormonal overproduction.

Before surgery, the patient (if able to comprehend) and her parents should be informed of the possibility of ovarian cancer, the surgical options, and the goal of preserving reproduction while giving appropriate care.

The general health of the patient is evaluated (allergies, asthma, surgical risk, etc.), together with the current status (vomiting, fluid balance, etc.). Preoperative chest radiography should be done on all patients. If there is concern about the possibility of malignancy, then a thorough bowel preparation is done and a gynecologic oncologist should be consulted preoperatively. Ideally, an expert pathologist should be available for frozen section.

IV. OPERATIVE MANAGEMENT

Malignant germ cell tumors have a tendency to present acutely with rupture or torsion (acute presentation occurs in 10% of cases of such tumors). As a result, it is not uncommon for the practitioner to find himself or herself faced with operating on a young patient with a malignant germ cell tumor in the middle of the night, when the availability of consultants (both from the pathology and oncology circles) may be limited. Thus, it is imperative that the clinician has a solid understanding of how to manage such a patient.

There are two important caveats to bear in mind when operating on a young patient with an ovarian malignancy. The first is that preservation of fertility is possible in the majority of cases. Ovarian malignancies in young women tend to be stage I and unilateral oophorectomy is acceptable treatment when the contralateral ovary is normal for women with germ cell, epithelial, and stromal cell malignancies.[13–15] The second is that if there is any question about the diagnosis from the histologic point of view, it is better not to proceed with irrevocable fertility-impacting surgery. Rather the abdomen should be closed and further surgery and staging can be done at a later point if needed.

If the diagnosis is clear prior to surgery, a vertical incision is preferred to allow adequate staging (and debulking, if necessary). If a lower abdominal transverse incision is done for the presumed diagnosis of a benign ovarian process and a malignancy is discovered, the following are options:

1. Cut the rectus abdominus muscles transversely in the line of incision thereby converting it into a Maylard incision
2. Cut the rectus abdominus muscles where they insert at the symphysis pubis, thereby converting it into a Cherney incision
3. If the above still does not give adequate access to the upper abdomen, extend the incision cephalad as a paramedian incision to form a "hockey stick," "J," or reserve "J" incision. The seemingly simple idea of a midline extension or "inverted T" results in a weak intersection. This is different from the "inverted T" uterine incision in Cesarean section where there is a rich blood supply.

At the time of initial entry into the abdomen of any young patient with a pelvic mass, a systematic exploration, including palpation of the diaphragms, omentum, upper abdominal viscera, small and large bowel, and aortic and pelvic lymph nodes should be undertaken. The site of origin of the mass should be determined. If the mass is ovarian in origin, the mass is closely inspected. The presence of a solid ovarian mass, particularly if it is large or necrotic (in the absence of torsion) raises the suspicion for malignancy, as does the presence of surface excresences. Clearly, if apparent metastases are present, the diagnosis is almost, but not definitely, certain. (Extensive, intra-abdominal endometriosis can mimic metastatic, malignant disease.) Similarly, the presence of ascites or enlarged lymph nodes suggests but does not confirm a malignant process.

In general, neither malignant germ cell tumors nor malignant stromal tumors tend to be bilateral. The exception is the dysgerminoma, which has been reported to be bilateral in 20–25% of cases. Juvenile granulosa cell tumors are bilateral in only 5% of cases.[16] Bilaterality in the case of Sertoli-Leydig cell tumors or the non-dysgerminomatous malignant germ cell tumors is exceedingly rare in the absence of widely metastatic disease. In the case of epithelial cancers, the serous subtype is the most likely to be bilateral. Approximately 25% of serous cancers are bilateral in the absence of metastatic disease.

An interesting phenomenon is the tendency for benign cystic teratomas to coexist with malignant germ cell tumors.[17, 18] Approximately 5–10% of patients with such tumors will have an ipsilateral or contralateral cystic teratoma. Misinterpretation of the nature of such tumors by the surgeon has been known to lead to unnecessary castration. When operating on a young patient with a pelvic mass, the surgeon should always be aware that bilaterality is the exception rather than the rule in the absence of metastatic disease and that, given the histologic entities that tend to occur in this age group, it is almost always possible to preserve at least part of one ovary.

The operative procedure begins with washings from the pelvis for cytology (or retrieval of ascites, if present). If the tumor appears to be benign, and a portion of normal ovary is identifiable, a cystectomy is done. Great care is taken to avoid rupture to avoid spill from a possible malignancy. If bilateral ovarian involvement is seen, the procedure is begun with the most impressive appearing ovary. A frozen section is done to establish the diagnosis. If the diagnosis is that of a malignant tumor, and the contralateral ovary is normal, no biopsies of the contralateral ovary are necessary, except in the case of the dysgerminoma. Approximately 10–15% of dysgerminomas will be associated with microscopic, contralateral disease. Thus, consideration should be given to an ovarian biopsy (and contralateral oophorectomy should a dysgenetic gonad be discovered) in this situation.

If the contralateral ovary is abnormal, an attempt should be made to perform a cystectomy. If it is not possible to completely remove malignant tumor from the contralateral ovary, and the diagnosis is that of a germ cell tumor, consideration can be given to leaving behind small volume ovarian disease in patients who will be receiving chemotherapy. Low *et al.* reported that of 74 patients receiving conservative (fertility-sparing) surgery for malignant germ cell tumors, 2 patients had bilateral ovarian involvement and both remained without evidence of disease.[15] At this point, such an approach should be considered experimental as data confirming that primary or metastatic ovarian germ cell tumors can be eradicated by chemotherapy are sparse. Contralateral ovarian preservation in young patients with LMP tumors and bilateral ovarian involvement is also a consideration. Limited data suggest that ovarian cystectomy for LMP tumors is feasible when the tumor is not multilocular and can be cleanly removed. Most recurrences that did occur were of LMP and were amenable to surgical removal. In the rare patient with a bilateral malignant epithelial tumor or stromal tumor, bilateral salpingo-oophorectomy is the standard of care.

The uterus should be left in place if it is uninvolved, even if bilateral oophorectomy is necessary, since pregnancy is now possible with hormone substitution and ovum donation. Uterine curettage should be performed in patients with stromal or epithelial malignancies (especially if the histology is endometrioid), if uterine preservation is contemplated. The former are at risk for endometrial hyperplasia as a result of hormone production, the latter are at risk for synchronous endometrial carcinomas and for endometrial metastases.

If the cancer seems limited to one or both ovaries, then traditional surgical staging is done to determine the stage, prognosis and management (see Chapter 25). Any suspicious peritoneal masses or enlarged pelvic or aortic nodes are removed. If no obvious metastases are seen, washings are taken from the pericolic gutters and right diaphragm. Multiple peritoneal biopsies are done at the sites predisposed to metastases, including the right diaphragm, pelvic sidewall peritoneum, anterior and posterior cul-de-sac, and right and left pericolic gutters. The infracolic omentum is sampled as are the pelvic and para-aortic lymph nodes.

Approximately 30% of germ cell tumors,[5] 3% of malignant stromal-cell tumors,[10, 11, 16] and 25% of LMP tumors [19] are at an advanced stage when first diagnosed (as compared to frankly invasive epithelial tumors, of which 75% tend to have metastasized at time of diagnosis). In patients with epithelial tumors, an attempt at debulking should be made as prognosis is clearly impacted by the amount of residual disease. In the case of malignant germ cell tumors, the role of debulking is not as clear. These tumors are inherently more sensitive to chemotherapy. Two studies from the Gynecologic Oncology Group [20, 21] reported that, in women with advanced malignant germ cell tumors, progression-free survival was superior in those with completely resected disease, especially in patients with non-dysgerminomatous tumors. The decision to proceed with aggressive, potentially risky, surgical debulking in patients with malignant germ cell tumors should be made by an experienced surgeon who is best able to weigh the risk versus benefit ratio in each individual case. In the case of malignant stromal tumors, there are no data confirming the impact of surgical debulking on prognosis. Most authorities support aggressive surgical debulking in these patients, given the benefit seen in women with epithelial tumors who are completely debulked.[22]

V. POSTOPERATIVE MANAGEMENT

A. Malignant Germ Cell Tumors

A major breakthrough occurred in the 1970s when multiagent chemotherapy, which had been found to be effective in testicular germ cell malignancies, was utilized for their ovarian counterparts. As a result, non-dysgerminomatous germ cell tumors, which had a terrible prognosis (less than a 20% patient survival rate, even in stage I), are now highly treatable. Prior to modern chemotherapy, metastatic dysgerminomas, being very radiosensitive, were treated with radiation with good results. At present, radiation (which destroys ovarian function) has been replaced with chemotherapy.

Postoperative chemotherapy is recommended for all patients with malignant germ cell tumors with the exceptions of the patient with a stage IA/B dysgerminoma and a stage IA, grade 1 immature teratoma. There is some controversy as to whether patients with higher grade, localized, immature teratomas require further treatment. Early data seeking to relate prognosis to tumor grade found that 45 and 67% of patients with grade 2 and 3 disease, respectively, recurred.[23] These data were collected during a time when surgical staging was not routine, thus it is possible that a number of patients with recurrences actually had metastatic disease at outset. More recent, nonrandomized data has suggested that surveillance may be a reasonable option for patients with stage IA, grade 2, and 3 pure immature teratomas because the majority of patients followed remain disease free.[23–25] Further studies on this issue are necessary before this approach can be considered standard.

The present standard chemotherapy for all malignant germ cell tumors that require chemotherapy is the combination of bleomycin, etoposide, and cisplatin (BEP). When used in an adjuvant setting, using three to four cycles, 96–100% of patients have remained disease free.[26, 27] For patients with advanced, incompletely resected disease, the MD Anderson Cancer Center reported an 83% progression-free survival using BEP.[26] Patients with incompletely resected dysgerminomas fare especially well with chemotherapy; failures in this group are uncommon.[28] Four cycles of BEP should be given and it is very important for the chemotherapy to be delivered on schedule, regardless of the hematologic parameters. Hematopoietic growth factors can be used if needed, particularly in those patients whose chemotherapy has been complicated by neutropenic sepsis.

Patients with early-stage disease that was completely resected should not undergo second-look laparotomy. If serum markers are normal, second-look surgery is usually negative.[29] Correspondingly, even in patients with incompletely resected germ cell tumor, there is usually no benefit to second-look laparotomy. Williams *et al.* reported that of 48 patients without teratomatous elements in their primary tumor, only 3 patients had a positive second-look laparotomy and all died despite further treatment.[29] The situation is different with incompletely resected tumor with teratomatous elements. At second-look, 4 of 24 such patients had immature teratoma and 16 had mature teratoma or gliosis, of which 7 had bulky residual tumor. Six of the seven patients with resected tumor have remained well, as have 14 of the 16 total patients. Such residual mature teratoma might cause serious complications or a late recurrence of malignancy. Thus second-look surgery is beneficial for incompletely resected immature teratoma.[29]

The outcome in patients with persistent or recurrent malignant germ cell tumors depends on whether the tumor retains sensitivity of the platinum agents (defined in this context as lack or progression for at least 6 weeks since the last chemotherapy cycle). The combination of cisplatin, vinblastine, and ifosfamide (VIP) is usually used, and if effective, there is evidence that further therapy with high-dose carboplatinum, etoposide, either cyclophosphamide or ifosfamide and stem cell rescue may be superior to VIP alone.[30] For patients who are truly platinum resistant, the outcome is dismal.

B. Sex Cord-Stromal Tumors

Juvenile granulosa cell tumors tend to be diagnosed at an early stage (90% are stage I at time of diagnosis).[31] Fortunately, the outcome for patients with stage I tumors is excellent (97% survival with a mean follow-up of 3.5 years).[31] Rupture of an otherwise localized juvenile granulosa cell tumor has not been found to worsen the prognosis.[31] For patients with advanced disease, the outcome is more bleak. Older studies have found that the majority (approximately 75%) of patients with advanced disease succumb to their disease.[31, 32] More recent data, entailing a limited number of patients, have suggested that disease remission can be obtained with the cisplatinum-based therapy.[33] It is as of yet unclear whether these remissions will be permanent.

Juvenile granulosa cell tumors tend to be more aggressive than the adult form of granulosa cell tumor. The adult form has a well-recognized latency phase and recurrences can occur 10–20 years after the diagnosis. Those juvenile granulosa cell tumors that do recur do so within three years.

The prognosis for Sertoli-Leydig cell tumors depends on the stage and grade. As noted previously, the vast majority of Sertoli-Leydig cell tumors will be limited to the ovary when diagnosed. Only 20% of stage I cases will behave in a malignant fashion. The major determinant of malignant behavior is differentiation. Approximately 10% of grade 2 tumors and over 50% of grade 3 tumors will recur.[10] Tumors that contain heterologous mesenchymal elements have a particularly poor prognosis.[10] Treatment with chemotherapy is indicated for patients with poorly differentiated tumors or with advanced disease. The optimal chemotherapy for treatment of Sertoli-Leydig cell tumors is not clear. Responses have been reported with the use of vincristine, actinomycin D, and cyclophosphamide (VAC) and cisplatin, doxorubicin, and cyclophosphamide.[34, 35] Chemotherapy with BEP and with paclitaxel and cisplatin is under evaluation.[17]

C. Epithelial Ovarian Cancer

Low malignant potential tumors tend to present at an early stage. Prognosis for stage I cases is excellent, with the vast majority of patients remaining disease free. Even in advanced stages, the usual 5-year survival is over 80%.[36] Chemotherapy does not appear to have an affect on the outcome of advanced disease and is reserved for those patients with invasive implants. Surgical cytoreduction is also an important tool for patients with metastatic tumors of LMP that clinically progress. Given the indolent nature of this tumor, surgical excision can result in a prolonged disease-free interval.

Patients with stage IA/B, grade 1 frankly invasive epithelial cancer can be treated with conservative surgery and without chemotherapy. The 5-year survival rate is 95%. For all other patients, postoperative platinum-based chemotherapy is recommended. The combination of paclitaxel with carboplatin is the present standard of therapy for invasive epithelial ovarian cancer. Intraperitoneal chemotherapy and chemotherapy with sequential doublets are under investigation.

VI. EFFECT ON FUTURE FERTILITY

Laparotomy and ovarian biopsy may result in adhesions. Ovarian failure is greatest in young adult women who had radiation therapy and alkylating agent chemotherapy. The prepubertal ovary is more resistant to chemotherapy.

Kanazawa *et al.* [14] reported that, of 20 women with malignant germ cell tumors who had undergone fertility-sparing surgery (most also received chemotherapy), 17 (85%) had normal menstruation and 8 (40%) had become pregnant. The majority of those who had not conceived had not attempted pregnancy. Low *et al.* [15] reported that, of 47 patients with early-stage malignant germ cell tumors who had undergone fertility-sparing surgery and chemotherapy, 43 (91.5%) had regular menses, 2 had irregular menses (4%) and two (4%) were premenarchal at ages 13 and 14. Of the 20 patients who attempted to conceive, 19 (95%) were successful. Presumably, although not documented, similar good results would be obtained for other malignancies. The overall available data do not suggest an increase in anomalies and malignancies in children of young cancer survivors.[17]

VII. CONCLUSION

In the young patient with ovarian cancer, conservative surgery allowing preservation of fertility is usually possible. In general, the outcome is favorable.

References

1. Killackey, M. A., and Neuwirth, R. S. (1988). Evaluation and management of the pelvic mass: A review of 540 cases. *Obstet. Gynecol.* 71, 319.
2. Hernandez, E., and Miyazawa, K. (1988). The pelvic mass: Patients' age and pathologic findings. *J. Reprod. Med.* 33, 361.
3. Lack, E. E., Young, R. H., and Scully, R. E. (1992). Pathology of ovarian neoplasms in childhood and adolescence. *In* "Pathology Annual," Vol 27, Part 2. (P. P. Rosen, and R. E. Fechner, eds.), pp. 281–356, Appleton and Lange, Norwalk, CT.
4. Carlson, J. A. (1985). Gynecologic neoplasms. *In* "Pediatric and Adolescent Obstetrics and Gynecology." (J. P. Lavery, and J. S. Sanfilippo, eds.), pp. 124–148, Springer-Verlag, New York.
5. Williams, S. D., Gershenson, D. M., Horowitz, C. J., and Scully, R. E. (2000). Ovarian germ-cell tumors. *In* "Principles and Practice of Gynecologic Oncology." (W. J. Hoskins, C. A. Perez, and R. C. Young, eds.), pp. 1059–1073, Lippincott, Williams & Williams, Philadelphia, PA.
6. Kurman, R. J., and Norris, H. J. (1977). Malignant germ cell tumors of the ovary. *Hum. Pathol.* 8, 551.
7. Plantaz, D., Flamant, F., Vassal, G. *et al.* (1992). Granulosa cell tumors of the ovary in children and adolescents. Multicenter retrospective study in 40 patients aged 7 months to 22 years. *Arch. Fr. Pediatr.* 49, 793.
8. Tamimi, H. K., and Bolen, J. W. (1984). Enchondromatosis (Ollier's disease) and ovarian juvenile granulosa cell tumor. *Cancer* 53, 1605.
9. Tanaka, Y., Sasaki, Y., Nishihira, H., Izawa, T., and Nishi, T. (1992). Ovarian juvenile granulosa cell tumor associated with Maffucci's syndrome. *Am. J. Clin. Pathol.* 97, 523.
10. Young, R. H., and Scully, R. E., (1983). Ovarian Sertoli-Leydig cell tumors with a retiform pattern: A problem in histopathologic diagnosis. A report of 25 cases. *Am. J. Surg. Pathol.* 7, 755.
11. Zaloudek, C., and Norris, H. J. (1984). Sertoli-Leydig tumors of the ovary. A clinicopathologic study of 64 intermediate and poorly differentiated neoplasms. *Am. J. Surg. Pathol.* 8, 405.
12. Roman, L. D., Muderspach, L. I., Stein, S. M., Laifer-Narin, S., Groshen, S., and Morrow, C. P. (1997). Pelvic examination, tumor marker level, and gray-scale and doppler sonography in the prediction of pelvic cancer. *Obstet. Gynecol.* 89, 493–500.
13. Zanetta, G., Chiari, S., Rota, S., Bratina, G., Maneo, A., Torri, V., and Mangioni, C. (1997). Conservative surgery for Stage I ovarian carcinoma in women of childbearing age. *Br. J. Obstet. Gynecol.* 104, 1030–1035.
14. Kanazawa, K., Suzuki, T., and Sakumoto, K. (2000). Treatment of malignant ovarian germ cell tumors with preservation of fertility. Reproductive performance after persistent remission. *Am. J. Clin. Oncol.* 23, 244–248.
15. Low, J. J. H., Perrin, L. C., Crandon, A. J., and Hacker, N. F. (2000). Conservative surgery to preserve ovarian function in patients with malignant ovarian germ cell tumors. A review of 74 cases. *Cancer* 89, 391–398.
16. Scully, R. E. (1970). Sex cord tumor with annular tubules: A distinction ovarian tumor of the Peutz-Jeghers syndrome. *Cancer* 25, 1107.
17. Gershenson, D. M. (1994). Conservative management of ovarian cancer. *In* "Current Problems in Obstetrics, Gynecology and Fertility," pp. 167–191, Mosby Year Book, St. Louis.
18. Fishman, D. A., and Schwartz, P. E. (1994). Current approaches to diagnosis and treatment of ovarina germ cell malignancies. Current opinion. *Obstet. Gynecol.* 6, 98–104.
19. Pettersson, F., ed. (1988). "Annual Report of the Results of Treatment in Gynecologic Cancer," Vol. 20, International Federation of Gynecology and Obstetrics. Panoramic Press, Stockholm.
20. Slayton, R. E., Park, R. C., Silverberg, S. G., Shingleton, H., Creasman, W. T., and Blessing, J. A. (1985). Vincristine, dactinomycin, and cyclophosphamide in the treatment of malignant germ cell tumors of the ovary: A Gynecologic Oncology Group study (a final report). *Cancer* 56, 243.
21. Williams, S. D., Blessing, J. A., Moore, D. H., Homesley, H. D., and Adcock, L. (1989). Cisplatin, vinblastine, and bleomycin in advanced and recurrent ovarian germ-cell tumors. *Ann. Intern. Med.* 111–122.
22. Muram, D., Gale, C., and Thompson, E. (1990). Functional ovarina cysts in patients cured of ovarian neoplasms. *Obstet. Gynecol.* 75, 680.
23. Norris, H. J., Zirkin, H. J., and Benson, W. L. (1976). Immature (malignant) teratoma of the ovary. *Cancer* 2359.
24. Bonazzi, C., Peccatori, F., Colombo, N., Lucchini, V., Cantu, M. G., and Mangioni, C. (1994). Pure ovarian immature teratoma a unique and curable disease: 10 year's experience of 32 prospectively treatment patients. *Obstet. Gynecol.* 84, 598.
25. Dark, C. G., Bower, M., Newlands, E. S., Paradinas, F., and Rustin, G. J. S. (1997). Surveillance policy for stage I ovarian germ cell tumors. *J. Clin. Oncol.* 15, 620.
26. Gershenson, D. M., Kavanaugh, J. J., Copeland, L. J. *et al.* (1990). Treatment of malignant germ cell tumors of the ovary with bleomycin, etoposide, and cisplatin. *J. Clin. Oncol.* 8, 715.
27. Williams, S., Blessing, J. A., Liao, S., Ball, H., and Janjani, P. (1994). Adjuvant therapy of ovarian germ cell tumors with cisplatin, etoposide and bleomycin: A trial of the Gynecologic Oncology Group. *J. Clin. Oncol.* 12, 701.
28. Williams, S. D., Blessing, J. A., Hatch, K. D., and Homesley, H. D. (1991). Chemotherapy of advanced dysgerminoma: Trials of the Gynecologic Oncology Group. *J. Clin. Oncol.* 9, 1950.
29. Loehrer, l. P. J., Williams, S. D., and Einhorn, L. H. (1989). Testicular cancer: The quest continues. *J. Natl. Cancer Inst.* 80, 1373.
30. Beyes, J., Kramar, A., Mandanas, R. *et al.* (1996). High-dose chemotherapy as salvage treatment in germ cell tumors: A multivariate analysis of prognostic variables. *J. Clin. Oncol.* 14, 2638.
31. Young, R. H., Dickersin, G. R., and Scully, R. E. (1984). Juvenile granulosa cell tumor of the ovary. A clinicopathological analysis of 125 cases. *Am. J. Surg. Pathol.* 8, 575.
32. Zaloudek, C., and Norris, H. J. (1982). Granulosa tumors of the ovary in children: A clinical and pathologic study of 32 cases. *Am. J. Surg. Pathol.* 6, 503.

33. Calaminus, G., Wessalowski, R., Harris, D., and Gobel, U. (1997). Juvenile granulosa cell tumors of the ovary in children and adolescents: Results from 33 patients registered in a prospective cooperative study. *Gynecol. Oncol.* 65, 447.

34. Gershenson, D. M., Copeland, L. J., Kavanagh, J. J., Stringer, C. A., Saul, P. B., and Wharton, J. T. (1987). Treatment of metastatic stromal tumors of the ovary with cisplatin, doxorubicin, and cyclophosphamide. *Obstet. Gynecol.* 70, 765.

35. Schwartz, P. E., and Smith, J. P. (1976). Treatment of ovarian stromal tumors. *Am. J. Obstet. Gynecol.* 125, 402.

36. Look, K. Y. (1994). Ovarian tumors of low malignant potential. *Contemp. Ob/Gyn* Vol. 39, pp. 55–56, 58, 60.

CHAPTER

30

Ovarian Carcinoma Complicating Pregnancy

HUGH R. K. BARBER

Department of Clinical Obstetrics and Gynecology
Cornell University Medical College
New York, New York 10021

An estimated 23,400 new cases of carcinoma of the ovary and 13,900 deaths are anticipated in 2001. It is estimated that one of every 600 newborn girls (1.4% or 1:70) will develop ovarian cancer during their lifetime. The neoplasm accounts for approximately 4% of all cancers among women and 27% of the cancers of the female reproductive system. Although the ovarian cancer rate ranks second in incidence among gynecologic cancer, it causes more deaths than any other cancer of the female reproductive system. Women executives are postponing pregnancy until their late thirties and early forties. Therefore, more women at this time have a greater chance of developing ovarian carcinoma complicating pregnancy than occurred in the first half of the 20th century.

Carcinoma complicating pregnancy provides an opportunity for the study of a control group (the pregnancy) and an uncontrolled growth (the malignancy) in the same host. The association represents a major physiologic process for the maintenance of race, a major pathologic process that accounts for numerous deaths. The result of this struggle leads to biologic immortality or destruction.[1]

The introduction of new concepts in preventative medicine, enlightened use of antibiotics, and the establishment of blood banks has brought about a sharp decline in such killers of pregnant women as heart disease, toxemia, hemorrhage, and infectious diseases, whereas cancer has assumed an increasingly important role in maternal mortality studies.[2]

Carcinoma of the ovary accounts for approximately 1 in 18,000 pregnancies. Malignancy rate is 2–5% in contrast to an 18–20% malignancy rate in the nonpregnant state.[3] Deaths from carcinoma of the ovary have significantly increased over the past 40 years and the rate is now three times that of 1930. Signs and symptoms are not basically different from the nonpregnant state. Usually an adnexal mass is found at the time of the first antepartum visit. If it regresses in follow-up, the diagnosis is that of a functional cyst (corpus luteum).

Carcinoma of the ovary is the leading cause of death from gynecologic cancer. Common epithelial ovarian cancer is usually seen in women over age 40, but there is an increasing number seen in younger women as well. Germ cell tumors of the ovary are most commonly seen from birth to age 20, gonadal stromal tumors are usually seen during the child-bearing years. Germ cell and gonadal stromal tumors are more often unilateral than are the common epithelial ovarian cancer. Therefore, if the tumor is confined to the ovary, and the other ovary is negative, unilateral salpingo-oophorectomy may be an acceptable treatment during that pregnancy.

I. THE SUPPORTING SIGNS AND SYMPTOMS

The signs and symptoms of ovarian neoplasm are not basically different from those seen in the nonpregnant state. The presenting symptoms, such as torsion, rupture, hemorrhage, or infection may be a complication of the tumor.

The pelvic findings are an important part in the decision of whether to operate immediately or to observe the patient until the second trimester. The unilateral, seemingly well-encapsulated, freely moveable mass of uniform consistency that is less than 10 cm in diameter can be kept under observation until the second trimester. If the mass decreases in size, presumably it represents a corpus luteum cyst. However, progressive growth requires exploration without further delay. On the other hand, a hard, knobby, fixed mass of variegated consistency, bilateral masses, and signs of ascites or peritoneal fluid are indications for surgical intervention regardless of the trimester of pregnancy.

Fortunately, most malignancies during pregnancy are diagnosed at an early stage (stage I) because the patient seeks medical advice prior to the occurrence of symptoms related to the tumor and is examined at her first antepartum visit. The survival rate, which is much the same as for the nonpregnant, is determined by the stage and type of tumor. If the tumor is diagnosed during the third trimester, surgery may be delayed until the fetus is viable, but to delay beyond that point cannot be justified. The patient must be counseled in detail as to her options before surgery is undertaken. Her questions must be answered.

II. DIAGNOSTIC WORKUP [4]

Diagnostic workup should include a Papanicolau smear, proctosigmoidoscopy, and rectovaginal examination and a careful search for extra-pelvic metastases. Ultrasound examination is acceptable during pregnancy, but CT scans should have very little use in the face of a pregnancy. The role of MRI in pregnancy remains to be fully evaluated. If there is hepatomegaly or gross ascites, the outlook for a long survival is grim. Only about 8% of patients with ascites live 5 years. The toll of cancer will be lowered only if physicians begin to suspect carcinoma in every persistently enlarged ovary.

The presenting symptom may be a complication of ovarian tumor, such as torsion, rupture, hemorrhage, or infection. The symptom may be accompanied by acute abdominal pain with vomiting and possible shock. Surgical intervention is indicated immediately. Cesarean section should be reserved for the usual obstetric indications. At all Cesarean sections, routine inspection of the tubes and ovaries is mandatory.

III. MANAGEMENT OF OVARIAN CARCINOMA COMPLICATING PREGNANCY [5]

- Treat as in the nonpregnant state
- Undertake exploratory laparotomy
- Aspirate fluid from the pelvis and the abdomen for cytologic assessment
- If tumor is low-grade, unilateral, and encapsulated, a unilateral salpingo-oophorectomy is performed and the opposite ovary is biopsied and, if negative, the treatment at this time is considered to be adequate and the pregnancy is allowed to go to term.
- If the tumor has extended beyond the ovary, undertake aspiration for cytology, total hysterectomy, bilateral salpingo-oophorectomy, appendectomy, omentectomy, node sampling and, later, chemotherapy as indicated. The patient must be counseled as to what options there are before surgery is undertaken.
- If pregnancy is allowed to continue, Cesarean section is done only for an obstetrical indication. The ovaries and tubes should be inspected at every Cesarean section. A decision must be arrived at with the patient about definitive surgery and management.

If the surgeon finds an ovarian tumor, cyst, or malignancy during abdominal exploration, the first obligation is to stage the disease, collect peritoneal fluid for cytology and cell block examination, and remove the lesion for immediate frozen section in order to obtain definitive diagnosis and documentation.[6] This procedure is followed by whatever other surgery is indicated depending on the type of tumor and cytologic rating and the degree of anatomic spread. Biopsies of omentum, peritoneum, or any other intra-abdominal area where one suspects carcinoma are indicated. The information may prove helpful for selecting the appropriate therapy and for future follow-up examinations and studies.

Papillary serous cystadenocarcinoma, the most common type of ovarian malignancy, has been considered by some authorities as probably an advanced histologic type of a benign serous cystadenoma. If it is contained so papillary processes are within an intact capsule, the prognosis is reasonably good. Once there is extension through the capsule with papillations on the exterior of the tumor, extension to the surrounding organs appear promptly with great diminution in the chance of a 5-year survival. General abdominal carcinomatosis soon follows with death. The treatment is total abdominal hysterectomy, bilateral salpingo-oophorectomy, appendectomy, omentectomy, and sampling of pelvic and para-aortic nodes. Currently, combination chemotherapy is a favored adjunct treatment. Treatment must be tailored to the needs of the patient and the extent of disease. When there is doubt about the type of tumor or that a malignancy is present, if the tumor has an intact capsule and is freely moveable, especially in a patient under age 30, it is better to perform a salpingo-oophorectomy on the side of the tumor. The pelvis should be aspirated prior to excision and aspirate sent for a cell block examination. If the tumor proves to be highly malignant or cell block results are positive, the abdomen must be re-opened and the remaining reproductive organs excised as outlined above, if the surgeon judges that to be the best course. For certain low-grade malignancies, previously performed treatment may be considered sufficient to insure a cure. The decision about exploration following the delivery depends on the judgment of the responsible physician.

Papillary mucinous cystadenocarcinoma is the next most common type of ovarian carcinoma. About 1 in 4 is bilateral. Clinical and operative findings depend on whether the tissues are contained in an intact capsule. The spread of the tumor is fortunately slower than the spread of the papillary serous variety, so the prognosis is better. Treatment is the same as that for the serous cystadenocarcinoma.[7]

The philosophy must be to attack the carcinoma and ignore the pregnancy. This statement may seem harsh, but, if the mother is not saved, there is no incubator for the baby to survive. The ideal is to have a live mother, a live baby, and a cure of the carcinoma. The obstetrician must strive to achieve this.

IV. SOLID ADENOCARCINOMA

The solid adenocarcinoma is a common epithelial ovarian cancer with the same cells as those found in papillary serous or mucinous carcinoma of the ovary. These tumors are solid and highly undifferentiated and they have a great potential to spread and metastasize. They are bilateral in more than 50% of patients and the prognosis is poor. Treatment is similar to that outlined above.

V. DYSGERMINOMA [8, 9]

Dysgerminoma is not aggressively malignant in young patients and, in fact, dysgerminoma has a surprisingly high 5-year cure rate. If the tumor is unilateral and still encapsulated, unilateral oophorectomy may be carried out if the remaining ovary is negative on biopsy, the peritoneal fluid is negative, the external, and common and para-aortic nodes are negative as well. Dysgerminoma in patients over age 35, and surely in those over age 40, should undergo a more aggressive attack. If the tumor is bilateral or the capsule is perforated, total abdominal hysterectomy and bilateral salpingo-oophorectomy, omentectomy, appendectomy, and consideration of a para-aortic node dissection combined with postoperative x-ray treatment must be carried out in any age group. The surgery may be delayed until viability of the fetus, if the time is short.

Other germ cell tumors, both extra-embryonic and embryonic carcinomas, are highly malignant. The treatment is generally excision of the uterus, tubes, ovaries, appendix, and omentum. Combination chemotherapy should be given at monthly intervals for 6–8 months and consideration given to a second-look operation. As a group, these tumors are relatively radio-resistant.

VI. GONADAL STROMAL TUMORS

Gonadal stromal tumors (Sertoli-Leydig) are rarely associated with pregnancy. However, if they are unilateral and encapsulated with a negative opposite ovary on biopsy, negative cytology, and no evidence of spread, unilateral salpingo-oophorectomy is usually adequate therapy. If there is any evidence of spread or the tumor is bilateral, it should be managed as outlined above. These tumors are characterized by local late recurrence and are radio-sensitive.

VII. SARCOMA

Sarcoma of the ovary, either primary or metastatic, is highly malignant and spreads quickly by local invasion and blood vessel and lymphatic extension. It is usually found before child-bearing age. Prompt therapy should be complete removal of the pelvic gynecologic organs. Combination chemotherapeutic and progesterone agents should be given for 6–8 months and a decision then made whether to re-explore the patient or to continue therapy for a longer period.

VIII. METASTATIC CARCINOMA

Metastatic carcinoma of the ovaries from the uterus, breasts, thyroid, stomach, or colon may occur, although it is rare. There is confusion over whether all or only certain secondary cancers are eponymically designated Krukenberg tumors. The signet ring cell type of carcinoma described by Krukenberg is most often metastatic to the ovary from the pyloric end of the stomach.[10] The ultimate prognosis is poor, but removal of uterus, ovary, and tubes will permanently control the pelvic manifestations of the problem. Bilateral tumors are the rule. Of course, removal of the primary focus of disease probably will not result in cure at this stage, but at least adequate palliation may be accomplished. Some Krukenberg tumors that occur during pregnancy are hormonally active. Reports of androgenicity as well as estrogen secretion affecting even the fetus can be found in the literature.

It should be noted that ovaries at the end of pregnancy are resting and are comparatively small. They often have shaggy eosinophilic, wispy material on the surface that is deciduous. Any enlargement of the ovaries in a term pregnancy should be suspect and it is in the best interest of the patient for the operating surgeon to obtain biopsy specimens and frozen sections as a guide to additional therapy.

Non-malignant ovarian tumors may be encountered during pregnancy. After they are diagnosed as benign, the question of their management is raised. A brief discussion is included to serve as a guide to management.

IX. THERAPY FOR NON-MALIGNANT OVARIAN TUMOR

There are eight basic principles for therapy for the non-malignant ovarian tumor:

1. If the tumor is cystic, less than 6–8 cm in diameter and suddenly diminishes in size as the pregnancy continues, it can simply be observed. Operation is not indicated unless there is a torsion or rupture. If the tumor becomes enlarged, however, operative intervention is mandatory. When cystic tumors do not regress, the ideal time for operation is during the early part of the second trimester (12–14 weeks). By this time the corpus luteum is no longer important for maintaining the pregnancy. In most instances, after the 60th day of pregnancy, removal of the corpus luteum does not materially affect the outcome. If the tumor is benign on frozen section, the cyst should be resected and as much of the normal portion of the ovary as possible left in place.
2. Solid or suspicious tumors should be removed at once regardless of the trimester of pregnancy. With evidence of torsion, hemorrhage, or necrosis, prompt surgery is mandatory.
3. The uterus should be handled as little and as carefully as possible in the very early months of pregnancy. Excessive manipulation contributes to an increased abortion rate. Although some advise prophylactic progesterone therapy postoperatively, it is generally unnecessary. The results do not justify the means.
4. After the 18th week, it may be more difficult to remove a tumor because of the enlarged uterus. It can be done, but there are technical problems. Also, the closer the patient is to term, the greater is the stress on the healing abdominal wall and by the enlarging uterus with possible weakening and herniation. The earlier that surgery is done, the greater is the time remaining for proper healing.
5. During the last trimester of pregnancy, the main problem is an unsuspected tumor that may be blocking delivery. The fetal and maternal complications make operation mandatory. If the diagnosis is made before the onset of labor, surgical intervention is indicated about one week before the anticipated delivery date or, if the date is unreliable, during early labor. The operation consists of low-flap Cesarean section and either ovarian resection or oophorectomy or any procedure deemed necessary, depending upon the pathology and stage of disease.
6. If the exit of the child is not blocked and the tumor lies above the inlet, the child should be delivered vaginally and the tumor removed abdominally as soon as the patient's condition, which is usually within the first 48 h postpartum. During the interval between delivery and operation, one must watch for acute torsion, because, as mentioned previously, torsion during the postpartum period is a likely complication.
7. A tumor above the inlet and evidence of pain, tenderness, or peritoneal reaction while the patient is in labor probably indicates torsion or rupture. Prompt surgery is indicated. Cesarean section plus oophorectomy is the surgery of choice.
8. If a tumor blocking the pelvis is first diagnosed when the patient is in advanced labor and full dilatation, the abdomen can be opened, the tumor dislodged, and the baby delivered vaginally by an assistant. The tumor is then removed and the abdomen closed. This maneuver is spectacular, but most obstetricians will not see one case of this type in a lifetime. It is really an indictment of the patient's medical care. At the very least, the diagnosis should have been made during early labor. In this litigious environment, most obstetricians would perform a Cesarean section and then tailor the operation to the needs of the patient and the extent of disease.
9. If the tumor is diagnosed during the postpartum period within 48 h, surgery is indicated. With torsion, immediate surgery is indicated.

X. SUMMARY

Carcinoma of the ovary accounts for approximately 5–6% of all cancers. Among women it occurs in about 1 out of every 18,000 pregnancies. The malignancy rate of ovarian tumors complicating pregnancy is 2–5% in contrast to an 18–20% malignancy rate in the nonpregnant state. Deaths from this disease have slowly increased over the last 40 years and the rate is now three times that of 1930. Signs and symptoms are not basically different from the nonpregnant state. Usually an adnexal mass is found at the time of the first antepartum visit. If it regresses on follow-up, then it can be assumed that diagnosis is that of a functional cyst (corpus luteum).

A unilateral encapsulated, freely moveable mass of uniform consistency that is less than 20 cm can be kept under observation until the second trimester. Surgical intervention is indicated if a complication occurs. A hard, knobby mass of variegated consistency bilaterally with signs of fluid are indications for surgical intervention despite the trimester of pregnancy. The presenting symptom may be a complication of the ovarian tumor, such as torsion, hemorrhage, or infection. There may be sudden, acute, abdominal pain with vomiting and possible shock.

While some advocate immediate attention to surgery despite the trimester, clinical judgment determines the plan of management.

The management of ovarian cancer during pregnancy is simple. Beware of the condition, have a high index of suspicion, make the diagnosis early, and tailor the treatment to the needs of the patient and the extent of disease. The patient often resists abdominal exploration during pregnancy because she fears that an abortion may follow or there may be danger to her fetus. The patient must have an explanation and be assured that an argument against operation is not valid and danger to the fetus is very low. Delay in surgery poses a potential danger to the mother that far exceeds the imagined danger to the fetus. Most of the failures in treating ovarian tumors in pregnancy are sins of omission rather than commission. If the patient does not follow advice after proper notification, the physician must withdraw from the case. The mortality rate from ovarian carcinoma can only be lowered by early diagnosis and aggressive management.

If a conservative operation is done in a localized stage I ovarian and the patient wants to have another baby, the pros and cons must carefully be explained to her. The patient may elect to take a calculated risk in her desire for another child. However, after the completion of the pregnancy, it is in her best interest to elect to have a hysterectomy with removal of tubes and ovaries, as well as the appropriate biopsies and node sampling.

The primary responsibility of the physician is to save the mother and the baby. The mother must be saved if the baby is to have a chance, since the mother provides the incubator. There is no way the baby can survive unless the mother is saved. Before undertaking surgery in the pregnant patient with possible ovarian cancer, it is mandatory that the problem be completely disclosed to the patient and informed consent obtained to allow the surgeon to proceed in any manner deemed necessary.

In most reported series about one-third of the patients are stage III or IV at surgery and one must be prepared for this contingency. The most aggressive lesions in terms of early spread are the solid adenocarcinomas and the serous cystadenocarcinomas.

The survival of pregnant patients with ovarian cancer is no different from survival in the nonpregnant group. The type of tumor and its anatomic spread determine the 5-year cure rate. Pregnancy has no affect on the tumor. Only aggressive early exploration can save the patient. Interruption of pregnancy has no beneficial effect on the future course of this disease.

With cancer of the ovary metastatic from the stomach, colon, liver, or breast, decisions about therapy must be made on an individual basis. Certainly nobody would quarrel with the decision to shoot the works and clean out the entire pelvis. In certain instances, expectant parents aware of the poor prognosis for the mother may elect to have the baby for whatever joy it may bring to the remaining time of the mother's life and to the father in the future. Under these circumstances, vaginal delivery (if there is no tumor blocking the pelvic canal) followed by pelvic surgery after the birth of the child may well be the most compassionate procedure. Cesarean section is performed if indicated for obstetric reasons and the uterus, ovaries, and tumors are removed at this time.

Carcinoma is a disease more common in the elderly, but 13% of cancers in women develop during the child-bearing years. Both in the U.S. and the U.K., about 1 in 1000 pregnancies are complicated by malignancy.

A thorough history and physical examination at the first prenatal visit can be used to convince the patient to have routine examinations. This is the height of professional integrity as far as practicing preventative medicine is concerned.

References

1. Barber, H. R. K., and Brunschwig, A. (1962). Gynecologic cancer complicating pregnancy. *Am. J. Obstet. Gynecol.* 85, 156.
2. Barber, H. R. K. (2001). Malignant disease in pregnancy. *J. Perinat. Med.* 79, 9.
3. Buscher, N. A., Buttery, B. W., Fortune, D. W., and Macafee, C. A. J. (1971). Growth and malignancy of ovarian tumors in pregnancy. *Aust. N. Z. J. Obstet. Gynecol.* 11, 208.
4. Chung, A., and Bernbaum, G. J. (1972). Ovarian cancer associated with pregnancy. *Obstet. Gynecol.* 41, 211.
5. Grendys, E. C., and Barnes, W. A. (1995). Ovarian cancer in pregnancy. *Surv. Clin. N. A.* 75 (No. 1), 3.
6. Ueda, M., and Ueki, M. (1996). Ovarian tumors associated with pregnancy. *Int. J. Gynecol. Obstet.* 55, 59.
7. Novak, E. R., Lambrou, C. D., and Woodruff, J. D. (1975). Ovarian tumors in pregnancy. An ovarian tumor registry review. *Obstet. Gynecol.* 46, 401.
8. Elit, L., Bocking, A., Kenyon, C., and Natale, R. (1999). An endodermal sinus tumor diagnosed in pregnancy: Case report and review of the literature. *Gynecol. Oncol.* 72, 123.
9. Bower, M., Fife, K., Holden, L., Paradinas, F. J., Rustin, G. L. S., and Newlands, E. S. (1996). Chemotherapy for ovarian germ cell tumors. *Eur. J. Cancer* 32 (No. 4), 593.
10. Singh, P., and Hancheran, A. (1998). "Cancer in Pregnancy: Essentials of Gynaecological Cancer. Electrodiagnostic Studies." (F. Lawton, M. Friedlander, and T. Gillian, eds.) Chapman and Hall Medical, London.

CHAPTER

31

Ovarian Cancer: The Initial Laparotomy

JAMAL RAHAMAN

Division of Gynecologic Oncology
The Mount Sinai School of Medicine and Hospital
New York, New York 10029

CARMEL J. COHEN

Division of Gynecologic Oncology
The Mount Sinai School of Medicine and Hospital
New York, New York 10029

I. INTRODUCTION

Surgical assessment and histologic evaluation are the only means by which a neoplasm can be classified as benign or malignant, primary or metastatic. When an early primary ovarian cancer is diagnosed, the next goal is determining the extent of disease or stage. Surgical staging is critical to define those patients in whom surgery alone may be curative and those who will require adjuvant therapy, and determine the modality, intensity, and duration of such treatment. Accurate surgical staging also permits assignment of prognosis, allows comparison of cure rates, and defines subsequent surveillance. In the 70–75% of patients who present with advanced ovarian cancer, the goal of laparotomy is also to remove as much tumor as possible through a process of surgical "cytoreduction" to maximize response to chemotherapy, and improve survival. We offer epithelial ovarian cancer as a model; the principles of treatment also apply to ovarian germ cell tumors, stromal tumors, and other primary ovarian cancers.

II. PREOPERATIVE PREPARATION

A thorough history is obtained, including age, parity, history of medication use including oral contraception, ovulation induction drugs, and treatment for endometriosis.

Patients with a family history or personal history of ovarian, breast, or colon cancer are at increased risk for developing ovarian cancer, although only 5–10% of patients with ovarian cancers have such histories.[1] The risk of developing ovarian cancer in the general female population is about 1 in 70 after the age of 40 years. A woman with 2 or more first-degree relatives with the disease has been assumed to have up to a 50% lifetime risk of developing ovarian cancer.[2] Current detection of the BRCA1 and BRCA2 genes adds precision to risk estimation.[3–5]

Complete physical examination determines suitability for extensive surgery and may reveal the extent of disease. A fixed pelvic mass, cul-de-sac nodularity, or upper abdominal mass requires appropriate preoperative planning for resection of bowel. Occult fecal blood should be explained by colonoscopy. Any woman over 40 who has not had previous colonoscopy should have this procedure prior to treatment for ovarian cancer.

Patients should have a thorough assessment of intercurrent medical illnesses, and deficits must be corrected preoperatively. Preoperative assessment of hemogram, electrolytes, and liver and renal function should be made. Serum markers for cancer should be measured.

Preoperative computerized (CT) scanning of the chest, abdomen, and pelvis is essential in identifying disease in the chest and abdominal retroperitoneal compartment, especially in the lymph nodes and along the ureters whose normal position might be distorted by disease. In addition, it allows assessment of the probability of achieving optimal cytoreduction in the epigastrium. When successful cytoreduction seems unlikely, or the patient is a poor surgical risk, neoadjuvant chemotherapy prior to attempted cytoreduction might have utility.[7] CT scan criteria predicting inability to achieve optimal cytoreduction have been published.[8, 9]

All patients with a suspicion of advanced ovarian cancer should have complete bowel preparation as resection is often necessary;[10, 11] and lack of adequate mechanical preparation is associated with higher infectious morbidity.[12] Ambulatory bowel preparation utilizing a combination of clear liquid diet with oral laxatives and enemas with or without antibiotics is an alternative to preoperative hospitalization.[13] Liquid electrolyte solutions (GOLYTELY) may be used to empty the bowel; however, these preparations are sometimes poorly tolerated by patients with ascites or upper abdominal disease. Currently we prefer the use of oral Fleet phospho-Soda or magnesium citrate which is better tolerated and provides an equivalent mechanical effect.

Detailed explanation about the anticipated surgical procedure, its risks, and the probability of finding cancer should be offered to the patient and her family.[14] Younger patients wishing to maintain child-bearing ability should be counseled about the possibilities and limitation of preserving fertility based on the operative findings and the current range of conservative options with the expanded role of artificial reproductive technologies (ARTs). Patients at low risk of having ovarian cancer undergoing laparoscopic removal of an adnexal mass should also be warned that a laparotomy may be necessary if unexpected cancer is found. Intraoperative discovery of cancer in an uninformed and uncounseled patient can have tragic consequences.

III. EARLY OVARIAN CANCER

A. Staging Laparotomy

Ovarian cancer is a surgically staged disease by mandate of The International Federation of Gynecology and Obstetrics (FIGO) (Table 31.1). Understanding the three main mechanisms of spread is important in staging of ovarian

TABLE 31.1 FIGO Staging Classification of Epithelial Ovarian Cancer

Stage	Description
Stage I	Growth limited to the ovaries
Stage IA	Growth limited to one ovary; no ascites containing malignant cells present; no tumor on the external surfaces; capsule intact
Stage IB	Growth limited to both ovaries; no ascites containing malignant cells present; no tumor on the external surfaces; capsule intact
Stage IC[a]	Tumor either stage IA or IB but with tumor on the surface of one or both ovaries; or with the capsule ruptured; or with ascites present containing malignant cells or with positive peritoneal washings.
Stage II	Growth involving one or both ovaries with pelvic extension
Stage IIA	Extension and/or metastasis to the uterus and/or tubes
Stage IIB	Extension to other pelvic tissues
Stage IIC	Tumor either stage IIA or IIB but with tumor on the surface of one or both ovaries; or with capsule(s) ruptures; or with ascites present containing malignant cells or with positive peritoneal washings
Stage III	Tumor involving one or both ovaries with peritoneal implants outside the pelvis and/or positive retroperitoneal or inguinal nodes; superficial liver metastasis equals stage III; tumor is limited to the true pelvis but with histologically verified malignant extension to small bowel or omentum
Stage IIIA	Tumor grossly limited to the true pelvis with negative nodes but with histologically confirmed microscopic seeding of abdominal peritoneal surfaces
Stage IIIB	Tumor of one or both ovaries; histologically confirmed implants of abdominal peritoneal surfaces, none exceeding 2 cm in diameter; nodes negative
Stage IIIC	Abnormal implants 2 cm in diameter and/or positive retroperitoneal or inguinal nodes
Stage IV	Growth involving one or both ovaries with distant metastasis; if pleural effusion is present, there must be positive cytologic test results to allot a case to stage IV; parenchymal liver metastasis equals stage IV

[a]In order to evaluate the impact on prognosis of the different criteria for allotting cases to stage; IC or IIC, it would be of value to know if rupture of the capsule was (1) spontaneous or (2) caused by the surgeon and if the source of the malignant cells detected was (1) peritoneal washings or (2) ascites.

From Hacker, N. F., Jonathan, S. B., Lagasse, L. D. *et al.* (1983). *Obstet. Gynecol.* 38, 203.

TABLE 31.2 Mechanisms of Spread in Ovarian Cancer

Direct extension
Exfoliation of malignant cells
Lymphatic spread

cancer (Table 31.2). Tumor may spread by direct extension to adjacent pelvic structures. Abdominal structures that come in contact with pelvic tumor may also be involved with disease. When the tumor is no longer confined by the ovarian capsule, tumor cells exfoliate into the peritoneal cavity and circulate with peritoneal fluid, flowing through the abdominal cavity, implanting on omentum, undersurfaces of the diaphragms, and mesenteric surfaces of the large and small bowel. The third mechanism of tumor spread is endolymphatic. Tumor cells travel through the rich lymphatic channels in the broad ligament to the iliac vessels and then ascend into the para-aortic lymph node chain. Para-aortic lymph nodes may also be the site of direct lymphatic spread by way of the infundibulopelvic ligaments.[15, 16] Surgical staging requires a meticulous examination of all peritoneal and retroperitoneal surfaces and structures at risk for tumor spread. Table 31.3 outlines the procedures necessary for a thorough staging laparotomy. An incision large enough to remove the pelvic mass and organs and to adequately assess and/or treat the upper abdomen is necessary (Table 31.4). We prefer a vertical midline incision. On entering the peritoneal cavity, pelvic fluid should be collected for cytology. If no fluid is present, pelvic washings should be obtained. The pelvis is then closely examined. The size of pelvic tumor masses should be recorded as should the presence of tumor on the surface of the ovarian capsule, adhesions, and direct extension to adjacent pelvic structures as well as pre- or intraoperative cyst rupture. Several of these factors affect prognosis in stage I cancers.[17–19] The upper abdomen, bowel serosa, mesenteric surfaces, and retroperitoneal structures are palpated. Removal of the uterus, and both tubes and ovaries should be completed unless the patient has an apparent early stage tumor and is a candidate for fertility conservation.[20] Para-aortic lymph node sampling should extend to the renal vessels as illustrated in Fig. 31.1.

There have been several reports of inappropriate incisions and inadequate staging.[21–25] Young *et al.* reported a 31% rate of upstaging of ovarian cancer patients presumed to have stage I or II at initial inadequate surgery. When properly staged 77% of upstaged patients actually had stage III disease. The importance of stage at presentation can be inferred by inspecting the 5-year survivals for patients with ovarian cancer in Table 31.5.[26] Overall 5-year survival for stage I disease approaches 89%, but when disease is found outside the pelvis it drops to less than 24%.[26] When patients are treated for presumed early-stage disease when in fact their disease is advanced, cure is prevented.

TABLE 31.3 Surgical Staging Procedure for Apparent Early Ovarian Cancer

Total abdominal hysterectomy[a]
Bilateral salpingo-oophorectomy[a]
Peritoneal washings
Pelvic
Paracolic gutters
Subdiaphragmatic surfaces
Pelvic biopsies
Pelvic sidewall peritoneum
Anterior and posterior peritoneum
Bladder and rectal serosa
Infracolic omentectomy
Bilateral pelvic lymph node biopsy
Para-aortic lymph node biopsy

[a]Unilateral salpingo-oophorectomy may be performed in select patient wishing to preserve fertility.

TABLE 31.4 Site of Metastatic Disease in Apparent Early Ovarian Cancer

Site	Positive (%)	Ref.
Cytology	17/92 (18)	[22, 81, 82]
Omentum	16/225 (6)	[22, 81–85]
Diaphragm	22/241 (9)	[22, 81, 82, 84, 86]
Pelvic tissue	16/112 (14)	[22, 81, 82]
Abdominal tissue	10/122 (8)	[22, 81, 82, 86]
Pelvic nodes	16/203 (8)	[22, 82, 83, 85, 87]
Para-aortic nodes	30/263 (11)	[22, 82–85, 88]

Disease confined to the ovary and with low histologic grade requires no further therapy to achieve survival.[27] Patients with poor prognosis stage I tumors have been shown to benefit from thorough surgical staging and platinum-based chemotherapy with improved disease-free intervals and extended survival.[28–30] The role of platinum-based chemotherapy in advanced disease has been documented,[31–33] and the current standard employs a taxane/platinum combination.[34–37] The negative prognostic implications of an inadequate staging operation can therefore be appreciated. The magnitude of this problem is reflected in a recent report using the NCI/SEER database, which indicated that only 10% of American women with apparent early-stage ovarian cancer had appropriate surgical staging.[38]

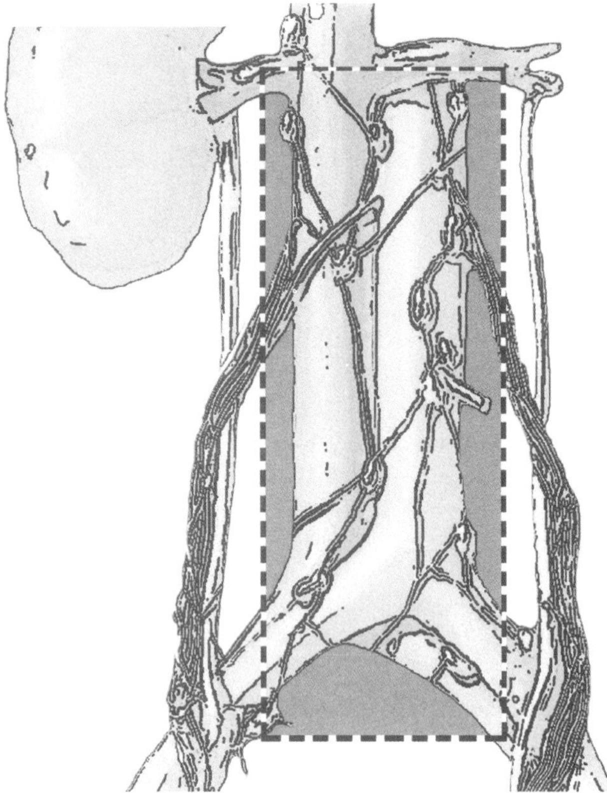

FIGURE 31.1 The para-aortic lymph node sampling extending to the renal vessels.

TABLE 31.5 5-Year Survival in Ovarian Cancer by Stage

Stage	5-year survival %
IA	92.1
IB	84.9
IC	82.4
IIA	69.0
IIB	56.4
IIC	51.4
IIIA	39.3
IIIB	25.5
IIIC	17.1
IV	11.6

B. Ovarian Tumors of Borderline or Low Malignant Potential

Ovarian tumors of borderline or low malignant potential (LMP) are a group of epithelial ovarian tumors having histologic features of cancer, but biologic features that don't show invasion. At presentation, approximately 80% of such cancers are confined to the pelvis. Conservative surgery to preserve fertility is an option in patients with disease confined to the ovaries. Patients with tumors of LMP, even those with widespread disease, can look forward to long disease-free intervals if left with no residual tumor. Adjuvant chemotherapy and radiotherapy have not been found to impact on disease-free interval and survival in most centers.[39, 40] In advanced disease the presence of invasive implants (22% of cases) is the most important prognostic indicator and such patients should be treated for invasive disease with adjuvant therapy. While survival of stage I tumors is virtually 100%, in advanced disease after 7.4 years of follow-up, patients with noninvasive implants have a 95.3% survival rate compared to only 66% in those with invasive implants.[41]

IV. ADVANCED OVARIAN CANCER

A. Role of Cytoreduction

The aim of the first surgery in patients with early epithelial ovarian cancer is staging. The goal of laparotomy in advanced disease is removal of all gross cancer so as to maximize the patient's response to adjuvant chemotherapy and improve survival. This is not always possible. Removal of all tumor greater than 1.0–1.5 cm results in improved survival after adjuvant treatment.[42, 43] While there are no prospective randomized data, there are abundant data to identify optimal cytoreduction as the most consistent independent prognostic variable affecting survival. The large series of reports studying the effect of cytoreduction is typified by the Danish Ovarian Cancer Group report on 361 advanced ovarian cancer patients which found a 10% risk of progression during chemotherapy and a 46% 5-year survival in optimally cytoreduced patients.[44] Suboptimaily cytoreduced patients had a 40% risk of progression and a 5-year survival of only 14%. At Mount Sinai, between 1985 and 1994, 230 stage III primary ovarian cancer patients underwent primary cytoreductive surgery and platinum-based chemotherapy (no paclitaxel was employed in this era). Patients achieving optimal primary cytoreduction to <1 cm (64.2%) had significantly improved survival ($p<0.0001$) with Kaplan-Meier 2-, 3-, and 5-year survivals of 82.5, 73.6, and 59.2%, respectively, versus 59.8, 38.8, and 18.8% in those with suboptimal primary cytoreduction.[45] Furthermore, a recent meta-analysis of 6848 patients with advanced ovarian cancer during the platinum era has identifed maximal cytoreduction as one of the most powerful determinants of cohort survival.[46] The ability optimally to cytoreduce is therefore critical, and the Mount Sinai Group have recently demonstrated that elderly patients with advanced disease who can be optimally cytoreduced enjoy similar survival benefits as their younger counterparts, and therefore should not be denied access to curative management options.[47]

While cytoreductive surgery is important, the biology of the disease itself has independent importance. Cancers that present as small-volume disease or can be successfully cytoreduced to small volume may be biologically different from those that cannot.[48] Cytoreduction may improve overall survival, however, it may not provide survival benefit equivalent to that of small-volume abdominal disease at presentation. These differences may reflect differences in the biologic activity of the tumor or a difference in the duration of disease. Tumors with more aggressive biologic behavior or those which have had more time to become entrenched may have a poorer prognosis regardless of the surgeon's ability to remove them. These notions still await scientific proof.

B. Cytoreduction Techniques

Primary cancer of the pancreas, colon, and stomach may present findings which are clinically indistinguishable from those of ovarian cancer, yet the value of cytoreduction is unproven for nonovarian cancer. Accurate histologic evaluation early in the surgery may avoid an unnecessary, lengthy surgical procedure when a palliative procedure is indicated instead, thus obtaining early intraoperative histologic analysis is essential.

An initial assessment should be made to determine resectability of the tumor. Disease may be considered unresectable when it involves the porta hepatis, extensive involvement of the base of the small bowel mesentery, and multiple liver parenchymal lesions.[49] However, cytoreduction of solitary accessible intraparenchymal liver lesions is feasible and should be attempted if it renders the patient surgically disease free. In fact, the ability to achieve optimal cytoreduction of the hepatic involvement has been demonstrated to be of independent prognostic value in improving survival.[50] Once the upper abdominal disease has been thoroughly evaluated and considered resectable; attention is turned to the pelvic disease. Extensive involvement of pelvic organs is usual in advanced ovarian cancer. The so-called "frozen pelvis" is often prematurely deemed inoperable, but with care and persistence cytoreduction is usually possible.[49, 51, 52] It is therefore important for patients to be cared for by specially trained clinicians.

Fortunately, ovarian cancer tends to spread over peritoneal surfaces allowing removal of large tumors by approaching avascular retroperitoneal planes and identifiable retroperitoneal structures. This requires complete understanding of retroperitoneal anatomy. By incising the peritoneum lateral to the external iliac vessels and the psoas muscles, access to the retroperitoneal space is gained. The round ligament can usually be identified in its retroperitoneal location and is ligated and cut. The peritoneal incision continues inferiorly over the bladder peritoneum, outside any peritoneal implants to remove as much tumor as possible. Using sharp dissection the peritoneum of the anterior cul-de-sac is dissected away from the bladder until it connects with the uterine serosa thus removing all of the involved anterior cul-de-sac peritoneum effecting an "anterior culdectomy." The bladder is then sharply dissected away from the lower uterine segment, anterior cervix, and vagina. The lateral peritoneal incision is extended superiorly to the level of the infundibulopelvic (IP) ligament. The ureter is identified on the medial leaf of the pelvic peritoneum and then the IP ligament can be safely ligated and divided. By dissecting the ureter off of the peritoneum and following it, the uterine artery is identified, ligated, and divided. If there is no rectosigmoid involvement a subtotal hysterectomy then completes the pelvic resection.

If the rectosigmoid colon is extensively involved with the pelvic tumor it can all be removed as an *en bloc* specimen by utilizing the avascular presacral space. The sigmoid colon is transected proximal to any disease with a mechanical stapler. Care should be taken to preserve as much colon as possible to allow a tension-free anastamosis. Sigmoid mesenteric vessels are individually identified and ligated. At the base of the sigmoid mesentery the presacral space can be entered and developed with blunt dissection. Care should be taken to avoid the anterior surface of the sacrum where trauma to perforating veins can produce tremendous blood loss. The rectal pillars and the lateral rectosigmoid attachments are clipped or ligated until the distal margin of the sigmoid resection is identified.

A subtotal hysterectomy is performed and the posterior cul-de-sac is mobilized with the specimen and the rectovaginal space is entered. The distal margin of the rectal resection is then transected with a mechanical stapler. Bowel continuity is re-established with an end-to-end stapler allowing low-rectal re-anastomosis without need for a protective colostomy.

The omentum is a common site of bulky upper abdominal disease.[43, 49, 51] A total (supracolic) or partial (infracolic) omentectomy should be performed so that no gross residual disease remains. Routine lymphadenectomy in obvious, advanced disease is not performed. The pelvic and para-aortic retroperitoneal lymph nodes should be palpated and palpable nodes removed, especially if such a maneuver results in complete cytoreduction.

These data suggesting that cytoreduction ("debulking") has a favorable impact on survival have influenced gynecologic surgeons to employ more radical surgical procedures to remove as much disease from adjacent pelvic structures as possible.[52] Mechanical stapling devices now commonly used to perform bowel resection and re-anastomosis seem to have a lower complication rate than suture anastamosis and certainly save operative time, blood loss, and length of hospital stay.[53] Many authors have confirmed that bowel resection in ovarian cancer cytoreduction is feasible with acceptable postoperative morbidity.[52–57]

Mechanical stapling devices allow *en bloc* resection of extensive pelvic disease with low anterior rectal resection and re-establishment of bowel continuity, virtually eliminating the need for colostomy in most patients.

Most well-trained gynecologic oncologists can perform these radical procedures to remove bulky tumor, however, the impact on overall survival of ovarian cancer patients is still being debated.[58, 59] Randomized trials to investigate the impact on survival of optimal cytoreduction with bowel resection or other radical debulking procedures are almost impossible to perform. In addition, bowel involvement with cancer may reflect a tumor biology that is different.

The importance of resecting other organs invaded by ovarian cancer to achieve optimal cytoreduction is less well defined. Splenectomy,[60, 61] lower urinary tract resection,[62] liver resection, and diaphragmatic [50, 63] resection have been performed in attempts to maximize patient response to postoperative chemotherapy.

V. ROLE OF THE GYNECOLOGIC ONCOLOGIST

Women with ovarian masses who have been identified preoperatively as having a significant risk of ovarian cancer should be given the option of having their surgery performed by a gynecologic oncologist (NIH Consensus Statement, 1994; 64). The importance is demonstrated in the report by McGowan *et al.* which evaluated 291 women with ovarian cancer and found that 97% of patients staged by gynecologic oncologist were properly staged, compared with only 52 and 35% of those cases operated on by obstetrician/gynecologists and general surgeons, respectively.[65] In addition, there are substantial data to indicate that patients operated upon by a gynecologic oncologist had a better prognosis than those treated by other surgeons.[66–68]

VI. CONCLUSION

The initial surgical approach to patients with epithelial ovarian cancer is a critical first step. The principles of management include assessment of preoperative risk of cancer, meticulous surgical staging to determine extent of disease and the need for further therapy in early disease, and removal of all tumor in patients with advanced disease. The adherence to these principles provides patients with the best chance for successful treatment.

The future of surgical management of primary ovarian cancer may already have arrived, as new, minimally invasive technologies have emerged. Laparoscopic staging of an apparent stage I ovarian cancer has been reported.[69] Since that report several highly skilled laparoscopic surgeons have described the technique of para-aortic lymph node dissection and have reported its feasibility and associated morbidity.[70–75] At present, surgical staging of early ovarian cancer by laparoscopy should be considered an evolving technique, and should be restricted to selected cases performed by appropriately trained surgeons. The initial surgical management of advanced ovarian cancer involves maximal cytoreduction. Laparoscopic techniques may prove to be more useful in surgical end staging and surveillance of patients responding to adjuvant chemotherapy.[76–80] Radical surgical techniques are now being employed to achieve optimal surgical debulking. Well-trained surgical subspecialists who understand the biology of ovarian cancer and possess the training and experience necessary to perform these procedures play an important role in ovarian cancer management.[65–68] However, all physicians caring for women should understand the importance of proper surgical management of ovarian cancer.

References

1. Piver, M. S., Baker, T. R., Jishi, M. F. *et al.* (1993). Familial ovarian cancer: A report of 658 families from the Gilda Radner Familial Ovarian Cancer Registry—1981–1991. *Cancer* 71(Suppl. 2), 582.
2. Perez, R., Godwin, A., Hamilton, T. *et al.* (1991). Ovarian cancer biology. *Semin. Oncol.* 15(3), 186.
3. Frank, T. S. (1999). Testing for hereditary risk for ovarian cancer. *Cancer Control* 6(4), 327.
4. Struewing, J. P., Hartge, P., Wacholder, S. *et al.* (1997). The risk of cancer associated with specific mutations of BRCA1 and BRCA2 among Ashkenazi Jews. *N. Engl. J. Med.* 336, 1401.
5. Boyd, J., Sonodo, Y., Federeci, M. G. *et al.* (2000). Clinicopathological features of BRCA-linked and sporadic ovarian cancer. *JAMA* 283(17), 2260.
6. Guidozzi, F., and Sonnendecker, E. (1991). Evaluation of preoperative investigations in patients admitted for ovarian primary cytoreductive surgery. *Gynecol. Oncol.* 40(3), 244.
7. Van der Burg, M. E. L., van Lent, M., Buyse, M. *et al.* (1995). The effect of debulking surgery after induction chemotherapy on the prognosis in advanced epithelial ovarian cancer. *N. Engl. J. Med.* 332, 629.
8. Nelson, B. E., Rosenfield, A. T., and Schwartz, P. E. (1993). Preoperative abdominal computed tomographic prediction of optimal cytoreduction in epithelial ovarian carcinoma. *J. Clin. Oncol.* 11(1), 166.
9. Bristow, R. E., Duska, L. R., Lambrou, N. C. *et al.* (2000). A model for predicting surgical outcome in patients with advanced ovarian carcinoma using computed tomography. *Cancer* 89(7), 1532.
10. Hammond, R., and Houghton, C. (1990). The role of bowel surgery in the primary treatment of epithelial ovarian cancer. *Aust. NZ. J. Obstet. Gynecol.* 30(2), 166.
11. Burghardt, E., Lahousen, M., and Stettner, H. (1990). The surgical treatment of ovarian cancer. *Geburtshilfe Frauenheilkd* 50(9), 670.
12. Donato, D., Angelides, A., Penalver, M. *et al.* (1992). Infectious complications after gastrointestinal surgery in patients with ovarian carcinoma and malignant ascites. *Gynecol. Oncol.* 44(1), 40.
13. Handelsman, J. C., Zeiler, S., Coleman, J. *et al.* (1993). Experience with ambulatory preoperative bowel preparation at the Johns Hopkins Hospital. *Arch. Surg.* 128, 441.
14. Helewa, M. E., Krepart, G. V., and Lotocki, R. (1986). Staging laparotomy in early epithelial ovarian carcinoma. *Am. J. Obstet. Gynecol.* 154(2), 282.
15. Eichner, E., and Bove, E. (1954). In vivo studies on the lymphatic drainage of the ovary. *Obstet. Gynecol.* 3, 287.

16. Feldman, G., and Knapp, R. (1994). Lymphatic drainage of the peritoneal cavity and its significance in ovarian cancer. *Am. J. Obstet. Gynecol.* 119, 991.
17. Vergote, I., De Brabanter, J., Fyles, A. *et al.* (2001). Prognostic importance of degree of differentiation and cyst rupture in stage I invasive epithelial ovarian carcinoma. *Lancet* 357, 176.
18. Ahmed, F. Y., Wiltshaw, E., A'Hern, B. *et al.* (1996). Natural history and prognosis of untreated stage I epithelial ovarian carcinoma. *J. Clin. Oncol.* 14, 2968.
19. Dembo, A. J., Day, M., Stenwig, A. E. *et al.* (1990). Prognostic factors in patients with stage I epithelial ovarian cancer. *Obstet. Gynecol.* 75(2), 263.
20. Navot, D., Fox, J. H., Williams, M. *et al.* (1991). The concept of uterine preservation with ovarian malignancies. *Obstet. Gynecol.* 78(3 Pt2), 566.
21. Piver, M. S., Lele, S., and Barlow, J. J. (1975). Preoperative and intraoperative evaluation in ovarian malignancy. *Obstet. Gynecol.* 48(3), 312.
22. Young, R. C., Decker, D. G., Wharton, J. T. *et al.* (1983). Staging laparotomy in early ovarian cancer. *JAMA* 250(22), 3072.
23. Hand, R., Fremgen, A., Chmiel, J. S. *et al.* (1993). Staging procedures, clinical management, and survival outcome for ovarian carcinoma. *JAMA* 269(9), 1119.
24. Helewa, M. E., Krepart, G. V., and Lotocki, R. (1986). Staging laparotomy in early epithelial ovarian carcinoma. *Am. J. Obstet. Gynecol.* 154, 282.
25. Trimbos, J. B., Schueler, J. A., van Lent, M. *et al.* (1990). Reasons for incomplete surgical staging in early ovarian carcinoma. *Gynecol. Oncol.* 37, 374.
26. Nguyen, H. N., Averette, H. E., Hoskins, W. *et al.* (1993). National survey of ovarian carcinoma VI: Critical assessment of current International Federation of Gynecologic and Obstetrics staging system. *Cancer* 72(10), 3007.
27. Young, R. C., Walton, L. A., Ellenberg, S. S. *et al.* (1990). Adjuvant therapy in stage I and stage II epithelial ovarian cancer: Results of two prospective randomized trials. *N. Engl. J. Med.* 322(15), 1021.
28. Dottino, P. R., Plaxe, S. C., and Cohen, C. J. (1991). A phase II trial of adjuvant cisplatin and duxorubicin in stage I epithelial ovarian cancer. *Gynecol. Oncol.* 43, 203.
29. Bolis, G., Colombo, N., Pecorelli, S. *et al.* (1995). Randomized multicenter clinical trial in stage I epithelial cancer. *Ann. Oncol.* 9, 887.
30. Colombo, N., Chari, S., Maggioni, A. *et al.* (1994). Controversial issues in the management of early epithelial ovarian cancer: Conservative surgery and the role of adjuvant therapy. *Gynecol. Oncol.* 55, 47.
31. Cohen, C. J., Goldberg, J., Holland, J. F. *et al.* (1983). Improved therapy with cis-platin regimens for patients with ovarian carcinoma (FIGO stages III and IV) as measured by surgical end-staging (second look operation). *Am. J. Obstet. Gynecol. Oncol.* 145, 955.
32. Advanced Ovarian Cancer Trialists' Group (1991). Chemotherapy in advanced ovarian cancer: An overview of randomised clinical trials. *Br. Med. J.* 303, 884.
33. Advanced Ovarian Cancer Trialists' Group (1998). Chemotherapy in advanced ovarian cancer: Four systematic meta-analysis of individual patientdata from 37 randomized trials. *Br. J. Cancer* 78(11), 1479.
34. McGuire, W. P., Hoskins, W. J., Brady, M. F. *et al.* (1996). Cyclophosphamide and cisplatin compared with paclitaxel and cisplatin in patients with stage III and stage IV ovarian cancer. *N. Engl. J. Med.* 334, 1.
35. Stuart, G., Bertelsen, K., Mangioni, C. *et al.* (1998). Updated analysis shows highly significant improved overall survival(OS) for cisplatin–paclitaxel as first-line treatment of advanced ovarian cancer: Mature results of the EORTC-GCCG, NOCOVA,NCIC,CTG, and Scottish intergroup trial. *Proc. Am. Soc. Clin. Oncol.* 17, 361.
36. Ozols, R. F., Bundy, B. N., Clarke-Pearson, D. *et al.* (1999). Randomized phase III study of cisplatin(CIS)/paclitaxel(PAC) versus carboplatin (CARBO)/PAC in optimal stage III epithelial ovarian cancer (OC) Gynecologic Oncology Group Trial (GOG 158). *Proc. Am. Soc. Clin. Oncol.* 18, 356a.
37. du Bois, A., Lueck, H. J., Meier, W. *et al.* (1999). Cisplatin/paclitaxel vs. carboplatin/paclitaxel in ovarian cancer: Update of an Arbeitsgemeinschaft Gynaekologische Onkologie (AGO) Study Group Trial. *Proc. Am. Soc. Clin. Oncol.* 18, 356a.
38. Munoz, K. A., Harlan, L. C., and Trimble, E. L. (1997). Patterns of care for women with ovarian cancer in the United States. *J. Clin. Oncol.* 15, 3408.
39. Fort, M., Pierce, V., Saigo, P. *et al.* (1988). Evidence for the efficacy of adjuvant therapy in epithelial ovarian tumors of low malignant potential. *Gynecol. Oncol.* 32, 69.
40. Koern, J., Trope, C. G., and Abeler, V. M. (1993). A retrospective study 370 borderline tumors of the tumor treated at the Norwegian Radium Hospital from 1970 to 1982. *Cancer* 71(5), 1810.
41. Seidman, J. D., and Kurman, R. J. (2000). Ovarian serous borderline tumors: A critical review of the literature with emphasis on prognostic indicators. *Hum. Pathol.* 31(5), 539.
42. Griffiths, C. T. (1975). Surgical resection of tumor bulk in the primary treatment of ovarian carcinoma. *Natl. Cancer Inst. Monogr.* 42, 101.
43. Hacker, N. F., Jonathan, S. B., Lagasse, L. D. *et al.* (1983). Primary cytoreductive surgery for epithelial ovarian cancer. *Obstet. Gynecol.* 61(4), 413.
44. Bertelsen, K. (1990). Tumor reduction and long-term survival in advanced ovarian cancer: A DACOVA study. *Gynecol. Oncol.* 38, 203.
45. Rahaman, J., Dottino, P., Jennings, T. S. *et al.* (1999). Second look operation improves survival in stage III ovarian cancer patients. *Int. J. Gynecol. Cancer* 9(1), 22.
46. Bristow, R. S., Tomacruz, D., Armstrong, E. *et al.* (2001). Survival impact of maximum cytoreductive surgery for advanced ovarian carcinoma during the platinum-era: A meta-analysis of 6848 patients. *J. Clin. Oncol.* 20(1), 202a.
47. Rahaman, J., Jennings, T. S., Dottino, P. *et al.* (2001). Impact of age on survival in advanced ovarian cancer: A re-examination. *J. Clin. Oncol.* 20(1), 217a.
48. Hoskins, W. J., Bundy, B. N., Thigpen, J. T. *et al.* (1992). The influence of cytoreductive surgery on recurrence free interval and survival in small-volume stage III epithelial ovarian cancer: A Gynecologic Oncology Group study. *Gynecol. Oncol.* 47, 159.
49. Heintz, A. P., Hacker, N. F., Berek, J. S. *et al.* (1986). Cytoreductive surgery in ovarian carcinoma: Feasibility and morbidity. *Obstet. Gynecol.* 67(6), 783.
50. Bristow, R. E., Montz, F. J., Lagasse, L. D. *et al.* (1999). Survival impact of surgical cytoreduction in stage IV epithelial ovarian cancer. *Gynecol. Oncol.* 72(3), 278.
51. Piver, M. S., and Baker, T. (1986). The potential for optimal (≤2 cm) cytoreductive surgery in advanced ovarian carcinoma at a tertiary medical center: A prospective study. *Gynecol. Oncol.* 24, l.
52. Berek, J. S., Hacker, N. F., and Lagasse, L. D. (1984). Rectosigmoid colectomy and reanastomosis to facilitate resection of primary and recurrent gynecologic cancer. *Obstet. Gynecol.* 64(5), 715.
53. Penalver, M., Averette, H., Sevin, B.-U. *et al.* (1987). Gastrointestinal surgery in gynecologic oncology: Evaluation of surgical techniques. *Gynecol. Oncol.* 28, 74.
54. Castaldo, T. W., Petrilli, E. S., Ballon, S. C. *et al.* (1981). Intestinal operations in patients with ovarian carcinoma. *Gynecol. Oncol.* 139, 80.
55. Soper, J. T., Couchman, G., Berchuck, A. *et al.* (1991). The role of partial sigmoid colectomy for debulking epithelial ovarian carcinoma. *Gynecol. Oncol.* 41, 239.
56. Eisenkop, S. M., Nalick, R. H., and Teng, N. N. H. (1991). Modified posterior exenteration for ovarian cancer. *Obstet. Gynecol.* 78(5), 879.
57. Tamussino, K., Lim, P. C., Webb, M. J. *et al.* (2001). Gastrointestinal surgery in patients with ovarian cancer. *Gynecol. Oncol.* 80, 79.

58. Potter, M. E., Partridge, E. E., Hatch, K. D. *et al.* (1991). Primary surgical therapy of ovarian cancer: How much and when. *Gynecol. Oncol.* 40(3), 195.
59. Partridge, E. E., Gunter, B. C., Gelder, M. S. *et al.* (1993). The validity and significance of substages of advanced ovarian cancer. *Gynecol. Oncol.* 48(2), 236.
60. Deppe, G., Zbella, E. A., Skogerson, K. *et al.* (1983). The rare indication of splenectomy as part of cytoreductive surgery in ovarian cancer. *Gynecol. Oncol.* 16, 282.
61. Sonnendecker, E. W. W., Guidozzi, F., and Margolius, K. (1989). Splenectomy during primary maximal cytoreductive surgery for epithelial ovarian cancer. *Gynecol. Oncol.* 35, 301.
62. Berek, J. S., Hacker, N. F., Lagasse, L. D. *et al.* (1982). Lower urinary tract resection as part of cytoreductive surgery for ovarian cancer. *Gynecol. Oncol.* 13, 87.
63. Kapnick, S., Griffiths, C., and Finkler, N. (1990). Occult pleural involvement in stage III ovarian carcinoma: Role of diaphragm resection. *Gynecol. Oncol.* 39(2), 135.
64. National Institutes of Health Censensus Development Conference Statement. (1994). *Gynecol. Oncol.* 55, S4–S14.
65. McGowan, L., Lesher, L. P., Norris, H. J. *et al.* (1985). Mistaging of ovarian cancer. *Obstet. Gynecol.* 65, 568.
66. Mayer, A. R., Chambers, S. K., Graves, *et al.* (1992). Ovarian cancer staging: Does it require a gynecologic oncologist? *Gynecol. Oncol.* 47, 223.
67. Eisenkop, S. M., Spirtos, N. M., Montag, T. G. *et al.* (1992). The impact of subspeciality training on the management of advanced ovarian cancer. *Gynecol. Oncol.* 47, 203.
68. Nguyen, H. M., Averette, H., Hoskins, W. *et al.* (1993). National survey of ovarian carcinoma part V: The impact of physician's specialty on patients survival. *Cancer* 72(12), 3663.
69. Reich, H., McGlynn, F., and Wilkie, W. (1990). Laparoscopic management of stage I ovarian cancer: A case report. *J. Reprod. Med.* 35(6), 601.
70. Herd, J., Fowler, J., Shenson, D. *et al.* (1992). Laparoscopic para-aortic lymph node sampling: Development of a technique. *Gynecol. Oncol.* 44, 271.
71. Querleu, D. (1993). Laparoscopic paraaortic node sampling in gynecologic oncology: A preliminary experience. *Gynecol. Oncol.* 49, 24.
72. Querleu, D., and Leblanc, E. (1994). Laparoscopic infrarenal para-aortic lymph node dissection for restaging of carcinoma of the ovary or fallopian tube. *Cancer* 73, 1467–1471.
73. Childers, J. M., Lang, J., and Surwit, E. A. (1995). Laparoscopic staging of ovarian cancer. *Gynecol. Oncol.* 59, 25–33.
74. Possover, M., Krause, N., Plaul, K., Kuhne-Heid, R., and Schneider, A. (1998). Laparoscopic para-aortic and pelvic lymphadenectomy: Experience with 150 patients and review of the literature. *Gynecol. Oncol.* 71, 19.
75. Dottino, P. R., Tobias, D. H., Beddoe, A. M., Golden, A. L., and Cohen, C. J. (1999). Laparoscopic lymphadenectomy for gynecologic malignancies. *Gynecol. Oncol.* 73, 383.
76. Bagley, C. M., Young, R. C., Schein, P. S., Chabner, B. A., and DeVita,V. (1973). Ovarian carcinoma metastatic to the diaphragm frequently undiagnosed at laparotomy. *Am. J. Obstet. Gynecol.* 116, 397.
77. Rosenoff, S. H., Young, R. C., Anderson, T., Bagley, C., Chabner, B., Schein, P. S., Hubbard, S., and DeVita, V. T. (1975). Peritoneoscopy: A valuable staging tool in ovarian carcinoma. *Ann. Intern. Med.* 83, 37.
78. Ozols, R. F., Fisher, R. I., Anderson, T., Makuch, R., and Young, R. (1981). Peritoneoscopy in the management of ovarian cancer. *Am. J. Obstet. Gynecol.* 140, 611.
79. Aburustum, N. R., Barakat, R. R., Siegel, P. L., Venkatraman, E., Curtin, J. P., and Hoskins, W. J. (1996). Second-look operation for epithelial ovarian cancer: Laparoscopy or laparotomy? *Obstet. Gynecol.* 88, 549.
80. Rahaman, J., Nezhat, F., Dottino, P. *et al.* (2001). The impact of second-look laparoscopy compared to standard second-look laparotomy on recurrence and survival in advanced stage ovarian cancer. *Gynecol. Oncol.* 80(2), 326.
81. Staging of gynecologic malignancies (1994). *In* "SGO Handbook," p. 29. Society of Gynecologic Oncologists.
82. Piver, M., Barlow, J., and Lele, S. (1978). Incidence of subclinical metastasis in stage I and II ovarian carcinoma. *Obstet. Gynecol.* 52, 100.
83. Soper, J. T., Johnson, P., Johnson, V. *et al.* (1992). Comprehensive restaging laparotomy in women with apparent early ovarian carcinoma. *Obstet. Gynecol.* 80(6), 949.
84. Knapp, R., and Friedman, E. (1974). Aortic lymph node metastasis in early ovarian cancer. *Am. J. Obstet. Gynecol.* 119, 1013.
85. Delgado, G., Chun, B., Caglar, H. *et al.* (1977). Paraaortic lymphadenectomy in gynecologic malignancies confined to the pelvis. *Obstet. Gynecol.* 50(4), 418.
86. Buschbaum, H. J., Brady, M. F., Delgado, G. *et al.* (1989). Surgical staging of carcinoma of the ovaries. *Surg. Gynecol. Obstet.* 169(9), 226.
87. Rosenoff, S. H., DeVita, V. T., Hubbard, S. *et al.* (1975). Peritoneoscopy in the staging and follow-up of ovarian cancer. *Semin. Oncol.* 2(3), 223.
88. Burghardt, E., Pickel, H., Lahousen, M. *et al.* (1986). Pelvic lymphadenectomy in operative treatment of ovarian cancer. *Am. J. Obstet. Gynecol.* 155(2), 315.
89. Knipscheer, R. J. J. L. (1982). Para-aortic lymph nodes dissection in 20 cases of primary epithelial ovarian carcinoma stage I (FIGO): Influence on staging. *Eur. J. Obstet. Gynecol. Reprod. Biol.* 13, 303.

CHAPTER

32

Surgical Management of Large Ovarian Carcinoma Tumor Masses

DANIEL DARGENT
Department of Gynecology
Hopital Edouard Herriot
69437 Lyon, France

PATRICE MATHEVET
Department of Gynecology
Hopital Edouard Herriot
69437 Lyon, France

The management of a large ovarian carcinoma relies on surgical removal of the visible tumor completed by so-called adjuvant chemotherapy (NIH consensus 1994). The standard operation is total hysterectomy and bilateral salpingo-oophorectomy (TAH, BSO) to which omentectomy and systematic lymphadenectomy, both pelvic and aortic, have to be added. This standard operation fits the tumors limited to the ovary(ies) even if extended to the uterus and tubes and even if associated with omental implants. Outside these presentations (which do not correspond to a continuum in the FIGO classification) the removal of the visible tumor masses and implants necessitates additional excision. This second situation is the only one we will consider in this chapter unfolding at first the technical problems then the strategical ones.

I. TECHNICAL ASPECTS

The technical problems one meets in the extended forms of ovarian cancer are linked with the particularities of extension of this cancer.

A. The Spreading of the Common Epithelial Cancer of the Ovary; Early Involvement of the Gastrointestinal Tract

Common epithelial cancer of the ovary is unique in killing the patient while being, in the vast majority of cases, enclosed in the anatomical area where it initially developed—the peritoneal cavity. Epithelial carcinoma can spread via the lymphatic route. Even with early localized cancer, lymph node metastases are not rare in either the pelvic or the aortic areas. Hematogeneous metastases can also occur (including parenchymatous liver metastases). However, in most of the cases death is due to intraperitoneal proliferation, ascites, protein loss, and cachexia.

The extension of the common epithelial cancer to the surface of the peritoneum is a very early phenomenon. The proliferation of the carcinomatous papillas leads almost immediately to detachment, transportation, and grafting everywhere in the peritoneal cavity, to the extent that the ovarian cancer might be considered a variety of mesothelioma.

Actually malignant mesothelioma is a disease whose epidemiology, clinical behavior, and morphological characteristics are completely different from those of common epithelial cancer of the ovary. But common epithelial ovarian carcinoma is the leading member of a spectrum of diseases which can be designated as "Mullerian Papillary Serous Carcinoma" (PSC) and which includes, besides ovarian

PSC (OPSC), peritoneal PSC (PPSC), and uterine PSC. The third entity is the less common. The second one accounts for 10–20% of the total.[1] It is characterized by the fact that ovaries are not enlarged (or enlarged by benign process), the involvement of the extra-ovarian sites is greater than the involvement of the surface of either ovaries and the ovarian component, microscopically, either absent, confined to the surface, or slightly infiltrative. PPSC seems to progress more slowly than OPSC but could have the same natural history in the sense that women submitted to prophylactic oophorectomy because of a genetic risk of ovarian cancer can be affected by PPSC.

Whatever its presentation, the spread of the Mullerian PSC, either ovarian or peritoneal, follows paths determined by gravity and by the streams of peritoneal fluid. The omentum, whose appetite for raw and unusual surfaces is high, is a very early site of the spread of the disease. That is the reason why the surgery should remove the uterus, ovaries, and omentum at the same time.

Omentectomy is easy if the roots of the omentum are not infiltrated. The removal of the other involved peritoneal surfaces includes more or less difficulties depending on the topography and more precisely on the thickness of the retroperitoneal cellulo-adipose tissues. There is no problem in the parietal area (anterior abdominal wall, posterior abdominal wall, and paracolic gutters). The resection is difficult in the dorso-median area, i.e., at the bottom of the Douglas cul-de-sac, and it becomes impossible along the anterior surface of the rectum.

Peritoneal removal is impossible in every area where the retroperitoneal tissue is very thin or does not exist. That is the case for the metastatic grafts developed on the wall of the gastrointestinal tract as well as on the surface of the liver and spleen or at the top of the diaphragmatic domes.

B. Excision of the Large Pelvic Masses: The Radical Oophorectomy

Except at the bottom of the pouch of Douglas and on the anterior surface of the rectum, the retroperitoneal cellular tissue is smooth and abundant everywhere in the pelvic cavity. For this reason the complete extirpation of large ovarian carcinoma pelvic masses is almost always possible even if these masses appear fixed to the pelvic wall. The key to success is passing behind the peritoneum and, considering the peritoneum as the capsule of the tumoral masses, use the retroperitoneal space as an extracapsular plane. This makes possible an operation which appeared impossible.

This technique was first described by Hudson [2] who named it "radical oophorectomy." It starts with the opening of the pararectal spaces which frees the dorsal part of the pelvic side wall. The presacral space is opened afterward which mobilizes "*en bloc*" the pelvic organs fused by the cancerous proliferation. The next step is separating the genital organs from the bladder and the rectum. This is done using "the front to back" technique of hysterectomy described by Delle Piane.[3] The detachment of the rectum is the very last step. It is made cranialward. If it appears impossible, the part of the intestine stuck to the ovarian masses is removed. The operation gets a "modified posterior exenteration."[4]

The operation starts with the incision of the peritoneum along the pelvic brim. The round ligaments are divided. The infundibulopelvic ligaments are also divided as high as possible with mobilization of the cecum on the right side, and of the left colon on the left side. The ligaments have to be divided at the level of the termination of the vena ovarica in the vena cava on the right side and at the level of the vena renalis on the left side. Then the pararectal spaces can be opened. The ureters are identified and one progresses along the lateral surfaces of the rectum up to the pelvic floor. The lateral freeing of the tumor mass is over.

The freeing of the posterior surface of the tumor mass cannot be performed due to the fact that it is attached to the anterior wall of the rectum. One has to work at a distance and use the retrorectal or presacral space. That is very easily done while dividing the pelvic peritoneum on the right side medially to the ureter, opening the presacral space at the level of the promontory and going forward with the hand up to the coccyx. The posterior surface of the tumor mass becomes mobile (Fig. 32.1).

The "front-to-back hysterectomy" begins with a transverse incision of the pelvic peritoneum parallel to the pubis. Detaching this peritoneum from the underlying muscle is usually very easy. It can be difficult at the bottom of the vesico-uterine cul-de-sac if the tumor grafts are numerous.

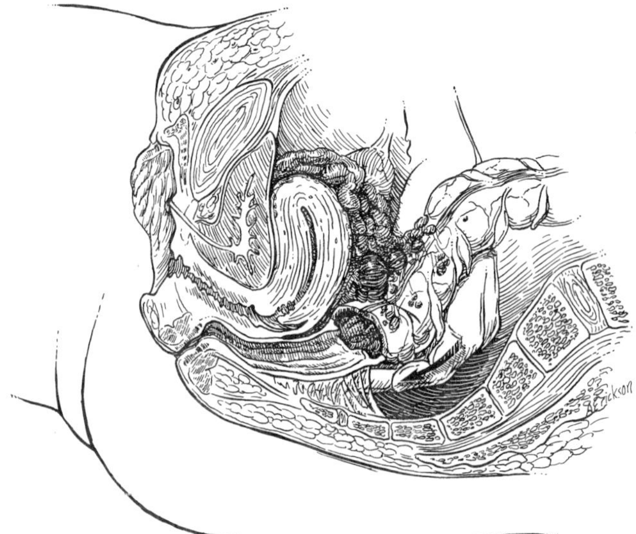

FIGURE 32.1 Hudson operation. The right hand of the surgeon slips along the posterior surface of the rectum in the presacral space which is always free of tumor involvement.

Griffiths recommends in these cases doing a cystotomy in order to identify the dissection plane with the aid of a guiding finger. It is very rare that a partial cystectomy, and even rarer that an anterior exenteration, should be done.

After detaching the bladder peritoneum, the bladder itself is mobilized caudally in the median line and the anterior surface of the vagina is exposed and then divided transversely. After opening the vaginal cavity the insertions of the cardinal ligaments are clamped at the same time as the lateral edges of the vagina. We have to use clamps of appropriate curvature (100–120°) in order not to endanger the terminal ureter whose course has to be controlled before the division of the ligaments. After the division of the ligaments the tumor mass becomes more mobile. The uterine arteries can be dissected and divided. Eisenkop *et al.* [4] recommend managing the uterine arteries and cardinal ligaments with the technique used in the Piver class 1 or 2 radical hysterectomy. This technique should be safer for ureters.

The next and last step of the retrograde hysterectomy is dividing the posterior surface of the vagina at the level of its insertion on the cervix uteri. The uterosacral ligaments have to be previously clamped and divided. A consecutive mobilization of the mass facilitates the following steps. After the sectioning of the vagina, the last thing is dividing the fascia of Denonvilliers which covers the posterior surface of the vagina (Fig. 32.2). This last section opens the space situated between the external face of the peritoneal cul-de-sac and the anterior surface of the rectum—it is the space to enter in order to attempt the separation between the tumor mass and the intestinal wall.

After carrying out all the previous divisions, the tumor block (adnexa, pelvic peritoneum, and uterus) is removed from the pelvis. The last adhesion, the adhesion to the rectum, can thus be treated more readily. It has to be treated from the bottom to the top using the fine Metzenbaum scissors. The external longitudinal layer of the rectal wall can be entered. But, if the circular layer is entered and the mucosa evidenced and, even more, opened, then performing a typical intestinal resection is, both from the surgical and oncological point of view, better than making an atypical stripping of the mucularis followed by an atypical suture of it.

When making the decision to perform an intestinal resection the rectal ampulla has to be prepared at 2–5 cm from the inferior pole of the tumoral attachment. This preparation is done from front to back—the rectal wall is bared while dividing, after dissection and clamping, all the vessels arriving obliquely at the surface of it. The dorsal vessels are the most developed.

After preparation, the rectal ampulla is clamped and divided (Fig. 32.3). The tumor block is now entirely free, being attached to the body only by the continuity of the left colon. The superior rectal vessels are prepared, clamped, and divided at their very beginning. The sigmoid vessels are also divided, taking into account the tumor extension. Then the colon is, at the right place, prepared, clamped, and divided. The resection is over.

The reconstruction of the bowel is always (or almost always) possible. As a matter of fact, the division of the rectum is done, even in the worse cases, at a long distance from the anus (8–10 cm), and it is always possible to pull down the lower extremity of the left colon (using, if necessary,

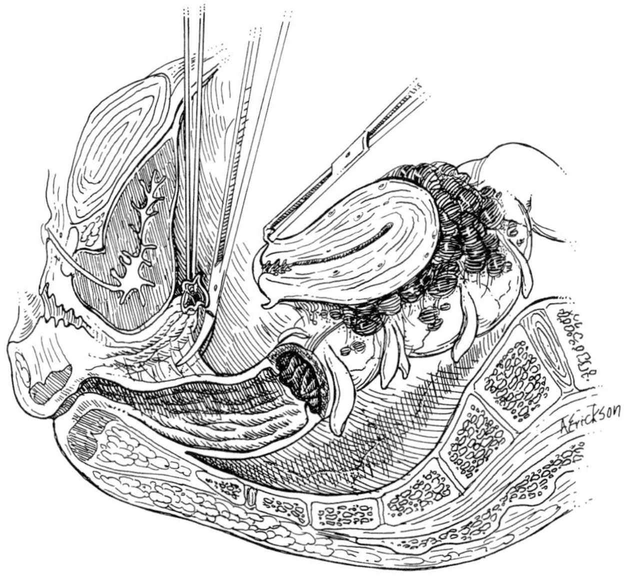

FIGURE 32.2 Hudson operation. After the hysterectomy performed from front to back, the surgeon trys to detach the inferior pole of tumor masses from the anterior surface of the rectum with scissors.

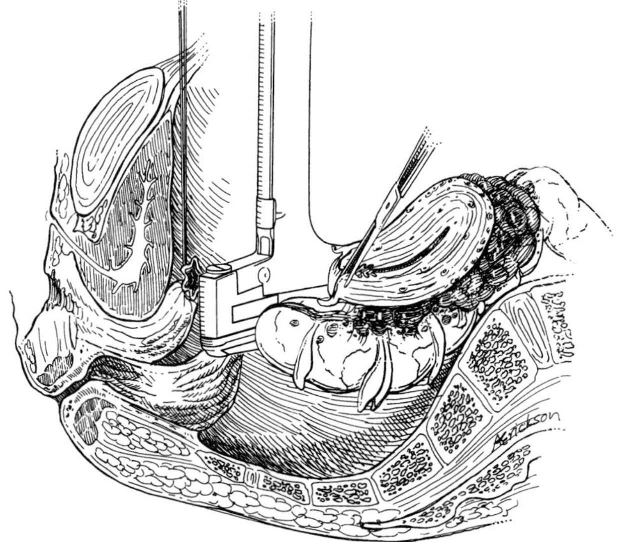

FIGURE 32.3 Hudson operation. If tumor masses are impossible to detach from the anterior surface of the rectum, the decision is made to do a resection. The rectum is divided using a stapler (TA 55® or similar device).

a large mobilization of the splenic curve). The indications to the terminal colostomy (Hartmann operation) are more than rare. The end-to-end anastomosis is done in almost all cases.

The intestinal anastomosis can be an end-to-end anastomosis done with a continuous suture of dexon. The contemporary surgeons have a preference for mechanical sutures and use the TA® stapler for clamping and suture of the rectal stump (Fig. 32.3) and then, through the staper line, do a sort of lateroterminal suture using the PCEEA® stapler (Fig. 32.4). Whichever technique is used, the permeability and the cohesion of the suture have to be assessed using a retrograde insufflation. The protective colostomy, in nonpreviously irradiated patients, is useless. Omental wrap and protective colostomy are recommended in irradiated patients. Suction drainage is mandatory.

The data concerning radical oophorectomy show that this surgery is in the same time feasible and efficient.[5–9] The study provided by Scarabelli [9] is the most informative because it relates to the cases only where the procedure was used with no additional visceral excision. In a series of 66 patients the rate of pre- and postoperative complications were low: 2 vessels injuries, 2 cystostomies, 3 severe hemorrhage (blood loss >1000), 10 prolonged ileus (more than 10 days), no anastomotic leackage, and one pulmonary embolism (32 days after the surgery). No postoperative death occurred. The median follow-up was 26 months. The estimated 2- and 5-year survival rates were 100% and 42.2%, respectively, for patients with no abdominal residual disease (24 out of 66) and 77.3 and 21.3%, respectively, for patients with abdominal residual disease less than 1 cm (28 out of 66). No patient with residual disease more than 1 cm was alive 2 years after surgery.

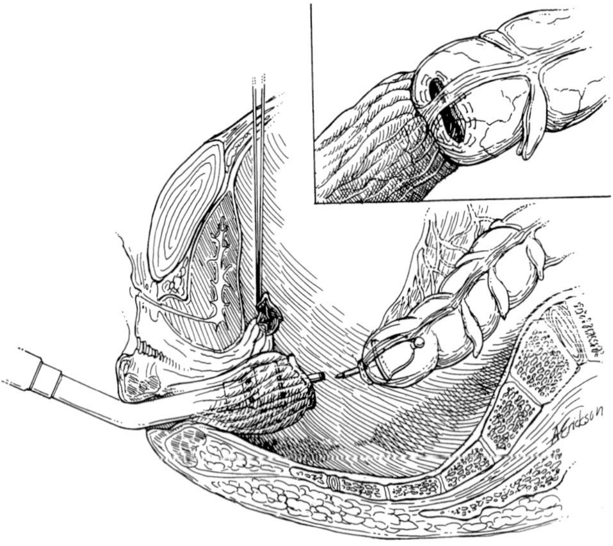

FIGURE 32.4 Hudson operation. If the recto-sigmoid junction has been resected, the low colo-rectal suture is made using an automatic circular stapler.

C. Removal and Destruction of the Peritoneal Implants

Peritoneal implants associated with ovarian cancer can either be removed or destroyed using ultrasonic aspiration argon beam destruction or loop electrosurgical excisions. If the implants are few, small destruction is the method of choice. If they are large the technique to choose depends to the topography.

Peritoneal implants developed onto the abdominal peritoneum and, to a certain extent, onto the diaphragmatic domes, can be removed by sharp striping. As far as the abdominal peritoneum, it is easy starting from the edge of the midline incision, to detach the peritoneum from the underlying abdominal muscles, then, to mobilize the colon in order to join the infundibulopelvic ligaments and divide them at the appropriate level before detaching the peritoneum covering the iliac area and going on with the pelvic step of the operation. As far as the diaphragm is concerned, the right side is the most commonly affected, and at the same time it is the most difficult to approach as sectioning of the triangular ligament and toppling of the liver have to be carried out. With the retroperitoneal cellular tissue being very thin, a muscular resection cannot be avoided in some patients. Tumor implants more than 5 cm large generally penetrate the muscle.[10]

For the implants penetrating the diaphragmatic muscle and for the implants developed on the capsule of Glisson, on the mesenteric and/on every surface where their number and volume precludes excision and repair, destructive tools can be elected. The Cavitron ultrasonic surgical aspirator (CUSA) has been advocated since the late 1980s.[11] This tool enables a rather selective destruction of the tumoral tissue which is more easily destroyed than the surrounding sound tissues because of its higher water content. However, the use of the CUSA seems to increase the chances for disseminated intravascular coagulation: 5 cases in about 19 operations versus 0 in about 14 in the Donovan series.[12] The mechanism of this induced coagulopathy could be more extensive endothelial cell trauma, collagen exposure, and release of thromboplastin from cellular fragmentation. On the other hand, in the retrospective case control study of Sert [13] the use of CUSA while not increasing the rate of complications (including severe hemorrhage) and improving the rate of optimal cytoreduction (69 versus 16%), did not increase the survival time of the patient. This will be discussed again in Section II. Tools other than CUSA seem to be equivalently efficient while less expansive and less expertise demanding. Lasers are not recommended because of the hazards they include both for the surgical team and for the patient (lack of control of the depth of destruction). Argon beam coagulation seems to be more appropriate.[14–16] Loop electrosurgical excision has the advantage of being mastered by all the gynecologists. It is likely to provide the same excellent results as CUSA (85% of reduction to no gross residual tissues in a series of

20 patients not optimally cytoreduced using the conventional instrumentation in the study by Fanning and Higers).[17]

Whatever the elected tool, destruction of the peritoneal implants is only possible if they are not too large and not penetrating the underlaying structures too deeply (two characteristics which are generally linked to each other). For the large implants whose destruction is theoretically the more interesting (see Section I.C) surgical resection is the only solution which includes the necessity of additional visceral excision.

D. Additional Visceral Excision

Outside the excision of the rectum which is often part of the radical oophorectomy, other excision of the intestine can appear necessary. The resection of the ileocecal junction or the right hemicolectomy is the most often performed adjunctive procedure (involvement of the intestinal wall at the contact of a massive infiltration of the omentum and/or gastrocolic ligament) and the left hemicolecotmy (spread of the tumor grafts lying in the left paracolic gutter) can also be considered. These procedures and even the total colectomy are not difficult to perform for the trained oncologic gynecologist (the pelvic procedure is much more difficult to perform). The ileectomies (involvement of ileal serosa and/or ileal mesentery) are also very easy to do. But the problem is recovery. One knows that very extensive intestinal resections may be done (50 cm of jejunum are enough if half of the colon is left in place and 150 cm if the colon has to be entirely resected). But the delay of total recovery is long (1–6 months of parenteral nursing depending on the length of the bowel) and poorly compatible with a dose-effective prompt chemotherapy.

Splenectomy and hepatectomy are very disputable additonal excisions. Splenectomy is perfectly accepted as treatment of the isolated splenic metastasis and even more if this event occurs at a distance from the initial treatment.[18–22] It can be performed using the hand-assisted laparoscopic approach.[22] Conversely splenectomy as part of the primary debulking is not usually accepted.[23–26] Partial hepatectomy is not often discussed. It is not often feasible due to the number and/or volume of the mestastases. In the Ucla series [30] 6 of 37 patients with liver metastases underwent sucessfull cytoreduction (both hepatic and extrahepatic lesions). The median survival was 50.1 months compared to 27 months for the 11 patients with optimal extrahepatic debulking and 7.6 months for the 20 patients suboptimally debulked both for the extrahepatic and hepatic lesions.

The feasability of the plurivisceral excision surgery is illustrated by a lot of recent papers.[27] Thanks to this heroic surgery the rate of optimal debulking which is between 25 and 55% in the general literature increases to more than 90%. However, the rate of complication is rather high including bleeding, with or without coagulopathy, bowel obstruction, and prolonged ileus (this may be linked to the lymphadenectomy), dehiscence of the wound, cardiac failure, bacteriemia, renal failures, and deep vein thrombosis. The postoperative casualities are 2 in about 30 in the Guidozzi and Ball series,[29] 3 in about 139 in the Eisenkop article,[30] and 2 in about 152 in the Michel series.[31] The rate of re-operation can be as high as 25%.[31] Major complications with or without re-operation can lead to a delay in the onset of adjuvant chemotherapy of which it has to be started less than 14 days after the surgery in order to prevent the regrowth of the disease.[32]

II. STRATEGICAL PROBLEMS

Management strategy, dealing with the extended forms of ovarian cancer, asks two questions: How to perform the surgery itself and how to combine it with the chemotherapy?

A. The Concept of Debulking Surgery

Complete removal of the tumor remains the gold standard in surgical oncology. In the forms of the ovarian cancer we are dealing with in this chapter, such a removal is not always possible or cannot be reached without excessively destructive surgery. An alternative to the complete removal is the so-called debulking or cytoreductive surgery combined with chemotherapy.

The concept of debulking surgery developed at the time chemotherapy was proposed as an effective, less toxic, and cheaper alternative to radiotherapy. As a matter of fact, debulking surgery's first goal is the inhibition of the vicious circle of malnutrition (nausea, vomiting, dyspepsia, and carcinomatous ileus due to the infiltration of the gastrointestinal tract and its mesentery). But debulking also has a curative aspect. If the tumor is very large, the time the antiblastic treatment needs to kill the last cell can be very long. On the other hand, as stressed by Griffiths, the growth fraction, i.e., the part of the tumor which is sensitive to the action of the cytotoxics is in the large tumors, less than in the small tumors. These are the reasons why debulking enhances the efficiency of the chemotherapy. The data of Griffiths [33] confirm the theory: the survival curve of the patients whose largest residual mass size was, after surgery, below the 1.5-cm limit is the same at the curve of the patients whose large metastatic lesions were below the 1.5-cm limit at the outset.

An important point concerning the debulking surgery is assessing the quantity of tumor residue starting from where the effect of debulking surgery is not effective anymore. This question has been adressed many times. The GOG protocol 97 [34] gives the answer. Patients affected by stage III ovarian cancer and submitted, after a suboptimal surgery, to platinum-based chemotherapy had a significantly improved survival if the tumor residue was less than 2 cm compared to the patients whose tumor residue was more than 2 cm. But no differences existed between the patients whose tumor residue was 2–4 cm,

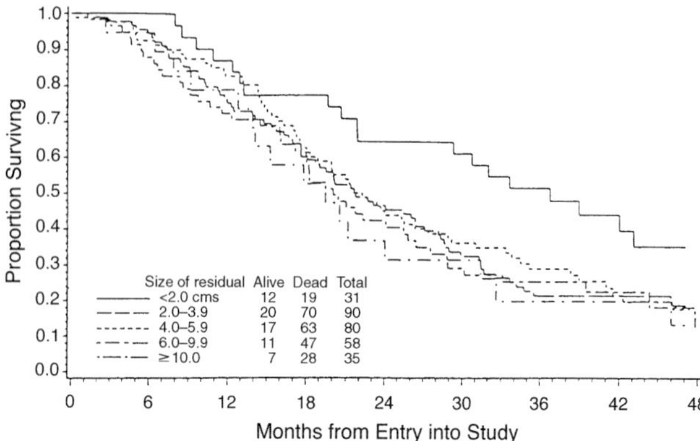

FIGURE 32.5 Survival by maximum diameter of residual disease in a reanalysis of GOG Protocol 97 by Hoskins et al. (From Hoskins, W. J. *et al.* (1992). *Gynecol. Oncol.* 47, 159–166. With permission.)

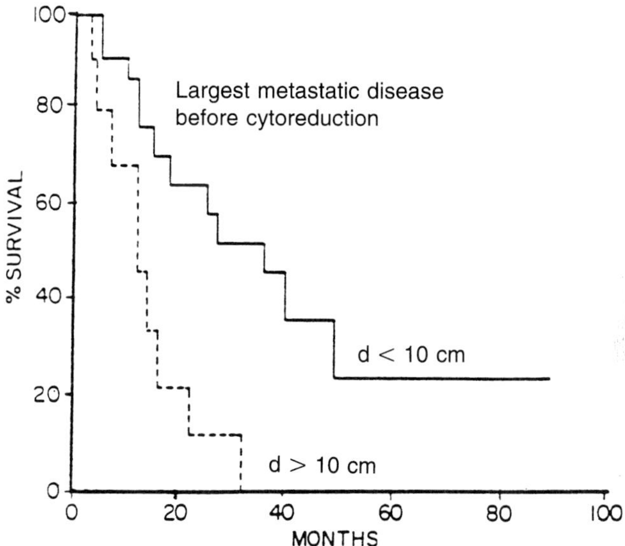

FIGURE 32.6 Chances of survival after primary optimal debulking, depending on the diameter of the largest metastatic disease.[42]

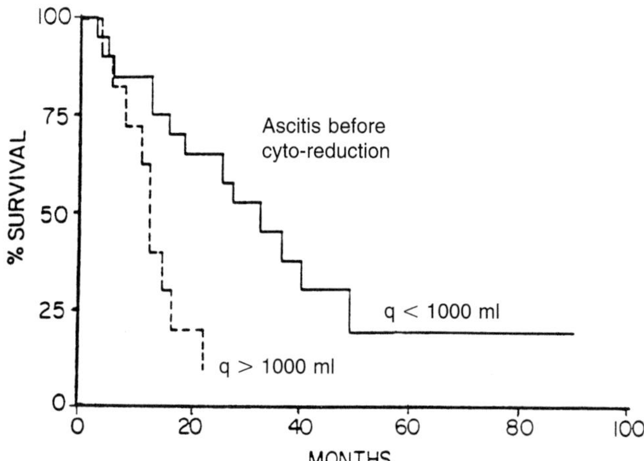

FIGURE 32.7 Chances of survival after primary optimal debulking, depending on the presence of ascites.[42]

4–6 cm, 6–10 cm, or more than 10 cm (Fig. 32.5). One can conclude that debulking surgery has no proven benefit if it cannot reduce the tumor implants to less than 2 cm.

Another conceptual dilemma concerns the role of preoperative status. First, opposite from the seminal data provided by Griffiths, it seems that the patients who are affected by large-volume disease even if cytoreduced to less than 1 cm, have a shorter recurrence-free time and global survival than the patients found at first exploration to have extrapelvic disease 1 cm or less. This was demonstrated by the GOG protocol 52.[35] Hacker, Berek, and Lagasse [36] had already shown that no patient could be salvaged by optimal cytoreduction if the largest metastatic disease had, before the cytoreductive surgery, a diameter more than 10 cm (Fig. 32.6.) and/or if an ascites more than 1000 ml existed (Fig. 32.7). That means that the concept "small is chemosensitive" is an oversimplified concept.

From the biological viewpoint one knows that the growth curve of experimental tumors is asymptotic at its two extremities, meaning that in very small tumors, as in the very big ones, the growth fraction, i.e., the chemosensitive fraction, is reduced. Another phenomenon is that drug-resistant tumor phenotypes can develop at any time as a result of a spontaneous or induced mutation. The risk of mutation is a direct function of the number of mitoses. That means that the biggest tumors, generally the result of a faster growth index, are the richest in drug-resistant phenotypes (this concept advocated by Goldie and Coldman [37] is illustrated by the molecular biology: p53 mutation and loss of heterozygoty are more frequent in the largest tumors), which obviously remain in the postsurgical residue and will be a source of recurrence whatever the size of the residue.

From the practical viewpoint, the meta-analysis performed in 1991 by Hunter,[38] confirms the doubts about the usefulness of debulking surgery. This meta-analysis included 58 publications encompassing 6962 patients submitted randomly to various regimens of adjuvant chemotherapy after primary debulking. The overall median survival and the proportion of patients undergoing maximum cytoreduction (mostly postsurgical tumor residue less than 2 cm) were known in all series. If maximum cytoreductive surgery is responsible for improving the prognosis, the median survival of the whole group should be greater in those series containing a high percentage of patients undergoing maximum cytoreductive surgery.

The addition of all the published data is likely to show that there is an association between the percentage of maximum cytoreductive surgery and median survival time (Fig. 32.8). Each 10-point increase in the percentage of maximum cytoreductive surgery is associated with an estimated 16.3% increase

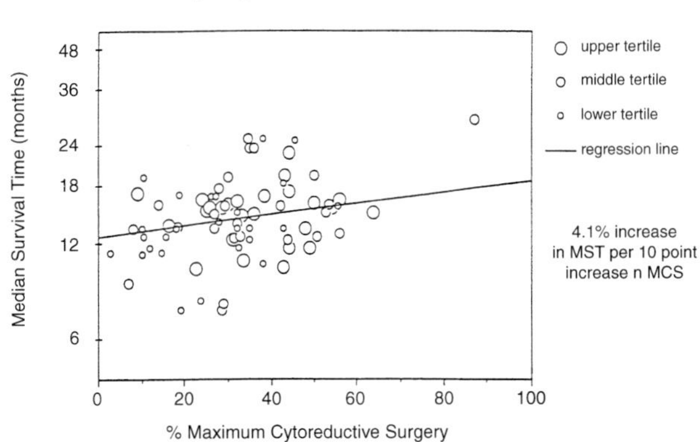

FIGURE 32.8 Median survival time and percent of maximum cytoreductive surgery. Metanalysis of 76 cohorts. Adjustment for effect of dose intensity, percent stage IV and platinum chemotherapy.[42]

in median survival time (+10.4 to −22.5%). But if a correction is done taking into account the percentage of stage IV, the use of platinum, and the dose intensity of chemotherapy, the 10-point increase in percent maximum surgery leads to an only 4.1% increase in median survival time. The 95% confidence interval is −0.63 to +9.1%. The difference is not significant (and it becomes less significant if, in the studies including more than 1 cohort, the only largest cohort is taken into account −2.5 to +8.1%). One has to conclude, with the authors, that cytoreductive surgery probably has only a small effect on the survival of women with advanced ovarian cancer. The type of chemotherapy used is more important.

Only a randomized trial comparing cytoreduction to no cytoreduction would provide an unequivocal answer to the question of the usefulness of debulking surgery. Such a trial never will be performed. Actually we do not have first level evidence enabling us to state that cytoreduction benefits all patients, we cannot deny it to them because we know "it can, for some of them, undoubtedly prolong survival."[39] The question is finally appropriately choosing the candidates, respecting the rules of a comprehensive surgery, and making as efficient as possible the combination of cytoreductive surgery and cytotoxic medical treatement.

B. The Practice of Debulking Surgery

Debulking surgery is only acceptable if it reduces all tumor implants to less than 2 cm. If some of them, developed in the upper abdomen, appear nonreduceable to such a dimension debulking surgery has to be dismissed. Conversely, if tumor implants less than 2 cm are present either in the upper or lower abdomen whose complete removal necessitates a plurivisceral excision, such a heroic surgery is not indicated, for the adjuvant chemotherapy theoretically is able to destroy these implants. This illustrates the necessity of a careful predecisional evaluation. Ideally the "undebulkability" should be forecast by the preoperative workup including plasmatic CA125 measurement and imaging.

As far as CA125 is concerned, Geisler *et al.* [40] reported that the mean initial CA125 level was 966 UI/ml in patients whose implants reduced to less than 2 cm tumor residue versus 3316 for other patients. Chi *et al.* [41] confirm that the probability of performing optimal cytoreduction decreased with increasing CA125 levels. With a CA125 less than 500 UI/ml 73% of the patients could be reduced to less than 1-cm tumor residues versus 22% for the patients with the CA125 level more than 500 UI/ml. As pointed out by Bereck [42] this threshold should be hightened to 1000 UI/ml, for the percentage of optimal debulking in the series of Chi was only 45% as it is higher in most of the recent published series which implicate that patients with a larger tumor bulk (and a higher CA125 level) can be optimally reduced.

The predictive value of a CT scan for ovarian cancer resectability is poorly documented. One knows that the sensitivity varies between 30 and 80% and the specificity between 80 and 100% in the detection of tumor residues after completion of surgery and adjuvant chemotherapy.[43–48] Actually the accuracy depends on the topography of the tumor implants (omentum, mesentery, diaphragm) and, obviously, on their diameter. As far as resectability is concerned the criteria depends on the philosophy and skills of the surgeon. If one takes into consideration the results collected in the same surgical context the number of patients considered falsely as inoperable is 6 in about 42 for Nelson [49] and 2 in about 42 in the article by Taieb.[50] It was 6 about 42 in a first series of Forstner,[51] but it can go down to zero.[52] Conversely the number of patients falsely considered as inoperable which is low in the first series (1 in about 13—Nelson—and 2 in about 23, Taieb) is high in the other ones (5 about 12—Meyer—and 3 about 6, Forstner). The main source of errors is the assessment of the diaphragmatic domes in the absence of ascities. MRI could have a better sensitivity (with less specificity). FDG positron emission tomography (FDG PET scan) could be a better tool as far as sensitivity is concerned.[54–55]

Adding laparoscopy to CA125 measurements and imaging is the last refinement in the predecisional workup. Vergote [56] was the first one to propose using laparoscopy in order to assess the resectability of extended ovarian cancer. In his series, 77 patients underwent open laparoscopy. In the subgroup of 31 patients who were estimated operable, a primary debulking surgery to less than 0.5-cm residual mass was feasible in 79% of the cases. The 46 other patients were submitted to neo-adjuvant chemotherapy. This predecisional laparoscopy does not jeopardize the chances for cure at the condition it is performed using the open technique. In a series of 104 patients [57] abdominal wall metastasis occurred in 9 (9%). In 12 cases the laparoscopy was carried out using the classical blunt procedure: 7 trocar sites with implantation metastasis (58%). In the remaining 92 patients an open laparoscopy was performed: 2 trocar sites with implantation metastasis (2%). The difference is attributed to the careful closure of the peritoneum, rectus abdominalis sheath, and skin which is performed in the second technique and not in the first one. At the condition of excising the trocar sites if cytoreductive surgery is undertaken immediately or, if neoadjuvant chemotherapy is given it as soon as possible, the open laparoscopy appears to be a safe procedure in patients with disseminated ovarian cancer. Nevertheless some limitations do exist. The assessment of the retrogastric cavity, of the deepest part of the mesenterium and, even more important, of the dorsal part of the right diaphragmatic dome is not possible. Therefore some patients will go on being submitted to a purely explorative laparotomy even if the predecisional workup, including the open laparoscopy, leads to seeing the debulking as possible.

The inaugural procedure must be then standardized. The laparotomy has to be drawn on the midline astride the umbilicus. After aspiration of the ascites or washing of the peritoneum and collection of the fluid (one sample in each of the four quadrants), the hand is introduced in the abdominal cavity. The upper abdomen is assessed at first. If tumor bulk is detected on the right-side diaphragmatic dome the falciform ligament is transected and the liver is toppled. If the tumor implants appear undebulkable the procedure is dismissed. The same if liver metastasis forcing unbearable sacrifices are present. The same as well if undebulkable lesions are present at the level of the gastrohepatic omentum either at the contact of the portal trial, at the contact of the pancreas, or at the contact of the stomach and/or the spleen. Large tumor plates located on the mesenterium are other contra-indications to further attempt debulking. As far as the other abdominal implants are concerned excision or surrender are a matter of debate. Everyone admits that tumor bulk developed on the omentum must be removed if it is possible to detach it from the intestine. If a partial colectomy is necessary (transverse colon, ileocecal junction, sigmoid loop) some surgeons do it [28–31] and others do not.[56–58] Total colectomy itself is acceptable provided it is not associated with a large ileectomy (as a matter of fact the rectum being generally preserved a restoration of the intestinal continuity can be made without excessive disability provided the ileon is long enough). Stripping of the peritoneum on the anterior abdominal wall and/or in the paracolic gutters is admitted by everybody. Finally it is only in the cases where abdominal lesions are less than 2 cm or can be reduced to less than 2 cm that pelvic debulking has to be attempted. It generally succeeds if the procedure described above (radical oophorectomy) is followed.

C. Primary and Secondary Debulking

Many biological and clinical arguments favor the concept of primary debulking surgery (see previous section). However, the cost-effectiveness of primary debulking surgery is prohibitive in an important number of cases. These patients are sent directly to chemotherapy. The response to chemotherapy can be clinically and even anatomically complete. However, in most of the cases the response is only partial. Progression and no response are not rare instances. On the other hand, one knows that even in the optimally cytoreduced patients recurrences can occur. These recurrences, of course, are even more frequent in the case of suboptimal cytoreduction. Persistent and/or recurrent disease question the effort of the secondary surgery done at the time of the so-called "second-look laparotomy." This second-look laparotomy and even moreso the second debulking attempted at this occasion are controversial.

The second-look laparotomy was introduced in the 1960s as a procedure enabling the assessment of the peritoneal cavity in cases of clinically complete remission after adjuvant chemotherapy. It is beyond the scope of this chapter to describe how the procedure is carried out in the cases where the apparently complete response is confirmed at open abdomen (or with the laparoscope which today tends to replace the laparotomy). We remember that in cases of complete anatomical response (no tumor cells in the multiple biopsies) recurrences occur in about 50% of the cases. Conversely, if unforeseable tumor implants are in evidence, the most common opinion is that no valuable solution can be offered to these patients. No efficient second-line chemotherapy exists and the second surgical effort is hopeless. But there are new drugs (topotecan, doxorubicin, taxotere, gemcitabine) and new protocols (intraperitoneal chemotherapy and intraperitoneal chemohyperthermia) available. They can be proposed to the patients found with microscopic residue. For the patient found with macroscopic residue the debulking is to be considered. Many retrospective surveys and one prospective and randomized assay [59] show there is no significant difference between the survival of patients who undergo second-look laparotomy and patients who did not. The cost-effectiveness of secondary debulking is disputable. The rate of postoperative complications varies between 11 and 67% [60] depending of the aggressiveness of the secondary ablative surgery, and not all patients submitted to this more or less aggressive surgery benefit from it. We know that some of them do. The challenge is identifying this subgroup of patients.

Actually 40% of patients submitted to second-look laparotomy will have macroscopic disease detected. Among them 40% are able to undergo complete resection (no macroscopic residual tumor), 30% are able to be partially but optimally debulked (residual disease less than 2 cm), and 30% are left with bulky residual disease. Most of the studies [61–63] demonstrate that the cytoreduced patients take advantage of this cytoreduction. This advantage is dependent on the amount of residual disease. Other studies [64–67] show that the benefit only exists if the macroscopic residual disease is zero. There is an agreement about the fact that patients reduced to only microscopic disease have the same prognosis as patients found with microscopic disease at the beginning of the second-look laparotomy, i.e., around 50% of 5-year survival. Other factors influence the result of the secondary debulking including the amount of initial tumor bulk, the amount of tumor residue left after the first surgical effort, and if the grade of the tumor after secondary surgery had the same value they had initially. Interestingly enough the aggressiveness of the first surgical effort is likely to play a sort of paradoxical negative role. In the article by Eisenkop,[68] where the rate of optimal debulking (no tumor residue more than 1 cm) after the first surgery was 100% and the rate of complete debulking (no visible residual disease) was 84%, 78 patients underwent second-look laparotomy. Among these 78 patients 15 were found to have macroscopically visible tumor residue. Ten of them were cytoreduced to a macroscpically disease-free state and five were not. No difference in survival was observed between the two subgroups. It is important to point that 11 of the 15 patients found to have macroscopically visible residue had resection of all visible disease at their primary operation. These data, in the same time they demonstrate the high value of an agressive primary surgery (in a series published later by the same group only 8 in about 151 (5.3%) patients had persistent disease in the pelvis) clearly illustrate that tumor aggressiveness and lack of chemosensibility are preeminent factors in prognosis. Finally a good candidate for secondary debulking is a patient with a moderate initial tumor bulk and low or intermediate histologic grade who did not receive an optimal debulking at first surgery and is apparently free of disease after the adjuvant chemotherapy, but is found with some residue at second-look laparotomy which can be reduced to no visible tumor.

Another field of application for secondary surgery is recurrent disease. Chemosensitivity is once again the best predictor of success in debulking surgery applied to recurrent disease. As a matter of fact the longer the interval between the initial treatment and the relapse the better are the chances for success. This rate can be as high as 77% of clinical complete response and 32% of anatomical complete response in patients recurring more than 24 months after the initial optimal treatment.[70] Vaccarello [71] confirmed that patients reduced to small or no residual disease for recurrent cancer had a significant survival benefit. These results are obviously linked to the surgical cytoreduction. However, it is significant that they are obtained using the same systemic chemotherapy or an intraperitoneal chemotherapy [72] using the same drugs which were used for the primary and, apparently successful, treatment. This could be interpreted as a consequence of the good chemosensitivity of the dormant cells left after the initial treatment. However, studies using molecular biologic techniques are likely to illustrate that recurrent cancer is in most of the instances of a different nature. Buller *et al.* [73] compared molecular genetic fingerprints of 13 paired primary and late (28–62 months) "recurrent" cancer. The fingerprints of 3 tumor pairs were identical but the allelotypes of the 10 other pairs were different, suggesting that the recurrent cancer actually was a second primary. In recurrent cancer being considered as the consequence of reproliferation of dormant cells or as expression of a "field cancerization" the attempt to debulk it as completely as possible is recommended.

D. Intervention Debulking

The intervention or interval cytoreductive surgery could be the answer to the question asked in the previous section: How aggressive should the initial debulking be? In case of suboptimal debulking does the surgical effort done after chemotherapy make sense? If yes, at what time must it be scheduled—after three courses, after six courses? At the time of clinically obvious recurrence? And is there a place for laparoscopy in the different steps of the management?

The trial carried out by the European Association for Research and Treatment of Cancer [74] in 1998 afforded the first data in this field. The patients included were affected by stage IIB–IV epithelial ovarian cancer who underwent primary cytoreductive surgery with suboptimal tumor residue. Three cycles of cisplatin (75 mg/m^2) and cyclophosphamide (750 mg/m^2) were given at 3-week intervals. The 319 patients with complete response, partial response, or stable disease were randomized either to "interval debulking surgery" (140 patients) or no surgery (58 patients). The median survival with no surgery arm was 20 months versus 19.4 months for the patients found after intervention surgery to have bulky disease and were not reduced, 26.6 months for the patients who were debulked to optimal status (less than 1 cm), and 41.6 months for the patients who were not to be debulked because they were found with either no macroscopic tumor residue or small-volume (less than 1 cm) residue. The intervention debulking clearly benefits the patients who has residual tumor bulk and who can be optimally reduced—they get the same chances of survival as the patients who had been given an optimal debulking at the time of the initial surgery. This was already shown in 1996 by a Dutch group.[75] It had been confirmed recently by other groups.

Most of the published series [58, 76–81] only illustrate the feasability of interval debulking surgery and demonstrate that it increases the rate of optimal debulking while reducing the peri-operative casualities and complications. In the French cooperative study [81] 54 patients affected by stage IIIC or IV epithelial cancer deemed impossible to reduce optimally at the first staging procedure were submitted to primary chemotherapy. The first staging procedure was laparoscopy in 33 patients (61%) and a laparotomy in 21 patients (39%). The median number of chemotherapy cycles was 4. Eight patients progressed during chemotherapy and were not re-operated on. Forty-six patients apparently responded and were submitted to intervention procedures among which three were not debulked at all and four were suboptimally debulked. Among the 39 patients who were optimally debulked, 32 were debulked at the price of the only "standard" procedure, i.e., TAH, BSO, infracolic omentectomy, and systematic pelvic, and aortic lymphadenectomy. As a consequence 22 patients were spared blood transfusion and no intensive care unit stay was necessary for the 39 optimally debulked patients. The patients were included between Janurary 1996 and March 1999. At the end point the medial overall survival was 22 months for these patients who where deemed undebulkable at the first staging procedure.

Vergote [56] compared 112 patients with stage III or IV ovarian cancer treated between 1980 and 1988 and 173 patients treated between 1989 and 1997. During the first period all patients underwent primary debulking surgery (cytoreduction to less than 0.5 cm in 82% of the cases) and adjuvant chemotherapy. During the second period the patients were, after surgical evaluation, either submitted to primary chemotherapy (43%) or to primary debulking surgery (57%). The postoperative mortality was 6.2% during the first period and 0% during the second one. The 3-year crude survival rates were 26%±4.3 and 42%±4.6 ($p=0.0001$), respectively.

As convincing as the data of Vergote are, they cannot definitely reverse the current opinion favoring primary debulking. Eisenkop, Spirtos, and Freedman stress it in a letter to the editor published [82] after the publication of Schwarz.[58] We absolutely need a randomized prospective assay. Such an assay is underway under the aegis of OERTC.[83] All stage IIIC and IV patients will be included. Knowing that some of them will progress under primary chemotherapy (in the French cooperative study 8 patients in about 54 did it and 3 died before the completion of the scheduled chemotherapy) it seems more ethical including only the patients who are surely risky candidates for primary debulking. The criteria of undebulkability proposed by Nelson [49] remain valuable: omentum implants developed at the contact of the spleen and implants more than 2 cm developed in the root of the mesentery at the contact of the superior mesenteric artery, in the liver or on the capsule of Glisson, on the diaphragmatic dome, on the gallbladder, in the suprarenal lymph nodes, and on the pericardic or on the pleural serosa. Vergote added volumetric criteria: estimated tumor load superior to 1000 g, uncontrollable—more than 100—peritoneal metastases and ascites of more than 5 liters.

III. CONCLUSION: HOW TO OPERATE ON THE PATIENTS AFFECTED BY EXTENDED OVARIAN CANCER AND WHO SHOULD DO IT ?

Until the moment the results of the ongoing prospective and randomized assay are released, it seems premature to renounce primary debulking of extended ovarian cancer. However, the preliminary data we have at our disposal are convincing enough to move to primary chemotherapy and intervention cytoreductive surgery in the cases where the primary optimal debulking cannot be obtained without excessive sacrifices. The criteria of inoperability have been listed previously. From a practical viewpoint an unofficial agreement exists for limiting the indications of primary debulking to the cases where it can be obtained at the price of the "standard operation," i.e., TAH, BSO, infracolic omentectomy, and pelvic and aortic lymphadenectomy while adding peritoneal stripping in the no-risk areas and/or peritoneal implant destruction in all areas they can develop at the condition they are not too deeply infiltrative. Whether or not excision of the rectum is part of the standard operation is a matter of debate. Our answer is yes. However, the "radical oophorectomy," which includes in most of the cases, rectal resection and immediate reconstruction is an operation reserved for skilled surgeons. This asks for important question of who should operate on these patients.

Surveys concerning the qualification of the surgeon who takes charge of ovarian cancer [84–86] demonstrate that the chances for survival are, at different levels, better if he or she is a gynecologic oncologist. The Scottish National Study [87] includes 1866 patients diagnosed in 1987, 1992, and 1994. No significant differences have been observed for patients with stage I, II, and IV. For stage III (44% of the cases) a 25% reduction of the rate of dying (relative hazard ratio: 0.75, $p=0.005$) was observed in the patients operated on by specialist gynecologists when compared to the patients operated on by general gynecologists. Specialist gynecologists, more often, debulked the tumor to less than 2 cm but even for the tumor left with residues more than 2 cm the survival was higher for patients treated by specialist gynecologists (Fig. 32.9).

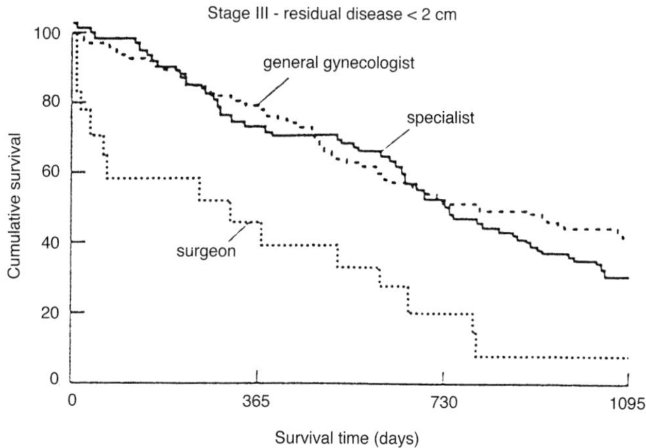

FIGURE 32.9 Kaplan-Meier survival curves in the management of stage III ovarian cancer by the speciality of the person performing the initial surgery. (From Junor, E. J. *et al.* (1999). *Br. J. Obstet. Gynaecol.* 106, 1130–1136. With permission.)

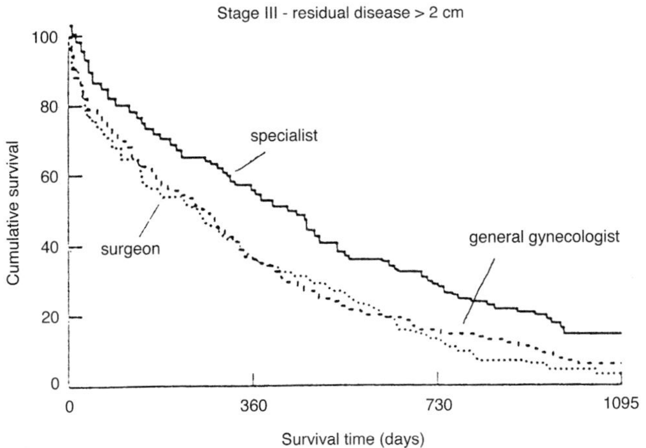

FIGURE 32.9 *(Continued)*

References

1. B. Piura, M. Meirovitz, M. Bartfeld *et al.* (1998). Peritoneal papillary serous carcinoma: Study of 15 cases and comparison with stage III-IV ovarian papillary serous carcinoma. *J. Surg. Oncol.* 68, 173–78.
2. C. N. Hudson (1968). A radical operation for fixed ovarian tumors. *J. Obstet. Gynaecol. Br. Cwlth* 75, 1155–1160.
3. G. Delle Piane (1967). Surgery in the modern treatment of ovarian carcinoma. 5th World Congress of Gynecology and Obstetrics. Sydney, Australia, pp. 473–496. Butterworth, Stoneham, MA.
4. S. M. Eisenkop, R. M. Nalik, and N. Teng (1991). Modified posterior exenteration for ovarian cancer. *Obstet. Gynecol.* 78, 879–885.
5. P. Benedetti-Panici, F. Maneschi, G. Scambia *et al.* (1996). The pelvic retroperitoneal approach in the treatment of advanced ovarian carcinoma. *Obstet. Gynecol.* 87, 532–538.
6. W. Barnes, J. Johnson, S. Waggoner *et al.* (1999). Reverse hysterocolposigmoidectomy (RHCS) for resection of pan-pelvic tumors. *Gynecol. Oncol.* 42, 151–155.
7. J. E. Bridges, Y. Leung, I. G. Hammond *et al.* (1993). *En bloc* resection of epithelial ovarian tumors with concomitant rectosigmoid colectomy The KEMH experience. *Int. J. Gynecol. Cancer* 3, 199–202.
8. R. S. Cuesta, A. Goodman, and S. S. Halverson (1996). *En bloc* pelvic peritoneal resection of the intraperitoneal pelvic viscera in patients with advanced epithelial ovarian cancer. *Cancer J.* 2, 152–157.
9. C. Scarabelli, A. Gallo, S. Franceschi *et al.* (2000). Primary cytoreductive surgery with rectosigmoid colon resection for patients with advanced epithelial ovarian carcinoma. *Cancer* 88, 389–397.
10. S. J. Kapnick, C. T. Griffiths, N. J. Finkler *et al.* (1990). Occult pleural involvement in stage III ovarian carcinoma : Role of diaphragm resection. Gynecol. Oncol. 39, 135–138.
11. M. D. Addelson, M. S. Baggish, D. B. Seifer *et al.* (1988). Cytoreduction of ovarian cancer with the Cavitron ultrasonic surgical aspirator. *Obstet. Gynecol.* 72, 140–143.
12. J. T. Donovan, D. K. Veronickis, J. L. Powell *et al.* (1994). Cytoreductive surgery for ovarian cancer with the Cavitron Ultrasonic Surgical Aspirator and the development of disseminated intravascular coagulation. *Obstet. Gynecol.* 83, 1011–1014.
13. M. B. Sert, F. M. Abbas, J. L. Currie *et al.* (2000). Use of the ultrasound surgical aspirator in ovarian cancer: A case-control study. *Eur. J. Gynaecol. Oncol.* 21, 24–27.
14. S. M. Eisenkop, R. H. Nalik, H. J. Wang, and N. N. Teng (1993). Peritoneal implant elimination during cytoreductive surgery for ovarian cancer: Impact of survival. *Gynecol. Oncol.* 51, 224–229.
15. E. Brand, and N. Pearlman (1990). Electrosurgical debulking of ovarian cancer: A new technique using the argon beam coagulator. *Gynecol. Oncol.* 39, 115–118.
16. T. Huff, and E. Brand (1992). Pseudomixoma peritoneii: Treatment with the argon beam coagulator. *Obstet. Gynecol.* 80, 569–571.
17. J. Fanning, and R. D. Higers (1995). Loop electrosurgical excision procedure for intensified cytoreduction of ovarian cancer. *Gynecol. Oncol.* 57, 188–190.
18. J. H. Malfetano (1986). Splenectomy for optimal cytoreduction in ovarian cancer. *Gynecol. Oncol.* 24, 392–394.
19. Y. Minagawa, Y. Kanamori, and H. Ishihara *et al.* (1991). Solitary metastatic ovarian carcinoma of the spleen: A case report. *Asia Oceania J. Obstet. Gynaecol.* 17, 45–48.
20. R. Farias-Eisner, P. Braly, J. S. Berek *et al.* (1993). Solitary recurrence metastasis of epithelial ovarian cancer in the spleen. *Gynecol. Oncol.* 48, 338–341.
21. M. L. Gemignani, D. S. Chi, C. C. Gurin *et al.* (1999). Splenectomy in recurrent epithelial ovarian cancer. *Gynecol. Oncol.* 72, 407–410.
22. P. J. Klinger, S. L. Smith, B. J. Abendstein *et al.* (1998). Hand-assisted laparoscopic splenectomy for isolated splenic metastasis from an ovarian carcinoma. A case report with review of the literature. *Surg. Laparosc. Endosc.* 8, 49–54.
23. J. L. Nicklin, L. J. Copeland, R. V. O'Toole *et al.* (1995). Splenectomy as part of cytoreductive surgery for ovarian carcinoma. *Gynecol. Oncol.* 58, 244–247.
24. E. W. W. Sonnendecker, F. Guidozzi, and K. A. Margolius (1989). Splenectomy during primary maximal cytoreductive surgery for epithelial ovarian cancer. *Gynecol. Oncol.* 35, 301–306.
25. M. Morris, D. M. Gershenson, T. W. Burke *et al.* (1991). Splenectomy in gynecologic oncology: Indications, complications and technique. *Gynecol. Oncol.* 43, 118–122.
26. M. Glezerman, I. Yanai-Inbar, I. Charuzi *et al.* (1988). Involvement of the spleen in ovarian adenosquamous carcinoma. *Gynecol. Oncol.* 30, 143–148.
27. R. E. Bristow, F. J. Montz, K. M. L. D. Lagasse *et al.* (1999). Survival impact of surgical cytoreduction in stage IV epithelial ovarian cancer. *Gynecol. Oncol.* 72, 278–287.
28. J. Dauplat, G. Le Bouedec, C. Pomel, and C. Scherer (2000). Cytoreductive surgery for advanced stages of ovarian cancer. *Semin. Surg. Oncol.* 19, 42–48.
29. F. Guidozzi, and J. H. S. Ball (1994). Extensive primary cytoreductive surgery for advanced epithelial ovarian cancer. *Gynecol. Oncol.* 53, 326–330.
30. S. M. Eisenkop, R. L. Friedman, and H. J. Wang (1998). Complete cytoreductive surgery is feasible and maximizes survival in patients with advanced epithelial ovarian cancer: A prospective study. *Gynecol. Oncol.* 69, 103–108.
31. G. Michel, P. De Iaco, D. Castaigne *et al.* (1997). Extensive cytoreductive surgery in advanced ovarian carcinoma. *Eur. J. Gynaec. Oncol.* 18, 9–15.
32. J. C. Schink (1999). Current initial therapy of stage III and IV ovarian cancer: Challenges for managed care. *Semin. Oncol.* 26, 2–7.
33. C. T. Griffiths (1985). Surgical tretament of advanced ovarian cancer. *In* "Ovarian Cancer," (C. N. Hudson, ed.), 213–238. Oxford Medical Publications, London.
34. W. J. Hoskins (1989). The influence of cytoreductive surgery on progression-free interval and survival in epithelial ovarian cancer. *Baill. Clin. Obstet. Gynaecol.* 37, 311–314.
35. W. J. Hoskins, B. N. Bundy, J. T. Thigpen, and G. A. Omura (1992). The influence of cytoreductive surgery on recurrence-free interval and survival in small-volume stage III epithelial ovarian cancer: A Gynecologic Oncology Group study. *Gynecol. Oncol.* 47, 159–166.
36. N. F. Hacker, J. S. Berek, K. M. L. D. Lagasse *et al.* (1968). Primary cytoreductive surgery for epithelial ovarian cancer. *Obstet. Gynaecol. Br. Cwlth* 75, 1155–1160.

37. J. H. Goldie, and A. J. Coldman (1979). A mathematic model for relating the drug sensitivity of tumors to their spontaneous mutation rate. *Cancer Treat. Rep.* 63, 1727–1733.
38. R. W. Hunter, N. D. Alexander, S. T. D. M. *et al.* (1992). Meta analysis of surgery in advanced ovarian cancer: Is maximum cytoreductive surgery an independant determinant of prognosis. *Am. J. Obstet. Gynecol.* 166, 504–511.
39. N. F. Haker (1996). Cytoreduction for advanced ovarian cancer in perspective. *Int. J. Gynecol. Cancer* 6, 159–160.
40. J. P. Geisler, G. A. Miller, T. H. Lee *et al.* (1996). Relationship of preoperative serum CA125 to survival in epithelial ovarian carcinoma. *J. Reprod. Med.* 41, 140–142.
41. D. S. Chi, E. S. Venkatraman, V. Masson, and W. J. Hoskins (2000). The ability of preoperative serum CA 125 to predict optimal primary tumor cytoreduction in Stage III epithelial ovarian carcinoma. *Gynecol. Oncol.* 77, 227–231.
42. J. S. Berek (2000). Preoperative prediction of optimal resectability in advanced ovarian cancer using CA125. *Gynecol. Oncol.* 77, 225–226.
43. P. G. Rose, K. L. Reuter, B. E. Nelson *et al.* (1996). The impact of CA125 on the sensitivity of abdominal pelvic CT scan before second-look laparotomy in advanced ovarian carcinoma. *Int. J. Gynecol. Cancer* 6, 213–218.
44. W. J. Hoskins *et al.* (1994). The effect of diameter of largest residual disease on survival after primary cytoreductive surgery in patients with suboptimal residual epithelial ovarian carcinoma. *Am. J. Obstet. Gynecol.* 170, 974–980.
45. G. Frasci, A. Contino, and R. Laffaioli (1994). Computerized tomography of the abdomen and pelvis with peritoneal administration of soluble contrast (IPC-CT) in detection of residual disease for patients with ovarian cancer. *Gynecol. Oncol.* 52, 154–160.
46. S. K. Stevens, H. Hricak, and J. L. Stern (1991). Ovarian lesions: Detection and characterization with gadolinium-enhanced MR images at 1, 5. *Radiol.* 181, 481–488.
47. R. N. Low, W. D. Carter, F. Saleh *et al.* (1995). Ovarian cancer: Comparison of findings with Perfluorocarbon-enhanced MR Imaging, in 111-CYT-103 Immunoscintigraphy, and CT. *Radiology* 195, 391–400.
48. M. W. Method, A. N. Serafini, H. E. Averette *et al.* (1996). The role of immunoscintigraphy and CT scan prior to reassessment laparotomy of patients with ovarian carcinoma. *Cancer* 77, 2286–2292.
49. B. E. Nelson, A. T. Rosenfield, and P. E. Schwartz (1993). Preoperative abdominopelvic computed tomographic prediction of optimal cytoreduction in epithelial ovarian carcinoma. *J. Clin. Oncol.* 11, 166–172.
50. S. Taieb, F. Bonodeau, E. Leblance *et al.* (2000). Valeur predictive du scanner abdominoèpelvien pour la chirurgie optimale des carcinomes de l'ovaire. *Bull. Cancer* 87, 265–272.
51. R. Forstner, H. Hricak, K. A. Occhipinti *et al.* (1995). Ovarian cancer: Staging with CT and MR imaging. *Radiology* 197, 619–626.
52. R. Forstner, H. Hricak, and S. White (1995). CT and MRI of ovarian cancer. *Abdom. Imaging* 20, 2–8.
53. J. L. Meyer, A. W. Kennedy, R. Friedman *et al.* (1995).Ovarian carcinoma: Value of CT predicting success of debulking surgery. *Am. J. Roentgenol.* 165, 875–878.
54. S. B. Kang, C. M. Lee, Y. B. Kim *et al.* (1999). Assessment of recurrent ovarian carcinoma by positron emission tomography (abstract). *Int. J. Gynecol Cancer* (Suppl.) 1, 31–32.
55. F. Raspagliesi, F. Crippa, and R. Fontanelli (1999). Whole body positron emission tomography with 2-(18F)–Fluoro 2-Deoxo-D-glucose for detecting recurrent ovarian carcinoma (Abstract). *Int. J. Gynecol. Cancer* (Suppl.) 1, 42.
56. I. Vergote, I. DE Wever, W. A. Tjalma *et al.* (1998). Neoadjuvant chemotherapy or primary debulking surgery in advanced ovarian carcinoma: A retrospective analysis of 285 patients. *Gynecol. Oncol.* 71, 431–436.
57. P. A. Van Dam, J. De Cloedt, W. A. Tjalma *et al.* (1999). Trocar implantation metastasis after laparoscopy in patients with advanced ovarian cancer: Can the risk be reduced? *Am. J. Obstet. Gynecol.* 181, 536–541.
58. P. E. Schwartz, T. J. Rutherford, J. T. Chambers *et al.* (1999). Neoadjuvant chemotherapy for advanced ovarian cancer: Long-term survival. *Gynecol. Oncol.* 72, 93–99.
59. M. O. Nicoletto, S. Tumolo, T. Talamini, L. Salvagno *et al.* (1997). Surgical second look in ovarian cancer: A randomized study in patients with laparoscopic complete remission: A Northeastern Oncology Cooperative Group—Ovarian cancer Cooperative Group Study. *J. Clin. Oncol.* 15, 994–999.
60. E. A. Sijmons, and A. P. Heintz (2000). Second-look and second surgery: Second chance or second best? *Semin. Surg. Oncol.* 19, 54–61.
61. S. M. Lippman, D. S. Alberts, D. J. Slymen *et al.* (1988). Second look laparotomy in epithelial ovarian cancer. 61, 2571–2577.
62. K. Bertelson (1990). Tumor reduction surgery and long-term survival in advanced ovarian cancer: DACOVA study. *Gynecol. Oncol.* 38, 203–209.
63. E. Podczaski, A. Manetta, P. Kaminski *et al.* (1990). Survival of patients with ovarian epithelial carcinomas after second-look laparotomy. *Gynecol. Oncol.* 36, 43–47.
64. K. C. Podratz, M. F. Schray, H. S. Wieand *et al.* (1988). Evaluation of treatment and survival after positive second-look laparotomy. *Gynecol. Oncol.* 31, 9–21.
65. A. P. M. Heintz, A. T. Van Oosterom, J. B. M. C. Trimbos *et al.* (1988). The treatment of advanced ovarian carcinoma (II): Interval reassessment operations during chemotherapy. *Gynecol. Oncol.* 30, 359–371.
66. W. J. Hoskins, S. C. Rubin, E. Dulaney *et al.* (1989). Influence of secondary cytoreduction at the time of second-look laparotomy on the survival of patients with epithelial ovarian carcinoma. *Gynecol. Oncol.* 34, 365–371.
67. M. E. Potter, K. D. Hatch, S. J. Soong *et al.* (1992). Second look laparotomy and salvage therapy: A research modality only? *Gynecol. Oncol.* 44, 3–9.
68. S. M. Eisenkop, R. L. Friedman, and N. M. Spirtos (2000). The role of secondary cytoreductive surgery in the treatment of patients with recurrent epithelial ovarian carcinoma. *Cancer* 88, 144–153.
69. N. M. Spirtos, S. M. Eisenkop, J. B. Schlaert, and S. C. Ballon (2000). Second look laprotomy after modified posterior exenteration: Patterns of persistence and recurrence in patients with stage III and stage IV ovarian cancer. *Am. J. Obstet. Gynecol.* 182, 1321–1327.
70. M. Markman, R. Rothman, T. Hakes, B. Richman *et al.* (1991). Second-line cisplatin therapy in patients with ovarian cancer previously treated by cisplatin. *J. Clin. Oncol.* 9, 389–393.
71. L. Vaccarello, S. C. Rubin, V. Vlamis, G. Wong *et al.* (1995). Cytoreductive surgery in ovarian carcinoma patients with a documented previously complete surgical response. *Gynecol. Oncol.* 57, 61–65.
72. M. Markman, B. Reichman, T. Hakes, J. J. Lewis *et al.* (1992). Impact on survival of surgically defined favorable responses to salvage intraperitoneal chemotherapy in small-volume residual ovarian cancer. *J. Clin. Oncol.* 10, 1479–1484.
73. R. E. Buller, J. S. Skilling, A. K. Sood, S. Plaxe *et al.* (1998). Field cancerization: Why late "recurrent" ovarian cancer is not recurrent? *Am. J. Obstet. Gynecol.* 178, 641–649.
74. M. E. Van Der Burg, M. Van Lent, M. Buyse, A. Kobierska *et al.* (1995). The effect of debulking surgery after induction chemotherapy on the prognosis in advanced epithelial ovarian cancer. Gynaecological Cancer Cooperative Group of the European Organization for Research and Treatment of Cancer. *N. Engl. J. Med.* 332, 629–634.
75. J. Wils, G. Blijham, A. Navs *et al.* (1986). Primary or delayed debulking surgery and chemotherapy consisting of cisplatin, doxorubicin and cydophosphamide in Stage III-IV epithelial ovarian cancer. *J. Clin. Oncol.* 4, 1068–1073.
76. E. Surwit, J. Childers, I. Atlas, M. Nour *et al.* (1996). Neoadjuvant chemotherapy for advanced ovarian cancer. *Int. J. Gynecol. Cancer* 6, 356–361.
77. F. Shapiro, J. Schneider, M. Markman, and S. Bonnie *et al.* (1997). High intensity intravenous cyclosphosphamide and cisplatin, interim

surgical debulking and intraperitoneal cisplatin in advanced ovarian carcinoma: A pilot trial with ten-year follow-up. *Gynecol. Oncol.* 67, 39–45.

78. A. de Gramont, A. Pigne, Ch. Louvet, A. Sezeur *et al.* (1997). La cytoreduction chirurgicale précoce après chimiothérapie dans le cancer de l'ovaire avancé. *Ann. Chir.* 51, 1069–1076.
79. S. Tingwei, and F. Yuzeng (1998). Evaluation of second cytoreductive surgery in the treatment of epithelial ovarian cancer. *Chin. Med. J.* 111, 272–274.
80. W. Meier, M. Gropp, A. Burges, and H. Hepp (1999). Sekundäres Debulking nach dosisintensivierter Chemotherapie beim Ovarialkarzinom Praxis. 88, 519–525.
81. Y. Ansquer, E. Leblanc, K. Clough, Ph. Morice *et al.* Neoadjuvant chemotherapy for unresectable ovarian cancer: A french multicenter study. ????
82. S. M. Eisenkop, N. M. Spirtos, R. L. Friedman (1999). Neoadjuvant chemotherapy for advanced ovarian cancer. *Gynecol. Oncol.* 74, 311–313.
83. I. Vergote, I. De Wever, W. Tjalma, M. Van Gramberen *et al.* (1999). Neoadjuvant chemotherapy in advanced ovarian cancer: Time for a prospective randomized study. *Int. Gynecol. Cancer* 9(Suppl.) 52–53.
84. H. N. N'guyen, H. E. Averette, W. Hoskins, M. Penalver *et al.* (1993). National survey of ovarian cancer-part V. The impact of physician's speciality on patients' survival. *Cancer* 72, 3663–3670.
85. S. M. Eisenkop, N. M. Spirtos, T. W. Montag, R. H. Nalick *et al.* (1992). The impact of subspeciality training onto the management of advanced ovarian cancer. *Gynecol. Oncol.* 47, 203–209.
86. A. R. Mayer, S. K. Chambers, E. Graves *et al.* (1992). Ovarian cancer staging: Does it require a gynaecologic oncologist? *Gynecol. Oncol.* 47, 223–227.
87. E. J. Junor, D. J. Hole, L. Mc Nulty, M. Masson *et al.* (1999). Specialist gynaecologists and survival outcome: A Scottish national study of 1966 patients. *Br. J. Obstet. Gynaecol.* 106, 1130–1136.

CHAPTER

33

The Long-Term Management of Ovarian Cancer

JAMAL RAHAMAN
Division of Gynecologic Oncology
The Mount Sinai School of Medicine and Hospital
New York, New York 10029

CARMEL J. COHEN
Division of Gynecologic Oncology
The Mount Sinai School of Medicine and Hospital
New York, New York 10029

I. INTRODUCTION

The gynecologist who undertakes the challenge of caring for patients with carcinoma of the ovary should be prepared to manage a chronic disease with a difficult course and often unsuccessful outcome. Epithelial ovarian cancer includes a wide spectrum of disease from early-stage tumor, cured by complete surgical extirpation; to very aggressive disease presenting in advanced stage with rapid progression and not amenable to any intervention. However, stage is not an infallible predictor of outcome, as early-stage can behave with unexpected fatal virulence and unresectable abdominal disease can occasionally be exquisitely sensitive to cytotoxic drugs. There is a wide variation in both host response and tumor biology.

This chapter will briefly present the approach of a single institution to the long-term care of the patient with epithelial ovarian cancer.

II. INITIAL APPROACH TO OVARIAN CARCINOMA

The treatment of ovarian carcinoma has evolved from an exercise in palliation to an aggressive effort.[1] Critical to this evolution has been the utilization of maximal surgical cytoreduction and platinum-coordination compounds. For the common presentation of widespread peritoneal carcinomatosis from an ovarian cancer, surgical excision of all tumor implants is often not feasible. Because active cytotoxic agents can eradicate small volumes of residual ovarian tumor, gross tumor can be left on the surfaces of important structures if such excision leaves only a relatively thin residuum of tumor, especially if complete resection would cause unacceptable morbidity. In this setting, debulking can reduce tumor load to a subclinical residual volume of less than 10^9 cells. Also called "cytoreduction," this surgical maneuver is distinctly different from the "radical" tumor resection attempted with other solid tumors in that there is no attempt to achieve free margins some distance from gross tumor. In several prospective studies of advanced epithelial ovarian carcinoma, the best survival was achieved for those patients in whom optimal cytoreduction was possible, defined as residual tumor remaining on pelvic and abdominal structures of less than 1 or 2 cm [2] depending on institutional definitions.

Most women diagnosed with ovarian cancer will have metastatic disease beyond the ovaries and not be curable by surgical extirpation alone. Adjuvant cytotoxic therapy has been proven useful in both early and advanced optimally cytoreduced ovarian cancer.[3] The most important modern advance in the treatment of ovarian cancer has been the development of chemotherapeutic regimens based on platinum-coordination compounds.[4] Long-term follow-up of patients with ovarian cancer has shown that response to cytotoxic treatment with platinum is a predictor of survival, with a 23% decrease in the relative death rate compared to those who did not receive platinum.[5] Adjuvant chemotherapy regimens based on organoplatinum compounds offer overall clinical response rates of 60–80%, with complete response rates as high as 50% in many series.[6–13] Platinum-based chemotherapy is therefore indicated for all patients with advanced disease (stage III and IV), and high-risk patients with early disease (stage IA and B grade 2 and 3, IC, and II).

The old standard of cisplatin/cyclophosphamide had been replaced as the "gold standard" by cisplatin/paclitaxel following the results of GOG 111 which compared these two regimens in suboptimally cytoreduced advanced stage patients. In this Phase III randomized clinical trial significant improvement was noted in the paclitaxel arm with higher overall response rates (73 versus 60%, $p=0.01$), complete clinical response rate (51 versus 31%, $p=0.01$), longer progression-free survival interval (18 versus 13 months, $p<0.001$), and longer median survival (38 versus 24 months, $p<0.001$).[14] Follow-up on this study now exceeds 60 months and there is a 20% reduction of risk of progression and a 34% reduction in risk of death in patients randomized to cisplatin 75 mg/m^2 and paclitaxel 135 mg/m^2 over 24 h. The European and Canadian (OV–10) Trial corroborated this finding, however, the paclitaxel was administered at 175 mg/m^2 over 3 h in this trial and although the therapeutic effect was similar there was a much higher incidence of grade 3 neurotoxicity (18%) in the paclitaxel arm compared to the cyclophosphamide arm (1%).[15] This increased neurotoxicity was attributed to the shorter infusion rate of paclitaxel in the European Trial compared to the GOG trial.

Carboplatin is a second generation platinum compound which is less nephrotoxic, neurotoxic, and emetogenic than cisplatin and can be easily administered in an outpatient setting without forced hydration. There have been at least 12 randomized trials comparing carboplatin and cisplatin as single agents or in combination regimens for advanced ovarian cancer. Two meta-analyses performed on these randomized trials have confirmed equivalence.[16, 17].

The GOG 158 was designed as an equivalency trial in which 840 patients with optimally cytoreduced advanced ovarian cancer were randomized to 6 cycles of paclitaxel/cisplatin at GOG 111 doses or paclitaxel 175 mg/m^2 and carboplatin at AUC=7.5. The preliminary results indicated no difference in progression-free survival in the two arms.[18] Virtually identical results were reported from a large trial in Germany (AGO) involving 776 patients,[19] and a smaller study from Denmark and The Netherlands (190 patients).[20] All three studies confirmed reduced nonhematologic toxicities with carboplatin. In addition the AGO trial demonstrated significant improvement in quality of life indices. Based on these trials which confirm ease of administration, decrease in toxicity without loss of efficacy, carboplatin plus paclitaxel is now considered the preferred regimen for patients with advanced ovarian cancer.

III. PROGNOSTIC INDICATORS

The most important clinical markers are primary tumor size, residual tumor after primary cytoreductive surgery, age, and presence of large-volume ascites, performance status, FIGO stage, and histological grade.[13, 21] Serum CA125 at the time of diagnosis is not predictive of survival.[22] The only identified factor that can be affected by the treating physician is residual tumor volume after primary cytoreductive surgery, with a small but real advantage to those patients who underwent aggressive primary surgical debulking.[23] However, many investigators suggest the ability to optimally debulk ovarian cancer is determined by the biological virulence of the cancer and not by the ability of the surgeon.

Other laboratory prognostic factors studied include DNA content, HER-2/neu oncogene amplification and expression, clonogenicity in soft agar, proliferative indices, progesterone and estrogen receptor measurement, and rate of decline of CA125 values.[21] Overexpression of the oncogene HER-2/neu is controversial [24–26] as well as epidermal growth factor receptor, c-fins, p53, c-myc, and erbB-1. Recent studies by investigators at The Mount Sinai Hospital have identified alterations in the *quantitative expression* of the HER-2/neu protein product in the normal peritoneum that are predictive of the presence of ovarian cancer, and may be predictive of survival as well.[27]

IV. SURVEILLANCE / EVALUATION OF RESPONSE TO TREATMENT

After surgical cytoreduction and the initiation of a platinum-based cytotoxic drug regimen, careful scrutiny of a patient's response to treatment is essential. Tumor response to cytotoxic therapy may be described as regression (or response), progression, stable disease, and relapse. Response can be further classified as complete or partial. To monitor the response of ovarian cancer to treatment, three methods are available: clinical measurement (including radiography), serologic markers, and surgical end staging (Table 33.1).

A. Clinical Evidence of Disease

If a patient is left with grossly measurable disease at the conclusion of the initial laparotomy, radiographic or clinical measure of the size of the residual tumor mass may accurately

TABLE 33.1 Surveillance Methods for Patients with Epithelial Ovarian Cancer Undergoing Adjuvant Cytotoxic Therapy

Surveillance methods
1. Clinical
Physical examination
X-ray Findings (pleural effusions)
Computed tomography sonography
Magnetic resonance imaging
Immunoscintography
PET Scanning
2. Serologic serum
CA125
M-CSF
OVX1
LPA
CA19-9
CA15-3
Carcinoembryonic antigen (CEA)
3. Surgical end staging
Second-look laparoscopy
Second-look laparotomy

reflect response to treatment. In standard oncologic descriptions, this disease may be followed by calculating the product of the two maximal dimensions of tumor deposits, and disease status may be expressed as percentage change with treatment. In patients with no measurable or detectable disease after surgical cytoreduction, the reappearance of any tumor during cytotoxic therapy must be considered disease progression, including the appearance of malignant effusions such as ascites or pleural effusions. It must be remembered that the reappearance of symptoms that originally brought the patient to medical attention can be an important suggestion of tumor recurrence.

B. Use of Serum Tumor Markers

Up to 80% of patients with advanced ovarian carcinoma may be left with residual tumor that is unmeasurable by standard radiographic or clinical methods after initial laparotomy. Serum-oncofetal markers carcinoembryonic antigen (CEA) and placental alkaline phosphatase are expressed in not more than 20–50% of ovarian carcinomas.[28, 29]

Three tumor-associated antigens: ovarian cystadenocarcinoma-associated antigen (OCAA), ovarian cancer-associated antigen (OCA), and NB/70K have limited usefulness.[30, 31] In 1981, Bast and associates described the first monoclonal antibody to have clinical utility in the management of ovarian carcinoma.[32] CA125 is found elevated in at least 80% of epithelial ovarian cancers. Other known monoclonal antibodies useful for the management of patients with ovarian cancer include CA19-9, CA15-3, and TAG 72.[33–36] A number of markers have been described with selectivity for certain germ cell tumors, including alpha-fetoprotein (AFP), chorionic gonadotropin (hCG), and lactate dehydrogenase (LDH). Serum inhibin has also emerged as the definitive marker for granulosa cell tumors.

Serum CA125 values correlate with tumor response in over 83% of patients treated for epithelial malignancies.[37] Preoperative CA125 values do not appear to be predictive of either chemotherapeutic response or survival, but both the rates of decline of CA125 and the absolute values of CA125 during therapy have been correlated with tumor response.[38, 39] In a more practical vein, investigators at The Mount Sinai Hospital in New York noted that the continued detection of serum CA125 after the third cycle of chemotherapy predicted a median survival of only 35 months, whereas complete absence of the serum antigen at this time predicted a median survival that was not reached at 54 months.[40] Other markers such as CA19-9 may be useful for mucinous tumors that are less likely to present with elevations of CA125.[41] When an elevated tumor marker such as CA125 is identified, it should be measured serially as a monitor of response. At our institution, all known elevated tumor markers are measured with each course of treatment; if no marker is known to be elevated, CA125 values are followed.

Not all subtypes of epithelial ovarian tumors secrete the carbohydrate marker OC125 [42] and absolute CA125 values after completion of chemotherapy often cannot be used to discriminate between patients with a complete pathological response and those with only small volumes of persistent disease.[43] Despite the achievement of an "optimal CA125 response" at the prescribed interval during treatment in the studies described above, nearly 50% of patients still succumb to recurrent tumor. Thus, serologic response to initial therapy is not an infallible predictor of ultimate survival.

Recently investigators have explored the possibility of utilizing multiple markers in various combinations to improve the predictive value of serum tumor markers in the diagnosis and follow-up of ovarian cancer. Macrophage-colony stimulating factor (M-CSF) is a growth factor that acts as a chemoattractant for monocytes and found in 70% of ascites or the serum of patients with epithelial ovarian cancer. Elevated M-CSF has been detected in patients with normal CA125 and clinical evidence of disease as well as in some patients with persistent disease at second-look laparotomy.[44, 45] OVX1 is another recently developed antibody that compliments CA125 and is useful as a predictor of residual disease at second-look. A panel of CA125, M-CSF, and OVX1 has shown high sensitivity (98%) and moderate specificity (49%) in identifying early-stage ovarian cancer in women screened for abnormal ovaries.[46]

Lysophosphatidic acid (LPA) is the most recent biomarker identified and elevated levels were found in nine of ten patients with early ovarian cancer in a preliminary study.[47]

C. Surgical End Staging (Second-Look Surgery)

Although controversial, the most accurate method for determination of tumor response is repeat surgical assessment at the completion of primary therapy. Following re-operation in patients treated for colon carcinoma,[48] surgical end staging was first applied to ovarian cancer in the 1960s.[49] Surgical end staging searches for tumor deposits, if such deposits are undetected by noninvasive means. Second-look laparotomy is usually performed via a midline vertical incision, with cytologic aspirations, a thorough evaluation of the peritoneal content, and liberal biopsies of suspicious peritoneal surfaces; attention is directed to the sites of previous tumor locations (stumps of the infundibulopelvic ligaments and lateral pelvic walls). Any residual omentum is routinely resected. If present, the appendix is removed. Sampling of pelvic and para-aortic nodal chains is completed. Typically, the specimens may be 25–75 in number if no grossly suspicious findings are noted. Frozen section evaluation of suspicious findings are requested during the procedure, which is terminated if any biopsies reveal persistent cancer unless secondary cytoreduction is indicated. In the past, laparoscopy was utilized to demonstrate gross tumor implants prior to the performance of second-look laparotomy in selected patients,[l] but at present some gynecologic oncologists have utilized operative laparoscopy as the only method of surgical end staging.[50–54]

Significantly longer survival has been found in patients noted to have no histologic or cytologic evidence of disease at second look.[55] Patients found to have only microscopic disease have survival rates of 71% at 5 years if further cytotoxic treatment is offered.[56] However, approximately 20–50% of patients with advanced ovarian cancer who undergo surgical end staging will relapse despite a "negative" second-look procedure.[57] Despite this, there is still no technique that is more predictive of favorable versus unfavorable prognosis after a complete clinical response to platinum-based chemotherapy.

Three advantages of surgical end staging may be seen: determination of tumor response with unequaled accuracy in predicting long-term remission and survival; the discontinuation of cytotoxic therapy for those patients without disease; and the possible therapeutic advantages of secondary cytoreduction prior to the development of larger symptomatic recurrences in patients destined for chemotherapeutic failure. *Up to one-half of women with normal radiographic and serologic studies prior to second-look procedures are found to have disease at laparotomy.* Conversely, there are three disadvantages of surgical end staging: (1) the potential morbidity of repeat surgical assessment, (2) the incidence of clinical relapse in patients after "negative" second-look procedures, and (3) the paucity of evidence that the surgical procedure itself may contribute to patient survival.

In the earliest reported series on second-look procedures, it was not possible to demonstrate any significant survival advantage for those patients who agreed to undergo this invasive method of detection of disease.[1, 57–61] Recent data from GOG 158 (see above) have critical importance with regard to this issue. In this Phase III study of 840 optimally cytoreduced advanced ovarian cancer patients, although not randomly allocated to second look, approximately half of the patients elected the procedure with no improvement in overall survival seen.[18] The Mount Sinai Group also recently reported their experience with second look in a retrospective cohort analysis of 230 stage III ovarian cancer patients treated from 1985–1994. All patients were managed by the same team of gynecologic oncologists from initial surgery to terminal care, and received platinum-based adjuvant chemotherapy (no taxol was given in this era). No consolidation chemotherapy was offered and all patients had access to the same range of subsequent treatment options. In the optimally cytoreduced group (62%) analogous to GOG 158, there was no difference in survival outcome between those electing second-look compared to those refusing. However, among the suboptimally cytoreduced group those receiving second-look (n=32) had a significantly improved survival (37% 5-year) compared to those refusing (n=15, 13% 5-year survival) with a relative risk of 0.209 (95% CI 0.063–0.686, $p<0.02$).[62] These findings would suggest that patients with advanced disease who have suboptimal primary cytoreduction should have second-look procedures because of the therapeutic and survival implications.

V. RECURRENCE AFTER PRIMARY PLATINUM THERAPY

Despite the high responses seen in patients treated with platinum-based cytotoxic therapy for advanced epithelial ovarian carcinoma, the majority of patients will eventually manifest recurrence. It may be due to tumor clones that are insensitive to cytotoxic therapy during the period of treatment, to the emergence of platinum-resistant tumor clones, or to the emergence of new disease.

A. Drug Resistance

Human solid tumors may have either intrinsic or acquired drug resistance. Many mechanisms of drug resistance have been described.[63, 64] Expression of the *MDR1* gene, that encodes the drug efflux protein known as P-glycoprotein, has been shown to confer the characteristic of multidrug resistance to clones of some cancers. Prior treatment with natural products such as paclitaxel, doxorubicin, etoposide, or vincristine may induce or allow selection of the *MDR1* gene.[63] The binding of antineoplastic drugs to this efflux pump can be inhibited by verapramil and other drugs, which restores cytotoxic sensitivity by increasing intracellular drug levels. [65] Fortunately *MDR1* over-expression has not been observed in patients treated with cisplatin and alkylating agents.[64]

In addition to *MDR1* gene, overexpression of the MDR-associated protein (MRP) has been implicated in the multidrug resistant phenotype. Novel agents capable of reversing both MRP and *MDR1* have entered clinical trial including the cyclosporine analog PSC-833 in combination with paclitaxel and carboplatin, and biricodar in combination with paclitaxel.[66]

Resistance to bifunctional alkylating agents and to platinum complexes is multifactorial. It has been associated with increased inactivation of detoxification of enzymes such as glutathione S transferase (GST), direct binding to nonprotein thiols such as glutathione (GSH), or to protein thiols such as metallothionein.[67] Resistance is also accounted for by increased removal of lethal DNA adducts by activated DNA repair enzymes. Several agents are in trials to reverse drug resistance, e.g., buthionine sulfoximine (BSO) which decreases GSH levels by inhibiting gamma glutamyl cysteine synthetase.[68] Ethacrynic acid inhibits GST and is been tested with thiotepa in drug resistant patients.[69]

B. Platinum Resistance

The most widely considered definition of platinum response is response to first-line platinum treatment and length of disease-free (or platinum-free) intervals.[70–72] Patients with relapses greater than six months after completion of first-line platinum-based chemotherapy are considered "platinum sensitive." "Platinum resistance" may be defined as any progression on treatment (also called refractory group) or relapse within six months of treatment completion. There is no absolute interval that completely separates these patients. It is clear that response rates for re-treatment with platinum increases over a continuum as the interval from previous therapy lengthens: platinum-free interval <6 months, 10%; 6–12 months, 27%; 13–24 months, 33%; >24 months, 59%.[70]

VI. TREATMENT OPTIONS FOLLOWING RELAPSE

A. Secondary Debulking

Secondary cytoreduction of intraperitoneal recurrences often decreases symptoms (palliation) and may significantly improve survival.[73–77]

It should be omitted if the patient is medically infirm or the recurrence appears to involve vital structures.

For patients in whom tumor is grossly detected at second-look procedures, there is a distinct survival advantage if tumor masses can be resected to microscopic volumes (43–51% survival at 5 years) over those with unresectable large tumors (less than 20% 5-year survival).[75–77] In our own experience at The Mount Sinai Hospital, patients who could be optimally secondarily cytoreduced (defined as tumor residual of less than 2 cm) survived a mean of 27 months versus only 9 months for those patients who were suboptimally treated.[73] While the success after secondary cytoreduction has not been confirmed by all investigators,[78] there are also data to substantiate improvement in subjective quality of life.[79]

B. Chemotherapeutic Options

Second-line treatment options are sharply stratified by the response and duration of response following primary chemotherapy. Data from at least one randomized clinical trial document that platinum-sensitive patients with recurrent disease have a greater than 50% chance of secondary response to platinum-based chemotherapy.[80] Thus this patient group is often treated by platinum containing regimens reserving alternatives for secondary failure.[81]

Platinum-resistant patients should be treated with non-platinum regimens which should include any of the most active agents not included in the primary regimen.

1. Platinum-Sensitive Patient

a. Intraperitoneal Chemotherapy

Patients with stage III ovarian cancer who are platinum sensitive and have minimal intraperitoneal (IP) disease are candidates for aggressive second-line chemotherapy with cisplatin and or paclitaxel.[81] Markman *et al.* reported higher pathologic complete response rates at third-look among platinum-sensitive patients (42%) treated intraperitoneally compared to the platinum-resistant group (7%). Other IP chemotherapy options include paclitaxel with or without cisplatin, etoposide and cisplatin, mitoxantrone, and floxuridine.[81–88].

b. Intravenous Chemotherapy

Platinum responders who relapsed after a disease-free interval of six months may also be retreated by IV platinum regimens. Carboplatin is the preferred platinum compound for IV treatment since it is as active as cisplatin but significantly less nephrotoxic, neurotoxic, and ototoxic.

2. Platinum-Resistant Patient

Patients with disease recurrence within 6 months of platinum plus paclitaxel primary therapy have a poor response when retreated with platinum- or paclitaxel-based regimens. For such patients there is a wide range of treatment options including standard agents and experimental therapies. Reported response rates for selected agents commonly used as second-line therapy for recurrent ovarian cancer are listed in Table 33.2, however, response data are not strictly comparable.

TABLE 33.2 Published Response Rates of Selected Agents in Recurrent Epithelial Ovarian Carcinoma

Agent	Overall response (%)	Ref.
Cisplatin, standard dose	31–50%	Bruckner [105]
Cisplatin, high dose	20–72%	Bruckner [106]
		Seltzer [107]
Carboplatin	21–31%	Ozols [108]
		Kjorstad [109]
		Kavanagh [110]
Paclitaxel (taxol)	20–37%	Thigpen [111]
		Einzig [112]
Topotecan	13–33%	McGuire [113]
		Bookman [114]
Doxorubicin (liposomal)	19.7–27%	Muggia [115]
		Campos [117]
Gemcitabine	13–22%	Shapiro [118]
		von Minckwitz [119]
Ifosfamide	7–20%	Sutton [120]
Docetaxel	23–35%	Verschraegen [121]
Vinorelbine	15–30%	Gershenson [122]
Etoposide	6–34%	Rose [123]
Altretamine	12–33%	Moore [124]
		Fields [125]
Methotrexate/leucovorin	5%	Parker [126]
Tamoxifen	0–17%	Jakobsen [127]
		Beecham [128]
		Markman [129]

VII. PATTERNS OF SURVIVAL

Although important improvements have been made in the treatment of advanced ovarian cancer in the last twenty years, it is difficult to measure significant changes in survival patterns because of widely varying treatment programs and complex institutional variables.[90]

Nonplatinum-based regimens prior to 1980 for advanced stages of ovarian cancer gave an estimated survival of only 9% at 8 years.[91] As platinum-based chemotherapy and surgical cytoreduction were adopted, modest improvements in survival were made,[92] including a 5-year survival in advanced (stages III and IV) disease from 16.5–20.7%. There was an associated 23% reduction in death due to cancer with the use of cisplatin.[5] More recently Trimble *et al.* reported a significantly improved 5-year survival rate in the U.S. based on SEER data for the periods 1983–1987 compared to 1988–1994. The 5-year survival rate for stage III increased from 29.9–37.45%, while stage IV increased from 18.05–25.47% ($p<0.01$).[93] After 1994 with the widespread availability of paclitaxel, further improvement in survival have been demonstrated. However, despite this real improvement in response to therapy and a significant improvement in 5-year survival rates, the patient with epithelial ovarian cancer is at risk for recurrence even after long periods of disease-free survival. Emerging evidence suggests that based on gene analysis of the tumors, after three years this pattern represents new disease.

VIII. LATE RECURRENCES

For the majority of solid tumors other than breast carcinoma, recurrences will happen within five years of diagnosis, after which time the risk of recurrence diminishes dramatically. However, recurrences after platinum-based therapy for advanced ovarian cancer may continue after five years.[94] Late recurrences are an important facet of care in ovarian carcinoma, a factor that was overlooked by investigators in the 1980s.

Late recurrences may differ in their anatomic location from the more typical IP sites of recurrence seen earlier. Isolated recurrences in atypical sites have been noted years after apparently successful cytotoxic therapy. Aberrant recurrences have been described in the cerebrum, cerebellum, meninges,[95–98] liver parenchyma, long bones, and supraclavicular lymph nodes. Central nervous system relapse has been suggested to be a "sanctuary site" due to the lower exposure to systemic cytotoxic therapy because of the blood-brain barrier.[98] We have found that such late recurrences in aberrant locations may require novel applications of multimodality therapy with irradiation, surgery, and salvage chemotherapy.[99]

IX. PALLIATIVE CARE

Comprehensive care of the women afflicted with ovarian carcinoma will require sensitive and timely correction of deficits in nutrition, hydration, pain, and relief of suffering in over two-thirds of patients originally diagnosed with advanced ovarian carcinoma, as well as some patients with early-stage disease.

Because in the majority of women progressive or recurrent disease occurs within the abdominal cavity, intestinal obstruction is frequent.[100] For inoperable patients percutaneous gastrostomy offers a more comfortable alternative to prolonged nasogastric tube drainage. Frequently bowel obstruction may be relieved by prolonged drainage, parenteral nutrition, and cytotoxic therapy.[101]

Relief from malignant effusion is particularly important given the frequency of this complication in end stage disease. Drainage is temporarily effective; IP administration of cisplatin, carboplatin, taxol, etoposide, mitoxantrone, cytosine arabinoside (ara-C), and other agents can slow or prevent the accumulation of ascites in many patients.[82–88] Malignant pleural effusions can be effectively managed by pleural installation of talc, platinum, tetracycline, or bleomycin.[103, 104]

X. CONCLUSION

In the last two decades, the aggressive treatment of epithelial ovarian cancer has seen remarkable improvements in the response rates of patients with advanced ovarian cancer. Indeed, ovarian cancer may be the most remarkable example of an adult solid tumor that is "almost" curable. Although the higher response rates of platinum compared to other agents may seem ephemeral as they often do not translate to long-term cure, the immediate response of almost all patients and the promise of new drugs and consolidation regimens augers well for expected improvement. Recognition of the importance of minimal residual disease, the superior response rates for platinum/taxane combination chemotherapy, the high incidence of late relapse despite a favorable response to platinum-based therapy, and the availability of new chemotherapy agents with high activity provides us with a map for future study.

References

1. Cohen, C. J., Goldberg, J. D., Holland, J. F. *et al.* (1983). Improved therapy with cisplatin regimens for patients with ovarian carcinoma as measured by surgical end staging. *Am. J. Obstet. Gynecol.* 145, 955–967.
2. Hoskins, W. J., McGuire, W. P., Brady, M. F. *et al.* (1994). The effect of diameter of largest residual disease on survival after primary cytoreductive surgery in patients with suboptimal residual epithelial ovarian carcinoma. *Am. J. Obstet. Gynecol.* 170, 974–980.
3. Smith, J. P., and Rutledge, F. N. (1975). Chemotherapy in advanced ovarian cancer. *NCI Monogr.* 42, 141.
4. Schilder, R. J., and Ozols, R. F. (1992). New therapies for ovarian cancer. *Cancer Invest.* 10, 307.
5. Omura, G., Brady, M. F., Homelsley, H. D. *et al.* (1991). Long-term follow up and prognostic factor analysis in advanced ovarian carcinoma: The Gynecologic Oncology Group Experience. *J. Clin. Oncol.* 9, 1138–1150.
6. Gruppo Interegionale Cooperativo Oncologico Ginecologia. Randomized comparison of cisplatin with cyclophosphamide/cisplatin and with cyclophosphamide/doxorubicin/cisplatin in advanced ovarian cancer. (1987). *Lancet* ii, 353.
7. Louie, K. G., Ozols, R. F., Flyers, C. E. *et al.* (1986). Long-term results of a cisplatin-containing combination chemotherapy regimen for the treatment of advanced ovarian carcinoma. *J. Clin. Oncol.* 4, 1579–1585.
8. Hand, R., Fremgen, A., Chmiel, J. S. *et al.* (1993). Staging procedures, clinical management, and survival outcome for ovarian carcinoma. *JAMA* 269, 1119.
9. Neijt, J. P., ten Bokkel Huinink, I., van der Burg, A. T. *et al.* (1987). Randomized trial comparing two combination chemotherapy regimens in advanced ovarian carcinoma. *J. Clin. Oncol.* 5, 1157–1168.
10. Edmonson, J. H., McCormack, G. W., and Wieand, H. S. (1990). Late emerging survival differences in a comparative study of HCAP vs. CP in stage III-IV ovarian carcinoma. *In* "Adjuvant Therapy of Cancer VI" (S. E. Salmon, ed.). W. B. Saunders, New York.
11. Sutton, G. P., Stehman, F. B., Einhorn, L. H. *et al.* (1989). Ten-year follow-up of patients receiving cisplatin, doxorubicin, and cyclophosphamide chemotherapy for advanced epithelial ovarian carcinoma. *J. Clin. Oncol.* 7, 223–229.
12. Hainsworth, J. D., Grosh, W. W., Burnett, L. S. *et al.* (1988). Advanced ovarian cancer: Long-term results of treatment with intensive cisplatin-based chemotherapy of brief duration. *Ann. Int. Med.* 108, 165–172.
13. Krag, K. J., Canellos, G. P., Griffiths, C. T. *et al.* (1989). Predictive factors for long-term survival in patients with advanced ovarian cancer. *Gynecol. Oncol.* 34, 88–93.
14. McGuire, W. P., Hoskins, W. J., Brady, M. F. *et al.* (1996). Cyclophosphamide and cisplatin compared with paclitaxel and cisplatin in patients with stage III and IV ovarian cancer. *N. Engl. J. Med.* 334, 1–6.
15. Stuart, G., Bertelson, K., Mangioni, C. *et al.* (1988). Updated analysis shows a highly significant improved overall survival (OS) for cisplatin-paclitaxel as first line treatment of advanced ovarian cancer: Mature results of the EORTC–GCCG, NOCOVA, NCTC, CT, and Scottish Intergroup Trial. *Proc. Am. Soc. Clin. Oncol.* 17, 361a.
16. Aabo, K., Adams, M., Adnitt, P. *et al.* (1998). Chemotherapy in advanced ovarian cancer: Four systematic meta-analysis of individual patient data from 37 randomized trials. *Br. J. Cancer* 78(11), 1479.
17. Stewart, L. A. (1991). For the Advanced Ovarian Cancer Trialist Group (AOCTG). Chemotherapy in advanced ovarian cancer: An overview of randomized clinical trials. *Br. Med. J.* 303, 884.
18. Ozols, R. F., Bundy, B. N., Clark-Pearson, D. *et al.* (1999). Randomized phase III study of cisplatin (CIS)/ paclitaxel (PAC) versus carboplatin (CARBO)/PAC in optimal stage III epithelial ovarian cancer (OC) Gynecologic Oncology Group Trial (GOG 158). *Proc. Am. Soc. Clin. Oncol.* 18, 356a.
19. du Bois, A., Lueck, H. J., Meier, W. *et al.* (1999). Cisplatin / paclitaxel vs. carboplatin/paclitaxel in ovarian cancer: Update of an Arbeitsgemeinschaft Gynaekologische Onkologie (AGO) Study Group Trial. *Proc. Am. Soc. Clin. Oncol.* 18, 356a.
20. Neijt, J. P., Hansen, M., Hansen, S. W. *et al.* (1997). Randomized phase III study in previously untreated epithelial ovarian cancer FIGO stage IIB, IIC, III, IV comparing paclitaxel-cisplatin and paclitaxel-carboplatin. *Proc. Am. Soc. Clin. Oncol.* 16, 352a.
21. de Souza, P. L., and Friedlander, M. L. (1992). Prognostic factors in ovarian cancer. *Hematol. Oncol. Clin. N. Am.* 6, 761.
22. Hoskins, W. J., McGuire, W. P., Copeland, L. *et al.* (1993). Serum CA 125 for prediction of progression in advanced epithelial ovarian carcinoma. *J. Clin. Oncol.* 11, 223 (abstract 707).
23. Hunter, R. W., Alexander, N. D. E., and Soutter, W. P. (1992). Meta-analysis of surgery in advanced ovarian carcinoma: Is maximum cytoreductive surgery an independent determinant of prognosis? *Am. J. Obstet. Gynecol.* 166, 504.
24. Slamon, D. J., Godolphin, W., Jones, L. A. *et al.* (1989). Studies of the HER-2/neu proto-oncogene in human breast and ovarian cancer. *Science* 244, 707.
25. Berchuck, A., Kamel, A., and Whittaker, R. (1990). Overexpression of the HER-2/neu is associated with poor survival in advanced epithelial ovarian cancer. *Cancer Res.* 50, 4087.
26. Rubin, S. C., Finstad, C. L., Wong, G. Y. *et al.* (1993). Prognostic significance of HER-2/neu expression in advanced epithelial ovarian cancer. *Am. J. Obstet. Gynecol.* 168, 1623.
27. Jennings, T. S., Dottino, P. R., Mandeli, J. P. *et al.* (1994). Growth factor expression in normal peritoneum of patients with gynecologic carcinoma. *Gynecol. Oncol.*
28. Stall, K. E., and Martin, E. W. (1981). Plasma carcinoembryonic antigen levels in ovarian cancer patients. *J. Reprod. Med.* 26, 73.
29. Nouwen, E. J., Pollet, D. E., Schelstraete, J. B. *et al.* (1985). Human placental alkaline phosphatase in benign and malignant ovarian neoplasia. *Cancer Res.* 45, 892.
30. Knauf, S., and Urbach, F. I. (1980). A study of ovarian cancer patients using a radioimmunoassay for human ovarian tumor-associated antigen OCA. *Am. J. Obstet. Gynecol.* 138, 1222–1223.

31. Knauf, S., and Urbach, F. I. (1981). Identification, purification and radioimmunoassay of NB/70K, a human ovarian tumor-associated antigen. *Cancer Res.* 41, 1351–1357.
32. Bast, R. C., Feeney, M., Lazarus, H. *et al.* (1981). Reactivity of a monoclonal antibody with human ovarian carcinoma. *J. Clin. Invest.* 68, 1331–1337.
33. Jacobs, I. J., Rivera, H., Oram, D. H., and Bast, R. C. (1993). Differential diagnosis of ovarian cancer with tumor markers CA 125, CA 15-3, and TAG 72.3. *Br. J. Obstet. Gynecol.* 100, 1120.
34. Einhom, N., Knapp, R. C., Bast, R. C. *et al.* (1989). CA 125 assay used in conjunction with CA 15-3 and TAG 72 assays for discrimination between malignant and non-malignant diseases of the ovary. *Acta Oncol.* 28, 655.
35. Bast, R. C., Knauf, S., Epenetos, A. *et al.* (1991). Coordinate elevation of serum markers in ovarian cancer but not in benign disease. *Cancer* 68, 1758–1763.
36. Soper, J. T., Hunter, V. L., Daly, L. *et al.* (1990). Preoperative serum tumor-associated antigen levels in women with pelvic masses. *Gynecol. Oncol.* 35, 249.
37. Cruickshank, D. J., Tern, P. B., and Fullerton, W. T. (1992). CA 125 response assessment in epithelial ovarian cancer. *Int. J. Cancer* 51, 58–61.
38. Rustin, G., Gennings, J. N., Nelstrop, A. E. *et al.* (1989). Use of CA-125 to predict survival of patients with ovarian carcinoma. *J. Clin. Oncol.* 7, 1667–1671.
39. Hawkins, R. E., Roberts, K., Wiltshaw, E. *et al.* (1989). The prognostic significance of the half-life of serum CA 125 in patients responding to chemotherapy for epithelial ovarian carcinoma. *Br. J. Obstet. Gynecol.* 96, 1395–1399.
40. Dottino, P. R., Segna, R. A., and Cohen, C. J. (1992). Early serum negativity of CA 125 is a prognostic variable in patients treated for epithelial ovarian cancer. Twenty-third Annual Meeting of the Society of Gynecologic Oncologists. Abstract #86.
41. Canney, P. A., Wilkinson, P. M., James, R. D. *et al.* (1985). CA 19-9 as a marker for ovarian cancer: Alone and in comparison with CA 125. *Br. J. Cancer* 52, 131–133.
42. Kabawat, S. E., Bast, R. C., Welch, W. C. *et al.* (1983). Immunopathologic characterization of a monoclonal antibody that recognizes common surface antigens of human ovarian tumors of serous, endometrioid, and clear cell types. *Am. J. Clin. Pathol.* 79, 98–104.
43. Patsner, B., Orr, J. W., Mann, W. J. *et al.* (1990). Does serum CA-125 prior to second-look laparotomy for invasive ovarian adenocarcinoma predict size of residual disease? *Gynecol. Oncol.* 38, 373–378.
44. Ramakrishnan, S., Xu, F. J., Brandt, S. J. *et al.* (1990). Elevated levels of Macrophage colony stimulating factor (MCS-F) in serum and ascites from patients with epithelial ovarian cancer. *Proc. SGO* 21, 40.
45. Kacinski, B. M., Stanley, E. R., Carter, D. *et al.* (1989). Circulating levels of CSF1 (MCS-F), a lymphohematopoietic cytokine, may be a useful marker of disease status in patients with malignant ovarian neoplasms. *Int. J. Radiat. Oncol. Biol. Phys.* 17, 159.
46. Woolas, R. P., Xu, F. J., Jacobs, I. J. *et al.* (1993). Elevation of multiple serum markers in patients with stage I ovarian cancer. *J. Natl. Cancer Inst.* 85, 1748.
47. Xu, Y., Shen, Z., Wiper, D. W. *et al.* (1998). Lysophosphatidic acid as a potential marker for ovarian and other gynecologic cancers. *JAMA* 280, 719.
48. Wangensteen, O. H., Lewis, F. J., and Tongen, L. A. (1951). The "second-look" in cancer surgery. *Lancet* 71, 303.
49. Smith, J. P., Delgado, G., and Rutledge, F. N. (1976). Second-look operation in ovarian carcinoma. *Cancer* 38, 1438–1442.
50. Canis, M., Chapron, C., Made, G. *et al.* (1992). Techneique et resultats preliminaires du second look percoelioscopique clans les tumeurs epitheliales malignes de l'ovarie. *J. Gynecol. Obstet. Biol. Reprod.* 21, 655.
51. Jennings, T. S., and Dottino, P. R. (1994). The application of operative laparoscopy to gynecologic oncology. *Curr. Opin. Ob/Gyn* 6, 80.
52. Jennings, T. S., Dottino, P., Rahaman, J., and Cohen, C. J. (1998). Results of selective use of operative laparoscopy in gynecologic oncology. *Gynecol. Oncol.* 70, 323–328.
53. Rahaman, J., Nezhat, F., Dottino, P. *et al.* (2001). The impact of second look laparoscopy compared to second look laparotomy on recurrence and survival in advanced stage ovarian cancer. *Gynecol. Oncol.* 80(2), 326.
54. Abu-Rustum, N. R., Barakat, R. R., Siegel, P. L. *et al.* (1996). Second-look operation for epithelial ovarian cancer: Laparoscopy or laparotomy. *Obstet. Gynecol.* 88, 549.
55. Gershensen, D. G., Copeland, L. J., Wharton, J. T. *et al.* (1985). Prognosis of surgically determined complete responders in advanced ovarian cancer. *Cancer* 55, 1129.
56. Copeland, L. J., Gershenson, D. M., Wharton, J. T. *et al.* (1985). Microscopic disease at second-look laparotomy in advanced ovarian cancer. *Cancer* 55, 472.
57. Luesley, D. M., Lawton, F. G., Blackledge, G. *et al.* (1988). Failure of second-look laparotomy to influence survival in epithelial ovarian cancer. *Lancet* ii, 599.
58. Creasman, W. T., Gall, S., Bundy, B. N. *et al.* (1989). Second-look laparotomy in the patient with minimal residual stage III ovarian cancer (a Gynecologic Oncology Group Study). *Gynecol. Oncol.* 35, 378.
59. Chambers, S. K., Chambers, J. T., Kohorn, E. L. *et al.* (1988). Evaluation of the role of second-look surgery in ovarian cancer. *Obstet. Gynecol.* 72, 404.
60. Ho, A. G., Beller, U., Speyer, J. L. *et al.* (1987). A reassessment of the role of second-look laparotomy in advanced ovarian cancer. *J. Clin. Oncol.* 5, 1316–1321.
61. Nicoletto, M. O., Tumolo, S., Talamini, R. *et al.* (1997). Surgical second-look in ovarian cancer: A randomized study in patients with laparoscopic complete remission-A Northeastern Oncology Cooperative Group-Ovarian Cancer Cooperative Group Study. *J. Clin. Oncol.* 15, 994–999.
62. Rahaman, J., Dottino, P., Jennings, T. S. *et al.* (1999). Second look operation improves survival in Stage III ovarian cancer patients. *Int. J. Gynecol. Cancer* 9(1), 22.
63. Fojo, A., Hamilton, T. C., Young, R. C., and Ozols, R. F. (1987). Multidrug resistance in ovarian cancer. *Cancer* 60, 2075.
64. Bourhis, J., Goldstein, L. J., Riou, G. *et al.* (1989). Expression of a human multidrug resistance gene in ovarian carcinomas. *Cancer Res.* 49, 5062.
65. Rogan, A., Hamilton, T., and Ozols, R. (1984). Reversal of adriamycin resistance by verapramil in human ovarian cancer. *Science* 224, 994–996.
66. Rowinsky, E. K., Smith, L., Wang, Y. M. *et al.* (1998). Phasel and pharmacokinetic study of paclitaxel in combination with biricodar, a novel agent that reverses multidrug resistance conferred by overexpression of both MDR1 and MRP. *J. Clin. Oncol.* 16(9), 2964.
67. Kelley, S. L., Basu, A., Teicher, B. A. *et al.* (1988). Overexpression of metallothionein confers resistance to anticancer drugs. *Science* 241, 1813.
68. O'Dwyer, P. J. (1992). Depletion of glutathione in normal and malignant human cells in vivo by buthionine sulfoximine: Clinical and biochemical endpoints. *J. Natl. Cancer Inst.* 84, 264–267.
69. O'Dwyer, P. J., La Creta, F. P., Nash, S. *et al.* (1991). Phase I study of thiotepa in combination with glutathione transferase inhibitor ethacrynic acid. *Cancer Res.* 51, 6059.
70. Blackledge, G., Lawton, F., Redman, C. *et al.* (1989). Response of patients in phase II studies of chemotherapy in ovarian cancer: Implications for patient treatment and design of phase II trials. *Br. J. Cancer* 59, 299.
71. Markman, M., Rothman, R., Hakes, T. *et al.* (1991). Second-line platinum therapy in patients with ovarian cancer previously treated with cisplatin. *J. Clin. Oncol.* 9, 389.
72. Markman, M., and Hoskins, W. (1992). Responses to salvage chemotherapy in ovarian cancer. A critical need for precise definitions of the treated population. *J. Clin. Oncol.* 10, 513.

73. Segna, R. A., Dottino, P. R., Mandeli, P. *et al.* (1993). Secondary cytoreduction for ovarian cancer following cisplatin therapy. *J. Clin. Oncol.* 11, 434.
74. Vogl, S. E. *et al.* (1980). Second-effort surgical resection for bulky ovarian cancer. *Cancer* 54, 2220.
75. Hoskins, W. J., Rubin, S. C., Dulaney, E. *et al.* (1989). Influence of secondary cytoreduction at the time of second-look laparotomy on the survival of patients with epithelial ovarian carcinoma. *Gynecol. Oncol.* 34, 365.
76. Lippman, S. M., Alberts, D. S., Slymen, D. J. *et al.* (1988). Second-look laparotomy in epithelial ovarian carcinoma. *Cancer* 61, 2571.
77. Podratz, K. C., Malkasian, G., Hilton, J. F. *et al.* (1985). Second-look laparotomy in ovarian cancer: Evaluation of pathologic variables. *Am. J. Obstet. Gynecol.* 152, 230.
78. Raju, K. S., McKina, M. A., Barker, G. H. *et al.* (1982). Second-look operations in the planned management of advanced ovarian carcinoma. *Am. J. Obstet. Gynecol.* 144, 650-654.
79. Blythe, J. G., and Wahl, T. P. (1982). Debulking surgery: Does it increase the quality of survival? *Gynecol. Oncol.* 14, 396.
80. Colombo, N., Marzola, M., Parma, G. *et al.* (1996). Paclitaxel vs. CAP (cyclophosphamide, adriamycin, cisplatin) in recurrent platinum sensitive ovarian cancer: A randomized phase II study. *Proc. Am. Soc. Clin. Oncol.* 15, 279.
81. Alberts, D. S. (1999). Treatment of refractory and recurrent ovarian cancer. *Semin. Oncol.* 26(1), 8–14.
82. Muggia, F. M., Liu, P. S., Alberts, D. S. *et al.* (1996). Intraperitoneal mitoxantrone or floxuridine: Effects on time-to-failure in survival in patients with minimal residual ovarian cancer after second-look laparotomy—A randomized phase II study by the Southwest Oncology Group. *Gynecol. Oncol.* 61, 395–402.
83. Markman, M. (1995). Intraperitoneal paclitaxel in the management of ovarian cancer. *Semin. Oncol.* 22, 86–87.
84. Dedrick, R. L., Myers, C. E., Bungay, P. M., and De Vita, V. T. (1978). Pharmacokinetic rationale for peritoneal drug administration in the treatment of ovarian cancer. *Cancer Treat. Rep.* 62, 1–9.
85. Cohen, C. J. (1985). Surgical considerations in ovarian cancer. *Semin. Oncol.* 12, 53.
86. ten Bokkel Huinink, W. W., Dubbelman, R., Aartsen, E. *et al.* (1985). Experimental and clinical results with intraperitoneal cisplatin. *Semin. Oncol.* 12, 43.
87. Markman, M., Reichman, B., Hakes, T. *et al.* (1992). Impact on survival of surgically defined favorable responses to salvage intraperitoneal chemotherapy in small-volume residual ovarian cancer. *J. Clin. Oncol.* 10, 1479–1484.
88. Howell, S. B., Zimm, S., Markman, M. *et al.* (1987). Long-term survival of advanced refractory ovarian carcinoma patients with small-volume disease treated with intraperitoneal chemotherapy. *J. Clin. Oncol.* 5, 160–167.
89. Gershenson, D. M., Kavanaugh, J. J., Copeland, L. J. *et al.* (1989). Re-treatment of patients with recurrent epithelial ovarian cancer with cisplatin-based chemotherapy. *Obstet. Gynecol.* 73, 798.
90. Bailar, J. C., and Smith, E. M. (1986). Progress against cancer? *N. Engl. J. Med.* 314, 1226.
91. Wharton, J. T., Edwards, C. L., and Rutledge, F. N. (1984). Long term survival after chemotherapy for advanced epithelial ovarian carcinoma. *Am. J. Obstet. Gynecol.* 148, 997.
92. Ries, L., Hankey, B., Miller, B., Hartman, A., Edwards, B., eds. (1991). "Cancer Statistics Review 1973–88 (NIH 91–2789)." National Institutes of Health, National Cancer Institute, Bethesda, MD.
93. Trimble, E. L., Kosary, C. A., Cornelison, T. L. *et al.* (1999). Improved survival for women with ovarian cancer. *Gynecol. Oncol.* 72, 324.
94. Sutton, G. P., Stehman, F. B., Einhorn, L. H. *et al.* (1989). Ten-year follow-up of patients receiving cisplatin, doxorubicin, and cyclophosphamide chemotherapy for advanced epithelial ovarian carcinoma. *J. Clin. Oncol.* 7, 223–229.
95. Hardy, J. R., and Harvey, V. J. (1989). Chemotherapy metastases in patients with ovarian cancer treated with chemotherapy. *Gynecol. Oncol.* 33, 296.
96. Bruzzone, M., Campora, E., Chiara, S. *et al.* (1993). Cerebral metastases secondary to ovarian cancer: Still an unusual event. *Gynecol. Oncol.* 49, 37.
97. Stein, M., Steiner, M., Klein, B. *et al.* (1986). Involvement of the central nervous system by ovarian carcinoma. *Cancer* 58, 2066.
98. Plaxe, S. C., Dottino, P. R., Lipsztein, R. *et al.* (1990). Clinical features and treatment outcome of patients with epithelial carcinoma of the ovary metastatic to the central nervous system. *Obstet. Gynecol.* 75, 278.
99. Bruckner, H. W., and Gorbaty, M. (1987). Management of apparent single foci of epithelial ovarian cancer. *J. Surg. Oncol.* 35, 204.
100. Rubin, S. C., Hoskins, W. J., Benjamin, I. *et al.* (1989). Palliative surgery for intestinal obstruction in advanced ovarian cancer. *Gynecol. Oncol.* 34, 16.
101. Malone, J. J., Koonce, T., Larson, D. M. *et al.* (1986). Palliation of small bowel obstruction by percutaneous gastrostomy in patients with progressive ovarian carcinoma. *Obstet. Gynecol.* 68, 431.
102. Qazi, R., and Savlov, E. D. Peritoneovenous shunt for palliation of malignant ascites. *Cancer* 49, 600.
103. Moores, D. (1991). Malignant pleural effusions. *Semin. Oncol.* 18(1), 59–61.
104. Figlin, R., Mendoza, E., Piantadosi *et al.* (1994). Intrapleural chemotherapy without pleurodesis for malignant pleural effusions. *Chest* 106(6), 363–366.
105. Bruckner, H. W., Cohen, C. J., Deppe, G. *et al.* (1981). Treatment of chemotherapy-resistant advanced ovarian cancer with a combination of cyclophosphamide, hexamethylmelamine, adriamycin and cis-diamminedichloroplatinum (CHAP). *Gynecol. Oncol.* 12, 150–153.
106. Bruckner, H. W., Wallach, R., Cohen, C. J. *et al.* (1981). High-dose platinum for the treatment of refractory ovarian cancer. *Gynecol. Oncol.* 12, 64–67.
107. Seltzer, V., Vogl, S., and Kaplan, B. (1985). Recurrent ovarian carcinoma: Retreatment utilizing combination chemotherapy including cis-diamminedichloroplatinum in patients previously responding to this agent. *Gynecol. Oncol.* 21, 167.
108. Ozols, R. F., Ostchega, Y., Curt, G., and Young, R. C. (1987). High-dose carboplatin in refractory ovarian cancer patients. *J. Clin. Oncol.* 5, 197.
109. Kjorstad, K., Bertelsen, K., Slevin, M. *et al.* (1986). Phase II trial of carboplatin in ovarian cancer. *Proc. Am. Soc. Oncol.* (abstr.) 5, 441.
110. Kavanagh, J., Tresukosol, D., Edwards, C. *et al.* (1995). Carboplatin re-induction after taxane in patients with platinum-refractory epithelial ovarian cancer. *J. Clin. Oncol.* 13, 1584.
111. Thigpen, T., Blessing, J., Ball, H. *et al.* (1990). Phase II trial of taxol as second-line therapy for ovarian carcinoma. *Proc. Am. Soc. Oncol.* (abstr.) 9, 604.
112. Einzig, A. I., Wiernik, P. H., Sasloff, J. *et al.* (1992). Phase 11 study and long-term follow-up of patients treated with taxol for advanced ovarian adenocarcinoma. *J. Clin. Oncol.* 10, 1748.
113. McGuire, W. P., Blessing, J. A., Bookman, M. A. *et al.* (2000). Topotecan has substantial antitumor activity as first-line salvage therapy in platinum-sensitive epithelial ovarian carcinoma: A Gynecologic Oncology Group Study. *J. Clin. Oncol.* 18(5), 1062.
114. Bookman, M. A., Malmstrom, H., Bolis, G. *et al.* (1998). Topotecan for the treatment of advanced epithelial ovarian cancer: An open label phase II study in patients treated after prior chemotherapy containing cisplatin or carboplatin and paclitaxel. *J. Clin. Oncol.* 16, 3345.
115. Muggia, F. M., Hainsworth, J. D., Jeffers, S. *et al.* (1997). Phase II study of liposomal doxorubicin in refractory ovarian cancer: Antitumor activity and toxicity modification by liposomal encapsulation. *J. Clin. Oncol.* 15(3), 987.

116. Gordon, A. N., Fleagle, J. T., Guthrie, D. *et al.* (2001). Recurrent epithelial ovarian carcinoma: A randomized phase III study of pegylated liposomal doxorubicin versus Topotecan. *J. Clin. Oncol.* 19(14), 3312–3322.
117. Campos, S. M., Penson, R. T., Mays, A. R. *et al.* (2001). The clinical utility of liposomal doxorubicin in recurrent ovarian cancer. *Gynecol. Oncol.* 81(2), 206.
118. Shapiro, J. D., Millward, M. J., Rischin, D. *et al.* (1996). Activity of gemcitabine in patients with advanced ovarian cancer: Responses seen following platinum and paclitaxel. *Gynecol. Oncol.* 63, 89.
119. von Minckwitz, G., Bauknecht, T., Visseren-Grul, C. M., and Neijt, J. P. (1999). Phase II study of gemcitabine in ovarian cancer. *Ann. Oncol.* 10(7), 853.
120. Sutton, G. P., Blessing, J. A., Homesly, H. D. *et al.* (1989). Phase II trial of ifosfamide and mesna in advanced ovarian carcinoma. *J. Clin. Oncol.* 7, 1672.
121. Verschraegen, C. F., Sittisomwong, T., Kudelka, A. P. *et al.* (2001). Docetaxel for patients with platinum resistant mullerian carcinomas. *J. Clin. Oncol.* 18, 2733.
122. Gershenson, D. M., Burke, T. W., Morris, M. *et al.* (1998). A phase I study of daily×3 schedule of intravenous vinorelbine for refractory epithelial ovarian cancer. *Gynecol. Oncol.* 70, 404.
123. Rose, P. G., Blessing, J. A., Mayer, A. R. *et al.* (1998). Prolonged oral etoposide as second line therapy for platinum-resistant and platinum-sensitive ovarian carcinoma: A Gynecologic Oncology Group study. *J. Clin. Oncol.* 16, 405.
124. Moore, D. H., Fowler, W. C., Jones, C. P., and Crumpler, L. S. (1991). Hexamethylmelamine chemotherapy for persistent or recurrent epithelial ovarian cancer. *Am. J. Obstet. Gynecol.* 165, 573.
125. Fields, A. L., Schink, J. C., Miller, D. S. *et al.* (1991). Oral hexamethylmelamine: An effective salvage therapy for recurrent ovarian cancer. 13th World Congress of Gynecology and Obstetrics, Singapore, (Abstr. #2048).
126. Parker, L. M., Griffiths, C. T., Yankee, R. A. *et al.* (1979). High-dose methotrexate with leucovorin rescue in ovarian cancer: A phase II study. *Cancer Treat. Rep.* 63, 275.
127. Jakobsen, A., Bertelsen, K., and Sell, A. (1987). Cyclic hormonal treatment in ovarian cancer. *Eur. J. Clin. Oncol.* 23, 15.
128. Beecham, B., Blessing, J., Creasman, W., and Hatch, K. (1988). Tamoxifen is effective as second line therapy for certain patients with advanced, chemotherapy-resistant epithelial ovarian cancer. *Proc. Am. Soc. Oncol.* (abstr.) 7, 135.
129. Markman, M., Iseminger, J. A., Hatch, K. D. *et al.* (1996). Tamoxifen in platinum-refractory ovarian cancer: A Gynecologic oncology ancillary report. *Gynecol. Oncol.* 62, 4.

C H A P T E R

34

The Laparoscopic Management of Adnexal Masses and Ovarian Cancer

FARR NEZHAT
Division of Gynecologic Oncology
The Mount Sinai School of Medicine and Hospital
New York, New York 10029

TANJA PEJOVIC
Division of Gynecologic Oncology
Yale University School of Medicine
New Haven, Connecticut 06520

During the past decade minimally invasive surgery has become a part of almost every field of surgery. The gynecologic surgeons were among the first to recognize the potentials of laparoscopic approach for management of various benign gynecologic problems. As the new techniques are being developed, the indications for use of laparoscopy in gynecologic oncology are emerging. The increasing number of publications report on feasibility, safety, and potential risks of this approach, indicating growing interest in endoscopic approach to gynecologic cancer.

The laparoscopic approach offers several advantages over laparotomy.[1] Pelvic and abdominal anatomy appear magnified under the laparoscope and on video camera, allowing precise diagnosis and treatment of the disease adjacent to vital organs, blood vessels, and nerve structures. Likewise, identification of subtle changes that may represent metastatic disease is improved. This particularly pertains to surfaces at risk for metastatic disease in ovarian and other gynecologic cancers: the upper abdomen, surfaces of the liver and diaphragm, the posterior cul-de-sac, broad ligament, and peritoneal and mesenteric surfaces (Fig. 34.1). Additional benefits of laparoscopy in gynecologic oncology include minimized bleeding from the small vessels afforded by pneumoperitoneum, the elimination of large abdominal incision, early ambulation, faster recovery and shorter hospital stay, and therefore lower cost, and earlier installment of postoperative chemotherapy and radiation if needed.

Numerous procedures in gynecologic oncology can be accomplished by endoscopic approach. These include pelvic and periaortic lymphadenectomy, laparoscopy-assisted vaginal hysterectomy with bilateral salpingo-oophorectomy, colostomy, intraperitoneal port placement, second-look surgery, radioactive needle implants, laparoscopic radical hysterectomy, staging for endometrial cancer, and limited ovarian debulking surgery.[2–4] In applying advanced laparoscopic techniques to gynecologic oncology, three critical principles must be respected: (1) the extent of necessary surgery must be adequate, (2) the safety must comparable to traditional laparotomy, and (3) prognosis and cure rate must be comparable with standard laparotomy approach. Having these criteria in mind, we have reviewed current literature on the role and risks of laparoscopy in treatment of adnexal masses and ovarian cancer.

I. LAPAROSCOPY FOR ADNEXAL MASSES

Surgical diagnosis remains the crucial step for adequate surgical management of adnexal mass. One of the major benefits of laparoscopic approach to all adnexal masses is avoiding overtreatment and unnecessary laparotomy. Most adnexal masses are benign with malignancy found in only 7–13% of

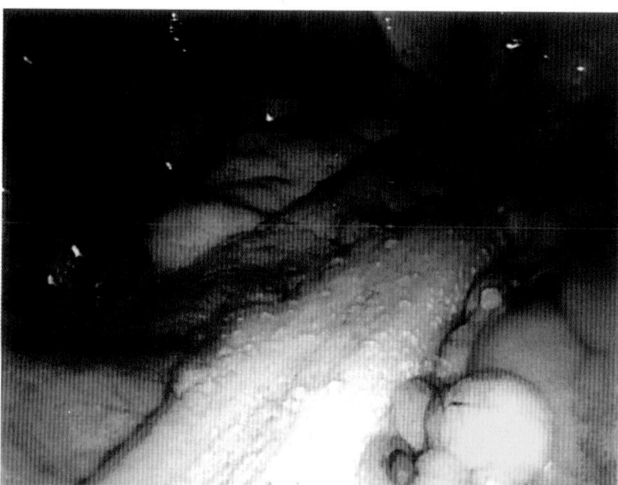

FIGURE 34.1 Macroscopical metastases on the surface of the recta-sigmoid colon during diagnostic laparoscopy.

premenopausal and 8–45% postmenopausal patients.[5] The incidence of unsuspected ovarian cancer at laparoscopy has been shown to be only 0.04% by Nezhat *et al.* [12] and in 1990 survey of American Association of Gynecologic Laparoscopists.[6] Further benefits of laparoscopic treatment of adnexal masses include shorter length of hospital stay,[7, 8] decreased postoperative pain and recovery time,[9] less adhesion formation,[10] and lesser cost to the patient and the hospital.[11] Accurate diagnosis at surgery is a key in management of adnexal masses. The availability of immediate histologic diagnosis on frozen sections is crucial. In the largest series of laparoscopically managed adnexal masses in reproductive age women, Nezhat *et al.* reported that the most reliable indicator of malignancy was the combination of laparoscopic visualization and frozen section analysis.[12] In most subsequent studies, both the sensitivity and accuracy of frozen section in detecting ovarian cancer have been greater than 92%.[13] In a prospective study of 160 patients with adnexal masses treated at gynecologic oncology service, Dottino *et al.* found discrepancy between frozen section and final pathology in 3% of the cases.[14] It seems therefore that laparoscopy is a safe and reliable tool in diagnosis of pelvic masses if performed cautiously and with the principles of cancer surgery kept in mind. Adequate procedure mandates careful inspection of the ovaries and the whole peritoneal cavity with frozen section analysis.[12] Aspiration of pelvic fluid or pelvic washings is necessary in all cases. Further treatment is tailored according to the age of the patient and intraoperative findings.

In reproductive age women, outcome of laparoscopically managed cysts no greater than 8–10 cm has been uniformly favorable. The principles of cancer surgery should apply to the treatment of benign-appearing cysts, as up to one-third of malignancies will retain a benign appearance.[15] Larger cysts, after excision from the ovary and placement in endobag, may be ruptured to facilitate their removal without peritoneal contamination. Even larger cysts, which exceed the size of intracorporeal sacs, may be removed through minilaparotomy or colpotomy with excellent results.[16, 17] Canis reported results of a 12-year study of laparoscopically managed benign ovarian cysts demonstrating a low complication rate of 1.5%, effectiveness of the procedure with recurrence rate of 1.8%, and preservation of fertility after laparoscopic management.[18]

The role of laparoscopy in the management of noncystic masses has been a subject of controversy over last decade.[19–22] According to the American Association of Gynecologic Laparoscopists, the majority of clinicians consider laparotomy to be the safest treatment of noncystic masses.[6] Maiman *et al.* reported that laparoscopic visualization may fail to identify cancer in one-third of the cases.[15] Wenzel *et al.* reported that 31 of 42 patients who underwent laparoscopic oophorectomy for malignancy had a residual disease at subsequent staging laparotomy.[23] However, in both studies the use of frozen section analysis was minimal and conversion to laparotomy was not performed in patients who were felt to have malignant or suspicious masses. On the other hand, in a French study conducted by Chapron *et al.* 11% of 228 masses evaluated preoperatively as "low risk" were found to have features of malignancy during laparoscopy; all 26 were spared unnecessary surgery by obtaining frozen section diagnosis of excised adnexa.[13] Dottino *et al.* reported on safe use of laparoscopy in 88% of 160 pre- and postmenopausal patients with suspicious adnexal masses.[14] All authors stress the importance of preoperative counseling, availability of immediate frozen section analysis, and surgical expertise.[13, 18]

Standard operative approach to adnexal mass in postmenopausal woman had been explorative laparotomy to ensure adequate exposure for the treatment of ovarian cancer. Reports beginning in the late 1980s started to question this approach observing that even in this group of patients there was propensity for benign lesions [24–26] and in some series up to 75% of tumors were histologically benign.[14, 21, 27] In the only prospective study Dottino *et al.* reported that nearly 90% of cases were managed laparoscopically without appreciable increase in morbidity.[14] The same principles of careful visualization of peritoneal cavity, obtaining the washings from the diaphragm, paracolic gutters, and pelvis prior to other surgical interventions has to be followed. Cystectomy in the postmenopausal woman is not recommend, instead removal of the entire adnexa with frozen section diagnosis is warranted. Removal of normal appearing contralateral ovary should be performed according to preoperative consultation and past medical and family history when pathology is benign.

II. EARLY OVARIAN CANCER

The staging procedure is a cornerstone of diagnosis, treatment, and prognosis of ovarian cancer. Standard surgical staging procedure according to FIGO includes: peritoneal washings, total abdominal hysterectomy (TAH), bilateral salpingo-oophorectomy (BSO), retroperitoneal lymphadenectomy, and omentectomy.[28] Surgical staging is of particular importance in presumed early-stage disease where it results in the detection of occult metastases in 24–28% of the patients.[29]

A few small series on role of laparoscopy on surgical staging of ovarian cancer have been reported. Querleu and LeBlanc reported adequate laparoscopic staging of 9 patients with ovarian carcinoma, 4 patients were staged for presumed stage I disease, and the remaining 5 either had borderline tumors or underwent second-look surgery.[30] There were no complications and average length of hospital stay was 2–8 days.

Nezhat *et al.* reported preliminary results of laparoscopic staging of 10 patients with ovarian cancer, 5 of whom had stage Ia-Ic disease.[31] In all but two patients who wanted to preserve fertility, full and adequate surgical staging was accomplished. There were no serious complications and all patients were discharged on postoperative day one. Childers *et al.* reported a series of 14 patients who underwent adequate laparoscopic staging for early ovarian cancer.[32] Metastatic disease was found in 8 of the 14 patients (57%). In their hands, there were no complications and the length of stay was 1–6 days. They concluded that laparoscopic staging is a safe and adequate procedure for presumed early ovarian cancer and that it affords detection of microscopic dissemination of the disease in the high-risk areas. Malik *et al.* reported on 11 patients who underwent laparoscopy for treatment of adnexal mass in whom pathology revealed malignant tumor.[33] Two of the 11 patients had borderline tumors stage Ia, one had malignant Brenner tumor stage Ia, and the fourth patient had malignant transitional cell carcinoma stage with "discrete peritoneal carcinomatosis"; all four were treated laparoscopically. The remaining seven patients underwent immediate or interval staging laparotomy. The authors underline the use of frozen section diagnosis, endobag for tumor removal, and other safety measures to avoid contamination of the peritoneal cavity.

Of particular interest is the prognostic significance of tumor rupture in early ovarian cancer. Spontaneous cystic tumor rupture has been suggested as an independent prognostic factor in several studies,[34, 35] but rupture during surgery was significant only in univariate analyses.[35, 36] Recently, Vergote *et al.*, in a large retrospective analysis of prognostic factors in 1545 patients with stage I ovarian cancer, identified the degree of tumor differentiation as the most powerful prognostic variable, followed by rupture before surgery (hazard ratio 2.65) and rupture during surgery (hazard ratio 1.64).[37] However, the results of this study should be taken with extreme caution, as the patients from different institutions did not undergo full and/or uniform surgical staging.

III. LAPAROSCOPY FOR "INADEQUATELY STAGED" OVARIAN CANCER

Several reports described the safe and efficient use of laparoscopy for management of previously inadequately staged ovarian cancer. The cases of inadequately staged cancer occur in the setting of the disease incidentally found during laparoscopic surgery performed by nongynecologic oncologists, or in rare cases when the disease is not recognized intraoperatively.

One of the first large series dates back to 1987, when Dagnini *et al.* reported on 45 patients undergoing laparoscopy for staging, follow-up, and restaging of ovarian carcinoma.[38] In 10 cases, remaining extraovarian disease was found. The authors underline the feasibility of the laparoscopic approach for completion staging and detection of peritoneal/diaphragmatic metastatic disease. Amara *et al.* described two cases where meticulous extensive laparoscopic completion staging procedure was performed.[39] The first patient underwent TAH, BSO for well-differentiated mucinous carcinoma of the ovary. The following laparoscopic procedure included omentectomy, appendectomy, washings, and pelvic and periaortic lymphadenectomy, and placement of intraperitoneal catheter. The duration of the procedure was 5 h and 10 min and blood loss was 300 cc. The second patient underwent TAH, BSO, appendectomy, and pelvic washings by general surgeon and was referred when final pathology showed granulosa cell tumor with positive washings. Subsequent laparoscopy included peritoneal washings, omental biopsies, and pelvic and para-aortic lymph node dissection. The operative time was 3 h and 10 min and blood loss 30 cc. GOG Trial #9302 has been designed to assess the role of laparoscopy in staging of inadequately staged ovarian cancer. Seventy patients have been entered into the trial since 1993 and although the results are eagerly awaited, no conclusions can be drawn at this time.

The completion staging laparoscopy seems to be an attractive concept for the patients who recently underwent the major surgical procedure, and it is safe and accurate if performed by a gynecologic oncologist trained in advanced laparoscopic techniques.

A. Laparoscopy in Advanced Stage Ovarian Cancer

Although laparoscopic techniques have been used for staging and treatment of advanced ovarian cancer, the reports are isolated, and the need for objective assessment of the procedure through prospective clinical trials is needed.[31, 39]

1. Laparoscopic Staging Technique for Ovarian Cancer

The full surgical staging by either laparotomy or laparoscopy includes careful inspection of the abdomen, cytologic assessment of the ascites or peritoneal washings, pelvic and para-aortic lymphadenectomy, infracolic omentectomy, debulking, and multiple biopsies.

A long suction-irrigator probe with lactated Ringer's solution with heparin is used to obtain peritoneal washings. Once ovarian mass is evaluated and decision made to proceed laparoscopically the mass is extirpated in a usual fashion. Care must be taken not to rupture the mass and to remove it without letting the tissue contaminate the abdominal wall. This is done by removing all possibly malignant tissue in a laparoscopic endobag A more durable Cook bag is recommended for larger masses which require aspiration or morcellation within the bag prior to the removal.

Peritoneal biopsies are obtained using CO_2 laser and hydrodissection, biopsy forceps, and endoshears, or combination of sharp dissection and electrocautery. Diaphragmatic biopsies are taken very superficially with a biopsy forceps or CO_2 laser. For infracoloic omentectomy, the patient is placed in a straight supine position and the omentum is excised from the inferior margin of the transverse colon, using a harmonic scalpel, endoshears and bipolar forceps, a linear stapler, or sutures. The harmonic scalpel is superior for omentectomy because the ease and speed of use, its shape, and minimal plume formation.

2. Pelvic Lymphadenectomy

Pelvic and para-aortic lymphadenectomy is accomplished after hysterectomy and bilateral oophorectomy. The initial approach is to expose the anterior and posterior leaves of the broad ligament by incising the round ligament and cutting the broad ligament in a cephalad fashion lateral and parallel to the infundibulopelvic ligament. Creating the avasular paravesical space helps identify the ureter, obturator nerve and vessels, and pelvic vessels (Fig. 34.2). The superior vesical artery identifies the medial border of the paravesical space. The spaces lateral to this vessel and medial to the external iliac vein and obturator internus muscle are created with blunt and sharp dissection. Electrocoagulation should not be necessary as these spaces are generally avascular. Once the spaces are created, the obturator internus muscle and bony lateral side wall, the levator plate posteriorly, and the obturator nerve and vessels anteriorly should be visible (Fig. 34.2). The pelvic lymph nodes can now be safely removed. Starting laterally over the psoas muscle and proceeding medially provides a safe approach that avoids the genitofemoral nerve. The external iliac nodes along the external iliac artery and vein are excised caudally to the level of the deep circumflex iliac vein seen crossing over the distal portion of the external iliac artery (Fig. 34.3). The obturator nerve is identified by blunt dissection

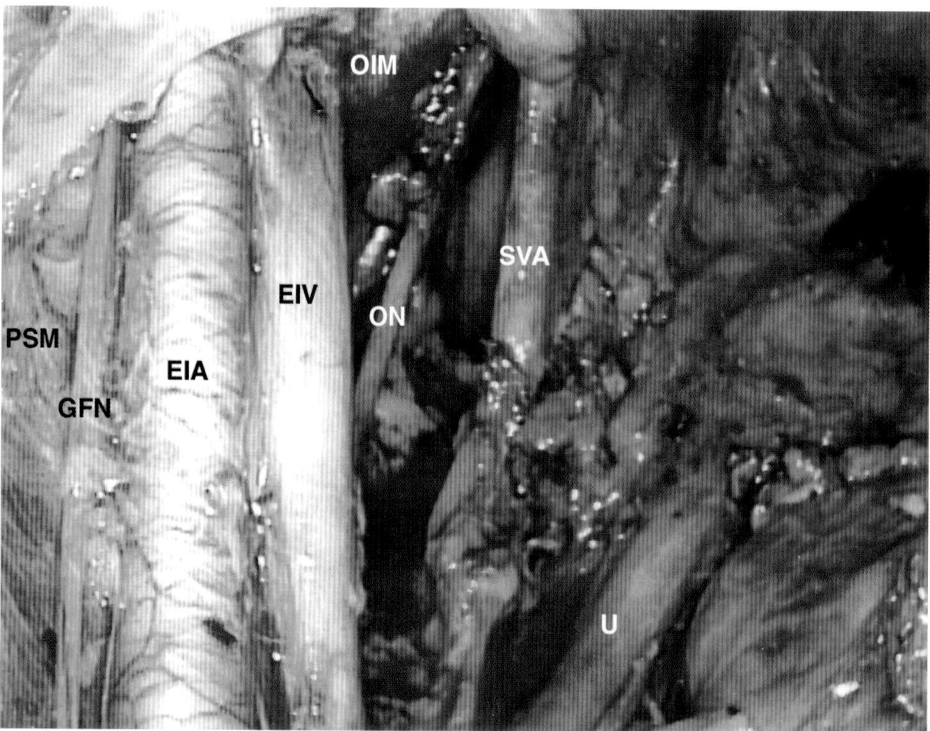

FIGURE 34.2 Left retro-peritoneal pelvic anatomy after laparoscopic pelvic left adenectomy. From left to right: PSM (psoas muscle), GFN (genitofemoral nerve), EIA (external iliac artery), EIV (external iliac vein), OIM (obturator internus muscle), ON (obturator nerve), SVA (superior vesicle artery), and U (ureter).

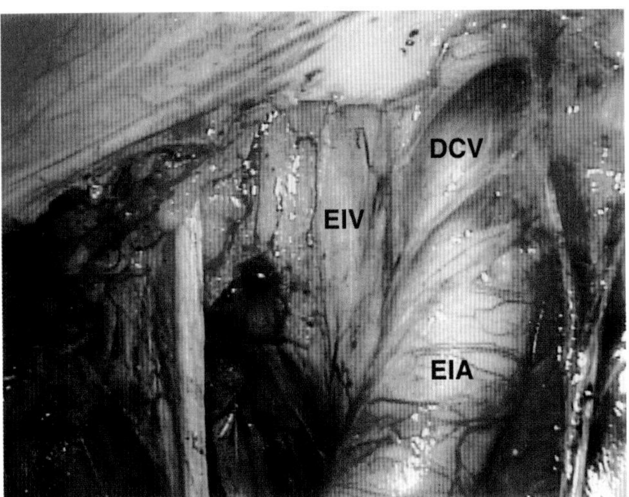

FIGURE 34.3 Deep circumflex vein crossing over the distal portion of the right external iliac artery. From right to left: EIA (external iliac artery), DCV (deep circumflex vein), and EIV (external iliac vein).

below and between the obliterated umbilical artery and the external iliac vein. Of note is that although the obturator vessels are usually posterior to the nerve, sometimes an aberrant obturator vein may arise from the external iliac artery and is anterior to the nerve. The nodal tissue anterior and lateral to the nerve and medial and inferior to the external iliac vein is removed by blunt and sharp dissection. Venous anastomosis between the obturator and the external iliac veins are saved from injury. The obturator nerve nodes are excised caudally to the pelvic sidewall where the obturator nerve exits the pelvis through the obturator canal and cephalad up to the bifurcation of the common iliac artery. Before the removal of each nodal bundle, each pedicle is ligated by electrocoagulation or endoscopic hemoclips, to prevent lymphocyst formation. The lymph node packets are removed in a bag through the largest trocar to avoid any contact between potentially malignant lymph node tissue and the abdominal wall.

To excise the lymph nodes around the common iliac artery, a plane is created between the posterior peritoneum and the adventitia overlying the common iliac artery. Another option is to extend the dissection over the common iliac vessels when removing the proximal portion of the external iliac nodes. Before the nodes are detached, the orientation of the ureter and ovarian vessels crossing the common iliac artery is identified. When one is performing a left pelvic lymph node dissection, it may be necessary to take down rectosigmoid colon from the left pelvic side wall to allow visualization of the pelvic vessels.

3. Para-Aortic Lymphadenectomy

There are several ways to begin the dissection: incising the peritoneum overlying the aorta, opening the peritoneum over sacral promontory, and extending the incision overlying the common iliac artery toward the aorta. Next, the retroperitoneal space is created by infusing this space with lactated Ringer's solution or using sharp and blunt dissection, to develop the space lateral to the aorta. Before cutting, it is essential to identifying the right ureter, separate it from underlying tissue, and retract it laterally. The nodal tissue overlying the aorta, right common iliac artery, and sacral promontory is removed laterally toward the psoas muscle. This maneuver allows the nodal tissue anterior to the vena cava to be detached. The dissection is continued cephalad to the level of the inferior mesenteric artery, removing all lymphatic tissue anterior to the aorta and inferior vena cava. Again, it is essential to identify the ureter along the inferior border of the dissection and the transverse duodenum along the superior margin of the dissection. Perforating vessels from the vena cava are electrocoagulated or ligated with hemoclips.

The removal of the left para-aortic nodes may be more difficult because of the location of the sigmoid colon. Attention is necessary to avoid injury to the inferior mesenteric artery, ovarian vessels, and the ureter. The left common iliac vein lies at the bifurcation of the aorta. The dissection proceeds from the aorta laterally toward the psoas muscle, excising the lymph nodes from above the inferior mesenteric artery to below the left common iliac artery (Fig. 34.4). This allows the surgeon to dissect laterally in a plane that is beneath the inferior mesenteric artery and the mesentery of the sigmoid colon. It is important not to dissect laterally until the adventitia of the aorta is incised to prevent entering the wrong plane.

In ovarian cancer, the para-aortic lymphadenectomy is extended to the level of the left renal vein and right ovarian vein (Fig. 34.5). The ovarian vessels are ligated, if necessary, to prevent bleeding. After the lymphadenectomy is completed, evaluation of the area under decreased pneumoperitoneal pressure is done to ensure hemostasis. As with pelvic lymphadenectomy, the peritoneum is not closed and the drains are not placed. Interceed can be applied to decrease postoperative adhesions.

IV. SECOND-LOOK LAPAROSCOPY

A second-look operation for ovarian cancer is the most accurate method of accessing the disease status in patients who have undergone staging/debulking procedure and primary chemotherapy. Traditionally, the operation is performed through a midline vertical abdominal incision as a second-look laparotomy. Candidates for surgery are the patients with advanced disease who achieved a complete clinical remission after initial treatment. The overall probability of finding persistent disease at the time of second-look is 50%.[40]

The second-look procedure can be accomplished laparoscopically. Although this procedure allows for better visualization of the diaphragm and the liver, the adequacy of

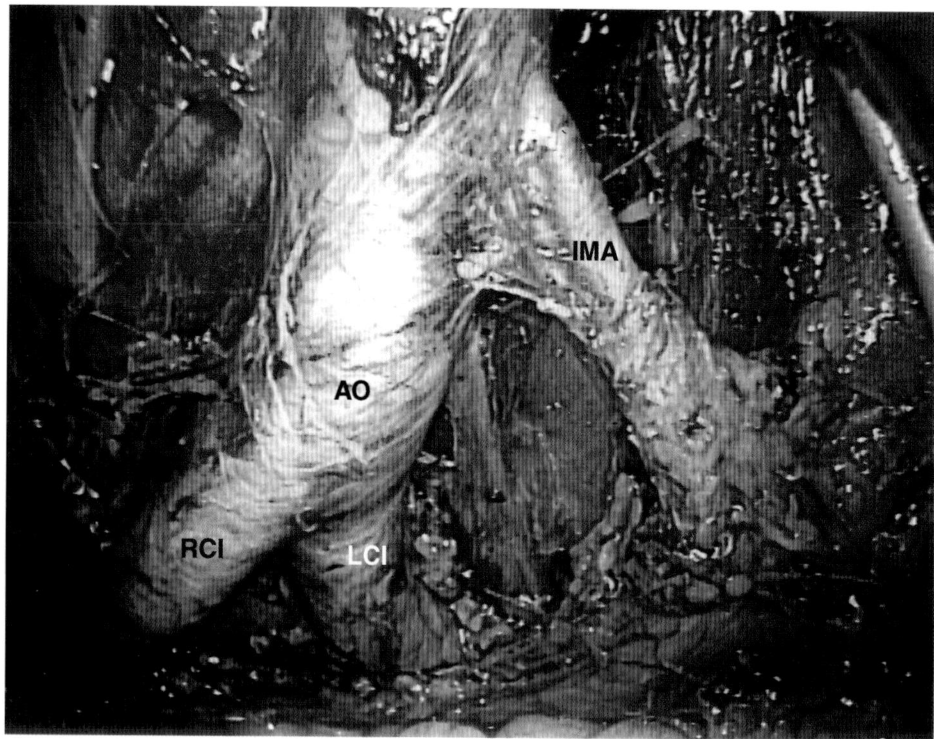

FIGURE 34.4 Bifurcation of the aorta and inferior mesenteric artery. From left to right IMA (inferior mensenteric artery), AO (aorta), LCI (left common iliac artery), and RCI (right common iliac artery).

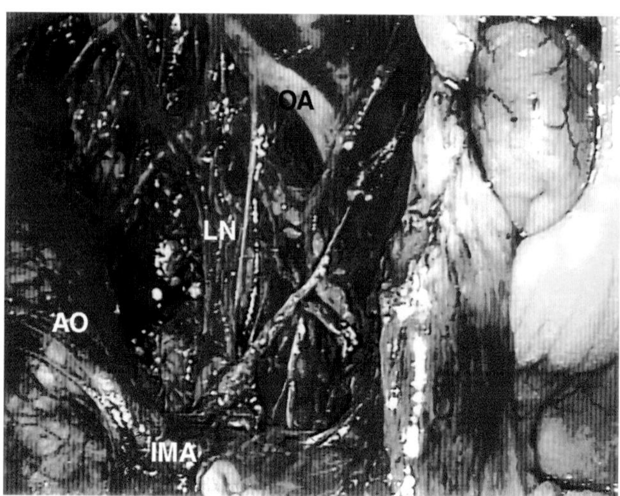

FIGURE 34.5 Left para-aortic lymph nodes above IMA. From left to right: OA (left ovarian artery), LN (lymph nodes), IMA (inferior mesenteric artery), and AO (aorta).

laparoscopic second-look in the presence of severe adhesions and in the evaluation of small bowel has been a topic of concern because the lack of tactile sensation in laparoscopy. It has been suggested that this would lead to higher false-negative rates for laparoscopic second-look compared with traditional approach. However, we and others believe that light touch palpation is achievable with laparoscopic instruments after proper training.[41] Even more, data from laparoscopic second-look surgery do not support this concern. Nezhat *et al.* in a series of 19 patients undergoing second-look surgery, found persistent disease in 9, the rate comparable to that of second-look laparotomies.[31] Similarly, Childers found persistent disease in 24 of 44 laparoscopic second-look procedures, 5 of whom had only microscopic disease.[42] In two of the patients metastatic disease was found only in periaortic lymph nodes above the level of inferior mesenteric artery where primary periaortic lympadenectomy ended. The mean operative time was 75.5 min in this study. Significant complications occurred in 6 of 44 patients (14%), 3 of whom required laparotomy because of trocar injury to transverse colon, vena cava injury during periaortic lymphadenectomy, and small bowel injury during adhesiolysis. Three remaining complications were managed laparoscopically: trocar liver injury, 6-mm perforation of the right external iliac vein, and laceration of the right hemidiaphragm. This complication rate compares favorably with staging using laparotomy in the setting of second-look.[43]

In a comparison of 57 laparoscopic and 69 traditional second-look procedures, laparoscopic procedures had significantly less blood loss (33.9 versus 164.9 cc), significantly shorter operative time (81.3 versus. 130.4 min), and shorter hospital stay (0.3 versus 6.8 days), and the direct cost per case was significantly reduced in cases managed laparoscopically

($2765 versus 5420).[44] Despite obtaining 50% fewer biopsies during laparoscopy, the ability to detect the disease was comparable: 52.6% for laparoscopy group versus 53.6% in the laparotomy group. There was no difference in morbidity between the groups.

These results were recently corroborated by a large study of 150 patients undergoing second-look laparoscopy.[45] The rate of positive second-look was 54%. The rate of conversion to laparotomy in this study was 12%, comparable to those reported by Casey *et al.* (10.6%) and Childers *et al.* (11.4%)[42, 44]. The overall rate of major complications was low 2.7%, remarkable for the population of patients who had undergone a prior major abdominal and pelvic surgery.

Several studies addressed the influence of laparoscopic approach to second-look on recurrence rate survival. Abu-Rustum and colleagues compared the results of 31 second-look laparoscopies with those of 70 second-look laparotomies.[46] Again, laparoscopy was associated with less blood loss, shorter hospital stay, and lower hospital charges. All intra- and immediate postoperative complications were found in laparotomy group. With a median follow-up time of 22 months, recurrence after a negative second-look operation was 14% for both laparoscopy and laparotomy. Nezhat *et al.* reported similar progression-free interval and survival in 25 patients undergoing second-look laparoscopy compared with 27 patients in second-look laparotomy arm.[47] On the other hand, in a multicenter Italian retrospective study of 192 patients with advanced ovarian cancer who underwent second-look surgery, Gadducci *et al.* reported higher recurrence rate and shorter survival after negative laparoscopy as compared with negative second look laparotomy.[48] However, there was no common therapy after negative second-look surgery in the group of 115 patients in the study and the choices of treatment were based on personal preference.

Although controversy still seems to exist about influence of second-look operations on survival, they have undoubtedly contributed immensely to our understanding of the biologic behavior of ovarian cancer and remain standard in clinical protocols determining the effectiveness of a specific treatment. Second-look laparoscopy seems to be as safe and effective as laparotomy. However, as it is one of the most difficult endoscopic procedures, it should be performed only by a surgeon with extensive experience in advanced laparoscopic techniques.

V. RISKS OF LAPAROSCOPY IN ONCOLOGY: ABDOMINAL WALL METASTASES AND PERITONEAL TUMOR DISSEMINATION

Abdominal wall metastases, also called port or wound site metastases, have been reported after both laparoscopy and laparotomy. The incidence of these complications has been 1% after laparotomy and 1–3% after laparoscopy.[49] The most likely mechanism for port site metastases seems to be a direct contamination by the surgical procedure. Ports are contaminated by tumor extraction or the postoperative withdrawal of contaminated ports and loss of abdominal insufflations. Chu *et al.* [50] described recurrence at port sites in a patient who underwent laparoscopic staging for cervical cancer. Similar port site recurrence was described by Wang *et al.* [51] Although port/wound site recurrences may be disfiguring and difficult to treat, there is no prospective evidence that port site metastases worsen prognosis.[49]

A number of animal studies suggest increased tumor dissemination after a CO_2 pneumoperitoneum.[52] Voltz *et al.* reported diffuse intraperitoneal tumor spread after laparoscopy in nude-mice model as well as the shortest survival time in that group.[53] Canis *et al.* [54] used immunocompetent rats injected intraperitoneally with rat ovarian carcinoma cells. There was a greater tumor growth after laparotomy than laparoscopy. In the high-pressure pneumoperitoneum group (10 mmHg) tumor was disseminated more diffusely than in the low-pressure pneumoperitoneum (4 mmHg) group. Wound metastases were larger and more frequent after laparotomy. As pointed by Canis *et al.* [52] one has to be cautious when interpreting results of animal studies. Important variables, which must be taken into consideration before reaching conclusions, include: animal model, choice of cell line for inoculation, postoperative immune situation, the pressure of pneumoperitoneum, and sample size (number of animals). Each detail of a model can influence results given that it is difficult to mimic clinical situation in any animal model.

However, a few clinical reports also raised concerns regarding possible intraperitoneal tumor dissemination following laparoscopy. Canis *et al.* reported a case of pelvic dissemination found at restaging procedure 3 weeks after initial adnexectomy for well-differentiated serous adenocarcinoma of the ovary.[55] Although one may argue that these findings are indicative of tumor biology more than a consequence of surgical approach, it would be prudent to introduce surgical measures to prevent tumor dissemination and port site contamination. Removal of all specimen using an endobag and removal of all ports while the abdomen is still insufflated to prevent possible contamination of port sites as well as the immediate local treatment of the ports with a cytotoxic agent is mandatory.

In the Division of Gynecologic Oncology at Mount Sinai School of Medicine in New York laparoscopy has been used liberally in evaluation and management of suspicious adnexal masses, second-look evaluation, and primary and end staging of ovarian cancer, when the disease is not extensive and bulky; and in a selected groups of patients with localized disease for secondary cytoreduction. In our experience, few trocar site metastases were observed and a single documented case of disseminated tumor metastases.

VI. CONCLUSIONS

The role of operative laparoscopy in the management of patients with benign and malignant ovarian masses is expanding, offering distinct advantages of lower morbidity, improved postoperative recovery, and reduced cost. Endoscopic approach can be used in management of benign or suspicious adnexal masses in pre- and postmenopausal women, staging of early ovarian cancer, as a completion staging of inadequately staged ovarian cancer, and staging of selected cases of advanced cancer of the ovary. It has been used for monitoring the effect of primary treatment for ovarian cancer, as seen during laparoscopic second-look surgery.

Advanced operative laparoscopy, when performed by a surgeon trained in advanced laparoscopic techniques and in adequately equipped centers, is as safe and effective as open techniques.[12, 21] However, most practicing gynecologic oncologists are not trained in advanced endoscopic techniques. Therefore, development of a formal training program within the subspecialty of gynecologic oncology is needed to establish and propagate skills necessary to perform advanced laparoscopic surgery. The competency of a larger number of gynecologic oncologists in operative laparoscopy would facilitate organization of large, prospective trials, which are needed to objectively assess the utility and safety of endoscopic procedures.

References

1. Nezhat, C., Siegler, A., Nezhat, F. *et al.* (2000). The role of laparoscopy in the management of gynecologic malignancy. *In* "Operative Gynecologic Laparoscopy—Principles and Techniques," 2nd Ed. (C. Nezhat, ed.), pp. 301–328, McGraw-Hill, New York.
2. Nezhat, C. R., Burrell, M. O., Nezhat, F. R. *et al.* (1992). Laparoscopic radical hysterectomy with paraaortic and pelvic lymph node dissection. *Am. J. Obstet. Gynecol.* 166, 864–865.
3. Querleu, D. (1993). Case report: Laparoscopy-assisted radical vaginal hysterectomy. *Gynecol. Oncol.* 51, 248–254.
4. Childers, J. M., Brzechffa, P. R., Hatch, K. *et al.* (1993). Laparoscopically assisted surgical staging (LASS) of endometrial cancer. *Gynecol. Oncol.* 51, 33–38.
5. Parker, W. H., and Berek, J. S. (1994). Laparoscopic management of the adnexal mass. *Obstet. Gynecol. Clin. N. Am.* 21, 79–92.
6. Hulka, J. T., Parker, W. H., Surrey, M. W. *et al.* (1992). American Association Gynecologic Laparoscopists. Survey of management of ovarian masses in 1990. *J. Reprod. Med.* 37, 599–602.
7. Mais, V., Ajossa, S., Guerriero, S. *et al.* (1996). Laparoscopic versus abdominal myomectomy: A prospective randomized trial to evaluate benefits in early outcome. *Am. J. Obstet. Gynecol.* 174, 654–658.
8. Mais, V., Ajossa, S., Piras, B. *et al.* (1995). Treatment of nonendometriotic benign adnexal cyst. A randomized comparison of laparoscopy and laparotomy. *Obstet. Gynecol.* 86, 770–774.
9. Davison, J., Park, W., and Penney, L. (1993). Comparative study of operative laparoscopy vs. laparotomy: Analysis of the financial impact. *Reprod. Med.* 38, 357–360.
10. Lundorff, P., Thorburn, J., Hahlin, M. *et al.* (1991). Adhesion formation after laparoscopic surgery in tubal pregnancy: A randomized trial versus laparotomy. *Fertil. Steril.* 55, 911–915.
11. Maruiri, F., and Azziz, A. (1993). Laparoscopic surgery for ectopic pregnancies: Technology assessment and public health implications. *Technol. Steril.* 59, 487–498.
12. Nezhat, F. R., Nezhat, C. H., Welander, C. E., and Benigno, B. (1992). Four ovarian cancers diagnosed during laparoscopic management of 1011 women with adnexal masses. *Am. J. Obstet. Gynecol.* 167, 790–796.
13. Chapron, C., Dubuisson, J. B., Kadoch, O. *et al.* (1998). Laparoscopic management of organic ovarian cysts: Is there a place for frozen section in the diagnosis. *Hum. Reprod.* 13, 324–329.
14. Dottino, P. R., Levine, D. A., Ripley, D. L., and Cohen, C. J. (1999). Laparoscopic management of adnexal masses in premenopausal and postmenopausal women. *Obstet. Gynecol.* 93, 223–228.
15. Maiman, M., Seltzer, V., and Boyce, J. (1991). Laparoscopic excision of ovarian neoplasms subsequently found to be malignant. *Obstet. Gynecol.* 77, 563–765.
16. Flyn Niloff, J. M. (1995). Minilaparotomy for the ambulatory management of ovarian cysts. *Am. J. Obstet. Gynecol.* 173, 1727–1730.
17. Teng, F. Y., Muzsnai, D., and Perez, R. (1996). A comparative study of laparoscopy and colpotomy for the removal of ovarian dermoid cysts. *Obstet. Gynecol.* 87, 1009–1013.
18. Canis, M., Pouly, J. L., Watticz, A. *et al.* (1997). Laparoscopic management of adnexal masses suspicious at ultrasound. *Obstet. Gynecol.* 89, 679–683.
19. Chi, D. S., Curtin, J. P., and Barakat, R. R. (1995). Laparoscopic management of adnexal masses in women with a history of nongynecologic malignancy. *Obstet. Gynecol.* 86, 964–968.
20. Nezhat, C. T., Kayoncus, S., Nezhat, C. H. *et al.* (1999). Laparoscopic management of ovarian dermoid cysts: Ten year's experience. *J. Soc. Laparosc. Surg.* 3, 179–184.
21. Childers, J. M., Nasseri, A., and Surwit, E. A. (1996). Laparoscopic management of suspicious adnexal masses. *Am. J. Obstet. Gynecol.* 175, 1171–1179.
22. Parker, W. H. (1995). The case for laparoscopic management of the adnexal mass. *Clin. Obstet. Gynecol.* 38, 362–369.
23. Wenzel, R., Lehner, R., Husslein, P., and Sevelda, P. (1996). Laparoscopic surgery in cases of ovarian malignancies: An Austrian-wide survey. *Gynecol. Oncol.* 63, 57–61.
24. Andolf, E., Jorgensen, C., Scalenius, E. *et al.* Ultrasound measurement of the ovarian volume. *Acta Obstet. Gynecol. Scand.* 66, 387–392.
25. Rulin, M. C., and Preston, A. L. (1987). Adnexal mass in postmenopausal women. *Obstet. Gynecol.* 70, 578–581.
26. Granberg, S., Wikland, M., and Jansson, I. (1989). Microscopic characterization of ovarian tumors and the relation to the histologic diagnosis: Criteria to be used for ultrasound evaluation. *Gynecol. Oncol.* 35, 139–144.
27. Shalev, E., Eliyahu, S., Peleg, D., and Tsabari, A. (1994). Laparoscopic management of adnexal cystic masses in postmenopausal women. *Obstet. Gynecol.* 83, 594–596.
28. FIGO Cancer Committee (1988). Annual report on the results of treatment in gynecologic cancer. Vol. 20, Radiumhemmet, Stockholm, Sweden.
29. Burghardt, E., Girardi, F., Lahousen, M. *et al.* (1991). Patterns of pelvic and para-aortic lymph node involvement in ovarian carcinoma. *Gynecol. Oncol.* 40, 103–106.
30. Querleu, D., and LeBlanc, E. (1994). Laparoscopic infrarenal paraaortic lymph node dissection for restaging of carcinoma of the ovary or fallopian tube. *Cancer* 73, 1467–1471.
31. Nezhat, C., Nezhat, F., Teng, N. H. *et al.* (1994). The role of laparoscopy in the management of gynecologic malignancy. *Semin. Surg. Oncol.* 10, 431–439.
32. Childers, J. M., Lang, J., Surwit, E. A. *et al.* (1995). Laparoscopic surgical staging of ovarian cancer. *Gynecol. Oncol.* 59, 25–33.
33. Malik, E., Bohm, W., and Stoz, F. (1998). Laparoscopic management of ovarian tumors. *Surg. Endosc.* 12, 1326–1333.

34. Sjovall, K., Nilsson, B., and Einhorn, N. (1994). Different types of rupture of the tumor capsule and the impact on survival in early ovarian carcinoma. *Int. J. Gynecol. Cancer* 4, 333–336.
35. Kodama, S., Tanaka, K., Tokunaga, A. *et al.* (1997). Multivariate analysis of prognostic factors in patients with ovarian cancer stage I and II. *Int. J. Gynaecol. Obstet.* 56, 147–153.
36. Webb, M. J., Decker, D. G., Mussey, E., and Williams, T. J. (1973). Factors influencing survival in stage I ovarian cancer. *Am. J. Obstet. Gynecol.* 116, 222–228.
37. Vergote, I., DeBrabanter, J., Fyles, A. *et al.* (2001). Prognostic importance of degree of differentiation and cyst rupture in stage I invasive epithelial ovarian carcinoma. *Lancet* 357, 176–182.
38. Dagnini, G., Marin, G., Caldroni, M. W. *et al.* (1987). Laparoscopy in staging, follow-up, and restaging of ovarian carcinoma. *Gastrointest. Endosc.* 33, 80–83.
39. Amara, P. D., Nezhat, C., Teng, N. N. H. *et al.* (1996). Operative laparoscopy in the management of ovarian cancer. *Surg. Laparosc. Endosc.* 6, 38–45.
40. Copeland, L. J., Gershenson, M., Wharton, J. T. *et al.* (1985). Miscroscopic disease at second-look laparotomy for advanced ovarian cancer. *Cancer* 5, 472–478.
41. Dargent, D. F. G. (1999). Current therapeutic issues in gynecologic cancer. *Hematol. Oncol. Clin. N. Am.* 13, 1–14.
42. Childers, J. M., Lang, J., Surwit, E. A., and Hatch, K. D. (1995). Laparoscopic surgical staging of ovarian cancer. *Gynecol. Oncol.* 59, 25–33.
43. Buschsbaum, H. J., Brady, M. F., Delgado, F. *et al.* (1989). Surgical staging of carcinoma of the ovaries. *Surg. Gynecol. Obstet.* 169, 226–232.
44. Casey, C. A., Farias-Eisner, R., Pisni, A. L. *et al.* (1996). What is the role of reassessment laparoscopy in the management of gynecologic cancers in 1995? *Gynecol. Oncol.* 60, 454–461.
45. Husain, A., Chi, D. S., Prasad, M. *et al.* (2001). The role of laparoscopy in second-look evaluations for ovarian cancer. *Gynecol. Oncol.* 80, 44–47.
46. Abu-Rustum, N. R., Barakat, R. R., Siegel, P. L. *et al.* (1996). Second-look operation for epithelial ovarian cancer: Laparoscopy or laparotomy. *Obstet. Gynecol.* 88, 549–553.
47. Nezhat, F. R., Rahaman, J., Dottino, P. *et al.* (1999). Accuracy of second-look laparoscopy compared with second-look laparotomy in predicting recurrence and survival in advanced ovarian cancer. Abstracts of the Global congress of Gynecologic Endoscopy, 28th Annual Meeting of the Amerian Association of Gynecologic Laparoscopists', S146.
48. Gadducci, A., Sartori, E., Maggino, T. *et al.* (1998). Analysis of failures after negative second-look in patients with advanced ovarian cancer: An Italian multicenter study. *Gynecol. Oncol.* 68, 150–155.
49. Kruitwagen, R. F. P. M., Swinkels, B. M., Keyser, K. G. G. *et al.* (1996). Incidence and effect on survival of abdominal wall metastases at trocar puncture sites following laparoscopy or paracentesis in women with ovarian cancer. *Gynecol. Oncol.* 60, 233–237.
50. Chu, K., Chang, S., Chen, F. *et al.* (1997). Laparoscopic surgical staging in cervical cancer-preliminary experience among Chinese. *Gynecol. Oncol.* 64, 49–53.
51. Wang, P. H., Yuan, C. C., Chao, K. C. *et al.* (1997). Squamous cell carcinoma of the cervix after laparoscopic surgery: A case report. *J. Reprod. Med.* 42, 801–804.
52. Canis, M., Botchorishvilli, R., Wattiez, A. *et al.* (2000). Cancer and laparoscopy, experimental studies: A review. *Eur. J. Obstet. Gynecol. Reprod. Biol.* 91, 1–9.
53. Voltz, J., Paolucci, V., Schaeff, B. *et al.* (1998). Laparoscopic surgery: The effects of insufflation gas on tumour-induced lethality in nude mice. *Am. J. Obstet. Gynecol.* 178, 793–795.
54. Canis, M., Botchorishvilli, R., Wattiez, A. *et al.* (1998). Tumor growth and dissemination after laparotomy and CO_2 pneumoperitoneum: A rat ovarian cancer model. *Obstet. Gynecol.* 92, 104–108.
55. Canis, M., Mage, G., Pouly, J. L. *et al.* (1994). Laparoscopic diagnosis of adnexal cystic masses: A 12-year experience with long-term follow-up. *Obstet. Gynecol.* 83, 707–712.

CHAPTER

35

Chemotherapy of Ovarian Cancer

MARTEE L. HENSLEY
Developmental Chemotherapy Service
Department of Medicine
Memorial Sloan-Kettering Cancer Center
New York, New York 10021
and
Novartis Pharma AG, Oncology
CH-4002 Basel, Switzerland

WILLIAM J. HOSKINS
Curtis & Elizabeth Anderson Cancer Institute
Memorial Health University Medical Center
Savannah, Georgia 31404

ABSTRACT

The chemotherapy for epithelial and nonepithelial tumors is discussed. The majority of patients with epithelial ovarian cancer will require post-cytoreductive surgery chemotherapy. Standard front-line therapy includes paclitaxel plus carboplatin or cisplatin. Intraperitoneal therapy with cisplatin may be appropriate for certain patients with very small-volume peritoneal disease. Clinical complete response rates are high, however the majority of patients relapse and require second-line therapy. Patients with potentially platinum-sensitive therapy are generally treated with platinum-based regimens. Patients with platinum-resistant disease may be treated with one of a number of noncross-resistant agents that have been identified in phase II trials in ovarian cancer.

Nonepithelial ovarian cancers occur in young patients and have a high likelihood of cure. Fertility-sparing surgery is appropriate for most patients. Following surgery, chemotherapy recommendations depend on the specific histology of the tumor. Patients with completely resected stromal tumors may not require chemotherapy, but are frequently treated at the time of relapse with cisplatin-based regimens. Patients with true stage IA dysgerminomas may be observed following complete staging surgery. Cisplatin-based, combination chemotherapy is recommended for patients with more advanced dysgerminomas, and patients with nondysgerminoma germ cell tumors.

Cancers of the ovary can be classified as epithelial and nonepithelial ovarian cancers. Epithelial ovarian cancer accounts for approximately 60% of ovarian cancers, germ cell tumors for approximately 30%, sex cord-stromal tumors for 10%, and mixed Mullerian tumors (carcinosarcomas) of the ovary for less than 1%.[1, 2] Careful histologic review of the pathological specimen is critical for determining best management of all ovarian cancers. Recommendations for chemotherapy will differ according to tumor histology and disease stage. The epidemiology, diagnostic evaluation, pathological classification, and surgical management of ovarian cancers are addressed in Chapters 6–8, 17, 19, 30, and 31. This chapter will focus on the specifics of chemotherapy for epithelial and nonepithelial ovarian cancers.

I. CHEMOTHERAPY FOR EPITHELIAL OVARIAN CANCER

Each year, epithelial ovarian cancer is diagnosed in approximately 25,000 women in the U.S., and accounts for over 14,000 deaths.[3] Early-stage epithelial ovarian cancer (stages I and II, in which disease is limited to the ovaries or to the ovaries and adjacent pelvic structures) is frequently curable, with 5-year survival rates over 80% for patients with stage II disease, and over 90% for patients with stage I disease.[4]

Only a subset of patients with early-stage disease will require chemotherapy following appropriate staging and debulking surgery. Unfortunately, nearly 70% of women with epithelial ovarian cancer have stage III or IV disease at the time of diagnosis. While over 80% of patients with advanced-stage ovarian cancer will respond to chemotherapy, the majority will ultimately succumb to their disease, with 5-year overall survival ranging from 5–30%.[5, 6]

A. Initial Management of Epithelial Ovarian Cancer

Comprehensive surgical staging by a gynecologic oncologist [7] should be considered for all patients with epithelial ovarian cancer, although initial treatment with chemotherapy may be appropriate for some patients with advanced disease who are not surgical candidates.[8] Complete surgical staging is important for prognosis and for chemotherapy treatment decisions. The bulk of residual disease that persists after comprehensive staging and debulking surgery has been consistently associated with survival.[9, 10] Patients in whom all residual tumor nodules are less than 1 cm in size have an approximately 22-month survival advantage over patients with bulkier residual disease.[11, 12] Following complete staging, most patients will be candidates for chemotherapy. Certain patients with stage I disease may not require chemotherapy, provided they have undergone comprehensive staging to assure that the disease is truly stage I, as up to 30% of patients with apparent stage I disease are upstaged at the time of complete surgical staging.[13]

1. Chemotherapy in Early-Stage Ovarian Cancer

Women with early-stage ovarian cancer can be classified as having a favorable or unfavorable prognosis, according to the specific substage criteria and tumor histology. Women with stage IA and stage IB, well- and moderately well-differentiated tumors have an excellent prognosis when treated with surgery alone. Five-year survivals exceed 90% in this favorable prognosis group. The role of adjuvant chemotherapy for this group of patients has been assessed in a randomized trial.[4] Eighty-one women with stage IA or stage IB, well- or moderately well-differentiated epithelial ovarian cancer were randomly assigned to receive adjuvant melphalan (0.2 mg/kg daily for 5 days, with treatment cycles repeated every 4–6 weeks for up to 12 cycles), or to receive no adjuvant chemotherapy. Disease-free survival was 91% in patients who received no chemotherapy versus 98% in the melphalan-treated patients ($P=0.41$); overall survival was 94 versus 98% ($P=0.43$). Women who meet these early-stage, favorable prognosis criteria do not require adjuvant chemotherapy and should be spared its associated toxicities.

Women with less favorable histologies (moderate to poorly differentiated tumors, all clear cell histologies) and those with more advanced stages of early ovarian cancer (stage IC, stage II) have a less favorable prognosis, with 5-year survivals estimated at 60–80%. These patients should be considered for adjuvant chemotherapy; however, it should be noted that randomized trials comparing the outcomes of patients receiving adjuvant chemotherapy to those of patients in a no-chemotherapy control arm have yet to show a clear survival benefit to adjuvant therapy in this less favorable prognosis group.

The Italian Inter-Regional Cooperative Group studied 85 women with stage IA or IB, grade 2 or 3 ovarian cancers in which patients were randomly assigned to receive adjuvant cisplatin (50 mg/m^2 every 28 days for 6 cycles) or to receive no adjuvant chemotherapy. In this study the 5-year disease-free survival was superior for patients who received adjuvant cisplatin (83 versus 63%); however, the overall survival rates were similar (88 versus 82%). One possible explanation for the observed difference in disease-free survival but lack of a difference in overall survival is that patients with recurrent disease in the observation arm may have been successfully salvaged with platinum therapy. In the second randomized trial, 161 women with stage IA or IB, grade 2, or stage IC ovarian cancer were randomly assigned to receive adjuvant cisplatin or adjuvant intraperitoneal phosphorous-32 (P-32). Again, disease-free survival at 5 years was superior for cisplatin-treated patients (85 versus 65%), but overall survival at 5 years was similar (80 versus 78%).[14]

Intraperitoneal P-32 was compared to intravenous melphalan in 141 patients with stage I or II ovarian cancer. Five-year disease-free survival was 80% in both treatment groups, and overall survival was 81% among the melphalan-treated patients versus 78% among patients who were assigned to receive P-32 ($P=0.48$).[4]

Adjuvant intravenous cisplatin (100 mg/m^2) plus cyclophosphamide (1 gm/m^2, delivered every 3 weeks for three cycles) was compared to intraperitoneal P-32 in a randomized trial conducted by the Gynecologic Oncology Group (GOG) in 205 patients with Stage IA or IB, grade 3, or Stage IC or IIA ovarian cancer (GOG 95). Five-year disease-free survival was 77% for patients in the cisplatin/cyclophosphamide arm versus 66% for patients in the P-32 arm ($P=0.075$), and overall survival was 84 versus 76%.[15] The relative risk of recurrence was 0.69 for patients receiving cisplatin/cyclophosphamide (90% confidence interval, 0.45–1.06). Although the disease-free survival difference did not achieve statistical significance, the authors concluded that platinum-based adjuvant therapy is preferred to P-32 because of the greater toxicity observed in the P-32 arm. Randomized clinical trial results in early-stage ovarian cancer are summarized in Table 35.1.

The high response rates observed among patients with advanced-stage ovarian cancer treated with paclitaxel plus platinum regimens prompted the adoption of this regimen for use in patients with early-stage but less favorable prognosis

TABLE 35.1 Adjuvant Chemotherapy in Early-Stage Ovarian Cancer

Favorable prognosis[a]								
	Melphalan vs.	Observation[c]						
DFS	98%	91%						
OS	98%	94%						
Unfavorable prognosis[b]								
	Cisplatin vs.	Observation[d]	Cisplatin vs.	P-32[e]	Melphalan vs.	P-32[f]	Cisplatin/CTX vs.	P-32[g]
DFS	83%	63%	83%	65%	80%	80%	77%	66%
OS	88%	82%	80%	78%	81%	78%	84%	76%

DFS: disease-free survival at 5 years; OS: overall survival at 5 years.
[a]Epithelial ovarian cancer, stage IA or IB, well- or moderately well-differentiated histology.
[b]Epithelial ovarian cancer, stage IA or IB, moderately to poorly differentiated or clear cell histology, or stage IC or stage II, any histology.
[c]Ref. 13. [d]Ref. 4. [e]Ref. 4. [f]Ref. 14. [g]Ref. 4.

ovarian cancer. The GOG has recently completed accrual to an adjuvant chemotherapy trial comparing 6 cycles of paclitaxel (175 mg/m^2) plus carboplatin (area-under-the-curve, AUC 6) to 3 cycles of paclitaxel and carboplatin at the same doses (GOG 157). Disease-free and overall survival results of this study are eagerly awaited. The GOG is currently conducting a study for patients with stage IA or IB, grade 3, or stage IC or stage II ovarian cancer in which patients are randomly assigned to receive either three cycles of paclitaxel/carboplatin or three cycles of paclitaxel/carboplatin followed by weekly treatment with paclitaxel (40 mg/m^2) for 24 weeks.

The relative rarity of early-stage ovarian cancer (few patients), and its relatively favorable prognosis (few relapses or "events") make the enrollment of eligible patients in clinical trials critical for improving the management of these cancers. Clinical trials will focus on maximizing disease-free and overall survival without causing untoward toxicity in this special group of ovarian cancer patients in which cure rates are high.

2. Chemotherapy in Advanced-Stage Ovarian Cancer

Systemic chemotherapy should be considered for all patients with advanced-stage epithelial ovarian cancer, following cytoreductive and staging surgery. Ovarian cancer is a highly chemotherapy-sensitive disease and response rates of 70–80% can be expected with platinum-paclitaxel-containing regimens.

a. Chemotherapy: Agents, Doses, and Combinations

Platinum-based therapy has long been the backbone of chemotherapy treatment for ovarian cancer. Paclitaxel was identified as a new chemotherapy agent with activity in patients with platinum-resistant disease, and was therefore adopted for testing in the front-line, postcytoreductive surgery setting. In study GOG 111, 386 patients with suboptimally debulked stage III or IV ovarian cancer were randomly assigned to receive either cyclophosphamide 750 mg/m^2 plus cisplatin 75 mg/m^2 or paclitaxel 135 mg/m^2 by 24-h infusion plus cisplatin 75 mg/m^2. Both regimens were given every 3 weeks for 6 cycles. The objective response rates, progression-free survival, and overall survival were superior in the paclitaxel plus cisplatin treatment arm, (median overall survival 38 months, paclitaxel/cisplatin versus 24 months, cyclophosphamide/cisplatin, $P<0.001$).[6] The paclitaxel-cisplatin-associated survival advantage was confirmed in a large randomized trial conducted in Europe and Canada (OV10) involving 680 women with advanced-stage ovarian cancer. In this study, the same doses and schedule of cyclophosphamide plus cisplatin were used; however, the paclitaxel was given as 175 mg/m^2 by 3-h infusion plus cisplatin 75 mg/m^2. Response rates, progression-free survival, and overall survival (35.6 versus 25.8 months, $P=0.0016$) were again superior in the paclitaxel/cisplatin treatment arm.[18]

An additional large randomized trial addressing the role of paclitaxel in front-line therapy has recently been completed, and preliminary data reported. In this multinational study, 2074 patients with stage I–IV epithelial ovarian cancer were randomly assigned to receive carboplatin (AUC 5) plus paclitaxel (175 mg/m^2 by 3-h infusion) or control therapy of either cisplatin (50 mg/m^2) plus doxorubicin (50 mg/m^2) plus cyclophosphamide (500 mg/m^2) (CAP) or carboplatin (minimum AUC 5) alone.[19] The choice of control arm (either CAP or carboplatin alone) was made prior to randomization, at the discretion of the institutional principal investigator. Twenty percent of the patient population had stage I or II disease. With median follow-up of 29 months, progression-free survival is 16.2 months in the control arm (carboplatin or CAP treatment) versus 16.8 months in the paclitaxel-carboplatin arm. Median overall survival is 36 months in the control arm versus 38.7 months in the paclitaxel-carboplatin arm. These results need to be interpreted carefully in light of the survival advantage to paclitaxel-cisplatin over cyclophosphamide-cisplatin demonstrated in GOG 111 and OV10. It is possible that the inclusion of patients at much lower risk of relapse (stage I and II patients) might obscure the benefit of paclitaxel in the front-line treatment setting. It is also possible that patients in the control arm were salvaged with paclitaxel, or received paclitaxel following treatment with carboplatin, obscuring a survival benefit. Given the results of this study, it is also possible that front-line therapy with paclitaxel-carboplatin may not be vastly superior to treatment with single-agent carboplatin followed by paclitaxel.[20]

Before the survival advantage of paclitaxel plus cisplatin over cyclophosphamide plus cisplatin was known, the GOG evaluated the efficacy of single-agent paclitaxel 200 mg/m^2 by 24-h infusion versus single-agent cisplatin 100 mg/m^2 versus the combination of paclitaxel 135 mg/m^2 by 24-h infusion plus cisplatin 75 mg/m^2 among 614 women with suboptimal stage III and IV ovarian cancer (GOG 132). Objective response rates were inferior for the single-agent paclitaxel arm compared with either of cisplatin regimens (42 versus 67%, respectively, $P<0.001$).[21] Overall survival was similar in all three arms of the study, likely due to salvage of many patients by crossover to the other regimen at time of disease progression. Since the combination therapy was tolerated best of the three treatment regimens, and response rates best in the cisplatin arms, the authors concluded that the combination of cisplatin plus paclitaxel was the preferred initial treatment for advanced ovarian cancer.

Prior to completion of the studies demonstrating the activity of paclitaxel in the front-line treatment of ovarian cancer, two other important questions were being addressed in randomized trials: whether the less-toxic platinum analog carboplatin, had efficacy similar to that of cisplatin; and whether higher doses of carboplatin were associated with improved response rates. Cisplatin plus cyclophosphamide was compared to carboplatin plus cyclophosphamide in two randomized trials. In both, carboplatin was associated with less nephrotoxicity, less nausea and vomiting, and less neurotoxicity, but greater myelosuppression. The efficacy of carboplatin was similar to that of cisplatin.[22, 23]

The dose-response relationship of carboplatin in ovarian cancer was investigated in two important studies. The Danish Ovarian Cancer Group randomly assigned 222 patients with stage II–IV ovarian cancer to receive carboplatin at an AUC of 4 or carboplatin AUC 8, in combination with cyclophosphamide 500 mg/m^2, delivered every 4 weeks for 6 cycles.[24] There was no difference in the percentage of patients achieving pathologic complete remission (confirmed at second-look surgical evaluation), and no difference in overall survival. There was significantly more myelosuppression in the carboplatin AUC 8 arm, with grade 3 or 4 thrombocytopenia observed in 6% of patients treated with AUC 4 versus 81% of patients treated with AUC 8. In a second study, conducted by the London Gynecological Oncology Group, 227 women with stage II–IV, or relapsed stage I ovarian cancer who had received no prior chemotherapy, were randomly assigned to receive carboplatin AUC 6 or carboplatin AUC 12, delivered every 4 weeks for 6 cycles.[25] There was no difference in progression-free or overall survival, whereas carboplatin AUC 12 was associated with greater toxicity and more treatment delays. The lack of a dose-response curve for carboplatin in ovarian cancer, at least within the range of doses that can be delivered with acceptable toxicity, supports the recommendations for use of carboplatin doses in the AUC 5–7 range in the front-line treatment of ovarian cancer.

Carboplatin's more favorable toxicity profile led to interest in testing it in front-line therapy in combination with paclitaxel.[26] Two large randomized trials compared paclitaxel plus carboplatin to paclitaxel plus cisplatin. GOG 158 compared 6 cycles of paclitaxel 135 mg/m^2 by 24-h infusion plus cisplatin 75 mg/m^2 to paclitaxel 175 mg/m^2 by 3-h infusion plus carboplatin AUC 7.5 in 840 patients with optimally cytoreduced stage III ovarian cancer.[27] Progression-free survival and overall survival were similar in both arms with median follow-up of 19 months. Patients in the cisplatin-containing arm experienced significantly more nausea, vomiting, and electrolyte abnormalities. Grade 3 or 4 thrombocytopenia was more common among patients in the carboplatin-paclitaxel arm (5% in the cisplatin arm versus 39% in the carboplatin arm). The frequency of grade 2 and 3 neurotoxicity was similar in both arms, perhaps due to the relatively high dose of carboplatin (AUC 7.5) used in combination with 3-h paclitaxel.

The Arbeitgemeinschaft Gynaekologische Onkologie (AGO) study group also conducted a randomized trial comparing carboplatin plus paclitaxel to cisplatin plus paclitaxel in 798 patients with stage II, III, or IV ovarian cancer.[28] The AGO study differed from GOG 158 in that paclitaxel 185 mg/m^2 was given over 3-h in combination with cisplatin 75 mg/m^2, and the carboplatin dose utilized in this study was lower, carboplatin AUC 6. Both regimens were delivered every 3 weeks for 6 cycles. As in GOG 158, no difference has been observed between the two treatment regimens in terms of progression-free or overall survival. The carboplatin-paclitaxel combination was associated with significantly less grade 3 or 4 neurotoxicity (8% in carboplatin arm versus 19% in cisplatin arm) and less grade 3 or 4 nausea and vomiting (7% in the carboplatin arm versus 19% in the cisplatin arm). Formal quality-of-life evaluation favored the carboplatin-paclitaxel regimen. Grade 3 or 4 thrombocytopenia occurred in 4% of patients in the carboplatin arm. The lower frequency of thrombocytopenia compared with that observed in GOG 158 may be due to the lower carboplatin dose used in the AGO study. The high frequency of neurotoxicity in the cisplatin-paclitaxel arm is likely due to the combined neurotoxic potential of the cisplatin combined with the short-infusion paclitaxel. Paclitaxel has greater potential for neurotoxicity when given by short infusion, compared with 24-h infusion paclitaxel.

Although survival data for both studies are not yet mature, the preliminary data suggest that it is highly unlikely that the carboplatin-paclitaxel regimen will be inferior to the control arm regimen of cisplatin-paclitaxel. The favorable toxicity profile, the ability to deliver carboplatin-paclitaxel on an outpatient basis, and the probable equivalency to cisplatin-paclitaxel has led many to recommend the combination of carboplatin AUC 5–6 plus paclitaxel 175 mg/m^2 by 3-h infusion as front-line treatment for advanced ovarian cancer.[29, 30] The recent major randomized, controlled trials on ovarian cancer are summarized in Table 35.2.

b. Intraperitoneal versus Intravenous Chemotherapy

The tendency of ovarian cancer to spread within the peritoneal cavity, the standard approach of initial cytoreductive surgery, and the ability to achieve high intraperitoneal drug concentrations, have made the use of intraperitoneal delivery of chemotherapy an attractive concept for the initial treatment of patients with ovarian cancer who have been cytoreduced to low-volume disease. Prior to completion of studies confirming the role of paclitaxel in front-line treatment of ovarian cancer, two important randomized trials were conducted using cisplatin plus cyclophosphamide-based therapy to determine whether initial intraperitoneal cisplatin treatment was superior to intravenous cisplatin treatment in patients with minimal bulk disease following cytoreductive surgery. In the first study, 654 patients with stage III ovarian cancer with no residual tumor mass larger than 2 cm were randomly assigned to receive cyclophosphamide (600 mg/m^2) plus intravenous cisplatin (100 mg/m^2) or cyclophosphamide plus intraperitoneal cisplatin (100 mg/m^2) for 6 cycles, starting within 4 weeks of cytoreductive surgery. Median survival was longer among patients in the intraperitoneal cisplatin arm than among patients in the intravenous cisplatin arm (49 versus 41 months); and the risk of death was lower in the intraperitoneal treatment arm (hazard ratio, 0.76; 95% confidence interval, 0.61–0.96; $P=0.02$).[31] A second study included 113 patients with stage II–IV ovarian cancer with residual disease <2 cm. Patients were randomly assigned to intraperitoneal cisplatin (50 mg/m^2) plus epidoxorubicin (60 mg/m^2) and cyclophosphamide (600 mg/m^2) or the same doses of epidoxorubicin and cyclophosphamide plus intravenous cisplatin (50 mg/m^2). No significant difference in pathologic response was observed between the two arms of the study among the 67 patients in the study who underwent second-look evaluation. Median progression-free survival was 42 months in the intraperitoneal cisplatin arm versus 25 months in the intravenous cisplatin arm, but this difference did not reach statistical significance ($P=0.13$). Similarly, overall survival was longer, but not significantly so, among patients assigned to intraperitoneal cisplatin (67 versus 51 months, $P=0.14$).[32] Because these trials were designed prior to the availability of paclitaxel for use in initial therapy, there is a need to determine whether intraperitoneal therapy offers a significant survival advantage when paclitaxel is incorporated in the front-line treatment regimen. This question is being addressed in GOG 172, a study for patient with optimally cytoreduced stage III ovarian cancer in which patients are randomly assigned to receive intravenous paclitaxel plus intravenous cisplatin versus intravenous paclitaxel plus intraperitoneal cisplatin and intraperitoneal paclitaxel. Preliminary data reported in abstract form from this study show that recurrence rates are lower with the intraperitoneally administered chemotherapy, although toxicity rates were somewhat higher. Survival data from this study are not yet mature.[32a] When progression-free and overall survival data are available, will substantially clarify the role of intraperitoneal therapy in the paclitaxel era for the subset of stage III ovarian cancer patients with minimal volume of cancer after cytoreductive surgery. In the meantime, these preliminary data and results from previous trials comparing intravenous with intraperitoneal-containing chemotherapy support the consideration of intraperitoneal

TABLE 35.2 Chemotherapy for Ovarian Cancer: Recent Randomized Clinical Trials

Group/trial	Regimens compared	Outcomes
GOG 111 [6]	P 135 mg/m^2 over 24 h + Cis 75 mg/m^2 vs. CTX 750 mg/m^2 + Cis 75 mg/m^2	Median OS 38 months (P/Cis) vs. 24 months (CTX/Cis)
OV10 [18]	P 175 mg/m^2 over 3 h + Cis 75 mg/m^2 vs. CTX 750 mg/m^2 + Cis 75 mg/m^2	Median OS 35.6 months (P/Cis) vs. 25.8 months (CTX/Cis)
ICON3 [19]	P 175 mg/m^2 over 3 h + Carbo AUC 5 vs. Cis/Dox/CTX or Carbo AUC 5	PFS 16.8 months (P/Carbo)/ vs. 16.2 months (Cis/Dox/CTX or Carbo)
GOG 132 [21]	P 200 mg/m^2 over 24 h vs. Cis 100 mg/m^2 vs. P 135 mg/m^2 over 24 h + Cis 75 mg/m^2	Response rate 67% with either Cis-containing regimen vs. 42% for P alone
GOG 158 [27]	P 135 mg/m^2 over 24 h + Cis 75 mg/m^2 vs. P 175 mg/m^2 over 3 h + Carbo AUC 7.5	No difference in PFS or OS at 19 months; P/Carbo better tolerated
AGO [28]	P 185 mg/m^2 over 3 h + Cis 75 mg/m^2 vs. P 185 mg/m^2 over 3 h + Carbo AUC 6	No difference in PFS or OS; P/Carbo associated with better quality of life

P: paclitaxel; Cis: cisplatin; CTX: cyclophosphamide; Dox: doxorubicin; AUC: area-under-the-curve; OS: overall survival; PFS: progression-free survival.

therapy as a standard treatment option for optimally debulked, stage III ovarian cancer.[32b]

c. Duration of Chemotherapy in Advanced Disease

The question of the optimal duration of therapy and optimal number of chemotherapy cycles has not been addressed since the introduction of paclitaxel to front-line therapy. However, at the time that cyclophosphamide and cisplatin combinations were considered standard of care, a randomized trial was conducted at Memorial Sloan-Kettering Cancer Center to determine whether 10 cycles of cyclophosphamide, cisplatin, and doxorubicin were superior to 5 cycles of the same drugs in terms of overall survival.[33] In that trial, continuing chemotherapy beyond 5 cycles did not improve survival. The majority of clinical trials incorporating paclitaxel have been designed to deliver 6 cycles of front-line chemotherapy.

3. Role of Neoadjuvant Chemotherapy

Ovarian cancer patients whose tumors can be cytoreduced to no tumor nodule >1 cm (optimally debulked) at the time of staging and cytoreductive surgery have a greater chance for long-term survival than patients with larger volume residual disease.[34] Indeed, patients with stage IIIC ovarian who cannot be optimally debulked have survival rates similar to that of patients presenting with stage IV disease (approximately 5–15% at 5 years).[35] The percentage of advanced ovarian cancer patients who can be optimally cytoreduced has not been definitely established, but reports from multiple series of patients puts the mean at approximately 35%, with a range of 24–87%.[36] Since many patients cannot be optimally debulked, and since some patients are poor surgical candidates due to comorbidities, there has been interest in treating patients with advanced disease with chemotherapy prior to surgical cytoreduction (neoadjuvant chemotherapy). To date, no randomized trial has been completed to assess whether neoadjuvant chemotherapy yields equivalent or superior outcomes to initial cytoreductive surgery followed by chemotherapy in advanced stage ovarian cancer. An ongoing study conducted by the EORTC Gynecologic Cancer Cooperative Group (Protocol 55971) is designed to address this question. The trial is currently accruing patients with stage IIIC or IV epithelial ovarian cancer. Participants are randomly assigned to upfront cytoreductive surgery versus neoadjuvant chemotherapy.

Pending results of this important randomized trial, available data regarding the role of neoadjuvant chemotherapy come from series of patients who were selected for treatment with neoadjuvant chemotherapy [37, 38] comparing their outcomes with those of patients treated with upfront cytoreductive surgery. In one of the larger studies, a retrospective analysis of 285 patients, overall survival in an earlier time period (1980–1998) when all patients underwent upfront cytoreductive surgery was compared to overall survival in a later time period (1989–1997) when 43% of the patients were selected for treatment with neoadjuvant chemotherapy. In general, patients with stage IV disease, large-volume disease that was likely to render optimal resection impossible (porta hepatis involvement, superior mesenteric artery involvement), or an "uncountable" number of mesenteric implants, large-volume ascites, and poor performance status were treated with neoadjuvant chemotherapy. In this study, the 3-year overall survival rate was 42% among patients treated in the later time period when neoadjuvant chemotherapy was incorporated in the management strategy, compared with 3-year overall survival of 26% in the time period when all patients had upfront cytoreductive surgery ($P=0.0001$).[39] The observed superior outcome in the group of patients in which neoadjuvant chemotherapy was available should be interpreted carefully in light of other potentially important differences between the groups that may explain the observed survival difference, such as better chemotherapy regimens and better supportive care in the later time period of the study.

Another large retrospective study compared the progression-free and overall survival of 56 patients with advanced ovarian cancer treated with neoadjuvant chemotherapy, to that of 206 consecutive patients who underwent upfront cytoreductive surgery.[40] The time period of the study spanned 17 years. All patients received platinum-based chemotherapy. The median overall survival was 2.18 years among the 206 patients who underwent upfront cytoreductive surgery versus 1.07 years among the 59 patients treated with neoadjuvant chemotherapy ($P=0.1578$). Although this survival difference did not meet statistical significance, it is possible that this retrospective study was underpowered to detect a meaningful difference in outcome.[41] The role of neoadjuvant chemotherapy in epithelial ovarian cancer will be clarified when results of the European randomized trial of neoadjuvant chemotherapy versus up-front cytoreductive surgery become available. Until such data are available, according to guidelines published by the National Comprehensive Cancer Network, neoadjuvant chemotherapy may be considered for patients who are poor surgical candidates.[8]

4. Major Side Effects of Paclitaxel-Platinum-Based Chemotherapy for Epithelial Ovarian Cancer

Treatment with paclitaxel and platinum agents for epithelial ovarian cancer is generally well tolerated. However, chemotherapy agents have narrow therapeutic windows, and close monitoring of patients is required. Treatment of patients with chemotherapy should be done by physicians who have specialized training and are experienced in the use of chemotherapy for ovarian cancer, usually either a gynecologic oncologist or a medical oncologist.

a. Hypersensitivity Reactions

Paclitaxel can cause acute hypersensitivity reactions [42] that may be severe enough to result in death. Premedication with dexamethasone plus histamine-1 and histamine-2 receptor antagonists can dramatically decrease the severity and frequency of hypersensitivity reactions,[43] and the use of such premedications is considered standard prior to paclitaxel infusions. Among 450 patients with gynecologic cancer treated at a single institution, 44 patients (9.7%) experienced 71 episodes of clinically relevant paclitaxel-associated hypersensitivity events.[44] The majority of severe hypersensitivity reactions occurred with the first or second paclitaxel infusion. Re-challenge after re-treatment with diphenhydramine and hydrocortisone (if there had been resolution of the signs and symptoms of hypersensitivity), was successful in 65 (93%) of the incidences. Nine remaining patients were treated with a longer desensitization protocol and were subsequently able to tolerate paclitaxel. Another study also reported the successful re-treatment of eight patients who had had severe hypersensitivity reactions, following desensitization that generally included several doses of dexamethasone plus diphenhydramine and histamine-2 receptor antagonists.[45]

Carboplatin may also be associated with hypersensitivity reactions. An important retrospective study reported carboplatin hypersensitivity reaction in 24 of 205 patients (12%) treated for gynecologic malignancies.[46] Carboplatin hypersensitivity reactions differ from paclitaxel reactions in several clinically important ways: carboplatin reactions are more likely to occur after many previously well-tolerated cycles (median number of prior platinum cycles prior to the carboplatin reaction was eight in the experience reported by Markman *et al.* [46]), carboplatin reactions may occur after more than half of the dose has been infused, and patients with carboplatin reactions are unlikely to be successfully re-challenged, even with desensitization regimens similar to those used for paclitaxel re-challenge.

b. Renal Insufficiency/Electrolyte Abnormalities

Renal clearance accounts for more than 90% of the clearance of platinum agents.[47] Cisplatin may cause nephrotoxicity ranging from reversible azotemia to chronic renal insufficiency. Cisplatin frequently causes impairments in proximal tubular function and distal tubule reabsorbtion, which lead to electrolyte abnormalities, particularly hypokalemia and hypomagnesemia.[48, 49] Intravenous hydration is required for patients receiving cisplatin to minimize toxicity. Patients with severe renal impairment (glomerular infiltration rate <30 ml/min) are generally not candidates for cisplatin therapy, and dose adjustment is necessary for patients with intermediate renal function (GFR 30–50 ml/min).[50]

Carboplatin rarely causes renal dysfunction at the doses used for treatment of ovarian cancer. However, since the clearance of carboplatin is linearly related to the GFR,[51] decreases in the GFR lead to high plasma levels of carboplatin, which may cause other toxicities. Thus, carboplatin should be dosed using the Calvert formula (dose, mg = target AUC × GFR + 25), which was developed to calculate the dose of carboplatin necessary to achieve a particular AUC.[52]

c. Neurotoxicity

Both cisplatin and paclitaxel may cause dose-related sensory neuropathies that may be irreversible. The risk of neuropathy is additive when paclitaxel and cisplatin are combined.[53] As discussed above, shorter paclitaxel infusions are associated with greater risk of neuropathy; thus, when paclitaxel is used in combination with cisplatin, many choose to deliver the paclitaxel by 24-h infusion. Ototoxicity may also occur, manifested by high-frequency hearing loss. Ototoxicity is more common with cisplatin, but has been reported in approximately 1% of patients treated with carboplatin.[54] Cisplatin-related hearing loss occurs less frequently with intraperitoneal delivery than with intravenous delivery of drug (5% among patients treated with intravenous cyclophosphamide plus intraperitoneal cisplatin versus 15% among patients treated with intravenous cyclophosphamide plus intravenous cisplatin, $P < 0.001$).[31]

d. Myelosuppression

Paclitaxel and carboplatin both cause dose-dependent bone marrow suppression. With carboplatin, thrombocytopenia is generally more pronounced than neutropenia, and effects may be cumulative.[55] Bleeding complications are unusual, however, despite grade 3 or 4 thrombocytopenia. Cisplatin is less marrow-suppressive, with severe leukopenia or thrombocytopenia occurring in 5–6% of patients when given as a single agent, although anemia is more common.[56]

Neutropenic fever is a potentially life-threatening complication of chemotherapy-related myelosuppression. Fortunately, even relatively severe neutropenia is infrequently complicated by neutropenic fever. For example, in the AGO randomized trial of paclitaxel plus carboplatin versus paclitaxel plus cisplatin, grade 3 or 4 neutropenia occurred in 14% of cycles of paclitaxel plus carboplatin versus 8% of cycles of paclitaxel plus cisplatin; however, neutropenic fever was observed in <1% of the cycles of treatment.[28]

e. Nausea/Vomiting

Cisplatin is associated with both acute (occurring within the first 24 h following treatment) and delayed (occurring >24 h and up to several days after treatment) nausea and vomiting. Carboplatin and paclitaxel at the doses utilized in the treatment of ovarian cancer are less emetogenic than cisplatin, and do not generally cause delayed emesis. The use of 5-hydroxytryptamine (5-HT3) receptor antagonists, particularly in combination with corticosteroids, prior to chemotherapy dramatically decreases the frequency and severity of acute nausea and vomiting,[57] but is less effective at preventing delayed nausea and vomiting.[58] In the ovarian cancer clinical trials comparing paclitaxel plus cisplatin to paclitaxel plus carboplatin, the frequency of severe nausea and vomiting was consistently higher among patients receiving cisplatin. In the AGO study, 19% of patients treated with paclitaxel plus cisplatin experience grade 3 or 4 nausea and vomiting versus 7% of patients treated with paclitaxel plus carboplatin.[28] In GOG 158, 23% of patients in the paclitaxel plus cisplatin arm experienced grade 3 or 4 gastrointestinal toxicity versus 10% of patients in the paclitaxel plus carboplatin arm.[27]

5. New Directions in Initial Therapy for Epithelial Ovarian Cancer

Although response rates and overall survival in advanced ovarian cancer have improved, the majority of patients will relapse and ultimately succumb to their disease. Research efforts are directed at improving the outcomes for women with ovarian cancer. One focus of research efforts is the incorporation of noncross-resistant chemotherapy agents such as topotecan,[59] gemcitabine,[60] or liposomal doxorubicin [61] into front-line treatment, either as triplet therapy or sequential doublet therapy. Triplet therapy is attractive because the tumor cells are constantly exposed to several agents with different mechanisms of anti-tumor activity, which may translate into the ability to overcome inherent drug resistance. Combination therapy may also allow for certain agents to potentiate the activity of other drugs. However, combined toxicities, particularly myelosuppression, may make it difficult to deliver effective doses of all agents. Sequential doublet treatment allows full doses of each agent to be delivered, but may not allow for constant exposure of the tumor to the most active agents.[62] The feasibility and efficacy of these approaches to ovarian cancer are being investigated in several clinical trials.[63–65] An international randomized trial is underway to assess the efficacy of five different doublet regimens in the front-line treatment of ovarian cancer. Other important research approaches include the investigation of vaccine therapy for women with minimal residual disease, and studies of the efficacy of agents with novel anti-tumor mechanisms such as anti-angiogenesis agents, signal transduction inhibitors, and matrix metalloproteinase inhibitors.

B. Chemotherapy for Refractory/Persistent/Recurrent Epithelial Ovarian Cancer

Patients who fail to achieve remission with front-line chemotherapy, and patients who relapse after achieving remission are unlikely to be cured. Treatment with chemotherapy may result in objective tumor responses, and may provide palliation of the symptoms of the cancer, but does not generally lead to prolonged, treatment- and disease-free survival. Patients with longer-duration first clinical remissions are more likely to achieve second clinical remissions that may be relatively durable. There are no randomized trials comparing second-line chemotherapy to best supportive care. Although tumor responses may be seen with many different chemotherapy agents, it is not clear that tumor response ultimately translates into longer overall survival. When considering second- and greater-line chemotherapy options for progressive/recurrent ovarian cancer, patients should be aware that, while cure is unlikely, the goals of treatment are control of tumor-related symptoms and improvement or maintenance of quality of life.

1. Management of Patients with Primary Refractory Disease

Approximately 20% of patients with ovarian cancer will fail to respond to front-line, paclitaxel-platinum-based chemotherapy. There are no identified, potentially curative interventions for this poor-prognosis group with primary refractory disease. If the patient's performance status and organ function are good, palliative therapy with one of the agents discussed below for platinum-refractory, recurrent disease may be considered, or participation in a clinical trial. Additional surgical intervention in patients with primary refractory disease has not been shown to alter the median survival of approximately 12 months.[66]

2. Chemotherapy for Patients with Persistent Disease

Patients with evidence of response to front-line chemotherapy (decreasing measurable disease in suboptimally cytoreduced patients, or declining serum CA125 levels in optimally cytoreduced patients), may not achieve complete clinical remission. Such patients may have a persistently elevated CA125 or be found to have small-volume or microscopic disease at the time of second-look laparotomy/laparoscopy. There is no standard chemotherapy approach for patients with persistent disease. Treatment options include continued systemic therapy or dose-intensive chemotherapy. The initial response to platinum-based therapy has been the rationale for continued paclitaxel-platinum-based therapy. The optimal number of additional cycles is not known, nor is it known if altering the drug delivery schedule (giving paclitaxel weekly, for example) will improve overall outcomes. An alternative systemic treatment strategy for patients with persistent disease is to treat with one of the nonplatinum agents. In other diseases it has been suggested that early use of noncross-resistant therapy may increase the number of patients achieving complete remission by overcoming inherent drug resistance.[67] Although this strategy may be feasible in patients with persistent ovarian cancer,[68] a disease-free or overall-survival benefit has not yet been demonstrated.

Treating patients with chemotherapy-responsive, low-volume disease with dose-intensive consolidation therapy is an attractive strategy. Unfortunately, the GOG randomized trial designed to test this strategy using high-dose chemotherapy with stem cell support in ovarian cancer patients with persistent disease at second-look laparotomy closed because of poor accrual. The intraperitoneal delivery of chemotherapy to patients with low-volume disease is an alternative dose-intense strategy for management of persistent ovarian cancer. Candidates for intraperitoneal therapy are those with microscopic disease, or with no tumor mass >1.0 cm in size, as drug delivery to the tumor tissue is by direct penetration. Intraperitoneal cisplatin has been demonstrated to achieve pathologic complete responses in 25–30% of patients with responsive, but persistent, microscopic or low-volume (all nodules ≤0.5 cm) disease.[69] Patients who did not respond to systemic platinum treatment are unlikely to respond to intraperitoneal platinum, even if the volume of persistent disease is low.[70]

3. Chemotherapy for Potentially Platinum-Sensitive Disease

Retrospective data have been used to identify which patients with recurrent ovarian cancer may respond to re-treatment with platinum-based therapy, the "platinum-sensitive" population. In general, the longer the duration of the first clinical remission from platinum-based therapy, the higher the likelihood of response to re-treatment with platinum for recurrent disease. Fewer than 10% of patients with a less than 6-month interval from the last platinum therapy will respond to re-treatment with platinum, while platinum responses may be seen in approximately 27% of patients with a 6- to 12-month platinum treatment-free interval, and in 33% of patients with a 13- to 24-month platinum treatment-free interval. Patients with an initial complete remission lasting greater than 24 months demonstrated a 77% response rate to platinum-based re-treatment.[71] The correlation between the platinum treatment-free interval and response to re-treatment with platinum-based therapy has also been demonstrated in patients who received platinum as front-line therapy, followed by paclitaxel for recurrent disease. The overall response rate to re-treatment with carboplatin was 21%. All responses were seen among the patients with a greater than 12-month interval from completion of prior platinum therapy.[72]

The response to nonplatinum agents is consistently higher in the potentially platinum-sensitive population, compared to the responses in platinum-refractory disease. This should be borne in mind when interpreting results of phase II trials of new agents in recurrent ovarian cancer. There are no data addressing the issue of whether survival in potentially platinum-sensitive patients is superior with platinum re-treatment as compared to treatment with a nonplatinum agent. The choice of whether to re-treat with platinum alone, platinum plus paclitaxel,[73] paclitaxel alone,[17, 74, 75] or a nonplatinum agent [76] is frequently guided by whether there are persistent toxicities (neuropathy or hearing loss from prior treatment) and the side effect profile of the drugs being considered.

TABLE 35.3 Chemotherapy Options for Patients with Recurrent Ovarian Cancer

Initial response to platinum, relapse >6 months after completion of treatment	**No complete response to platinum, or relapse <6 months after completion of treatment**
Carboplatin ± paclitaxel	Oral etoposide
Cisplatin ± paclitaxel	Topotecan
Paclitaxel	Liposomal doxorubicin
	Gemcitabine
	Tamoxifen
	Ifosfamide
	Vinorelbine
	Docetaxel
	Paclitaxel

4. Chemotherapy for Platinum-Resistant Disease

Numerous chemotherapy agents have been identified in phase II studies that demonstrate objective tumor responses in platinum-resistant ovarian cancer (Table 35.3). Response rates are generally in the 15–30% range. Data come from phase II studies, and comparisons across trials are unlikely to be valid due to differences in patient populations and sample sizes. Although clinical responses may be observed, there are no data that demonstrate a survival benefit to chemotherapy treatment in the platinum-refractory setting compared with best supportive care. Complete response rates are low, and cure of the patient with platinum-resistant ovarian cancer is highly unlikely. The goal of chemotherapy treatment is generally symptom control; thus, the potential benefits and toxicities, and the patient's quality of life, should be carefully considered. Some patients may achieve stable disease with limited drug toxicity, which is a reasonable clinical goal.[77]

a. Specific Agents for Platinum-Resistant Ovarian Cancer

Topotecan achieves objective responses in approximately 20–33% of platinum-sensitive patients, and in 13–17% of platinum-refractory patients.[76, 78–80] Response rates in patients who are resistant to both platinum and paclitaxel are generally lower.[81] Significant myelosuppression is common, although the severity of the myelosuppression may not be cumulative.

Liposomal doxorubicin, studied in patients who had failed paclitaxel- and platinum-based treatment, has demonstrated objective responses in 17–26% of patients. Nausea, vomiting, alopecia, and severe myelosuppression are uncommon with liposomal doxorubicin. Skin and mucosal toxicities (palmar-plantar erythrodysesthesia) occurred in more than one third of patients treated at 50 mg/m^2 every 3 weeks, but were less common with doses of 40 mg/m^2 [83] or with dosing intervals of 4–5 weeks.

Oral etoposide dosed at 50 mg/m^2/day for 21 days, delivered in 28-day cycles resulted in objective responses in 26.8% of 82 patients with platinum-resistant disease, and 34% of patients with platinum-sensitive disease.[84] The major side effect of oral etoposide is myelosuppression, which may be cumulative. Rarely, prolonged exposure to etoposide has been associated with myelodysplasia and acute leukemia.

Gemcitabine, dosed at 800–1000 mg/m^2 weekly for 3 weeks followed by a 1-week break, has demonstrated response rates of 13–20%.[85] The major side effect is dose-related myelosuppression, although skin toxicity and drug fever may also be observed. Vinorelbine, administered weekly at 25–30 mg/m^2, resulted in an overall response rate of 15–29% among patients with recurrent ovarian cancer, with the higher response rates observed among patients who were potentially platinum-sensitive. Potential side effects include myelosuppression and worsening of preexisting neurotoxicity.[86, 87]

Docetaxel achieves response rates of 20–35% of patients with platinum-resistant disease,[88, 89] which is similar to the response rates expected with paclitaxel in platinum-resistant patients. However, recent data suggest that docetaxel may have activity in patients that are resistant to paclitaxel. Among 30 patients with evaluable, paclitaxel-resistant Mullerian tumors, objective responses were seen in 23%. Responses were higher among patients with a longer time period from prior paclitaxel therapy.[90] Docetaxel's side effects include myelosuppression and fluid retention.

Because paclitaxel is so frequently employed in combination with platinum as front-line therapy for ovarian cancer, patients with disease that has recurred less than 6 months after completing front-line therapy are often thought to be resistant to both platinum and paclitaxel. However, the mechanisms of drug resistance are likely to be different for paclitaxel and platinum, and some platinum-resistant patients may still have paclitaxel-sensitive disease. A partial response rate of 15% was observed among a small number of patients who have progressed less than 6 months after paclitaxel therapy who were subsequently treated with weekly paclitaxel.[91] Doses of 60–80 mg/m^2/week by 1-h infusion are well tolerated in terms of myelosuppression, but may be associated with peripheral neurotoxicity.

Ifosfamide is associated with response rates of 10–20% among patients previously treated with platinum,[92–94] and with response rates of 15% among patients who have received both platinum and paclitaxel.[95] Ifosfamide is generally delivered over several consecutive days. Toxicities include significant myelosuppression, renal and central nervous system toxicity, and hemorrhagic cystitis.

Tamoxifen is a hormonal agent with a favorable side-effect profile, compared to the side effects commonly encountered with most cytotoxic chemotherapy agents. Tamoxifen has been reported to have activity in approximately 15% of patients with platinum-resistant ovarian cancer.[96, 97] Whether this level of response can be expected in patients that have received both platinum and paclitaxel is not known. Tamoxifen's favorable side-effect profile makes it a reasonable choice for use in patients with relapsed ovarian cancer manifested only by a rising CA125, or those with asymptomatic, low-volume relapses.

Few randomized trials have been conducted in the relapsed ovarian cancer setting; thus, it is not possible to determine which treatment regimen for relapsed, platinum-resistant ovarian cancer is best. One recent large study compared liposomal doxorubicin to topotecan in 474 patients with relapsed ovarian cancer. Patients were randomly assigned to receive liposomal doxorubicin 50 mg/m^2 every 4 weeks or topotecan 1.5 mg/m^2 daily for 5 days every 3 weeks. In the report of the preliminary data, response rates and median time-to-progression were similar in both arms. Among platinum-sensitive patients, responses were seen in 28.4% of patients treated with liposomal doxorubicin versus 28.8% of patients treated with topotecan. Among platinum-refractory patients, responses were 12.3% with liposomal doxorubicin versus 6.5% with topotecan. Despite similar response rates, median survival was 23 weeks longer among patients treated with liposomal doxorubicin. Longer-term follow-up is required to determine whether this slight advantage to liposomal doxorubicin is maintained.[98] Participation in clinical trials should be strongly encouraged for patients with relapsed ovarian cancer in order to identify new agents and to improve our understanding of which of the available agents results in the best outcomes in terms of survival and quality of life.

II. CHEMOTHERAPY FOR NONEPITHELIAL OVARIAN CANCERS

Ovarian cancers may arise from nonepithelial elements, and include the mixed Mullerian tumors, stromal tumors, and germ cell tumors. Careful histologic review is important, as the treatment and prognosis of these tumors is highly dependent on histology.

A. Mixed Mullerian Tumors of the Ovary

Mixed Mullerian tumors (MMT) of the ovary comprise less than 1% of primary ovarian cancers.[1] Like MMT of the uterus, MMT of the ovary contains malignant epithelial and sarcomatous elements. The disease is frequently widespread at the time of diagnosis, and in case series, optimal debulking is achieved in less than half of patients.[99, 100] Median survival is approximately 8–18 months.[101, 102] Because of the high-grade nature of the tumor and tendency for aggressive behavior, most patients with MMT of the ovary are offered chemotherapy after surgical debulking of the tumor.

Few prospective clinical trials have been conducted specifically for MMT of the ovary. Retrospective studies have reported activity of several chemotherapy agents. Because most of these are single-institution studies with variable patient populations, it is not possible to draw comparisons across studies to determine the best front-line chemotherapy regimen for MMT of the ovary. Agents and combinations of agents that have been reported in the more recent literature to have response rates (ranging from 27–85%, often in very small patient series) include cisplatin plus doxorubicin,[103] cisplatin plus doxorubicin plus cyclophosphamide,[104] paclitaxel plus carboplatin, ifosfamide plus cisplatin,[105] and single-agent ifosfamide. The GOG completed an important prospective phase II trial of second-line therapy using ifosfamide plus mesna in patients with MMT of the ovary who had previously received platinum-based therapy. Among 28 patients evaluable for response, 1 patient achieved complete response, and 4 had partial responses, for an overall response in this pretreated population of 17.9%.[106] The optimal front-line regimen for MMT of the ovary remains to be determined. Platinum-based therapy is reasonable, and most reported studies have used combination therapy. Prospective trials are needed to determine whether the addition of doxorubicin, paclitaxel, or ifosfamide to the platinum backbone improves outcomes in this rare tumor.

B. Sex Cord-Stromal Tumors

The sex cord-stromal tumors are nonepithelial ovarian cancers that include the granulosa cell tumors (70% of ovarian stromal tumors), the Sertoli-Leydig cell tumors, and unclassified sex cord-stromal tumors. Treatment of these tumors is primarily surgical. The majority of granulosa cell tumors are stage I at diagnosis, and 5-year survival for patients with completed resected stage I tumors is approximately 90%.[107, 108] Fertility-sparing surgery may be appropriate in many cases, and chemotherapy is not generally recommended for early-stage, completely resected disease. Recurrence rates are 10–33%, with late recurrences (5–20 years after initial diagnosis) being characteristic of these tumors. Patients presenting with disease spread beyond the pelvis (stage III disease) have a poorer prognosis, with 5-year survivals of 0–22%.[109, 110]

The optimal management of patients with advanced sex cord-stromal tumors and patients with recurrent disease has not been defined. Data are limited by the rarity of the tumors. Serum inhibin levels may be elevated in patients with sex cord-stromal tumors, and may be useful for monitoring response to treatment. Several chemotherapy agents and combinations have been reported to have activity in these cancers. The GOG reported three responses among 13 patients with advanced granulosa cell tumors treated with dactinomycin, 5-fluorouracil, and cyclophosphamide.[111] Case reports and small case series [112–115] reporting the activity of cisplatin in this disease led to a study of the combination of cisplatin, vinblastine, and bleomycin in 11 patients with advanced granulosa cell tumors. Objective responses were seen in 9 of the 11 patients (6 complete responses and 3 partial responses), with the 6 complete responses confirmed by second-look laparotomy.[116] The activity of cisplatin, vinblastine, and bleomycin was confirmed in a larger study of 38 patients with recurrent or advanced granulosa cell tumors. Response rates were 52% among 25 patients treated after surgery alone, and 77% among 13 patients who had received prior postoperative radiation therapy and/or chemotherapy.[117]

The combination of cisplatin, etoposide, and bleomycin achieved a response rate of 83% in 9 patients with sex cord-stromal tumors.[118] The GOG further established the activity of cisplatin, etoposide, and bleomycin in ovarian stromal tumors in an important study involving 57 women with incompletely resected stage II–IV granulosa cell, Sertoli-Leydig, unclassified sex cord-stromal, or malignant thecoma cancers or with recurrent ovarian stromal tumors.[119] The rationale for the substitution of etoposide for vinblastine was the experience reported in testicular germ cell tumors in which this substitution preserved efficacy with less toxicity.[120] In this GOG study, there were two early deaths related to bleomycin toxicity, and the dose of bleomycin was reduced for all subsequent patients. The final treatment regimen was bleomycin 20 mg/m^2 day 1 every week for 4 weeks, etoposide 75 mg/m^2 days 1–5 every 3 weeks for 4 weeks, and cisplatin 20 mg/m^2 days 1–5 every 3 weeks for 4 weeks. Of the 38 patients that had second-look laparotomy to confirm response, 14 (37%) had no residual tumor. Grade 3 or 4 granulocytopenia occurred in 79% of patients, although there were no hospitalizations for neutropenic fever. Patients with measurable disease at the time of enrollment on study were more likely to progress and had shorter survivals than patients with no measurable disease.

The rarity of the sex cord-stromal tumors and the relatively good prognosis for patients with early-stage granulosa cell tumors has made it difficult to design and complete randomized trials to define optimal therapy. Recommendations for management are based on retrospective data and prospective phase II data. For early-stage, completely resected granulosa cell tumors, adjuvant chemotherapy is not generally recommended. For patients with recurrent disease, or incompletely resected advanced disease, platinum-based chemotherapy may be considered. While there are no data comparing single-agent treatment to combination, the most active regimen reported is the combination of bleomycin, etoposide, and cisplatin. Patients treated with this regimen require careful monitoring for bleomycin-related pulmonary toxicity with serial lung diffusion capacity testing and careful monitoring for myelosuppression. Some researchers have suggested that the deliverable dose of bleomycin in the GOG trial was so low as to suggest that bleomycin may not be necessary for the treatment of sex cord-stromal tumors,[121] although confirmation of this would require further study.

C. Germ Cell Tumors

Germ cell tumors of the ovary are nonepithelial ovarian cancers that include the dysgerminomas, endodermal sinus tumors, embryonal carcinomas, choriocarcinomas, teratomas (mature and immature), and mixed germ cell tumors. Most malignant germ cell tumors occur in young women. Fertility-sparing surgery is feasible in most patients. Since disease-free survival rates are high following chemotherapy for germ cell tumors, physicians and researchers must be concerned with late effects of chemotherapy. Ovarian function is frequently maintained with the chemotherapy agents recommended for treatment of germ cell tumors. Secondary malignancies may occur, particularly etoposide-related acute monocytic or myelomonocytic leukemias. The risk may be lower with lower cumulative doses of etoposide.[122, 123]

1. Dysgerminomas

Dysgerminomas may be considered the female equivalent of the male testicular germ cell tumor, seminoma. Dysgerminomas appear unilateral in approximately 90% of cases. After complete surgical staging approximately two thirds of patients will be confirmed to have stage I, unilateral disease. Dysgerminomas that are shown, after careful surgical staging, to be limited to one ovary, can be managed with unilateral oophorectomy and observed closely after surgery.[124–126] Relapse may occur in 15–25% of patients, but nearly all will be successfully salvaged with chemotherapy.

Patients with dysgerminomas that are incompletely resected, or are completely resected but have higher than stage IA tumors, require postsurgical therapy.[127] Although the tumors are radiosensitive, the desire to maintain ovarian function has led to the increased use of chemotherapy,[128] rather than radiation therapy, as postoperative treatment for dysgerminomas.[129]

Most patients with dysgerminoma have been treated with the combination of bleomycin, cisplatin, and either vinblastine or etoposide. Patients in a more recent GOG study were treated with bleomycin, etoposide, and cisplatin (BEP) followed by vincristine, dactinomycin, and cyclophosphamide (VAC). Among 20 patients with incompletely resected disease treated with these agents on two GOG studies, 19 patients remained disease-free at 26 months median follow-up, and among the 14 patients who had second-look surgical evaluations, all were pathologically confirmed disease-free.[129] In another report, BEP treatment of 26 patients with dysgerminoma greater than stage IA resulted in disease-free survival of 96%.[130] In this study, 16 of the 26 patients had fertility-sparing surgery. Among 14 patients evaluable for menstrual functioning follow-up, 13 (93%) maintained or resumed normal menstrual functioning.

While cisplatin-based, combination chemotherapy is a standard approach for patients with greater than stage IA dysgerminoma, the optimal treatment regimen has not been defined. The GOG has studied etoposide plus carboplatin, in an effort to minimize the toxicities associated with cisplatin, although results are not yet reported. The optimal number of treatment cycles is not known, although patients are generally treated with 3–4 cycles of BEP.

2. Nondysgerminoma Germ Cell Tumors

Patients with mature teratoma are generally managed with surgical resection alone, and have an excellent prognosis. There is small risk of malignant germ cell tumor occurring in the opposite ovary. The prognosis in immature teratoma is related to tumor grade.[131] Grade 1 immature teratomas are associated with a low risk of relapse (80–85% of patients remain disease-free after complete resection); however, relapses occur in more than 70% of patients with grade 3 immature teratoma.

Endodermal sinus tumors, embryonal carcinomas, and choriocarcinomas are rare tumors that demonstrate aggressive behavior. The high rate of recurrence after surgical resection of these tumors means that adjuvant chemotherapy is frequently recommended.

Serum levels of human chorionic gonadotropin (hCG) and alpha-fetoprotein (AFP) may be elevated in patients with germ cell tumors, and may be used to monitor response to chemotherapy. The diagnosis of dysgerminoma requires that the AFP level be normal (as in pure seminoma of the testis, the male equivalent of dysgerminoma), but hCG may be elevated. The serum AFP is always elevated in endodermal sinus tumors, and may be elevated in patients with immature teratoma or embryonal carcinoma. hCG is elevated in patients with choriocarcinoma.

Combination, cisplatin-based chemotherapy is recommended for patients with advanced endodermal sinus tumors, embryonal carcinomas, choriocarcinomas, and immature teratomas. The GOG treated 89 patients with germ cell tumors of varying histologies, about one third of whom had had prior chemotherapy, with cisplatin, vinblastine, and bleomycin. With median follow-up of 52 months, 47 (53%) of patients remained disease free.[132] Eight patients who relapsed had durable remissions to second-line therapy. An important observation was that 27% of patients with no measurable disease relapsed, evidence of the aggressive nature of the nondysgerminoma germ cell tumors.

Because of the successful substitution of etoposide for vinblastine in patients with advanced testicular germ cell tumors,[120] the combination of bleomycin, etoposide, and cisplatin was used in several studies of ovarian germ cell tumors. In these phase II trials, disease-free, long-term survival is achieved in 60–80% of patients.[133, 134] The GOG assessed the use of adjuvant treatment with three cycles of BEP for completely resected nondysgerminoma ovarian germ cell tumors in 93 patients. In this study, 89 patients remained free of germ cell cancer. Two patients had small foci of immature teratoma at second-look laparotomy. Although acute toxicity was moderate, there were two patients with late malignancies: one acute myelomonocytic leukemia, and one malignant lymphoma. The high disease-free survival rate and overall acceptable toxicity profile of the regimen led to the recommendation that all patients with completely resected, ovarian germ cell tumors be offered adjuvant treatment with BEP.[135] Because of the aggressive nature of these tumors, it is generally recommended that adjuvant therapy be initiated within 1–2 weeks of surgery, if possible.[136] It is possible that certain patients with completely resected, early-stage immature teratoma may not require adjuvant chemotherapy, and that patients with relapsed immature teratoma could be successfully salvaged with chemotherapy at the time of relapse. One study included 44 patients (median age 10 years) with immature teratoma (31 tumors confirmed on pathologic review to be immature teratoma, grade 1 in 17, grade 2 in 12, grade 3 in 2). Thirteen patients had immature teratoma plus yolk sac tumor; alpha-fetoprotein was elevated in 34% of patients with immature teratoma, and in 83% of patients with immature teratoma plus yolk sac elements. Event-free and overall survival at 4 years following surgery without adjuvant chemotherapy was 97.7% in patients with ovarian immature teratoma, and 100% in patients with immature teratoma plus yolk sac tumor. One patient relapsed but was successfully treated with BEP.[137] Larger, prospective trials are required before omission of adjuvant chemotherapy is recommended as standard of care for patients with completely resected immature teratoma.

References

1. Dehner, L. P., Norris, H. J., and Taylor, H. B. (1971). Carcinosarcomas and mixed mesodermal tumors of the ovary. *Cancer* 27, 207–216.
2. Robboy, S. J., Duggan, M., and Kurman, R. T. (1988). The female reproductive system. *In* "Pathology" (E. Rubin, and J. Farber, eds.), 2nd ed. J. B. Lippincott, Philadelphia, PA.
3. Landis, S. H., Murray, T., Bolden, S., and Wingo, P. A. (1999). Cancer Statistics, 1999. *CA Cancer J. Clin.* 49, 8–31.
4. Young, R. C., Walton, L. A., Ellenberg, S. S., Homesley, H. D., Wilbanks, G. D., Decker, D. G., Miller, A., Park, R., and Major, F. (1990). Adjuvant therapy in stage I and II epithelial ovarian cancer. Results of two prospective randomized trials. *N. Engl. J. Med.* 322, 1021–1027.
5. Bonnefoi, H., A'Hern, R. P., Fisher, C., Macfarlane, V., Barton, D., Blake, P., Shepherd, J. H., and Gore, M. E. (1999). Natural history of stage IV epithelial ovarian cancer. *J. Clin. Oncol.* 17, 767–775.
6. McGuire, W. P., Hoskins, W. J., Brady, M. F., Kucera, P. R., Partridge, E. E., Look, K. Y., Clarke-Pearson, D. L., and Davidson, M. (1996). Cyclophosphamide and cisplatin compared with paclitaxel and cisplatin in patients with stage III and stage IV ovarian cancer. *N. Engl. J. Med.* 334, 1–6.
7. McGowan, L., Lesher, L. P., Norris, H. J., and Barnett, M. (1985). Mis-staging of ovarian cancer. *Obstet. Gynecol.* 65, 568–572.
8. Ozols, R. F., Morgan, R. J., Copeland, L., Gershenson, D., Locker, G., McIntosh, D., and Teng, N. (1997). Update of the NCCN ovarian cancer practice guidelines. *Oncology* 11, 95–105.
9. Hoskins, W. J., McGuire, W. P., Brady, M. F., Homesley, H. D., Creasman, W. T., Berman, M., Ball, H., and Berek, J. S. (1994). The effect of diameter of largest residual disease on survival after primary cytoreductive surgery patients with suboptimal residual epithelial ovarian carcinoma. *Am. J. Obstet. Gynecol.* 170, 974.
10. Bristow, R., Moritz, F., Lagasse, L., Leuchter, R., and Karlan, B. (1999). Survival impact of surgical cytoreduction in stage IV epithelial ovarian cancer. *Gynecol. Oncol.* 72, 278–287.
11. Piver, M. S., Lele, S. B., Marchetti, D. L., Baker, T. R., Tsukada, Y., and Emrich, L. J. (1988). The impact of aggressive debulking surgery and cisplatin-based chemotherapy on progression-free survival in stage III and IV ovarian carcinoma. *J. Clin. Oncol.* 6, 989.
12. Sutton, G. P., Stehman, F. B., Einhorn, L. H., Roth, L. M., Blessing, J. A., and Ehrlich, C. E. (1989). Ten-year follow-up of patients receiving cisplatin, doxorubicin, and cyclophosphamide chemotherapy for advanced epithelial ovarian carcinoma. *J. Clin. Oncol.* 7, 223.
13. Young, R. C., Decker, D. G., Wharton, J. T., Piver, M. S., Sindelar, W. F., Edwards, B. K., and Smith, J. P. (1983). Staging laparotomy in early ovarian cancer. *JAMA* 250, 3072.
14. Pecorelli, S., Bolis, G., Colombo, N. *et al.* (1994). Adjuvant therapy in early ovarian cancer. *Proc. SGO* A14.
15. Young, R. C., Brady, M. F., Nieberg, R. M., Long, H. J., Mayer, A., Lentz, S. S., Hurteau, J., and Alberts, D. S. (1999). Randomized clinical trial of adjuvant treatment of women with early (FIGO I-IIA high risk) ovarian cancer—GOG#95. *Proc. ASCO* 18, A1376.
16. Kohn, E. C., Sarosy, G., Bicher, A., Link, C., Christian, M., Steinberg, S. M., Rothenberg, M., Adamo, D. O., Davis, P., Ognibene, F. P. *et al.* (1994). Dose-intense Taxol: High response rates in patients with platinum-resistant recurrent ovarian cancer. *J. Natl. Cancer Inst.* 86, 18.
17. Thigpen, J. T., Blessing, J. A., Ball, H., Hummel, S. J., and Barrett, R. J. (1994). Phase II trial of paclitaxel in patients with progressive ovarian carcinoma after platinum-based therapy. A Gynecologic Oncology Group study. *J. Clin. Oncol.* 12, 1748–1753.
18. Piccart, M. J., Bertelsen, K., James, K., Mangioni, C., Simonsen, E., Stuart, G., Kaye, S., Vergote, I., Blom, R., Grimshaw, R., Atkinson, R. J., Swenerton, K. D., Trope, C., Nardi, M., Kaern, J., Tumolo, S., Timmers, P., Ro, J. A., Lhoas, F., Lindvall, B., Bacon, M., Biert, A., Anderson, J. E., Zee, B., Paul, J., Baron, B., and Pecorelli, S. (2000). Randomized intergroup trial of cisplatin-paclitaxel vs. cisplatin-cyclophosphamide in women with advanced epithelial ovarian cancer: Three-year results. *J. Natl. Cancer Inst.* 92, 699–708.
19. Harper, P. on behalf of the ICON Collaborators. (1999). A randomized trial of paclitaxel (T) and carboplatin (J) versus a control arm of single-agent carboplatin or CAP (cyclophosphamide, doxorubicin and cisplatin): 2075 patients randomized into the 3rd International Collaborative Ovarian Neoplasm Study (ICON3). *Proc. ASCO* 18, 356a.
20. Seiden, M. (2000). Highlights in ovarian cancer. *Oncologist* 5, 267–273.
21. Muggia, F. G., Braly, P. S., Brady, M. F., Sutton, G., Nieman, T. H., Lentz, S. L., Alvarez, R. D., Kucera, P. R., and Small, J. M. (2000). Phase III randomized trial of cisplatin v. paclitaxel versus cisplatin and paclitaxel in patients with suboptimal stage III or IV ovarian cancer: A Gynecologic Oncology Group study. *J. Clin. Oncol.* 18, 106–115.

22. Alberts, D. S., Green, S., Hannigan, E. V., O'Toole, R., Stock-Novack, D., Anderson, P., Surwit, E. A., Malvlya, V. K., Nahhas, W. A., and Jolles, C. J. (1992). Improved therapeutic index of carboplatin plus cyclophosphamide versus cisplatin plus cyclophosphamide: Final report by the Southwest Oncology Group of a phase III randomized trial in stages III and IV ovarian cancer. *J. Clin. Oncol.* 10, 706–717.
23. Swenerton, K., Jeffrey, J., Stuart, G., Roy, M., Krepart, G., Carmichael, J., Drouin, P., Stanimir, R., O'Connell, G., MacLean, G. *et al.* (1992). Cisplatin-cyclophosphamide versus carboplatin-cyclophosphamide in advanced ovarian cancer: A randomized phase III study of the National Cancer Institute of Canada Clinical Trials Group. *J. Clin. Oncol.* 10, 718–726.
24. Jakobsen, A., Bertelsen, K., Andersen, J. E., Havsteen, H., Jakobsen, P., Moeller, K. A., Nielson, E., Sandberg, E., and Stroeyer, I. (1997). Dose-effect study of carboplatin in ovarian cancer: A Danish Ovarian Cancer Group Study. *J. Clin. Oncol.* 15, 193–198.
25. Gore, M., Mainwaring, P., A'Hern, R., A'Hern, R., MacFarlane, V., Slevin, M., Harper, P., Osborne, R., Mansi, J., Blake, P., Wiltshaw, E., and Shepherd, J. (1998). Randomized trial of dose-intensity with single-agent carboplatin in patients with epithelial ovarian cancer. *J. Clin. Oncol.* 16, 2426–2434.
26. Neijt, J. P., Engelholm, S. A., Tuxen, M. K., Sorensen, P. G., Hansen, M., Sessa, C., deSwart, C. A. M., Hirsch, F. R., Lund, B., and van Houselingen, H. C. (2000). Exploratory phase III study of paclitaxel and cisplatin versus paclitaxel and carboplatin in advanced ovarian cancer. *J. Clin. Oncol.* 18, 3084–3092.
27. Ozols, R. F., Bundy, B. N., Fowler, J., Clarke-Pearson, D., Mannel, R., Hargenbach, E. M., and Baergen, R. (1999). Randomized phase III study of cisplatin(CIS)/paclitaxel(PAC) versus carboplatin/PAC in optimal stage III epithelial ovarian cancer (OC): A Gynecologic Oncology Group trial (GOG 158). *Proc. ASCO* 18, 356a.
28. duBois, A., Lueck, H. J., Meier, W., Moebus, V., Costa, S. D., Bauknecht, T., Richter, B., Warm, M., Schroeder, W., Olbricht, S., Nitz, U., and Jackisch, C. (1999). Cisplatin/paclitaxel vs carboplatin/paclitaxel in ovarian cancer: Update of an Arbeitgemeinschaft Gynaekologische Onkologie (AGO) study group trial. *Proc. ASCO* 18, 356a.
29. duBois, A., Neijt, J. P., and Thigpen, J. T. (1999). First-line chemotherapy with carboplatin plus paclitaxel in advanced ovarian cancer—a new standard of care? *Ann. Oncol.* 10 (Suppl. 1) 35–41.
30. Ozols, R. F. (2000). Paclitaxel (Taxol)/carboplatin combination chemotherapy in the treatment of advanced ovarian cancer. *Semin. Oncol.* 27, 3 (Suppl. 7), 3–7.
31. Alberts, D. S., Liu, P. Y., Hannigan, E. V., O'Toole, R., Williams, S. D., Young, J. A., Franklin, E. W., Clarke-Pearson, D. L., Malviya, V. K., DuBeshter, B, Adelson, M. D., and Hoskins, W. J. (1996). Intraperitoneal cisplatin plus intravenous cyclophosphamide versus intravenous cisplatin plus intravenous cyclophosphamide for stage III ovarian cancer. *N. Engl. J. Med.* 335, 1950–1955.
32. Gadducci, A., Carnino, F., Chiara, S., Brunetti, I., Tanganelli, L., Romanini, A., Bruzzone, M., and Conte, P. R., for the GONG Collaborative Centers. (2000). Intraperitoneal versus intravenous cisplatin in combination with intravenous cyclophosphamide and epidoxorubicin in optimally cytoreduced advanced epithelial ovarian cancer: A randomized trial of the Gruppo Oncologico Nord-Ovest. *Gynecol. Oncol.* 76, 157–162.
32a. Armstrong, D. K., Bundy, B. N., Baergen, R. *et al.* (2002). Randomized phase III study of intravenous (IV) paclitaxel and cisplatin versus IV paclitaxel, intraperitoneal (IP) cisplatin and IP paclitaxel in optimal stage III epithelial ovarian cancer (OC): Gynecological Oncology Group trial (GOG 172). *Proc. Am. Soc. Clin. Oncol.* 21, 201a (abstr. 803).
32b. Alberts, D. S., Markman, M., Armstrong, D., Rothenberg, M. L., Muggia, F., and Howell, S. B. (2002). Intraperitoneal therapy for stage III ovarian cancer: A therapy whose time has come! *J. Clin. Oncol.* 20, 3944–3946.
33. Hakes, T. B., Chalas, E., Hoskins, W. J., Jones, W. B., Markman, M., Rubin, S. C., Chapman, D., Almadrones, L., and Lewis, J. L. (1992). Randomized prospective trial of 5 versus 10 cycles of cyclophosphamide, doxorubicin and cisplatin in advanced ovarian carcinoma. *Gynecol. Oncol.* 45, 284–289.
34. Hoskins, W. J. (1993). Surgical staging and cytoreductive surgery of epithelial ovarian cancer. *Cancer* 71, 1534–1540.
35. Cannistra, S. (1993). Cancer of the ovary. *N. Engl. J. Med.* 329, 1550–1559.
36. Ozols, R. F., Rubin, S. C., Thomas, G., and Robboy, S. (1997). Epithelial ovarian cancer. *In* "Principles and Practice of Gynecologic Oncology," 2nd ed. (W. J. Hoskins, C. A. Perez, and R. C. Young, eds.), pp. 919–986. Lippincott-Raven Publishers, Philadelphia.
37. Jacob, H. H., Gershenson, D. M., Morris, M., Copeland, L, Burke, T. W., and Wharton, J. T. (1991). Neoadjuvant chemotherapy and interval debulking surgery for advanced ovarian cancer. *Gynecol. Oncol.* 42, 146–150.
38. Schwartz, P. E., Chambers, J. T., and Makuch, R. (1994). Neoadjuvant chemotherapy for advanced ovarian cancer. *Gynecol. Oncol.* 53, 33–37.
39. Vergote, I., DeWever, I., Tjalma, W., van Gramberen, M., Decloedt, J., and van Dam, P. (1998). Neoadjuvant chemotherapy or primary debulking surgery in advanced ovarian carcinoma: A retrospective analysis of 285 patients. *Gynecol. Oncol.* 71, 431–436.
40. Schwartz, P. E., Ruthereford, T. J., Chambers, J. T., Kohorn, E. I., and Thiel, R. P. (1999). Neoadjuvant chemotherapy for advanced ovarian cancer: Long-term survival. *Gynecol. Oncol.* 72, 93–99.
41. Eisenkop, S. M., Spiritos, N. M., and Friedman, R. L. (1999). Neoadjuvant chemotherapy for advanced ovarian cancer (letter). *Gynecol. Oncol.* 74, 311–312.
42. Weiss, R. B., Donehower, R. C., Wiernik, P. H., Ohnuma, T., Gralla, R. J., Trump, D. L., Baker, J. R., Van Echo, D. A., Von Hoff, D. D., and Leyland-Jones, B. (1990). Hypersensitivity reactions from Taxol. *J. Clin. Oncol.* 8, 1263–1268.
43. Eisenhauer, E. A., ten Bokkel Huinink, W. W., Swenerton, K. D., Gianni, L., Myles, J., van der Burg, M. E., Kerr, I., Vermorken, J. B., Buser, K., Colombo, N. *et al.* (1994). European-Canadian randomized trial of paclitaxel in relapsed ovarian cancer. High-dose versus low-dose and long versus short infusion. *J. Clin. Oncol.* 12, 2654–2666.
44. Markman, M., Kennedy, A., Webster, K., Kulp, B., Peterson, G., and Belinson, J. (2000). Paclitaxel-associated hypersensitivity reactions: Experience of the Gynecologic Oncology Program of the Cleveland Clinic Cancer Center. *J. Clin. Oncol.* 18, 102–105.
45. Peereboom, D. M., Donehower, R. C., Eisenhauer, E. A., McGuire, W. P., Onetto, N., Hubbard, J. L., Piccart, M., Gianni, L., and Rowinsky, E. K. (1993). Successful re-treatment with Taxol after major hypersensitivity reactions. *J. Clin. Oncol.* 11, 885–890.
46. Markman, M., Kennedy, A., Webster, K., Elson, P., Peterson, G., Kulp, B., and Belinson, J. (1999). Clinical features of hypersensitivity reactions to carboplatin. *J. Clin. Oncol.* 17, 1141–1145.
47. Reed, E., Dabholkar, M., and Chabner, B. A. (1996). Platinum analogues. *In* "Cancer Chemotherapy and Biotherapy: Principles and Practice" (B. A. Chabner, and D. L. Longo, eds.), pp. 357–378. Lippincott-Raven, Philadelphia, PA.
48. Daugaard, G., Abildgaard, U., Holstein-Rathlou, N. H., Leyssac, P. P., Amtorp, O., and Off, T. G. (1986). Acute effect of cisplatin on renal hemodynamics and tubular function in dog kidneys. *Renal Physiol.* 9, 308–316.
49. Daugaard, G., and Abildgaard, U. (1989). Cisplatin nephrotoxicity. *Cancer Chemother. Pharmacol.* 25, 1–9.
50. Kintzel, P. E., and Doff, R. O. (1995). Anticancer drug renal toxicity and elimination. Dosing guidelines for altered renal function. *Cancer Treat. Rev.* 21, 33–64.

51. Egorin, M. J., Van Echo, D. A., Tipping, S. J., Olman, E. A., Whitacre, M. Y., Thompson, B. W., and Aisner, J. (1984). Pharmacokinetics and dosage reduction of cis-diammine (1,1-cycloburanedicarboxylato)-platinum in patients with impaired renal function. *Cancer Res.* 44, 5432–5438.
52. Calvert, A. H., Newell, D. R., Gumbrell, L. A., O'Reilly, S., Burnell, M., Boxall, F. E., Siddik, Z. H., Judson, I. R., Gore, M. E., and Wiltshaw, E. (1989). Carboplatin dosage: Prospective evaluation of a simple formula based on renal function. *J. Clin. Oncol.* 7, 1748–1756.
53. Rowinsky, E. K., Gilbert, M. R., McGuire, W. P., Noe, D. A., Grochow, L. B., Forastiere, A. A., Ettinger, D. S., Lubejko, B. G., Clark, B., Sartorius, S. E. *et al.* (1991). Sequences of Taxol and cisplatin: A phase I and pharmacologic study. *J. Clin. Oncol.* 9, 1692–1703.
54. Canetta, R., Goodlow, J., Smaldone, L. *et al.* (1990). Pharmacologic characteristics of carboplatin. Clinical experience. *In* "Carboplatin (JM-8): Current Perspective and Future Directions" (P. A. Bunn, R. Canetta, and R. F. Ozols, eds.) WB Saunders, Philadelphia, PA.
55. Go, R. S., and Adjei, A. A. (1999). Review of the comparative pharmacologic and clinical activity of cisplatin and carboplatin. *J. Clin. Oncol.* 17, 409–422.
56. Von Hoff, D. D., Schilsky, R., Reichert, C. M., Reddick, R. L., Rozencweig, M., Young, R. C., and Muggia, F. M. (1979). Toxic effects of cis-dichlorodiammineplatinum (II) in man. *Cancer Treat. Rep.* 63, 1527–1531.
57. Marty, M., Pouillart, P., Scholl, S., Droz, J. P., Azab, M., Brion, N., Pujade-Lauraine, E., Paule, B., Paes, D., and Bons, J. (1990). Comparison of the 5-hydroxytryptamine3 (serotonin) antagonist ondansetron (GR 38032F) with high-dose metoclopramide in control of cisplatin-induced emesis. *N. Engl. J. Med.* 322, 816–821.
58. Morrow, G. R., Hickok, J. T., and Rosenthal, S. N. (1995). Progress I reducing nausea and emesis. Comparisons of ondansetron (Zofran), granisetron (Kytril), and tropisetron (Navoban). *Cancer* 76, 343–357.
59. Creemers, G. J., Bolis, G., Gore, M., Scarfone, G., Lacave, A. J., Guastalla, J. P., Despax, R., Favalli, G., Kreinberg, R., Van Belle, S., Hudson, I., Verweij, J., and ten Bokkel Huinink, W. W. (1996). Topotecan, an active drug in the second-line treatment of epithelial ovarian cancer: Results of a large European phase 11 study. *J. Clin. Oncol.* 14, 3056–3061.
60. Lund, B., and Neijt, J. P. (1996). Gemcitabine in cisplatin-resistant ovarian cancer. *Semin. Oncol.* 23, 72–76.
61. Muggia, F. M., Hainsworth, J. D., Jeffers, S., Miller, P., Groshen, S., Tan, M., Roman, L., Uziely, B., Muderspach, L., Garcia, A., Burnett, A., Greco, F. A., Morrow, C. P., Paradiso, L. J., and Liang, L.-J. (1997). Phase II study of liposomal doxorubicin in refractory ovarian cancer: Antitumor activity and toxicity modification by liposomal encapsulation. *J. Clin. Oncol.* 15, 987–993.
62. Cannistra, S. (1999). Back to the future: Multiagent chemotherapy in ovarian cancer revisited. *J. Clin. Oncol.* 17, 741–743.
63. Du Bois, A., Lück, H. J., Bauknecht, T., Meier, W., Richter, B., Kuhn, W., Quaas, J., and Pfisterer, J. (1999). First-line chemotherapy with epirubicin, paclitaxel, and carboplatin for advanced ovarian cancer: A phase I/II study of the Arbeitsgemeinschaft Gynakologische Ondologie Ovarian Study Group. *J. Clin. Oncol.* 17, 46–51.
64. Herben, V. M. M., Nannan Panday, V. R., Richel, D. J., Schellens, J. H. M., van der Vange, N., Rosing, H., Beusenberg, F. D., Hearn, S., Doyle, E., Beijnen, J. H., and ten Bokkel Huinink, W. W. (1999). Phase I and pharmacologic study of the combination of paclitaxel, cisplatin, and topotecan administered intravenously every 21 days as first-line therapy inpatients with advanced ovarian cancer. *J. Clin. Oncol.* 17, 747–755.
65. Rose, P. G., Rodriguez, M., Waggoner, S., Greer, B. E., Horowitz, I. R., Fowler, J. M., and McGuire, W. P. (2000). Phase I study of paclitaxel, carboplatin and increasing days of prolonged oral etoposide in ovarian, peritoneal, and tubal carcinoma: A Gynecologic Oncology Group study. *J. Clin. Oncol.* 18, 2957–2962.
66. Morris, M., Gershenson, D. M., and Wharton, J. T. (1989). Secondary cytoreductive surgery in epithelial ovarian cancer: Nonresponders to first-line therapy. *Gynecol. Oncol.* 33, 1–5.
67. Norton, L. (1997). Evolving concepts in the systemic drug therapy of breast cancer. *Semin. Oncol.* 24, s3–s10.
68. Bolis, G., Scarfone, G., Tateo, S., Mangili, G., Antonella, V., and Parazzini, F. (2001). Response and toxicity to topotecan in sensitive ovarian cancer cases with small residual disease after firstline treatment with carboplatinum and paclitaxel. *Gynecol. Oncol.* 80, 13–15.
69. Markman, M. (1991). Intraperitoneal chemotherapy. *Semin. Oncol.* 18, 248–254.
70. Markman, M., Reichman, B., Hakes, T., Jones, W., Lewis, J. L., Rubin, S., Almadrones, L., and Hoskins, W. (1991). Responses to second-line cisplatin-based intraperitoneal therapy in ovarian cancer: Influence of a prior response to intravenous cisplatin. *J. Clin. Oncol.* 9, 1801–1805.
71. Markman, M., Rothman, R., Hakes, T., Reichman, B., Hoskins, W., Rubin, S., Jones, W., Almadrones, L., and Lewis, J. L. (1991). Second-line platinum therapy in patients with ovarian cancer previously treated with cisplatin. *J. Clin. Oncol.* 9, 389–393.
72. Kavanagh, J., Tresukosol, D., Edwards, C., Freedman, R., de Leon, C. G., Fishman, A., Mante, R., Hord, M., and Kudelka, A. (1995). Carboplatin reinduction after taxane in patients with platinum-refractory ovarian cancer. *J. Clin. Oncol.* 13, 1584–1588.
73. Rose, P. G., Fusco, N., Fluellen, L., and Rodriguez, M. (1998). Second-line therapy with paclitaxel and carboplatin for recurrent disease following first-line therapy with paclitaxel and platinum ovarian or peritoneal carcinoma. *J. Clin. Oncol.* 16, 1494–1497.
74. Zannotti, K. M., Belinson, J. L., Kennedy, A. W., Webster, K. D., and Markman, M. (2000). Treatment of relapsed carcinoma of the ovary with single-agent paclitaxel following exposure to paclitaxel and platinum employed as initial therapy. *Gynecol. Oncol.* 79, 211–215.
75. Abu-Rustum, N. R., Aghajanian, C., Barakat, R., Fennelly, D., Shapiro, F., and Spriggs, D. (1997). Salvage weekly paclitaxel in recurrent ovarian cancer. *Semin. Oncol.* 24, s62–s67.
76. McGuire, W. P., Blessing, J. A., Bookman, M. A., Lentz, S. S., and Dunton, C. J. (2000). Topotecan has substantial antitumor activity as first-line salvage therapy in platinum-sensitive epithelial ovarian carcinoma: A Gynecologic Oncology Group study. *J. Clin. Oncol.* 18, 1062–1067.
77. Markman, M., and Bookman, M. A. (2000). Second-line treatment of ovarian cancer. *Oncologist* 5, 26–35.
78. Creemers, G. J., Bolls, G., Gore, M., Scarfone, G., Lacave, A. J., Guastalla, J. P., Despax, R., Favalli, G., Kreinberg, R., Van Belle, S., Hudson, I., Verweij, J., and ten Bokkel Huinink, W. W. (1996). Topotecan, an active drug in the second-line treatment of epithelial ovarian cancer: Results of a large European phase 11 trial. *J. Clin. Oncol.* 14, 3056–3061.
79. Kudelka, A. P., Tresukosol, D., Edwards, C. L., Freedman, R. S., Levenback, C., Chantarawiroj, P., Gonzalez de Leon, C., Kim, E. E., Madden, T., Wallin, B., Hord, M., Verschraegen, C., Raber, M., and Kavanagh, J. J. (1996). Phase II study of intravenous topotecan as a 5 day infusion for refractory epithelial ovarian carcinoma. *J. Clin. Oncol.* 14, 1552–1557.
80. Ten Bokkel Huinink, W. W., Gore, M., Carmichael, J., Gordon, A., Malfetano, J., Hudson, I., Broom, C., Scarabelli, C., Davidson, J., Spanczynski, M., Bolis, G., Malmstrom, H., Coleman, R., Rields, S. C., and Heron, J.-F. (1997). Topotecan versus paclitaxel for the treatment of recurrent epithelial ovarian cancer. *J. Clin. Oncol.* 15, 2183–2193.
81. Bookman, M. A., Malmstrom H., Bolis, G., Gordon, A., Lissoni, A., Krebs, J. B., and Fields, S. Z. (1998). Topotecan for the treatment of advanced epithelial ovarian cancer: An open-label phase 11 study in patients treated after prior chemotherapy containing cisplatin or carboplatin and paclitaxel. *J. Clin. Oncol.* 16, 3345–3352.
82. Gordon, A. X., Granai, C. O, Rose, P. G., Hainsworth, J., Lopez, A., Weissman, C., Rosales, R., and Sharpington, T. (2000). Phase 11 study

of liposomal doxorubicin in platinum- and paclitaxel-refractory epithelial ovarian cancer. *J. Clin. Oncol.* 18, 3093–3100.

83. Markman, M., Kennedy, A., Webster, K., Peterson, G., Kulp, B., and Belinson, J. (2000). Phase 2 trial of liposomal doxorubicin (40 mg/m^2) in platinum/paclitaxel-refractory ovarian and fallopian tube cancers and primary carcinoma of the peritoneum. *Gynecol. Oncol.* 78, 369–372.
84. Rose, P. G., Blessing, J. A., Mayer, A. R., and Homesley, H. D. (1998). Prolonged oral etoposide as second-line therapy for platinum-resistant and platinum-sensitive ovarian carcinoma. A Gynecologic Oncology Group study. *J. Clin. Oncol.* 16, 405–410.
85. Shapiro, J. D. Millward, M. J., Rischin, D., Michael, M., Walcher, V., Francis, P. A., and Toner, G. C. (1996). Activity of gemcitabine in patients with advanced ovarian cancer: Responses seen following platinum and paclitaxel. *Gynecol. Oncol.* 63, 89–93.
86. Bajetta, E., Di Leo, A., Biganzoli, L., Mariani, L., Cappuzzo, F., Di Barolomeo, M., Zilembo, N., Artale, S., Magnani, E., Celio, L., Buzzoni, R., and Carnaghi, C. (1996). Phase II study of vinorelbine in patients with pretreated advanced ovarian cancer: Activity in platinum-resistant disease. *J. Clin. Oncol.* 14, 2546–2551.
87. Burger, R. A., Di Saia, P. J., Roberts, J. A., O'Rourke, M., Gershenson, D. M., Homesley, H. D., Lichtman, S. M., Barnes, W., Moore, D. H., and Monk, B. J. (1999). Phase II trial of vinorelbine in recurrent and progressive epithelial ovarian cancer. *Gynecol. Oncol.* 72, 148–153.
88. Francis, P., Schneider, J., Hann, L., Balmaceda, C., Barakat, R., Phillips, M., and Hakes, T. (1994). Phase II trial of docetaxel in patients with platinum-refractory advanced ovarian cancer. *J. Clin. Oncol.* 12, 2301–2308.
89. Piccart, M. J., Gore, M., ten Bokkel Huinink, W. W. *et al.* (1995). Docetaxel: An active new drug for treatment of advanced epithelial ovarian cancer. *J. Natl. Cancer Inst.* 87, 676–681.
90. Verschraegen, C. F., Sittisomwong, T., Kudelka, A. P., de Paula Guedes, E., Steger, M., Nelson-Taylor, T., Vincent, M., Rogers, G., Atkinson, E. N., and Kavanagh, J. J. (2000). Docetaxel for patients with paclitaxel-resistant Mullerian carcinoma. *J. Clin. Oncol.* 18, 2733–2739.
91. Fennelly, D., Aghajanian, C., Shapiro, F., O'Flaherty, C., McKenzie, M., O'Connor, C., Tong, W., Norton, L., and Spriggs, D. (1997). Phase I and pharmacologic study of paclitaxel administered weekly inpatients with relapsed ovarian cancer. *J. Clin. Oncol.* 15, 187–192.
92. Sutton, G. P., Blessing, J. A., Homesley, H. D., Berman, M. L., and Malfetano, J. (1989). Phase II trial of ifosfamide and mesna in advanced ovarian carcinoma: A Gynecologic Oncology Group study. *J. Clin. Oncol.* 7, 1672–1676.
93. Sorenson, P., Pfeiffer, P., and Bertelsen, K. (1995). A phase 2 trial of ifosfamide/mesna as salvage therapy in patients with ovarian cancer refractory to or relapsing after prior platinum-containing chemotherapy. *Gynecol. Oncol.* 56, 75–78.
94. Markman, M., Hakes, T., Reichman, B., Lewis, Jr., J. L., Rubin, S., Jones, W., Almadrones, L., Pizzuto, F., and Hoskins, W. (1992). Ifosfamide and mesna in previously treated advanced epithelial ovarian cancer: Activity in platinum-resistant disease. *J. Clin. Oncol.* 10, 243–248.
95. Markman, M., Kennedy, A., Sutton, G., Hurteau, J., Webster, K., Peterson, G., Kulp, B., and Belinson, J. (1998). Phase 2 trial of single agent ifosfamide/mesna in patients with platinum/paclitaxel refractory ovarian cancer who have not previously been treated with an alkylating agent. *Gynecol. Oncol.* 70, 272–274.
96. Hatch, K. D., Beecham, J. B., Blessing, J. A., and Creasman, W. T. (1991). Responsiveness of patients with advanced ovarian carcinoma to tamoxifen. A Gynecologic Oncology Group study of second-line therapy in 105 patients. *Cancer* 68, 269–271.
97. Ahlgren, J. D., Ellison, N. M., Gottlieb, R. J., Laluna, F., Lokich, J. J., Sinclair, P. R., Ueno, W., Wampler, G. L., Yeung, K. Y., Alt, D. *et al.* (1993). Hormonal palliation of chemoresistant ovarian cancer: Three consecutive phase II trials of the Mid-Atlantic Oncology Program. *J. Clin. Oncol.* 11, 1957–1968.
98. Gordon, A. X., Fleagle, J. T., Guthrie, D., Parkin, D. E., Gore, M., Lacave, A. J., and Mutch, D. (2000). Interim analysis of a phase III randomized trial of Doxil/Caelyx versus Topotecan in the treatment of patients with relapsed ovarian cancer. *Proc. ASCO* 19, 380a.
99. Muntz, H. G., Jones, M. A., Goff, B. A., Fuller, A. F., Jr., Nikrui, N., Rice, L. W., and Tarraza, H. M. (1995). Malignant mixed mullerian tumors of the ovary: Experience with surgical cytoreduction and combination chemotherapy. *Cancer* 76, 1209–1213.
100. Le, T., Krepart, G. V., Lotocki, R. J., and Heywood, M. S. (1997). Malignant mixed mesodermal ovarian tumor treatment and prognosis: A 20-year experience. *Gynecol. Oncol.* 65, 237–240.
101. Morrow, C., d'Ablaing, G., Brady, L., Blessing, J., and Hreschyshyn, M. (1984). A clinical and pathologic study of 30 cases of malignant mixed mullerian epithelial and mesenchymal ovarian tumors: A Gynecologic Oncology Group study. *Gynecol. Oncol.* 18, 278–282.
102. DiSilverto, P., Gajewski, W., Lukwig, M., Kourea, H., Sung, J., and Granai, C. (1995). Malignant mixed mesodermal tumors of the ovary. *Obstet. Gynecol.* 86, 780–782.
103. Plaxe, S. C., Dottino, P. R., Goodman, H. M., Deligdisch, L., Idelson, M., and Cohen, C. J. (1990). Clinical features of advanced ovarian mixed mesodermal tumors and treatment with doxorubicin and cisplatin-based chemotherapy. *Gynecol. Oncol.* 37, 244–249.
104. Andersen, W. A., Young, D. E., Peters, W. A., Smith, E. B., Bagley, C. M., and Taylor, P. T. (1989). Platinum based combination chemotherapy for malignant mixed mesodermal tumours of the ovary *Gynecol. Oncol.* 32, 319–322.
105. Sit, A. S. Y., Price, F. V., Kelley, J. L., Comerci, J. T., Kunschner, A. J., Kanbour-Shakir, A., and Edwards, R. P. (2000). Chemotherapy for malignant mixed Mullerian tumors of the ovary. *Gynecol. Oncol.* 79, 196–200.
106. Sutton, G. P., Blessing, J. A., Homesley, H. D., and Malfetano, J. H. A phase II trial of ifosfamide and mesna in patients with advanced or recurrent mixed mesodermal tumors of the ovary previously treated with platinum-based chemotherapy: A Gynecologic Oncology Group study. *Gynecol. Oncol.* 53, 24–26.
107. Ayhan, A., Tuncer, Z. S., Tuncer, R., Mercan, R., Yuce, K., and Ayhan, A. (1994). Granulosa cell tumor of the ovary: A clinicopathological evaluation of 60 cases. *Eur. J. Gynaecol. Oncol.* 15, 320–324.
108. Segal, R., DePetrillo, A. D., and Thomas, G. (1995). Clinical review of adult granulosa cell tumors of the ovary. *Gynecol. Oncol.* 56, 338–344.
109. Evans, M. P., Webb, M. J., Gaffey, T. A., Katzmann, J. A., Suman, V. J., and Hu, T. C. (1995). DNA ploidy of ovarian granulosa cell tumors. *Cancer* 75, 2295–2298.
110. Biorkholm, E., and Silfverward, C. (1981). Prognostic factors in granulosa cell tumors. *Gynecol. Oncol.* 11, 261–274.
111. Slayton, R., Brady, L., Johnson, G., and Blessing, J. A. (1980). Radiotherapy or chemotherapy in malignant stromal tumors of the ovary. *Proc. ASCO*, abstr. C444.
112. Jacobs, A. J., Deppe, G., and Cohen, C. J. (1982). Combination chemotherapy of ovarian granulosa cell tumor with cisplatin and doxorubicin. *Gynecol. Oncol.* 14, 294–297.
113. Kaye, S. T., and Davies, E. (1986). Cyclophosphamide, adriamycin, and cis-platinum for the treatment of advanced granulosa cell tumor, using serum estradiol as a tumor marker. *Gynecol. Oncol.* 24, 261–264.
114. Neville, A. J., Gilchrist, K. W., and Davis, T. E. (1984). The chemotherapy of granulosa cell tumors of the ovary: Experience of the Wisconsin Clinical Cancer Center. *Med. Pediatr. Oncol.* 12, 397–400.
115. Zambetti, M. A., Pilotti, S., and DePalo, G. (1990). Ciplatinum/vinblastine/bleomycin combination chemotherapy in advanced or recurrent granulosa cell tumors of the ovary. *Gynecol. Oncol.* 36, 317–320.

116. Colombo, N., Sessa, C., Landoni, F., Sartori, E., Pecorelli, S., and Mangiom, C. (1986). Cisplatin, vinblastine, and bleomycin combination chemotherapy in metastatic granulosa cell tumor of the ovary. *Obstet. Gynecol.* 67, 265–268.

117. Pecorelli, S., Wagenaar, H. C., Vergote, I. B., Currant, D., Beex, L. V. A., Wiltshaw, E., and Vermorken, J. B. (1999). Cisplatin (P), vinblastine (V), and bleomycin (B) combination chemotherapy in recurrent or advanced granulosa (-theca) cell tumors of the ovary. And EORTC Gyneacologic Cancer Cooperative Group study. *Eur. J. Cancer* 35, 1331–1337.

118. Gershenson, D. M., Morris, M., Burke, T. W., Levenback, C., Matthews, C. M., and Wharton, J. T., (1996). Treatment of poor-prognosis sex cord-stromal tumors of the ovary with the combination of bleomycin, etoposide, and cisplatin. *Obstet. Gynecol.* 87, 527–531.

119. Homesley, H. D., Bundy, B. N., Hurteau, J. A., and Roth, L. M. (1999). Bleomycin, etoposide, and cisplatin combination therapy of ovarian granulosa cell tumors and other stromal malignancies: A Gynecologic Oncology Group study. *Gynecol. Oncol.* 72, 131–137.

120. Williams, S. D., Birch, R., Einhorn, L. H., Irwin, L., Greco, F. A., and Loehrer, P. J. (1987). Treatment of disseminated germ-cell tumors with cisplatin, bleomycin, and either vinblastine or etoposide. *N. Engl. J. Med.* 316, 1435–1440.

121. Colombo, N., Parma, B., and Franchi, D. (1999). An active chemotherapy regimen for advanced ovarian sex cord-stromal tumors. *Gynecol. Oncol.* 72, 129–130.

122. Pedersen-Bjergaard, J., Daugaard, G., Hansen, S. W., Philip, P., Larsen, S. O., and Rorth, M. (1991). Increased risk of myelodysplasia and leukaemia after etoposide, cisplatin, and bleomycin for germ-cell tumors. *Lancet* 338, 359–363.

123. Nichols, C. R., Breeden, E. S., Loehrer, P. J., Williams, S. D., and Einhorn, L. H. (1993). Secondary leukemia associated with a conventional dose of etoposide: Review of serial germ cell tumor protocols. *J. Natl. Cancer Inst.* 85, 36–40.

124. Thomas, G. M., Dembo, A. J., Hacker, J. T., and DePetrillo, A. D. (1987). Current therapy for dysgerminoma of the ovary. *Obstet. Gynecol.* 70, 268–275.

125. Ayhan, A., Bildirici, I., Gunlap, S., and Yuce, K. (2000). Pure dysgerminoma of the ovary: A review of 45 well-staged cases. *Eur. J. Gynaecol. Oncol.* 21, 98–101.

126. Dark, G. G., Bower, M., Newlands, E. S., Paradinas, F., and Rustin, G. J. S. (1997). Surveillance policy for stage I ovarian germ cell tumors. *J. Clin. Oncol.* 15, 620–624.

127. Culine, S., Lhomme, C., Kattan, J., Duvillard, P., Michel, G., Gerbaulet, A., and Droz, J.-P. (1995). Cisplatin-based chemotherapy in dysgerminoma of the ovary: Thirteen-year experience of the Institut Gustave Roussy. *Gynecol. Oncol.* 58, 344–348.

128. Gershenson, D. M., Wharton, T., Kline, R. C., Larson, D. M., Kavanagh, J. J., and Rutledge, F. N. (1986). Chemotherapeutic complete remission in patient with metastatic ovarian dysgerminoma. Potential for cure and preservation of reproduction capacity. *Cancer* 58, 2594–2599.

129. Williams, S. D., Blessing, J. A., Hatch, K. D., and Homesley, H. D. (1991). Chemotherapy of advanced dysgerminoma: Trials of the Gynecologic Oncology Group. *J. Clin. Oncol.* 9, 1950–1955.

130. Brewer, M., Gershenson, D. M., Herzog, C. E., Mitchell, M. F., Silva, E. G., and Wharton, J. T. (1999). Outcome and reproductive function after chemotherapy for ovarian dysgerminoma. *J. Clin. Oncol.* 17, 2670–2675.

131. Norris, H. J., Zirkin, H. J., and Benson, W. L. (1976). Immature (malignant) teratoma of the ovary. *Cancer* 37, 2359–2372.

132. Williams, S. D., Blessing, J. A., Moore, D. H., Homesley, H. D., and Adcock, L. (1989). Cisplatin, vinblastine, and bleomycin in advanced and recurrent ovarian germ-cell tumors. *Ann. Int. Med.* 111, 22–27.

133. Gershenson, D. M., Morris, M., Cangir, A., Kavanagh, J. J., Stringer, C. A., Edwards, C. L., Silva, E. G., and Wharton, J. T. (1990). Treatment of malignant germ cell tumors of the ovary with bleomycin, etoposide, and cisplatin. *J. Clin. Oncol.* 8, 715–720.

134. Segelov, E., Campbell, J., Ng, M., Tattersall, M., Rome, R., Free, K., Hacker, N., and Friedlander, M. L. (1994). Cisplatin-based chemotherapy for ovarian germ cell malignancies: The Australian experience. *J. Clin. Oncol.* 12, 378–384.

135. William, S., Blessing, J. A., Liao, S. Y., Ball, H., and Hanjani, P. (1994). Adjuvant therapy of ovarian germ cell tumors with cisplatin, etoposide, and bleomycin: A trial of the Gynecologic Oncology Group. *J. Clin. Oncol.* 12, 701–706.

136. Williams, S. D. (1998). Ovarian germ cell tumors: An update. *Semin. Oncol.* 25, 407–413.

137. Cushing, B., Giller, G., Ablin, A., Cohen, L., Cullen, J., Hawkins, E., Heifetz, S., Krailo, M., Lauer, S. J., Marina, N., Rao, P. V., Rescorla, F., Vinocor, C. D., Weetman, R. M., and Castleberry, R. P. (1999). Surgical resection alone is effective treatement for ovarian immature teratoma in children and adolescents: A report of the pediatric oncology group and the children's cancer group. *Am. J. Obstet. Gynecol.* 181, 353–358.

C H A P T E R

36

Intraperitoneal Chemotherapy

MAURIE MARKMAN

The Cleveland Clinic Taussig Cancer Center
Department of Hematology/Medical Oncology
The Cleveland Clinic Foundation
Cleveland, Ohio 44195

ABSTRACT

The delivery of antineoplastic agents directly into the peritoneal cavity as treatment of malignancies principally confined to this body compartment (e.g., ovarian cancer) is based on sound pharmacokinetic and anatomic principles. Over the past two decades investigators have defined both the potential benefits, and limitations, associated with this unique method of drug delivery in the treatment of ovarian cancer. Recently, two large well-designed and conducted randomized phase III trials have confirmed a survival advantage associated with the administration of cisplatin by the intraperitoneal route in the initial treatment of advanced small volume residual advanced ovarian cancer, compared to the systemic delivery of the same cytotoxic drug. In several clinical settings involving patients with ovarian cancer, fallopian tube cancer, or primary peritoneal carcinoma it is appropriate to consider intraperitoneal treatment (generally with either cisplatin or carboplatin) as a rationale management option. These include: (1) patients who achieve a major response following therapy with systemic platinum-based treatment, but who persist in having microscopic or very small volume residual macroscopic disease (largest tumor nodule <0.5–1 cm in maximal diameter) at the time of a second-look laparotomy/laparoscopy; (2) patients with large volume intraperitoneal disease, or those with grade 3 tumors, who achieve a surgically-documented complete response following systemic chemotherapy ("consolidation therapy"); and (3) previously untreated patients with stage 3A (microscopic disease only in the upper abdomen) or those with stages 3B or 3C disease who have no visible macroscopic cancer following initial surgical cytoreduction.

I. INTRODUCTION

The concept of delivering drugs directly into the peritoneal cavity as therapy for ovarian cancer was initially tested clinically more than four decades ago.[1] However, it has only been within the past 15–20 years that a firm scientific basis for this method of drug delivery has been established.[2, 3] Of note, randomized controlled phase III trials have now demonstrated the use of intraperitoneal cisplatin-based chemotherapy as initial treatment of small-volume residual advanced ovarian cancer can result in an improvement in survival in the malignancy.[4, 5]

The focus of this chapter will be on intraperitoneal drug delivery in the management of ovarian cancer. However, existing data strongly suggest statements made regarding treatment of this malignancy are also relevant for patients with both primary carcinoma of the peritoneum and cancer of the fallopian tube.

II. RATIONALE FOR INTRAPERITONEAL THERAPY

The basic aim of intraperitoneal chemotherapy is to expose tumor present within the cavity to *higher concentrations* of drug for *longer periods of time* than can be achieved with systemic delivery of the agent.[2, 3, 6] The specific characteristics of an antineoplastic agent that would make it attractive to consider for regional delivery are outlined in Table 36.1. Drugs for which there are experimental data to demonstrate the degree of cytotoxicity against the cancer within the cavity can be enhanced by increased exposure (higher peak levels or prolonged contact) would be of particular interest to examine for intraperitoneal administration.[7]

TABLE 36.1 Characteristics of the "Ideal" Antineoplastic Agent for Intraperitoneal Administration

1. Not toxic to the peritoneal lining (i.e., does not cause pain or adhesion formation)
2. Slowly exists the peritoneal cavity, maximizing differences in the concentration between the body compartment and systemic circulation (e.g., large and water-soluble agents are more slowly absorbed than small or lipid-soluble drugs)
3. Rapidly metabolized during initial passage through the portal circulation, as drugs administered intraperitoneally enter the portal vein prior to reaching the systemic compartment.
4. Highly active against the tumor type being treated (e.g., cisplatin in ovarian cancer)
5. Experimental evidence the cytotoxicity of the agent against the particular tumor type is enhanced by increasing either the concentration or duration of exposure

It is important to note there are a number of both theoretical and practical issues that must be addressed before considering a regional chemotherapy approach in the management of ovarian cancer, or other gynecologic malignancy. These are briefly outlined in Tables 36.2 and 36.3. However, data to be presented in this chapter clearly demonstrate patients can be safely and effectively treated by the intraperitoneal route if they are appropriately selected and carefully observed for the potential toxicities of treatment.

III. PHASE I TRIALS OF INTRAPERITONEAL ANTINEOPLASTIC DRUG DELIVERY

A number of cytotoxic and biological agents have been examined in phase I trials for their safety and pharmacokinetic advantage when delivered by the intraperitoneal route (Table 36.4).[6] Of note, several of these agents have known activity in the management of gynecologic malignancies, particularly ovarian cancer.

IV. CISPLATIN-BASED INTRAPERITONEAL CHEMOTHERAPY OF OVARIAN CANCER

It should come as no surprise that cisplatin has undergone the most extensive evaluation for regional treatment of ovarian cancer, due to its central role in the management

TABLE 36.2 Theoretical Concerns Associated with Intraperitoneal Therapy of Gynecologic Cancers

1. Inadequate distribution of the antineoplastic agent when administered directly into the peritoneal cavity
2. Limited penetration of the agent directly into tumor tissue
3. Decreased delivery of the antineoplastic agent to tumor by *capillary flow* following regional drug administration

TABLE 36.3 Practical Considerations Associated with Intraperitoneal Antineoplastic Drug Delivery

1. Local toxicity of the agent(s) (e.g., abdominal pain, adhesion formation leading to bowel dysfunction and obstruction)
2. Requirement to develop a safe and convenient method of access to the peritoneal cavity for treatment delivery
3. Additional costs associated with regional therapy (e.g., catheter placement, time required for drug delivery)
4. Potential for infectious complications associated with intraperitoneal delivery devices (e.g., semi-permanent indwelling catheters or percutaneous catheter placement with each course)

TABLE 36.4 Pharmacokinetic Advantage Associated with Intraperitoneal Delivery of Selected Antineoplastic Agents

	Peak peritoneal cavity/plasma concentration ratio
Cisplatin	20
Carboplatin	18
Paclitaxel	1000
Doxorubicin	474
Mitoxantrone	620
Methotrexate	92
5-Fluorouracil	298
Melphalan	93
Alpha-interferon	100

TABLE 36.5 Summary of Experience with Second-Line Cisplatin-Based Intraperitoneal Chemotherapy of Ovarian Cancer

Maximum tumor diameter	Surgically defined complete response rate
Microscopic disease only	30–40%
<0.5–1 cm	15–25%
>1 cm	<10%

of the malignancy. Phase I trials have revealed the drug can be safely delivered into the peritoneal cavity, with a 10- to 20-fold pharmacokinetic advantage being observed for exposure of the cavity compared to that of the systemic circulation.[8–11]

Despite the major difference in the degree of exposure, significant concentrations of active cisplatin reach the systemic compartment following regional delivery. This is due to the fact that this agent is not metabolized in the liver and does not cause significant abdominal pain or adhesion formation after intraperitoneal delivery. This important feature allows for escalation of the cisplatin dose delivered regionally permitting adequate drug concentrations to leave the body compartment and enter the systemic circulation. Thus, the dose-limiting toxicities of intraperitoneally administered cisplatin are the systemic effects of the agent (e.g., nephrotoxicity, neurotoxicity, emesis).

A. Phase II Trials of Second-Line Cisplatin-Based Intraperitoneal Chemotherapy

Phase II trials of second-line cisplatin-based intraperitoneal therapy of ovarian cancer, following platinum-based (cisplatin or carboplatin) systemic treatment, have revealed objective responses can be achieved, including surgically documented complete responses (Table 36.5).[6, 12–15] Overall, approximately 20–40% of women with ovarian cancer considered for a cisplatin-based regional treatment approach will respond to the treatment program.

It is important to note responses are essentially limited to patients with microscopic or small-volume residual macroscopic disease (e.g., largest tumor nodule <0.5–1 cm in maximal diameter) at the time of initiation of the regional strategy.[6, 12] This finding is not surprising, as there is limited penetration of the drug directly into tumor tissue. In fact, experimental data have revealed the depth of penetration of cisplatin into the peritoneal lining or tumor following regional delivery is only 1–2 mm from the peritoneal surface.[16]

There was a second important observation that resulted from these second-line phase II cisplatin-based intraperitoneal chemotherapy trials.[12, 17] It was noted that the 10- to 20-fold higher concentrations of drug achievable within the peritoneal cavity following regional delivery could be translated into objective tumor regression only in patients whose cancers had exhibited evidence of a clinical or surgically documented response to the previously administered platinum-based systemic therapy ("relative tumor resistance"). In striking contrast, individuals whose cancer had essentially failed to respond to initial therapy ("absolute tumor resistance") rarely showed any evidence of a response to the intraperitoneal treatment program.

(It is important to mention here that the implications of these results are highly relevant for all second-line *dose-intensive* antineoplastic drug treatment strategies considered in management of gynecologic malignancies. Tumors shown to be *inherently resistant* to specific cytotoxic chemotherapeutic agents are extremely unlikely to exhibit clinically meaningful objective responses to the drugs at dose levels which are achievable in patients, regardless of the "intensity" utilized. In this clinical setting alternative therapeutic approaches will need to be employed.)

Unfortunately, there have been *no* reported randomized phase III trials of second-line cisplatin-based intraperitoneal chemotherapy, compared to systemic treatment, in the management of ovarian cancer. Thus, it is not possible to make a definitive statement regarding the impact of this approach on either progression-free or overall survival in this clinical setting.

However, several *retrospective studies* have documented the potential for women with small-volume persistent ovarian cancer (i.e., microscopic disease only, largest remaining tumor nodules <0.5–1 cm in maximum diameter) documented at the time of a second-look laparotomy to achieve extended survival (e.g., >4–5 years) (Table 36.6).[18–20] On the basis of these data, and the documented relative safety of intraperitoneal cisplatin-based treatment, it is appropriate to suggest specific clinical characteristics where a second-line intraperitoneal cisplatin-based treatment approach is a reasonable therapeutic option (Table 36.7).

TABLE 36.6 Prolonged Survival Associated with Second-Line Cisplatin-Based Intraperitoneal Therapy of Ovarian Cancer

Institution	Results
University of California San Diego (Ref. 18)	Median survival >4 years (patients with <2 cm maximal residual disease)
Memorial Sloan-Kettering Cancer Center (Ref. 19)	Median survival >4 years (patients with microscopic disease achieving a surgically defined complete response)
Roswell Park Cancer Institute (Ref. 20)	36% 5-year survival (patients with ≤0.5 cm maximal residual disease)

TABLE 36.7 Candidates for Cisplatin-Based Intraperitoneal Chemotherapy as Second-Line Therapy of Ovarian Cancer

1. Documented response to initial platinum-based systemic chemotherapy
2. Microscopic disease only or small volume macroscopic residual disease (<0.5–1 cm maximal diameter) documented at the time of the performance of a second-look laparotomy/laparoscopy
3. Minimal intra-abdominal adhesions
4. Ability to tolerate systemic toxicities of cisplatin (e.g., emesis, nephrotoxicity, neurotoxicity) (an alternative approach would be to employ intraperitoneal carboplatin)

B. Intraperitoneal Cisplatin as a *Consolidation Strategy* Following a Surgically Defined Complete Response

Despite the major activity of platinum-based systemic therapy in individuals with ovarian cancer, the majority of patients with advanced disease ultimately relapse and die of complications of their malignancy. In fact, for women with high grade (grade 3) tumors who achieve a *surgically documented* complete response, the ultimate relapse rate approaches 50–60%.[21]

Thus, it is reasonable to ask whether it is possible for some form of "consolidation therapy," administered after a patient achieves an optimal response, to favorably impact both progression-free and, ultimately, overall survival in this disease.

In limited, nonrandomized studies, intraperitoneal cisplatin has been examined for this clinical indication. Perhaps the most provocative report regarding the potential therapeutic benefit of this innovative strategy has come from investigators at the Memorial Sloan-Kettering Cancer Center (New York).[22] Over a period of several years patients achieving a surgically defined complete response were offered a consolidation treatment strategy (phase II trial) of three courses of intraperitoneal cisplatin plus etoposide (total of 36 patients).

During the identical time period a number of patients treated at the same institution by the same surgeons who also achieved a surgically documented complete response did not receive the intraperitoneal consolidation treatment (total of 46 patients). There were a number of reasons patients did not undergo intraperitoneal therapy, including both patient and physician choice.

The Memorial Sloan-Kettering investigators subsequently elected to examine and compare the outcomes of the two treatment groups.[22] It is important to recognize the inherent difficulty in comparing results of patient populations for whom treatment was *not* selected by random chance. A particular concern is for conscious or unconscious *favorable* selection bias associated with the experimental treatment arm.

However, in this setting, there actually appeared to be selection bias in favor of the "control" (untreated) group. For example, the 'control' population consisted of more patients who initially presented with stage II disease (39 versus 8%), compared to the treated group. Further, the experimental population included a greater percentage of women who initiated systemic therapy with suboptimal residual cancer (33 versus 20%). This "grouping of patients" is not surprising as it might be anticipated physicians would be more likely to recommend, and patients more likely to agree to receive, the consolidation approach if it "was perceived they had a *greater risk* for developing disease recurrence."

Despite this fact, patients undergoing the experimental intraperitoneal treatment program experienced a *lower risk* of relapse compared to the population that did not undergo the consolidation strategy (39 versus 54%, with a median follow-up of 36 months from second-look surgery). Of interest, in the 28 patients who received all three of the initially planned consolidation intraperitoneal courses, the relapse rate was only 28%.

It is important to note these results cannot be considered definitive as the study did not employ a randomized phase III trial design. However, this experience, along with other data presented in this section, provide a *strong rationale* to consider intraperitoneal platinum-based consolidation therapy in carefully selected women with advanced ovarian cancer who achieve a surgically defined complete response to initial systemic chemotherapy (Table 36.8).

TABLE 36.8 Candidates for Cisplatin-Based Intraperitoneal Therapy as a "Consolidation Strategy" in Ovarian Cancer Following a Surgically Documented Complete Response

1. Presence of significant intra-abdominal disease at the initiation of systemic platinum-based chemotherapy (stage IIIB, stage IIIC), *or*
2. Advanced disease with high grade (grade 3) tumor histology (risk of relapse >50–60%)
3. Minimal intra-abdominal adhesions

V. INTRAPERITONEAL THERAPY WITH OTHER AGENTS ACTIVE IN GYNECOLOGIC MALIGNANCIES

A number of other cytotoxic drugs have been examined as single agents and in combination regimens, when administered by the intraperitoneal route in the management of ovarian cancer.[6, 23] Unfortunately, several of these drugs, despite achieving objective clinical responses, have been shown to produce rather severe local toxicity (e.g., doxorubicin,[24, 25] mitoxantrone [26]) and have not been pursued further in clinical trials. Novel biological agents, such as interferon-alpha [27, 28] and interleukin-2,[29] have also been evaluated in small phase II studies, but a role for these drugs in standard clinical management remains to be defined.

Two agents, carboplatin and paclitaxel, have undergone more extensive testing, and are worthy of further discussion.

A. Carboplatin

Due to its more favorable toxicity profile, carboplatin has largely replaced cisplatin in the systemic treatment of ovarian cancer and primary carcinoma of the peritoneum.[30, 31] This is particularly relevant in patients receiving a platinum agent and paclitaxel, due to the potential for neurotoxicity associated with the two drug combination chemotherapy regimen.[32, 33]

Despite this fact, in the case of intraperitoneal drug delivery, there remains far less experimental and clinical data with carboplatin than cisplatin. There are several reasons for this observation.

First, during the period of time where the platinum agents were initially investigated for intraperitoneal use, there was less experience with carboplatin as a therapeutic option in ovarian cancer, and far less certainty the agent was therapeutically equivalent to cisplatin. Second, there exist preclinical *in vitro* data which suggest the concentration of platinum *within tumor cells* following *direct diffusion* from the cavity (in contrast to delivery by capillary flow) is superior with cisplatin, compared to carboplatin.[34]

Finally, a retrospective examination of a single institution nonrandomized trial experience has suggested patients with small-volume *macroscopic residual* ovarian cancer receiving second-line intraperitoneal therapy achieved a higher surgically defined complete response rate when treated with cisplatin, as compared to carboplatin.[35] In contrast, in this same analysis, there was no difference in the surgical response rate in women with *microscopic disease only*, suggesting a potential difference in the degree of penetration or retention of the two platinum agents when administered regionally.

However, it is well established that the use of intraperitoneal carboplatin is associated with a favorable side effect profile, with limited local toxicity being observed.[36, 37] As with cisplatin, the dose-limiting toxicity is the systemic effects of the agent (principally bone marrow suppression). A pharmacokinetic advantage for peritoneal cavity exposure similar to that of cisplatin has been observed in several phase I studies.[36, 37] Finally, objective responses, including surgically defined complete responses, have been documented in patients receiving intraperitoneal carboplatin as second-line treatment of advanced ovarian cancer.[38, 39]

These data strongly support the argument that the use of intraperitoneal carboplatin should be further examined as a management strategy in women with ovarian cancer. In addition, it is reasonable to substitute carboplatin for cisplatin in individual patients being considered for regional therapy (e.g., microscopic disease at second-look surgery) where the toxicity of the older platinum agent is excessive (e.g., emesis).

B. Paclitaxel

Based on its demonstrated activity in platinum-resistant ovarian cancer, paclitaxel has been examined for its potential use when delivered by the intraperitoneal route in both phase I and II clinical trials. A major pharmacokinetic advantage for regional drug delivery (>1000-fold increased exposure for the peritoneal cavity compared to the systemic compartment) has been demonstrated.[40, 41] In contrast to the platinum agents, the dose-limiting toxicity of intraperitoneal paclitaxel is abdominal pain, which limits the concentration of the agent that can be safely delivered directly into the peritoneal cavity.

There are several features of paclitaxel that make the drug particularly appealing to administer by the intraperitoneal route. First, as noted above, there is a truly profound pharmacokinetic advantage associated with exposure of the peritoneal cavity, compared to the systemic compartment, following regional administration. This is particularly apparent when contrasting the pharmacokinetic advantage of paclitaxel (i.e., 1000-fold) to that of either cisplatin or carboplatin (i.e., 10- to 20-fold).

Second, as experimental data have strongly suggested the cytotoxicity of paclitaxel is *cycle specific*,[42] prolonged exposure of ovarian cancer cells present within the peritoneal cavity to the agent following regional delivery may be associated with far greater tumor cell kill. In fact, phase I data have revealed cytotoxic concentrations of paclitaxel persist within the peritoneal cavity for more than *one* week following a single intraperitoneal administration.[41]

Finally, as paclitaxel has now been demonstrated to be an important component of the initial chemotherapy program for advanced ovarian cancer,[43] it is reasonable to suggest the intraperitoneal administration of both paclitaxel *and* cisplatin (or carboplatin) has the potential to improve survival in this clinical setting.

It should be noted that following the regional delivery of paclitaxel there are limited concentrations of the agent measured in the systemic compartment.[40] This is due to the fact that the amount of drug that can be safely administered by the intraperitoneal route is limited by the development of local toxicity (e.g., abdominal pain). These data strongly suggest that the "optimal use" of paclitaxel in the management of small-volume residual ovarian cancer may be to treat patients by *both* the systemic and intraperitoneal routes of drug delivery.

Support for this conclusion is provided by the results of a phase II trial of single agent intraperitoneal paclitaxel (no systemic drug delivery) employed as second-line treatment for women with small volume residual ovarian cancer following initial systemic chemotherapy.[44] Individuals with *microscopic residual* disease only at the initiation of the regional paclitaxel program experienced a high surgically documented complete response rate (61%; n=28). In contrast, for patients with any macroscopic disease present when intraperitoneal therapy was begun, the surgically documented complete response rate was only 3% (n=31).

These data suggest there was limited penetration of drug directly into even the smallest tumor nodules or into the systemic circulation following regional treatment. In contrast, the extremely high concentrations of paclitaxel bathing the tumor cells present on the surface of the peritoneal lining were effective in producing a major cytotoxic effect.

However, it is important to acknowledge that while these theoretical considerations and results of the phase II trial are of interest, it will only be through the conduct of well-designed randomized clinical trials that the potential benefits of regional therapy employing paclitaxel can be appropriately evaluated.

VI. PHASE III TRIALS OF INITIAL TREATMENT OF SMALL-VOLUME RESIDUAL ADVANCED OVARIAN CANCER EMPLOYING CISPLATIN-BASED INTRAPERITONEAL CHEMOTHERAPY

The concept of regional drug delivery as initial treatment of ovarian cancer is supported by the observation that the clinical manifestations of the disease are principally (although not exclusively) confined to the peritoneal cavity for the majority of its natural history.[45] This fact, and considerable preclinical and clinical data, provide a strong rationale for considering intraperitoneal cytotoxic drug delivery in the initial treatment of ovarian cancer. Unfortunately, the absence of data from randomized controlled clinical trials makes it inappropriate to draw any firm conclusions regarding a potential role for this unique method of drug delivery in the standard management of this malignancy.

A. Phase III Trial: Intraperitoneal Cisplatin versus Intravenous Cisplatin (Plus Intravenous Cyclophosphamide)

A landmark study, conducted by the Southwest Oncology Group (SWOG) and the Gynecologic Oncology Group (GOG), comparing a regimen of intravenous cisplatin to intraperitoneal cisplatin (both delivered at a dose of 100 mg/m^2) established for the first time the potential superiority of the regional route of drug delivery in the management of ovarian cancer.[4] In this trial all patients received intravenous cyclophosphamide (600 mg/m^2) in addition to cisplatin.

The study found a lower incidence of severe neutropenia, tinnitus, clinical hearing loss, and neuromuscular toxicity in patients receiving intraperitoneal cisplatin, compared to intravenous drug delivery. While patients receiving regional treatment experienced more abdominal discomfort, this was generally mild or moderate in severity, and rarely interfered with continuation of the treatment program. Of note, there was no difference in treatment-related deaths between the study arms.

However, patients treated by the *intraperitoneal route* experienced a *statistically significant improvement in survival*, compared to standard systemic cisplatin drug delivery ($p=0.02$) (Table 36.9). The median survival for patients receiving intravenous cisplatin-based therapy was 41 months, in contrast to 49 months for women randomized to the intraperitoneal cisplatin study arm.

The relative risk of death for patients treated with intraperitoneal cisplatin was 24% lower than in the systemic cisplatin treatment arm. To put this "relative risk reduction" into the context of other strategies commonly employed as "standard of care" in the management of malignant disease, the magnitude of this difference was similar to that observed when tamoxifen is administered as adjuvant treatment of node-positive breast cancer.[46]

TABLE 36.9 Phase III Randomized Trials of Cisplatin-Based Intraperitoneal Therapy as Initial Treatment of Small Volume Residual Advanced Ovarian Cancer

	Median progression-free survival (months)		**Median overall survival (months)**	
	IP	**IV**	**IP**	**IV**
IP versus IV cisplatin (plus IV cyclophosphamide) (Ref. 4)	—		49	41 ($p=0.02$)
IP versus IV cisplatin (plus IV paclitaxel)[a] (Ref. 5)	28	22 ($p=0.01$)	63	52 ($p=0.05$)

[a]Experimental arm received two courses of carboplatin (AUC 9) prior to IP cisplatin.

B. Phase III Trial: Intraperitoneal Cisplatin versus Intravenous Cisplatin (Plus Intravenous Paclitaxel)

A limitation of the above-noted study was the failure to include paclitaxel in the control and experimental regimens. This was due to the fact the SWOG/GOG study was initiated in the mid-1980s, prior to the demonstration that addition of paclitaxel to cisplatin favorably impacted survival in advanced ovarian cancer.[43] As a result, many questioned whether the use of intraperitoneal cisplatin would provide any benefit beyond that already achieved by the incorporation of paclitaxel into the initial chemotherapy regimen in the disease.

Therefore, a second randomized controlled trial was initiated by the GOG and SWOG to directly address this important clinical issue.[5] Women with "small-volume residual" advanced ovarian cancer (i.e., largest residual tumor nodule <1 cm in maximal diameter) following an attempt at maximal surgical tumor cytoreduction were eligible for treatment on this phase III intergroup trial.

Patients either received a standard treatment regimen consisting of intravenous cisplatin (75 mg/m^2) and paclitaxel (135 mg/m^2 delivered over 24 h), or an "experimental program" consisting of two courses of moderately high dose intravenous carboplatin (AUC 9) followed by 6 cycles of intraperitoneal cisplatin (100 mg/m^2) and intravenous paclitaxel (135 mg/m^2 delivered over 24 h). The initial two carboplatin courses were designed to rapidly "chemically debulk" any residual tumor nodules, theoretically optimizing the chances for a favorable impact associated with the intraperitoneal cisplatin.[47]

Unfortunately, the initial two intravenous cycles were associated with fairly severe bone marrow toxicity, particularly thrombocytopenia. This resulted in considerable difficulty with the subsequent ability to deliver the intraperitoneal therapy. For example, approximately 20% of patients randomized to the experimental regimen were given two or fewer courses of intraperitoneal treatment.

Despite the failure of a substantial percentage of individuals to be able to receive an optimal intraperitoneal regimen, patients treated with this program experienced a statistically significant improvement in progression-free survival (28 versus 22 months, $p=0.01$), and a borderline improvement in overall survival (63 versus 52 months, $p=0.05$).

These survival figures translate into a 22% relative risk reduction for disease progression, and 19% for death, associated with intraperitoneal cisplatin treatment. It should be noted these figures are remarkably similar to that observed in the previously discussed randomized intraperitoneal chemotherapy trial.

Unfortunately, as a result of the considerable toxicity associated with this specific combination intraperitoneal and intravenous treatment regimen, it could not be recommended for further investigation or for use in standard clinical practice. However, the study again demonstrated the potential for a regional treatment strategy to have a significant impact on survival in advanced ovarian cancer.

C. Phase III Trial: Intraperitoneal Cisplatin Plus Both Intravenous and Intraperitoneal Paclitaxel versus Intravenous Cisplatin and Paclitaxel

The GOG has recently completed a phase III trial which may represent the "ideal" evaluation of the potential of regional cytotoxic drug delivery in the management of advanced ovarian cancer. Patients randomized to the experimental study arm received both cisplatin and paclitaxel by the intraperitoneal route, in addition to intravenous paclitaxel. The "control arm" was again the GOG "gold standard" of intravenous cisplatin and paclitaxel.

Thus, the experimental intraperitoneal regimen included both the most active drug in the management of ovarian cancer (i.e., a platinum compound), and a second active agent in the cancer that maximizes the differences in the potential for tumor-drug interactions between systemic and regional drug delivery (i.e., profound increase in peak and AUC concentrations in the peritoneal cavity and prolonged exposure of tumor within the body compartment). The results of this study will be awaited with interest.

VII. FUTURE DIRECTIONS WITH INTRAPERITONEAL THERAPY OF GYNECOLOGIC MALIGNANCIES

Despite the demonstrated ability of cisplatin-based intraperitoneal treatment of small-volume residual advanced ovarian cancer to expert a favorable impact on survival, few oncologists currently employ this approach in routine clinical practice. Several reasons can be provided to explain this apparent lack of interest in the favorable results of two randomized controlled trials.

Clinicians may be concerned about the potential for increased morbidity associated with the regional treatment approach. However, the findings of the two previously noted randomized studies,[4, 5] as well as the reports from numerous single institutions that have evaluated intraperitoneal drug delivery, have provided no evidence for excessive toxicity associated with this regional management approach.[6, 17] This conclusion assumes appropriate care is taken in patient selection (e.g., absence of severe intra-abdominal adhesions) and in preventing infectious complications (e.g., use of meticulous sterile technique).

It is perhaps more likely that oncologists are not inclined to utilize intraperitoneal treatment due to the apparent

TABLE 36.10 When It Is Appropriate to Consider Intraperitoneal Chemotherapy as a Component of Standard Clinical Care of Ovarian and Fallopian Tube Cancers and Primary Carcinoma of the Peritoneum?

1. Second-line therapy of very small volume residual disease, following the documentation of a response to initial platinum-based systemic chemotherapy
2. Consolidation strategy in patients achieving a surgically defined complete response to platinum-based systemic chemotherapy
3. Initial chemotherapy for patients with microscopic residual disease (stage IIIA or completely surgically resected stage IIIB and stage IIIC)
4. Minimal intra-abdominal adhesion

requirement to employ cisplatin, rather than carboplatin, with its associated greater systemic toxicity (e.g., emesis, neurotoxicity, nephrotoxicity).[30, 31] This observation provides further justification for a formal evaluation of a carboplatin-based intraperitoneal program as initial treatment of small-volume residual advanced ovarian cancer. It can be hoped such a study will be initiated at some point in the future.

Other novel strategies are worthy of exploration employing the intraperitoneal route of drug delivery, including biological and antimetastatic agents and gene therapy.

VIII. CONCLUSION

Over the past two decades the use of intraperitoneal drug delivery has evolved from a theoretical concept into a rational strategy that may be considered an appropriate management approach for several carefully selected subsets of women with advanced ovarian cancer, primary carcinoma of the peritoneum, and fallopian tube cancer (Table 36.10).

In the future it can be anticipated newer cytotoxic drugs, and novel antineoplastic agents, will be explored for their safety and efficacy when delivered by the intraperitoneal route. Until highly effective systemic antineoplastic therapy is developed for the treatment of ovarian cancer, it is likely regional drug delivery will continue to play an important role in disease management.

References

1. Weisberger, A. S., Levine, B., and Storaasli, J. P. (1955). Use of nitrogen mustard in treatment of serous effusions of neoplastic origin. *J. Am. Med. Assoc.* 159, 1704–1707.
2. Dedrick, R. L., Myers, C. E., Bungay, P. M., and DeVita, V. T., Jr., (1978). Pharmacokinetic rationale for peritoneal drug administration in the treatment of ovarian cancer. *Cancer Treat. Rep.* 62, 1–9.
3. Dedrick, R. L. (1985). Theoretical and experimental bases of intraperitoneal chemotherapy. *Semin. Oncol.* 12 (3;Suppl. 4), 1–6.
4. Alberts, D. S., Liu, P. Y., Hannigan, E. V., O'Toole, R., Williams, S. D., Young, J. A., Franklin, E. W., Clarke-Pearson, D. L., Malviya, V. K., DuBeshter, B., Adelson, M. D., and Hoskins, W. J. (1996). Intraperitoneal cisplatin plus intravenous cyclophosphamide versus intravenous cisplatin plus intravenous cyclophosphamide for stage III ovarian cancer. *N. Engl. J. Med.* 335, 1950–1955.
5. Markman, M., Bundy, B. N., Alberts, D. S., Fowler, J. M., Clarke-Pearson, D. J., Carson, L. F., Wadler, S., and Sickel, J. (2001). Phase III trial of standard dose intravenous cisplatin plus paclitaxel versus moderately high dose carboplatin followed by intravenous paclitaxel and intraperitoneal cisplatin in small volume stage III ovarian carcinoma: An intergroup study of the Gynecologic Oncology Group, Southwestern Oncology Group, and Eastern Cooperative Oncology Group. *J. Clin. Oncol.* 19, 1001–1007.
6. Markman, M. (1993). Intraperitoneal therapy for treatment of malignant disease principally confined to the peritoneal cavity. *Crit. Rev. Oncol. Hematol.* 14, 15–28.
7. Alberts, D. S., Young, L., Mason, N., and Salmon, S. E. (1985). In vitro evaluation of anticancer drugs against ovarian cancer at concentrations achievable by intraperitoneal administration. *Semin. Oncol.* 12 (3; Suppl. 4), 38–42.
8. Howell, S. B., Pfeifle, C. E., Wung, W. E., Olshen, R. A., Lucas, W. E., Yon, J. L., and Green, M. (1982). Intraperitoneal cisplatin with systemic thiosulfate protection. *Ann. Intern. Med.* 97, 845–851.
9. Casper, E. S., Kelsen, D. P., Alcock, N. W., and Lewis, J. L. (1983). Ip cisplatin in patients with malignant ascites: Pharmacokinetics evaluation and comparison with the iv route. *Cancer Treat. Rep.* 67, 325–328.
10. Lopez, J. A., Krikorian, J. G., Reich, S. D., Smyth, R. D., Lee, F. H., and Issell, B. F. (1985). Clinical pharmacology of intraperitoneal cisplatin. *Gynecol. Oncol.* 20, 1–9.
11. Pretorius, R. G., Hacker, N. F., Berek, J. S., Ford, L. C., Hoeschele, J. D., Butler, T. A., and Lagasse, L. D. (1983). Pharmacokinetics of Ip cisplatin in refractory ovarian carcinoma. *Cancer Treat. Rep.* 67, 1085–1092.
12. Markman, M., Reichman, B., Hakes, T., Jones, W., Lewis, J. L., Jr., Rubin, S., Almadrones, L., and Hoskins, W. (1991). Responses to second-line cisplatin-based intraperitoneal therapy in ovarian cancer: Influence of a prior response to intravenous cisplatin. *J. Clin. Oncol.* 9, 1801–1805.
13. Hacker, N. F., Berek, J. S., Pretorius, G., Zuckerman, J., Eisenkop, S., and Lagasse, L. D. (1987). Intraperitoneal cis-platinum as salvage therapy for refractory epithelial ovarian cancer. *Obstet. Gynecol.* 70, 759–764.
14. Kirmani, S., Lucas, W. E., Kim, S., Goel, R., McVey, L., Morris, J., and Howell, S. B. (1991). A phase II trial of intraperitoneal cisplatin and etoposide as salvage treatment for minimal residual ovarian carcinoma. *J. Clin. Oncol.* 9, 649–657.
15. Morgan, R. J., Jr., Braly, P., Leong, L., Shibata, S., Margolin, K., Somlo, G., McNamara, M., Longmate, J., Schinke, S.., Raschko, J., Nagasawa, S., Kogut, N., Najera, L., Johnson, D., and Doroshow, J. H. (2000). Phase II trial of combination intraperitoneal cisplatin and 5-fluorouracil in previously treated patients with advanced ovarian cancer: Long-term follow-up. *Gynecol. Oncol.* 77, 433–438.
16. Los, G., Mutsaers, P. H. A., van der Vijgh, W. J. F., Baldew, G. S., de Graaf, P. W., and McVie, J. G. (1989). Direct diffusion of cis-diamminedichloroplatinum(II) in intraperitoneal rat tumors after intraperitoneal chemotherapy: A comparison with systemic chemotherapy. *Cancer Res.* 49, 3380–3384.
17. Markman, M. (1999). Intraperitoneal chemotherapy. *Crit. Rev. Oncol. Hematol.* 31, 239–246.
18. Howell, S. B., Zimm, S., Markman, M., Abramson, I. S., Cleary, S., Lucas, W. E., and Weiss, R. J. (1987). Long-term survival of advanced refractory ovarian carcinoma patients with small-volume disease treated with intraperitoneal chemotherapy. *J. Clin. Oncol.* 5, 1607–1612.
19. Markman, M., Reichman, B., Hakes, T., Lewis, J. L., Jr., Jones, W., Rubin, S., Barakat, R., Curtin, J., Almadrones, L., and Hoskins, W. (1992).

Impact on survival of surgically defined favorable responses to salvage intraperitoneal chemotherapy in small-volume residual ovarian cancer. *J. Clin. Oncol.* 10, 1479–1484.

20. Recio, F. O., Piver, M. S., Hempling, R. E., and Driscoll, D. L. (1998). Five-year survival after second-line cisplatin-based intraperitoneal chemotherapy for advanced ovarian cancer. *Gynecol. Oncol.* 68, 267–273.
21. Rubin, S. C., Hoskins, W. J., Saigo, P. E., Hakes, T. B., Markman, M., Cain, J. M., Chapman, D., Almadrones, L., Pierce, V. K., and Lewis, J. L., Jr. (1988). Recurrence following negative second-look laparotomy for ovarian cancer: Analysis of risk factors. *Am. J. Obstet. Gynecol.* 159, 1094–1098.
22. Barakat, R. R., Almadrones, L., Venkatraman, E. S., Aghajanian, C., Brown, C., Shapiro, F., Curtin, J. P., and Spriggs, D. (1998). A phase II trial of intraperitoneal cisplatin and etoposide as consolidation therapy in patients with stage II-IV epithelial ovarian cancer following negative surgical assessment. *Gynecol. Oncol.* 69, 17–22.
23. Markman, M. (1985). Intracavitary chemotherapy. *CRC Crit. Rev. Oncol. Hematol.* 3(3), 205–233.
24. Ozols, R. F., Young, R. C., Speyer, J. L., Sugarbaker, P. H., Green, R., Jenkins, J., and Myers, C. E. (1982). Phase 1 and pharmacological studies of adriamycin administered intraperitoneally to patients with ovarian cancer. *Cancer Res.* 42, 4265–4269.
25. Markman, M., Howell, S. B., Lucas, W. E., Pfeifle, C. E., and Green, M. R. (1984). Combination intraperitoneal chemotherapy with cisplatin, cytarabine, and doxorubicin for refractory ovarian carcinoma and other malignancies principally confined to the peritoneal cavity. *J. Clin. Oncol.* 2, 1321–1326.
26. Markman, M., George, M., Hakes, T., Reichman, B., Hoskins, W., Rubin, S., Jones, W., Almadrones, L., and Lewis, J. L., Jr. (1990). Phase 2 trial of intraperitoneal mitoxantrone in the management of refractory ovarian carcinoma. *J. Clin. Oncol.* 8, 146–150.
27. Berek, J. S., Hacker, N. F., Lichtenstein, A., Jung, T., Spina, C., Knox, R.M., Brady, J., Greene, T., Ettinger, L. M., Lagasse, L., Bonnem, E. M., Spiegel, R. J., and Zighelboim, J. (1985). Intraperitoneal recombinant alpha-interferon for "salvage" immunotherapy in stage III epithelial ovarian cancer: A Gynecologic Oncology Group study. *Cancer Res.* 45, 4447–4453.
28. Berek, J. S., Markman, M., Stonebraker, B., Lentz, S. S., Adelson, M. D., DeGeest, K., and Moore, D. (1999). Intraperitoneal interferon-α in residual ovarian carcinoma: A phase II Gynecologic Oncology Group study. *Gynecol. Oncol.* 75, 10–14.
29. Edwards, R. P., Gooding, W., Lembersky, B. C., Colonello, K., Hammond, R., Paradise, C., Kowal, C. D., Kunschner, A. J., Baldisseri, M., Kirkwood, J. M., and Herberman, R. B. (1997). Comparison of toxicity and survival following intraperitoneal recombinant interleukin-2 for persistent ovarian cancer after platinum: Twenty-four-hour versus 7-day infusion. *J. Clin. Oncol.* 15, 3399–3407.
30. Alberts, D. S., Green, S., Hannigan, E. V., O'Toole, R., Stock-Novack, D., Anderson, P., Surwit, E. A., Malviya, V. K., Nahhas, W. A., and Jolles, C. J. (1992). Improved therapeutic index of carboplatin plus cyclophosphamide versus cisplatin plus cyclophosphamide: Final report by the Southwest Oncology Group of a phase III randomized trial in stages III and IV ovarian cancer. *J. Clin. Oncol.* 10, 706–717.
31. Swenerton, K., Jeffrey, J., Stuart, G., Roy, M., Krepart, G., Carmichael, J., Drouin, P., Stanimir, R., O'Connell, G., MacLean, G., Kirk, M. E., Canetta, R., Koski, B., Shelley, W., Zee, B., and Pater, J. (1992). Cisplatin-cyclophosphamide versus carboplatin-cyclophosphamide in advanced ovarian cancer: A randomized phase III study of National Cancer Institute of Canada Clinical Trials Group. *J. Clin. Oncol.* 10, 718–726.
32. Connelly, E., Markman, M., Kennedy, A., Webster, K., Kulp, B., Peterson, G., and Belinson, J. (1996). Paclitaxel delivered as a 3-hour infusion with cisplatin in patients with gynecologic cancers: Unexpected incidence of neurotoxicity. *Gynecol. Oncol.* 62, 166–168.
33. Piccart, M. J., Bertelsen, K., James, K., Cassidy, J., Mangioni, C., Simonsen, E., Stuart, G., Kaye, S., Vergote, I., Blom, R., Grimshaw, R., Atkinson, R. J., Swenerton, K. D., Trope, C., Nardi, M., Kaern, J., Tumolo, S., Timmers, P., Roy, J-A., Lhoas, F., Lindvall, B., Bacon, M., Birt, A., Andersen, J. E., Zee, B., Paul, J., Baron, B., and Pecorelli, S. (2000). Randomized intergroup trial of cisplatin-paclitaxel versus cisplatin-cyclophosphamide in women with advanced epithelial ovarian cancer: Three-year results. *J. Natl. Cancer Inst.* 92, 699–708.
34. Los, G., Verdegaal, E. M. E., Mutsaers, P. H. A., and McVie, J. G. (1991). Pentetration of carboplatin and cisplatin into rat peritoneal tumor nodules after intraperitoneal chemotherapy. *Cancer Chemother. Pharmacol.* 28, 159–165.
35. Markman, M., Reichman, B., Hakes, T., Rubin, S., Lewis, J. L., Jr., Jones, W., Barakat, R., Curtin, J., Almadrones, L., and Hoskins, W. (1993). Evidence supporting the superiority of intraperitoneal cisplatin compared to intraperitoneal carboplatin for salvage therapy of small volume residual ovarian cancer. *Gynecol. Oncol.* 50, 100–104.
36. DeGregorio, M. W., Lum, B. L., Holleran, W. M., Wilbur, B. J., and Sikic, B. I. (1986). Preliminary observations of intraperitonal carboplatin pharmacokinetics during a phase I study of the Northern California Oncology Group. *Cancer Chemother. Pharmacol.* 18, 235–238.
37. Elferink, F., van der Vijgh, W. J. F., Klein, I., ten Bokkel Huinink, W. W., Dubbelman, R., and McVie, J. G. (1988). Pharmacokinetics of carboplatin after intraperitoneal administration. *Cancer Chemother. Pharmacol.* 21, 57–60.
38. Speyer, J. L., Beller, U., Colombo, N., Sorich, J., Wernz, J. C., Hochster, H., Green, M., Porges, R., Muggia, F. M., Canetta, R., and Beckman, E. M. (1990). Intraperitoneal carboplatin: Favorable results in women with minimal residual ovarian cancer after cisplatin therapy. *J. Clin. Oncol.* 8, 1335–1341.
39. Pfeiffer, P., Bennedbaek, O., and Bertelsen, K. (1990). Intraperitoneal carboplatin in the treatment of minimal residual ovarian cancer. *Gynecol. Oncol.* 36, 306–311.
40. Markman, M., Rowinsky, E., Hakes, T., Reichman, B., Jones, W., Lewis, J. L., Jr., Rubin, S., Curtin, J., Barakat, R., Phillips, M., Hurowitz, L., Almadrones, L., and Hoskins, W. (1992). Phase I trial of intraperitoneal taxol: A Gynecologic Oncology Group study. *J. Clin. Oncol.* 10, 1485–1491.
41. Francis, P., Rowinsky, E., Schneider, J., Hakes, T., Hoskins, W., and Markman, M. (1995). Phase I feasibility and pharmacologic study of weekly intraperitoneal paclitaxel: A Gynecologic Oncology Group Pilot Study. *J. Clin. Oncol.* 13, 2961–2967.
42. Rowinsky, E. K., Donehower, R. C., Jones, R. J., and Tucker, R. W. (1988). Microtubule changes and cytotoxicity in leukemic cell lines treated with taxol. *Cancer Res.* 48, 4093–4100.
43. McGuire, W. P., Hoskins, W. J., Brady, M. F., Kucera, P. R., Partridge, E. E., Look, K. Y., Clarke-Pearson, D. L., and Davidson, M. (1996). Cyclophosphamide and cisplatin compared with paclitaxel and cisplatin in patients with stage III and stage IV ovarian cancer. *N. Engl. J. Med.* 334, 1–6.
44. Markman, M., Brady, M. F., Spirtos, N. M., Hanjani, P., and Rubin, S. C. (1998). Phase II trial of intraperitoneal paclitaxel in carcinoma of the ovary, tube, and peritoneum: A Gynecologic Oncology Group Study. *J. Clin. Oncol.* 16, 2620–2624.
45. Bergman, F. (1966). Carcinoma of the ovary: A clinicopathological study of 86 autopsied cases with special reference to mode of spread. *Acta Obstet. Gynecol. Scand.* 45, 211–231.
46. Early Breast Cancer Trialists' Collaborative Group. (1998). Tamoxifen for early breast cancer: An overview of the randomised trials. *Lancet* 351, 1451–1467.

CHAPTER

37

Prevention of Ovarian Serous Epithelial Carcinoma

ALBERT ALTCHEK

Department of Obstetrics, Gynecology and Reproductive Science
The Mount Sinai School of Medicine and Hospital
New York, New York 10029

ABSTRACT

Ovarian cancer has no early signs or symptoms, and is usually discovered in an advanced stage with a poor prognosis. Screening is not recommended for the general population and is not very effective for the high-risk group.

There are only two standard methods of reducing the chance of ovarian cancer—oral contraceptives pills (OCs) and prophylactic oophorectomy (PO). Oral contraceptives (OCs) give a 50% reduction of ovarian cancer risk. Prophylactic oophorectomy (PO) has a small chance of discovering an occult cancer, has a moderate chance of a minor complication, a very small chance of a dangerous complication, and causes surgical menopause problems. It is the only method which prevents ovarian cancer. There remains a life-long small chance of a new primary peritoneal cancer in high-risk women for which there is no prevention at present. This clarifies the confusing standard theory that PO has about a 95% chance of reducing deaths from "ovarian" (really combined ovarian and primary peritoneal) cancer. Premenopausal PO also reduces the later chance of breast cancer by about 50% in high-risk women however continuous surveillance in required. PO has now been replaced by prophylactic salpingo-oophorectomy because the tube is part of the hereditary ovarian cancer syndrome and may develop carcinoma with the same histology. The site where the tube develops carcinoma has ramifications concerning the unsubstantiated suggestion for prophylactic hysterectomy. Women with hereditary ovarian cancer syndrome should have a PO beginning at 35 and after completing childbearing. Breast cancer survivors with BRCA1 and BRCA2 (BRCA1/2) mutations have an increased risk of a second breast cancer and of ovarian cancer and therefore should consider PO. BRCA2 mutation carriers have to keep in mind also the increased risk of general cancers including pancreatic. Male BRCA1/2 mutation carriers are at increased risk for breast (although less than women), prostate, pancreatic and other general cancers. Women with HNPCC should have PO and hysterectomy.

Speculation about peritoneal carcinogenesis may be related to unappreciated constant stimulation to protect the non-stick peritoneal surface necessary to all life forms with an intestine.

The new report of combined estrogen and progestin hormone replacement therapy (EPHRT) showing risks exceeding benefits requires rethinking of standard care.

I. SEMANTICS OF "AT RISK." WHAT DOES "AT RISK" MEAN?

In medical practice we tend to use labels to convey an understood concept, however, they may be misunderstood by the general public. Every woman with ovaries is "at risk" for ovarian cancer. The at risk phrase has various meanings. Understanding of a chance or risk is the essential factor. The intended meaning of 'at risk' is an increased risk compared to other women of the same group (age, parity, etc.)

II. RISKS

A. What Is the Risk for the General Population?

Ovarian cancer has no early signs or symptoms. Most cases are discovered with advanced disease with poor prognosis. Surgical debulking and chemotherapy usually give good initial remission but often within two years there is a relapse. Most ovarian carcinoma is serous epithelial papillary carcinoma. The general population lifetime risk ("sporadic") is about 1.6% with a median age of diagnosis about 63. Risk factors include age, nulliparity, early menarche, late menopause, and anovulatory infertility. Risk decreases with pregnancy, lactation, the use of oral contraceptives (OCs), bilateral tubal ligation (BTL), and hysterectomy.[1]

Risk increases with age. It is remote before age 30, and then it increases lineally from 30 to 50 after which the increase slows. The highest incidence is in the eighth decade with a rate of 57/100,000 women age 75–79, compared to 16/100,000 in the 40–44 group.[2] The overall incidence is 13.3/100,000. In Sweden it is 14.9 and in Japan 2.7. American women of Japanese ancestry have a rate that approaches the U.S. average, thereby implicating environmental factors.[3]

The standard concept is that "incessant ovulation" with the need for monthly repair of the ovarian surface increases risk and that any reduction of ovulation reduces ovarian cancer. It does not explain the reduction found in excess of the expected reduction, nor does it explain BTL and hysterectomy.

About 90% of ovarian cancer is "sporadic" being unexpected without any particular family history. Since it is infrequent, usually nothing special is done. Sometimes apprehensive women request screening. Screening has not been recommended for the general population because of low prevalence, and the cost in dollars and resources (not "cost-effective"). Furthermore screening is not very effective and often misleading.

Screening, or in its intensive form "surveillance," involves: (1) clinical evaluation which usually discovers cancer only when advanced, (2) serum tumor marker CA125 which will only detect half of early cancer and false-positives are frequent especially premenopausally, and (3) transvaginal ultrasound which at best can detect small enlargements of the ovary that rarely may be cancer (which sometimes has already spread) or usually a benign enlargement possibly requiring surgery to decide (reasonable sensitivity, poor specificity). With menstruating women, radiologists usually suggest that ultrasound be repeated in about 6 weeks for ovarian enlargements.

A reasonable approach for the apprehensive woman would be genetic consultation. A problem is lack of family history because of adoption or because of the Holocaust. Eastern European Jewish ancestry (Ashkenazi) carries an increased chance of hereditary ovarian cancer, thus genetic testing might be considered. A nonspecific approach is to consider OC use during menstrual life.

B. What Is the Risk for Hereditary Ovarian Cancer (HOC)?

Efforts to reduce ovarian cancer are focused on women with an increased risk due to HOC. Previously thought to be about 5%, hereditary (genetic, familial) ovarian cancer is now considered to represent about 10% of cancer cases. The mean age for hereditary cancer is 48–51 (some report 54), and as early as the fourth decade, compared to age 63 for the general population.[4, 5]

HOC was recognized before discovery of the BRCA1 and BRCA2 (BRCA1/2) germline mutations (1994, 1995) and therefore risk estimates were based on family history. Such estimates may have been underestimated because they averaged the mutation carrier and noncarrier (50% chance of first-degree relatives being a carrier). Noncarriers have no unusual or very little risk.

HOC had been divided into two syndromes: mainly hereditary breast/ovarian, and less frequently site-specific ovarian. Both have been found to be variations of the same basic syndrome caused by germline BRCA1/2 gene mutations and therefore the original names have been discontinued or replaced with hereditary breast/ovarian cancer (HBOC syndrome). Germplasm BRCA1 gene mutations cause 70% of the cases and BRCA2 gene mutations cause 20%. These are highly penetrant, autosomal, dominant mutations. HBOC syndrome causes about 75–90% of all hereditary ovarian cancer and 30–70% of all breast cancer.[6]

Germplasm genetic mutations of invasive epithelial carcinoma are not involved with borderline epithelial carcinoma or invasive mucinous carcinoma.

Family history gives the clue to HOC. The lifetime baseline risk for the general population is estimated by some to be 1.4% or 1/70. The odds ratio for developing ovarian cancer compared to the general population is 2.9 for second-degree relatives and 3.1–3.6 for first-degree relatives giving the latter a 5.0% lifetime probability. With two or three relatives the odds ratio increased to 4.6, giving a 7.2% lifetime probability. There is a tendency to familial clustering.[5, 7]

Germline mutations of BRCA1 and BRCA2 occur in 1/345 in the general population in the U.S., but in 1/40 Ashkenazi Jews, making a total of about one million persons.[8] BRCA1/2 mutants have a ninefold lifetime increase in ovarian cancer.[9] In addition, there are about 100,000 breast cancer survivors with BRCA mutations having a 16% risk for a subsequent ovarian cancer.[10]

Hereditary ovarian and breast cancer family syndromes are inherited in an autosomal dominant mode, therefore each child has a 50% chance of inheriting the mutant gene from either parent. Distant family members can also carry the mutations.[11]

The original studies of BRCA1 mutation carriers indicated a cumulative risk of cancer by age 70 of 87% for breast and 44% for ovary. BRCA2 mutants had lower risks of 84% breast risk by age 80 and a 27% ovarian risk by age 70. These data were unwittingly selected from strong positive family history groups. Recent reviews indicate lower rates of BRCA1 mutations with about a 45–68% risk of breast cancer and with about 36% of ovarian cancer.[5, 6] BRCA2 ovarian cancer occurs at a later age and has about a 20% risk.[5, 6, 12, 13]

In a surveillance group of 89 BRCA1/2 mutants, of mean age 46.8 years, followed for a mean of 17.0 months, 5 (5.6%) were found to have ovarian or primary peritoneal cancer. Two were stage I, one stage II, one was tubal, and one incompletely staged.[8]

Jewish women with BRCA1/2 mutations and with intact ovaries were found to have a 10-year risk of peritoneal or ovarian cancer of 16%.[14] Clinically serous ovarian cancer, primary peritoneal cancer, and primary fallopian tube cancer have a similar presentation and pathology. The latter is often misdiagnosed as ovarian.[5]

Breast cancer is more common and appears earlier than ovarian cancer. Breast cancer is usually diagnosed at an earlier stage because of accessible physical examination by physician and patient self-examination and routine mammography. The latter alone may miss 10% of carcinoma cases, and not infrequently many of these are discovered by breast self-examination (BSE). The prognosis of breast cancer is much better than ovarian cancer. Aside from earlier detection, breast cancer is probably slower growing and does not readily disturb vital life functions.

BRCA1/2 hereditary breast cancer has an increased chance of a secondary breast cancer and of primary ovarian cancer (16% by age 70).[15]

Whereas breast cancer has only germline BRCA1/2 mutations, germplasm HOC can acquire additional somatic mutations. Even sporadic ovarian cancer occasionally acquires germline BRCA1/2 mutations.

Very rarely breast cancer is part of the Li-Fraumeni multiple cancer syndrome (TP53 gene).[16]

About 2% of ovarian cancer is due to hereditary non-polyposis colorectal cancer syndrome (HNPCC), previously referred to as Lynch Syndrome type II. It is associated with early–onset proximal colon cancer (70–80%), endometrial cancer (20–25%), and ovarian cancer (12%). HNPCC increases other cancer risks including stomach, kidney, ureter, brain, small intestine, and biliary tract. HNPCC is an inherited, autosomal dominant syndrome with DNA mismatch repair germline gene mutations of mainly MLH1 and MSH2, but also of PMS1 and PMS2.[6, 11, 17, 18]

III. GENETIC COUNSELING

A. Who Should be Referred for Genetic Counseling?

Ideally any patient who is concerned about a family or personal history of malignancy, especially with ovarian or breast cancer, and who wishes to should be referred for counseling.

This does not necessarily mean that testing should be done. Counseling is a multistep on-going process involving patient interaction which includes a detailed multigeneration family history, consideration of the appropriateness of genetic testing, and if testing is planned, pre- and post-test counseling. The family history must include both sides of the family since half of all women with BRCA1 and BRCA2 mutations have inherited it from their fathers.[6]

Autosomal dominant inheritance of cancer predisposition is suggested by vertical transmission via female or male, with each child having a 50% chance of inheritance. Suggestions of familial BRCA1/2 mutation include: early or bilateral breast cancer, breast and ovarian cancer in the same individual, males with breast cancer, two primary cancers in the same individual, and Ashkenazi Jewish ancestry especially with early-onset breast cancer. Although early ovarian cancer histories are suspicious for hereditary cancer appearing before age 50, this is true for BRCA1 mutations, however, most hereditary cancers over 60 years are due to hereditary BRCA2 mutation. "Past studies may have underestimated the contribution of BRCA2 to ovarian cancer, because mutations in this gene cause predominantly late-onset cancer."[9]

B. Who Should have Genetic Testing?

Genetic testing requires signed informed consent. There are various shades of opinion regarding testing related to the year, experiences, ethnic selection incidence, and new findings. The indications have been liberalized from formerly when there was great concern over emotional impact, technologic skill, and laboratory volume capability.

In 1995 the American Society for Clinical Oncology recommended that cancer predisposition testing be offered only when:

1. The likelihood of a positive result is over 10%
2. The test can be adequately interpreted
3. The results will influence the medical care of the patient or family member [19]

At present testing should be considered for suggestive family history such as:

1. Many family members in a single lineage
2. Two or more with early-onset breast cancer (before age 50)
3. Ovarian cancer at any age
4. Breast and ovarian cancer in the same individual
5. Male breast cancer at any age
6. Extra suspicion for Ashkenazi Jewish women (or any other ethnic group or families with increased mutations) especially with early-onset breast cancer or ovarian cancer at any age
7. Women who already have early-onset breast cancer; if a BRCA1/2 mutation carrier she may be at increased risk for a second primary breast cancer or an ovarian cancer
8. Women who already have ovarian invasive epithelial cancer at any age even without a family history [9]

Unselected, clinic-based ovarian cancer patients have germline BRCA1 mutations in 12/258 (4.6%) with a strong correlation with family history of breast and/or ovarian cancer. This indicated "...that these women are most likely to benefit from genetic susceptibility testing."[20]

"...It is reasonable to offer genetic testing to any woman diagnosed with invasive, nonmucinous, epithelial ovarian cancer,"[5] especially since 6.5% of women with a negative family history tested positive,[9] and especially in Jewish women. "In the event that a mutation is found in the index case, then other female relatives should be offered testing."[5] Presumably this is with permission of the index case. Each first-degree relative has a 50% chance of having it as well.

Prior to prophylactic oophorectomy genetic testing should be offered. "In the event that a mutation is present in a family member, but is not found in the woman herself, then preventive surgery is not indicated."[5] Nevertheless some are more flexible with a strong family history, the possibility that a mutation may not be detectable, or be an unrecognized unique isolated familial BRCA1/2 mutation not tested for because other affected family members were not tested, or the emotional need of the patient.

The three founder mutations cause 90% of HBOC in 90% of Ashkenazi Jewish women with cancer. "It is important to bear in mind that mutations other than BRCA1 and BRCA2 may cause disease in the remaining 10% of these families, so that genetic testing alone will not detect all predisposing mutations."[11] A recent report described two Jewish women with a positive family history and negative comprehensive

BRCA1/2 testing who developed breast and ovarian cancers.[14] In addition about 8% of HOC cases have unknown putative gene mutations.[6] Isolated non-Jewish populations in The Netherlands, Iceland, and Switzerland may have unique BRCA1/2 mutations.[11, 21]

C. What Tests Should be Done?

It is unsettling to find that there are differences of opinion regarding which tests to do. Although there is agreement that most hereditary ovarian and breast cancers are related to germline BRCA1/2 mutations, each gene has numerous possible mutation errors. The most precise test for BRCA1 and BRCA2 gene mutations is a complete gene sequence analysis of the complete coding sequence. One problem is the technical difficulty. Another problem is the discovery of mutations of uncertain significance such as at splice sites and in noncoding intron sequences. Furthermore, most disease-associated BRCA1/2 mutations are rare among total mutations.

Germline BRCA1/2 mutations are frequent in non-Ashkenazi families especially with a member having a double primary breast and ovarian cancer, similar to Ashkenazi families, however, the specific mutations are different than the usual Ashkenazi Jewish founder mutations and comprehensive sequencing is required. There are hundreds of separate unique BRCA1/2 mutations reported in non-Ashkenazi women brought to light by family history. "For this reason, non-Ashkenazi Jewish women with family histories suggestive of an inherited syndrome for developing breast and ovarian cancer warrant comprehensive sequencing of BRCA1 and BRCA2."[22] BRCA1 dysfunction in ovarian cancer is common and occurs by multiple mechanisms. Testing for BRCA1 mutations in large populations, especially non-Ashkenazi Jewish is impractical. The loss of heterozygosity (LOH) at the BRCA1 locus rather than a family history of ovarian cancer is a good screening strategy followed by a protein truncation test.[23] Researchers have used different testing methods including for protein-truncating mutations in BRCA1 by single-strand conformation polymorphism analysis.[20] A Swedish report of a low estimate of mutation carriers of familial cancer might be due to the method of sequencing for two exons and single-strand conformation polymorphisms (SSCPs) or denaturing high-performance liquid chromatography (d HPLC) which "...may well have missed many deleterious mutations."[24]

For women with ovarian cancer "it also appears worthwhile to test all women with invasive nonmucinous ovarian cancer for the three common Ashkenazi Jewish founder mutations, since they occur not infrequently in other ethnic groups." "In addition, testing should include examination of the BRCA1 exon 1 3 6-kb duplication mutation, which is missed by standard assay methods, including direct sequencing."[9] About 2.5% of Ashkenazi Jewish women whose ancestry is Eastern European carry a common BRCA1/2 gene mutation pattern referred to as "founder" mutations. This suggests a small original group with these originally spontaneous mutations which become maintained by hereditary germplasm and whose population increased relatively more than other Jewish communities. Other ethnic groups have other "founder" mutations of BRCA1/2 especially when in isolated communities. This explains the increased incidence of breast and ovarian cancer. The usual BRCA1 mutations in Ashkenazi Jews is 185 del AG and 5382 ins C. The BRCA2 mutation is 617 del T. Moroccan and Spanish families have 185 del AG founder mutations also and Russians have 5382 ins C. The standard laboratory procedure (Myriad Genetic Laboratories) tests for the sequence of the protein-coding regions of the BRCA1 and BRCA2 genes where almost all of the clinically significant mutations occur. It is 99% sensitive and specific.[25]

There could still be a 1% chance of technical error, as well as overlooking a rare other mutation. A practical approach is to: (1) include testing for Jewish "founder" mutations, (2) discover the family pattern of germplasm gene mutations if possible and test the patient for that specific pattern.

HNPCC is often overlooked. It may be suggested by early, high-grade proximal right colon carcinoma, premenopausal endometrial carcinoma, ovarian carcinoma, and other related cancers in both sides of the family. Women with a 10% probability of hereditary ovarian cancer syndrome based on family and personal history should be tested for BRCA1, BRCA2, and MLH1 and MSH2 (HNPCC) gene mutations.[11] It increases the risk of colorectal cancer to 70–82% by age 70, in contrast to the 2% of the general population. It causes a risk of endometrial cancer of 42–60% by age 70. It increases the risk of colorectal or endometrial cancer to 20–25% before age 50, compared to 0.2% in the general population. It carries a 50% risk of a second cancer within 15 years. It gives a 12% risk of ovarian cancer by age 70. Other cancer-increased risk includes stomach, kidneys, ureter, brain, small intestine, and biliary tract.[6, 18]

D. Explanation of Test Results for BRCA1/2

There are three possible results for BRCA1/2 testing—positive, negative, or indeterminate.

1. Positive Test Result

This indicates a mutation of the BRCA1 or BRCA2 gene which prevents the translation of a specific functioning protein. Regardless of ethnicity or family history this implies a lifetime risk of increased breast cancer to 56–85%, as well as an increased ovarian cancer risk of about 20–40%.[6] The risks should be broken down into risk of having a mutation, whereas the risk of cancer is less. Each first-degree relative has a 50% chance of having the same mutation. Nevertheless an accurate assessment of genetic risk may be difficult because "rates of positive tests from a population-based study can be very different from those measured in high-risk genetic counseling clinics." The former have scientific significance. The latter are more clinically relevant.[24]

About 10% of all ovarian cancers are hereditary and associated with highly penetrant cancer susceptibility genes. About 70% are due to BRCA1 and 20% to BRCA2 gene mutations. Either gene mutation increases the chance of ovarian and/or breast cancer and cause the clinical "breast-ovarian cancer syndrome" and "site-specific ovarian cancer." Both syndromes are variations of BRCA1/2 mutations and are no longer separately identified. There are more than 600 different BRCA1 and 450 BRCA2 germline mutations, and each family group has its unique mutation. "Founder" mutations are common in defined groups (Ashkenazi Jewish descent). The BRCA1/2 mutations are mainly associated with breast and ovarian cancers. Whereas in breast cancer all the mutations are hereditary, in sporadic ovarian cancers 5–10% have somatic mutations which developed after birth. A positive test may help to establish a family pattern. Men with BRCA1/2 mutations have a 3–6% risk of breast cancer and an 8% risk of prostate cancer by age 70 and 20% by age 80. Both sexes have a 2–3% risk of pancreatic cancer.[6]

2. Negative Test Result

This requires interpretation with the patient's history and family history. The significance is easy if there is a known specific mutation in family members with cancer and if the patient (who is usually tested only for it) is negative. The interpretation is that the patient has no greater cancer risk than the general population and that it will not be passed on. This is understandable since for breast cancer BRCA1/2 mutations are only germline transmitted, and not acquired in somatic cells. Accordingly the negative testing brings emotional relief, however, there is still background risk for sporadic cancer. Ovarian cancers are different than breast because ovarian somatic cells can acquire BRCA1/2 mutations as part of 5–10% of sporadic cancers and a negative test may be less reassuring. If there is no family identified BRCA1/2 mutation it reduces the chance of hereditary ovarian/breast cancer, "...but does not rule it out entirely."[6] There might be an unidentified mutation of BRCA1/2. Of a group of 290 Jewish women with HOC there were 2 who developed cancer (one incident ovarian, one incident breast) and yet were negative for the three common "founder" Jewish mutations and even negative for rare BRCA1/2 mutations.[14] Thus there must be an undetected BRCA1/2 mutation. In addition, there may be unrecognized susceptibility loci, restriction fragment-linked polymorphisms, loss of chromosome genetic material with multiple tumor-suppressor gene mutations, and LOH especially at loci in 3p, 6q, 11p, 13q, 17p, and 17q.

Since Ashkenazi Jewish women if affected have "founder" mutations, even with lack of identification of a family mutation, a negative test result "substantially reduces the likelihood of hereditary cancer risk." It is also possible that one relative might have had a BRCA1/2 mutation because of "sporadic" ovarian cancer acquisition. About 2% of HOC is associated with HNPCC due to DNA mismatch genes, and not due to BRCA1/2 mutations. About 8% of HOC is due to as yet unidentified gene mutations.[6]

3. Indeterminate Test Result

This occurs about 12% of the time. It is usually due to missence mutations (single-base pair change) not in critical functional domains, or those that cause only minimal protein change may not be associated with cancer, but are of unknown cancer risk. If feasible other family cancer members should be tested for this.

Of 258 women with primary ovarian epithelial cancer, 12 had polymorphism mutations of unknown significance of BRCA1. Since the polymorphisms were present in higher frequency among women without a family history of cancer compared to those with a positive history, it is suggested that they are associated with a reduced risk.[20] Without a positive family history, some gene mutations may be difficult to interpret.

E. How to Use the Test Results

If the patient tested positive for BRCA1/2 and does not have cancer, then various options are discussed with the advantages and disadvantages of each. This is helpful for informed consent background. The decision is up to the patient. Should the patient request it the counselor may give a personal opinion. If the patient had a positive test it should be compared to other family members with cancer and positive testing to establish the family pattern. If the patient had a positive test and is the first in the family to be tested, it would be desirable to have other family members tested, especially first-degree relatives who should have a 50% chance of a positive test if it is a germplasm mutation. It is possible for the patient to have a sporadic ovarian carcinoma with an acquired BRCA1/2 mutation. Thus a positive test for the patient may be of value to other family members. If the patient already had a breast cancer, a positive test would increase the chance of a second primary cancer in the opposite breast and of a new primary cancer of the ovary. There are great variations in patient response to testing. It may be related to case selection differences in counseling and the desire to remain well to care for children. In a prospective observational study of women in breast-ovarian cancer families one year following BRCA1/2 testing, only 21% had prophylactic oophorectomy and only 21% reported a CA125 and 15% reported a transvaginal ultrasound. There was no increase in rate of mammography. Thus despite the vast majority not having prophylactic oophorectomy or prophylactic mastectomy (only 3%), "many do not adhere to surveillance recommendations."[26]

On the other hand, in Rotterdam women with a high-risk family history requested BRCA testing at a young age, especially those with children. Of those with positive tests 51% (35 of 68) opted for bilateral mastectomy and 64% (24 of 45) for oophorectomy. Parenthood was a predictor for prophylactic mastectomy while age was associated with prophylactic oophorectomy. Thus this population had a high demand for testing and for prophylactic surgery.[27] Mastectomy is a disfiguring operation while oophorectomy, especially with laparoscopy is not noticeable. With mastectomy there are often small areas which cannot be removed. In addition breast cancers are often discovered in an early stage and have a better prognosis than ovarian tumors. Thus, even though breast cancer is more common, prophylactic mastectomy is not done frequently.

F. New Concepts

The "...most accurate description of BRCA1 and BRCA2 associations in ovarian cancer that has thus far been published" suggested that the location of mutations of the BRCA1 gene may affect penetrance.[9] This is based on new findings that breast cancer penetrance increases with more downstream mutations in the BRCA1 coding sequence. If confirmed it implies that prophylactic mastectomy may be less indicated for certain upstream mutations. The study did not find a BRCA1 mutation location effect on penetrance of ovarian cancer but there were only a small number of cases. Nevertheless, ovarian penetration with BRCA1 mutations is great enough to warrant prevention strategy. Regarding BRCA1 mutations there was a significant excess of breast cancer with nonovarian cancer-cluster region (OCCR) mutations, and some have reported that only non-OCCR mutations are associated with increased risk of breast cancer.[9]

It is interesting that first-degree relatives of cases with BRCA1 mutations had increased risks of ovarian, breast, and stomach cancers and leukemia/lymphomas; while risk of colorectal cancer was increased for relatives with BRCA2 mutations.

"Ovarian, colorectal, stomach, pancreatic, and prostate cancer occurred in first-degree relatives of carriers of BRCA2 mutations only when mutations were in the OCCR of exon 11, whereas an excess of breast cancer was seen when mutations were outside the OCCR." In the future mutation location may be found to have a "significant impact on treatment decisions for BRCA1 carriers."[9] Among 649 unselected incident cases of ovarian cancer in Ontario, Canada, who were tested for 11 of the most common mutations of BRCA1/2, none were found in 134 with borderline tumors. Of the 515 with invasive cancer, 60 (11.7%) had mutations. This was higher than previous estimates, perhaps because 11 rather than the usual 3 "foundation" mutations were studied. "It is possible, however, that some mutations could have been missed in this screen and that the hereditary fraction could thus be somewhat higher, perhaps 10–15% greater for BRCA1 and 20–25% greater for BRCA2." Of those who were diagnosed at under age 50 with ovarian cancer, 83% were due to BRCA1, while 60% of those over age 60 were due to BRCA2. BRCA2-associated ovarian cancer occurs at the same ages as sporadic, the majority at age 50–70. Ovarian cancers with BRCA1 mutations are diagnosed about 4–7 years earlier than without mutations or sporadic, in the age group 40–60. Women with first-degree relatives with breast or ovarian cancer had 19% mutations, while without relatives there were 6.5%.[9]

If confirmed for all site cancers that the penetrance of OCCR BRCA2 mutations is high in males as in females, males should have genetic testing for suspicion of BRCA2 mutations.

IV. THE BREAST—SURVEILLANCE, CHEMOPREVENTION, AND PROPHYLACTIC BILATERAL MASTECTOMY

Breast surveillance includes:

1. Monthly BSE starting about age 18–21 years
2. Clinical breast examinations, annual, semiannual, or quarterly
3. Annual mammography beginning at age 25–35 years, sometimes with ultrasound and/or MRI

Tamoxifen, a selective estrogen receptor modulator (SERM) may reduce the risk of breast cancer by 45% [28] or after breast cancer reduce the risk of contralateral breast cancer by 50–75%.[29, 30] Unfortunately tamoxifen may increase endometrial carcinoma (usually discovered early), uterine sarcoma (very rare but aggressive), and venous thromboembolism especially over age 50. Aromatase inhibitors may be replacing tamoxifen to reduce unwanted side effects.[31] Prophylactic bilateral mastectomy will reduce the chance of breast cancer in high-risk women by more than 90% even though not all breast tissue is usually removable.[32, 33] Nevertheless, the vast majority of high-risk mutation carrier women do not have mastectomy because of mutilation, problems of surgical reconstruction, the frequent early diagnosis of breast cancer, and generally good prognosis. Of course, prophylactic mastectomy has no beneficial effect on later possible ovarian cancer, unlike prophylactic oophorectomy.[5, 6]

V. CHOICES FOR THE PATIENT REGARDING RISK REDUCTION OF OVARIAN CANCER

The choices to be made by the patient include:

1. Surveillance
2. OCs

3. Prophylactic BTL
4. Prophylactic hysterectomy (as part of another indication)
5. Prophylactic oophorectomy (PO)
   - The general population
   - The hereditary ovarian cancer woman
   - The question of additional hysterectomy
5. Do nothing except routine check-ups and lifestyle change

VI. PSYCHOLOGICAL REACTIONS OF PATIENTS

Women need additional education about ovarian cancer risk and "…most women over estimated their risk…." Some of the general population get screening even though it is not recommended. Women with a single affected relative often report "…high levels of perceived risk" and have screening. "A significant percentage… at high risk fail to get recommended screening."[34] Women who had positive testing did not regret their decision, however, they complained of the lengthy wait for results and felt that a support group would be helpful. Prophylactic oophorectomy was more acceptable than prophylactic mastectomy.[35]

An exploratory study of 14 women, between 4 months and 7 years after PO, revealed that all but one were satisfied with their decision to undergo oophorectomy. They emphasized that it had decreased their anxiety about developing ovarian cancer. Postmenopausal women reported no negative impact on their libido. All but 1 of 6 premenopausal women started hormone replacement therapy (HRT) following surgery. It was a psychologically acceptable risk reduction strategy.[36] Of course these women must have been fully informed, prepared, and highly motivated.

Women who have had PO had more menopausal symptoms (especially premenopausal), but had no difference in sexual functioning or cancer worry. Laparoscopic cases did better than laparotomy cases.[37] The most common concerns of 30 women before prophylactic oophorectomy were the discomfort of surgery and recovery (40%) and concerns of immediate menopause and hormone replacement (37%). Two (7%) expressed regret about the decision for PO. The remaining 28 (93%) had no regret. Of 30 who selected surveillance, half had regrets and three were frankly dissatisfied. Nearly half did not know about the option of PO.[38] There is great interest in PO among high-risk women and physicians although there is great concern about complications of premature menopause.[4]

Patient satisfaction regarding choices of PO versus surveillance depends on patient understanding of the benefits and risks of each. A high percent of women would have liked more information before hand. Most women who were adequately informed in advance and had surgery do well emotionally especially when placed on HRT immediately postoperatively especially if premenopausal, if desired. The essential factors are motivation, emotional stability, basic intelligence, and expert continuous counseling before and after testing. Even after PO the patient realizes that there is a chance of breast cancer (although reduced) and a small irreducible chance of primary peritoneal cancer (which has a poor prognosis) forever.

VII. SURVEILLANCE FOR OVARIAN CANCER

The standard screening tests for ovarian cancer are

1. History and physical examination
2. Serum CA125
3. Transvaginal ultrasound

Screening for the general population is not recommended because of low prevalence, low positive predictive value, and high cost. Clinical evaluation usually does not discover cancer until it is advanced with ascites and a large pelvic mass. Serum CA125 does not detect half of all early-stage carcinoma. "Annual or semiannual measurement of serum CA125 is widely regarded as an unreliable screen for ovarian cancer..."[6] Serial long-term CA125 testing is being studied but even if helpful it probably would not have benefit for the individual patient. A new experimental serum proteonomic pattern analysis is promising but requires verification.[39]

Transvaginal ultrasound has good sensitivity in detecting ovarian enlargement but lacks specificity. It cannot detect ovarian cancer until after the ovary has enlarged, and most enlargements are benign.

Nevertheless high-risk women with family history and with BRCA1/2 mutations should be followed carefully with all three tests once or twice yearly, hence we use the word "surveillance" with the hope of making it more reliable.

Unlike what the public may believe surveillance does not prevent or reduce the risk of ovarian carcinoma. Previously there was a theory that ovarian carcinoma developed from a preexisting large benign ovarian neoplasm and therefore discovery and removal of benign neoplasms would prevent ovarian cancer. It is now recognized that the vast majority of ovarian epithelial carcinomas arise *de novo*, or from microscopic putative dysplasia. Therefore there cannot be a significant reduction of ovarian carcinoma by removal of benign neoplasms.[40] The most that surveillance might accomplish is detection of small ovarian enlargements which might be due to early-stage ovarian carcinoma, which presumably would result in improved therapy prognosis. Unfortunately surveillance not infrequently detects carcinoma after it is in advanced stage, despite a negative ultrasound within the preceding few months. Additional problems of surveillance include (1) false suspicious findings requiring unnecessary surgical exploration, (2) failure of the patient to continue periodic testing,[26] (3) constant anxiety, and (4) the discovery of occult carcinoma already present with negative testing at the time of PO indicating the unreliability of testing. "Intensive surveillance by use of CA125 and ultrasound does not seem to be an effective means of diagnosing early-stage ovarian cancer..." in high-risk women.[14] High-risk women who prefer surveillance not infrequently have unnecessary surgical exploration for suspicious or persistent abnormalities for benign conditions. The general consensus is that surveillance by itself is not recommended for high-risk women.

Another prospective study showed that despite intense surveillance of 290 motivated Jewish women that of the eight cases of ovarian/peritoneal cancers, six were found with advanced stage III cancer diagnosed by pain and ascites. Only 3/8 had one increased CA125. Of the eight, five had normal ultrasounds. Only one early-stage ovarian cancer was discovered. Thus the surveillance was essentially similar to no screening. Since it was prospective it was possible to find that of the eight cases, six were primary peritoneal serous papillary carcinomas with 185 del AG mutations, with a cumulative risk of 20% at 10 years.[14]

"Because there is no effective way to screen for early-stage ovarian cancer, we recommend PO to all postmenopausal women with hereditary susceptibility to the disease."[6]

The possible reason for the failure of serum CA125 to detect early stage I ovarian cancer is that elevated serum levels "...were closely related to the presence of serosal fluids and serosal involvement whatever the origin is."[41] This conforms to previous cell cultures where the peritoneum was more efficient in secreting CA125 than ovarian cancer."[42] When not due to ovarian cancer in postmenopausal women, serum CA125 elevation may be due to breast or lung cancer.[43]

Unfortunately "...a significant percentage of women at high risk fail to get recommended screening" while some of the general population get screening, although it is not recommended, because of the low risk and "...there are potentially significant negative consequences of a false-positive result..."[34]

A single prospective report, from a leading institution, of 89 women found 5 with early-stage ovarian or primary peritoneal cancer detected by semiannual ultrasound and CA125. They wrote that this "...supports the efficacy of their approach in genetically defined high-risk populations."[8] (However, there were five cases with unnecessary surgical explorations because of false-positive ultrasound and/or CA125 determinations.) The editorial comment to the report had the opposite conclusion: "...these data provide valuable insight into the severe limitations of both current screening approaches (transvaginal ultrasound and CA125) and of the evaluation of the efficacy of screening." The claimed sensitivity of ovarian cancer screening of 71% and specificity of 91% was questioned. The editorial also boosted the role of BSEs. The goal of reduction of cancer mortality in women with BRCA1/2 mutations will require a prospective precise, multicenter approach.[44]

An expert opinion is that "currently we do not support the position that screening is a viable alternative to preventive surgery." This is based on screening which at best can only detect early-stage ovarian carcinoma which may not necessarily be curable and with limited data on BRCA mutants.[5]

Surveillance for HNPCC includes:

1. Colonoscopy begun 5–10 years before the youngest diagnosed family member or at age 25 repeated within 3 years, and annually after age 40. If a polyp is found screening is done at 6-month to 1-year intervals.
2. Transvaginal ultrasound to detect endometrial thickening and ovarian enlargements, periodic (annual) endometrial biopsy, and serum CA125 starting at age 25.[6, 11, 18]

VIII. A POSSIBLE SIMPLE UNEXPECTED METHOD TO REDUCE OVARIAN CANCER RISK

Lifetime leisure time physical activity is associated with a reduced risk of epithelial ovarian cancer with an odds ratio of 0.73 with a range from 0.64–0.78, even after adjustments for parity, OC, family history, and body mass index (BMI).[45] Of course there might be associated, unrecognized socioeconomic, environmental, or cultural factors.

IX. ORAL CONTRACEPTIVES

Oral contraceptives (OCs) give a 50% risk reduction of ovarian carcinoma in the general population. The longer the use of OCs, the greater the ovarian cancer risk reduction. The preferred specific OC formulation and the age to start are unknown. There may be a 10% decrease in risk after one year of OCs, and a 50% after five years, both in nulliparous and parous women with older high-dose OCs. The beneficial effect persists for 10–15 years after OCs have been discontinued. Women with a positive family history (mother or sister) and therefore with an increased chance of ovarian cancer had a risk reduction of from 4 to 2 women per 100 women from the use of OCs for 4–8 years.[46]

The extent of OC reduction of ovarian cancer in BRCA1/2 mutants was similar to that in the general population. There was a 20% reduction for up to 3 years of use and a 60% for 6 years or more. The protective effect was not affected by parity, tubal ligation, and ages at delivery of a first and last child. OC use reduces the risk of later ovarian cancer both sporadic and with BRCA mutations by at least 50%.[47] The risk reduction begins after 2 years and increases with duration of use with 6 years having a 60% reduction. Expert opinion is "...that five years of oral contraceptive pills will significantly reduce the risk of ovarian cancer, without appreciably increasing the risk of breast cancer."[5]

OCs are recommended for contraception in women for high risk of ovarian cancer, and some researchers has suggested that OCs "...be used as a primary preventive measure."[46]

"Our data suggest that the administration of an oral contraceptive agent should be considered as part of a program of prevention for women with BRCA1 or BRCA2 mutations who have not had ovarian cancer. However, our data do not allow us to address the specific formulation to be recommended or the age at which treatment should begin."[46]

There is no FDA recommendation or approval for prophylactic use of OCs to prevent ovarian cancer. Nevertheless, the physician is permitted to prescribe any off label use of medication depending on personal judgment and with the knowledge of the patient. If there are no contraindications it would seem reasonable to prescribe current low-dose OCs to prevent ovarian cancer to women who are at increased risk, who do not wish oophorectomy at the time (or who might with it at a later time), especially if they wish contraception, or even if there is no need for contraception. There are no data on when to stop the OC since women generally have stopped the OC at menopause.

Oral contraceptives taken during menstrual life in the average population for contraception reduce by one-third or more the chance of ovarian cancer later in life. This was true for original formulations which contained 50 μg or more of estrogen as well as high doses of progestin. Since 1972 lower dose pills (estrogen and progestin) have been used with an "identical" (actually 40%) reduction in ovarian cancer which continues for at least 30 years after discontinuation. The protection began after 1–4 years. The age of onset of OCs was not different. The longer the use the greater the risk reduction.[48, 49]

There was a suggestion that while risk reduction of ovarian cancer with OCs agreed well with observed rates in women ages 30–49, the observed risk reduction rates were lower in women age 50–64.[50] Oral contraceptives may protect against benign ovarian tumors.[51]

A report suggesting a slight risk (relative risk 1.24) of breast cancer associated with long-term use of OCs may have been related to increased detection because the discovered cancers were less advanced.[52]

A recent retrospective study of women with a first-degree relative with breast cancer who ever took OCs during or prior to 1975 (when formulations had higher dosages of estrogen and progestins) "...may be at particularly high risk for breast cancer" with an increased relative risk of 3.3. (This has not been reported by others perhaps due to case selection and overlooking family history.) There was apparently no increased breast cancer risk with OCs since 1975, however, the numbers were too small to be reliable.[53]

There seems to be a small risk of breast cancer in young and older women associated with OC use. Current use relative risk is 1.2 and with past use is 1.1. "However, there was no increased risk in the subgroup of women with a family history of breast cancer (defined as having a mother or sister affected)."[5] A recent study confirmed no effect of OC use on breast cancer in BRCA1/2 mutants.[47] OCs should be considered as part of a program of prevention of ovarian cancer for BRCA1/2 mutants. OCs during menstrual life will reduce the later incidence of ovarian cancer. The original interpretation was prevention of "incessant ovulation," since repeated proliferation stimulus probably increases the chances of spontaneous somatic mutation of ovarian surface epithelium. In addition, the longer the use of OC the greater the benefit. The traditional explanation was reinforced by *in vitro* experiment of malignant tumors developing from rat surface epithelium forced to rapidly recolonize new repeated reculturing.[54] Although this may be an experimental mechanism in the rat, it overlooks putative physiologic *in vivo* stromal stimulation, and the slower time sequence of the woman. It also does not explain the later life cancer risk.

Based on the number of ovulations prevented it was found that OCs had an even greater than expected cancer risk reduction possibly by direct effect.[11]

All methods of contraception reduce ovarian cancer risks in multigravid women. The odds ratios for ever-use compared to never-use were: oral contraceptives 0.6, intrauterine device 0.8, barrier methods 0.8, tubal ligation 0.5, and vasectomy 0.8. Nulligravid women were not protected by any of these contraceptive methods. "The results imply mechanisms other than hormonal or ovulatory by which ovarian cancer risk is reduced."[55] Retrospective human investigation found that combination estrogen and progestin OCs with high-progestin potency had greater reduction in risk of ovarian cancer than those with low-progestin potency.[56] The progestin effect is thought to be related to a direct effect which increases apoptosis of DNA damaged cells.

If this hypothesis is correct then there was already an unknown acquired accumulative gene change which the body defense mechanisms could not detect or control. This also implies that ovarian epithelial carcinoma takes decades to develop with the only abnormal histology of dysplasia appearing relatively shortly before invasive carcinoma.

Levonorgestrel in macaque monkeys showed a marked decrease in the expression of transforming growth factor—β1 (TGF-β1) and in increase in TGF—β2/3 isoforms together with an increase in apoptosis. It was thought that the progestin acted directly on the ovarian epithelium to affect TGF-β which caused the apoptosis. Interestingly TGF-β is related to Mullerian inhibitory factor. TGF-β may be a "...potent tumor-suppressor and cancer preventive agent."[57, 58] Peptide growth factors may also be affected by retinoids and vitamin D compounds.

Theoretically short-term use of high-dose progestin might also cause apoptosis. This awaits further long-term prospective human epidemiological study.

There is a need for retrospective studies on women who have been given progestin such as:

1. IUD containing progestin
2. IM progestin (Depo-Provera) for contraception

3. Oral progestin alone or as part of hormone replacement therapy

"It is interesting to speculate that the combination of a progestin, which regulates TGF-β in the ovarian epithelium, and a retinoid and/or vitamin D might achieve synergistic or additive effects on TFG-β pathways in the ovarian epithelium, leading to a powerful cancer preventive agent."[58] In the general population the risk of ovarian cancer is reduced by parity. As with OCs the traditional explanation was reduction of "incessant" ovulation, however, pregnancy is a high progestin state and the protection might be due to apoptosis.

X. BTL

Interval laparoscopic tubal sterilization is considered safe, with nondangerous complication rates from 1.17–1.95, and one life-threatening event among 9475 cases. Predictors of complications include diabetes mellitus, general anesthesia, previous abdominal or pelvic surgery, and obesity.[59–61] Of course this is a select group of younger multiparous women.

Although tubal ligation reduces ovarian cancer with a relative risk between 0.2 and 0.9, it does not change the risk for breast cancer. Tubal ligation by unknown mechanism decreases ovarian cancer risk in BRCA1 mutation carriers (but not BRCA2) and in the general population with an adjusted relative risk of 0.39 and reduction of 61%. With added contraceptive pills the relative risk was further reduced to 0.28 with 72% protection.[5, 61, 62] Others report a relative risk reduction of 0.52 in the general public.[63] Hysterectomy has a weaker decrease risk.[64]

"Tubal ligation is a feasible option to reduce the risk of ovarian cancer in women with BRCA1 mutations who have completed childbearing."[59] For high-risk women who do not wish to take oral contraceptive pills, who wish to avoid or delay oophorectomy and who do not wish to be pregnant then tubal ligation (sterilization) is an alternative.[5]

The main value would seem to be for the general population. It reduces risk in hereditary ovarian cancer, however, it is not as effective as oophorectomy, which is preferred.

In stage III cancer a previous sterilization is an adverse independent prognostic factor. This suggests such cases have a relatively strong predisposition to cancer which overcomes the sterilization protection.[65]

XI. PO AT THE TIME OF OTHER SURGERY FOR THE GENERAL POPULATION

In the general population all agree that "...there is no role for surgery solely for prophylaxis." It is customary practice to remove ovaries at the time of hysterectomy for benign disease to prevent later ovarian cancer development.

A contrary opinion is: "While this may seem reasonable at first glance, there is little evidence to support such practice." The reason is at age 40 the subsequent lifetime risk is about 1% in the general population.[66] After hysterectomy the risk is reduced to less than 0.5% [64] and probably 0.25%.[67]

Nevertheless, most surgeons still advise incidental removal of ovaries with approaching menopause at about 45 when abdominal hysterectomy is done and with vaginal hysterectomy if feasible. About 10% of women with ovarian cancer had a previous hysterectomy after age 40.[64, 68] and this would prevent ovarian (but not primary peritoneal cancer). With the current trend of vaginal hysterectomy rather than of abdominal hysterectomy there has been a reduction of incidental oophorectomy from 63–18%. If laparoscopy-assisted vaginal hysterectomy (LAVH) is done there is an increase in oophorectomy.[68] In high-risk families or with two first-degree relatives with ovarian cancer even without genetic testing, prophylactic oophorectomy is recommended incident with nongynecologic surgery.[69] When abdominal hysterectomies are done for benign conditions in postmenopausal women concomitant oophorectomy is done in 61%, or odds ratio (OR) of 11.42. With laparoscopy-assisted vaginal hysterectomy the OR was 11.34. At vaginal hysterectomy there is less chance of oophorectomy being done, presumably for technical reasons, although greater among those who perform many such operations. Oophorectomy did not increase morbidity.[70]

Dublin consultants do not do prophylactic oophorectomies at the time of abdominal hysterectomy up to age 39, from 40–44 6% are done, from 45–49 43%, and over 49, 68%.[71]

XII. RECOMMENDATION FOR SELECTIVE PO FOR THE HIGH-RISK WOMAN AND INFORMED CONSENT

Recommendation for selective prophylactic oophorectomy for the high-risk woman is considered for:

1. BRCA1/2 gene mutation carriers
2. Women with breast cancer
3. Women with HNPCC (together with hysterectomy)

Special individualized situations for consideration include:

1. Women with a strong family history of breast/ovarian cancer who have not been tested or who have negative tests (or unidentifiable mutations)
2. Women with any type of colon cancer to discover or prevent metastases for quality of life

In 1995 an NIH consensus panel stated that "... the risk of ovarian cancer from families with hereditary ovarian cancer syndromes is sufficiently high to recommend prophylactic oophorectomy in these women at 35 years of age, or after childbearing is completed."[72]

Hereditary ovarian cancer occurs at a younger age than sporadic cancer with the mean in the mid-40s and 17% by age 40.[73, 74] PO is recommended before the end of the fourth decade after childbearing. With BRCA1 mutations PO is considered from the age of 35. PO also reduces the risk of later breast cancer.[5]

With BRCA2 mutations ovarian cancer occurs later, often over age 50 and therefore prophylactic oophorectomy is recommended between age 45 and 50.[74] Some believe that with BRCA2 mutations oophorectomy may not reduce breast cancer risk.[5, 9, 73, 75] Nevertheless, even patients over 60 are candidates for prophylactic oophorectomy because 44% with BRCA1 mutations and 71% with BRCA2 mutations occurred after age 60.

BRCA2 mutation carriers may have a more generalized predisposition to cancer, aside from breast/ovarian cancers, such as nongynecologic cancer of the pancreas, gallbladder, bile duct, stomach, male breast, prostate, and malignant melanoma.[73]

PO for BRCA1/2 mutation carriers gives a dramatic 90–98% chance of reduction of "ovarian" (which includes ovarian/peritoneal) carcinoma with hazard ratios ranging from 0.04–0.15.[76, 77]

PO for BRCA1/2 mutation carriers gives a 50% reduction of later breast cancer with hazard ratios of 0.32–0.47, especially if done prior to menopause and despite later HRT.[4, 78–80] In anticipating that prophylactic oophorectomy in high-risk women gives at least 75% (probably 90–95%) reduction in ovarian cancer risk and 50% reduction in breast cancer risk, there was predicted a dramatic increase in life expectancy of approximately six years.[81] HRT did not reduce the benefit. To put it another way "...the projected proportion of women who will be free of breast cancer or BRCA-related gynecologic cancer five years from the time of salpingo-oophorectomy or the beginning of surveillance is 94% in the salpingo-oophorectomy group and 69% in the surveillance group.[80]

Other potential benefits of PO are

1. There might be discovered an occult ovarian carcinoma already present
2. A potential substitution for lack of diligent surveillance

Women who are survivors of breast cancer and carriers of BRCA1/2 mutations should consider PO. There is a significant chance of later ovarian cancer, which is more lethal than breast cancer and usually not discovered until advanced. Additional potential benefits include removal of an estrogen source in young women, and discovery or prevention of ovarian metastases.

Women with BRCA1/2 associated cancer are at increased risk for contralateral breast cancer and ovarian cancer. Compared to surveillance alone, a 30-year-old early-stage breast cancer patient theoretically would have life expectancy (LE) extension probabilities of 0.4–1.3 years from tamoxifen therapy, 0.2–1.8 years from bilateral oophorectomy, and 0.6–2.1 years from prophylactic contralateral mastectomy. With low-penetrance mutations there is least gain of LE based on assumed contralateral breast cancer risk of 24% and ovarian cancer risk of 6%. The greatest gain of LE is for those with high-penetrance mutations of assumed risk of breast cancer of 65% and ovarian 40%.[82]

With HNPCC there is a lifetime increase of various cancers which require surveillance:

Colon/rectum 82% (general population 2%)
Endometrium 60% (1.5%)
Stomach 13% (<1%)
Ovary 12% (<1%)
Small intestine 5% (<1%)
Brain 3.7% (<1%)
Biliary tract 2% (<1%)

Endometrial surveillance may be done by transvaginal ultrasound and endometrial biopsy beginning at age 30–35 and done every 1–2 years. Ovarian surveillance may be done at age 30–35 at 1–2 year intervals.[83] Gynecologic cancer presents at a mean of 49.3 years, while colorectal cancer presents at 51.2 years. Surveillance is recommended beginning at age 25. There were 5 gynecologic cancers (7.1%) by age 35 among 64 women. Considerations should be given for prophylactic hysterectomy and oophorectomy after childbearing and over age 35 with colectomy.[18] Special situations: women with strong family histories of ovarian and breast cancer without identifiable gene mutations.

Theoretically in BRCA1/2 families if the patient does not have the mutation she does not have increased cancer risk despite a strong family history and PO has not been recommended.[6, 84] This is true especially in Jewish women whose BRCA1/2 gene mutations are supposedly only the classic "founder" mutations.

Nevertheless, despite the fact that BRCA1/2 mutations are autosomal dominant and that there is a 50% chance of inheritance, some still consider "...reliance solely on genetic testing as a major predictor of breast and ovarian cancer is not supported by the science. An accurate evaluation of family history remains essential in assessing breast and ovarian cancer risk. Analysis has shown that multiple affected first- and second-degree relatives, both maternal and paternal, particularly with early onset disease, may significantly alter an individual's risk for breast and ovarian cancer." "...genetic testing for BRCA1 mutations (are) and uncertain and incomplete science." And "... a negative test result for the BRCA1 185 del AG mutation alone would have little meaning in the presence of a strong family history of breast and ovarian cancer."

Thus, although this is a minority review, it may be reasonable under certain circumstances because of the possibility of rare unrecognized BRCA1/2 mutations, which may be present, to consider PO. Hereditary familial cancer clusters in different groups may have unusual BRCA1/2 gene mutations. If the usual familial pattern mutations are known then it is simple to test the patient. A single BRCA1 185 del AG gene mutation is characteristic in high-risk families and in 1% or Eastern European Jews. "There is a possibility that other BRCA1 mutations exist within the same population. For this reason, a negative test result for the BRCA1 185 del AG mutation alone would have little meaning in the presence of a strong family history of breast and ovarian cancer."[85]

Two Jewish women from high-risk families who had negative "founder" BRCA1/2 gene mutations developed ovarian cancer in a surveillance study at a leading center. This, together with a 30% incidence of cancers other than ovarian/breast of the same group suggests a new, unrecognized syndrome.[14]

Another minority authoritative opinion is: "Not all patients will have undergone genetic testing and it may be reasonable to perform prophylactic surgery in patients who have a strong family history, such as those with two or more first-degree relatives with ovarian cancer, or in women with early-onset breast cancer with a direct lineage of breast or ovarian cancer."[66]

At primary resection for colorectal cancer PO should be considered to prevent later symptomatic ovarian metastases and/or primary ovarian cancer.[86] Theoretically PO might give a survival advantage if the patient is surgically disease free.[87]

Ideally when considering prophylactic salpingo-oophorectomy the patient should be informed of the:

1. Diagnosis
2. Contemplated treatment
3. Inherent risks
4. Other alternative methods
5. Prognosis with treatment
6. Prognosis without treatment[88]

Additional cancer concerns include: (1) the small possibility of the discovery of an already present occult carcinoma, the need for surgical staging, possible additional surgery, and possible chemotherapy; and (2) the later possible 2–11% (some report less than 5%) chance of primary peritoneal cancer in BRCA1/2 mutation carriers over many years.[68]

There may be other concerns including:

1. Premature menopause
2. Menopausal symptoms, hot flashes, HRT, cardiovascular status
3. Potential osteoporosis
4. Possible psychological reactions

For most women the deciding factor for PO is breast/ovarian cancer anxiety, rather than objective risk.[89]

XIII. PROPHYLACTIC SURGERY FOR THE HIGH-RISK WOMAN

A. What Surgery Should be Done?

An almost overnight change of standard care occurred with the report that 7 of 44 (16%) of unselected fallopian tube carcinoma cases had germline BRCA mutations, of which 5 (11%) were BRCA1, and 2 (5%) were BRCA2.[90] Since BRCA testing was not complete probably the 16% is an underestimate. Thus "...fallopian tube cancer is a component of the hereditary breast and ovarian cancer syndrome." This concept is reinforced by molecular evidence of association with BRCA1/2 germline mutations. Therefore bilateral salpingo-oophorectomy is the "...minimal procedure of choice."[75] An added advantage of adding salpingectomy is that it reduces the risk of leaving ovarian remnants in the mesovarium.[91, 92] Ovarian cancer has developed from ovarian remnants.[93]

Some institutions use the phrase "risk reduction prophylactic salpingo-oophorectomy" rather than "preventive" prophylactic surgery.[80, 94] This would make the patient's expectation more realistic and be a better description.

B. Surgical Technique

The prophylactic procedure of choice is laparoscopic ambulatory salpingo-oophorectomy with removal of as much of the fallopian tube as feasible.[75, 94] General endotracheal anesthesia is customary to keep the lungs properly inflated. Video control is standard so that the assistants can help. Without video only the surgeon can see the operative field with the telescope. Three or more puncture sites are made; infraumbilical for the telescope, suprapubic, and lateral. For hemostasis a GIA staple and cutting device is often used because it is fast, however, it is expensive, requires careful placement, and does not always give good hemostasis. Bipolar electric (Kleppinger forceps) coagulation and cutting is less expensive but takes longer. It depends on operator preference. The tube and ovary are partially skeletonized, incising the median leaf of the broad ligament to release any adherent underlying ureter and the infundibulopelvic ligament (IP) transected with concern for hemostasis and avoiding the close ureter. Care is taken for the broad ligament in which there may be many irregular distended veins (especially in multiparas and premenstrual). The extension of the uterine vessels irregularly spread into the broad ligament to anastomose with the IP vessel extensions. Additional laparoscopic procedures may be done at the same time if feasible. This would include inspection of the pelvis and upper abdomen for gross evidence of tumor, and if possible the paracolic gutters, bowel, undersurface of the diaphragm and omentum. Another procedure recommended is peritoneal lavage cytology. Of 35 cases of PO with grossly normal ovaries, 3 cases had malignant cells of whom 2 (BRCA1 positive) were found to have occult adenocarcinoma *in situ* of the ovary and tube. In one case the source was unknown and the patient was given chemotherapy,[95] presumably it was an occult primary peritoneal carcinoma. Although peritoneal washings fail to identify 66% of gross disease and 78% of microscopic disease, lavage is recommended with PO.[96] Some also advocate swabbing cytology of the diaphragm, and random multiple systematic peritoneal and omental biopsies [91, 97] but this adds risks. In practice most surgeons only do salpingo-oophorectomy with inspection of the pelvis.

If there are dense adhesions of the adnexa to the lateral side walls of the pelvis then it is reasonable to perform a laparotomy to avoid ureter, large vessel, or bowel injuries. This may occur with old pelvic inflammatory disease, endometriosis, previous surgery (appendectomy, ectopic tubal pregnancy, etc.), or severe diverticulitis.

The disadvantage of ambulatory surgery is the brief postoperative observation. Although minor complications are not unusual, there may be rare serious complications. The patient should be instructed to report any undue persistent pain, distention, fever, other adverse symptoms, or failure to progressively feel better. Ideally there should be careful histology by experts of serial sections of all tissue removed at 2- to 3-mm intervals. Tissue must be handled gently to avoid surface abrasion.[97] Previous negative reports based on a few random sections have been repeated with serial sections which have revealed occult carcinoma.[98]

C. The Question of Hysterectomy at the Same Time

Some have recommended hysterectomy at the time of PO in order to remove the uterine intramural portion of the fallopian tube.[99] Additional advantages would be: (1) avoiding possible increase of endometrial carcinoma (and now also uterine sarcoma) if tamoxifen is used later to reduce the risk of breast cancer or of contralateral breast cancer for BRCA mutation carriers; (2) avoiding possible uterine bleeding from later HRT; and (3) avoiding progestin (and estrogen) of HRT which might increase the risk of breast cancer and cause premenstrual-like symptoms.[4] Some have embraced this concept since 1955 prior to this reason. "...we have long advocated laparoscopy-assisted vaginal hysterectomy bilateral salpingo-oophorectomy (LAVH-BSO) as the procedure of choice for women at increased risk of gynecological cancers because of the HBOC and HNPCC syndromes."[68] Some indicated that the indication for hysterectomy is not clear [5, 75] and if done it should be for another reason. Most feel that hysterectomy is not recommended because germline BRCA mutations do not increase endometrial cancer, as well as the increased risk, morbidity, hospitalization, recovery time, and cost.[92, 100] An expert opinion is that, "There is no proven benefit in removing the uterus except in patients who are members of an HNPCC kindred."[66]

XIV. ADVANTAGES OF PROPHYLACTIC SALPINGO-OOPHORECTOMY (PSO)

A. Risk Reduction of Ovarian Cancer

Logic indicates that after PSO, if there is no occult ovarian cancer there will not be any new ovarian cancer. Any new epithelial cancer with the histology of primary ovarian cancer has to develop from primary peritoneal cancer. The precise risk is not known but has been estimated as 3–4% [66] or 2–11%.[101] Confusion has occurred because of similar histology especially with control cases who did not have PSO. It is thought that about 10% or more of all "ovarian" cancer is in fact primary peritoneal cancer.[5] Because of this confusion some authors lump both together as "ovarian," "coelomic," or "gynecologic" cancer. The main advantage of PSO is prevention of future ovarian cancer. Subsequent cancer is of primary peritoneal origin. Because ovarian cancer is more common than peritoneal cancer and appears earlier, combined data show dramatic reduction of "ovarian" (actually ovarian and peritoneal) cancer. It should be ovarian 0% and any cancer listed as peritoneal. Since peritoneal cancer appears later than ovarian (sometimes 20 or 30 years), usual follow-up studies are usually not long enough. Other data problems are the possible further delay in mean age and/or reduction of peritoneal cancer after PSO. "When the analysis was limited to new ovarian, fallopian tube, and primary peritoneal cancers, the time to a diagnosis of cancer was longer in the salpingo-oophorectomy group than in the surveillance group."[80] Long-term investigation is required, additional significant data would be the precise locations of the BRCA1/2 gene mutations, and the fact that BRCA2 cancers usually occur later than BRCA1. PSO prevents ovarian cancer but does not prevent, but might possibly reduce or cause even later appearance of primary peritoneal cancer. When the infrequent occult ovarian or tubal cancer is discovered at PSO it is understandably usually stage I.

When surveillance cases are discovered to have ovarian-peritoneal cancer because of signs or symptoms or testing, it is often advanced. PSO reduces new "coelomic" epithelium BRCA1/2 cancer risk by 96% and of breast cancer by 53%.[102] At surgery or by histology after PSO 3.1% were found to have occult ovarian or papillary serous peritoneal carcinoma (PSPC) versus 19.9% of surveillance controls. Of the 8 occult ovarian cancers, six were stage I. After PO there was at least a 5-year follow-up. In 37/292 controls with surveillance who developed ovarian cancer (with a known stage) 11% had stage I, 16% stage II, 65% had stage III and 9% had stage IV. Excluding 6/259 (2.3%) who had occult stage I ovarian carcinoma, PO reduced the risk of "coelomic" epithelial cancer to a hazard ratio of 0.04% with 2 cases of papillary serous peritoneal carcinoma at 3.8% and 8.6 years later. Breast cancer developed in 21.2% after PO, contrasted to 42.3% in the control group.[102]

In another report there was a 94% projection of absence of breast or BRCA-related "gynecologic" cancer for 5 years after PSO but only 69% in the surveillance group. There were 3/170 who were discovered to have occult stage I ovarian carcinoma at PSO.[80]

Bilateral prophylactic oophorectomy (BPO) gives a significant reduction in ovarian and breast cancer risk (HR reduction 0.46%) with BRCA1/2 mutations. Ovarian cancer risk reduction was HR = 0.02, excluding 5/248 at the time of BPO, with only 1/248 (0.4%) with later "ovarian" (presumably primary peritoneal) cancer in a 9.4 year average follow-up. Subsequent breast cancer developed in 25 women (10.1%).[76]

B. Risk Reduction of Breast Cancer

The first study to show a statistical difference in breast cancer risk among BRCA1 mutation carriers found hazard ratio (HR) of 0.53 (almost a 50% reduction). Risk reduction was even greater (HR = 0.28) for women who were followed 5–10 years. In addition "use of HRT did not negotiate the reduction of breast cancer risk after surgery." The presumed mechanism was reduction of ovarian hormone exposure.[78]

Further study showed that oophorectomy gave an OR for subsequent breast cancer of 0.42, with a reduction in both BRCA1 and BRCA2 mutation carriers. Risk reduction was maximum if performed before age 40 (OR = 0.24), intermediate for 40–44 (OR = 0.60), and least for after 50.[103] PO reduces the risk of breast cancer by 53%. The mean age was 40.1 (range 21.3–66.4) of PO was thereby creating an early surgical menopause. Reduction occurred despite any HRT in 83.8% with BRCA1 mutations and in 18.2% with BRCA2 mutations.[80, 102, 103]

Among 99 women who had PO and who were followed for breast cancer, it developed in 21 (21.2%) compared to 60 (42.3%) in the control group, thereby reducing the HR to 0.4%. Of interest is that the PO group was significantly older at the time of diagnosis (52.5 versus 46.7), and the mean time for PO cases to develop breast cancer was 11.4 years and 8 for control.[102, 103] Another report confirmed that the time to breast cancer or "gynecologic" cancer was longer in the salpingo-oophorectomy group with an HR of 0.25.[80]

These reports suggest that PSO reduces the risk and delays the onset of breast cancer and peritoneal cancer.

C. Other Advantages: Reduction of Anxiety, Need for Intensive Surveillance, and the Elimination of Unnecessary Surgical Exploration for Suspicious Benign Conditions

In the surveillance group 7/72 had surgical exploration for benign conditions.[80] Nevertheless, although there is a reduced risk there must continue breast cancer surveillance with mammography, clinical examination and BSE. In addition BRCA2 mutation carrier women still have to keep alert to pancreatic, bile duct, and general cancer, and BRCA2 mutation carrier men have to be alert to prostate, breast, pancreatic, and general cancers.

XV. SURGICAL RISKS OF PROPHYLACTIC LAPAROSCOPIC SALPINGO-OOPHORECTOMY (PLSO)

A. Introduction—Not Innocuous

There is a general agreement among experts that even "...diagnostic laparoscopy is not an innocuous operation..." [104] despite the popular public concept of simple "band-aid" or "minimally invasive" surgery, and that patients should be informed. Complications can occur even in "experience hands" and increase with the complexity of the procedure.[105] Although complications are not unusual most are minor. Major complications are rare. Large blood vessel injury is an immediate threat to life, while bowel injury is often overlooked and can result in delayed sepsis and fatality.

B. No Reliable Data—Underreporting

There are no reliable data on the surgical risks of laparoscopic PSO. The procedure has only been done recently. In addition there is underreporting because: (1) of omissions with voluntary reporting; (2) different institutions have different definitions and study design, for example, conversion to laparotomy may or may not be considered a complication, minor complications may not be reportable, and PLSO has been considered as both minor and major surgery; (3) only favorable series tend to be published; (4) a significant percent of complications are overlooked at surgery and are not recognized until after the patient is discharged. The patient may go elsewhere for further care or even if she returns it might not be recorded; (5) the relative percentages of simple observation versus complex operative laparoscopies may not be given in general laparoscopy complications; (6) data from day-care ambulatory facilities may reflect favorable patient selection factors; (7) reports from large institutions "... may give a false sense of security to those working in a less favorable environment."[106]

Bowel injury is a major cause of morbidity and mortality in gynecologic laparoscopy. There is wide variation in reports. It "...is likely to be under-reported" because of late (among other things) diagnosis after discharge, and the ratio of diagnostic/minor procedures to advanced procedures. For the minor surgery, bowel injury was 1 in 1652 while it was 1 in 280 in advanced procedures. [106]

Despite reports of insignificant complications with laparoscopic hysterectomy, a report of all 760 procedures in Adelaide, Australia (done mainly with disposable staples) revealed significant complications in 14% of the patients.

"Hemorrhage, hematoma, and laparotomy rates were higher then published data suggest..." and "...urinary tract injuries were significantly elevated in comparison with published data."[107] Most trocar injuries are abdominal wall vessel injury (0.15–10.5%), major vascular injury (under 0.15%), visceral trauma (2.5%), and incisional hernia (up to one-third). "It is believed that the actual rate of such injuries is at least three times the published rate."[108]

C. Reports of PLSO

The current recommendation is laparoscopic bilateral salpingo-oophorectomy rather than the previous oophorectomy. Removal of the fallopian tube would increase the potential surgical risk. The mesosalpinx has many irregular blood vessels, often has markedly dilated veins especially in multipara, is extremely delicate, and is just above the ureter. The IP vessels are large and very close to the ureter. Although not always transected with oophorectomy they are cut routinely with salpingo-oophorectomy. A recent report of a U.S. hospital indicated that laparoscopic prophylactic oophorectomy "...is a safe and effective outpatient method for primary prevention of ovarian cancer in women at risk for HOC."[8] The surgical technique was (customary) video laparoscopy, examination of the entire abdominal cavity, triple puncture technique, surgical stapling, and presumably salpingo-oophorectomy rather than oophorectomy. Nevertheless the abstract reported that of 131 cases of laparoscopic oophorectomy from 1995–2000, there were 10 operative complications in 9 women (6.9%), including 3 uterine perforations, and 1 each of hemorrhage, conversion to laparotomy/wound cellulitis, cystotomy, (small) bowel obstruction, enterocolitis, and metabolic abnormality. There were 32 women (24.4%) who had only laparoscopy prophylactic oophorectomy and required a one-day admission for nausea, urinary retention, pain, or anxiety.[94] The true total complication rate was 31.3%. Nevertheless all would agree that it is a recommended procedure.

A later paper by the same group indicated only 4/80 complications with risk-reducing salpingo-oophorectomy without hysterectomy. One had a laparotomy because of adhesions from previous surgery with a postoperative wound infection. A second had a bladder perforation requiring a Foley catheter for 5 days. Another had distal small bowel obstruction 8 weeks later which resulted from adhesions between the distal ileum and staples on the right ovarian vessels, and the last had a perforation of the uterus.[80] Although the authors felt that the complication rate is "...similar to those reported in other studies of laparoscopic gynecologic procedures...," in fact most reports have a lower incidence of complications. Possibly the prospective analysis as contrasted to retrospective studies reveals more of the complications. In addition it was not clear what the actual complications were. It is generally agreed that when laparoscopy is difficult due to adhesions then liberal conversion to laparotomy should be considered. With major extensive adhesiolysis the complication rate increases to 8.4 per 1000.[109]

A different institution reporting laparoscopic prophylactic oophorectomy concluded it "... is feasible and safe...", and "...associated with low blood loss...." Nevertheless in 62 cases, 2 (3.2%) were converted to laparotomy because of dense adhesions and stayed for 7 and 9 days postoperatively because of fever and ileus. One patient (1.6%) had a vascular intraoperative complication secondary to bleeding or opening the broad ligament peritoneum with a 1500 ml blood loss and transfusion of 2 units of packed red blood cells. There were minor complications in 10 cases (16.1%). There was one major complication with a 6 point drop in hematocrit requiring 2 units transfusion due to retroperitoneal hematoma from an IP ligament that had been stapled.[110] Thus the complication rate was in fact 6.4%. Although 15 of the cases were LVH-BSO, the complications were all laparoscopic.

D. Risks of Other Laparoscopic Surgery

The closest approximations are those of general gynecologic laparoscopy. In salpingo-oophorectomy for adnexal masses, laparoscopy could be used in 70.8% (121/171) of cases for benign masses. Bilateral adnexectomy was done in 37 (30.6%), and unilateral in 84 (69.4%). Mean hospitalization was 2.8 days. Postoperative complication occurred in 8.3% (10 cases), including 6 with infections, 1 with transient bowel occlusion after lysis adhesions, 2 (1.69%) required re-operation, one with eventration at 10-cm port, and one with epiploic evisceration at the trocar invasion site. There was one major complication of severe adhesions to the sigmoid colon and later peritonitis requiring bowel repair. Bipolar coagulation was recommended.[111]

The success rate for PSO is expected to be better because the ovaries are not enlarged. It is difficult to get reliable comparable data.

A report of 11,448 consecutive laparoscopies done by 15 gynecologists from one center in Australia was flawed because: (1) it was a free-standing day surgical center (which implies preselection of simple cases); (2) there was no separation of diagnostic versus operative laparoscopies and salpingectomy and oophorectomy were considered as "...complex operative procedures...", and therefore probably only few were done; (3) major complication was defined as one which required laparotomy; (4) a voluntary questionnaire was relied upon; and (5) minor complications were not recorded. There were 0.78 major complication per 1000. Their literature review showed a variation of complication from rates of 2.2 to 5 per 1000.[112] Other large French series also did not record minor complications.[113]

Laparoscopic complications vary with the complexities of the surgery as would be expected. Thus for observation diagnostic laparoscopy, tubal sterilization, or other minor procedures the risk is usually about 0.1% while major procedure complications are about 0.5%.[109] The complication rate for advanced complex procedures such as laparoscopic hysterectomy is about 11% even when done by experts.[104, 109] Some large European series report total complication rates between 3.6 and 5.7 per 1000 with laparotomy being required for 3.3/1000.[113]

A large Netherlands series of all 25,764 laparoscopies found 5.7 per 1000 complications, 2 deaths, and laparotomy was required in 3.3 per 1000. The most frequent complications were epigastric vein hemorrhage and intestinal injuries requiring laparotomy in 90%. The complication rate was 2.7 per 1000 for diagnostic laparoscopy, 4.5 per 1000 for sterilization, and 17.9 per 1000 for operative laparoscopy, especially with previous laparotomy and laparoscopic hysterectomy.[114]

In a series of 7064 general laparoscopies, there was a rate of 2.76 per 1000 complications requiring laparotomy. It was 1.67 per 1000 for diagnostic laparotomies, 0.42 for minor laparoscopic surgery, and 4.46 for major surgery. Half of the cases requiring laparotomy were intestinal injuries and half of the intestinal injuries were missed until later peritonitis developed. There was one fatality.[115, 116]

A multicenter study from seven "top" French centers of all diagnostic and operative gynecologic laparoscopies (29,966 over 9 years) found an overall complication rate of 4.64 per 1000 with a mortality rate of 3.33 per 100,000. The complication rate was correlated with the complexity of the procedure. The complication rate which required laparotomy was 3.20 per thousand.[104]

The low complication rates in part might be related to their ratios of diagnostic laparoscopy (19.9%), and minor surgery (19.8%), while major surgery was 48.8% and laparoscopic surgery 11.5%. Of significant concern were the facts that one-third of the complications occurred in the initial phase ("setting up") and 28.6% were not diagnosed during the operation.[104] Conversion to laparoscopy of itself was not recorded as a complication. Unfortunately there was no description of methodology and data collection.

Reports from U.S. hospitals are not as favorable as from European centers. A one year review of all laparoscopic surgeries (843 cases) other than tubal ligation at Brigham and Women's Hospital during 1994 gave an overall major complication rate of 1.9%, a 5% unintended laparotomy rate, and a combined bowel and urinary injury rate of less than 1%. The difficulty of the procedure was the strongest predictor of complications. Fourteen percent of oophorectomies were converted to laparotomies, however, these included malignancies. LAVH-BSO had the highest complication rate and 90% were admitted postoperatively. There were increased complications with low BMI, possibly because the viscera are closer to the abdominal wall. Salpingo-oophorectomies and salpingectomies had high rates of postoperative admissions, perhaps because ectopic pregnancy was the most common indication.[97]

Aside from laparoscopic hysterectomy another new advanced complex procedure is lymphadenectomy in cervix cancer. The conclusion was that laparoscopic bilateral aortic lymph node sampling appeared to be reasonably safe and feasible. Laparoscopic therapeutic bilateral pelvic lymphadenectomy had a "...reasonable complication rate." Despite this optimistic conclusion the conversion rate to laparotomy was 14.5% (10 of 67). There were 7 major vascular injuries (10.4% of 67), all by experienced surgeons.[117]

"In a retrospective review of the literature and the author's experience, data revealed 15 deaths in 501,779 laparoscopic procedures, a death rate of 3 per 100,000."[109] Variations include smaller series with none and others with 5.4 per 100,000. A U.S. report of 3.6 deaths per 100,000 disclosed 29 associated with tubal sterilization (which is usually considered a simple procedure). Anesthesia caused 11, unrecognized bowel injury caused sepsis in 7, major blood vessel laceration caused 4, myocardial infarction caused 3, and other causes were 4.[109]

E. The Inherent Unappreciated Risk of All Laparoscopies Is Due to the Trocar and Insufflation Needle

Analysis of complications indicates that there are two aspects. One is the obvious complexity of the surgery. However, there is an unappreciated additional risk component present in all laparoscopies both minor and major in the preparation, "set-up," phase involving the piercing of the abdomen with the primary and secondary trocars to establish ports and the Veress needle for instillations of gas. This is a significant almost unavoidable baseline risk. The major risk is passage of the main trocar in order to create a port to pass the laparoscope. The most common injury is damage to the bowel which is frequently overlooked and several days later (or longer) may result in peritonitis with a high risk of fatality. A less frequent injury is of the large retroperitoneal blood vessels which may be an immediate threat to life. Urologic injuries (bladder, ureters) are infrequent but may be serious. "...laparoscopy has small risks which cannot be completely eliminated, for about half of the complications are due to the laparoscopic approach."[114]

One-third of complications (34.1% n = 43) were secondary to creation of the pneumoperitoneum or installation of the trocars. It was divided into 13.1% (n = 5) for urologic, 32.5% (n = 14) for bowel, and 48.9% (n = 24) for hemorrhagic. This was despite expert surgeons in excellent hospitals. It occurs with the blind penetration into the abdomen. The complications relating to the actual surgical procedure were kept to a minimum by controlled surgery under observation. However, equally disconcerting was that 28.6% (n = 36) of complications went unnoticed during the surgical procedure and were only diagnosed subsequently. These included 23.7% urological, 20.0% vascular, and 41.8% bowel. This occurred despite expertise and observations.[118]

Some believe that with expert surgeons there is a greater percent (or even most) of complications occurring in the preliminary phase with the Veress needle and trocar insertion than from the actual operative procedure.[109]

F. Bowel Injury Is the Most Common Injury, and When Unrecognized May Cause Late Peritonitis and Death

The most common gynecologic laparoscopy complication is gastrointestinal injury. It causes 20–46% of all complications, with an incidence of 0.6–1.6 per thousand.[118] The diagnosis was made intraoperatively in only 20 cases (35.7%) while in 36 (64.3%) it was made in the following week or two because of peritonitis.[116] In a voluntary report, a series of 62 gastrointestinal injuries showed 32.1% occurred during the "set-up" phase, especially during passage of the umbilical trocar (16.1%), and of the pneumoperitoneum needle (10.7%). During the operative phase there were 57% especially with sharp dissection (46.5%) and unipolar electrosurgery (10.7%), another 10.7% were of unknown cause. "The fact that bowel injuries in the experience group were as common during access as during surgery indicated that blind access remains a risk even in experienced hands."[106]

A high percent of bowel injury is associated with adhesions from previous surgery during access (primary trocar, Veress needle) while adhesions from endometriosis were the problem during the surgical procedure (forceps, scissors, electro- and laser surgery). "In experienced hands trauma occurred as frequently during access as during the surgical procedure" because access is blind. In one series of 45 bowel injuries, it was diagnosed and treated during surgery in 38 cases, of 7 cases (15%) with delayed diagnosis, 2 died seven days later (28%).[106] Many reviews indicated underreporting of bowel injuries.[88] French reports of bowel injury was not considered a complication when laparoscopic repair was done. Another series was based on only a 24% response from a questionnaire.[106] A voluntary French questionnaire review, without knowing the incidence, reported 56 women with 62 gastrointestinal injuries. There had been 66.1% with previous surgical procedures (and presumably) with adhesions.[118]

Five of the cases were diagnostic laparoscopy, 7 were sterilization, although most (44 cases 78.6%) occurred in major or advanced laparoscopy. Thus it may occur even with simple minor procedures, presumably because "...one-third of the injuries occurred during the set-up phase." In 64.3% the gastrointestinal injury went unnoticed during the surgery.[118]

G. Major Vascular Injury (MVI)—A Rare Emergency, Sometimes Fatal

Major vascular injuries are rare but are serious emergency situations usually diagnosed during the laparoscopy and usually managed by immediate laparotomy and a vascular surgeon.[118]

Literature reviews indicate that MVI are rare. About 0.22% of laparoscopic gynecologic operations had major vascular injury, 75% which were caused by trocars or Veress needles. Others report an incidence of such complication as little as 0.1%, however, a prospective report found 1.4% with trocar complications of which 0.9% were vascular. [119] On the other hand, a mail survey of certified Canadian gynecologists with a response rate of 50.9% (407/800) revealed that one-quarter had at least one case of sharp trocar or needle injury and of these one-half required laparotomy for correction. This is an unexpectedly high rate. Such divergent reports suggest underreporting.[120]

Of 24 with 31 MVI three of 4 MVIs (79.2%, 19 cases) occurred during the setting-up phase of laparoscopy with 15 due to the umbilical trocar and 4 due to the needle. In 5 cases (20.8%) MVI occurred during the laparoscopic surgical procedure. Five (20.8%) women died and 4 others (12.5%) had serious complications.[118] Others also give a 20% death rate.[108]

Of 629 trocar injuries of all types of laparoscopies reported from 1993–1996 to the Food and Drug Administration in which disposable trocars with safety shields were used, there were 408 with major blood vessels, 182 bowel, and 30 abdominal wall hematomas. Of the 32 deaths, 81% were from vascular injury mainly aorta and inferior vena cava which were 38% of fatal injuries and 19% from bowel injury. The diagnosis of bowel injury was initially unrecognized in 10% and in this group the mortality was 21%. The most common vascular injury reported was the common iliac artery or vein. Unfortunately the total number of cases was not reported and therefore the incidence of omplications was not known.In addition of the 30 cases of abdominal wall bleeding, all were significant with 8 being re-operated, 9 with blood transfusions, and 6 requiring a laparotomy to control the bleeding. Therefore logically none of the minor complications were reported. Despite theoretical advantages neither "safety-shields" nor "direct-view" trocars "cannot prevent serious injuries." [119] "Injuries associated with trocar and pneumoperitoneum needle insertion during laparoscopy still occur in spite of increasing physician expertise and the use of safeguards."[120]

H. Urologic Injury

"The main complications of laparoscopy are hemorrhage and perforation of the bladder and bowel by the Veress needle and trocar." Literature reviews indicate bladder injuries from 0.01–8.3% especially with previous surgery. "A frequent and known cause of bladder injury is the second trocar insertion, with an incidence of approximately 1.6% of all laparoscopic procedures." A possible treatment is a minilaparotomy with a 2 or 3 layer purse-string closure leaving the trocar in place for identification and an indwelling Foley catheter for 10 days.[121]

A review of 15 cases of ureteral injury found 4 with laparoscopic sterilization (usually considered a minor procedure), and 7 with endometriosis with uterosacral involvement. Although sterilization bipolar coagulation is considered relatively safe there may be ureteral injury directly or indirectly by vascular supply damage. There may be a delay of a week for symptoms of a ureteral fistual due to electric surgery current or adjacent heat injury.[121]

Laparoscopic assisted hysterectomy may have a 1% risk of ureteral injury usually due to thermal damage and necrosis. Literature review indicates 0.12–0.25% ureteral injury with laparoscopic surgery. The ureter is susceptible because of its proximity and difficult visualization at the uterosacral ligament.[121]

I. Port Site Spread of Ovarian Cancer

An unappreciated risk is port site metastases from an unsuspected occult or small gross size ovarian cancer. Such cases may not have signs, symptoms, or abnormal examination. Although not emphasized, preoperative transvaginal sonography should be considered as a routine for PLSO. In addition the specimen should be contained in an endobag without morcellation to avoid possible tumor dissemination.

The incidence of port site metastases is unknown. Laparoscopies for endometrial and general surgical malignancies have less than 1% port site metastases, similar to laparotomy. Ovarian tumors being intraperitoneal presumably have a higher incidence of spread.[122]

Implantation metastases from unsuspected cancer may be at the port sites or abdominal wall and may be related to the laparoscopy and tumor aggressiveness.[108]

Although thought to be rare, laparoscopy port sites may show upward of 16% metastases,[123] however, these are usually advanced cases with ascites.[124] Interestingly recurrent ovarian cancer may appear in port sites or operative incision prior to the initial cancer surgery.[125] There were 3 cases reported with apparent intraperitoneal spill in which occult low malignant potential cancer was removed by laparoscopy (2 oophorectomies, 1 cystectomy) in whom within 3 weeks re-exploration found tumor implantation at the port site and intraperitoneal tumor spread. It was suggested that at surgical staging at the port site should be excised in a full-thickness fashion. In addition care should be taken to avoid spillage even though the cyst appears grossly benign. The apparent increased risk of cancer metastases in port sites compared to laparotomy incision might be related to pneumoperitoneal pressure, carbon dioxide environment, or lack of port site irrigation.[126]

XVI. CONCERNS WITH PSO

A. Discovery of Occult Carcinoma

Although previously considered by some to be a "complication" early discovery of occult carcinoma can only be helpful. It cannot be detected by surveillance just as stage I is usually not detected clinically. Essentially all series of PSO for BRCA1/2 mutation carriers report discovery of occult carcinoma rates from 1.7–17% in the ovary and fallopian tube. Rarely occult carcinoma is found to be primary peritoneal (separate from the tube which is also considered part of primary peritoneal) and presumed primary peritoneal because of positive washings. I believe the higher incidence is more reliable. The tenfold difference is probably related to:

1. Serial sections of all tissue removed by experienced pathologists; overlooking microscopic cancer may explain subsequent peritoneal cancer
2. Whether all the cases are BRCA1/2 mutation carriers
3. Age—PSO may precede the development of occult cancer since it is done before most cancer develops, in addition BRCA2 mutation carriers develop cancer later than BRCA1, primary peritoneal cancer also develops later
4. Careful inspection and washings of the peritoneum for primary peritoneal cancer
5. Parity
6. Previous OCs, tubal ligation, or even any contraception
7. Strong family history especially of unusual BRCA1/2 mutations

In compiling 10 recent series of PSO there were 33 cases of occult ovarian and tubal cancers in 945 cases.[8, 76, 80, 91, 97, 102, 127–130] These were not detected by ultrasound. In 2/4 cases occult cancer of one series there were microscopic multiple poorly differentiated surface cancers on both ovaries and peritoneum.[97] This might be due to metastases or to two separate simultaneous primary ovarian carcinomas. Molecular testing was not done for unifocal or multifocal origin. In one case 5 died of abdominal carcinometastasis within a 4-year follow-up.[129] Series with high percent of occult carcinoma of 8,[129] 12,[97] and 17% [130] are explained by serial sectioning of the ovary and tube, avoiding specimen bruising, and limited study cases to BRCA1/2 mutation carriers rather than only family history. "No case of occult carcinoma at the time of PO has been reported in any BRCA-negative patient, even though there may have been a significant risk as assessed by family history."[129] Of the highest series of 5/30 (17%) occult cancer, 1 had gross primary peritoneal carcinoma, 3 had peritoneal carcinoma, 3 had primary fallopian tube malignancy (2 *in situ* and 1 early invasion), and 1 ovarian. (These could easily be overlooked.) Three had BRCA1 mutations, one had a BRCA2 mutation, and 1 was not tested. "The high rate of occult malignancy... is relatively common." In most the cancer was not recognized at the time of surgery. "Laparoscopy or laparotomy are the surgical modalities of choice to allow inspection of the peritoneal surfaces at the time of prophylactic oophorectomy...."[130]

After this chapter was written a new paper appeared.[130a] In 30 women with mutations of BRCA1, BRCA2, or a suggestive family history had prophylactic oophorectomy. Five (17%) had clinically occult malignancy. Four of the five were found only on histology. One had a grossly apparent primary peritoneal carcinoma. Three had primary fallopian tube malignancy. Three of the 5 were BRCA1 mutation carriers, one had a BRCA2 mutation, and one was not tested. Recalculation showed that in this small series 21% of BRCA carriers and 33% of BRCA2 carriers had malignant findings.

The mean age was 46. It was emphasized that:

1. The fallopian tubes and ovaries should be serially sectioned and be evaluated by an expert oncology gynecologic pathologist
2. Laparoscopy and/or laparotomy should be used to inspect peritoneal surface and do peritoneal washing
3. BRCA1 and BRCA2 mutation carrier may be at increased risk for tubal cancers
4. BRCA1 and BRCA2 mutation carriers should be offered the option of bilateral salpingoophorectomy. The recommendation for simultaneous hysterectomy was not explained

Discovery of an occult stage I ovarian carcinoma suggests a prompt gynecologic oncology consultation and traditional surgical staging including hysterectomy, omentectomy, and pelvic and para-aortic node sampling.[91]

With stage I carcinoma the most powerful prognostic indicator of disease-free survival is the degree of differentiation (grade) which should be used in deciding therapy. The important factors are rupture before and during surgery and age. "None of the following were of prognostic value: histological type, dense adhesions, extracapsular growth, ascites, FIGO stage 1988, and size of tumor."[131] Not all would agree on the lesser factors. Grade would be the clue to biologic aggressiveness. Avoiding rupture is critical.

If primary occult ovarian cancer (which is unifocal) is treated and cured it is not known how this would affect the chance of later primary peritoneal cancer which is multifocal.

Of interest are 35 reproductive-age women of the general population with stage IA or IC ovarian carcinoma who wished to retain fertility, 18 had unilateral adnexectomy and 17 had adjuvant chemotherapy. The differentiation was 31 cases of grade 1, 10 grade 2, and 3 grade 3. Median follow-up was 67.5 months. Four had recurrences 8–78 months later—in the contralateral ovary (2), contralateral ovary and tube (1), and lung (1). Eight had subsequent contralateral oophorectomy and hysterectomy. At present 43 are without evidence of disease and 1 died after 97 months. The disease-free survival rate was 95.2% at 5 years and 86.3% at 10 years. Twelve patients had 16 normal deliveries without anomalies. "The long-term survival of patients with stage IA and IC epithelial ovarian cancer treated with unilateral adnexectomy is excellent."[132]

After this chapter was written the complete paper was published.[132a] There were now 52 women with stage I epithelial ovarian cancer, 42 with stage IA, and 10 with stage IC cancers. Twenty had adjuvant chemotherapy. Eight cases had second-look laparotomies and all were negative. The median follow-up was 68 months. Five had tumors recurrence (contralateral ovary (3), peritoneum (1), and lung (1). Fifty were alive without disease, 2 died of disease (13 and 97 months after initial treatment). The estimated survival was 98% at 5 years and 93% at 10 years.

Of 24 who attempted pregnancy 17 conceived and of these there were 26 term deliveries (without congenital anomalies) and 5 had spontaneous abortions. The original conclusion was verified and in addition "Fertility-sparing surgery should be considered as a treatment option in women with Stage I epithelial ovarian cancer who desire further child bearing."

Among 25 premenopausal women with breast cancer of the general population, therapeutic prophylactic laparoscopic oophorectomies were done. Twelve women (32%) were found to have breast micrometastases. It was apparently safe because at a mean follow-up of 38.1 months none developed metastases of the abdominal wall or at the puncture sites.[133] Although they were from the general population, the premenopausal selection probably indicated an increased hereditary risk.

B. Discovery of Ovarian Preneoplastic Dysplasia

Not all investigators have agreed that there is such a thing as dysplasia. These are putative preneoplastic histologic changes of ovarian surface epithelium on the geographic surface but usually in inclusion cysts which originate on the surface. Dysplasia may be independent, close to carcinoma, or occasionally found to be evolving into carcinoma. A recent retrospective slide review from a leading institution of 33 cases of PO for BRCA1/2 mutation carriers did not find any histologic evidence of an ovarian precursor lesion.[134] The report was flawed because:

1. Only "one to six H&E stained slides were available from each case" (divided among two ovaries)
2. The slides came from "several" institutions without any special handling to avoid bruising and questions as to where to take the sections from
3. The fallopian tubes were not removed or examined
4. There was no record of the pathology report of the original hospital

5. There was no clinical information such as
   - Parity, OC use, or tubal ligation
   - Inspection of the peritoneal cavity or of peritoneal cytology washings
   - Subsequent clinical history

The chance of ovarian epithelial dysplasia being reported may depend on experience of the pathologist (who has not been trained to identify it and whose focus is usually "cancer or no cancer"), the use of new technology, serial sections, BRCA1/2 mutation carriers, risk selection factors, and age of the patient. Reports vary from none [134] to 77.6%.[128] The latter might be related to patient selections (Ashekenazi Jewish Israeli women) with strong family history, mean age of 51.2 which is older than other series and closer to the time of cancer, expert pathologist, and novel morphometric analysis. In addition there were 3 with dysplasia who had no recognized BRCA mutations, suggesting an undiagnosed rare mutation. This phenomenon was also noticed in California Jewish women who developed ovarian cancer.[14] One series found 23/26 with "benign atypical histologic alterations."[91]

A report of no cancer precursors [135] was followed by another from the same group [135a] which eloquently described and named dysplasia evolving into cancer in ovarian inclusion cysts and indicated it is short lived before it evolves into cancer. Therefore, timing may be critical. The practical application is that finding microscopic dysplasia may be a clue to adjacent microscopic occult cancer. Removal of the ovary with dysplasia should be curative. It is not known whether dysplasia has implications regarding possible later primary peritoneal cancer. Our ongoing study has found that without (before) dysplasia, there is an apparent increase in the number of inclusion cysts, and even more prominent is that they tend to occur in clusters. The inclusion cyst lining cells have a relatively large nucleus and a relatively small cytoplasmic volume which suggests that they are young cells and presumably are proliferating. Some inclusion cysts show pseudostratification and overgrowth. This proliferation may be the first histologic stage of carcinogenesis between normal and dysplasia. This provides histologic accord of increased proliferation of surface epithelial cells to match our finding of the grossly visible "brain-like" surface of the ovary due to increased surface area. Histologic mitoses were not observed.

C. Premature Menopause Problems, Hot Flashes, HRT

There are conflicting theories about HRT further increasing the risk of breast cancer in BRCA1/2 mutation carriers which is already increased above the general population. These are the women who have had surgical menopause with PO or PSO, often premenopausal, and complain of hot flashes. To begin with such women may have a 50% reduced risk for breast cancer,[4, 78] which would reduce the risk close to that of the general population.

In the general population there are conflicting reports. A meta-analysis indicated a relative risk of breast cancer with HRT of 1.35 for women who took HRT for 5 or more years after menopause. After discontinuation the excess risk disappeared within 5 years. Since the cancers were less advanced it is possible that the excess risk was the result of increased detection.[136]

Some report no effect, while others report a slight effect, which increases with duration of years of use and with an OR of 1.24 at 5 years.[137] Despite the traditional concept that estrogen is the culprit (as with the endometrium), some suggest that it was the progestin of HRT.[138] "These data refute the notion that progestins are protective against breast cancer development and, in fact, suggest that progestins may substantially increase the small ERT (estrogen replacement therapy) related increase in breast cancer risk."[137] Combined estrogen/progestin (HRT) is associated with greater increase in breast cancer than estrogen alone (ERT). The relative risk increased by 0.08 per year for the former, and 0.01 per year with the latter.[139] Others have agreed.[140]

The data studies to date are retrospective and may be biased by patient recall. Until unequivocal data from ongoing long-term trials are completed, "... we will likely continue to see data and debate on both sides of the battle."[137]

There is no consensus on HRT for high-risk women with intact breasts. An expert opinion is "...if HRT is to be used, we believe that progesterone should be avoided if possible," "...because the progesterone component significantly increases breast cancer risk."[5] Gynecologists recommend progestin as part of HRT to reduce the chance of estrogen stimulation of endometrial cancer. There is great variation in customary practice regarding HRT for high-risk women without PO and especially after PO with surgical menopause. Some avoid HRT completely, some prescribe it for a few months varying up to 5 years. Some use progestin at 3-month intervals. Most feel that it is relatively safe to use HRT for hot flashes for a short time. The dose is less than that of physiologic estrogen. It is often routinely prescribed immediately at surgery even before hot flashes appear. General menopausal issues should be addressed including hot flashes, vaginal atrophy, psychological aspects, osteoporosis, routine mammography, clinical examination, BSE, family history of hypertension, cardiovascular problems, diabetes, malignancy, serum lipids, cardiac status, weight, lifestyle, exercise, colonoscopy, etc.

The in-progress Women's Health Initiative study of HRT (estrogen and progestin) in the general population suggests a slight increase in the risk of heart attacks, strokes, and blood clots which begins immediately and a slight risk of breast cancer which appears at about 4 years of HRT. It is possible that women with vascular complications have a predisposing undiagnosed factor. Estrogen-only HRT is still being studied.

XVII. PRIMARY PERITONEAL SEROUS CARCINOMA (PPSC) ALSO REFERRED TO AS PRIMARY PERITONEAL CARCINOMA (PPC) AND PRIMARY FALLOPIAN TUBE CARCINOMA (PFTC) ALSO REFERRED TO AS FALLOPIAN TUBE CARCINOMA (FTC)

There is no known method to reduce the risk of PPC. Research therapeutic suggestions include short-term progestin (which apparently is the active ingredient of OC and has a direct effect by apoptosis of abnormal cells), however, it might stimulate breast cancer and vitamin A and its derivative retinoids.[141] Surveillance for primary peritoneal cancer is the same as for ovarian cancer: (1) serum CA125; (2) for ovarian surveillance usually only transvaginal ultrasound is done, but one should consider abdominal and pelvic ultrasound in addition to check for ascites, masses and (even though not ideal) for pancreatic tumors; and (3) clinical history and examination, alerting patients to possible symptoms and signs. Some recommend surveillance at 6 month intervals or annually. Some do not recommend any screening at all,[5] probably because primary peritoneal cancer is infrequent and because it is usually diagnosed first clinically (before screening discovers it) because of ascites and an abdominal mass. Nevertheless, the prepared patient understands the unreducible risk and having gone through PSO probably would wish screening at least initially for emotional reasons. Since the peritoneum is more potent than ovarian cancer in elevating serum CA125, theoretically it might be a better indication for early cancer.

Usual risk estimates of primary peritoneal cancer in BRCA1/2 mutation carriers varies from about 3–4% but some go from 0–10%. "Prophylactic oophorectomy will prevent the development of an ovarian cancer and reduce the incidence of breast carcinoma, but will not prevent the subsequent development of primary peritoneal cancer, histologically indistinguishable from epithelial ovarian cancer." A report of 6/234 (1.8%) who had PO for a strong family history developed PPC 1, 2, 5, 13, 15, and 27 years later.[142] Since these cases did not have BRCA1/2 testing, because of 50% inheritance risk, the true incidence might be twice 1.8 or 3.6%. It does show that PPC may appear many years later.

In a group of 248 who had PO for BRCA1/2 mutations, only one (0.4%) developed PPC. This suggested that PO reduces the risk of PPC,[76] however, the observation time may have been too short. Similarly, in another report of 98 who had PSO there was only one later PPC, however, the follow-up was only a mean of 24.2 months. Among 72 under surveillance ovarian cancer developed in 4 and 1 developed PPC,[80] thus PSO did not reduce the incidence of PPC. The overall statistics were misleading regarding PPC (because ovarian and PPC were lumped together) in that the HR after risk-reducing PSO was 0.15 for ovarian fallopian tube or primary peritoneal cancer.

A retrospective study of 259 BRCA mutation carriers found that two developed papillary serous peritoneal cancers at 3.8 and 8.6 years after surgery, with an average follow-up of 8.2 years. Strangely "no cases of papillary serous peritoneal cancer were diagnosed in controls with intact ovaries."[102] This suggests that PO increases the chance of later PPC. Yet the overall conclusion was "the HR for cancer of the coelomic epithelium after prophylactic oophorectomy was 0.04%."[102] Obviously these data from reduction of ovarian cancer hid the facts of peritoneal cancer. Therefore these reports are misleading regarding PO reducing PPC. Perhaps this may be part of the reason that one institution refers to "risk-reducing salpingo-oophorectomy" while most use the traditional "prophylactic" surgery. Theoretically if there is no occult carcinoma in a removed ovary with no microscopic spread there should not be later new ovarian carcinoma. Risk-reduction salpingo-oophorectomy would be applicable to risk reduction for later breast carcinoma but not for PPC. Of course all agree that PO should be done or seriously considered because of the dramatic reduction of subsequent ovarian cancer and reduction of breast cancer. A prospective study of 8 cases of ovarian/peritoneal cancer in Jewish women revealed 6 to be primary peritoneal which would have not been prevented by prophylactic oophorectomy.[14] There is a suggestion that PO might reduce the incidence of later primary papillary serous peritoneal cancer in high-risk families,[12] but even if correct it would still be greater than in the general population. There is no reliable long-term data.

It is not known whether the risk of peritoneal cancer is affected by OCs, or tubal ligation.[5] Personal speculation is that if these cancers are part of the same syndrome then OCs might also reduce risk as with ovarian cancer since there should be a similar risk reduction by apoptosis of abnormal cells.

Later peritoneal carcinomatosis is not a complication of prophylactic surgery but is actually the biologic history of the BRCA mutant woman. It is known to occur later than primary ovarian cancers. The incidence of later peritoneal carcinomatosis depends on age and length of follow-up. The reported incidence varies from 0.6% (16 months follow-up) to 10.7% and probably is about 3.8% (12 of 380 cases).

PSPC, also called PPC tends to appear at about 63.8 years of age (versus ovarian cancer of 55), has a later onset of menarche (13.3 versus 12.8), and is not related to parity, OCs or hormone use.[143] Whereas papillary serous ovarian carcinoma (PSOC), also called epithelial carcinoma, is uniclonal from 1 cancer cell, PSPC is multiclonal, each different and multicentric because of a field effect.

Although PSPC and PSOC are histologically similar and have similar 80% overexpression of p53 and contain shared genetic events on 4 chromosome arms, there are molecular differences. LOH occurs less frequently in PSPC on 4 chromosome arms compared to PSOC on 18 chromosome arms with higher median LOH frequency. The highest frequency of loss was in the BRCA1 area. The lower LOH frequencies of PSPC compared to PSOC suggest a reduced tendency toward carcinogenesis. "In addition, PSPC may be a more homogeneous malignancy with fewer carcinogenic pathways than PSOC."[144] Nevertheless PSPC is still polyclonal, suggesting that the relatively huge surface is the reason it starts many individual polyclonal cancers simultaneously but with less individual variation than between individual PSOC. PSPC has occurred after PO for BRCA mutations and PSPC cases may have germline mutations. "To date, germline BRCA2 mutations have not been identified in PSPC."[144]

Among Ashkenazi Jewish (AJ) women with PPC having BRCA founder mutations (41%) is similar in incidence of mutation in AJ patients with epithelial ovarian cancer. The incidence of mutations in AJ cases with FTC is lower (18%) than in AJ cases with epithelial ovarian cancer (EOC) (40%) but similar to the reported incidence of all cases with FTC. Women with BRCA founder mutations had a lower mean age of 61 versus 70 for both cancers.[145] This confirms that PPC is part of the hereditary ovarian cancer syndrome (HOCS). The small number of cases could have underrated the BRCA mutation incidence of FTC. Most believe that PTC is part of the HOCS. "... an estimated 7–15% of all cases of PSOC could be reclassified as PSPC."[144]

Since tubal cancer is now considered to be part of the BRCA mutation syndrome along with ovarian and breast cancer, presumably the risk is greater than in the general population. It is uncertain if primary peritoneal cancer risk is increased with BRCA mutation. It is unknown whether tubal cancer is more common than primary peritoneal cancer. Some consider tubal cancer to be part of primary peritoneal cancer. This raises the question of whether a unit area of tubal epithelium has a higher risk than the same unit area of peritoneum. If it did it might be related to proximity to the ovary with its stromal stimulation and/or embryologic proximity, and/or "incessant" tubal changes related to ovulation. Even if it did the total risk would increase with peritoneal cancer because of the vastly larger surface area. There is speculation that the incidence of tubal carcinoma has been underestimated, as well as primary peritoneal carcinoma, and attributed to ovarian cancer because all have ovarian histology.

A. What Is the Site of Origin of FTC? Implications for Hysterectomy

Although the uterus is a Müllerian derivative of the embryonic coelomic cavity "...the relative risk of this (endometrial) malignancy in BRCA mutation carriers is not significantly elevated over that of the general population."[5] This might be expected because the endometrium is thicker and glandular and therefore with unique specialization and different from the single cuboidal cell layer of the surface peritoneum. Correspondingly the inner layer of its extension in the fallopian tube might also not have the predisposition to malignancy, and BRCA-associated FTC might originate from the peritoneum covering of the outer tube. Logically the uterine serosal peritoneal surface should have the same BRCA-associated increased risk of primary peritoneal cancer as the general peritoneum. The site of origin of FTC should be carefully investigated histologically. If the above deductive reasoning is correct it cancels the rationale for hysterectomy to remove the intramural tube because that tubal segment has no serosa. It may also be possible that PFTC which forms in the endosalpinx lining might not be related to BRCA mutation but might be associated with chronic endosalpingitis. A theory about ovarian cancer risk reduction of tubal ligation is that it prevents ascent of carcinogens from the vagina and uterus.

What is the risk of primary FTC? Theoretical calculations indicate that the relative risk for primary tubal carcinoma is increased in BRCA1/2 mutation carriers, however, the absolute lifetime risk is low, perhaps 3–5%. In the general population the absolute lifetime risk of primary tubal carcinoma is about 0.0246%.[146]

Tubal carcinoma would be more readily identified than general peritoneal carcinoma especially because of serial sectioning of PSO specimens. General peritoneal primary carcinomas may be multifocal, in different stages, each with a different genome, and difficult to visualize in an early stage.

B. Speculation about Peritoneal Carcinogenesis

Whereas there is a theory of "incessant ovulation" with consequent repetitive repair being the mechanism of ovarian carcinoma, "no comparable model has been described to account for the development of PSPC."[144]

Why should the peritoneum produce a primary carcinoma although usually later than ovarian carcinoma? Ovarian carcinoma derives from surface epithelial coelemic serosa similar to peritoneum, however, the ovarian serosa is directly affected by stromal growth factors. This would make carcinoma develop faster.

Traditionally peritoneal lining was assumed to have very little physiologic activity and was mainly a placid lining analogous to the putative inactivity of the thin endothelium. The latter is now understood to have vital regulatory functions including nitric oxide secretion to relax arteriole muscle walls and affecting the coagulation process. Deductive reasoning suggests that the peritoneum should secrete (or by passive transfer) peritoneal fluid and lubricating substances to maintain a smooth "Teflon" nonadhesive surface to permit intestinal motility. Significant adhesions could be fatal. Thus all animals with coelomic or peritoneal cavities have had such nonadhesive surfaces since early in evolution. In addition surgical or accidental trauma heals rapidly and within hours a protective adhesion forms to cover any raw surface followed by rapid cell repair. Therefore there must be a continuous, alert, life-long stimulation of the peritoneum, which has not been appreciated because of its apparently simple sleepy one-cell lining. The peritoneum has to remain vigorous. It performs a vital role just as does the cardiovascular pulmonary and renal systems. Possibly the constant stimulation and self-repair from unrecognized trauma increases the risk of malignancy analogous to the theory of "incessant ovulation." It is also interesting that peritoneum reaction produces more CA125 than ovarian epithelial carcinoma.

XVIII. THE NEW REPORT OF ESTROGEN WITH PROGESTIN HRT (EPHRT) SHOWING RISKS EXCEEDING BENEFITS

Since preparation of this chapter a report of a large trial of healthy women aged 50–79 taking conjugated equine estrogen 0.625 mg and medroxyprogesterone acetate 2.5 mg daily was discontinued after 5.2 years because the health risks exceeded the benefits.[147] The HR (relative risk, normal baseline 1.00) was coronary heart disease (CHD) 1.29, breast cancer 1.26, stroke 1.4, pulmonary embolism (PE) 2.13, while colorectal cancer was reduced to 0.63, endometrial cancer 0.83, hip fracture 0.66, and death due to other causes 0.92.

The absolute excess risks per 10,000 person-years were 7 more CHD events, 8 more strokes, 8 more PE, 8 more invasive breast cancers, 6 fewer colorectal cancers, and 5 fewer hip fractures. The absolute excess risks of the global index was 19 per 10,000. However "all-cause mortality was not affected during the trial." The conclusion was that it was not "... a viable intervention for primary prevention of chronic disease..." and it should not be used for primary prevention of CHD.

The cumulative HR for breast cancer increased at 4 years. There was no increase of *in situ* breast cancer. The risk of CHD and stroke began soon after beginning EPHRT. The risk of stroke increased between 1 and 2 years. "This trial did not address short-term risks and benefits of hormones for the treatment of menopausal symptoms." A parallel trial of only estrogen in women with a previous hysterectomy is being continued until March 2005 with an 8.5 year follow-up.

The companion editorial [148] observed that 38% of postmenopausal women in the U.S. use HRT. The original HRT was the estrogen Premarin which apparently reduced the risk of cardiovascular disease. HRT has been FDA approved for relief of menopausal symptoms and prevention of osteoporosis. Progestin was added to prevent estrogen-induced endometrial carcinoma. There were suggestions that both hormones together might increase the chance of breast cancer with long-term use and that there was an increased risk of CHD in the first year. Both adverse effects were attributed to progestin. It was noted that the risk for stroke and venous thromboembolism continued through the 5-year trial, while increased coronary artery disease was largely limited to the first year. Although "...the absolute risk of harm to an individual woman is very small," when accumulated over the 5.2 years the excess number of events was 100 per 10,000 or 1%. Since the purpose "...is to preserve health and prevent disease," "...we recommend that clinicians stop prescribing this combination for long-term use."

Regarding short-term use (up to one year) for menopausal symptoms the comment was that there was a suggestion that combination HRT has risks for CHD and thromboembolic disease. "The possibility of these small absolute risks must be balanced against the severity of symptoms and benefit of treatment."

The editorial did not point out that the experimental group on conjugated equine estrogens 0.625 mg with medroxyprogesterone acetate 2.5 mg daily (Prempro) did not include women with hot flashes since this would destroy the plan of unknown medication ("double-blind"). Thus the group was older than the usual early menopausal woman who might have less chance of adverse cardiovascular incidents. The mean age at initial screening was 63.2 which is at least 10 years older than the usual age of menopause. In practice most HRT is prescribed for hot flashes of early menopause.

Apparently progestin is the culprit regarding the increase in CHD, stroke, PE, and breast cancer. Since PSO is recommended over age 35 and after childbearing is completed, a significant percent of candidates will still be premenopausal. This has the advantage of being done before the small chance of the development of occult cancer and to obtain the greatest risk reduction in later breast cancer, especially in those with BRCA1 (as opposed to BRCA2 mutations which may cause cancer later) gene mutations. The disadvantage is the high probability of surgical menopause causing hot flashes which can be very distressful. Automatic start of estrogen with progestin HRT (EPHRT) with prophylactic surgery has been used for hot flashes effectively, and makes the surgery more acceptable. The study did not determine whether those who developed breast cancer had BRCA1/2 mutations or a family history of hereditary breast/ovarian cancer. Thus it is unknown whether such women with an inherent breast cancer risk (although reduced by 50% by PSO) would have further increased (and by what magnitude) risk from EPHRT. Previous reports focused on BRCA1/2 mutations suggested that reduction of later breast cancer risk was not diminished by EPHRT.[4, 5, 78–80] The study showed that breast cancer with EPHRT increased at 4 years, although cardio-circulatory complications started immediately. The increased risk of EPHRT above the control group is relatively small. The estrogen-only trial continues and presumably has not had dramatic adverse events. Prior to the addition of progestin to EHRT, in order to prevent unopposed estrogen stimulation causing endometrial cancer, estrogen alone apparently had less adverse effects regarding vascular problems and breast cancer. In fact it was thought to have a possible beneficial effect on prevention of coronary artery problems. Previous studies have suggested that the addition of progestin to EHRT was associated with increase of breast cancer in the general population.[5]

Progestin has an adverse effect on serum lipids. Progestin added to estrogen in combination may cause bleeding and mood disturbances. Thus progestin should be avoided. The danger of endometrial cancer may be monitored by bleeding, transvaginal ultrasound to test for endometrial thickening, and endometrial biopsy.

Estrogen has been used to prevent or treat hot flashes (and sometimes associated emotional disturbances). It has also been considered the first choice to prevent osteoporosis. It tends to improve lipid profile. It was thought to possibly help retard CHD and Alzheimer's disease.

The most effective treatment for hot flashes is estrogen. It might be of benefit for associated disturbances, and possibly theoretically by helping endothelium, circulation, and serum lipids. Unfortunately it might predispose to venous thrombosis which might be related to the first passage (when taken orally) through the liver with stimulation of thrombogenic factors. Thus a tendency to thrombosis might be a contraindication such as history (or family history) of PE, thrombophlebitis, smoking, etc. Although up to the present EPHRT has been the "gold standard" or first-line therapy to prevent osteoporosis, with the new report its chronic use for such purpose is now contraindicated.

How might the new report affect clinical practice or what to do? The physician might consider:

1. Patient education
2. Discussion of options
3. Patient participation in decision making
4. Customized individualization
5. Why is the patient considering HRT?
6. Avoiding progestin
7. If estrogen is to be used, use the lowest dose
8. Do not use chronic EPHRT to prevent or treat osteoporosis or CHD

Dr. Nathan Kase (personal communication) has suggested that if estrogen is to be used it should be as a transdermal skin patch of estradiol. This will bypass the liver which might be stimulated to produce thrombogenic factors by "first pass" estrogen. Thus there would be a risk reduction while maintaining benefit.

Most physicians feel that if there are no contraindications that estrogen should be prescribed for disturbing hot flashes. The main reason for EHRT is to prevent or treat hot flashes. It might be started with prophylactic surgical menopause to prevent it or wait and see whether hot flashes develop and then treat. Once begun it might be gradually reduced and discontinued after several months with the hope that hot flashes will stop, or continued (in part pending the later expected report in progress). Some women just feel better with EHRT and insist on continuing especially if there are emotional disturbances with hot flashes. Flexible individualization is important with concern for strong preferences of the patient and her medical background with risk factors for CHD, stroke, PE, and breast cancer. Risk factors for osteoporosis might suggest consideration of bisphosphonates as well as vitamins, calcium, and exercise. Menopause gives the opportunity to improve lifestyle and general health including weight, smoking, alcohol, exercise, control of blood pressure, recreational drugs, serum lipids, routine mammography, BSE, possible breast MRI or ultrasound, routine eye examination, routine colonoscopy, thyroid tests, and blood chemistries.

XIX. THE MOOT CONCERN OF EHRT AND INCREASE OF OVARIAN CANCER

A new study reported that women who used estrogen-only hormone replacement therapy especially for 10 or more years had a significantly increase risk of ovarian cancer with a rate ratio of 1.8. However "...much of the long-term ERT use likely included higher average daily doses of estrogen than what is currently recommended." Another problem was that in 29% of the cohort family history was unavailable. Of the available 71%, "...one quarter of women who developed ovarian cancer reported breast or ovarian cancer in first-degree relatives."[149] Furthermore the type of ovarian cancer was not specified.

The accompanying editorial observed that "... the association between estrogen use and ovarian cancer should be worrisome enough for clinicians to consider carefully whether to suggest EHRT.[150]

Neither mentioned the deduction that ovarian and breast tissues react differently to estrogen and progestin. In the breast progestin promotes growth (as would be expected in pregnancy) and is thought to predispose to malignancy. In the ovary the progestin of OCs is considered the essential ingredient which reduces the later risk of ovarian epithelial cancer presumably by increasing the rate of apoptosis of cells with abnormal DNA. In general, estrogen is thought to increase endothelial cells, blood flow, and cell growth especially in the endometrium.

Since this chapter deals with PSO there are no ovaries and there will not be subsequent ovarian cancer. The study made no mention of EHRT and later primary peritoneal epithelial carcinoma.

ADDENDUM

A retrospective hospital-based case-control study conducted in Mexico and Thailand found that Depot-Medroxyprogesterone Acetate (DMPA) for contraception did not reduce the risk of epithelial ovarian cancer in later life.[151] If valid it indicates that different progestins have different protective effects.

References

1. Tortolero-Luna, G., and Mitchell, M. F. (1995). The epidemiology of ovarian cancer. *J. Cell Biochem.* Suppl., 23, 200–207.
2. Amos, C. I., and Struewing, J. P. (1993). Genetic epidemiology of epithelial ovarian cancer. *Cancer* 71, 566–572.
3. Heintz, A. P., Hacker, N. F., and Lagasse, L. D. (1985). Epidemiology and etiology of ovarian cancer: A review. *Obstet. Gynecol.* 66, 127–135.
4. Eisen, A., Rebbeck, T. R., Wood, W. C., and Weber, B. L. (2000). Prophylactic surgery in women with a hereditary predisposition to breast and ovarian cancer. *J. Clin. Oncol.* 18, 1980–1995.
5. Narod, S. A., and Boyd, J. (2002). Current understanding of the epidemiology and clinical implications of BRCA1 and BRCA2 mutations for ovarian cancer. *Curr. Opin. Obstet. Gynecol.* 14, 19–26.
6. American Medical Association CME Advisory Committee. Identifying and managing hereditary risk for breast and ovarian cancer (2001).
7. Kerlikowske, K., Brown, J. S., and Grady, D. G. (1992). Should women with familial ovarian cancer undergo prophylactic oophorectomy? *Obstet. Gynecol.* 80, 700–707.
8. Scheuer, L., Kauff, N., Robson, M., Kelly, B., Barakat, R., Satagopan, J. *et al.* (2002). Outcome of preventive surgery and screening for breast and ovarian cancer in BRCA mutation carriers. *J. Clin. Oncol.* 20, 1260–1268.
9. Risch, H. A., McLaughlin, J. R., Cole, D. E., Rosen, B., Bradley, L., Kwan, E. *et al.* (2001). Prevalence and penetrance of germline BRCA1 and BRCA2 mutations in a population series of 649 women with ovarian cancer. *Am. J. Hum. Genet.* 68, 700–710.
10. Burstein, H. J., and Winer, E. P. (2000). Primary care for survivors of breast cancer. *N. Engl. J. Med.* 343, 1086–1094.
11. Schilder, J. M., and Holladay, D. V. (2001). Hereditary ovarian cancer: Clinical syndromes and management. *In*: "Ovarian Cancer," (S. C. Rubin and G. P. Sutton), pp. 181–200. Lippincott Williams & Wilkins, Philadelphia, PA.
12. Struewing, J. P., Hartge, P., Wacholder, S., Baker, S. M., Berlin, M., McAdams, M. *et al.* (1997). The risk of cancer associated with specific mutations of BRCA1 and BRCA2 among Ashkenazi Jews. *N. Engl. J. Med.* 336, 1401–1408.
13. Ford, D., Easton, D. F., Stratton, M., Narod, S., Goldgar, D., Devilee, P. *et al.* (1998). Genetic heterogeneity and penetrance analysis of the BRCA1 and BRCA2 genes in breast cancer families. The Breast Cancer Linkage Consortium. *Am. J. Hum. Genet.* 62, 676–689.
14. Liede, A., Karlan, B. Y., Baldwin, R. L., Platt, L. D., Kuperstein, G., and Narod, S. A. (2002). Cancer incidence in a population of Jewish women at risk of ovarian cancer. *J. Clin. Oncol.* 20, 1570–1577.
15. Cancer risks in BRCA2 mutation carriers.The Breast Cancer Linkage Consortium. (1999). *J. Natl. Cancer Inst.* 91, 1310–1316.
16. Malkin, D., Li, F. P., Strong, L. C., Fraumeni, J. F., Jr., Nelson, C. E., Kim, D. H. *et al.* (1990). Germ line p53 mutations in a familial syndrome of breast cancer, sarcomas, and other neoplasms. *Science* 250, 1233–1238.
17. Salovaara, R., Loukola, A., Kristo, P., Kaariainen, H., Ahtola, H., Eskelinen, M. *et al.* (2000). Population-based molecular detection of hereditary nonpolyposis colorectal cancer. *J. Clin. Oncol.* 18, 2193–2200.
18. Brown, G. J., St John, D. J., Macrae, F. A., and Aittomaki, K. (2001). Cancer risk in young women at risk of hereditary nonpolyposis colorectal cancer: Implications for gynecologic surveillance. *Gynecol. Oncol.* 80, 346–349.
19. Statement of the American Society of Clinical Oncology: Genetic testing for cancer susceptibility, Adopted on February 20, 1996. (1996). *J. Clin. Oncol.* 14, 1730–1736.
20. Smith, S. A., Richards, W. E., Caito, K., Hanjani, P., Markman, M., DeGeest, K. *et al.* (2001). BRCA1 germline mutations and polymorphisms in a clinic-based series of ovarian cancer cases: A Gynecologic Oncology Group study. *Gynecol. Oncol.* 83, 586–592.
21. Schoumacher, F., Glaus, A., Mueller, H., Eppenberger, U., Bolliger, B., and Senn, H. J. (2001). BRCA1/2 mutations in Swiss patients with familial or early-onset breast and ovarian cancer. *Swiss. Med. Wkly.* 131, 223–226.
22. Schorge, J. O., Mahoney, N. M., Miller, D. S., Coleman, R. L., Muller, C. Y., Euhus, D. M. *et al.* (2001). Germline BRCA1-2 mutations in non-Ashkenazi families with double primary breast and ovarian cancer. *Gynecol. Oncol.* 83, 383–387.
23. Geisler, J. P., Hatterman-Zogg, M. A., Rathe, J. A., and Buller, R. E. (2002). Frequency of BRCA1 dysfunction in ovarian cancer. *J. Natl. Cancer Inst.* 94, 61–67.
24. Berry, D. A., Parmigiani, G., Sanchez, J., Schildkraut, J., and Winer, E. (1997). Probability of carrying a mutation of breast-ovarian cancer gene BRCA1 based on family history. *J. Natl. Cancer Inst.* 89, 227–238.
25. Li, A. J., Cass, L., and Karlan, B. Y. (2001). BRCA1 and BRCA2: Genetic testing and intervention strategies. *Contemp. OB/GYN,* 83–95.
26. Lerman, C., Hughes, C., Croyle, R. T., Main, D., Durham, C., Snyder, C. *et al.* (2000). Prophylactic surgery decisions and surveillance practices one year following BRCA1/2 testing. *Prev. Med.* 31, 75–80.
27. Meijers-Heijboer, E. J., Verhoog, L. C., Brekelmans, C. T., Seynaeve, C., Tilanus-Linthorst, M. M., Wagner, A. *et al.* (2000). Presymptomatic DNA testing and prophylactic surgery in families with a BRCA1 or BRCA2 mutation. *Lancet* 355, 2015–2020.
28. Fisher, B., Costantino, J. P., Wickerham, D. L., Redmond, C. K., Kavanah, M., Cronin, W. M. *et al.* (1998). Tamoxifen for prevention of breast cancer: Report of the National Surgical Adjuvant Breast and Bowel Project P-1 Study. *J. Natl. Cancer Inst.* 90, 1371–1388.
29. Narod, S. A., Brunet, J. S., Ghadirian, P., Robson, M., Heimdal, K., Neuhausen, S. L. *et al.* (2000). Tamoxifen and risk of contralateral breast cancer in BRCA1 and BRCA2 mutation carriers: A case-control study. Hereditary Breast Cancer Clinical Study Group. *Lancet* 356, 1876–1881.
30. Tamoxifen for early breast cancer: An overview of the randomised trials. Early Breast Cancer Trialists' Collaborative Group. (1998). *Lancet* 351, 1451–1467.
31. Bentrem, D. J., and Jordan, V. C. (2002). Role of antiestrogens and aromatase inhibitors in breast cancer treatment. *Curr. Opin. Obstet. Gynecol.* 14, 5–12.
32. Hartmann, L. C., Schaid, D. J., Woods, J. E., Crotty, T. P., Myers, J. L., Arnold, P. G. *et al.* (1999). Efficacy of bilateral prophylactic mastectomy in women with a family history of breast cancer. *N. Engl. J. Med.* 340, 77–84.
33. Hartmann, L. C., Schaid, D. J., Sellers, T. A., *et al.* (2000). Bilateral prophylactic mastectomy (PM) in BRCA1/2 mutation carriers. *Proc. Am. Assoc. Cancer. Res.* 41, 222–223.
34. Andersen, M. R., Peacock, S., Nelson, J., Wilson, S., McIntosh, M., Drescher, C. *et al.* (2002). Worry about ovarian cancer risk and use of ovarian cancer screening by women at risk for ovarian cancer. *Gynecol. Oncol.* 85, 3–8.
35. Di Prospero, L. S., Seminsky, M., Honeyford, J., Doan, B., Franssen, E., Meschino, W. *et al.* (2001). Psychosocial issues following a positive result of genetic testing for BRCA1 and BRCA2 mutations: Findings from a focus group and a needs-assessment survey. *CMAJ.* 64, 1005–1009.
36. Meiser, B., Tiller, K., Gleeson, M. A., Andrews, L., Robertson, G., and Tucker, K. M. (2000). Psychological impact of prophylactic oophorectomy in women at increased risk for ovarian cancer. *Psychooncology* 9, 496–503.
37. Fry, A., Busby-Earle, C., Rush, R., and Cull, A. (2001). Prophylactic oophorectomy versus screening: Psychosocial outcomes in women at increased risk of ovarian cancer. *Psychooncology* 10, 231–241.

38. Swisher, E. M., Babb, S., Whelan, A., Mutch, D. G., and Rader, J. S. (2001). Prophylactic oophorectomy and ovarian cancer surveillance. Patient perceptions and satisfaction. *J. Reprod. Med.* 46, 87–94.
39. Petricoin, E. F., Ardekani, A. M., Hitt, B. A., Levine, P. J., Fusaro, V. A., Steinberg, S. M. *et al.* (2002). Use of proteomic patterns in serum to identify ovarian cancer. *Lancet* 359, 572–577.
40. Scully, R. E. (2000). Influence of origin of ovarian cancer on efficacy of screening. *Lancet* 355, 1028–1029.
41. Topalak, O., Saygili, U., Soyturk, M., Karaca, N., Batur, Y., Uslu, T. *et al.* (2002). Serum, pleural effusion, and ascites CA-125 levels in ovarian cancer and nonovarian benign and malignant diseases: A comparative study. *Gynecol. Oncol.* 85, 108–113.
42. Zeimet, A. G., Marth, C., Offner, F. A., Obrist, P., Uhl-Steidl, M., Feichtinger, H. *et al.* (1996). Human peritoneal mesothelial cells are more potent than ovarian cancer cells in producing tumor marker CA-125. *Gynecol. Oncol.* 62, 384–389.
43. Sjovall, K., Nilsson, B., and Einhorn, N. (2002). The significance of serum CA 125 elevation in malignant and nonmalignant diseases. *Gynecol. Oncol.* 85, 175–178.
44. DeMichele, A., and Weber, B. L. (2002). Risk management in BRCA1 and BRCA2 mutation carriers: Lessons learned, challenges posed. *J. Clin. Oncol.* 20, 1164–1166.
45. Cottreau, C. M., Ness, R. B., and Kriska, A. M. (2000). Physical activity and reduced risk of ovarian cancer. *Obstet. Gynecol.* 96, 609–614.
46. Walker, G. R., Schlesselman, J. J., and Ness, R. B. (2002). Family history of cancer, oral contraceptive use, and ovarian cancer risk. *Am. J. Obstet. Gynecol.* 186, 8–14.
47. Narod, S. A., Risch, H., Moslehi, R., Dorum, A., Neuhausen, S., Olsson, H. *et al.* (1998). Oral contraceptives and the risk of hereditary ovarian cancer. Hereditary Ovarian Cancer Clinical Study Group. *N. Engl. J. Med.* 339, 424–428.
48. Ness, R. B., Grisso, J. A., Klapper, J., Schlesselman, J. J., Silberzweig, S., Vergona, R. *et al.* (2000). Risk of ovarian cancer in relation to estrogen and progestin dose and use characteristics of oral contraceptives. SHARE Study Group. Steroid Hormones and Reproductions. *Am. J. Epidemiol.* 152, 233–241.
49. Sanderson, M., Williams, M. A., Weiss, N. S., Hendrix, N. W., and Chauhan, S. P. (2000). Oral contraceptives and epithelial ovarian cancer. Does dose matter? *J. Reprod. Med.* 45, 720–726.
50. Gnagy, S., Ming, E. E., Devesa, S. S., Hartge, P., and Whittemore, A. S. (2000). Declining ovarian cancer rates in U.S. women in relation to parity and oral contraceptive use. *Epidemiology* 11, 102–105.
51. Westhoff, C., Britton, J. A., Gammon, M. D., Wright, T., and Kelsey, J. L. (2000). Oral contraceptive and benign ovarian tumors. *Am. J. Epidemiol.* 152, 242–246.
52. Breast cancer and hormonal contraceptives: Collaborative reanalysis of individual data on 53,297 women with breast cancer and 100,239 women without breast cancer from 54 epidemiological studies. Collaborative Group on Hormonal Factors in Breast Cancer (1996). *Lancet* 347, 1713–1727.
53. Grabrick, D. M., Hartmann, L. C., Cerhan, J. R., Vierkant, R. A., Therneau, T. M., Vachon, C. M. *et al.* (2000). Risk of breast cancer with oral contraceptive use in women with a family history of breast cancer. *JAMA* 284, 1791–1798.
54. Godwin, A. K., Testa, J. R., Handel, L. M., Liu, Z., Vanderveer, L. A., Tracey, P. A. *et al.* (1992). Spontaneous transformation of rat ovarian surface epithelial cells: Association with cytogenetic changes and implications of repeated ovulation in the etiology of ovarian cancer. *J. Natl. Cancer Inst.* 84, 592–601.
55. Ness, R. B., Grisso, J. A., Vergona, R., Klapper, J., Morgan, M., and Wheeler, J. E. (2001). Oral contraceptives, other methods of contraception, and risk reduction for ovarian cancer. *Epidemiology* 12, 307–312.
56. Schildkraut, J. M., Calingaert, B., Marchbanks, P. A., Moorman, P. G., and Rodriguez, G. C. (2002). Impact of progestin and estrogen potency in oral contraceptives on ovarian cancer risk. *J. Natl. Cancer Inst.* 94, 32–38.
57. Rodriguez, G. C., Walmer, D. K., Cline, M., Krigman, H., Lessey, B. A., and Whitaker, R. S. *et al.* (1998). Effect of progestin on the ovarian epithelium of macaques: Cancer prevention through apoptosis? *J. Soc. Gynecol. Invest.* 5, 271–276.
58. Rodriguez, G. C., Nagarsheth, N. P., Lee, K. L., Bentley, R. C., Walmer, D. K., Cline, M. *et al.* (2002). Progestin-induced apoptosis in the Macaque ovarian epithelium: Differential regulation of transforming growth factor-beta. *J. Natl. Cancer Inst.* 94, 50–60.
59. Rioux, J. E., and Daris, M. (2001). Female sterilization: An update. *Curr. Opin. Obstet. Gynecol.* 13, 377–381.
60. Jamieson, D. J., Hillis, S. D., Duerr, A., Marchbanks, P. A., Costello, C., and Peterson, H. B. (2000). Complications of interval laparoscopic tubal sterilization: Findings from the United States Collaborative Review of Sterilization. *Obstet. Gynecol.* 96, 997–1002.
61. Narod, S. A., Sun, P., Ghadirian, P., Lynch, H., Isaacs, C., Garber, J. *et al.* (2001). Tubal ligation and risk of ovarian cancer in carriers of BRCA1 or BRCA2 mutations: A case-control study. *Lancet* 357, 1467–1470.
62. Narod, S., Sun, P., and Risch, H. (2002). Effects of parity and use of oral contraceptives on the risk of ovarian cancer among carriers and non-carriers of BRCA1/2. *N. Engl. J. Med.* (In Press).
63. Cornelison, T. L., Natarajan, N., Piver, M. S., and Mettlin, C. J. (1997). Tubal ligation and the risk of ovarian carcinoma. *Cancer Detect. Prev.* 21, 1–6.
64. Hankinson, S. E., Hunter, D. J., Colditz, G. A., Willett, W. C., Stampfer, M. J., Rosner, B. *et al.* (1993). Tubal ligation, hysterectomy, and risk of ovarian cancer. A prospective study. *JAMA* 270, 2813–2818.
65. Naik, R., Nordin, A., Cross, P. A., Hemming, D., de Barros, Lopes A., and Monaghan, J. M. (2000). Risk factors in stage III epithelial ovarian cancer: Previous sterilisation is an adverse independent prognostic indicator. *Eur. J. Gynaecol. Oncol.* 21, 357–361.
66. Barakat, R. R., and Rubin, S. C. (2002). Perspective: Should we remove a woman's ovaries to prevent ovarian cancer? *Contemp. OB/GYN* 47, 69–78.
67. Schwartz, P. E. (1992). The role of prophylactic oophorectomy in the avoidance of ovarian cancer. *Int. J. Gynaecol. Obstet.* 39, 175–184.
68. Lynch, H. T., and Casey, M. J. (2001). Current status of prophylactic surgery for hereditary breast and gynecologic cancers. *Curr. Opin. Obstet. Gynecol.* 13, 25–30.
69. Piver, M. S., and Rosen, B. (1998). The role of prophylactic oophorectomy. *In* "Ovarian Cancer: Controversies in Management," (D. M. Gershenson, and W. P. McGuire, eds.), pp. 17–40. Churchill Livingstone, New York.
70. Gross, C. P., Nicholson, W., and Powe, N. R. (1999). Factors affecting prophylactic oophorectomy in postmenopausal women. *Obstet. Gynecol.* 94, 962–968.
71. Geary, M., Geoghegan, A., and Foley, M. (1997). Prevention of ovarian cancer: A survey of the practice of prophylactic oophorectomy by consultant gynaecologists in Ireland. *Ir. Med. J.* 90, 186–187.
72. NIH consensus conference (1995). Ovarian cancer. Screening, treatment, and follow-up. NIH Consensus Development Panel on Ovarian Cancer. *JAMA* 273, 491–497.
73. Struewing, J. P., Watson, P., Easton, D. F., Ponder, B. A., Lynch, H. T., and Tucker, M. A. (1995). Prophylactic oophorectomy in inherited breast/ovarian cancer families. *J. Natl. Cancer Inst. Monogr.* 33–35.
74. Boyd, J., Sonoda, Y., Federici, M. G., Bogomolniy, F., Rhei, E., Maresco, D. L. *et al.* (2000). Clinicopathologic features of BRCA-linked and sporadic ovarian cancer. *JAMA* 283, 2260–2265.
75. Boyd, J. (2001). BRCA: The breast, ovarian, and other cancer genes. *Gynecol. Oncol.* 80, 337–340.
76. Weber, B. L., Punzalan, C., Eisen, A. *et al.* (2000). Ovarian cancer risk reduction after bilateral prophylactic oophorectomy (BPO) in BRCA1 and BRCA2 mutation carriers. *Am. J. Hum. Genet.* 67(S2), 59.

77. Grann, V. R., Panageas, K. S., Whang, W., Antman, K. H., and Neugut, A. I. (1998). Decision analysis of prophylactic mastectomy and oophorectomy in BRCA1-positive or BRCA2-positive patients. *J. Clin. Oncol.* 16, 979–985.

78. Rebbeck, T. R., Levin, A. M., Eisen, A., Snyder, C., Watson, P., Cannon-Albright, L. *et al.* (1999). Breast cancer risk after bilateral prophylactic oophorectomy in BRCA1 mutation carriers. *J. Natl. Cancer Inst.* 91, 1475–1479.

79. Rebbeck, T. R. (2000). Prophylactic oophorectomy in BRCA1 and BRCA2 mutation carriers. *J. Clin. Oncol.* 18, 100S–103S.

80. Kauff, N. D., Satagopan, J. M., Robson, M. E., Scheuer, L., Hensley, M., Hudis, C. A. *et al.* (2002). Risk-reducing salpingo-oophorectomy in women with a BRCA1 or BRCA2 mutation. *N. Engl. J. Med.* 346, 1609–1615.

81. Randall, T. C., Armstrong, K., Sanford Schwartz, J., Weber, B., and Rubin, S. C. (2002). Hormone replacement and survival following prophylactic oophorectomy for women with BRCA1 mutations: A decision analysis. *Gynecol. Oncol.* 76, 263.

82. Schrag, D., Kuntz, K. M., Garber, J. E., and Weeks, J. C. (2000). Life expectancy gains from cancer prevention strategies for women with breast cancer and BRCA1 or BRCA2 mutations. *JAMA* 283, 617–624.

83. Powell, M. A., and Mutch, D. G. (2001). Identifying and treating hereditary colon and endometrial cancer. *Contemp. OB/GYN*, 85–90.

84. Ponder, B. (1997). Genetic testing for cancer risk. *Science* 278, 1050–1054.

85. ACOG committee opinion. (2001). Breast-ovarian cancer screening. Number 239, August 2000. American College of Obstetricians and Gynecologists. Committee on genetics. *Int. J. Gynaecol. Obstet.* 75, 339–340.

86. Schofield, A., Pitt, J., Biring, G., and Dawson, P. M. (2001). Oophorectomy in primary colorectal cancer. *Ann. R. Coll. Surg. Engl.* 83, 81–84.

87. Huang, P. P., Weber, T. K., Mendoza, C., Rodriguez-Bigas, M. A., and Petrelli, N. J. (1998). Long-term survival in patients with ovarian metastases from colorectal carcinoma. *Ann. Surg. Oncol.* 5, 695–698.

88. Borton, M., and Friedman, E. A. (1989). Informed consent and counseling. *In* "Legal Principles and Practice in Obstetrics and Gynecology," (M. Borten, and E. A. Friedman, eds.), p. 418. Year Book Medical Publishers, Chicago.

89. Meiser, B., Butow, P., Barratt, A., Friedlander, M., Gattas, M., Kirk, J. *et al.* (1999). Attitudes toward prophylactic oophorectomy and screening utilization in women at increased risk of developing hereditary breast/ovarian cancer. *Gynecol. Oncol.* 75, 122–129.

90. Aziz, S., Kuperstein, G., Rosen, B., Cole, D., Nedelcu, R., McLaughlin, J. *et al.* (2001). A genetic epidemiological study of carcinoma of the fallopian tube. *Gynecol. Oncol.* 80, 341–345.

91. Morice, P., Pautier, P., Mercier, S., Spatz, A., Lhomme, C., Duvillard, P. *et al.* (1999). Laparoscopic prophylactic oophorectomy in women with inherited risk of ovarian cancer. *Eur. J. Gynaecol. Oncol.* 20, 202–204.

92. Morice, P., Pautier, P., and Delaloge, S. (2001). Prophylactic surgery in patients with inherited risk of ovarian cancer. *Gynecol. Oncol.* 83, 445–447.

93. Narayansingh, G., Cumming, G., Parkin, D., and Miller, I. (2000). Ovarian cancer developing in the ovarian remnant syndrome. A case report and literature review. *Aust. N. Z. J. Obstet. Gynaecol.* 40, 221–223.

94. Barakat, R. R., Hensley, M., Bhaskaran, D., Rastogi, P., Korytowsky, B., Boyd, J., Robson, M., and Offit, K. (2002). Prophylactic oophorectomy in women at risk for hereditary ovarian carcinoma. *Gynecol. Oncol.* 84, 482.

95. Colgan, T. J., Boerner, S. L., Murphy, J., Cole, D. E., Narod, S., and Rosen, B. (2002). Peritoneal lavage cytology: An assessment of its value during prophylactic oophorectomy. *Gynecol. Oncol.* 85, 397–403.

96. Rubin, S. C. (2002). Prophylactic oophorectomy comes of age. *Gynecol. Oncol.* 85, 395–396.

97. Lu, K. H., Garber, J. E., Cramer, D. W., Welch, W. R., Niloff, J., Schrag, D. *et al.* (2000). Occult ovarian tumors in women with BRCA1 or BRCA2 mutations undergoing prophylactic oophorectomy. *J. Clin. Oncol.* 18, 2728–2732.

98. Agoff, S. N., Mendelin, J. E., Grieco, V. S., and Garcia, R. L. (2002). Unexpected gynecologic neoplasms in patients with proven or suspected BRCA-1 or -2 mutations: implications for gross examination, cytology, and clinical follow-up. *Am. J. Surg. Pathol.* 26, 171–178.

99. Paley, P. J., Swisher, E. M., Garcia, R. L., Agoff, S. N., Greer, B. E., Peters, K. L. *et al.* (2001). Occult cancer of the fallopian tube in BRCA-1 germline mutation carriers at prophylactic oophorectomy: A case for recommending hysterectomy at surgical prophylaxis. *Gynecol. Oncol.* 80, 176–180.

100. Ansink, A. C., Burger, C. W., and Seynaeve, C. (2001). Occult cancer in the fallopian tube in patients with a BRCA-1 germline mutation. *Gynecol. Oncol.* 83, 445.

101. Castiel, M., Hensley, M., Marcelli, A. R., Aggarwal, K., Brown, C., Stier, E. *et al.* (2002). Gynecologic care of the cancer patient. *OBG Manag.* 2.

102. Rebbeck, T. R., Lynch, H. T., Neuhausen, S. L., Narod, S. A., Van't Veer, L., Garber, J. E. *et al.* (2002). Prophylactic oophorectomy in carriers of BRCA1 or BRCA2 mutations. *N. Engl. J. Med.* 346, 1616–1622.

103. Eisen, A., Rebbeck, T. R., Lynch, H., Lerman, C., Ghadirian, P., Dube, M. P., Weber, B. L., and Narod, S. (2000). Reduction in breast cancer risk following bilateral prophylactic oophorectomy in BRCA1 and BRCA2 mutation carriers. *Am. J. Hum. Genet.* 67(S2), 58.

104. Chapron, C., Querleu, D., Bruhat, M. A., Madelenat, P., Fernandez, H., Pierre, F. *et al.* (1998). Surgical complications of diagnostic and operative gynaecological laparoscopy: A series of 29,966 cases. *Hum. Reprod.* 13, 867–872.

105. Donnez, J., Chantraine, F., and Nisolle, M. (2001). Complications of laparoscopic surgery in gynecology. *In* "An Atlas of Operative Laparoscopy and Hysteroscopy," J. Donnez, and M. Nisolle, eds.), pp. 373–387. Parthenon Publishing Group, New York.

106. Brosens, I., and Gordon, A. (2001). Bowel injuries during gynecological laparoscopy: A multinational survey. *Gynecol. Endosc.* 10, 141–145.

107. O'Shea, R. T., and Petrucco, O. (1996). Adelaide laparoscopic hysterectomy audit. *J. Am. Assoc. Gynecol. Laparosc.* 3, S35–S36.

108. Rein, H. (2001). Complications and litigation in gynecologic endoscopy. *Curr. Opin. Obstet. Gynecol.* 13, 425–429.

109. Nezhat, C. R., Siegler, A., Nezhat, F., Nezhat, C., Seidman, D., and Luciano, A. (2000). Complications. *In* "Operative Gynecologic Laparoscopy: Principles and Techniques," (C. R. Nezhat, ed.), pp. 365–390. McGraw-Hill, Health Professions Division, New York.

110. Eltabbakh, G. H., Piver, M. S., Hempling, R. E., Recio, F. O., and Paczos, T. (1999). Laparoscopic management of women with a family history of ovarian cancer. *J. Surg. Oncol.* 72, 9–13.

111. Chapron, C., Dubuisson, J. B., and Capella-Allouc, S. (1997). Salpingo-oophorectomy for adnexal masses. Place and results for operative laparoscopy. *Eur. J. Obstet. Gynecol. Reprod. Biol.* 73, 43–48.

112. Tsaltas, J., Healy, D. L., and Lloyd, D. (2001). Complications of laparoscopy: A tautological audit. *Gynecol. Endosc.* 10, 17–19.

113. Querleu, D., Chapron, C., Chevallier, L., and Bruhat, M. A. (1993). Complications of gynecologic laparoscopic surgery—a French multicenter collaborative study. *N. Engl. J. Med.* 328, 1355.

114. Jansen, F. W., Kapiteyn, K., Trimbos-Kemper, T., Hermans, J., and Trimbos, J. B. (1997). Complications of laparoscopy: A prospective multicentre observational study. *Br. J.Obstet. Gynaecol.* 104, 595–600.

115. Chapron, C., Querleu, D., Mage, G., Madelenat, P., Dubuisson, J. B., Audebert, A. *et al.* (1992). Complications of gynecologic laparoscopy. Multicentric study of 7,604 laparoscopies. *J. Gynecol. Obstet. Biol. Reprod.(Paris)* 21, 207–213.

116. Chapron, C., Pierre, F., Harchaoui, Y., Lacroix, S., Beguin, S., Querleu, D. *et al.* (1999). Gastrointestinal injuries during gynaecological laparoscopy. *Hum. Reprod.* 14, 333–337.

117. Schlaerth, J. B., Spirtos, N. M., Carson, L. F., Boike, G., Adamec, T., and Stonebraker, B. (2002). Laparoscopic retroperitoneal lymphadenectomy followed by immediate laparotomy in women with cervical cancer: A gynecologic oncology group study. *Gynecol. Oncol.* 85, 81–88.
118. Chapron, C., Pierre, F., Querleu, D., and Dubuisson, J. B. (2001). Complications of laparoscopy in gynecology. *Gynecol. Obstet. Fertil.* 29, 605–612.
119. Bhoyrul, S., Vierra, M. A., Nezhat, C. R., Krummel, T. M., and Way, L. W. (2001). Trocar injuries in laparoscopic surgery. *J. Am. Coll. Surg.* 192, 677–683.
120. Yuzpe, A. A. (1990). Pneumoperitoneum needle and trocar injuries in laparoscopy. A survey on possible contributing factors and prevention. *J. Reprod. Med.* 35, 485–490.
121. Donnez, J., Jadoul, P., Chantraine, F., and Nisolle, M. (2001). Ureteral and bladder injury during laparoscopic surgery. *In* "An Atlas of Operative Laparoscopy and Hysteroscopy," (J. Donnez, and M. Nisolle, eds.), pp. 363–372. Parthenon Publishing Group, New York.
122. Canis, M., Rabischong, B., Botchorishvili, R., Tamburro, S., Wattiez, A., Mage, G. *et al.* (2001). Risk of spread of ovarian cancer after laparoscopic surgery. *Curr. Opin. Obstet. Gynecol.* 13, 9–14.
123. Kruitwagen, R. F., Swinkels, B. M., Keyser, K. G., and Doesburg, W. H., and Schijf, C. P. (1996). Incidence and effect on survival of abdominal wall metastases at trocar or puncture sites following laparoscopy or paracentesis in women with ovarian cancer. *Gynecol. Oncol.* 60, 233–237.
124. Neuhaus, S. J., Texler, M., Hewett, P. J., and Watson, D. I. (1998). Port-site metastases following laparoscopic surgery. *Br. J. Surg.* 85, 735–741.
125. Carlson, N. L., Krivak, T. C., Winter, W. E., III, and Macri, C. I. (2002). Port site metastasis of ovarian carcinoma remote from laparoscopic surgery for benign disease. *Gynecol. Oncol.* 85, 529–531.
126. Hopkins, M. P., von Gruenigen, V., and Gaich, S. (2000). Laparoscopic port site implantation with ovarian cancer. *Am. J. Obstet. Gynecol.* 182, 735–736.
127. Salazar, H., Godwin, A. K., Daly, M. B., Laub, P. B., Hogan, W. M., Rosenblum, N. *et al.* (1996). Microscopic benign and invasive malignant neoplasms and a cancer-prone phenotype in prophylactic oophorectomies. *J. Natl. Cancer Inst.* 88, 1810–1820.
128. Deligdisch, L., Gil, J., Kerner, H., Wu, H. S., Beck, D., and Gershoni-Baruch, R. (1999). Ovarian dysplasia in prophylactic oophorectomy specimens: Cytogenetic and morphometric correlations. *Cancer* 86, 1544–1550.
129. Colgan, T. J., Murphy, J., Cole, D. E., Narod, S., and Rosen, B. (2001). Occult carcinoma in prophylactic oophorectomy specimens: Prevalence and association with BRCA germline mutation status. *Am. J. Surg. Pathol.* 25, 1283–1289.
130. Leeper, K., Garcia, R. L., Swisher, E. M., Goff, B. A., Greer, B. E., and Paley, P. J. (2002). Pathologic findings in prophylactic oophorectomy specimens in high-risk women. *Gynecol. Oncol.* 87, 52–56.
130a. Leeper, K., Garcia, B., Swisher, E., Goff, B., Greer, B., and Paley, P. (2002). Pathologic findings in prophylactic oophorectomy specimens in high-risk women. *Gynecol. Oncol.* 87, 52–56.
131. Vergote, I. (2001). Prognostic factors in stage I ovarian carcinoma. *Verh. K. Acad. Geneeskd. Belg.* 63, 257–271.
132. Schilder, J. M., Thompson, A. M., De Priest, P. D., Ueland, F. R., Cibull, M. L., Kryscio, R. J., Modesitt, S. C., Geisler, J. P., *et al.* (2002). Outcome of reproductive-age women with stage IA or stage IC invasive epithelial ovarian cancer treated with fertility sparing surgery. *Gynecol. Oncol.* 87, 1–7.
132a. Schilder, J. M., Thompson, A. M., De Priest, P. D., Ueland, F. R., Cibull, M. L., Kryscio, R. J., Modesitt, S. C., Lu, K. H., Geisler, J. P. *et al.* (2002). Outcome of reproductive age women with stage 1A or 1C invasive epithelial ovarian cancer treated with fertility-sparing therapy. *Gynecol. Oncol.* 87, 1–7.
133. Mueller, M. D., Dreher, E., Eggimann, T., Linder, H., Altermatt, H., and Hanggi, W. (1998). Is laparoscopic oophorectomy rational in patients with breast cancer? *Surg. Endosc.* 12, 1390–1392.
134. Casey, M. J., Bewtra, C., Hoehne, L. L., Tatpati, A. D., Lynch, H. T., and Watson, P. (2000). Histology of prophylactically removed ovaries from BRCA1 and BRCA2 mutation carriers compared with noncarriers in hereditary breast ovarian cancer syndrome kindreds. *Gynecol. Oncol.* 78, 278–287.
135. Barakat, R. R., Federici, M. G., Saigo, P. E., Robson, M. E., Offit, K., and Boyd, J. (2000). Absence of premalignant histologic, molecular, or cell biologic alterations in prophylactic oophorectomy specimens from BRCA1 heterozygotes. *Cancer* 89, 383–390.
135a. Pothuri, B., Leitano, M., Barakat, R. R., Akram, M., Bogomolniv, F. *et al.* (2001). Genetic analysis of ovarian carcinoma histogenesis. *Gynecol. Oncol.* 80, 277.
136. Breast cancer and hormone replacement therapy: Collaborative reanalysis of data from 51 epidemiological studies of 52,705 women with breast cancer and 108,411 women without breast cancer. (1997). Collaborative Group on Hormonal Factors in Breast Cancer. *Lancet* 350, 1047–1059.
137. Mahavni, V., and Sood, A. K. (2001). Hormone replacement therapy and cancer risk. *Curr. Opin. Oncol.* 13, 384–389.
138. Ross, R. K., Paganini-Hill, A., Wan, P. C., and Pike, M. C. (2000). Effect of hormone replacement therapy on breast cancer risk: Estrogen versus estrogen plus progestin. *J. Natl. Cancer Inst.* 92, 328–332.
139. Schairer, C., Lubin, J., Troisi, R., Sturgeon, S., Brinton, L., and Hoover, R. (2000). Menopausal estrogen and estrogen-progestin replacement therapy and breast cancer risk. *JAMA* 283, 485–491.
140. Clavel-Chapelon, F., and Hill, C. (2000). Hormone replacement therapy in menopause and risk of breast cancer. *Presse Med.* 29, 1688–1693.
141. Veronesi, U., and Decensi, A. (2001). Retinoids for ovarian cancer prevention: Laboratory data set the stage for thoughtful clinical trials. *J. Natl. Cancer Inst.* 93, 486–488.
142. Piver, M. S. (2002). Hereditary ovarian cancer. Lessons from the first twenty years of the Gilda Radner Familial Ovarian Cancer Registry. *Gynecol. Oncol.* 85, 9–17.
143. Eltabbakh, G. H., Piver, M. S., Natarajan, N., and Mettlin, C. J. (1998). Epidemiologic differences between women with extraovarian primary peritoneal carcinoma and women with epithelial ovarian cancer. *Obstet. Gynecol.* 91, 254–259.
144. Cass, I., Baldwin, R. L., Fasylova, E., Fields, A. L., Klinger, H. P., Runowicz, C. D. *et al.* (2001). Allelotype of papillary serous peritoneal carcinomas. *Gynecol. Oncol.* 82, 69–76.
145. Levine, D. A., Yee, C., Marshall, D. S., Olvera, N., Bogolmolniv, F., Barakat, R. R., Soslow, R. A., and Boyd, J. (2002). Frequency of BRCA founder mutations among Ashkenazi Jewish patients with primary peritoneal and fallopian tube adenocarcinoma. *Gynecol. Oncol.* 84, 493.
146. Quillin, J. M., Boardman, C. H., Bodurtha, J., and Smith, T. (2001). Preventive gynecologic surgery for BRCA1/2 carriers—information for decision-making. *Gynecol. Oncol.* 83, 168–170.
147. Writing Group for the Women's Health Initiative Investigators. (2002). Risks and benefits of estrogen plus progestin in healthy postmenopausal women: Principal results from the Women's Health Initiative randomized controlled trial. *JAMA* 288, 321–333.
148. Fletcher, S. W., and Colditz, G. A. (2002). Failure of estrogen plus progestin therapies for prevention. *JAMA* 288, 366–368.
149. Lacey, J. V., Mink, P. J., Lubin, J. H., Sherman, M. E., Troisi, R., Hartge, P., Schatzin, A., and Schairer, C. (2002). Menopausal hormone replacement therapy and risk of ovarian cancer. *JAMA* 288, 334–341.
150. Noller, K. L. (2002). Estrogen replacement therapy and risk of ovarian cancer. *JAMA* 288, 369.
151. WHO Collaborative Study of Neoplasia and Steroid Contraceptives. (1991). Depot-Medroxyprogesterone Acetate (DMPA) and risk of epithelial ovarian cancer. *Int. J. Cancer* 49, 191–195.

CHAPTER

38

Psychological Aspects of Ovarian Cancer and BRCA Testing

JENNIFER LIU

San Francisco Veteran's Affairs Medical Center
University of California, San Francisco
San Francisco, California 94121

JIMMIE C. HOLLAND

Department of Psychiatry
Memorial Sloan-Kettering Cancer Center
New York, New York 10021

I. INTRODUCTION

Approximately one-third of patients with newly diagnosed or recurrent cancer have been found to experience psychological distress.[1] While each person's concept of cancer, death, and dying varies depending on the person's societal, philosophical, spiritual, and religious beliefs, cancer disrupts all aspects of life, work, and finances as well as family and friends. As the fifth leading cause of cancer mortality overall and the leading cause of cancer mortality among gynecologic cancers, ovarian cancer presents circumstances that are particularly challenging, both physically and psychologically. The doctor-patient relationship is vital in helping the woman with ovarian cancer and her family negotiate these challenges. In addition, however, the team of nurses, social workers, mental health professionals, and clergy as well as community resources are important in providing the optimal emotional support.

Symptoms of anxiety and depression are experienced by a significant number of patients with cancer, either due to the direct effects of the cancer, treatments given for the cancer, or as a manifestation of the psychological distress experienced in response to being given a diagnosis of cancer. This chapter reviews psychosocial issues related to the diagnosis, management, and palliative care of ovarian cancer, as well as the most common psychiatric diagnoses of anxiety, depression, and delirium. In addition, this chapter reviews the psychiatric impact of genetic testing. Although only 5–10% of ovarian cancers are inherited, individuals with BRCA1/BRCA2 mutations are at significantly at higher risk of developing cancer. A unique set of psychosocial issues arises from the availability of genetic susceptibility testing for those individuals with a family history of breast and ovarian cancer, as well as for their siblings and offspring. Finally, as patient dissatisfaction with the doctor-patient relationship has been associated with noncompliance with medical advice and treatment, "doctor-shopping," poorer coping, and general dissatisfaction, issues related to the doctor-patient relationship are discussed.[2]

II. PSYCHOLOGICAL ISSUES RELATED TO THE DIAGNOSIS AND TREATMENT OF OVARIAN CANCER

The woman who is given a diagnosis of ovarian cancer may experience a range of emotions, from shock and despair, anxiety and sadness, to helplessness in the face of uncertainty and her own mortality. However, over a period of several months, the majority of individuals adjust to the vicissitudes of having cancer and to what is often described as a "roller coaster." In addition to the common responses to a diagnosis of cancer described, a woman's age, stage in life, and type of ovarian cancer influence her reaction. This varies with age, but the most common is epithelial, predominantly affecting peri- and postmenopausal women. In general, germ cell tumors account for only 20–25% of ovarian cancers in the U.S., but they constitute over 70% of ovarian cancers in young women, and one-third are malignant. While the younger woman will more likely have a germ cell tumor and more likely a good prognosis, she will be confronted with loss of fertility. Since current technology cannot successfully preserve ova, women who would like children are left with the options of adoption, egg donation, and surrogacy. However, for those in which conservative, fertility-sparing surgery is possible, miscarriage rates have been found to be in the range expected for the general population with only a slightly increased rate of malformations.[3] Even for those women with children who do not desire more children, loss of their reproductive organs still affects body image, self-worth, and feminine identity.

The shock of hearing the diagnosis of ovarian cancer and the initial treatment results in feeling overwhelmed, with anxiety that makes rational decision making difficult. It is helpful for the patient to have a family member or friend to go to visits with the doctor to provide emotional support and to have someone with whom to discuss the information later. If the initial treatment is surgical, it is important to answer questions about practical details, such as the nature of the procedure, time in the hospital, and rehabilitation that is possible based on body parts or functions lost or impaired. Misconceptions and expectations should be clarified. Common fears that arise in anticipation of surgery are an increased sense of vulnerability, fears of loss of control and fears of death while under anesthesia, fears of being partially awake during surgery, and fears of damage to pelvic organs.[4] A relatively inexpensive and effective aid in helping the patient gain a sense of control over her anxiety is relaxation training by audiocassette, which has been shown to reduce use of analgesics and length of stay in abdominal surgery patients.[5] In addition to relaxation techniques, the induction of pleasant imagery, distraction, and the substitution of positive, coping statements for negative thoughts can also be useful. Those individuals who are too anxious to make use of such techniques may benefit from pharmacological assistance with moderate to longer acting benzodiazepines such as lorazepam and clonazepam peri- and postoperatively. Dosing regimens for benzodiazepines will be discussed in detail in Section IIIB.

Following initial surgery for staging and debulking, chemotherapy is the standard treatment. In a small study evaluating the impact of ovarian cancer and its management on quality of life, alopecia was the most stressful or disruptive side effect of treatment, followed by the anxiety experienced in anticipation of treatment, and the pain and dysfunction due to peripheral neuropathy related to cisplatin.[6] In addition to feelings of helplessness, vulnerability, and a damaged body image, the debilitating side effects of chemotherapy may cause the patient to have to contend with feelings of dependency and alienation. And while the patient may eagerly anticipate the completion of treatment, it also commonly increases fears of recurrence. Given the high rate of recurrence, anxiety is high at the time of follow-up visits, especially fears related to changes in CA125, whose elevation is an early sign of recurrence, as well as at second-look surgery. She may be faced with yet more uncertainty and disability with progression on standard treatment and the option of second-line therapy or a clinical trial. In Kornblith and colleagues' study of quality of life of women with ovarian cancer, physical disability was the most important predictor of psychological distress, suggesting the need for more frequent monitoring of their psychological function as their physical functioning declines.[7]

Ideally, sexual function should be assessed before the initiation of treatment, but in practice, preoccupation with the progress of treatment will supercede concerns about sexual function until treatment is completed. Inquiring about sexual function may be an awkward topic for the physician to broach, and good rapport is helpful as well as approaching it like any another routine activity of daily living. In addition to inquiring about relationship status, a sexual history should include questions about the nature of sexual activity before and after cancer, such as frequency of activity with a partner, frequency of masturbation, who initiates partner sex, and cancer myths related to sexual functioning of both the woman and her partner, as well as an evaluation of each phase of the woman's sexual response for any dysfunction. Interviewing the woman and her partner separately may allow either individual to disclose issues related to abuse or sexually transmitted diseases more openly.

Sexual function is an integral component in an individual's quality of life that should not be overlooked or minimized, as rehabilitation may be possible. Anxiety about pain, fear of transmitting cancer to one's partner, or being reminded of one's cancer with the thought of sex is a common cause of loss of desire. Methyl testosterone is often used in combination with estrogen for decreased libido, dyspareunia, or lack of vaginal lubrication. Sildenafil also may be beneficial in the treatment of anorgasmia in women.[8] Dyspareunia is the most common sexual problem following cancer treatment, and is helped by marital counseling with advice about adjusting positions and use of a water-based lubricant and a vaginal dilator. The American Cancer Society's (1-800-227-2345) pamphlet, "Sexuality and Cancer: For the Woman who has Cancer and her Partner," is helpful. There are several sexual therapy techniques that may be beneficial and that should be provided by a trained sex therapist. The American Association of Sex Educators, Counselors, and Therapists (AASEC) can provide members who have had specific training in sex therapy.

III. ISSUES RELATED TO PALLIATIVE CARE

As ovarian cancer is often asymptotic in its early stages, most women have disease that is no longer localized at the time of diagnosis. With a 5-year survival rate of less than 10% in suboptimally debulked stage III and IV patients, palliative care is a vital component in the management of advanced ovarian cancer.[9] Palliative care includes any treatment whose goal is not curative. The benefits of palliative chemotherapy on symptom control and the quality of life (QOL) of ovarian cancer patients have been little studied. It is clear that many patients accept chemotherapy with actual chance of benefit. The same is true for second and third line regimens. The power of hope is crucial in determining patients' participation in conventional and therapies.

Given its location and the tendency for ovarian cancer to spread locally, death from ovarian cancer often may result from metastases causing bowel obstruction. This is often preceded by months of intermittent partial bowel obstruction requiring hospitalization and treatment. This incidence has been estimated to occur in 5–51% of patients. Options for the management of bowel obstruction range from surgical (resection, bypass, or colostomy), the placement of a drainage PEG tube, to supportive care, including the option of parenteral nutrition. In addition to a widening girth due to the bulk of the disease, having an ostomy or PEG tube heightens issues about altered body appearance and self-image.

The place of surgery and parenteral nutrition in malignant bowel obstruction remains controversial and deserves further discussion. Feuer and colleagues performed an extensive meta-analysis of the surgical management of malignant bowel obstruction due to gynecologic and gastrointestinal cancer.[10] All but one study was retrospective in nature, and there was significant variation in symptom assessment, definitions of symptom control, and outcome measures. The majority defined symptom control as the ability to tolerate an oral diet, with success ranging from 42% to over 80%, with high re-obstruction rates ranging from 10–50%, without mention of time to re-obstruction. Post operative mortality ranged from 5–32%. Given the retrospective nature of the studies, none included any QOL measures. Clearly, more rigorous, prospective studies with QOL measures are needed to assess the benefit of surgical intervention and establish management guidelines in this population. Regarding the use of parenteral nutrition in obstructed patients, again studies are lacking, but the available information suggests that parenteral support may be of benefit in preventing dehydration and therefore avoiding hospitalization as well as maintaining nutrition in patients with abdominal carcinomatosis without other impending organ failure.[11]

Pain control is a critical component of palliative care. In a study of patients with gynecologic cancer at various stages, fear of pain was cited as the most frequent source of fear.[12] In another study, two-thirds of ovarian cancer patients experienced pain that substantially interfered with functioning.[13] Pain control should be guided by the etiology of the pain and its associated pain syndrome (tumor-related nocioceptive, tumor-related neuropathic, treatment-related). In addition to the direct suffering caused by uncontrolled pain, anxiety and depression are increased in the presence of uncontrolled pain.

For the patient with advanced disease, pain control and symptom management are the primary goals of treatment. Initiating discussion about end-of-life issues may be difficult and often occurs late. The SUPPORT study, involving more than 9000 seriously ill patients, found that 46% of Do-Not-Resuscitate (DNR) orders were written two days before death, and only 47% of physicians knew patients' DNR preferences.[14] Multiple factors contribute to the avoidance of talking about end-of-life care, including societal values, physician fears that this will be perceived as "giving up" if they talk about dying, the difficulty in presenting an absence of treatment options and hospice care, and the uncertainty about prognosis. However, failure to provide appropriate information about prognosis and palliative care can contribute to unnecessary pain and suffering. Quill has suggested topics and questions for initiating discussions about these topics regarding end-of-life issues (Table 38.1).[15]

Beyond pain control and symptom management, terminally ill patients value personal care, such as being kept physically clean, having a positive relationship with caregivers, maintaining a sense of dignity, and control and for many, but not all, anticipating the end of life.[16] Some people wish to discuss what they can expect during the dying process and wish to arrange a leave-taking and care for family after their death. However, others are threatened by this; their wish not to prepare must be equally respected.

Another common fear terminally ill patients experience is abandonment by medical staff. This sometimes happens because physicians are inadequately taught about end-of-life care and feel a sense of professional failure in the face of a dying patient.[17, 18] Physicians and staff ideally should continue contact after referral to hospice care to diminish the sense of abandonment.

A. Depression

Twenty to twenty-five percent of cancer patients will manifest symptoms of depression at some point in the course of their illness, with those suffering higher levels of disability and pain at greater risk, as well as those with a personal or family history of depression.[19] Only two studies have focused specifically on depression in ovarian cancer patients, and they found similar rates to those found in cancer patients overall.[20] There is also growing evidence that depression is associated with increased mortality in patients with medical illness, including cancer.[21, 22] Despite its high incidence and associated mortality, depression is often underdiagnosed.

TABLE 38.1

Domain	Representative questions
Goals	Given the severity of your illness, what is most important for you to achieve? How do you think about balancing quality of life with length of life in terms of your treatment? What are your most important hopes? What are your biggest fears?
Values	What makes the most worth living for you? Would there be any circumstances under which you would find life not worth living? What do you consider your quality of life to be like now? Have you seen or been with someone who had a particularly good death or particularly difficult death?
Advance directives	If with future progression of your illness you are not able to speak for yourself, who would be best able to represent your views and values (health-care proxy)? Have you given any thought to what kinds of treatment you would want (and not want) if you become unable to speak for yourself in the future (living will)?
Do-Not-Resuscitate order	If you were to die suddenly, that is, you stopped breathing or your heart stopped, we could try to revive you by using cardiopulmonary resuscitation (CPR). Are you familiar with CPR? Have you given thought as to whether you would want it? Given the severity of your illness, CPR in all likelihood will be ineffective. I would recommend that you choose not to have it, but that we continue all potentially effective treatments. What do you think?
Palliative care (pain and other symptoms)	Have you ever heard of hospice? Tell me about your pain. Can you rate it on a 10-point scale? What is your (breathing) like when you feel at your best? How about when you are having trouble?
Palliative care ("unfinished business")	If you were to die sooner rather than later, what would be left undone? How is your family handling your illness? What are their reactions? Has religion been an important part of your life? Are there any spiritual issues you are concerned about at this point?

This in part due to women not revealing psychological symptoms out of embarrassment or a fear of being stigmatized. It is also related to the difficulty in distinguishing depression in women with advanced ovarian cancer from the physical symptoms due to cancer. For instance, loss of energy, insomnia, and anorexia are side effects of chemotherapy, radiotherapy, advanced disease, and chronic pain. And of course, depressed patients may often present with somatic symptoms. Several approaches to the diagnosis of depression have been suggested for use in the medical population, including what have been termed "exclusive" and "substitutive" approaches.[23, 24] The exclusive approach eliminates anorexia and fatigue from the criterion symptoms. The substitutive or Endicott criteria replace those symptoms more likely to be confused with medical illness, such as loss of energy, weight loss, decreased concentration, and psychomotor changes, with mood and depressive thoughts and behavior, such as irritability, and tearfulness.

Both preserve and emphasize negative, depressive thinking, such as worthlessness, excessive guilt, and thoughts of death, as well as anhedonia, or lost of interest or pleasure, one of the key symptoms of depression that is less affected by disease- and treatment-related factors.

Similar to the primary care population, physicians have been found to recognize depression in cancer patients about half of the time.[25] In a study conducted by Passik *et al.* involving 12 oncologists and 1109 patients given the Zung Self-Rating Depression Scale, oncologists correctly classified one-third of mildly depressed patients and only one-eighth (13%) of moderate to severely depressed patients. Physician depression ratings were most highly correlated with their ratings of the patients' anxiety, and to a lesser extent, pain. Of note, 36% of the patients in this study reported clinically significant depressive symptoms, and about half were diagnosed with early-stage disease.[26] In addition to the issues of patient fear and embarrassment and the complicated nature of diagnosis due to overlapping symptoms related to cancer and depression, Passik also suggests two areas that merit further study regarding the underrecognition of depression in patients with cancer, namely that staff may minimize a patient's level of distress as an emotional safeguard and that there also may be "hard to read" patients.

Ideally, the management of depression in cancer patients should include a combination of supportive psychotherapy, using crisis intervention and cognitive-behavioral techniques, along with antidepressants. However, antidepressants remain the mainstay in the treatment of the significant depression seen in these women, particularly the selective serotonin reuptake inhibitors due to their favorable side-effect profiles (see Table 38.2). Selective serotonin reuptake inhibitors are equally effective but vary according to their side effect profile. Citalopram has the added benefit of having no drug-drug interactions, which is important for those individuals on medications such as warfarin, digoxin, carbamazepine, and type IC antiarrhythmics.

Up to half of patients experience sexual side effects from the selective serotonin reuptake inhibitors, which may respond to sildenafil.[27, 28] For those whom sildenafil is ineffective or do not find this option acceptable, alternative antidepressants are bupropion, nefazodone, mirtazapine, and venlafaxine (see Table 38.3). Bupropion has energizing effects that may be related to having a chemical structure similar to the psychostimulants. It should be noted that bupropion has a slight increase of seizure risk compared with the other antidepressants and therefore should be avoided in those patients with CNS disease or a previous history of CNS injury. In contrast, nefazodone is more sedating, and this may help patients with an anxious component to their depression. Others may not tolerate it due to being over-sedated. Mirtazapine also tends to be more sedating; this is helpful for depressed women with insomnia. In addition, it increases appetite and is of particular value in cachexic women. There has been one case series using mirtazapine to treat depression in women with breast or gynecologic cancer, and given its 5HT-3 receptor blockade properties, a follow-up study to investigate the antiemetic effects of mirtazapine is underway[29]. Venlafaxine, another antidepressant in its own class, is a norepinephrine-serotonin reuptake inhibitor. It tends to be more energizing and is generally well tolerated.

It is important to obtain a psychiatric consultation for women with concurrent medical problems on multiple medications, who do not respond or have sexual dysfunction on a selective serotonin reuptake inhibitor, or are severely and/or psychotically depressed. Other psychopharmacologic options for the treatment of depression in the cancer patient include the tricyclic antidepressants and psychostimulants: methylphenidate, dextroamphetamine, and pemoline. Psychostimulants are also useful in treating cancer-related fatigue and opiate sedation. Occasionally it is necessary to consider electroconvulsive therapy in ovarian cancer patients who have depression associated with psychotic features or who are refractory to antidepressants. However, psychotic depression is extremely rare in patients with cancer and should be evaluated for medical causes, particularly brain metastases.

TABLE 38.2

Drug	Dose range	Typical side effects
Citalopram (Celexa)	20–40 mg	Mild sedation
Fluoxetine (Prozac)	20–80 mg	Anxiety
Paroxetine (Paxil)	20–50 mg	Moderate sedation, constipation
Sertraline (Zoloft)	50–200 mg	Diarrhea

TABLE 38.3

Drug	Dose range	Characteristics and typical side effects
Bupropion (Wellbutrin)	200–450 mg	Energizing, not for anxiety; slight increased seizure risk
Mirtazapine (Remeron)	15–45 mg	Sedating, weight gain, possible antiemetic
Nefazodone (Serzone)	300–600 mg	Sedating, helps with anxiety; orthostatic hypotension
Venlafaxine (Effexor)	150–375 mg	Energizing; slight increase in blood pressure

B. Anxiety

One study involving 246 women with ovarian cancer at various stages found that they experienced more anxiety than depression.[30] As is typical of cancer patients in general, various factors contribute to anxiety or experiencing a worsening of a preexisting anxiety disorder or depression with anxious features—stress of having a life-threatening disease, response to pain or dypsnea—due to illness or treatment. Women during treatment for ovarian cancer have increased anxiety at the time of diagnosis, before the first-look procedure, anticipating diagnostic tests or procedures that might identify recurrence, before second-look surgery, and anticipating chemotherapy treatment and outcome. Support groups help women cope with these concerns by talking with others with the same problems and finding information. ACS (1-800-ACS-2345), the National Ovarian Cancer Coalition (1-888-OVARIAN), and SHARE are reliable sources of information. If anxiety disrupts an individual's ability to function or causes an intolerable degree of distress, a psychiatric consultation should be considered to diagnose the source of anxiety and reduce it through supportive psychotherapy and behavioral interventions, such as meditation, guided imagery, and relaxation techniques, particularly to reduce insomnia and daytime tension. Table 38.4 outlines the anti-anxiety drugs and doses.

Some considerations about choice are that lorazepam, oxazepam, and temezapam are metabolized by conjugation in the liver and therefore are safer than alprazolam or clonazepam in patients with liver disease. Low-dose antipsychotics (see Table 38.5) are useful for women whom benzodiazepines are ineffective or relatively contraindicated, either due to a

TABLE 38.4

Drug	Approximate dose equivalents for Bz	Route of administration	Usual dosage range (mg/day)
Benzodiazepines			
Alprazolam (Xanax)	0.25	0.25, 0.5, 1, 2 mg tablets	0.5–4
Clonazepam (Klonopin)	0.5	0.5, 1, 2 mg tablets	0.5–6
Diazepam (Valium)	5	2, 5, 10 mg; IV	2–40
Lorazepam (Ativan)	1	0.5, 1, 2 mg; IV	1–4
Midazolam (Versed)	1.25–1.7	IV only	1–5
Oxazepam (Serax)	15	10, 15, 30 mg	30–120
Temezapam (Restoril)	5	15, 30 mg tablets	15–30
Chlordiazepoxide (Librium)	10	5, 10, 25 mg; IM, IV	15–100
Buspirone	N/A	5, 10, 15 mg tablets	15–60

Adapted from Kaplan, H. I., and Sadock, B. J. (1988). *Clinical Psychiatry: From Synopsis of Psychiatry*, New York, Lippincott.

TABLE 38.5

Drug	Route of administration	Typical dose range
Haloperidol (Haldol)	0.5, 1, 2, 5, 10, 20 mg tablets; IM; IV	0.5–20
Chlorpromazine (Thorazine)	10, 25, 50, 100 mg tablets; IM; IV; PR	25–100
Olanzapine (Zyprexa)	2.5, 5, 10, 15 mg tablets; IM	2.5–20
Risperidone (Risperdal)	1, 2, 3, 4 mg tablets	0.5–2

history of substance abuse, or due to their medical condition, particularly those with respiratory compromise or cognitive impairment. For those women with chronic anxiety, antidepressants and buspirone are effective and have a good safety profile. The doses of antidepressants used to treat anxiety are generally the same as those used to treat depression, except for those individuals who have obsessive-compulsive disorder, who require greater doses.

C. Delirium

Delirium involves alterations in consciousness and cognition and is a very common problem in the treatment of cancer. Up to 51% of postoperative patients, 25% of all cancer patients, and 75% of all terminally ill cancer patients seen in psychiatric consultation have been found to have a delirium.[31] It may be associated with psychotic symptoms, such as hallucinations and paranoia, and intermittent disorientation, impaired attention, memory and judgment, and an altered sleep-wake cycle. Delirium is classified as hyperactive, hypoactive, or mixed, based on psychomotor activity. Hypoactive delirium is often misdiagnosed as depression, as the decrease in psychomotor activity can be mistaken for the social withdrawal and psychomotor retardation of depression. Differentiating dementia from delirium involves assessing the patient's alertness, which is not affected in demented patients; therefore, demented patients do not exhibit waxing and waning of consciousness. Corticosteroids, given to minimize the side effects of chemotherapy, may cause a mood change or occasionally confusion. Although this typically occurs with higher doses and within the first two weeks of steroid use, it can occur at any dose at any time, even during a taper of the steroid.[32] Neutropenic fevers, anemia, dehydration, and electrolyte disturbances, which are complications of some chemotherapy agents, can cause delirium at times. Metastatic CNS involvement may produce delirium, as well as organ failure in advanced disease.

In general, the appropriate management of delirium is directed at identifying the underlying causes and managing the symptoms. Antipsychotics help to relieve confusion and disruptions in the sleep-wake cycle in addition to psychotic symptoms (see Table 38.5). Haloperidol is the antipsychotic of choice due to its low incidence of cardiovascular and anticholinergic effects as well as being available in parenteral form, which is twice as potent as the oral form. For agitated patients who do not respond to haloperidol, chlorpromazine may be an alternative, but it can cause significant decreases in blood pressure and should not be used in women with cardiac arrhythmias. While the atypical antipsychotic, olanzapine, is equally effective and has fewer extrapyramidal symptoms, it may be given only orally and intramuscularly.[33] Risperidone is another atypical antipsychotic that has been used to manage delirious patients at Memorial Sloan-Kettering Cancer Center. For women requiring opiates for pain management, delirium may become a limiting factor for a particular opiate. If adjusting the dose or switching agents does not resolve the symptoms, it may be necessary to add an antipsychotic, since they are used as adjuvant analgesics. While benzodiazepines may be used in the management of the extremely agitated patient, they should not be used alone.[34]

IV. PATIENT-PHYSICIAN ISSUES

Women with ovarian cancer, and patients with cancer in general, express a desire for more information and involvement in decision making about treatment choices. Stewart and colleagues studied decision making among women with ovarian cancer. They found that, at the time of diagnosis, slightly more women with ovarian cancer wanted to hear the "best possible" rather than the "most likely" outcome. As they dealt with their feelings of shock and despair, they shifted to wanting to know the "most likely" outcome during treatment and post-treatment.[35] Two-thirds of patients wanted information about physical and psychological aspects of their health, while one-third wanted information about physical aspects of their health only. Involvement in decision making may assist the individual dealing with cancer in maintaining a sense of control and gaining a sense of empowerment. However, it is helpful to adjust the amount of information to an individual's preferences and coping style, as information-seeking "monitors" will want to know more details than those who prefer to cope by avoidance or "blunting." Overall, most patients saw decision making as a joint partnership between themselves and their physician. A little over 60% wanted to share decision making with their doctors, about 15% wanted to make their own decisions after seriously considering the doctor's opinion, and a little over 20% wanted to take a passive role and have their physician decide for them.

The importance of the doctor-patient relationship cannot be overestimated in regard to both patient and physician satisfaction. Satisfaction with care affects both compliance and coping. Satisfaction is determined in part by the communication with the doctor, the quality of information provided, and having the opportunity to ask questions.[36] One study of the physician-patient interaction during morning rounds found that patients' perceptions of physician behavior were better predictors of satisfaction than actual behavior.[37] Conversely, the factor foremost in oncologists' satisfaction was feeling that they deal with patients and relatives. However, only 56% felt that they had received sufficient training in communication skills. Those who felt insufficiently trained in communication skills experienced significantly greater stress in dealing with patients' suffering.[38]

V. GENETIC TESTING FOR BRCA1 AND BRCA2

Psychological distress is highly prominent among women who fear they are at genetic risk. They often must deal with the knowledge of ovarian or breast cancer in family members and thus, their own risk. Between 5–10% of ovarian cancers are related to mutations in BRCA1 and BRCA2 genes, with a 15–60% lifetime risks of developing ovarian cancer.[39, 40] Screening programs for women at increased risk are available in some cancer centers; contact the National Cancer Institute's Cancer Information Service (1-800-4-CANCER, www.cancernet.nci.nhi.gov). Counseling about whether to undergo genetic testing is important, as well as counseling about the meaning of the results. Groups have proved helpful in coping for these women. Surveillance is by using the marker CA125, combined with transvaginal ultrasound, chemoprevention with oral contraceptives, and prophylactic oophorectomy. Management guidelines have been established by the American Society of Clinical Oncology and by the Cancer Genetics Studies Consortium.[41, 42]

Several studies have assessed the complex psychological issues raised by the availability of genetic testing, from the motivations and expectations of those pursuing testing to the impact of declining testing. BRCA1 carriers experienced higher levels of anger and worry than they had anticipated, which was associated with a significant increase in general psychological distress six months afterward.[43] One study of 65 women at risk found that 33% had depression at baseline and 38% at follow-up, while 16% had elevated anxiety at baseline and only 6% at follow-up. The one predictor that accounted for higher depression scores at follow-up was concern of the women for their daughter's risk.[44] They feel guilty about passing on a high risk of cancer. Another interesting finding of this study, which has been corroborated by others, is the overestimation of risk as compared to the level of risk given to them.[45] Furthermore, the difficulties women experience assimilating risk estimates run deeper than these distortions, as those who accurately recalled their estimated risk continued to estimate their risks as 100%.[46]

Prophylactic oophorectomy will reduce but not eliminate the risk for the development of ovarian cancer, with a reported frequency of primary peritoneal cancer even after oophorectomy of about 2–10%.[47] Interest in prophylactic oophorectomy has been found to be associated with a woman's increased anxiety about developing ovarian cancer rather than her objective risk.[48] This suggests another important role psychiatric consultation may have in helping a woman with a BRCA1 or BRCA2 mutation, by assisting her to clarify her emotions so that she may more thoughtfully weigh the various risks and benefits of her treatment options.

In premenopausal women, bilateral oophorectomy produces menopause, which is associated with an increased risk of depression, heart disease, and osteoporosis.[49] Hormone replacement therapy (HRT) may be recommended, but noncompliance is common, with only one-third to one-half of women complying with treatment.[50] When likely long-term compliance with HRT is lacking, prophylactic oophorectomy may be recommended, but it leads to short life expectancy prior to the age of 45.[51] In those women where HRT is not clinically indicated, or for those who do not wish to take HRT, several antidepressant medications, including fluoxetine, paroxetine, and venlafaxine, have been found to be useful in treating the symptoms of menopause, particularly hot flashes but also libido, sleep disturbance, depressed mood, and quality of life.[52, 53] Only venlafaxine has been studied regarding dosage, with a recommended starting dose of 37.5 mg that may be increased to 75 mg after one week, if necessary. Women treated with 150 mg daily experienced increased toxicity with no additional benefit.

Choosing not to be tested does not protect one from its psychological impact. In one study, those women who belonged to hereditary breast and ovarian cancer families and were invited but declined testing were more likely to have depressive symptoms than those who underwent testing.[54] In a survey of genetic counselors regarding their personal decisions if they were to undergo testing, the majority (57%) responded that they would seek professional psychological support to cope with the result.[55] The high rates of psychological distress throughout the testing process highlight the importance of psychosocial support in this evolving area of clinical service.

VI. SUMMARY

Ovarian cancer patients must contend with difficult physical symptoms and psychological problems throughout their clinical course; anxiety and depressive symptoms are present throughout, but increase in severity in advanced stages. The oncologist may help the woman with ovarian cancer maneuver the challenges by being aware of the emotions and issues related to diagnosis, treatment, and survival and by adjusting his communication style to accommodate to her coping style and informational preferences. Symptoms of depression and anxiety should be managed, in consultation with a psychiatrist providing the appropriate pharmacological and psychotherapeutic support. Other mental health professionals need to be available to provide counseling, individual support and groups for women and their families. Delirium is an under-diagnosed disorder, resulting often from cancer treatment that causes much distress and can be minimized with the appropriate pharmacological management. In general, psychosocial issues in ovarian cancer have not been well studied. Sexual dysfunction, quality of life, and the management of the psychological issues in of genetic testing are all in need of study.

References

1. Zabora, J., Brintzenhofeszoc, K., Curbow, B. *et al.* (2001). The prevalence of psychological distress by cancer site. *Psycho-Oncology* 10, 19–28.
2. Botow, P. N., Tattersall, H. N., and Goldstein, D. (1997). Communication with cancer patients in culturally diverse societies. *Ann. N. Y. Acad. Sci.* 809, 317–319.
3. Zanetta, G., Bonazzi, C., Cantu, M. G. *et al.* (2001). Survival and reproductive function after treatment of malignant germ cell ovarian tumors. *J. Clin. Oncol.* 19, 1015–1020.
4. Strain, J., and Grossman, S. (1975). "Psychological Care of the Medically Ill." Appleton-Century-Crofts, New York.
5. Wilson, J. F. (1981). Behavioral preparation for surgery: Benefit or harm. *J. Behav. Med.* 4, 79–102.
6. Guidozzi, F. (1993). Living with ovarian cancer. *Gyn. Oncol.* 50, 202–207.
7. Kornblith, A. B. *et al.* (1995). Quality of life of women with ovarian cancer. *Gyn. Oncol.* 59, 132–242.
8. Berman, J. R., Berman, L., and Goldstein, I. (1999). Female sexual dysfunction: Incidence, pathophysiology, evaluation, and treatment options. *Urology* 54, 385–391.
9. Omura, G. A., Brady, M. F., Homesley, H. D. *et al.* (1991). Long-term follow-up and prognostic factor analysis in advanced ovarian carcinoma the Gynecologic Oncology Group experience. *J. Clin. Oncol.* 9, 1138–1150.
10. Feuer, D. J., Broadley, K. E., Shepherd, J. H., and Barton, D. P. J. (1999). Systematic review of surgery in malignant bowel obstruction in advanced gynecological and gastrointestinal cancer. *Gynecol. Oncol.* 75, 313–322.
11. Loprinzi, C. L. (Arbiter). (1998). Should cancer patients with incurable disease receive parenteral or enteral nutritional support? *Eur. J. Cancer* 34, 279–285.
12. Roberts, J. A. *et al.* (1997). Factors influencing views of patients with gynecologic cancer about end-of-life decisions. *Am. J. Ob. Gyn.* 176, 166–172.
13. Portenoy, R. K. *et al.* (1994). Pain in ovarian cancer patients. *Cancer* 74, 907–915.
14. A controlled trial to improve care for seriously ill hospitalized patients: The study to understand prognoses and preferences for outcomes and risks of treatments (SUPPORT). (1995). *JAMA* 274, 1591–1598.
15. Quill, T. E. (2000). Initiating end-of-life discussions with seriously ill patients: Addressing the "elephant in the room." *JAMA* 284, 2502–2507.
16. Steinhauser, K. E., Christakis, N. A., Clipp, E.C. *et al.* (2000). Factors considered important at the end of life by patients, family, physicians, and other care providers. *JAMA* 284, 2476–2482.
17. Hill, T. P. (1995). Treating the dying patient: The challenge for medical education. *Arch. Intern. Med.* 155, 1265–1269.
18. Block, S. D., and Sullivan, A. M. (1998). Attitudes about end-of-life care: A national cross-section studey. *J. Palliat. Med.* 1, 347–355.
19. Massie, M. J., and Holland, J. C. (1990). Depression and the cancer patient. *J. Clin. Psychol.* 51, 12–17.
20. Bodurka-Bevers, D., Basen-Engquist, K., Carmack, C. L. *et al.* (2000). Depression, anxiety, and quality of life in patients with epithelial ovarian cancer. *Gynecol. Oncol.* 78, 302–308.
21. Ganzini, L., Smith, D. M., Fenn, D. S., and Lee, M. A. (1997). Depression and mortality in medically ill older adults. *J. Am. Geriatr. Soc.* 45, 307–312.

22. Von Ammon Cavanaugh, S., Furlanetto, L. M., Creech, S. D., and Powell, L. H. (2001). Medical illness, past depression, and present depression: A predictive triad for in-hospital mortality. *Am. J. Psychol.* 158, 43–48.
23. Bukberg, J., Penman, D., and Holland, J. (1984). Depression in hospitalized cancer patients. *Psychosom. Med.* 46, 199–212.
24. Endicott, J. (1984). Measurement of depression in patients with cancer. *Cancer* 53, 2243–2247.
25. Hardman, A., Maguire, P., Crowther, D. *et al.* (1989). The recognition of psychiatric morbidity on a medical oncology ward. *J. Psychosom. Res.* 33, 235–239.
26. Passik, S. D., Dugan, W., McDonald, M. V. *et al.* (1998). Oncologists' recognition of depression in their patients with cancer. *J. Clin. Oncol.* 16, 1594–1600.
27. Shen, W. W., Urosevich, Z., and Clayton, D. O. (1999). Sildenafil in the treatment of female sexual dysfunction induced by selective serotonin reuptake inhibitors. *J. Reprod. Med.* 44, 535–542.
28. Nurnberg, H. G. *et al.* (1999). Sildenafil for women patients with antidepressant-induced sexual dysfunction. *Psych. Serv.* 50, 1076–1078.
29. Thompson, D. S. (2000). Mirtazapine for the treatment of depression and nausea in breast and gynecological oncology. *Psychosomatics* 41, 356–357.
30. Bodurka-Bevers, D. *et al.* (2000). Depression, anxiety, and quality of life in patients with epithelial ovarian cancer. *Gynecol. Oncol.* 78, 302–308.
31. Breitbart, W., and Cohen, K. R. (1998). Delirium. *In* "Psycho-oncology." (J. C. Holland, ed.), pp. 564–575. Oxford University Press, New York.
32. Breitbart, W. (1995). Identifying patients at risk for, and treatment of major psychiatric complications of cancer. *Support. Care Cancer* 3, 45–60.
33. Sipahimalani, A., and Masand, P. (1998). Olanzapine in the treatment of delirium. *Psychosomatics* 39, 422–430.
34. Breitbart, W., Platt, M., Marotta, R. *et al.* (1991). Low-dose neuroleptic treatment for AIDS delirium (abstract). 144th Annual Meeting, American Psychiatric Association, 11–16 May.
35. Stewart, D. E., Wong, F., Cheung, A. M. *et al.* (2000). Information needs and decisional preferences among women with ovarian cancer. *Gynecol. Oncol.* 77, 357–361.
36. Wiggers, J. H. *et al.* (1990). Cancer patient satisfaction with care. *Cancer* 66, 610–616.
37. Blanchard, C. G., Labrecque, M. S., Ruckdeschel, J. C., and Blanchard, E. B. (1990). Physician behaviors, patient perceptions, and patient characteristics as predictors of satisfaction of hospitalized adult cancer patients. *Cancer* 65, 186–192.
38. Ramirez, A. J. *et al.* (1995). Burnout and psychiatric disorder among cancer clinicians. *Br. J. Cancer* 71, 1263–1269.
39. Holschneider, C. H., and Berek, J. S. (2000). Ovarian cancer: Epidemiology, biology, and prognostic factors. *Semin. Surg. Oncol.* 19, 3–10.
40. Matloff, E. T., Shappell, H., Brierley, K. *et al.* (2000). What would you do? Specialists' perspectives on cancer genetic testing, prophylactic surgery, and insurance discrimination. *J. Clin. Oncol.* 18, 2484–2492.
41. Statement of the American Society of Clinical Oncology: Genetic testing for cancer susceptibility (1996). Adopted February 20, 1996. *J. Clin. Oncol.* 14, 1730–1740.
42. Burke, W., Daly, M., Garber, J. *et al.* (1997). Recommendations for follow-up care of individuals with an inherited disposition to cancer. AA. BRCA1 and BRCA2. Cancer Genetics Studies Consortium. *JAMA* 277, 997–1003.
43. Dorval, M., Patenaude, A. F., Schneider, K. A. *et al.* (2000). Anticipated versus actual emotional reactions to disclosure of results of genetic tests for cancer susceptibility: Findings from p53 and BRCA1 testing programs. *J. Clin. Oncol.* 18, 2135–2142.
44. Ritvo, P., Robinson, G., Irvine, J. *et al.* (1999). A Longitudinal study of psychological adjustment to familial genetic risk assessment for ovarian cancer. *Gynecol. Oncol.* 74, 331–337.
45. Lloyd, S., Watson, M., Waites, B. *et al.* (1996). Familial breast cancer: A controlled study of risk perception, psychological morbidity and health beliefs in women attending for genetic counseling. *Br. J. Cancer* 74, 482–487.
46. Hopwood, P. (1997). Psychological issues in cancer genetics: Current research and future priorities. Patient Education Counsel. 32, 19–31.
47. Piver, M. S., Jishi, M. F., Tsukada, Y. *et al.* (1993). Primary peritoneal carcinoma after prophylactic oophorectomy in women with a family history of ovarian cancer. A report of the Gilda Radner Familial Ovarian Cancer Registry. *Cancer* 71, 2751–2755.
48. Meiser, B., Botow, P., Barratt, A. *et al.* (1999). Attitudes toward prophylactic oophorectomy and screening utilization in women at increased risk of developing hereditary breast/ovarian cancer. *Gynecol. Oncol.* 75, 122–129.
49. Gottlirb, W. H., Baruch, G. B., and Friedman, E. (2000). Prophylactic oophorectomy: Clinical considerations. *Semin. Surg. Oncol.* 19, 20–27.
50. Hammond, C. B. (1994). Women's concerns with hormone replacement therapy—compliance issues. *Fertil. Steril.* 62 (6 Suppl. 2), 157s–160s.
51. Speroff, T., Dawson, N. V., Speroff, L., and Haber, R. J. (1991). A risk-benefit analysis of elective bilateral oophorectomy: Effect of changes in compliance with estrogen therapy on outcome. *Am. J. Obstet. Gynecol.* 164 (1 Pt 1), 165–174.
52. Loprinzi, C. L. *et al.* (2000). Venlafaxine in management of hot flashes in survivors of breast cancer: A randomised controlled trial. *Lancet* 356, 2059–2063.
53. Stearns, V. *et al.* (2000). A pilot trial assessing the efficacy of paroxetine hydrochoride (Paxil) in controlling hot flashes in breast cancer survivors. *Ann. Oncol.* 11, 17–22.
54. Lerman, C., Hughes, C., Lemon, S. J. *et al.* (1998). What you don't know can hurt you: Adverse psychologic effects in members of BRCA1-linked and BRCA2-linked families who decline genetic testing. 16, 1650–1654.
55. Matloff, E. T. *et al.* (2000). What would you do? Specialists' perspectives on cancer genetic testing, prophylactic surgery, and insurance discrimination. *J. Clin. Oncol.* 18, 2484–2492.

Index

C

D

E

F

J

K

L

M

N

O

P

Q

R

S

T